MAYO INTERNAL MEDICINE
BOARD REVIEW
1994 - 95

MAYO
INTERNAL MEDICINE
BOARD REVIEW
1994 - 95

Udaya B. S. Prakash, M.D.

Editor-in-Chief

Mayo Foundation for Medical Education and Research

Rochester, Minnesota

DEDICATED TO

Residents and Fellows, past and present,

of

Mayo Clinic and Mayo Foundation

and

Mayo Graduate School of Medicine

FOREWORD

We are pleased to introduce *Mayo Internal Medicine Board Review 1994-95* for physicians preparing to take the American Board of Internal Medicine Certification and Recertification Board Examinations.

This book reflects Mayo's strong commitment to education. Through medical education, we hope to contribute to improved standards and to broader availability of medical care in this country and in other countries.

One of the strengths of this book is that it uses the multidisciplinary nature of Mayo by enlisting authors from all subspecialties of internal medicine. This exemplifies the teamwork approach to the practice and teaching of medicine here at Mayo.

On behalf of everyone at Mayo, we wish you the best in preparing for and taking the board examination and hope you continue to use this book often as a reliable reference source for internal medicine. Our hope is that, now and in the future, Mayo will serve as a resource for you in your practice.

Robert R. Waller, M.D.
President and Chief Executive Officer
Mayo Foundation

EDITORIAL AND PRODUCTION STAFF

CONTRIBUTORS

Charles F. Abboud, M.D.
Consultant, Division of Endocrinology/ Metabolism and Internal Medicine,* Associate Professor of Medicine†

Thomas F. Bugliosi, M.D.
Consultant, Division of Emergency Medical Services and Internal Medicine,* Instructor in Medicine†

Darryl S. Chutka, M.D.
Consultant, Section of Internal Medicine,* Assistant Professor of Medicine†

William W. Douglas, M.D.
Consultant, Division of Thoracic Diseases and Internal Medicine,* Assistant Professor of Medicine†

William F. Dunn, M.D.
Consultant, Division of Thoracic Diseases and Internal Medicine,* Assistant Professor of Medicine†

William W. Ginsburg, M.D.
Consultant, Division of Rheumatology,‡ Associate Professor of Medicine†

Thomas M. Habermann, M.D.
Consultant, Division of Hematology and Internal Medicine,* Assistant Professor of Medicine†

Philip T. Hagen, M.D.
Consultant, Division of Preventive Medicine and Internal Medicine,* Instructor in Medicine†

Stephen C. Hammill, M.D.
Consultant, Division of Cardiovascular Diseases and Internal Medicine,* Professor of Medicine†

Lynn C. Hartmann, M.D.
Consultant, Division of Medical Oncology,* Assistant Professor of Oncology†

James T. Li, M.D.
Consultant, Division of Allergic Diseases and Internal Medicine,* Assistant Professor of Medicine†

Scott C. Litin, M.D.
Consultant, Division of Area General Internal Medicine,* Assistant Professor of Medicine†

William F. Marshall, M.D.
Senior Associate Consultant, Division of Infectious Diseases and Internal Medicine,* Instructor in Medicine†

Marian T. McEvoy, M.D.
Consultant, Department of Dermatology,* Assistant Professor of Dermatology†

Virginia V. Michels, M.D.
Chair, Department of Medical Genetics,* Professor of Medical Genetics†

Deborah C. Newman, M.D.
Consultant, Section of Psychiatry,* Assistant Professor of Psychiatry†

*Mayo Clinic and Mayo Foundation, Rochester, Minnesota.
†Mayo Medical School, Rochester, Minnesota.
‡Mayo Clinic Jacksonville, Jacksonville, Florida.

Rick A. Nishimura, M.D.
Consultant, Division of Cardiovascular Diseases and Internal Medicine,* Professor of Medicine†

Douglas R. Osmon, M.D.
Senior Associate Consultant, Division of Infectious Diseases and Internal Medicine,* Instructor in Medicine†

Margot S. Peters, M.D.
Consultant, Department of Dermatology,* Associate Professor of Dermatology and of Pathology†

Steve G. Peters, M.D.
Consultant, Division of Thoracic Diseases and Internal Medicine,* Associate Professor of Medicine†

John J. Poterucha, M.D.
Senior Associate Consultant, Division of Gastroenterology and Internal Medicine,* Assistant Professor of Medicine†

Udaya B. S. Prakash, M.D.
Consultant, Division of Thoracic Diseases and Internal Medicine,* Professor of Medicine†

Thom Rooke, M.D.
Consultant, Division of Cardiovascular Diseases and Internal Medicine,* Assistant Professor of Medicine†

Edward C. Rosenow III, M.D.
Chair, Division of Thoracic Diseases and Internal Medicine,* Professor of Medicine†

Frank A. Rubino, M.D.
Consultant, Department of Neurology,‡ Associate Professor of Neurology†

Thomas R. Schwab, M.D.
Consultant, Division of Nephrology and Internal Medicine,* Assistant Professor of Medicine†

Gary L. Schwartz, M.D.
Consultant, Division of Hypertension and Internal Medicine,* Assistant Professor of Medicine†

Robert M. Valente, M.D.
Consultant, Division of Rheumatology and Internal Medicine,* Instructor in Medicine†

Thomas R. Viggiano, M.D.
Consultant, Division of Gastroenterology and Internal Medicine,* Associate Professor of Medicine†

Carole A. Warnes, M.D.
Consultant, Division of Cardiovascular Diseases and Internal Medicine,* Associate Professor of Medicine†

*Mayo Clinic and Mayo Foundation, Rochester, Minnesota.
†Mayo Medical School, Rochester, Minnesota.
‡Mayo Clinic Jacksonville, Jacksonville, Florida.

TABLE OF CONTENTS

1. **THE BOARD EXAMINATION** 1
   Udaya B. S. Prakash, M.D.

2. **ALLERGY** 5
   James T. Li, M.D.

3. **BLOOD GASES** 27
   William W. Douglas, M.D.

4. **CARDIOLOGY I** 39
   Rick A. Nishimura, M.D.

5. **CARDIOLOGY II** 69
   Stephen C. Hammill, M.D.

6. **CARDIOLOGY III** 97
   Carole A. Warnes, M.D.

7. **CHEST X-RAYS** 123
   Edward C. Rosenow III, M.D.

8. **CLINICAL PHARMACOLOGY AND TOXICOLOGY** 145
   Thomas F. Bugliosi, M.D.

9. **CRITICAL CARE MEDICINE** 161
   Steve G. Peters, M.D.

10. **DERMATOLOGY** 177
    Marian T. McEvoy, M.D.
    Margot S. Peters, M.D.

11. **ENDOCRINOLOGY** 203
    Charles F. Abboud, M.D.

12. **ETHICS IN MEDICINE** 301
    Udaya B. S. Prakash, M.D.
    William F. Dunn, M.D.

13. **GASTROENTEROLOGY I** 309
    Thomas R. Viggiano, M.D.

14. **GASTROENTEROLOGY II** 357
    John J. Poterucha, M.D.

15. **GENERAL INTERNAL MEDICINE** 375
    Scott C. Litin, M.D.

16. **GENETICS** 391
    Virginia V. Michels, M.D.

17. **GERIATRICS** 419
    Darryl S. Chutka, M.D.

18. **HEMATOLOGY** 433
    Thomas M. Habermann, M.D.

19. **HYPERTENSION** 479
    Gary L. Schwartz, M.D.

20. **INFECTIOUS DISEASES** 501
    Douglas R. Osmon, M.D.
    William F. Marshall, M.D.

21. **NEPHROLOGY** 585
    Thomas R. Schwab, M.D.

22. **NEUROLOGY** 613
    Frank A. Rubino, M.D.

23. **ONCOLOGY** 643
    Lynn C. Hartmann, M.D.

24. **PREVENTIVE MEDICINE** 665
    Philip T. Hagen, M.D.

25. **PSYCHIATRY** 679
    Deborah C. Newman, M.D.

26. **PULMONARY DISEASES** 697
    Udaya B. S. Prakash, M.D.

27. **RHEUMATOLOGY I** 775
    William W. Ginsburg, M.D.

28. **RHEUMATOLOGY II** 799
    Robert M. Valente, M.D.

29. **VASCULAR DISEASES** 841
    Thom Rooke, M.D.

Answers to Chapter Questions 859

PREFACE

For more than 2 decades, the staff of the Mayo Clinic and faculty of the Mayo Graduate School of Medicine have provided in-house didactic presentations for residents and fellows preparing for the internal medicine certifying examination administered by the American Board of Internal Medicine (ABIM). The extreme popularity of the Mayo "board reviews" among the residents and fellows and other physicians prompted the initiation of "Mayo Internal Medicine Board Review" courses in August 1992 to all physicians. Nearly 200 physicians in 1992 and twice that number in August 1993 attended the courses offered in Rochester, Minnesota. The popularity and the great demand for the course syllabus inspired us to write this book for candidates preparing for the ABIM examinations in internal medicine. This book, *Mayo Internal Medicine Board Review 1994-95*, will be used as the course syllabus for the "Mayo Internal Medicine Board Review" courses to be held in 1994 (July 24-30) and 1995 (July 23-29) in Rochester, Minnesota.

This is not a comprehensive textbook of medicine. It is rather analogous to a guide or a notebook containing selected topics deemed important for candidates preparing for the certifying or recertifying examinations offered by the ABIM in 1994 and 1995. The authors of this book assume that the candidates preparing for the board examinations will have studied at length a standard textbook of medicine before reading this review. The chapters are divided by subspecialty topics. As a means of underscoring the important clinical points for the boards, many paragraphs are followed by selected "pearls." Some of these pearls may seem repetitious, but this approach is intentional. We hope this format will aid readers in recapitulating the salient points of the topic under discussion. The questions at the end of each chapter are intended to familiarize the candidates with the format of the ABIM examination. Answers to these questions and their explanations are at the end of the book.

My coauthors and I are truly pleased to present this book and anticipate that it will be valuable to anyone preparing for the certifying and recertifying examinations in internal medicine of the ABIM. We look forward to hearing comments and suggestions from readers.

Udaya B. S. Prakash, M.D.
January 1994

CHAPTER 1
THE BOARD EXAMINATION

Udaya B. S. Prakash, M.D.

THE EXAMINATION

The American Board of Internal Medicine (ABIM) has stated that the certifying examination tests the breadth and depth of the candidate's knowledge in internal medicine (IM) to ensure that the candidate has attained the necessary proficiency required for the practice of IM. The questions cover a broad area of IM, including allergy, immunology, cardiology, critical care medicine, dermatology, endocrinology, epidemiology, gastroenterology, geriatrics, gynecology, hematology, infectious disease, medical ethics, nephrology, neurology, nutrition, oncology, otorhinolaryngology, preventive medicine, psychiatry, pulmonary diseases, rheumatology, and substance abuse. Even though a certain percentage of questions are allotted to each of these disciplines, the information sent to the candidates by the ABIM does not specify the details.

The examination dates are as follows: August 23-24, 1994, August 22-23, 1995, August 20-21, 1996, August 19-20, 1997, August 25-26, 1998, August 24-25, 1999, and August 22-23, 2000. More detail regarding the examination, training requirements, application forms, and other details can be obtained from the American Board of Internal Medicine, 3624 Market Street, Philadelphia, PA 19104 (telephone numbers: 215-243-1500 or 800-441-2246).

THE FORMAT

During four sessions (sessions A and C are 4 hours each and B and D are 3 1/2 hours each), the candidate answers several hundred questions. The bulk of the questions are based on patient presentation and management, mostly in the setting of outpatient or emergency room situations. The ABIM information booklet for 1993 states

that questions are based on patients of all age groups. It also states that the questions testing strict knowledge are in the minority and that the test is written to test the ability of the candidate to recognize patterns of disease and to demonstrate clinical judgment. Furthermore, the questions are reported to have been reviewed by practicing internists. A list of normal laboratory values is provided, and illustrative materials (electrocardiograms, chest radiographs, and photomicrographs) are used to test the candidate's ability to interpret diagnostic tests.

CORE AND NON-CORE QUESTIONS

Candidates who are preparing for or have appeared for the ABIM examination commonly want to know the difference between core and non-core questions. The reason for the interest is that scores are generated separately for the core and non-core segments of the examination. Candidates must achieve a passing score in both core and non-core questions to become ABIM-certified. Those who pass only one or the other will have to take both portions in the subsequent examination. The following is a verbatim statement contained in the ABIM information booklet for 1993.

> To appropriately reflect the contributions of each item format (one-best-answer and multiple true-false) counts are made of the number of correct answers for each format; the counts then are weighed by the amount of testing time devoted to each format. A composite score is formed for each portion by summing the weighted scores and dividing the results by the total amount of testing time.

The ABIM distinguishes core questions as those that encompass material that is critical to the practice of IM in terms of patient health outcome and of situations that are regularly encountered by internists. Non-core questions include a broad range of topics in all aspects of IM. Because the core and non-core questions are not labeled as such, it is difficult to differentiate them during the examination. Candidates should know that several questions are included for experimental purposes only (field questions). These cannot be identified during the examination, and the answers to these will not be scored. Because there is no penalty for guessing the answers, candidates should answer every question.

TYPES OF QUESTIONS

Two types of questions are used: multiple-choice (with a single correct answer) and multiple true/false (any or all answers can be true or false) formats. In both formats, the question may be in the form of a case history, a brief statement, an illustration, or a graph. The multiple-choice question has five possible answers, and the candidate has to identify the single best answer. The multiple true/false question has five answers, and any or all answers may be true or false. Examples of these are shown.

Multiple-Choice Question

A 56-year-old white woman has had a 25-year history of a dry, burning, and gritty sensation in the eyes, a dry mouth, and Raynaud's phenomenon. Examination confirms these findings in addition to enlarged parotid glands. Which of the following complications is most likely to occur in this patient?

a. Necrobiotic subcutaneous nodules
b. Transudative pleural effusion
c. Proximal myopathy
d. Desiccation of tracheobronchial tree
e. Aspiration pneumonia

Multiple True/False Question

Pneumonia caused by *Pneumocystis carinii* in adult patients with AIDS demonstrates the following differences in contrast to *Pneumocystis carinii* pneumonia in immunosuppressed patients without AIDS:

a. Longer duration of symptoms
b. Higher arterial oxygen tension
c. Greater incidence of side effects from trimethoprim-sulfamethoxazole
d. Recurrence or persistence of *P. carinii* infection
e. The number of organisms seen microscopically is usually scanty

The single best answer to the multiple-choice question is d, and in the multiple true/false question, a, b, c, and d are true statements.

Preparation for the Test

Each candidate has his or her own preparation method for the examination. Certain general suggestions, however, are as follows:

- Preparation starts at the beginning of the residency training in IM.
- Most candidates, however, require a minimum of 6 to 8 months of intense preparation for the examination.
- Any of the standard textbooks on IM should provide a good basic knowledge in all areas of IM. Ideally, the candidate should read one good textbook and not jump from one to another, except for reading certain chapters that are outstanding in a particular textbook (see below).
- Formation of study groups, three to five candidates per group, permits study of different textbooks and review articles in journals. It is important that the group meet regularly and that each candidate be assigned reading materials.
- Selected review papers and state-of-the-art articles on common and important topics in IM should be included in the study materials. Indiscriminate reading of articles from many journals should be avoided. In any case, most candidates who begin preparation 6 to 8 months before the examination will not find time for extensive study of journal materials.
- Notes and other materials the candidates have gathered during their residency training are also good sources of information. These clinical "pearls" gathered from mentors will be of help in remembering certain important points.
- This book and similar "board review" syllabi are also good tools for "brushing up" knowledge several weeks before the examination. They, however, cannot take the place of comprehensive textbooks of medicine.
- The Medical Knowledge Self-Assessment Program (MKSAP) prepared by the American College of Physicians is valuable to obtain practice in answering multiple-choice questions and multiple true/false questions. The text contents, however, are uneven in the coverage of topics. By design, the MKSAP is prepared for the continuing medical education of practicing (presumably ABIM-certified) internists rather than for those preparing for initial certification by the ABIM. For recertification purposes, MKSAP is a rea-

sonable aid.

- Certain diseases are more important because they are topical (for example, AIDS, tuberculosis, lipid disorders, and recent increase in asthma morbidity and mortality, to name a few).
- Try to remember some of the uncommon manifestations of the most common diseases (e.g., polycythemia in common obstructive pulmonary disease) and common manifestations of uncommon diseases (e.g., pneumothorax in eosinophilic granuloma).
- Certain diseases, many peculiar and uncommon, are eminently "board-eligible," meaning that they may appear in the board examinations more frequently than in clinical practice. Most of these are covered in this book.
- Certain formulas and points should be memorized (e.g., the alveolar gas equation).
- Most significantly, the clinical training and regular study habits during residency training are the most important aspects of preparing for the boards.

DAY OF THE BOARD EXAMINATION

- There will be plenty of time to cover all the questions; therefore, there is no need to rush or get anxious.
- Start by answering the first question and continue sequentially (do not skip too many--see below).
- Do not be alarmed by lengthy questions; look for the salient points in the question.
- When faced with a lengthy or confusing question, do not become distracted by that question. Mark it so you can find it later, then go to the next question and come back to the unanswered ones at the end.
- Extremely lengthy or confusing stem statements in the past were apparently intended to test the candidate's ability to separate the essential from the unnecessary or unimportant information. It is unclear whether such questions continue to appear on the examination.
- It is also my understanding that the questions no longer use double-negatives (this was common in the past). Nevertheless, look for phrases such as "all of the following except" or "which of the following is not…."
- Carry a simple ruler (make sure it is allowed) to the examination. It can be used for estimating P50 point on oxyhemoglobin dissociation curve or for drawing nomograms from memory.
- Ideally, good questions are supposed to test and educate the candidate simultaneously. In other words, the answers in a good question will contain more true statements than false ones. Whether the ABIM follows this approach is unclear.
- Use your basic fund of knowledge in IM and clinical experience to solve the questions. Approaching the questions as "real-life" patient encounters is far better than trying to second-guess the examiners or trying to analyze whether the question is "tricky."

CONNECTIONS

Associations, causes, complications, and other relationships between a phenomenon or disease and clinical features are important to remember and recognize. I call these "connections." For example, the following are some of the "connections" in infectious and occupational entities in pulmonary medicine. Each subspecialty has many similar connections, and candidates for the ABIM and other examinations may want to prepare lists like this in different areas.

Etiologic factor	Agent, disease
Cattle, swine, horses, wool, hide	Anthrax
Abattoir worker, veterinarian	Brucellosis
Travel to Southeast Asia, South America	Melioidosis
Squirrels, chipmunks, rabbits, rats	Plague
Rabbits, squirrels, infected flies, or ticks	Tularemia
Birds	Psittacosis, histoplasmosis
Rats, dogs, cats, cattle, swine	Leptospirosis
Goats, cattle, swine	Q-fever
Soil, water-cooling tower	Legionellosis
Military camps	Mycoplasmosis
Chicken coop, starling roosts, caves	Histoplasmosis
Soil	Blastomycosis

Travel in Southwestern United States	Coccidioidomycosis
Ohio and Mississippi river valleys	Histoplasmosis
Decaying wood	Histoplasmosis
Gardeners, florists, straw, plants	Sporotrichosis
Progressive, massive fibrosis	Silicosis, coal, hematite, kaolin, graphite, asbestosis
Autoimmune mechanism	Silicosis, asbestosis, berylliosis
Monday morning sickness	Byssinosis, bagassosis, metal fume fever
Metals and fumes producing asthma	Baker's asthma, meat wrapper's asthma, printer's asthma, nickel, platinum, toluene diisocyanate (TDI), cigarette cutter's asthma
Increased incidence of tuberculosis	Silicosis, hematite lung
Increased incidence of carcinoma	Asbestos, hematite, arsenic, nickel, uranium, chromate
Welder prone to develop	Siderosis, pulmonary edema, bronchitis, emphysema
Centrilobar emphysema	Coal, hematite
Generalized emphysema	Cadmium, bauxite
Silo filler's lung produced by	Nitrogen dioxide
Farmer's lung produced by	*Thermoactinomyces, Micropolyspora*
Asbestos exposure	Mesothelioma, bronchogenic carcinoma, gastrointestinal cancer
Eggshell calcification	Silicosis, sarcoid
Sarcoid-like disease	Berylliosis
Diaphragmatic calcification	Asbestosis (also ankylosing spondylitis)
Nonfibrogenic pneumoconioses	Tin, emery, antimony, titanium, barium
Minimal pathology in lungs	Siderosis, baritosis, stannosis
Bullous emphysema	Bauxite lung

NOTE

Each chapter is followed by a set of questions. These questions were used for the electronic response session during the course "Mayo Internal Medicine Board Review" in August 1993. A new set of questions will be used in the courses in July 1994 and July 1995.

For multiple-choice questions, select one best answer. For true/false questions, indicate whether each statement is true or false (see page 2).

The answers and explanations to answers begin on page 859.

CHAPTER 2
ALLERGY

James T. Li, M.D.

ASTHMA

History

Allergic asthma can be mild and self-limiting or potentially debilitating, but intrinsic asthma tends to be progressive, to result in hospitalization for status asthmaticus, and to require continuous steroid therapy for suppression. Some patients have both intrinsic and allergic asthma. You can be reasonably certain someone has allergic asthma if symptoms are sporadic and consistently related to exposure to animal dander (e.g., visiting house of someone who has cats) or are seasonal (e.g., correspond to hay fever season). You can be reasonably certain someone does not have it if allergy skin test results are negative.

- In allergic asthma, symptoms are sporadic and consistently related to exposure or are seasonal.

If a patient has either form of asthma, nonspecific bronchial hyperresponsiveness tends to blur distinctions between allergic and intrinsic aspects, with allergic patients likely responding also to many nonimmunologic triggers, e.g., airborne particulates (however inert), temperature change, air pollutants, and strong odors (including "fragrances"). Cold dry air is very provocative, especially under conditions of hyperpnea, e.g., physical exercise.

- Allergic patients likely to respond to many nonimmunologic triggers.
- Cold dry air is very provocative.

Assessment of Severity

Asthma is mild if symptoms are sporadic, continuous treatment is not needed, and the flow-volume curve during formal pulmonary function testing is normal between episodes of symptoms. Even in patients fitting this description, inflammation (albeit patchy) in airways is significant, and glucocorticoid inhaled on regular basis diminishes bronchial hyperresponsiveness.

- Glucocorticoid inhaled on regular basis diminishes bronchial hyperresponsiveness.

Asthma is moderate when 1) symptoms occur with some regularity or daily, 2) there is some nocturnal occurrence of symptoms, or 3) medication is required on regularly scheduled basis for asthma control. For many of these patients, the flow-volume curve is rarely normal, and complete pulmonary function testing may show evidence of hyperinflation, as indicated by increased residual volume or increase above expected levels for diffusing capacity of lung for CO_2.

Asthma is severe when symptoms are present almost continuously and when upper end of dose range of usual medications is needed to control the asthma. Most patients require either large doses of inhaled glucocorticoids or oral prednisone daily for adequate control. Most of them have been hospitalized more than once and for more than overnight observation. Occasionally, patients move from one form of asthma to another. Someone may have severe asthma for a couple years which finally is adequately controlled. Their status then changes to moderate asthma. Note that one of the first signs that asthma is not well-controlled is emergence of the nocturnal symptoms.

- Nocturnal symptoms suggest asthma is worsening.

Pathophysiology

Asthmatics tend to have abnormalities in β-adrenergic responsiveness throughout the body, not just the lung. Peripheral blood leukocytes and adrenergic neural pathways behave as though signal transduction is impaired in adrenergic receptors. How this relates to histologic changes in asthma is unclear.

- Abnormalities in β-adrenergic responsiveness.

Common to all forms of asthma is bronchial hyperresponsiveness. Bronchial hyperresponsiveness is measured by assessing pulmonary function before and after exposure to methacholine, histamine, cold air, or exercise. Prolonged glucocorticoid therapy reduces bronchial hyperresponsiveness. Prolonged therapy with certain other anti-inflammatory drugs, e.g., sodium cromolyn, also reduces bronchial hyperresponsiveness, as shown in study of long-term (1-year) therapy with nedocromil, a cromolyn congener. Note that although cromolyn and nedocromil both were originally touted as "antiallergic" (they inhibited mast cell activation), they affect most cells involved in inflammation; also the effects on these cells occur at lower doses than those that inhibit mast cell activation.

- Bronchial hyperresponsiveness generally present in all forms of asthma.
- Prolonged glucocorticoid therapy reduces bronchial responsiveness.
- Cromolyn and nedocromil affect most cells involved in inflammation.

Asthmatics with allergic asthma probably have mast cell and basophil mediators that play significant roles in development of the endobronchial inflammation and smooth muscle changes that occur after acute exposure to allergen. Polymorphonuclear leukocytes are prominent during the immediate reaction.

- In the immediate-phase reaction, mast cells and basophils are important.

In the so-called late-phase reaction to allergen exposure, bronchi have histologic features of chronic inflammation, and eosinophils become prominent in the reaction.

- In the late-phase reaction, eosinophils become prominent.

Patients with negative allergy skin test results and chronic asthma seem to have purely round-cell inflammatory infiltrate in the bronchi and a histologic picture dominated by eosinophils when asthma is active.

Various hypotheses explain development of nonallergic asthma. One proposal is that initial inflammation represents an autoimmune reaction arising from viral or other microbial infection in the lung and, for reasons unknown, inflammation becomes chronic and characterized by lymphocyte cytokine profile in which interleukin-5 (IL-5) is prominent. The intense eosinophilic inflammation is thought to come from IL-5 influence of T cells in the chronic inflammatory infiltrate. Consistent with this hypothesis is recent evidence implicating chlamydial infection as an inciting factor in several postinfectious adult-onset asthmatics. Airway macrophages and platelets have low-affinity IgE receptors on their membranes and are activated by cross-linking of these receptors by allergen, suggesting that some phases of lung inflammation in allergy may involve the macrophage as a primary responder cell.

- IL-5 stimulates eosinophils.
- Airway macrophages and platelets have low-affinity IgE receptors.

Spirometry

Peak flow rate (PFR) changes little during loss of a large fraction of expiratory flow rate in mid-regions of the flow-volume curve. PFR occurs when little more than anatomical dead space volume has been expired and is only an approximate measure of airway obstruction.

Asthma chiefly affects medium- and small-sized airways; expired air from these airways generates the mid-expiratory flow rates. The flow-volume curve of asthmatics is often concave.

- Medium- and small-sized airways are affected in asthma.
- The flow-volume curve in asthmatics is often concave.

As asthma progresses, the flow-volume curve declines and for the same reason that PFR eventually declines: hyperinflation induces acute restrictive change in pulmonary function. Because of air-trapping, there is no room to expire normal volume of air.

- As asthma progresses, flow-volume curve declines.
- Hyperinflation is secondary to air-trapping.

Pathology

Pathologic features of asthma have been studied chiefly in fatal cases; some bronchoscopic data are available about mild and moderate asthmatics. The amount of variation between mild and fatal asthma is unknown but probably is not large.

Histologic hallmarks of asthma are listed in Table 1.

- Histologic hallmarks of asthma: mucus gland hypertrophy, mucus hypersecretion, epithelial desquamation, widening of basement membrane, infiltration by eosinophils.

Table 2-1.--Histologic Hallmarks of Asthma

Mucus gland hypertrophy
Mucus hypersecretion
Alteration of tinctorial and viscoelastic properties of mucus
Widening of basement membrane zone of bronchial epithelial membrane
Increased number of intraepithelial leukocytes and mast cells
Round cell infiltration of bronchial submucosa
Intense eosinophilic infiltration of submucosa
Widespread damage to bronchial epithelium
Large areas of complete desquamation of epithelium into airway lumen
Mucus plugs filled with eosinophils and their products

Airway Inflammation

Glucocorticoids applied topically to asthmatic bronchi can decrease inflammation and control the disease. Glucocorticoids given systemically prevent eosinophil release from bone marrow, making them unavailable for the inflammatory response. This mechanism is not operative with topical therapy because topical therapy has little or no systemic effect.

- Inhaled glucocorticoids decrease airway inflammation.
- Inhaled glucocorticoids have little systemic effect.

The maintenance of round-cell lymphocyte/monocyte inflammatory infiltrate in bronchial submucosa likely depends on lymphokine secretory patterns. Glucocorticoids may interfere at several levels in the lymphokine cascade.

- Glucocorticoids reduce airway inflammation by modulating cytokines.

Finally, monocytes or platelets may be important in the asthmatic process. Glucocorticoids modify self-activation pathways for monocytes and activation properties of platelets (probably by modulating arachidonate metabolism).

- Glucocorticoids can inhibit the inflammatory properties of monocytes and platelets.

Furthermore, glucocorticoids have vasoconstrictive properties, which reduce vascular congestive changes in mucosa, and they tend to reduce mucus gland secretion (principally, proteoglycan components).

- Glucocorticoids have vasoconstrictive properties.
- Glucocorticoids reduce mucus gland secretion.

Corticosteroid Therapy

Because of long-term benefits in reduced bronchial hyperresponsiveness with little or no side effects, the trend is to prescribe inhaled glucocorticoids earlier in mild asthma, sometimes as the only therapeutic agent, even without antecedent bronchodilators. Long-term use of β-agonist bronchodilators may adversely affect asthma, hastening irreversible obstruction; this also argues for earlier use of inhaled glucocorticoids. Certainly, asthmatics with regularly recurring symptoms probably should have inhaled steroid (or cromolyn) as part of the treatment. When the steroid requirement is unknown, it is reasonable to start with two puffs of beclomethasone (Beclovent or Vanceril, 84 μg per puff) or triamcinolone acetonide (Azmacort, 200 μg per puff) four times daily, or flunisolide (Aerobid, 250 μg per puff) twice daily. In very mild cases, starting with inhaled steroid alone may be reasonable.

- Prescribe inhaled glucocorticoids earlier in mild asthma.
- Long-term use of β-agonist bronchodilators may worsen asthma.

In patients with significant symptoms, it probably is best to induce as complete a remission in airway inflammation as possible with 10-day course of oral prednisone concomitant with initiating inhaled steroid. If patient has not taken steroid in last 3 months or more, a reasonable prednisone course is 10 mg four times daily for first 7 days, tapering by 10 mg daily for next 3 days. If patient has taken steroid recently, particularly systemic steroid, then starting dose of inhaled steroid should be increased to four puffs four times daily, and oral prednisone dose schedule needs to be increased. Commonest cause of poor results in asthma therapy is poor inhaler technique by patients in taking inhaled steroid. Poor technique can make a powerful and effective therapy worthless.

- Commonest cause of poor results is poor inhaler technique.

Goals of Asthma Management

The goals of asthma management are listed in Table 2-2.

Table 2-2.--Goals of Asthma Management

Patient understands the disease

Hospitalizations for asthma are rare because patient understands step-care and has plan for responding to flares of the disease

Physician fosters independence of patient and accurate/appropriate self-care

Asthma has low impact on patient's life-style

Patient micromanages and physician provides guidance on broad issues and in setting goals

Treatment program makes adequate use of glucocorticoids and appropriately de-emphasizes β_2-agonist drugs

Pulmonary function test results are normal, nearly normal, or at patient's best documented level

---

Medications for Asthma

Medications for asthma are listed in Table 2-3. Currently, only anticholinergic drug available in U.S.A. for treating asthma is ipratropium bromide (Atrovent). Many β-adrenergic compounds are available, but albuterol (Proventil, Ventolin) and metaproterenol (Alupent) are probably prescribed most. Both agents are available in oral rather than inhaled form, and more side effects occur when they are given orally. Nebulized β-agonists are infrequently used chronically in adult asthma, although they may be life-saving in acute attacks. For home use, the metered-dose inhaler is the preferred delivery system. Theophylline is effective for asthma with narrow therapeutic index. Note drug interactions (cimetidine, erythromycin, and quinolone antibiotics).

- Theophylline has a narrow therapeutic index.
- β-agonists are best delivered by the inhaler route.

Table 2-3.--Medications for Asthma

Bronchodilator compounds
 Anticholinergic drugs (ipratropium bromide)
 β_2-agonist drugs
 Methylxanthines (theophylline + congeners)
"Anti-allergic" compounds
 Cromolyn
 Nedocromil
Glucocorticoids
 Systemic
  Prednisone
  Methylprednisolone
  Hydrocortisone
  Triamcinolone
  Dexamethasone
 Topical
  Triamcinolone acetonide
  Beclomethasone
  Flunisolide

Asthma-Provoking Drugs

It is important to recognize the potentially severe adverse response asthmatics may show to β-blocking drugs; propranolol leads list of agents causing severe adverse responses. Severe asthma can be provoked in some asthmatics who have been asymptomatic for long periods, so vigilance is necessary in all clinical circumstances. These remarks apply to asthmatics with glaucoma treated with ophthalmic preparations of timolol and betaxolol (betaxolol is much less likely to cause problems but is not completely innocent).

- β-blocking drugs, including eyedrops, can cause severe adverse responses.
- Note that so-called B-1 selective agents such as atenolol may also provoke asthma.

A significant fraction of asthmatics *cough* when given angiotensin converting enzyme (ACE) inhibitor drugs, and the asthma of some worsens. Because pulmonary function testing does not show decrement in many of these asthmatics and many nonasthmatics may also cough after taking ACE inhibitors, the coughing may not be additional bronchospasm, as it often seems to be when asthmatics cough.

- ACE inhibitors can cause coughing.

Aspirin ingestion can cause acute, severe, and fatal asthma in a small subset of asthmatics. The cause of the reaction is unknown. Most of the affected patients have nasal polyposis and hyperplastic pansinus mucosal disease and are steroid-dependent for control of asthma. However, not all asthmatics with this reaction to aspirin fit the profile; thus, physicians should be aware of this possibility. Many nonsteroidal anti-inflammatory drugs can trigger the reaction to aspirin; the likelihood of a drug causing the reaction correlates with its potency of inhibiting cyclooxygenase enzyme in vitro. Structural aspects of the drug seem unrelated to its tendency to provoke the reaction. Thus, enolic acid agents and carboxylic acids are capable of provoking reactions. Table 2-4 lists specific drugs. Only nonacetylated salicylates such as choline salicylate (a weak cyclooxygenase inhibitor) seem not to provoke the reaction.

● Aspirin and other nonsteroidal anti-inflammatory agents can cause acute, severe asthma.
● Asthma, nasal polyposis, and aspirin sensitivity form the aspirin triad.

Traditionally, asthmatics have been warned not to use antihistamines, because anticholinergic activity of some antihistamines was thought to cause drying of lower respiratory tract secretions, further worsening the asthma. However, antihistamines do not worsen asthma. Often, we specifically prescribe antihistamine for allergic asthmatics, because the drug may have some beneficial effect on asthmatic inflammation.

● Antihistamines are not contraindicated in asthma.

Occupational Asthma

Every patient interviewed about a history of allergy or asthma must also provide an adequate occupational history. A large fraction of occupational asthma probably escapes diagnosis because physicians obtain an inadequate (or no) history. An enormous range of possible industrial circumstances may lead to exposure and resultant disease. Table 2-5 lists the most widely recognized types of occupational asthma.

● Inquiry into a possible occupational cause of asthma is important in all asthmatics.

As new industrial processes and products evolve, occupational asthma may become more common. Example

Table 2-4.--Common Nonsteroidal Anti-Inflammatory Drugs That Can Provoke Bronchospasm in Aspirin-Sensitive Asthmatics

	Generic (Tradename)
Enolic acid	Piroxicam (Feldene)
Carboxylic acid	
Acetic group	Indomethacin (Indocin)
	Sulindac (Clinoril)
	Tolmetin (Tolectin)
Propionic acid group	Ibuprofen (Advil, Rufen)
	Naproxen (Naprosyn, Anaprox)
	Fenoprofen (Nalfon)
Fenamate group	Meclofenamate (Meclomen)
	Mefenamic acid (Ponstel)

of a potentially huge problem is latex-induced asthma among medical workers, with widespread use in last 3-4 years of gloves for medical workers. Another new problem is asthma in airline pilots exposed to cockpit communications equipment that uses TDI-based inks. Incidence of occupational asthma is estimated to be 6%-15% of all adult-onset asthmatics.

● Allergy to latex is a newly discovered cause of occupational asthma.

Gastroesophageal Reflux and Asthma

Role of gastroesophageal reflux in asthma is not known. Two mechanistic hypotheses are 1) reflux bronchospasm from acid in distal esophagus and 2) recurrent aspiration of gastric contents. A well-documented reflex in dogs links acid in distal esophagus to vagally mediated bronchospasm, but no such reflex had been identified in humans. Thus, hypothesis that gastric contents reach tracheobronchial tree by ascending to hypopharynx is apparently mechanism by which gastroesophageal reflux causes human asthma (if it does).

Table 2-5.--Industrial Agents That Can Cause Asthma

Metals
    Salts of platinum, nickel, chrome
Wood dusts
    Mahogany
    Oak
    Redwood
    Western red cedar (plicatic acid)
Vegetable dusts
    Castor bean
    Cotton dust
    Cottonseed
    Flour
    Grain (mite, weevil antigens)
    Green coffee
    Gums
Industrial chemicals and plastics
    Ethylenediamine
    Phthalic and trimellitic anhydrides
    Polyvinyl chloride
    Toluene diisocyanate
Pharmaceutical agents
    Phenylglycine acid chloride
    Penicillins
    Spiramycin
Food industry agents
    Egg crackers' disease
    Meat-wrappers' disease
Biologic enzymes
    Bacillus subtilis (laundry detergent workers)
    Pancreatic enzymes
Animal emanations
    Canine or feline saliva
    Horse dander (racing workers)
    Rodent urine (laboratory animal workers)

Methacholine Bronchial Challenge

Do not perform a methacholine challenge in patients with severe expiratory obstruction.

Stringent cutoff values for the percentage fall in 1-second forced expiratory volume (FEV_1) after methacholine were established by and are useful mainly in epidemiologic studies. Usually, a 20% decrease in FEV_1 is considered a positive result.

A patient with a history suggestive of episodic asthma but who on the day of the examination has normal pulmonary function test results is reasonable candidate for study. Much has been made of "cough" variant asthma, but its pathophysiology is uncertain, as is its rela-

tionship to typical asthma. The methacholine bronchial challenge is useful in evaluating patients for cough in whom baseline pulmonary function appears normal. However, negative results have to be interpreted carefully because of the test's lack of sensitivity and specificity in typical asthma. Positive results do not always mean asthma but represent more information to be weighed in the clinical evaluation. Some consider isocapneic hyperventilation with subfreezing dry air (by either exercise or breathing CO_2/air mixture) or exercise as alternatives to methacholine challenge.

- Patients with suspected asthma and normal results on pulmonary function tests can benefit from methacholine testing.

Cigarette-Smoking and Asthma

Combination of asthma and cigarette smoking leads to accelerated chronic obstructive pulmonary disease. Because of accelerated decline in irreversible obstruction, all asthmatics who smoke should be told to stop smoking.

Differential Diagnosis

The differential diagnosis of wheezing is given in Table 2-6.

Allergy Testing

Standard allergy testing relies on identifying the allergen-specific IgE antibody. Two classic means of doing this are immediate wheal-and-flare skin test (small amount of antigen introduced into skin and evaluated at 15 minutes for presence of an immediate wheal-and-flare reaction) and in vitro testing. The skin test identifies the presence of allergen-specific IgE antibody but *does not indicate whether the person with a positive cutaneous reaction has a mucosal immune response to the same antigen under natural conditions.*

Allergy practices without a clear scientific basis include cytotoxic testing, provocation-neutralization testing or treatment, "yeast allergy," and sublingual immunotherapy.

In Vitro Allergy Testing

In vitro allergy testing (RAST) involves chemically coupling allergen protein molecules to a solid-phase substance (e.g., microcrystalline cellulose) or to activated biologic membranes (e.g., nitrocellulose). The test is conducted by incubating a serum (from patient) that may contain IgE antibody specific for the allergen that has

Table 2-6.--Differential Diagnosis of Wheezing

Pulmonary embolism
Cardiac failure
Foreign body
Central airway tumors
Aspiration
Carcinoid syndrome
Chondromalacia/polychondritis
Loeffler's syndrome
Bronchiectasis
Tropical eosinophilia
Hyperventilation syndrome
Laryngeal edema
Vascular ring affecting trachea
Factitious (including psychophysiologic vocal cord adduction)
α_1-antitrypsin deficiency
Immotile-cilia syndrome
Bronchopulmonary dysplasia
Bronchiolitis (including bronchiolitis obliterans), croup
Cystic fibrosis

been immobilized to the membrane for a standard period of time. The solid phase is then washed free of non-binding materials from the serum and incubated in a second solution containing a signal reagent (e.g., radiolabeled anti-IgE antibody). The various wells are counted and the radioactivity is correlated directly with the preparation of a standard curve in which known amounts of allergen-specific IgE antibody were incubated with a set of standard preparations of a solid phase. RAST uses the principles of radioimmunoassay.

It is important to understand that this test only identifies the presence of allergen-specific IgE antibody in the same way that allergen skin test does. Generally, RAST is not as sensitive as any form of skin testing and has some limitations because of the potential for chemical modification of the protein while coupling it to the solid phase by means of covalent reaction. The advantage of RAST is its use in research as a specific quantifier of allergen-specific IgE antibody. Also, RAST is easier to follow over time than skin tests are. RAST generally is much more expensive than allergen skin tests and has no advantage in routine clinical work. RAST has the substantial liability of requiring about 3 days to be reported from our laboratory, but allergen skin testing results are available within 15 minutes of application to patient. RAST may be useful clinically for patients 1) who have been taking antihistamines and in whom no positive histamine responsiveness can be induced in the skin and 2)

who have primary cutaneous diseases that make allergen skin testing impractical or inaccurate (e.g., severe atopic eczema with most of the skin involved in a flare).

- Skin testing is more sensitive and less expensive than RAST.

Patch Tests and Prick (Cutaneous) Tests

Many people seem confused about the concept of patch testing of skin as opposed to immediate wheal-and-flare skin testing. Patch testing is used to investigate contact dermatitis, a type IV hypersensitivity reaction. Patch tests require about 96 hours for complete evaluation (similar to tuberculin skin reactivity that requires 72 hours). Patch testing is useful only for investigating type IV hypersensitivity reactions leading to contact dermatitis. Most substances that cause contact dermatitis are small organic molecules that can penetrate various barriers inherent in the skin surface. Mechanisms of hypersensitivity postulated to explain these reactions usually involve haptenation of endogenous dermal proteins.

Inhalant allergens generally are sizable intact proteins in which each molecule can be multivalent with respect to IgE binding. Such molecules penetrate skin poorly and are seldom involved in cutaneous type IV hypersensitivity reactions. The exception appears to be house dust mite allergen in damaged skin of patients with severe atopic dermatitis. These patients mount a positive patch test to house dust mite allergen and an immediate wheal-and-flare cutaneous response with prick testing of allergen solutions.

- Patch testing is used to investigate contact dermatitis.
- Prick (immediate) skin testing is used to investigate respiratory allergy to pollens and molds.

Practical Skin Testing

Prick, scratch, and intradermal testing involve introducing allergen to skin layers below external keratin layer. Each of these techniques is increasingly sensitive (but less specific) as allergen is introduced more closely to responding cells and at higher doses. We perform allergen skin tests by the prick technique because it adequately identifies patients with significant clinical sensitivities without unduly identifying a large number of those with minimal levels of IgE antibody and no clinical sensitivity. We use scratch or intradermal testing in selective cases, including the protocol for evaluating stinging insect venoms.

- Intradermal skin tests are more sensitive but less specific than prick skin tests.

Double-Blind Placebo-Controlled Food Challenge

Historically, double-blind placebo-controlled food challenges are the standard for evaluating food allergy. We rarely use this challenge for patients with routine complaints of food allergy. Most patients with food allergy are aware of foods that are significant allergens and avoid them, without needing further therapy. Usual end points in food challenge testing are nausea, vomiting, diarrhea, abdominal cramps, and urticaria. Normally, we do not use this test for patients who have had anaphylaxis.

- The double-blind challenge is the standard test for food allergy.

Three other primary types of clinical challenge testing used in allergy are conjunctival challenge in the eye, allergen challenge in the nose, and bronchial challenge by inhalation of allergen aerosols. Common principles of good challenge testing include 1) blinding the tests, 2) using both positive and negative controls (usual positive control is histamine and negative control is bland diluent without allergen), and 3) choosing a time course for challenge that allows adequate return of challenged tissue to baseline before a subsequent challenge. For bronchial challenges, basal conditions may not be regained for 3-6 weeks after a positive challenge. Thus, in most instances, investigating sensitivities by direct tissue challenge is a lengthy process.

CHRONIC RHINITIS

History

Vasomotor rhinitis is defined as nasal symptoms occurring in response to nonspecific (in the sense of immunologic specificity) stimuli. One cause is pre-existing inflammation in nasal mucosa; thus, allergic rhinitis can cause vasomotor rhinitis. However, vasomotor rhinitis does not cause allergic rhinitis. All patients with allergic rhinitis likely have nasal congestion and other nasal symptoms provoked by change in air temperature, inert particulates, irritants, and strong odors (even pleasant ones, e.g., fragrances). For patients with allergic rhinitis who have symptoms caused by such immunologically nonspecific stimuli, we say their allergic rhinitis is complicated by vasomotor rhinitis. Patients who have nasal symptoms but no allergy have (pure) vasomotor rhinitis.

- Vasomotor rhinitis is nasal symptoms in response to nonspecific stimuli.
- Vasomotor rhinitis does not cause allergic rhinitis.

Historical factors favoring allergic rhinitis include a history of nasal symptoms that have a recurrent seasonal pattern (e.g., every August and September) or seem to be provoked by being near animals. Factors favoring vasomotor rhinitis include weather, soap aisle in supermarkets, strong odors, humidity and temperature changes (independent of "weather," i.e., air conditioning is a potent trigger), and lack of response to previous therapeutic trials of topical glucocorticoid medications flunisolide (Nasalide), beclomethasone (Vancenase, Beconase), or triamcinolone (Nasacort).

- Allergic rhinitis has a recurrent season pattern and is provoked by being near animals.
- Triggers of vasomotor rhinitis include weather, humidity and temperature changes, supermarket soap aisle, and strong odors.

Factors favoring both allergic rhinitis and vasomotor rhinitis (thus, without differential diagnostic value) include perennial symptoms, intolerance of cigarette smoke, and history of "dust" sensitivity. Although "dust" is a widely recognized allergen, allergists and other professionals use the term to mean allergens of a specific arthropod, the house dust mite. These allergens cause allergic rhinitis when in airborne concentrations far below levels necessary for casual observers to detect a particulate load in the air. Therefore, patients are unlikely to offer historical observations that correlate with house dust mite allergen exposure. When patients offer a history of "dust" sensitivity, they mean that when symptoms are provoked the particulate load in atmosphere is enough to scatter light, appearing grossly "dusty." Because all particulates (inert or otherwise) can trigger vasomotor rhinitis, the observation that "dusty" places cause symptoms is nonspecific. Factors that suggest fixed nasal obstruction (which should prompt physicians to consider other diagnoses) include unilateral nasal obstruction, unilateral facial pain, unilateral nasal purulence, nasal voice but no nasal symptoms, disturbances of olfaction without any nasal symptoms, unilateral nasal bleeding, and reflux of swallowed materials through the nose.

- Perennial symptoms, intolerance of cigarette smoke, and history of dust sensitivity are common to allergic and vasomotor rhinitis.
- Dust mite sensitivity is a common cause of perennial allergic rhinitis.

Allergy Skin Tests

Allergy skin tests ask an artificial question: "Does patient have allergen-specific IgE antibody sensitizing cutaneous mast cells?" Even if the answer is "yes," no allergic disease may arise from the biologic phenomenon represented by the positive skin test. Many persons in the general population (15%) have positive allergy skin tests to one or more allergens and may not have symptoms of an allergy. Because of the statistical frequency of both positive allergy skin tests and chronic nonallergic rhinitis (also called vasomotor rhinitis) in the population, some patients with only vasomotor rhinitis as a clinical problem will also have positive allergy skin tests. How can this be sorted out?

- In the general population, 15% have positive allergy skin tests.

The interpretation of allergy skin test results must be tailored to the unique features of each patient.

1. For patient with perennial symptoms and negative results on allergy skin tests, diagnosis is vasomotor rhinitis.

2. For patient with seasonal symptoms and appropriately positive allergy skin tests, diagnosis is seasonal allergic rhinitis.

3. For patient with perennial symptoms and allergy skin tests positive to tree and ragweed pollens, two major possibilities are: a) skin tests are coincidental and unrelated to the perennial symptoms; thus, diagnosis is vasomotor rhinitis; b) skin tests indicate clinical sensitivity to tree and ragweed pollens.

4. For patient with perennial symptoms, allergy skin tests positive for house dust mite suggest house dust mite allergic rhinitis. Another way to decide whether house dust mite allergen is clinically important is to conduct a clinical trial of dust mite allergen avoidance, e.g., have patient encase bedding appropriately (because the bed probably provides greatest amount of house dust mite allergen exposure--but wet carpet on concrete is worse).

5. For patient with seasonal (spring and fall) nasal symptoms and negative allergy skin test results, diagnosis is vasomotor rhinitis.

Use Sinus Radiography Judiciously

Reasons for obtaining sinus radiographs in patients with rhinitis are listed in Table 2-7.

Table 2-7.--Reasons for Obtaining Sinus Radiographs in Patients With Rhinitis

History of facial pain, especially if positional[*]
Fever
Swelling of malar eminence, nasal bridge, or brow
Proptosis
Unilateral nasal purulence, especially if pus streams from sinus ostium
Fetid breath with any of the above
Change in voice resonance
Nasal polyps[†]
Unexplained leukocytosis

[*]Some physicians include headache, but the kind of headache to be included must be defined carefully, because it is an unspecified symptom in most patients with rhinitis.

[†]High percentage of patients with nasal polyps have diffuse hyperplastic inflammatory sinus mucosal disease.

Some physicians think the sensitivity of plain film radiographs of the sinuses is poor compared with that of computerized tomographic (CT) scanning (using coronal sectioning technique). Good-quality CT scans with coronal technique do reveal greater detail about sinus mucosal surfaces, but it is debated whether the additional time and cost of CT scans can be justified. However, CT scanning probably is reasonable for patients being considered for sinus surgery and for those failing standard treatment for sinusitis. Be aware that patients with extensive dental restorations that contain metal may generate too much artifact for CT to be useful. For these patients, magnetic resonance imaging (MRI) techniques are better.

- Sinus imaging is indicated for suspected sinusitis.
- Sinus CT is preferred to sinus radiography for complicated sinusitis.

Steroid Therapy for Rhinitis

The need for systemic steroid treatment for rhinitis is minimal. Occasionally patients with severe symptoms of hay fever may benefit greatly from 5 days of 10-mg prednisone (10 mg four times daily by mouth for 5 days).

This may induce sufficient improvement so that topical steroids can penetrate the nose and satisfactory levels of antihistamine can be established in the blood. Taper of such a course is usually not necessary. Some physicians inject intramuscularly a parenteral steroid preparation (such as triamcinolone, 40 mg) that is long-acting; this can be helpful in patients unresponsive to other standard treatment. Proper dose is important if good results are to be obtained, but often too low a dose is given for the treatment to succeed. Patients with nasal polyposis may warrant 2 weeks of oral prednisone at 10 mg four times daily, because a significant fraction of them have near-miraculous "melting away" of nasal polyps on such a course. Subsequently, their condition may be controllable with topical steroids alone. Some physicians believe that all patients with nasal polyposis contemplating surgical treatment of the polyps should undergo a trial of oral prednisone at this dosage schedule preoperatively, because some of them will have such satisfactory results that surgery is unnecessary. The percentage of polyposis patients who will benefit has not been reliably estimated, and the practice remains controversial among ENT surgeons.

- Need for systemic steroids in rhinitis is minimal.
- For very severe hay fever symptoms, 40-mg oral prednisone daily for 5 days.
- Nasal polyposis may warrant oral prednisone followed by topical corticosteroids.

Physicians proposing courses of systemic steroid at these dose schedules need to counsel patients carefully. The likelihood of any significant side effect is low for these short durations of therapy, but the side effects that are seen can be catastrophic. The following must be specifically mentioned to patients and this disclosure **must** be documented in each patient's record: acute steroid psychosis, aseptic necrosis of the femoral head(s), acute glaucoma, mania, depression, weight gain (both fluid retention and real fat expansion due to appetite stimulation as well as specific pharmacologic effects on certain fat tissues), acceleration of any pre-existing tendency to ocular cataract, and renal stone formation. It is also a good idea to make a summary comment to the patient emphasizing the importance of contacting the physician immediately if anything unusual or unexpected (in the way of medical symptoms) should occur during the course of steroid therapy, just in case a catastrophic complication should occur and not be recognized by the patient.

- Know the important adverse effects of systemic glucocorticoid therapy.

In contrast with systemic steroid therapy, topical steroid agents for the nose are easy to use. The only agents considered herein are beclomethasone (available as Beconase and Vancenase), flunisolide (Nasalide), and triamcinolone (Nasacort). The only other steroid marketed specifically for use in the nose is dexamethasone (Decadron Turbinaire), which has significant systemic effects when used as directed and no therapeutic advantage over beclomethasone and flunisolide.

- Intranasal beclomethasone, flunisolide, and triamcinolone have few if any systemic effects.

When should topical steroids be prescribed for rhinitis? They are successful in treating hay fever and are safe to use. If therapy is initiated about a week before start of the relevant pollen season, many patients can be free of allergic rhinitis symptoms for entire pollen season. In challenge laboratories, these agents are most potent protection for inhibiting mucosal responses to allergen, even when given only 1 hour before allergen exposure.

- Topical steroids are successful for hay fever.
- Initiate therapy about 1 week before start of relevant pollen season.

When intranasal corticosteroids are used in combination with an oral antihistamine, nearly 90% of hay fever patients are satisfied with the relief. However, many patients seek medical advice only after pollen season has started. They must be counseled that nasal spray works slowly and its full benefits will not be realized for 3 weeks. Recall that most people's experience with nasal sprays is that marked change occurs within 5 to 10 minutes after spraying; thus, if patients are not adequately counseled, they may abandon the spray after 2 or 3 doses, because it did nothing to help their symptoms. (These patients may become angry with the physician because of the expense of the spray.)

- When used with antihistamine, 90% of hay fever patients are satisfied.

Most people are aware that treatment with nasal sprays is a bad idea because of "addictive" potential (vicious cycle of rhinitis medicamentosa caused by topical vasoconstrictors is common knowledge). Reassure patients that topical steroid does not induce any dependence.

● Unlike decongestant nasal sprays, topical intranasal steroid does not induce tachyphylaxis and rebound congestion.

A significant number of patients with vasomotor rhinitis also have a good response to topical aerosol steroid therapy, especially if patient has nasal eosinophilia and/or nasal polyposis form of vasomotor rhinitis. Without eosinophils on nasal smears and nasal polyps, the response is unpredictable. Only nasal smears and nasal polyps permit distinguishing eosinophilic and non-eosinophilic types of vasomotor rhinitis, so a therapeutic trial is the simplest therapeutic approach for nonallergic rhinitis. Some physicians think the answer to "Who should have topical steroid sprays prescribed for rhinitis" is "everyone." Although others think this answer fosters an uncritical attitude and shotgun therapy, it is not inappropriate if the implications of response and nonresponse to therapeutic trials are considered.

● Many patients with vasomotor rhinitis have a good response to topical aerosol steroid therapy.

If hay fever patient does not receive adequate relief with topical steroid plus antihistamine therapy, it may indicate need for systemic steroid and for initiating immunotherapy in winter so patient is prepared for next pollen season.

● Allergy immunotherapy should be considered for patients with allergic rhinitis who fail pharmacologic management.

The only important side effect of intranasal glucocorticoids is nasal septal perforation. Dry powder spray cannisters deliver a powerful jet of particulates (Beconase, Vancenase, Nasacort), and a few patients have misdirected the jet to the nasal septum. Septal perforation occurred because of mechanical irritation. Aqueous preparations (Beconase AQ., Vancenase AQ., Nasalide) avoid this minor complication.

● Nasal topical steroid sprays can cause nasal septal perforation.

For all the foregoing reasons, it appears that rhinitis

patients with perennial symptoms can use topical steroids year-round without concern about side effects. There is no evidence that topical steroids adversely affect the natural history of viral upper respiratory tract infections, so such infections are not a reason to discontinue steroid therapy.

● Topical intranasal steroids do not adversely affect the natural history of viral upper respiratory tract infections.

If air-fluid levels are seen on the films and clinical picture suggests sinusitis, antibiotic therapy is warranted.

● If air-fluid levels are seen on sinus films, antibiotic therapy is warranted.

The important point is that internists, when acting as consultants to primary care physicians in cases of recurrent rhinitis, can make a more sophisticated evaluation of patients and make substantial contribution to understanding of the nature of the clinical condition. In such cases, any course of antibiotic therapy should have a clear evidential rationale.

Antihistamines and Decongestants

Antihistamines antagonize interaction of histamine with its receptors. If histamine is the cause of the nasal vascular congestion, antihistamines may diminish nasal congestion. However, in cases of rhinitis other than allergic rhinitis, the role of histamine is unclear, and effective antagonism may appear to have little impact on symptoms. Histamine may be more effective than other mediators for nasal itch and sneezing. These are symptoms most often responsive to antihistamine therapy. Almost all the nasal effects of histamine are mediated by H_1 receptors (H_2 receptors are mainly but not exclusively in the gut). More traditional antihistamines also have anticholinergic effects in many patients (mediated mostly via central nervous system rather than directly in periphery); the "drying" effects of antihistamines occur primarily by this mechanism rather than by antagonism of histamine receptors locally in respiratory tract. This is important in considering several newer antihistamines that are designed not to cross the blood-brain barrier. These agents have little or no anticholinergic effect and thus no "drying" effect. Previously, the "drying" effect of some antihistamines was thought useful in managing "wet" nose. Currently, patients are informed through advertising about nondrowsiness properties of newer antihistamines and usually request them. Terfenadine and astemizole can cause serious cardiac arrhythmias (prolonged QT and torsades de pointes) in patients taking erythromycin or ketoconazole or who have significant liver disease. These adverse effects are rare, but patients should be informed.

- Histamine is an important mediator in allergic rhinitis.
- Nasal effects of histamine are mediated by H_1 receptors.
- Terfenadine and astemizole can cause serious cardiac arrhythmias in patients taking erythromycin or ketoconazole or who have significant liver disease.

Two decongestants, pseudoephedrine and phenylpropanolamine, are commonest agents in nonprescription drugs for treating cold symptoms/rhinitis and usually are active agents in widely used proprietary prescription agents. A large number of legend and nonlegend combination agents combine antihistamine and decongestant. You cannot be familiar with all of them but should be aware that combination drugs dominate the nonprescription market. Decongestant preparations are often the only therapeutic option for patients with vasomotor rhinitis unresponsive to topical glucocorticoids, and they are often helpful for those patients in whom headache is a dominant feature of the symptom complex.

- Pseudoephedrine and phenylpropanolamine are commonest decongestant agents in nonprescription preparations.

Note that middle-aged and older men may have urinary retention caused by antihistamines (principally the older drugs that have anticholinergic effects) and decongestants; these patients should be alerted. Although there has been concern for years that decongestants may exacerbate hypertension because they are α-adrenergic agonists, no clinically significant hypertensive response has been seen in stable medicated patients with hypertension. Nevertheless, keep this possibility (or idiosyncrasy) in mind.

- Antihistamines and decongestants may cause urinary retention in men middle-aged and older.

For antihistamines with anticholinergic activity, elderly patients should be warned about exposure to warm summer days, because the elderly seem more sensitive to anticholinergically mediated failure of sweating, thus increasing danger of heat stroke. Extremely athletic individuals of all ages also should be aware of this potential complication.

- Elderly seem more sensitive to anticholinergically mediated failure of sweating.

Immunotherapy for Allergic Rhinitis

Until topical nasal glucocorticoid sprays were introduced, allergen immunotherapy was considered "first-line" therapy for allergic rhinitis when relevant allergen was seasonal pollen of grass, trees, or weeds. Immunotherapy became "second-line" therapy after topical steroids were introduced because: 1) immunotherapy has no greater efficacy than steroids (either in number of responders per 100 cases or in degree of symptom relief in individual cases), 2) steroids are less expensive (in both time and dollars), and 3) immunotherapy has small but irreducible risk of serious reaction (anaphylaxis) that may cause death, but topical steroids have no serious potential complications. However, immunotherapy for allergic rhinitis can be appropriate first-line therapy in selected patients.

- Immunotherapy is about as effective as intranasal glucocorticoids.
- Anaphylaxis is a risk of immunotherapy.
- Immunotherapy for allergic rhinitis is first-line therapy in selected patients.

Immunotherapy is usually reserved for patients who get no satisfactory relief with topical steroids or who cannot tolerate nasal sprays. Occasionally, patients who had salutary response to immunotherapy but for some reason interrupted it, want to resume it. A trial of topical steroid is often recommended for such patients to make more informed decisions, but immunotherapy may be appropriate for those explicitly requesting it because compliance with nasal steroids is often poor. Immunotherapy is not given for food allergy and not usually for animal dander allergy. Practice is less uniform with respect to mold allergens, with endorsement divided in the subspecialty.

- Immunotherapy is reserved for patients who get no relief with intranasal glucocorticoids or who cannot tolerate nasal spray.

Environmental Modification

House Dust Mite

House dust mites are so small they cannot maintain their own internal water unless ambient conditions are high humidity. They eat all kinds of organic matter but seem to favor mold and shed human epidermal scale. They occur in all human habitations, although the population size varies with local conditions. The only geographic areas free of house dust mites are those at great elevations with extreme dryness.

- House dust mites require high humidity.
- They are found in all human habitations.

Areas in the home harboring most significant mite populations are bedding and fabric-upholstered furniture (heavily used), and any area where carpeting is on concrete (when concrete is in contact with grade). Although carpeting is often cited as a significant mite-related problem, carpet on wooden floors in the superstructure of a house usually harbors a small population. Dispersion of allergen from this source is not great compared with that from bedding and furniture. To prevent egress of allergen when mattress and pillows are compressed by occupancy of the bed, encase bedding (and sometimes, when practical, furniture cushions) in plastic encasements. To some degree, this also prevents infusion of water vapor into bedding matrix. These two factors combine to significantly reduce the amount of airborne allergen.

- Dust mite is an important respiratory allergen.
- Most significant mite population is in bedding and fabric-upholstered furniture.
- Plastic encasements prevent egress of allergen.

Recently, fluid sprays capable of either killing mites or denaturing the protein allergens from them have been marketed. Despite immunochemical evidence that the allergen is denatured by denaturant and mites are killed by acaricides, neither one is substantially helpful when applied in the home.

Pollens

Air conditioning, which enables the warm-season home to remain tightly closed, is principal defense against pollinosis. Most masks purchased at local pharmacies are **not** capable of excluding pollen particles and thus not worth the expense. Some masks can protect the wearer from allergen exposure, such as industrial-quality respirators designed specifically to pass rigorous testing by OSHA and NIOSH that qualify them capable of excluding a wide spectrum of particulates, including radioactive dusts. These masks allow allergic patients to mow the lawn and do yard work otherwise intolerable because of exposure to pollen allergen.

- Only industrial-quality masks are capable of excluding pollen particles.

Animal Danders

No measure can compare with getting the animal completely out of the house. No air filtration scheme feasible for average homeowners to install can eliminate allergen from an actively elaborating animal. If complete removal is not tenable, some partial measure must be considered.

If the home is heated or cooled by forced-air system with ductwork, confining the pet to a single room in the home is only partially effective in reducing overall exposure, because air from every room is collected through the air-return ductwork and redistributed through central plenum. If air return ducts are sealed in room where animal is kept and air can escape from room only by infiltration, exposure may be reduced. The room selected for this measure should be as far as possible from the bedroom of the allergic patient. Naturally, allergic patient should avoid close contact with the animal and should consider using a mask if animal handling or entry into room where animal is kept is necessary. Most animal danders have little or nothing to do with animal hair, so its shedding status is irrelevant. Bathing cats about once every other week may reduce allergen load in the environment, but overbathing (daily) may cause dry skin and enhance allergen dispersal.

- Complete avoidance is the only entirely effective way to manage allergy to household pets.

URTICARIA AND ANGIOEDEMA

The distinction between acute and chronic urticaria is arbitrary and based on duration of the urticaria. If it has been present for 6 weeks or more, it is called chronic.

Secondary Urticaria

The only reason any disease associations were recognized for urticaria is that the disease came first. Urticaria is rarely the presenting sign of more serious internal disease. Most patients simply have urticaria as a skin disease. Urticaria is part of the clinical syndrome of lupus erythematosus and other connective tissue diseases, particularly of more difficult to categorize "overlap" syndromes. Internal malignancy, mainly of gastrointestinal tract, and lymphoproliferative diseases are associated with urticaria, as occult internal infection may be, particularly of gallbladder and dentition. Immune-complex disease has been associated with urticaria, usually with urticarial vasculitis, and only hepatitis B virus has been identified as antigen in the cases of immune-complex disease.

- Urticaria is associated with lupus erythematosus and other connective tissue diseases, internal malignancy, internal infection, immune-complex disease.

Commonest cause of urticaria and angioedema other than idiopathic variety probably is drug reaction. This is uncommon on a chronic basis without offending drug being recognized and stopped.

- Chronic urticaria and angioedema are often idiopathic.
- Commonest secondary cause of urticaria and angioedema is drug reaction.

Relationship Between Urticaria and Angioedema

There probably is no fundamental difference between urticaria and angioedema. The critical factor is in what type of tissue the capillary leak and mediator release occur. Urticaria occurs when capillary events are in the tightly welded tissue wall of skin--the epidermis. Angioedema occurs when capillary events affect vessels in loose, areolar connective tissue of deeper layers--the dermis. Virtually all patients with common, idiopathic type of urticaria also have angioedema from time to time. When urticaria is caused by allergic reactions, angioedema nearly always occurs, too. The only exception is with hereditary angioneurotic edema type of disease (HANE), which is not related to mast cell mediator release but is a complement disorder. Patients with this form of angioedema rarely have urticaria. Why the molecular events seem confined to the vessels in deeper tissues is unknown.

- Virtually all patients with urticaria also have angioedema from time to time.

C1 Esterase Inhibitor Deficiency

A number of significant clinical differences usually suggest the diagnosis of hereditary angioedema. If HANE is strongly suspected, the diagnosis should be proved by the appropriate measurement of complement factors (C1 esterase inhibitor, quantitative and functional, and C4 [also, C2, if seen during episode of swelling]).

- C1 esterase inhibitor levels and C4 are decreased in hereditary angioedema.

Duration of individual swellings is quite different. Typical idiopathic urticaria and angioedema swellings last 2-6 hours in usual cases and commonly up to 18 hours; HANE-related swellings last 3-5 days. Most HANE patients have had at least one hospitalization for what appeared to be intestinal obstruction. If they avoided laparotomy on these occasions, the obstruction resolved in 3-5 days. Cramps and diarrhea are the usual intestinal symptoms in patients with idiopathic urticaria and angioedema; 3-5 days of obstruction is rare. In common idiopathic urticaria, the lesions itch intensely because histamine is one of the causes of wheal formation.

- Typical urticarial lesions last 2-18 hours and are pruritic.

Lesions in the HANE-type do not itch. Response to epinephrine is a useful differential point: HANE lesions do not respond to epinephrine, but common angioedema usually melts away in ≤15 minutes. Laryngeal edema almost never occurs in common idiopathic type disease (although it occurs in allergic episodes with measurable frequency, most often in insect-sting anaphylaxis cases); however, it is relatively common in HANE (earlier papers quoted 30% mortality in HANE, with all deaths due to laryngeal edema). Finally, HANE episodes are traceable to local tissue trauma in high percentage of occurrences, with dental work often regarded as classic precipitating factor.

- In HANE, swelling lasts 3-5 days.
- Most HANE patients have been hospitalized for "intestinal obstruction."
- HANE lesions do not respond to epinephrine.
- In HANE, laryngeal edema is relatively common.
- Dental work is classic precipitating factor for HANE.

The common idiopathic form of urticaria and angioedema is usually unrelated to antecedent trauma except in special cases of delayed-pressure urticaria, in which hives and angioedema follow minor trauma (e.g., to the hands while playing golf) of soft tissues. Duration of the lesions distinguishes this special form of physical urticaria from HANE.

Thus, only a small fraction of all cases with episodic swelling are not easily categorized as HANE-like or not, and assays for serum complement factors may be reserved for the few doubtful cases or to prove the diagnosis in cases with a suggestive history.

The five types of HANE-like disorders are: 1. Classic HANE is a genetic dysregulation of gene function for C1 inhibitor in which one allele appears to suppress expression of the other allele (i.e., autosomal dominant). Therapy with androgens (testosterone, stanozolol, danazol) reverses the dysregulation and allows expression of otherwise normal gene, resulting in half-normal plasma levels of C1, which is sufficient to eliminate clinical manifestations of the disease.

- Classic HANE is a genetic dysregulation (autosomal dominant).
- Testosterone, stanozolol, and danazol reverse the dysregulation.

2. In some cases of HANE the gene for C1 inhibitor mutates, rendering the molecule functionally ineffective. However, plasma levels of the C1 inhibitor molecule may be normal in these cases. This is basis for requesting immunochemical and functional measures of serum C1 inhibitor (with immunochemical measures only, the diagnosis is missed in cases of normal levels of an inactive molecule). Both classic HANE (low levels of C1 esterase inhibitor) and classic HANE with mutated gene for C1 inhibitor (nonfunctional C1 esterase inhibitor) are inherited forms of the disease (although both may be seen wherein the proband is also the sport that starts the mutational line, so the family history is not invariably positive even in these forms).

- Hereditary angioedema with normal levels of C1 esterase inhibitor but nonfunctional (by esterase assay) indicates a gene mutation.

3. C1 esterase inhibitor deficiency is seen as an acquired disorder with carcinoma or lymphoproliferative disease. It can only be suspected if associated neoplasm is recognized--it is not worthwhile to search for occult neoplasm if angioedema is diagnosed. The molecular tip for the presence of the disease is that plasma levels for C1 and for C1 esterase inhibitor are low. The hypothesis for pathogenesis of this form of HANE is that the tumor has or releases determinants that fix complement, and with constant *consumption*, a point is reached wherein biosynthesis of C1 inhibitor cannot keep up with consumption rate and relative deficiency of C1 inhibitor allows episodes of swelling.

- C1 esterase inhibitor deficiency can be an acquired disorder in carcinoma or lymphoproliferative disease.
- C1 levels are low in acquired C1 esterase inhibitor deficiency.

4. and 5. Basically, these two types are autoimmune disorders in which antibody to catalytic site on C1 inhibitor or to binding site for C1 inhibitor on C1q interferes with function of C1 inhibitor, hastening its destruction.

Physical Urticaria

Heat, light, cold, vibration, trauma/pressure have been reported to cause hives in susceptible persons. Getting the history is the only way to suspect the diagnosis, which is established by applying each of the stimuli to patient's skin in the laboratory (with the history guiding selection of stimuli; we do not routinely do any of these tests in all patients with urticaria). Heat can be applied by placing coins (soaked in hot water for a few minutes) on patient's forearm. Cold can be applied with coins kept in freezer or with ice cubes. For vibration, use laboratory vortex mixer or any common vibrator. A pair of sandbags connected by strap can be draped over patients to create enough pressure to cause symptoms in most susceptible ones. Note that unlike most common idiopathic urticaria (in which lesions affect essentially all skin surfaces), many cases of physical urticarias seem to involve only certain areas of skin. Thus, challenges will be positive only in the areas usually involved and negative in other areas. Directing challenges to the appropriate area depends on the history.

- For physical urticaria, the history is only way to suspect diagnosis, which is established by applying stimuli to patient's skin.

Food Allergy in Chronic Urticaria

Food allergy almost never causes chronic urticaria. Although urticaria can be an acute manifestation of true food allergy, gastrointestinal consequences of food allergy or anaphylactic phenomena usually predominate and urticaria is considered a minor feature. Most patients with chronic urticaria do not have gastrointestinal symptoms or the symptoms are vague dyspepsias that a huge fraction of population has occasionally and are probably unrelated to the urticaria.

Conversely, food allergy may cause acute urticaria, angioedema, or anaphylaxis.

- Food allergy almost never causes *chronic* urticaria.
- Food allergy may cause *acute* urticaria, angioedema, or anaphylaxis.

Histopathology of Chronic Urticaria

Chronic urticaria is characterized by mononuclear cell perivascular cuffing around dermal capillaries, particularly involving capillary loops interdigitating with the rete pegs of epidermis. This mononuclear cell cuff is mostly helper T cells, with some monocytes, macrophages, B cells, and mast cells. This is the usual histologic location for most skin mast cells. It appears there is about a tenfold increase in number of mast cells in the cuff compared with the normal value. However, the number of mast cells is still small compared with that of other round cells in the cuff. This histologic picture is consistent throughout skin, regardless of recent active urtication. Most pathologists consider "vasculitis" to indicate actual necrosis of blood vessel structural elements; thus, the typical picture of chronic urticaria does not meet criteria for vasculitis. Immunofluorescence studies on chronic urticaria biopsy samples for fibrin, complement, and immunoglobulin deposition in blood vessels are negative.

Urticarial vasculitis occurs, usually with histologic features of leukocytoclastic vasculitis. A few cases have intermediate features, i.e., leukocytoclastic features (in terms of cells seen in tissue) occur with little or no visible vessel damage.

- Characteristic of chronic urticaria is a mononuclear cell perivascular cuff around capillaries.

Management of Urticaria

The history is of utmost importance if the 2%-4% of urticarial cases actually due to allergic causes are to be discovered. Complete physical examination is needed, with particular attention to skin (including some test for dermatographism), to evaluate for vasculitic nature of the lesions, and to liver, lymph nodes, and mucous membranes. Laboratory testing need not be exhaustive: complete blood cell count with differential to discover eosinophilia; liver enzymes; erythrocyte sedimentation rate; serum protein electrophoresis to assess acute phase reactants; hepatitis-B serologies; antinuclear antibody; urinalysis; stool exam for parasites; and chest radiography. Only if patient seems to have strong allergic diathesis and some element in the history suggests an allergic cause is allergy skin testing indicated medically. However, patients with urticaria often have fixed ideas about allergy causing their problem and skin testing often helps to dissuade them of this idea.

- The history is of utmost importance in diagnosing allergic urticaria.
- Laboratory testing may include eosinophils, liver enzymes, erythrocyte sedimentation rate, serum protein electrophoresis, hepatitis-B serologies, stool exam for parasites.

Management of urticaria and angioedema is usually with H_1 antagonists; addition of H_2 antagonists may be helpful. Tricyclic antidepressants, e.g., doxepin, have potent antihistamine effects and are useful.

- Management is with H_1 antagonists.

FOOD ALLERGY

Clinical History

The clinical syndrome of food allergy should prompt patients to provide a history containing some or all the following: For very sensitive individuals, some tingling, itching, and metallic taste in the mouth occurs while the food is still in the mouth. Within 15 minutes after swallowing the food, some epigastric distress should occur; it may be nonspecific. There may be nausea and, occasionally with marked sensitivity, vomiting. Abdominal cramping is felt chiefly in periumbilical area (small bowel phase), and lower abdominal cramping and watery diarrhea should occur. Urticaria may occur in any distribution or there may be only itching of the palms and soles. With increasing clinical sensitivity to offending allergen, anaphylactic symptoms may emerge, including tachycardia, hypotension, generalized flushing, and alterations of consciousness.

In extremely sensitive individuals, generalized flushing, hypotension, and tachycardia may occur before the other symptoms. Nonspecific dyspepsia, which does not emerge as a stereotypic syndrome, chronic rhinitis, and chronic asthma are not part of the natural history of food allergy, nor are chronic fatigue, tingling in limbs, and aching in muscles and joints. Most patients with food allergy know the offending allergenic foodstuffs, so diagnosis entails confirmation by skin testing or other methods for measuring allergen-specific IgE antibody.

- Allergic reactions to food usually include urticaria.

Common Causes of Food Allergy

Table 2-8 lists items considered the most common allergens.

Table 2-8.--Common Causes of Food Allergy

Eggs
Milk
Nuts
Peanuts
Shellfish
Soybean
Wheat

Food-Related Anaphylaxis

Food-induced anaphylaxis is the same process involved in acute hypersensitivity to food allergens except the severity of reaction is greater in anaphylaxis. Relatively few foodstuffs are involved in food-induced anaphylaxis; the main ones are peanuts, shellfish, and true nuts.

- Anaphylaxis to food can be life-threatening.

Allergy Skin Testing in Food Allergy

In actual practice, if a patient has positive results on one or more skin tests to foodstuffs (reasonable candidates based on clinical history), an open challenge with the foodstuff may be conducted under physician observation. If that challenge is positive, the most compelling evidence is obtained with a double-blind placebo-controlled food challenge. With comparison of double-blind placebo-controlled food challenge with open food challenge, the frequency of positive reactions falls by half. It is reasonable to conduct allergy skin tests on patients with vague symptoms who think they have a food allergy, because the negative test results can be used to assure them that food allergy is not the root of the problem. Patients with food anaphylaxis should strictly avoid offending foods and carry an epinephrine kit.

- Positive results on skin tests and double-blind food challenges can confirm the diagnosis of food allergy.
- If results of food skin tests are negative, food allergy is unlikely.
- Patients with anaphylaxis to food should strictly avoid the offending food and carry an epinephrine kit.

STINGING INSECT ALLERGY

In patients clinically sensitive to stinging Hymenoptera, reactions to a sting are either the large local or the anaphylactic variety. In the large local sting reaction, swelling at the sting site may be dramatic but there are no symptoms distant from that site. Stings of head, neck, and dorsum of hands are particularly prone to large local reactions.

Clinical phenomena of stinging insect anaphylaxis are similar to all other forms of anaphylaxis. With stinging insects, antigen is injected parenterally. Thus, onset of anaphylaxis may be very rapid, often within 1-2 minutes. Pruritus of palms and soles is commonest initial manifestation and frequently is followed almost immediately by generalized flushing and hypotension. The reason for attaching importance to whether a stinging insect reaction is a large local or a generalized one is that allergy skin testing and, if positive, allergen immunotherapy are recommended only for generalized reactions. A large local reaction is not a harbinger of future anaphylaxis.

- Two varieties of reaction to sting: large local and anaphylactic.

Bee and Vespid Allergy

Yellow jackets, wasps, and hornets are vespids and their venoms cross-react to substantial degree. Venom of honeybees (order Apidaea) does **not** cross-react with that of vespids. Unless the patient actually captures the insect delivering the sting, uncertainty will likely attend many cases of insect-stinging anaphylaxis. Thus, we usually conduct skin testing to honeybee and each of the vespids. To interpret skin tests accurately, it is helpful to know which insect caused the sting producing the generalized reaction. Often, the circumstances of the sting can help determine the type of insect responsible. Multiple stings received while mowing grass or doing other landscape jobs that may disturb yellow-jacket burrows in ground are likely causes of yellow-jacket stings. A single sting received while near picnic tables or refuse containers at picnic areas is likely from a yellow jacket or possibly a hornet. Stings received while working around house exterior (painting, cleaning eaves and gutters, attic work) are most likely from wasps.

- Yellow jackets, wasps, hornets are vespids and their venoms cross-react.
- Venom of bees does not cross-react with that of vespids.
- It is helpful to know which insect caused the sting.

Allergy Testing

Patients who have had generalized reaction warrant allergen skin testing. Patients who have had a large local reaction to one of the Hymenoptera stings do **not** warrant allergen skin testing because they are not at increased risk for future anaphylaxis.

- Generalized reaction warrants allergen skin testing.
- Large local reaction does not warrant allergen skin testing.

Skin testing should be delayed at least 1 month after sting-induced general reaction, because tests conducted closer to time of sting have a substantial risk of being falsely negative. Positive results on skin test that correlate with clinical history are sufficient evidence for considering Hymenoptera venom immunotherapy. If the patients are selected appropriately for skin testing, results of tests should not be ambiguous. However, random testing of general population turns up positive results in patients without history of anaphylaxis.

- Skin testing should be delayed at least 1 month after sting-induced general reaction.
- Patients with clinical anaphylaxis and positive results on venom skin tests may benefit from venom immunotherapy.

Venom Immunotherapy

Decision to undertake venom immunotherapy can only be reached after a discussion between patient and physician. General indications for venom immunotherapy are listed in Table 2-9. Patients must understand that once initiated the immunotherapy injection schedule has to be maintained and that there is a small risk of the immunotherapy inducing anaphylaxis. It is important that patients understand that despite receiving allergy immunotherapy, **they must carry epinephrine when outdoors** because of 2%-10% possibility that immunotherapy will not provide suitable protection.

- There is a small risk that immunotherapy will induce anaphylaxis.
- There is a 2%-10% chance immunotherapy will not provide protection.

Table 2-9.--Indications for Venom Immunotherapy

History of anaphylaxis to a sting
Positive results on skin tests to venom implicated historically in the anaphylactic reaction
Patient's level of anxiety disrupts usual habits and activities in warm months
Occupational--higher than usual risk of sting
House painters
Outdoor construction workers
Forestry workers

Avoidance

Table 2-10 lists the warnings that every patient with stinging-insect hypersensitivity should receive.

The circumstances of each patient may provide additional entries to the list in Table 2-10. Also, patients need to know how to use self-injectable epinephrine in its several forms. Many patients wear an anaphylaxis identification bracelet.

- All patients with stinging-insect sensitivity should carry an epinephrine kit.

DRUG ALLERGY

Anaphylaxis

Anaphylaxis is a generalized allergic reaction whose clinical hallmarks are flushing, hypotension, and tachycardia. Urticaria and angioedema may occur in many cases, and in patients with moderate to severe asthma or rhinitis as preexisting condition, the asthma and rhinitis can be made worse. This definition of anaphylaxis is

Table 2-10.--Do's and Don'ts for Patients With Hypersensitivity to Insect Stings

Avoid looking or smelling like a flower
  Avoid flowered prints for clothes
  Avoid cosmetics and fragrances, especially ones derived from flowering plants
Never drink from a soft-drink can out-of-doors during the warm months--a yellow jacket can land **on** or **in** the can while you are not watching and go inside the can and sting the inside of your mouth (one of the most dangerous places for a sensitive patient to be stung) when you take a drink
Avoid doing outdoor maintenance and yard work
Never reach into a mailbox without first looking in it
Never go barefoot
Always look at the underside of picnic table benches and park benches before sitting down
Never attempt physically to eject a stinging insect from the interior of an automobile but pull over, get out, and let someone else remove the insect

based on its clinical phenomena. A cellular and molecular definition of anaphylaxis is "a generalized allergic reaction in which large quantities of both preformed and newly synthesized mediators are released from activated basophils and mast cells." The dominant mediators of acute anaphylaxis are histamine and prostaglandin D_2. Physiologically, the hypotension of anaphylaxis is caused by peripheral vasodilatation and not by an impaired cardiac contractility. In anaphylaxis patients placed flat or in reverse Trendelenburg position and in whom blood pressure may be extremely low, cardiac output is elevated and circulatory system is characterized by hyperdynamic low-volume, high-flow state. Also, heparinemia may result from heparin release from mast cell granules (heparin provides polyanionic complex partner for polycationic histamine storage in mast cell granules); this further helps prevent vascular stasis and thrombosis due to low-flow states. For these reasons, anaphylaxis is usually fatal in patients with preexisting fixed vascular obstructive disease in whom a fall in proximal perfusion pressure leads to critical reduction in flow (stroke) or in patients in whom laryngeal edema develops and completely occludes the airway.

- Clinical hallmarks of anaphylaxis are flushing, hypotension, and tachycardia.
- Urticaria and angioedema may be present.
- Histamine and prostaglandin D_2 are dominant media-

tors of acute anaphylaxis.
- Peripheral vasodilatation causes hypotension of anaphylaxis.

Classes of Drug Allergy

Drug Allergy Not Involving IgE or Immediate-Type Reactions

Stevens-Johnson Syndrome

Stevens-Johnson syndrome is bullous skin and mucosal reaction; very large blisters appear over much of skin surface, in the mouth, and along gastrointestinal tract. Because of propensity of the blisters to break down and become infected, the reaction often is life-threatening. Treatment consists of stopping the drug causing the reaction, giving systemic steroids, and providing intense supportive care. The patients are often treated in burn units. Penicillin, sulfonamides, barbiturates, diphenylhydantoin, warfarin, and phenothiazines are well-known causes (it seems any drug may be etiologic agent in a particular patient). A drug-induced Stevens-Johnson reaction is an absolute contraindication to giving a causative drug to the patient, i.e., there are **no** circumstances in which the indications for giving the drug outweigh the hazard.

- Stevens-Johnson syndrome is life-threatening and is an absolute contraindication for rechallenge with the drug.

Toxic Epidermal Necrolysis Syndrome

Clinically, toxic epidermal necrolysis syndrome is almost indistinguishable from Stevens-Johnson syndrome. Histologically, the cleavage plane for the blisters is deeper than in Stevens-Johnson. Cleavage plane is *at* the basement membrane of the epidermis, so even basal cell layer is lost. This makes toxic epidermal necrolysis syndrome slightly more devastating than Stevens-Johnson, because healing occurs with much scarring. Often, healing cannot be accomplished without skin grafting, so mortality is even higher than in Stevens-Johnson. Patients with toxic epidermal necrolysis are always cared for in a burn unit because of full-thickness burns over 80%-90% of skin. Mortality is very high, as in burn patients with damage of this extent.

- Toxic epidermal necrolysis syndrome is a life-threatening exfoliative dermatitis.

Macular "Drug Red" Syndrome

Macular "drug red" syndrome is a generalized skin rash that is fairly characteristic because it is intensely bright red. It is nonpruritic, flat (macular), and (except for its frightening appearance) usually causes patient no significant discomfort. It cannot be predicted, and because it potentially is related to the serious syndromes above, most physicians regard this type of rash as strong contraindication to giving the drug anytime in the future.

- Macular "drug red" rash is intensely bright red, non-pruritic, and flat (macular).

Ampicillin-Mononucleosis Rash

Ampicillin-mononucleosis rash is unique drug rash occurring when ampicillin is given to acutely ill febrile patient who has mononucleosis (a viral illness). The rash is papular, nonpruritic, rose-colored, usually on the abdomen, and has a granular feel when the fingers brush lightly over surface of involved skin. It is not known why the rash is specific for ampicillin and mononucleosis. The rash does not portend penicillin anaphylaxis or any of the above syndromes.

- Ampicillin-mononucleosis rash is papular, nonpruritic, rose-colored, and on abdomen.

Fixed Drug Eruptions

Fixed drug eruptions are red to red-brown macules that appear on a certain area of patient's skin; any part of the body can be affected. The macules do not itch or have other signs of inflammation, although fever is associated with their appearance in a few patients. The unique aspect of this allergic phenomena is that if a patient is given the drug of cause in the future, exactly the same skin areas have the rash. Resolution of the macules often includes postinflammatory hyperpigmentation. Except for cosmetic problems due to skin discolorations, the phenomenon does not seem serious. Antibiotics and sulfonamides are most frequently recognized causes. How a systemically distributed drug causes something so sharply restricted anatomically is a mystery. Bilateral symmetry has been seen in patients with noncontiguous areas of disease.

- In fixed drug eruptions the same area of skin is affected.

Erythema Nodosum

Erythema nodosum is a characteristic rash of red nodules about size of a quarter, usually nonpruritic and appearing only over anterior lower legs. Histopathologically, nodules are plaques of infiltrating mononuclear cells. Erythema nodosum is associated with several connective tissue diseases, viral infections, and drug allergy. This drug allergy is a relative contraindication to re-administration of drug.

- Erythema nodosum rash is usually nonpruritic, appearing only over anterior lower legs.
- It is associated with several connective tissue diseases, viral infections, and drug allergy.

Contact Dermatitis

Contact dermatitis can occur with various drugs. Commonly, it is a form of drug allergy that is an occupational disease in medical or healthcare workers. Some patients receiving topical drugs on skin develop allergy to the drug or various elements in its pharmaceutical formulation, e.g., excipients, fillers, stabilizers, antibacterials, and emulsifiers. Contact dermatitis is manifestation of type IV hypersensitivity, and clinically appears as area of reddening on skin which progresses to granular weeping eczematous eruption of skin, with some dermal thickening and plaque-like quality of surrounding skin. Histopathologically, affected area is infiltrated by mononuclear cells. Giant cells and granulomata are usually absent, except in specialized cases, e.g., reactions to emulsions of particulates of metals. When patients receiving treatment for some kind of dermatitis develop contact hypersensitivity to steroid or other drug used in treatment, a particularly difficult diagnostic problem arises, unless physician is alert to this possibility. When contact hypersensitivity to drug occurs, it does not increase probability of acute type I hypersensitivity developing and is not harbinger of the above serious exfoliative syndromes. However, patients can develop exquisite cutaneous sensitivity of this type so that almost no avoidance technique in the workplace completely eliminates dermatitis. Thus, it can be occupationally disabling.

- Contact dermatitis is a form of drug allergy.
- It is a manifestation of type IV hypersensitivity.

Penicillin Allergy

Penicillin can cause anaphylaxis in sensitive individuals. It is IgE-mediated process that can be evaluated by skin testing to penicillin major and minor determinants. Patients with positive results on skin testing and clinical history of penicillin allergy can be desensitized to penicillin (usually orally) but procedure may be hazardous.

- Penicillin can cause anaphylaxis.
- It is an IgE-mediated process diagnosed by penicillin skin testing.
- Patients can be desensitized but procedure may be hazardous.

Radiographic Contrast Media Reactions

Radiographic contrast media can cause reactions that have the clinical appearance of anaphylaxis. Estimates of frequency of these reactions are 2%-6% of procedures involving intravenous contrast media. Incidence of intra-arterial contrast-induced reactions is lower. The anaphylactoid reactions **do not** involve IgE antibody (reason for term "anaphylact**oid**" reactions). Radiocontrast media appears to induce mediator release on basis of some other property intrinsic to contrast agent. The tonicity or ionic strength of the media seems particularly related to anaphylactoid reactions. With availability of low ionic strength media, incidence of reactions has been low.

- Frequency of contrast reactions is 2%-6% of procedures.
- Reaction does not involve IgE antibody.
- Nonionic or low osmolar contrast media cause fewer anaphylactoid reactions than standard contrast media.

Radiocontrast media reactions can be prevented with use of low ionic strength media in patients with history of asthma or atopy. Patients with reactions who subsequently need radiographic contrast media procedures can be pretreated with protocol of 50-mg oral prednisone every 6 hours for three doses, with last dose 1 hour before procedure. At time of last dose, also give 50-mg diphenhydramine and 25-mg ephedrine orally.

- Patients with a history of systemic reactions to radiocontrast media a) should be pretreated with prednisone, diphenhydramine, and ephedrine and b) should be offered nonionic contrast agents.

QUESTIONS
(See "Answers" section)

Multiple Choice

1. Airways of patients with fatal asthma generally show which of the following:
   a. Mucosal infiltration with eosinophils
   b. IgE immune complex deposition
   c. Extracellular deposition of mast cell histamine
   d. Airway smooth muscle atrophy
   e. Pollen in airway lumen

2. Which of the following is an important adverse effect of aerosol corticosteroids:
   a. Aseptic necrosis
   b. Diplopia
   c. Seizures
   d. Dysphonia
   e. Tremor

3. Immunotherapy is effective in asthmatic patients allergic to which of the following:
   a. *Candida*
   b. Smoke
   c. Bacteria
   d. *Trichophyton*
   e. Grass pollen

4. Asthmatic patients allergic to dust mite should not do which of the following:
   a. Encase pillows and mattress in dust-proof casings
   b. Remove carpeting, particularly when laid on concrete
   c. Add high-efficiency air filter to furnace fan
   d. Run humidifier in the winter
   e. Wash bedding and linen in hot water (>130°F)

5. Increased risk for fatal asthma is associated with:

a. Tapering inhaled glucocorticoids
b. Overuse of β-agonist inhalers
c. Allergy to animal dander
d. Recent allergy skin tests
e. Use of anticholinergic drugs

6. A patient with past anaphylaxis to honeybee stings should do which of the following:
   a. Carry an epinephrine kit
   b. Have total serum IgE measured
   c. Take up beekeeping
   d. Receive immunotherapy with honeybee whole body extract
   e. Receive immunotherapy with yellow jacket venom

7. Which of the following is not a cause of perennial chronic rhinitis:
   a. Dust mite allergy
   b. Nasal septal deformity
   c. Ragweed pollen allergy
   d. Rhinitis medicamentosa
   e. Nasal polyps

8. A patient describes a history of exfoliative dermatitis involving the palms, soles, and mucous membranes after taking sulfamethoxazole. This patient:
   a. Should avoid β-lactam antibiotics
   b. Could safely take sulfamethoxazole if pretreated with steroids and antihistamine
   c. Should be skin tested to sulfamethoxazole
   d. Should avoid all sulfa agents
   e. Should avoid sulfamethoxazole but not other sulfa antibiotics

9. Peripheral blood eosinophilia is not associated with which of the following:
   a. Asthma
   b. *Strongyloides* infection
   c. Radiocontrast media reactions
   d. Allergic bronchopulmonary aspergillosis
   e. Churg-Strauss vasculitis

10. Which of the following can cause increased susceptibility to infection with *Neisseria*:
    a. Hypereosinophilia syndrome
    b. Terminal component (C5, C6, C7, C8) deficiencies
    c. Allergic bronchopulmonary aspergillosis
    d. Cl esterase inhibitor deficiency
    e. Systemic mastocytosis

True/False

11. The late phase bronchial response is reduced by pretreatment with:
    a. Albuterol
    b. Terbutaline
    c. Cromolyn sodium
    d. Beclomethasone
    e. Pirbuterol
    f. Triamcinolone

12. Asthmatics sensitive to aspirin:
    a. Should avoid indomethacin
    b. Can be successfully desensitized to aspirin
    c. Show increased prevalence of nasal polyps
    d. Can safely take ibuprofen
    e. Should wear a medical alert bracelet
    f. Should have skin tests to aspirin

13. Indicate whether or not the following are associated with nasal polyps:
    a. Chronic nasal congestion
    b. Recurrent sinusitis
    c. Cystic fibrosis
    d. Tonsillitis
    e. Asthma and aspirin sensitivity
    f. Contact dermatitis

14. Indicate whether the following are true or false about patients with selective IgA deficiency:
    a. Are less common than those with IgG deficiency
    b. May also have IgG subclass deficiency
    c. Should receive gamma globulin
    d. Are often asymptomatic
    e. Are at risk for transfusion reactions
    f. Should carry an epinephrine kit

CHAPTER 3
BLOOD GASES

William W. Douglas, M.D.

ASSUMPTIONS FOR BOARD EXAMINATIONS

Most board questions will provide you with specific values for Pa_{O_2}, Sa_{O_2}, pH, Pa_{CO_2}, and actual bicarbonate; sometimes electrolyte values will be included. To determine when the lung is not functioning normally as an oxygenator, you should be able to calculate the $P_{(A-a)O_2}$, especially when the Pa_{CO_2} is abnormal. You must be able to utilize values for actual bicarbonate because you will probably not be provided with values for base excess. You will be expected to calculate your own anion gap when electrolyte values are available. You must be able to construct an O_2-Hb dissociation curve to compare Pa_{O_2} and Sa_{O_2}. You must be able to estimate the appropriate compensations for simple disturbances of acid-base balance. You must know the differential diagnosis for each of the simple acid-base disturbances.

ABBREVIATIONS

The abbreviations used in this chapter are as follows:

CO-Hb	Carboxyhemoglobin
$FEF_{25\%-75\%}$	Forced expired flow over 25%-75% of vital capacity (liter/second)
FEV_1	Forced expired volume in 1 second (liters)
FI_{O_2}	Inspired oxygen fractional concentration
H^+	Hydrogen ion
Hb	Hemoglobin concentration, g/dL
HCO_3	Serum bicarbonate concentration, mEq/L
Ionized Ca^{++}	Serum ionized calcium concentration, mg/dL
K^+	Serum potassium concentration, mEq/L
MHb	Methemoglobin
O_2-Hb	Oxygen-hemoglobin
P_{50}	Oxygen tension at which hemoglobin is 50% saturated
$P_{(A-a)O_2}$	Alveolar to arterial oxygen tension difference, mm Hg
Pa_{CO_2}	Arterial carbon dioxide tension, mm Hg
Pa_{O_2}	Arterial oxygen tension, mm Hg
PA_{O_2}	Alveolar oxygen tension, mm Hg
pH	"Puissance hydrogen" (the logarithm of the reciprocal of the hydrogen ion activity)
PI_{O_2}	Inspired oxygen tension, mm Hg
Sa_{O_2}	Oxygen saturation, %

DISTURBANCES OF OXYGENATION

Abnormal Pa_{O_2} or Sa_{O_2} should be evaluated together with FI_{O_2}, Pa_{CO_2}, and Hb. The most common causes for abnormalities include hypoventilation and hyperventilation, ventilation-perfusion mismatch or diffusion impairment, right-to-left shunt, and abnormal Hb. Other causes include venous samples, "leukocyte larceny," high altitude, low FI_{O_2}, and laboratory errors. Erythrocytosis suggests that arterial hypoxemia has been present for at least several weeks.

- Causes of oxygenation disturbances: hypoventilation, hyperventilation, ventilation-perfusion mismatch or diffusion impairment, right-to-left shunt, abnormal Hb value.

CALCULATION OF THE P(A-a)O$_2$

The PAO$_2$ can be calculated by the following simplified bedside calculation:

$$PAO_2 = PIO_2 - 1.2\, PaCO_2 \quad (PIO_2 = 150 \text{ mm Hg at sea level})$$

The P(A-a)O$_2$ is obtained by subtracting the measured PaO$_2$ from the calculated PAO$_2$:

$$P(A\text{-}a)O_2 = PAO_2 \text{ (calculated)} - PaO_2 \text{ (measured)}$$

This calculation is required only when the FIO$_2$ is other than 0.21 or when the PaCO$_2$ is abnormal. The P(A-a)O$_2$ is abnormal when it exceeds 20 mm Hg in the supine position in persons <45 years old or in the erect position in persons <62 years old. The P(A-a)O$_2$ is abnormal if it is >30 mm Hg in the supine position in persons >45 years old or in the erect position in persons >62 years old. The P(A-a)O$_2$ is abnormal if it is >50 mm Hg when the patient is breathing 100% oxygen (FIO$_2$ = 1.0).

- P(A-a)O$_2$ is abnormal when:
  >20 mm Hg: patient supine and <45 years old, or erect and <62 years old
  >30 mm Hg: patient supine and >45 years old, or erect and >62 years old
  > 50 mm Hg breathing 100% oxygen.

CAUSES OF ARTERIAL HYPOXEMIA

Arterial hypoxemia may be present when the P(A-a)O$_2$ is normal, when the barometric pressure is low (high altitude), when the FIO$_2$ is low (in closed systems such as refrigerator entrapment, submarines and spacecraft, and closed anesthesia circuits), and when the PaCO$_2$ is elevated with respiratory acidosis or alveolar hypoventilation. Arterial hypoxemia may be present when the P(A-a)O$_2$ is increased as a result of lung diseases that cause ventilation-perfusion mismatching, ventilation-diffusion mismatching, or perfusion-diffusion mismatching. These diseases include mild-to-moderate asthma, mild pneumonitis, interstitial lung diseases, mild pulmonary edema, and pulmonary emboli. In all of these conditions, the arterial hypoxemia is corrected by oxygen therapy. Arterial hypoxemia that persists despite therapy with oxy-

gen sufficient to raise the FIO$_2$ to approximately 0.6 represents a right-to-left shunt, which may be either intracardiac or intrapulmonary.

- Causes of arterial hypoxemia: low barometric pressure; elevated PaCO$_2$; lung diseases that cause ventilation-perfusion, ventilation-diffusion, or perfusion-diffusion mismatching.
- Oxygen therapy is used for arterial hypoxemia.
- If arterial hypoxemia persists, right-to-left shunt is present.

Intracardiac shunts are usually caused by septal defects with elevated right-sided pressures. Intrapulmonary shunts may reflect abnormal anatomic pathways such as arteriovenous fistulas, but most commonly they represent perfused but unventilated alveoli (alveoli filled with liquids such as pus, blood, aspirated liquid, cardiogenic edema, or noncardiogenic edema) or atelectasis (bronchial obstructing lesions, endotracheal tubes in the main bronchus, or alveolar collapse due to impaired surfactant function such as adult or infant respiratory distress syndrome).

COMPARING THE PaO$_2$ WITH THE SaO$_2$

You should be able to compare the PaO$_2$ and SaO$_2$ to clinically relevant points on a normal O$_2$-Hb dissociation curve. You can construct one of these curves yourself quickly. Some of the easy-to-remember points are given in Table 3-1.

If the PaO$_2$ and SaO$_2$ points do not match on a normal O$_2$-Hb dissociation curve, then one of three conditions is likely to be present. First, the measurements may be in error. Clinically, this is the most likely cause, but this is usually not asked in board questions. Second, an abnormal Hb such as a congenitally right- or left-shifted Hb or methemoglobinemia may be present. Congenitally left-shifted curves present with hereditary erythrocytosis; congenitally right-shifted curves present with either hereditary cyanosis or anemia. Third, the O$_2$-Hb dissociation curve may have shifted to the right or to the left. A right-shifted curve means that oxygen is given up more freely in the tissues and oxygen delivery is improved. The O$_2$-Hb dissociation curve shifts to the right in the presence of increased PaCO$_2$, increased hydrogen ion (acidemia), increased temperature, and increased 2,3-diphosphoglycerate concentration. Remember that oximeters vary; pulse and ear oximeters analyze only two wavelengths of transmitted light and thus overlook car-

Table 3-1.--Points to Remember for Comparison of PaO_2 With SaO_2

PaO_2, mm Hg	SaO_2, %	Comment
20	35	Lowest level tolerated by most tissues
26	50	P_{50} of normal Hb
40	75	Normal mixed venous oxygen, at rest
55	88	Medicare standard for continuous O_2 therapy
60	90	"Knee" of the O_2-Hb dissociation curve; hypoxic drive and erythrocytosis are expected below this level
80	95	Lower normal arterial range
100	97	Upper normal arterial range

boxyhemoglobinemia; when methemoglobin is present, desaturation is suggested. The CO-oximeter, model 282, evaluates four different wavelengths and reports all four species (O_2-Hb, Hb, CO-Hb, and MHb) accurately.

- Always compare PaO_2 with SaO_2.
- If PaO_2 and SaO_2 points do not match, consider:
    error in measurements
    abnormal Hb
    O_2-Hb dissociation curve may have shifted.

IS ERYTHROCYTOSIS PRESENT?

Erythrocytosis is anticipated when arterial hypoxemia (PaO_2 <60 mm Hg, SaO_2 <90%) has been present for >3 weeks. Erythrocytosis may be the only clue to intermittent hypoventilation, such as obstructive sleep apnea or bilateral diaphragmatic paralysis with nocturnal hypoventilation, because the arterial blood gas study done with the patient in the erect position when awake may be normal.

- Erythrocytosis anticipated when arterial hypoxemia present for >3 weeks.

TYPICAL QUESTIONS REGARDING OXYGENATION PROBLEMS

What conditions are indicated by the following findings? (Answers follow the list of questions.)

1. Arterial hypoxemia present, $PaCO_2$ 45-50 mm Hg, pulse oximetry normal
2. PaO_2 high, $PaCO_2$ low, $P(A-a)O_2$ normal
3. PaO_2 low, $PaCO_2$ high, $P(A-a)O_2$ normal
4. PaO_2 normal or low, $PaCO_2$ low, $P(A-a)O_2$ high
5. PaO_2 and SaO_2 normal, but Hb elevated
6. PaO_2 normal, $PaCO_2$ high, $P(A-a)O_2$ low or negative
7. PaO_2 and SaO_2 low, $PaCO_2$ normal or slightly low, $P(A-a)O_2$ high, PaO_2 improves on O_2 therapy
8. PaO_2 and SaO_2 low, $PaCO_2$ normal or slightly low, $P(A-a)O_2$ high, PaO_2 does not improve with O_2 therapy
9. PaO_2 and SaO_2 low, $PaCO_2$ high, $P(A-a)O_2$ high
10. PaO_2 normal, SaO_2 low, patient is cyanotic
11. PaO_2 low, SaO_2 low in the laboratory but pulse oximetry normal and patient is not cyanotic
12. PaO_2 normal, SaO_2 by pulse oximeter normal, lactic acidosis present

Answers to questions listed above:

1. Venous sample
2. Respiratory alkalosis with normal lungs
3. Respiratory acidosis with normal lungs
4. Respiratory alkalosis with abnormal lungs
5. Erythrocytosis could be due to nocturnal hypoxemia with obstructive sleep apnea; when patient is awake and erect, the blood gases are normal
6. Respiratory acidosis; the patient is receiving oxygen
7. Arterial hypoxemia due to ventilation-perfusion or ventilation-diffusion mismatch without right-to-left shunt
8. Right-to-left shunt, either intracardiac or intrapulmonary
9. Respiratory acidosis with abnormal lungs
10. Methemoglobinemia or congenital right-shifted hemoglobin
11. Leukocyte larceny due to leukemia
12. Carboxyhemoglobinemia, cyanide poisoning, malignant hyperthermia, status epilepticus, strychnine poisoning

ACID-BASE DISTURBANCES

When evaluating disturbances of acid-base balance, always first consider the clinical context. Next look at the pH, which usually indicates which disturbance is the primary one. Normal values and the boundaries for disturbances of pH are listed in Table 3-2.

$Paco_2$ reflects alveolar ventilation relative to CO_2 production (the respiratory component of an acid-base disturbance) and changes rapidly. In outpatients, normal range is usually considered to be 35-45 mm Hg. In the hospital, wider boundaries, such as 30-50 mm Hg, are often favored. A value <35 (or 30) mm Hg indicates respiratory alkalosis, reflecting hyperventilation relative to CO_2 production, and one > 45 (or 50) mm Hg defines respiratory acidosis or alveolar hypoventilation relative to CO_2 production.

- $Paco_2$ reflects alveolar ventilation relative to CO_2 production.
- Normal range: 35-45 mm Hg.

Table 3-2.--Normal Values and Boundaries for pH Disturbances

pH value	Condition
<6.90	Death imminent
<7.15	Metabolic: therapy indicated
<7.20	Respiratory: endotracheal intubation and mechanical ventilation are justified
<7.35	Acidemia
7.35-7.45	Normal
>7.45	Alkalemia
>7.60	Severe alkalemia, therapy indicated
>7.90	Death imminent

Actual bicarbonate reflects the nonrespiratory component of an acid-base disturbance and usually changes over hours to days, except in the case of lactic acidosis and some organic poisons. Unfortunately, the actual bicarbonate also changes with changes in the $Paco_2$. A normal actual bicarbonate value is 22-26 mEq/L. Metabolic acidosis is present when the actual bicarbonate value is <22 mEq/L, and metabolic alkalosis is present when the actual bicarbonate is >27 mEq/L. To use actual bicarbonate, rather than standard bicarbonate or base excess, one must know not only that the normal value is 24 mEq/L but also that the value increases by 1 mEq/L for every 10-mm Hg increase in the $Paco_2$ above 40 mm Hg; also, the actual bicarbonate decreases by 2 mEq/L for every 10-mm Hg decrease in the $Paco_2$ below 40 mm Hg.

- Actual bicarbonate reflects nonrespiratory component of acid-base disturbance.
- Normal value: 24 mEq/L.
- Value increases by 1 mEq/L for every 10-mm Hg increase in $Paco_2$ above 40 mm Hg.
- Actual HCO_3 decreases by 2 mEq/L for every 10-mm Hg decrease in $Paco_2$ below 40 mm Hg.

COMPENSATIONS FOR PRIMARY DISTURBANCES

Compensations for simple disturbances may be calculated without resorting to an acid-base map and are useful in helping to decide whether an acid-base disturbance is simple or complex. Many systems have been used, but the simplest one in clinical practice may be the following:

1. Acute respiratory acidosis: HCO_3 increases 1 mEq/L above 24 for every 10-mm Hg increase in $Paco_2$ over 40
2. Chronic respiratory acidosis: HCO_3 increases 3 mEq/L above 24 for every 10-mm Hg rise in $Paco_2$ over 40
3. Acute respiratory alkalosis: HCO_3 decreases 2 mEq/L below 24 for every 10-mm Hg decrease in $Paco_2$ below 40
4. Chronic respiratory alkalosis: HCO_3 decreases 5 mEq/L below 24 for every 10-mm Hg decrease in $Paco_2$ below 40
5. Metabolic acidosis: $Paco_2$ should be roughly equal to the last 2 digits of the pH, but will not go below 10-15 mm Hg
6. Metabolic alkalosis: $Paco_2$ should be roughly equal to the last 2 digits of the pH, but will be limited (overridden) by arterial hypoxemia (the Pao_2 will decrease to <60 mm Hg when the $Paco_2$ rises to >65 mm Hg, when breathing air with normal lungs at sea level)

ANION GAP

An increased anion gap defines the presence of metabolic acidosis. When electrolyte values are given in a clinical problem, it is usually wise to calculate the anion gap to exclude the presence of an otherwise unsuspected high anion gap metabolic acidosis. The anion gap is calculated as follows:

$$Na - (HCO_3 + Cl) = <13 \text{ mEq/L (normal)}$$

IS THE SERUM POTASSIUM LEVEL CONSISTENT WITH THE ALTERED pH?

With acidemia, H^+ shifts into skeletal muscle and K^+ shifts into the blood. This effect is dependent on skeletal muscle mass and may not occur in, for example, quadriplegics. The amount of shift averages about 0.5 mEq/L per 0.1-unit change in pH and is reciprocal in a person with average musculature (i.e., if the pH decreases to 7.20, the K^+ should increase by about 1.0 mEq/L).

PRIMARY DISTURBANCES OF ACID-BASE BALANCE

Respiratory Acidosis

Respiratory acidosis is present when the $PaCO_2$ is >46 mm Hg and the pH is <7.35. Respiratory acidosis reflects alveolar hypoventilation relative to CO_2 production. CO_2 diffuses into cells and cerebrospinal fluid, where it is poorly buffered. The effect on the brain is therefore more dramatic than that with metabolic acidosis with a similar pH. The effect on the central nervous system is to cause cerebral vasodilatation with increased cerebral blood flow and cerebral edema, which may lead to papilledema and neurologic findings. The levels of circulating catecholamines also increase, producing sweating, flushing, and hypertension. The presenting symptoms and signs include headache, confusion, obtundation, flushing, sweating, and neurologic abnormalities including hemiparesis. Papilledema may be present.

- Respiratory acidosis: $PaCO_2$ is >46 mm Hg and pH is <7.35.
- Reflects alveolar hypoventilation relative to CO_2 production.
- Effects on central nervous system: cerebral vasodilatation, cerebral edema.
- Circulating catecholamines increase.

The most common cause of respiratory acidosis is acute or chronic airway obstruction. Most frequently this is chronic obstructive lung disease, usually with an FEV_1 <0.9 liter and an $FEF_{25\%-75\%}$ ≤0.4 liter/sec. An elevated $PaCO_2$ is used often to define the presence of status asthmaticus in patients with asthma. Major airway obstruction, especially foreign bodies, may lead to acute respiratory acidosis. With restrictive lung disease, such as kyphoscoliosis or fibrothorax, the vital capacity is usually <1.0 liter. In neuromuscular disease, such as Guillain-Barré syndrome, the maximal inspiratory pressure that the diaphragm can exert is usually more than -20 cm H_2O (i.e., the patient cannot generate a subatmospheric pressure lower than -20 cm H_2O). When respiratory acidosis is due to central hypoventilation, the patient usually either is in coma or has findings suggesting a brain stem lesion on neurologic examination. Respiratory acidosis may occur in only certain positions, such as tracheal compression due to an anterior mediastinal mass when the patient lies supine, in obstructive sleep apnea during rapid eye movement (REM) sleep (worse supine), or with loss of voluntary accessory muscle function during sleep in patients with bilateral diaphragmatic paralysis. When respiratory acidosis occurs in patients with cardiogenic or noncardiogenic pulmonary edema or in patients with pulmonary fibrosis, it is usually a preterminal event. Ventilator malfunction is another common cause of respiratory acidosis in the intensive care unit in intubated patients.

- Most common cause of respiratory acidosis is acute or chronic airway obstruction.
- If it is due to central hypoventilation, patient usually in coma or has findings of brain stem lesion.
- Ventilator malfunction is another common cause of respiratory acidosis.

Remember that there is a reciprocal relationship between the PaO_2 and the $PaCO_2$ when patients are breathing air (see Calculation of the $P(A-a)O_2$, page 28). In these patients, the PaO_2 should decrease by at least 1 (usually 1.2) mm Hg for every 1 mm Hg of increase in the $PaCO_2$ above 40 mm Hg. Because of the buffering of CO_2 by blood, the actual HCO_3 should increase by 1 mEq/L for every 10-mm Hg increase in $PaCO_2$ from 40 in acute respiratory acidosis and by 3 mEq/L for every 10-mm Hg increase in $PaCO_2$ from 40 in chronic respiratory acidosis.

- There is reciprocal relationship between PaO_2 and $PaCO_2$ when patients breathe air.

Respiratory Alkalosis

Respiratory alkalosis is present when the $PaCO_2$ is <35 mm Hg and the pH is >7.45. Respiratory alkalosis reflects alveolar hyperventilation relative to CO_2 production. It leads to cerebral vasoconstriction and decreased brain volume, an effect that is used therapeutically in patients with cerebral edema. Respiratory alkalosis causes a decrease in serum ionized calcium, which may lead to tetany and paresthesias. Respiratory alkalosis often provokes adrenaline release with associated tachycardia, pallor, and sweating, the usual symptoms associated with a panic attack and hyperventilation syndrome.

- Respiratory alkalosis: $Paco_2$ <35 mm Hg, pH >7.45.
- Reflects alveolar hyperventilation relative to CO_2 production.
- Leads to cerebral vasoconstriction and decreased brain volume.
- Causes decrease in serum ionized calcium (can lead to tetany).

The causes of respiratory alkalosis include anxiety and pain, but respiratory alkalosis can also accompany shock, sepsis, and endotoxinemia. Early salicylate poisoning, hepatic failure, arterial hypoxemia, and severe anemia also are associated with respiratory alkalosis. Maladjusted mechanical ventilators also may cause inadvertent respiratory alkalosis in intubated patients in the intensive care unit.

- Causes of respiratory alkalosis: anxiety, pain, shock, sepsis, endotoxinemia, early salicylate poisoning, hepatic failure, arterial hypoxemia, severe anemia, maladjusted mechanical ventilators.

With respiratory alkalosis, the Pao_2 should increase by at least 1 (usually 1.2) mm Hg for each 1-mm Hg decrease in the $Paco_2$. Actual Hco_3 should decrease by 2 mEq/L for every 10-mm Hg increase in $Paco_2$ in acute respiratory alkalosis and should decrease by 5 mEq/L for every 10-mm Hg decrease in $Paco_2$ in chronic respiratory alkalosis.

Metabolic Alkalosis

Metabolic alkalosis is present when the pH is >7.45 and the actual Hco_3 is >28 mEq/L. Metabolic alkalosis is usually initiated by the administration of sodium bicarbonate or the loss of chloride, such as occurs with vomiting, use of nasogastric tubes, administration of diuretics, or potassium depletion. Metabolic alkalosis persists because of endogenous aldosterone excess with paradoxic aciduria when patients are volume-depleted and potassium-depleted. The signs and symptoms include weakness, skeletal muscle cramps, ileus, seizures, and ventricular arrhythmias. The initiating causes include the administration of sodium bicarbonate, lactate, citrate, or acetate. Loss of chloride from the gut is caused by vomiting, use of nasogastric tubes, cologastric fistulas, diarrhea, villous adenomas, and tumors secreting vasoactive intestinal peptide. Renal loss of chloride with retention of bicarbonate is promoted by the administration of diuretics, salt-retaining corticosteroids, or licorice and is enhanced by potassium depletion.

- Metabolic alkalosis: pH >7.45, actual Hco_3 >28 mEq/L.
- Usually initiated by administration of $NaHco_3$ or loss of chloride.
- Persists because of endogenous aldosterone excess with paradoxic aciduria.

A simple rule for remembering what the respiratory compensation should be is to recall that the $Paco_2$ should equal the last two digits of the pH. This response will be limited (when the patient is breathing air) by hypoxemia, which will override the tendency to hypoventilation. This effect is enhanced at higher altitudes when lung disease is present and is limited in normal lungs at sea level to a $Paco_2$ of 65 mm Hg unless oxygen is administered.

Metabolic Acidosis

Metabolic acidosis is present when the pH is <7.35 and the actual Hco_3 is <22 mEq/L. It is useful to separate patients with metabolic acidosis into two groups: those with a normal anion gap and those with an increased anion gap. A normal anion gap in metabolic acidosis is associated with carbonic anhydrase inhibitor therapy, ureterosigmoidoscopy, long ileal conduits, diarrhea, and renal tubular acidosis. It may also be present, usually with hyperkalemia, after the administration of ammonium chloride, calcium chloride, amino acid hydrochlorides, and hydrochloric acid. It may also occur with hypoaldosteronism and renal tubular acidosis type IV. An increased anion gap in metabolic acidosis is usually due to lactic acidosis, azotemic renal failure, ketoacidosis, ingestion of exogenous acids, or D-lactic acidosis. Lactic acidosis usually reflects a combination of hypoperfusion of muscle and poor perfusion of the liver, such as occurs with shock, status epilepticus, and strychnine poisoning. Carbon monoxide or cyanide poisoning, administration of dinitrophenol or phenformin, and advanced leukemia are rare causes.

- Metabolic acidosis: pH <7.35, actual HCO_3 <22 mEq/L.
- Lactic acidosis usually reflects combination of hypoperfusion of muscle and poor perfusion of liver.

With azotemic renal failure, the offending anions are sulfate and phosphate. With ketoacidosis, the cause may be diabetes, starvation, or withdrawal from alcohol. Exogenous acids include formic acid from ingestion of methyl alcohol, glycolic acid from ingestion of ethylene glycol, and salicylic acid plus organic acids from ingestion of salicylates. With metabolic acidosis, the respiratory compensation is such that the $Paco_2$ should be the same as the last two digits of the pH. Because of the mechanical properties of the respiratory system, this compensatory respiratory alkalosis is limited to a $Paco_2$ of about 10 mm Hg in children and 15 mm Hg in adults.

- Ketoacidosis may be caused by diabetes, starvation, withdrawal from alcohol.
- Exogenous acids: formic acid (ingestion of methyl alcohol), glycolic acid (ingestion of ethylene glycol), salicylic acids plus organic acids (ingestion of salicylates).

The treatment of metabolic acidosis depends on the cause. Note that lactic acidosis resolves rapidly if the cause is removed so that therapy should focus on the treatment of shock in most cases. In patients with tetanic muscle spasm, muscle paralysis with intubation and mechanical ventilation may be indicated. Therapy with sodium bicarbonate or tris(hydroxymethyl)-aminomethane (THAM) is indicated when the pH is <7.15, but the volume administered is limited by hyperosmolality. With metabolic acidosis, one must anticipate potassium depletion early by calculating the anticipated potassium at pH 7.40 using the formula described on page 31.

- Potassium depletion must be anticipated early in metabolic acidosis.

COMBINED DISTURBANCES OF ACID-BASE BALANCE

Metabolic and Respiratory Acidosis

Combined metabolic and respiratory acidosis is a true medical emergency and constitutes the basis for cardiopulmonary resuscitation. Untreated, it is rapidly fatal.

Severe hyperkalemia is likely. The most usual causes are cardiorespiratory arrest, advanced shock states, and status epilepticus or strychnine poisoning with tetanic spasm of muscles interfering with respiration.

- Metabolic and respiratory acidosis: true medical emergency.
- Untreated, it is rapidly fatal.
- Severe hyperkalemia is likely.

Metabolic Alkalosis and Respiratory Acidosis

This combination is most frequent in patients with chronic obstructive pulmonary disease and associated chronic respiratory acidosis who are treated with diuretics. The $Paco_2$ may be significantly higher during sleep at night and clearly represents the primary disturbance; but when blood gases are measured during the day, the $Paco_2$ may be lower, such that the pH is on the alkalemic side, a finding incorrectly suggesting that the primary disturbance is metabolic alkalosis.

- Metabolic alkalosis and respiratory acidosis: most frequent in chronic obstructive pulmonary disease and chronic respiratory acidosis treated with diuretics.

Metabolic Acidosis and Respiratory Alkalosis

This combination is common with salicylate poisoning, which causes both primary disturbances. It may also occur with a combination of hepatic and renal failure and in sepsis and endotoxinemia.

- Metabolic acidosis and respiratory alkalosis: common with salicylate poisoning, which causes both primary disturbances.

Metabolic and Respiratory Alkalosis

This combination is also dangerous and commonly provokes seizures or ventricular arrhythmias. It most commonly occurs in the intensive care unit when a patient with chronic compensated respiratory acidosis is treated with overzealous mechanical ventilation. It may rarely occur in other combination disturbances, such as liver disease or central nervous system disease when nasogastric suction or vomiting are superimposed or sodium bicarbonate has been administered.

- Metabolic and respiratory alkalosis: dangerous and commonly provokes seizures or ventricular arrhythmias.

● Most commonly occurs in intensive care unit.

ILLUSTRATIVE CASES

Case 1

18-year-old woman in emergency room (ER); dyspneic, tachypneic, breathing air.

PaO_2 123	SaO_2 99	Hb 14
pH 7.70	$PaCO_2$ 15	HCO_3 19
Na 140	K 3.5	Cl 105

This patient has straightforward, uncomplicated primary respiratory alkalosis with alveolar hyperventilation. Note that the PaO_2 has increased by at least the same number of millimeters of mercury as the $PaCO_2$ has decreased from 40 and that the bicarbonate has decreased by 5 mEq/L. In addition, the serum potassium level has decreased in proportion to the change in pH. Assuming that inspired PaO_2 is 150 mm Hg (sea level, breathing air), then the alveolar PO_2 would be 132 mm Hg and the alveolar to arterial O_2 difference would be 9 mm Hg, which is normal.

Case 2

18-year-old acutely anxious woman in ER: on birth control pills, recent stress, breathing air.

PaO_2 85	SaO_2 98	Hb 13
pH 7.60	$PaCO_2$ 20	HCO_3 21
Na 140	K 3.5	Cl 105

This patient has primary respiratory alkalosis with increased alveolar to arterial oxygen tension difference. Note that even though the PaO_2 is normal, it is considerably lower than in the first example. The alveolar PO_2 here would be 126 mm Hg, so the alveolar to arterial O_2 tension difference would be 41 mm Hg. This patient should be evaluated for the usual causes of mild arterial hypoxemia, including asthma and pulmonary embolism.

Case 3

24-year-old man in ER after auto accident: chest pain, breathing air.

PaO_2 90	SaO_2 94	Hb 15
pH 7.40	$PaCO_2$ 40	HCO_3 24
Na 140	K 4.5	Cl 105

These values are normal. The saturation is, however, a bit low and should be about 97% for a PaO_2 of 90 mm Hg.

Case 4

19-year-old woman in ER after auto accident: somnolent, breathing air.

PaO_2 60	SaO_2 90	Hb 14
pH 7.44	$PaCO_2$ 35	HCO_3 23
Na 140	K 4.5	Cl 105

This patient has mild arterial hypoxemia, as might occur with mild asthma, pneumonitis, pulmonary fibrosis and other interstitial lung diseases, mild pulmonary edema or pulmonary emboli, and mild atelectasis.

Case 5

48-year-old woman in postanesthesia recovery room after laparotomy for small bowel obstruction: reintubated because of respiratory distress, $FIO_2 = 0.6$.

PaO_2 60	SaO_2 90	Hb 14
pH 7.45	$PaCO_2$ 35	HCO_3 23
Na 140	K 4.5	Cl 105

This patient has severe arterial hypoxemia with right-to-left shunt uncorrected by oxygen therapy. The differential diagnosis would probably exclude an intracardiac shunt but should include various types of intrapulmonary shunt, which include an endotracheal tube in the right main bronchus, other obstruction of a bronchus, or alveoli filled with fluid (in this case, most likely due either to left-sided heart failure with pulmonary edema or to adult respiratory distress syndrome caused by either aspiration of fecal gastric content or a leukoagglutinin transfusion reaction).

Case 6

49-year-old man, immediately after bronchoscopy for postoperative atelectasis: cyanotic, intubated, $FIO_2 = 0.6$.

PaO_2 382	SaO_2 51	Hb 12
pH 7.40	$PaCO_2$ 40	HCO_3 24
Na 140	K 4.5	Cl 105

This patient has methemoglobinemia; note the discrepancy between the PaO_2 and the saturation. In clinical practice, a laboratory error might be more likely, except that the patient is cyanotic.

Case 7

28-year-old fireman in ER after smoke inhalation: coughing, dyspneic, no burns, bilateral rhonchi, breathing air.

PaO_2 85	SaO_2 95	Hb 15
pH 7.15	$PaCO_2$ 15	HCO_3 5
Na 140	K 5.8	Cl 105

This patient has primary metabolic acidosis with an increased anion gap and an increase in the alveolar to arterial oxygen tension difference. The findings suggest some degree of lung injury from smoke inhalation together with the presence of lactic acidosis, which in this context could be due to either carboxyhemoglobinemia or cyanide poisoning. Carbon monoxide poisoning would be far more commonly associated with smoke inhalation. The saturation is 95% because the measurement was made on an unsophisticated oximeter, which samples only two wavelengths of light (red and blue) for oxygenated and deoxygenated hemoglobin. The detection of carbon monoxide requires a more sophisticated oximeter, which evaluates multiple wavelengths such as the CO-oximeter, model 282. Pulse oximeters evaluate only two wavelengths.

Case 8

55-year-old man with acute myelogenous leukemia: leukocyte count 230,000/mm^3, chest radiographs suggest infiltrates, breathing air.

PaO_2 48	SaO_2 73	Hb 12.1
pH 7.40	$PaCO_2$ 40	HCO_3 24
Na 140	K 4.5	Cl 105

This patient has leukocyte larceny. The nucleated cells in the blood sample are consuming oxygen at such a rapid rate that the oxygen is significantly depleted during the time it takes to transport the blood to the electrodes. Repeat blood gas determinations would show different degrees of hypoxia and, depending on which sample is run through which machine first, there may be a discrepancy between the PaO_2 and the SaO_2. In these examples, most of the patients are neither dyspneic nor cyanotic, and a pulse oximeter shows normal readings unless there is some other associated lung disease.

Case 9

19-year-old man left on steps of ER in coma: breathing air.

PaO_2 45	SaO_2 70	Hb 14
pH 7.15	$PaCO_2$ 80	HCO_3 28
Na 140	K 5.7	Cl 105

This patient has primary respiratory acidosis, causing arterial hypoxemia by hypoventilation, an increase in bicarbonate by buffering, and hyperkalemia due to acidosis. The alveolar PO_2 is 54 mm Hg, so the alveolar to arterial oxygen tension difference is 9 mm Hg, which is normal. Therefore, there is no evidence for primary lung injury, and the respiratory acidosis could all be central in origin. The hyperkalemia and bicarbonate concentrations are completely appropriate for the change in pH and $PaCO_2$. The anion gap is normal.

Case 10

58-year-old man with chronic obstructive pulmonary disease and cor pulmonale: chest cold for 10 days, somnolent for 4 days, barely arousable, breathing air.

PaO_2 32	SaO_2 50	Hb 19
pH 7.25	$PaCO_2$ 80	HCO_3 34
Na 140	K 3.5	Cl 93

This patient has primary respiratory acidosis with some (about 6 mEq/L) renal compensation consistent with the clinical history of acute and chronic respiratory acidosis. Patients with chronic, completely compensated respiratory acidosis usually have a pH between 7.32 and 7.35. The PaO_2 is lower than anticipated for the $PaCO_2$ (the alveolar to arterial O_2 tension difference is increased), consistent with his known lung disease. The potassium value is inappropriately low, suggesting that he may have been taking diuretics and steroids. The anion gap is normal.

Case 11

58-year-old man with acute and chronic respiratory failure due to chronic obstructive pulmonary disease: breathing O_2 via mask at 6 liters/min.

PaO_2 88	SaO_2 94	Hb 19
pH 7.18	$PaCO_2$ 110	HCO_3 40
Na 140	K 4.8	Cl 90

This patient has severe primary respiratory acidosis. This is the same patient described in case 10, who has been given excessive oxygen, suppressing his hypoxic drive to breathe and aggravating his hypoventilation. The pH is now into a range at which intubation and mechanical ventilation are justifiable. The correct treatment for primary respiratory acidosis with arterial hypoxemia is low-flow oxygen with an aim to correct the Pa_{O_2} to between 55 and 60 mm Hg.

Case 12

58-year-old man with acute and chronic respiratory failure 4 hours after intubation and mechanical ventilation: $FI_{O_2} = 0.3$.

Pa_{O_2} 72	Sa_{O_2} 92	Hb 18
pH 7.66	Pa_{CO_2} 30	H_{CO_3} 33
Na 140	K 3.8	Cl 90

This patient has combined respiratory and metabolic alkalosis producing severe alkalemia. This is the same patient described in case 10 and case 11, who has received overzealous mechanical ventilation. The goal of mechanical ventilation in a patient with respiratory acidosis is a normal pH, not a normal Pa_{CO_2}, together with correction of the arterial hypoxemia.

Case 13

58-year-old man with chronic obstructive pulmonary disease and cor pulmonale: chest cold for 10 days, somnolent for 4 days, barely arousable, breathing air.

Pa_{O_2} 28	Sa_{O_2} 46	Hb 18
pH 7.15	Pa_{CO_2} 80	H_{CO_3} 27
Na 140	K 6.0	Cl 88

This patient has primary acidosis, similar to that noted in case 10. Note, however, that the pH and bicarbonate are in a range anticipated for acute respiratory acidosis alone, but the history suggests that there may have been chronic respiratory acidosis predating the acute deterioration. Calculation of the anion gap provides the answer: lactic acidosis is also present with an anion gap of 25 mEq/L. In most patients, this is caused by a combination of arterial hypoxemia and a low cardiac output and suggests a more urgent situation than that noted in case 10. This patient should probably have immediate intubation and mechanically assisted ventilation together with measures designed to augment cardiac output.

Case 14

58-year-old man with chronic obstructive pulmonary disease and cor pulmonale: receiving furosemide and prednisone therapy, breathing air.

Pa_{O_2} 45	Sa_{O_2} 80	Hb 19
pH 7.55	Pa_{CO_2} 60	H_{CO_3} 51
Na 140	K 2.0	Cl 79

This patient has metabolic alkalosis with (probably primary) respiratory acidosis, hypokalemia and hypochloremia, arterial hypoxemia with an increased alveolar to arterial O_2 tension difference, and erythrocytosis. These findings are not uncommon in patients with chronic obstructive pulmonary disease who are treated with diuretics and corticosteroids and who are not given potassium chloride replacement.

Case 15

50-year-old man transferred 4 weeks after operation for small bowel obstruction: nasogastric drainage, O_2 via nasal cannula at 2 liters/min.

Pa_{O_2} 76	Sa_{O_2} 97	Hb 12
pH 7.60	Pa_{CO_2} 60	H_{CO_3} 57
Na 140	K 2.0	Cl 75

This patient has metabolic alkalosis with respiratory acidosis, which may be only compensation or may be a separate primary disturbance. As a general rule, the Pa_{CO_2} will not increase higher than the last two digits of the pH, unless there is associated primary respiratory acidosis. In this example, pH and Pa_{CO_2} were normal in 4 days after treatment with potassium chloride for the hypokalemic-hypochloremic metabolic alkalosis caused by the nasogastric drainage.

Case 16

60-year-old woman with ureterosigmoidostomy and recent chest pain: breathing air.

Pa_{O_2} 90	Sa_{O_2} 96	Hb 14
pH 7.25	Pa_{CO_2} 25	H_{CO_3} 9
Na 140	K 5.2	Cl 118

This patient has primary metabolic acidosis with a normal anion gap consistent with ureterosigmoidostomy.

Case 17

75-year-old man collapsed after complaining of lower abdominal pain: blood pressure unobtainable, breathing air.

Pa_{O_2} 105	Sa_{O_2} 98	Hb 12
pH 7.25	Pa_{CO_2} 25	H_{CO_3} 9
Na 140	K 5.2	Cl 105

This patient has primary metabolic acidosis with an increased anion gap consistent with lactic acidosis due to a ruptured abdominal aortic aneurysm. Note that the Pa_{CO_2} in cases 16 and 17 is the same as the last two digits of the pH, suggesting that the respiratory compensation for the acidosis is appropriate.

Case 18

62-year-old man with ventricular fibrillation in coronary care unit during cardiopulmonary resuscitation: awake, breathing air.

Pa_{O_2} 45	Sa_{O_2} 70	Hb 14

pH 7.00	Pa_{CO_2} 80	H_{CO_3} 18
Na 140	K 6.2	Cl 105

This patient has primary respiratory acidosis and primary metabolic acidosis with an increased anion gap consistent with cardiorespiratory failure and associated lactic acidosis. The arterial hypoxemia is consistent with hypoventilation alone, suggesting that pulmonary edema has not yet developed.

Case 19

3-year-old child found stuporous, with labored breathing: in ER, breathing air.

Pa_{O_2} 120	Sa_{O_2} 99	Hb 13
pH 7.40	Pa_{CO_2} 15	H_{CO_3} 9
Na 140	K 4.5	Cl 105

This patient has primary respiratory alkalosis and primary metabolic acidosis with an increased anion gap, the combination resulting in a normal pH. The Pa_{O_2} is appropriate for the Pa_{CO_2}, suggesting that there is no significant lung injury. These findings in a child are most frequent with aspirin poisoning.

QUESTIONS
(See "Answers" section)

Multiple Choice
1. A 56-year-old woman is admitted because of dyspnea. Arterial blood gas values, obtained with her breathing air at sea level, are:

Pa_{O_2} 56	Sa_{O_2} 88	Hb 13.4
pH 7.44	Pa_{CO_2} 33	H_{CO_3} -23
Na 140	K 4.5	Cl 106

O_2 at 4 L/min via nasal cannula is given. Arterial blood gas values obtained after 30 minutes are:

Pa_{O_2} 120	Sa_{O_2} 99	Hb 13.4
pH 7.44	Pa_{CO_2} 33	H_{CO_3} -23
Na 140	K 4.5	Cl 106

Diagnostic possibilities include all but which of the following?
a. Pulmonary embolus
b. Pneumonitis
c. Mild asthma
d. Pulmonary fibrosis, early
e. Atrial septal defect with right-to-left shunt

2. A 78-year-old woman is brought from a nursing home after vomiting caused by a bowel obstruction. Laparotomy is done with lysis of adhesions. Postoperatively, she is extubated but develops cyanosis and respiratory distress. She is reintubated, and mechanical ventilation is begun using $F_{IO_2} = 0.6$. Arterial blood gas values are:

Pa_{O_2} 40	Sa_{O_2} 75	Hb 12.5
pH 7.42	Pa_{CO_2} 42	H_{CO_3} 24

| Na 140 | K 4.1 | Cl 105 |

The likely possibilities include all but which of the following?
a. The endotracheal tube is in the right main bronchus
b. Overdose of narcotic with hypoventilation
c. Retained secretions causing atelectasis
d. A myocardial infarction with pulmonary edema
e. Aspiration of gastric contents with adult respiratory distress syndrome

3. A 62-year-old man is transferred from another hospital because of a persistent small bowel obstruction after elective cholecystectomy. He has a nasogastric tube attached to suction and has been on O_2 at 2 L/min via nasal cannula. Arterial blood gas values are:

Pao_2 96	Sao_2 99	Hb 14.0
pH 7.60	$Paco_2$ 60	HCO_3 57
Na 140	K 2.6	Cl 73

The most probable cause of the elevated $Paco_2$ is:
a. Respiratory muscle weakness due to hypokalemia
b. Impaired O_2 transport due to hypophosphatemia
c. Unrecognized chronic obstructive pulmonary disease with respiratory failure aggravated by O_2 therapy
d. Metabolic alkalosis with appropriate compensation
e. Obstructive sleep apnea

4. A 3-year-old child is brought to the emergency room unresponsive. Arterial blood gas values, obtained breathing air, are:

Pao_2 125	Sao_2 99	Hb 13.0
pH 7.40	$Paco_2$ 15	HCO_3 8
Na 142	K 4.2	Cl 104

The most relevant test to order next is:
a. Type and crossmatch for transfusion
b. Salicylate level
c. Blood cultures
d. Blood lactate level
e. Creatinine and blood urea nitrogen

True/False

5. A 35-year-old firefighter comes to the emergency room after being exposed to fire smoke. He is coughing and is somewhat confused. Arterial blood gas values, obtained breathing air, are:

Pao_2 105	Sao_2 99	Hb 13.5
pH 7.25	$Paco_2$ 25	HCO_3 11
Na 140	K 5.2	Cl 102

Are the following statements true or false?
a. The patient most likely has lactic acidosis
b. The most likely culprit is carboxyhemoglobinemia
c. Oxygen therapy is urgently indicated

6. An 18-year-old woman is brought to the emergency room because of dyspnea. She has been under great stress, is taking birth control pills, appears anxious, and is breathing at 36 breaths/min. Arterial blood gas values, obtained breathing air, are:

Pao_2 82	Sao_2 99	Hb 14.0
pH 7.60	$Paco_2$ 22	HCO_3 20
Na 140	K 3.6	Cl 108

This patient is hyperventilating. Her lungs are normal. She can be reassured and dismissed from the emergency room. True or false?

7. A 29-year-old man is dumped at the steps of the emergency room. He is unresponsive, has tiny pupils, and is breathing at 8 breaths/min. Arterial blood gas values, obtained breathing air, are as follows:

Pao_2 50	Sao_2 95	Hb 15.4
pH 7.15	$Paco_2$ 80	HCO_3 28
Na 140	K 5.7	Cl 103

Are the following statements true or false?
a. The arterial hypoxemia is most likely due to an associated lung injury such as aspiration pneumonia or pulmonary edema
b. The hyperkalemia in this patient is most likely due to renal failure or rhabdomyolysis
c. The elevated bicarbonate concentration represents renal compensation of the primary disturbance rather than buffering alone

CHAPTER 4
CARDIOLOGY I

Rick A. Nishimura, M.D.

PART I
CORONARY ARTERY DISEASE

INTRODUCTION

Coronary artery disease, principally myocardial infarction, accounts for approximately one of three deaths in the U.S., or nearly 600,000 deaths annually. The substantial reductions in the death rate from acute myocardial infarction that have occurred in the last 2 decades (Fig. 4-1) are attributed to efforts in primary prevention and new interventions in the treatment of myocardial infarction. The variable presentation of myocardial infarction includes asymptomatic patients; ones with angina, silent ischemia, unstable angina, or myocardial infarction; and sudden death.

- About 1/3 of deaths annually in U.S. are due to myocardial infarction.
- Substantial decrease in last 2 decades in death from acute myocardial infarction is due to primary prevention and new treatments of myocardial infarction.

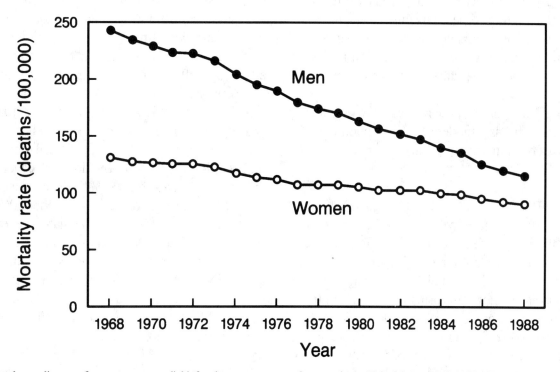

Fig. 4-1. Annual mortality rates from acute myocardial infarction among men and women in the United States, 1968-1988. (From Manson JE, Tosteson H, Ridker PM, Satterfield S, Hebert P, O'Connor GT, Buring JE, Hennekens CH: The primary prevention of myocardial infarction. N Engl J Med 326:1406-1416, 1992. By permission of the journal.)

PRIMARY PREVENTION OF CORONARY ARTERY DISEASE IN MYOCARDIAL INFARCTION

The known risk factors for coronary artery disease are tobacco abuse, serum cholesterol level, a lower serum HDL cholesterol level, serum LDL cholesterol level, hypertension, physical activity, obesity, diabetes, estrogens, and alcohol. Primary prevention includes modification of the following risk factors (N. Engl. J. Med. 326:1406-1416, 1992):

- Smoking more than doubles the incidence of coronary artery disease and increases mortality by 70%.
- The relative risk of smokers who have quit smoking decreases rapidly, approaching levels of nonsmokers within 2-3 years.
- A 1% reduction in total serum cholesterol yields a 2%-3% reduction in the risk of coronary artery disease.
- The estimated reduction risk of myocardial infarction is 2%-3% for each 1-mm Hg decrease in diastolic blood pressure.
- The estimated reduction in the risk of myocardial infarction with maintenance of an active compared with sedentary lifestyle is 35%-55%.
- The adjusted mortality rates for coronary artery disease are two to three times higher in diabetic men and three to seven times higher in diabetic women.
- In postmenopausal women, the reduction in risk of coronary artery disease attributable to estrogen therapy is 44%.
- Although heavy alcohol use increases the risk of cardiovascular disease, moderate consumption reduces the risk of heart disease.

MECHANISM OF ATHEROSCLEROSIS

The response to injury hypothesis is the most prevalent explanation of atherosclerosis (N. Engl. J. Med. 326:242-250, 1992). According to this hypothesis, chronic minimal injury to the arterial endothelium is caused mainly by a disturbance in the pattern of blood flow (type I injury), potentiated by high cholesterol levels, infections, and tobacco smoke. Type I injury leads to accumulation of lipids and macrophages. Release of toxic products by macrophages produces type II injury, which is characterized by adhesion of platelets. Macrophages and platelets with endothelial-release growth factors cause migration and proliferation of smooth muscle cells, which form a fibrointimal lesion or lipid lesion. Disruption of a lipid lesion with a thin capsule causes type III damage, with thrombus formation. The thrombus may organize and contribute to the growth of the atherosclerotic lesion or become totally occluded, culminating in unstable angina or myocardial infarction (Fig. 4-2).

- The most prevalent explanation for atherosclerosis is the response to injury hypothesis.
- Type II injury is characterized by adhesion of platelets.
- Type III damage is disruption of a lipid lesion leading to thrombus formation.
- Lipid-laden coronary artery lesions with less severe angiographic stenosis are more prone to rapid progression due to atherosclerotic plaque disruption.
- In up to two-thirds of cases of unstable angina or myocardial infarction, the lesion is a vessel with <50% stenosis.

CHRONIC STABLE ANGINA

Pathophysiology

In chronic stable angina, myocardial ischemia is caused chiefly by increased myocardial oxygen demand of the heart. Less important factors are perfusion pressure (aortic-to-right-atrial gradient), autoregulation (maintenance of coronary blood flow through a physiologic range of perfusion pressures), autonomic tone, and compressive effect (high left ventricular end-diastolic pressure decreases subendocardial flow). Normally, coronary blood flow can increase up to five times to meet myocardial oxygen demands of the heart. Ischemia occurs when flow reserve is inadequate, usually the result of fixed coronary artery disease. Resting blood flow does not cause ischemia unless vessel stenosis is >95%. However, a decrease in flow reserve begins to occur with about 60% stenosis, which is the mechanism for ischemia with exercise. The four factors that determine myocardial oxygen consumption are heart rate, afterload, contractility, and wall tension [wall tension = (left ventricular radius) x (left ventricular pressure)]. With a dilated, poorly contractile left ventricle, the contribution of wall tension to myocardial oxygen consumption outweighs the other factors. The temporal sequence of events includes ischemia $\rightarrow$ diastolic dysfunction $\rightarrow$ regional wall motion abnormalities $\rightarrow$ electrocardiographic changes $\rightarrow$ pain.

- In chronic stable angina, myocardial ischemia is caused by increased myocardial oxygen demand.

- Normally, coronary blood flow can increase up to five times to meet myocardial oxygen demands.
- Resting blood flow does not cause ischemia unless stenosis is >95%.
- Four factors of myocardial oxygen consumption--heart rate, afterload, contractility, wall tension.
- The temporal sequence of events: ischemia → diastolic dysfunction → regional wall motion abnormalities → electrocardiographic changes → pain.

Symptomatic Chronic Coronary Artery Disease

Many patients have symptoms of angina pectoris during physical activity. The pain is described variously as "pressure," "burning," "stabbing," "ache," "hurt," or "shortness of breath." It can be substernal or epigastric and can radiate to the neck, jaw, shoulder, elbow, or wrist. In chronic stable angina, the pain lasts 2-30 minutes and is usually relieved by rest. It is generally precipitated by any activity that increases myocardial oxygen consumption. The physical signs occurring with the pain include onset of a fourth heart sound and mitral regurgitant murmur due to papillary muscle dysfunction. ST-segment depression may be found on electrocardiogram (ECG), indicating subendocardial ischemia. The double product [(heart rate) x (systolic blood pressure)] is useful for defining myocardial oxygen demand. Nocturnal angina can be caused by unstable angina and also by increased wall tension with left ventricular dysfunction.

- The pain of angina pectoris during physical exercise is described in various ways.
- Physical signs occurring with the pain are fourth heart sound and mitral regurgitant murmur due to papillary muscle dysfunction.
- The double product [(heart rate) x (systolic blood pressure)] is useful for defining myocardial oxygen demand.

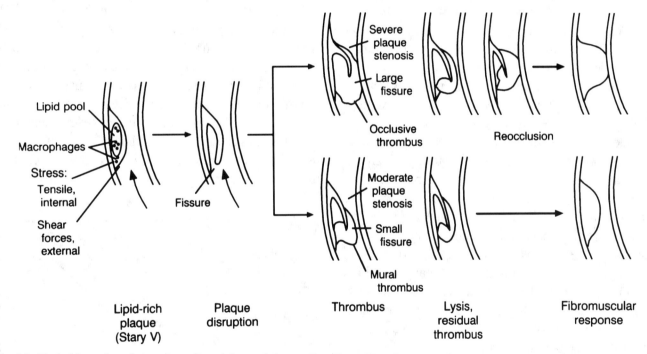

Fig. 4-2.--Typical dynamic evolution of complicated disrupted plaque. (From Fuster V, Badimon L, Badimon JJ, Chesebro JH: The pathogenesis of coronary artery disease and the acute coronary syndromes [First of two parts]. N Engl J Med 326:242-250, 1992. By permission of the journal.)

Silent Ischemia

Silent ischemia is common in patients with symptomatic stable coronary artery disease, unstable angina, or after myocardial infarction. It is diagnosed by the presence of ST-segment depression in the absence of symptoms. Silent ischemia can occur either with an increase in myocardial oxygen consumption or at rest. The treatment is similar to that for chronic unstable angina; nitrates, β-blockers, and calcium channel blockers are effective agents. Whether percutaneous transluminal coronary angioplasty or coronary artery bypass grafting should be performed for silent ischemia alone is debated. The prognosis for this condition is the same as for symptomatic ischemia.

- Silent ischemia is common in patients with symptomatic stable coronary artery disease, unstable angina, or after myocardial infarction.

- Silent ischemia diagnosed by presence of ST-segment depression in the absence of symptoms.
- Treatment is similar to that for chronic unstable angina.
- Nitrates, β-blockers, and calcium channel blockers are effective therapeutic agents.
- Whether coronary angioplasty or bypass grafting should be performed for silent ischemia is debated.
- Prognosis is same for silent ischemia and symptomatic ischemia.

Ancillary Testing

Ancillary tests for coronary artery disease include measurement of left ventricular function, stress testing, and coronary angiography. Left ventricular function is the most important predictor of prognosis and should be measured in all patients by two-dimensional echocardiography, radionuclide angiography, or left ventricular angiography. Exercise testing is performed with treadmill or bicycle exertion test in conjunction with ECG monitoring, thallium scanning (perfusion of myocardium), radionuclide angiography (left ventricular function), or echocardiography (left ventricular function) to check for ischemia. During standard treadmill test, i.e., exercise with stepped increases in workload every 2-3 minutes, heart rate, blood pressure, and onset of subjective symptoms are monitored. Continuous monitoring of cardiac rhythm and 12-lead ECG at 1-minute intervals are performed. ECG is positive for ischemia if flat ST-segment depression is ≥1 mm. ECG response is uninterpretable on treadmill exertion test when there are resting T-wave abnormalities, left bundle branch block, left ventricular hypertrophy, paced rhythm, digoxin therapy, or mitral valve prolapse. For interpreting the results of this test, Bayes' theorem is important. According to this theorem, the predictive value of a test depends on prevalence of the disease in the population studied.

- The most important predictor of prognosis is left ventricular function.
- ECG is positive for ischemia if flat ST-segment depression is ≥1 mm.
- T-wave abnormalities, left bundle branch block, left ventricular hypertrophy, paced rhythm, digoxin therapy, or mitral valve prolapse make ECG response to treadmill exertion test uninterpretable.
- Bayes' theorem--the predictive value of a test depends on the prevalence of the disease in the population studied.

As indicated on Figure 4-3, sensitivity and specificity of ECG treadmill exertion testing are about 70% and 75%, respectively. Thus, a young patient with atypical chest pain and no risk factors (A in Fig. 4-3) has a low pretest probability (5%) of coronary artery disease. If the test results are negative, the probability decreases to 3%. However, if the results are positive, the probability is <15%. In comparison, an older man (B in Fig. 4-3) with typical chest pain and multiple risk factors has a high pretest probability (90%) of coronary artery disease, and even with negative test results, the probability is >70%. Treadmill exertion test should not be used to make the *diagnosis* of coronary artery disease.

Several different types of cardiac imaging modalities add to sensitivity and specificity of ECG treadmill exertion testing. In thallium imaging, thallium-201 injected at peak exercise labels areas of perfusion; "cold spots" are nonperfused regions. Scanning is repeated 3 to 24 hours later. Persistent cold spots indicate previous infarction, and reperfused areas indicate ischemia. SPECT thallium scanning (use of multiple tomographic planes) is more accurate than planar thallium scanning. In patients with left bundle branch block and severe left ventricular hypertrophy, thallium scanning gives false-positive results. In radionuclide angiography (MUGA), red blood cells are labeled with technetium-99m and the left ventricular cavity is imaged during the cardiac cycle to measure, at rest and at peak exercise, left ventricular volume, ejection fraction, and regional wall motion abnormalities.

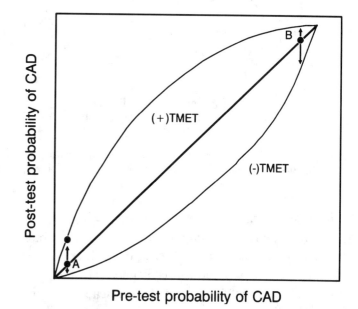

Fig. 4-3. The effect of Bayes' theorem on the ability of treadmill exertion testing (TMET) to diagnose coronary artery disease (CAD). Representative patients A and B are described in text.

MUGA is positive if ejection fraction decreases (>5%-7%) and/or new regional wall motion abnormalities appear. Because multiple cycles are gated, MUGA cannot be used with irregular rhythms. In exercise echocardiography, two-dimensional echocardiography is performed at rest and at peak exercise. Digital acquisition allows side-by-side comparisons of images from the same view. The test is positive for ischemia if global systolic function decreases and/or new regional wall motion abnormalities appear.

- Sensitivity and specificity of ECG treadmill exertion testing are about 70% and 75%, respectively.
- Treadmill exertion test should not be used to make diagnosis of coronary artery disease.
- Thallium scanning gives false-positive results in patients with left bundle branch block and severe left ventricular hypertrophy.
- MUGA is positive if ejection fraction decreases (>5%-7%) and/or new regional wall motion abnormalities appear.
- Two-dimensional echocardiography is positive for ischemia if global systolic function decreases and/or new regional wall motion abnormalities appear.

All these imaging modalities are more expensive than ECG treadmill exertion test. Because Bayes' theorem applies, imaging modalities should not be used for diagnosis of coronary artery disease over ECG treadmill testing except in cases of an uninterpretable ECG, or false-positive ECG results, or for localizing specific regions of ischemia (for future revascularization procedures).

Pharmacologic stress tests that provoke ischemia have been developed for patients who cannot exercise. These tests include use of dipyridamole thallium, which redistributes flow away from ischemic myocardium. Adenosine thallium works in the same way as dipyridamole. In dobutamine echocardiography, the myocardial oxygen demand is increased. Pacing echocardiography increases heart rate.

Treadmill exertion testing identifies high-risk patients. High-risk patients are identified if following are obtained on testing: less than stage I of the Bruce protocol, heart rate of <120 beats per minute, ST-segment depression >2 mm, ST-segment depression greater than 6 minutes' duration after stopping, decreased blood pressure, multiple perfusion defects, and ejection fraction decrease >20%. In patients with poor prognostic factors, it is reasonable to proceed with coronary angiography to define anatomy of coronary arteries and need for intervention.

However, in patients who achieve a good work load without significant ST-segment depression and have appropriate blood pressure and heart rate responses, medical management is indicated because of excellent prognosis.

- Major usefulness of stress testing is to identify high-risk patients, not diagnose coronary artery disease.
- Treadmill exertion test should not be performed on patients with either unstable angina or severe aortic stenosis.

Coronary Angiography

Although coronary angiography has many limitations, it is the standard method for defining severity of coronary artery disease. Subjective visual estimation of percentage of stenosis may grossly underestimate severity of the disease, especially if it is diffuse, because angiography outlines only the vessel lumen. The risk of serious complications of coronary angiography is about 1%; they include vascular complications (1.0%), myocardial infarction (0.5%), stroke (0.5%), ventricular fibrillation (0.5%), and death (0.1%). Risk is greater in older patients or those with severe left ventricular dysfunction, left main coronary artery disease, or other coexistent medical diseases.

- Coronary angiography is the standard method for defining severity of coronary artery disease.
- Visual estimation of percentage of stenosis may grossly underestimate disease severity.
- The risk of serious complications in coronary angiography is about 1%.

Medical Therapy

The medical treatment for chronic stable angina should be given in a step-wise manner according to symptoms. Initial therapy is sublingual nitroglycerin as needed. Long-acting nitrates, calcium channel blockers, or β-blockers should be added sequentially if symptoms continue. First drug should be increased to optimal dosage before second or third drug is added. Nitrates relieve angina mainly by producing venodilatation, which decreases wall tension. Calcium channel blockers relieve angina by decreasing afterload, heart rate, and contractility. Different calcium channel blockers have different relative effects (Table 4-1). β-Blockers relieve angina mainly by lowering heart rate, reducing contractility, and decreasing (long-term) blood pressure (renin effect). β-Blockers are the most effective drugs for reducing the double product (heart rate x blood pressure) with exercise.

Table 4-1.--Relative Effects of Calcium Channel Blockers

	Verapamil	Nifedipine	Diltiazem
Decrease heart rate	+++	±	+
Decrease blood pressure	++	+++	++
Decrease contractility	+++	+	++
Side effects	Constipation	Edema	Least
	AV block	Hypotension	
Lowest effective dose	120 mg tid	30 mg tid	90 mg tid

+, effective; ++, more effective; +++, most effective; ±, little effect.
AV, atrioventricular; tid, three times daily.

Nitrate tolerance can occur with continuous exposure (use nitrate-free interval with dosing three times daily). Isosorbide dinitrate (at least 20-30 mg three times a day) needs to be used. β-Blockers should not be used if patient has significant bronchospastic disease, congestive heart failure, or bradycardia. β-Blockers should be given at a dosage that keeps the resting heart rate <70 beats per minute. Always look for treatable underlying factors contributing to ischemia (anemia, thyroid abnormalities, hypoxia). In patients with left ventricular dysfunction and nocturnal angina, diuretics and angiotensin converting enzyme (ACE) inhibitors may be helpful in reducing wall tension.

- Initial therapy for chronic stable angina is sublingual nitroglycerin as needed.
- Add long-acting nitrates, calcium channel blockers, or β-blockers sequentially if symptoms continue.
- Nitrates relieve angina by producing venodilatation, which decreases wall tension.
- Calcium channel blockers relieve angina by decreasing afterload, heart rate, and contractility.
- β-Blockers relieve angina by lowering heart rate, reducing contractility, and decreasing blood pressure.
- β-Blockers are most effective drugs for reducing the double product.
- Nitrate tolerance can occur with continuous exposure.
- Do not use β-blockers if patient has significant bronchospastic disease, congestive heart failure, or bradycardia.
- β-Blockers should be given at a dosage to keep resting heart rate <70 beats per minute.
- Look for treatable underlying factors contributing to ischemia.
- Diuretics and ACE inhibitors may be helpful in patients with left ventricular dysfunction and nocturnal angina.

Antiplatelet agents may be helpful in patients with chronic stable angina pectoris. A low dose of aspirin probably does not prevent progression of atherosclerosis but may prevent acute myocardial infarction in patients with coronary artery disease. In two large primary prevention trials, aspirin produced a 33% reduction in the risk for first, nonfatal myocardial infarction in men (no convincing data exist about the use of aspirin in women). The role of aspirin in primary prevention of stroke or overall cardiovascular mortality is uncertain.

- Low dose of aspirin probably does not prevent progression of atherosclerosis but may prevent acute myocardial infarction in patients with coronary artery disease.
- No convincing data exist about use of aspirin in women.
- Role of aspirin in primary prevention of stroke or overall cardiovascular mortality is uncertain.

Catheter-Based Treatment

Percutaneous transluminal coronary angioplasty (PTCA) is most common catheter-based intervention. PTCA is a combination of "splitting" the atheroma and stretching the noninvolved segment of artery. In experienced laboratories, the success rate is usually >90%. However, the risk of complete abrupt closure, myocardial infarction, and death is as much as 4%-6%. These risks are increased in long, tubular, eccentric, and calcified lesions and also in older women. Restenosis is a major problem (30%-45% restenosis at 6 months). Antiplatelet agents given before PTCA may reduce the rate of acute closure but do not prevent restenosis. PTCA does not prevent myocardial infarction or sudden death. Indication for PTCA in chronic stable angina is limiting symptoms unresponsive to medical therapy. Other catheter-based therapies (atherectomy, laser, stent) have high restenosis rates similar to those of

PTCA. These therapies have no proven benefit over PTCA. No medical therapy has proven effective in preventing restenosis after PTCA or other catheter-based therapies. In single-vessel disease, medical therapy is comparable to PTCA for prognosis and for prevention of myocardial infarction.

- PTCA is a combination of splitting the atheroma and stretching the noninvolved segment of artery.
- Initial success rate is usually >90%.
- Restenosis is a major problem (30%-45% restenosis at 6 months).
- Antiplatelet agents do not prevent restenosis.
- PTCA does not prevent myocardial infarction or sudden death.
- No medical therapy is effective in preventing restenosis after PTCA.
- In single-vessel disease, medical therapy is comparable to PTCA for prognosis and for prevention of myocardial infarction.

Surgical Treatment

The surgical therapy for severely symptomatic patients with chronic stable angina is coronary artery bypass grafting (CABG) with either saphenous vein or internal mammary artery grafts. CABG provides excellent relief from symptoms (partial relief in >90% of patients and complete relief in >70%). In-hospital mortality after CABG varies widely from 2%-30%. Mortality increases with age, poor ventricular function, female gender, left main coronary artery disease, unstable angina, and diabetes mellitus. Complications of CABG include sternal wound infection (especially in diabetics), severe left ventricular dysfunction (from inadequate cardioprotection), and late constrictive pericarditis. The procedure is not without latent problems. Closure rates of saphenous vein grafts are 20% and 50% at 1 year and 5 years, respectively. The patency rate is higher in internal mammary arteries, possibly up to a 90% patency at 5 years.

- CABG provides excellent relief from symptoms.
- CABG gives partial relief in >90% of patients and complete relief in >70%.
- In-hospital mortality after CABG varies widely from 2%-30%.
- Mortality increases with age, poor ventricular function, female gender, left main coronary artery disease, unstable angina, and diabetes mellitus.

- Closure rates of saphenous vein grafts are 20% and 50% at 1 year and 5 years, respectively.

All the data about efficacy of CABG come from three major randomized trials.

- CABG does not prevent myocardial infarction.
- CABG does not uniformly improve left ventricular function.
- CABG does not decrease ventricular arrhythmias.
- CABG only improves survival in patients with 1) left main coronary artery disease, 2) three-vessel disease and moderately depressed left ventricular function, and 3) three-vessel disease and severe symptoms of ischemia at a low work load. In all other subsets of patients, CABG should not be performed to improve survival.
- The only indications for CABG are 1) relief of symptoms in patients who have limiting symptoms unresponsive to medical management and 2) prolonging life in subsets of patients listed above.
- Role of CABG in silent ischemia is unknown.

Postcardiotomy Syndrome

Postcardiotomy syndrome occurs 2 weeks-2 years postoperatively and consists of fever, pericarditis, and elevated sedimentation rate. It rarely can present as pericardial tamponade. It is probably an autoimmune process (associated with antimyocardial antibodies); treatment is with aspirin and nonsteroidal anti-inflammatory agents. Postperfusion syndrome is also characterized by fever and pericarditis but is associated with elevated values on liver function tests and atypical lymphocytes, presumably due to cytomegalovirus syndrome. In patients with fever and pleuritic chest pain postoperatively, perform sedimentation rate and special blood smear to check for postperfusion or postcardiotomy syndrome.

- Postcardiotomy syndrome occurs 2 weeks-2 years postoperatively.
- It consists of fever, pericarditis, and elevated sedimentation rate.
- It is probably an autoimmune process (associated with antimyocardial antibodies).
- Treatment--aspirin and nonsteroidal anti-inflammatory agents.
- Postperfusion syndrome: fever, pericarditis, elevated values on liver function tests, and atypical lymphocytes.
- Perform sedimentation rate and special blood smear

in patients with fever and pleuritic chest pain postoperatively to check for postcardiotomy or postperfusion syndrome.

UNSTABLE ANGINA

The definition of unstable angina is 1) accelerating pattern of angina, 2) rest pain or prolonged episodes of pain, 3) new onset of rapidly progressive angina, or 4) nocturnal angina. The mechanism is probably plaque rupture, with platelet aggregation and subsequent thrombus formation. Coronary artery spasm may have a role. Vasomotor response of coronary artery is regulated by endothelial-relaxing and endothelial-constricting factors, which are activated partly by platelets. Diagnosis of unstable angina is made on basis of medical history, ST-segment changes on ECG, and absence of elevated creatine kinase-MB fraction. It is important to diagnose unstable angina because it may be the prelude to acute myocardial infarction.

- Unstable angina is 1) accelerating pattern of angina, 2) rest pain or prolonged episodes of pain, 3) new onset of rapidly progressive angina, or 4) nocturnal angina.
- Mechanism is probably plaque rupture, with platelet aggregation and subsequent thrombus formation.
- Coronary artery vasomotor response is regulated by endothelial-relaxing and endothelial-constricting factors.
- Diagnosis is made on basis of medical history, ST-segment changes, absence of elevated creatine kinase-MB fraction.

Treatment of unstable angina consists of immediate hospitalization with ECG monitoring. It is important to decrease the myocardial oxygen demand. First and foremost, unstable angina is treated with sedation (to decrease anxiety and catecholamine stimulation of the heart). β-Blockers, nitrates, and calcium channel blockers are effective in decreasing myocardial oxygen demand (see Chronic Stable Angina, page 40). Antiplatelet agents, such as aspirin, are effective in reducing incidence of progression to myocardial infarction and should be used in all patients. Heparin given intravenously also reduces the incidence of progression to myocardial infarction and should be used in all patients without any contraindication.

- For unstable angina, immediate hospitalization with ECG monitoring.
- Decrease myocardial oxygen demand with β-blockers, nitrates, and calcium channel blockers.

- Antiplatelet agents are effective in reducing incidence of progression to myocardial infarction and should be used in all patients.
- Heparin given intravenously should be used in all patients without any contraindication.

Work-up for unstable angina is controversial. However, most cardiologists usually recommend coronary angiography to define coronary anatomy. Exercise testing is usually not performed because it may cause myocardial infarction. PTCA or CABG has not been shown to prevent myocardial infarction or to prolong longevity. However, even with optimal medical therapy, there is a high crossover to revascularization therapy in the following 6 months. Therefore, in certain clinical situations, it is reasonable to proceed with revascularization in patients with unstable angina and suitable coronary artery anatomy.

- Most cardiologists usually recommend coronary angiography for patients with unstable angina.
- Exercise testing usually is not performed.
- PTCA or CABG has not been shown to prevent myocardial infarction or to prolong longevity in patients with unstable angina but are highly effective in relieving pain.

CORONARY ARTERY SPASM

Vasomotor tone of coronary arteries is important in pathogenesis of coronary artery disease. Coronary artery vasoconstriction can be seen as a response to arterial injury. The endothelium affects vascular tone by releasing relaxing factors, e.g., prostacyclin and endothelium-derived relaxing factor, that prevent vasoconstriction and platelet deposition. With dysfunctional endothelium, these factors are absent and coronary arteries may be more prone to spasm. Most clinical episodes of coronary artery spasm occur superimposed on atherosclerotic plaques. However, patients may have primary coronary artery spasm and angiographically normal coronary arteries.

- Endothelium affects vascular tone by releasing relaxing factors, e.g., prostacyclin and endothelium-derived relaxing factor.
- With dysfunctional endothelium, coronary arteries may be more prone to spasm.
- Most episodes of spasm occur superimposed on atherosclerotic plaques.

- Patients may have primary coronary artery spasm and angiographically normal coronary arteries.

The typical presentation of coronary artery spasm consists of recurrent episodes of rest pain in association with ST-segment elevation, which reverses with administration of nitrates. Coronary angiography with ergonovine challenge has been used to diagnose these patients, but its sensitivity and specificity are unknown. ST-segment elevation on the resting 12-lead ECG during an episode of rest pain is the standard criterion for diagnosing coronary artery spasm. Coronary artery spasm is treated with long-acting nitrates and/or calcium channel blockers.

- Typical presentation of coronary artery spasm is recurrent episodes of rest pain and ST-segment elevation that is reversed with nitrates.
- Standard criterion for diagnosis: spontaneous ST-segment elevation on resting 12-lead ECG during rest pain.

MYOCARDIAL INFARCTION

Background

Myocardial infarction accounts for a large percentage of morbidity and mortality in U.S. in the 1990s. Over 500,000 people are admitted annually for myocardial infarction. However, >50% of people with myocardial infarction die before reaching the hospital. With the advent of coronary care units 3 decades ago, mortality from myocardial infarction was trimmed from 30% to 15% by treating ventricular arrhythmias. Beta-blockade has further reduced in-hospital and post-hospital mortality by 30%-40%. In the late 1980s, reperfusion therapy was shown to further improve survival and has become standard care for selected patients with myocardial infarction. Currently, overall in-hospital mortality is 5%-10%. After myocardial infarction, another 2%-10% die in the ensuing year.

- More than 50% of people with myocardial infarction die before reaching the hospital.
- By treating ventricular arrhythmias, mortality was trimmed from 30% to 15%.
- β-Blockade has reduced in-hospital and post-hospital mortality by 30%-40%.
- Thrombolytic therapy has reduced overall mortality to 5%-10%.

Pathogenesis

Acute transmural myocardial infarction is usually caused by sudden complete occlusion of a coronary artery. The mechanism of myocardial infarction is usually plaque rupture, leading to platelet aggregation and thrombus formation. Without collateral circulation, 90% of the myocardium supplied by an occluded artery is infarcted within 3 hours.

- Usual cause of acute transmural myocardial infarction is sudden complete occlusion of a coronary artery.
- Usual mechanism is plaque rupture, leading to platelet aggregation and thrombus formation.

Currently, two categories of myocardial infarction used clinically are based on ECG. "Q-wave myocardial infarction" is diagnosed on basis of chest pain with ST-segment elevation and subsequent development of Q waves. (This term replaces "transmural myocardial infarction" because not all myocardial layers are necessarily involved.) The likelihood of occlusive coronary artery thrombus at early coronary angiography is high (>85%). "Non-Q-wave myocardial infarction" is diagnosed by two of following three criteria: 1) prolonged chest pain, 2) persistent ST-segment changes >24 hours, and 3) elevated creatine kinase-MB fraction. (This term replaces "subendocardial myocardial infarction.") The likelihood of occlusive coronary artery thrombus is about 30%-40%. In these patients, multivessel disease is likely, because long-standing multivessel disease provides collaterals that prevent transmural injury.

- Q-wave myocardial infarction is diagnosed on basis of chest pain with ST-segment elevation and subsequent Q waves.
- Q-wave myocardial infarctions are associated with larger infarctions and higher in-hospital mortality than non-Q-wave myocardial infarctions.
- Non-Q-wave myocardial infarctions have a higher risk for reinfarction, continued angina, and even posthospital death.
- Some advocate predismissal coronary angiography for all patients with non-Q-wave myocardial infarction.

Several new concepts have been developed in the past decade for examining patients with myocardial infarction. "Stunned myocardium" occurs when a coronary artery is completely occluded and then opened. If reperfusion occurs early enough, systolic contraction of affected myocardium may remain reduced after the event, although the myocardium remains viable. Systolic contraction then returns hours to days later. Currently, no clinical test differentiates "stunned myocardium" from infarcted, dead myocardium. "Ischemia at a distance" occurs when infarction is in distribution of one coronary vessel and ischemia with subsequent hypokinesis occurs in distribution of a second vessel in which there is high-grade stenosis. When this is seen on echocardiography, prognosis is poor because of recurrent myocardial infarction and increased mortality. "Infarct remodeling" occurs mainly after large anteroapical myocardial infarctions. An area of infarction may undergo thinning, dilatation, and dyskinesis. This is associated with a higher incidence of congestive heart failure and posthospital mortality. ACE inhibitors may help prevent infarct remodeling.

- Stunned myocardium--coronary artery is completely occluded and then opened and transient akinesis of the myocardium occurs.
- Ischemia at a distance--infarction is in distribution of one coronary artery, and ischemia and subsequent hypokinesis are in distribution of a second vessel in which there is high-grade stenosis.
- Infarct remodeling--occurs after large anteroapical myocardial infarctions.
- ACE inhibitors may help prevent infarct remodeling.

Presentation and Diagnosis

Typical presentation of myocardial infarction is anginal-sounding pain lasting >30-45 minutes associated with ECG changes and elevated creatine kinase-MB fraction. However, >25%-30% of infarctions are silent and present later as new ECG abnormalities or regional wall motion abnormalities. Silent myocardial infarctions occur especially in patients with diabetes and in the elderly. Increased incidence of myocardial infarction in early morning is perhaps related to increased platelet aggregation. The pain of myocardial infarction mimics that of other diseases, e.g., gastrointestinal or pericardial disease, or musculoskeletal pain. Remember that myocardial infarction may occur without ECG changes. Thus, all patients with ischemic-sounding pain should be hospitalized despite lack of ECG changes. In these patients, echocardiography or radionuclide angiography showing regional wall motion abnormalities may help confirm the clinical diagnosis of myocardial infarction.

- More than 25%-30% of infarctions are silent.

- Silent infarctions occur especially in patients with diabetes and in the elderly.
- Increased incidence of myocardial infarction in early morning, perhaps related to increased platelet aggregation.
- Pain of myocardial infarction mimics that of other diseases.
- Myocardial infarction may occur without ECG changes.
- All patients with ischemic-sounding pain should be hospitalized.

Elevated creatine kinase-MB fraction, indicative of myocardial necrosis, confirms clinical diagnosis of myocardial infarction. The peak values are at 12-20 hours. Thus, negative creatine kinase-MB fraction at admission does not rule out myocardial infarction. Any creatine kinase-MB peak occurring earlier than 12 hours may indicate reperfusion. (SGOT and LDH levels, used in the past, have later peaks but are usually not required for diagnosis of myocardial infarction.)

- Elevated creatine kinase-MB fraction indicates myocardial necrosis.
- Negative creatine kinase-MB fraction at admission does not rule out myocardial infarction.

Basic and Drug Treatments

Bed rest and sedation are essential and are beneficial in the acute stage of myocardial infarction for decreasing myocardial oxygen demand. Analgesics, particularly morphine, is beneficial for recurrent pain. Currently, prolonged bed rest is not recommended, and the effort to shorten hospitalization is increasing. Many physicians recommend gradual increase in activity level over 5-6 days for an uncomplicated myocardial infarction. During the acute 3-4-day period, ECG monitoring is recommended for both tachyarrhythmias and bradyarrhythmias. Oxygen has no benefit unless hypoxia is present. However, modest hypoxemia is not uncommon, even with uncomplicated myocardial infarction, and is due to ventilation/perfusion lung mismatch.

- Prolonged bed rest is not recommended.
- Oxygen has no benefit unless hypoxia is present.

Heparin is important in treating acute myocardial infarction. It prevents 1) recurrent infarction, especially after thrombolytic therapy, 2) deep venous thrombosis, and 3) intracardiac thrombus formation. Intracardiac thrombus formation occurs in 40% of patients with anterior myocardial infarction, and almost 50% of these patients have a systemic embolic event. Thus, heparin therapy is especially indicated in these patients. The benefits of subcutaneous versus intravenous heparin are unsettled. Aspirin reduces recurrent infarction by 49% in patients not receiving thrombolytic therapy. It also reduces mortality when given in addition to thrombolytic therapy.

- Heparin is important in treating acute myocardial infarction.
- Heparin prevents recurrent infarction, deep venous thrombosis, and intracardiac thrombus formation.
- Intracardiac thrombus formation occurs in 40% of patients with anterior myocardial infarction.
- Benefits of subcutaneous versus intravenous heparin are unsettled.
- Aspirin reduces recurrent infarction by 49% in patients not receiving thrombolytic therapy.

Nitroglycerin is useful for a subset of patients with myocardial infarction--for those with heart failure (by decreasing wall tension) and for those with continued pain. In early stages of myocardial infarction, nitroglycerin given intravenously should be used instead of long-acting nitrates given orally to prevent acute decreases in blood pressure. Intravenous nitroglycerin may reduce infarct size by lowering wall tension and affecting "remodeling." Also, it may decrease susceptibility to ventricular fibrillation. If mean blood pressure is >80 mm Hg, intravenous nitroglycerin may reduce mortality by 10%-25%, specifically in patients with anterior myocardial infarction and poor left ventricular function. However, in patients with low blood pressure and those with inferior and right ventricular infarctions, nitroglycerin may decrease blood pressure too much and may cause increased mortality. The dosage of intravenous nitroglycerin is a 15-μg bolus and an initial infusion of 10 μg/min. Intravenous infusion should be increased every 5-10 minutes until the blood pressure decreases 10%-15%, up to a maximum of 150-200 μg/min. Mean blood pressure should be kept at >80 mm Hg. Nitrate intolerance occurs with infusions lasting >24 hours. Do not use intravenous nitroglycerin in patients with low blood pressure or right ventricular infarction. Intravenous nitroglycerin may improve mortality in patients with large anterior myocardial infarctions and congestive heart failure.

- Nitroglycerin is useful for patients with heart failure and those with continued pain.
- Intravenous nitroglycerin may reduce infarct size by lowering wall tension and affecting remodeling.
- Nitroglycerin may decrease susceptibility to ventricular fibrillation.
- Nitrate intolerance occurs with infusions >24 hours.
- Do not use intravenous nitroglycerin in patients with low blood pressure or right ventricular infarction.
- Intravenous nitroglycerin may improve mortality in patients with large anterior myocardial infarctions and congestive heart failure.

β-Blockers are useful both in acute myocardial infarction and postmyocardial infarction setting. If given early, they decrease infarction size and in-hospital mortality. If given after myocardial infarction is completed, β-blockers can reduce posthospital reinfarction and mortality. In acute setting, typical dosage of metoprolol is 5 mg given intravenously three times, 5 minutes apart, followed by 100 mg given orally twice daily. β-Blockers will also reduce the incidence of ventricular fibrillation and decrease pain. The beneficial effects are probably multifactorial but include 1) decreased myocardial oxygen demand, 2) increased threshold for ventricular fibrillation, 3) decreased platelet aggregability, and 4) decreased sympathetic effects on myocardium. β-Blockers are most beneficial in patients with large infarctions, i.e., those at higher risk of complications. Acute intravenous β-blockers are also beneficial in those patients undergoing thrombolytic therapy. β-Blockers are especially useful for patients with hyperdynamic circulation and continued postinfarction pain and should be given to patients presenting <12 hours of pain who do not have contraindications, especially those with anterior myocardial infarction.

- Acute intravenous β-blockers reduce infarction size and in-hospital mortality.
- Acute intravenous β-blockers reduce incidence of ventricular fibrillation.
- Contraindications to β-blockers are bradycardia, atrioventricular block, hypotension, severe heart failure, and inferior myocardial infarction with high vagal tone.

Calcium channel blockers have been used to treat patients with myocardial infarction, but their routine use has *no* proven benefit. Routine use of verapamil and nifedipine has no benefit and may increase mortality. Diltiazem, 60-90 mg given every 6 hours within 72 hours of myocardial infarction, may prevent later reinfarction and recurrent angina in patients with non-Q-wave myocardial infarction; however, it probably increases mortality in patients with Q-wave myocardial infarction and depressed left ventricular function. Because most patients with non-Q-wave myocardial infarction at risk for later events will probably be identified and have a revascularization procedure performed, routine use of calcium channel blockers is not indicated. However, by producing coronary vasodilatation and decreasing myocardial oxygen demand, calcium channel blockers may be beneficial in treating postinfarction angina.

- Routine use of calcium channel blockers for myocardial infarction has no proven benefit.
- Routine use of verapamil and nifedipine may increase mortality.
- Calcium channel blockers may be beneficial for patients with postinfarction angina and those with non-Q-wave myocardial infarction.

Treatment of Arrhythmias (See Chapter 5)

Treatment--Reperfusion Therapy

Early reperfusion therapy has had tremendous impact on the treatment of acute myocardial infarction. Overall, mortality is decreased $27 \pm 3\%$ when reperfusion is given early. In >50,000 patients in ISIS-3 and GISSI-2 studies, the 35-day in-hospital mortality was only 10% with thrombolytic therapy. Time is of the essence when giving reperfusion therapy. The faster the reperfusion, the better the extent of myocardial salvage and the better the effect on mortality. Without collaterals, 90% of the myocardium at risk is infarcted within 3 hours of occlusion. Very early reperfusion has a major effect on direct myocardial salvage. In a study in which thrombolysis was given <90 minutes after pain onset, the mortality was 1%. In most U.S. studies, average time from pain onset to artery opening is 3.7 hours. The delay is in patient presentation (22%), transport (21%), in-hospital institution of the drug (35%), and reperfusion drug time (19%). Reperfusion at 2-6 hours salvages the peri-infarction zone, depending on degree of collateral circulation. Thus, there is a lesser effect on myocardial salvage but an important effect on survival. The "open artery concept" describes a benefit in improvement in posthospital mortality in the presence of an open artery after thrombolytic therapy, which is not reflected in improved ventricular function. The reason for this is unclear but may be related to improved electrical stability or prevention of ventricular remodeling.

- Overall, mortality is decreased $27 \pm 3\%$ when reperfusion is given early.
- In >50,000 patients, 35-day in-hospital mortality was 10% with thrombolytic therapy.
- Faster the reperfusion, better the extent of myocardial salvage.
- Without collaterals, 90% of the myocardium at risk is infarcted within 3 hours of occlusion.

Controversy exists about the effectiveness of intravenous thrombolytic therapy versus emergency PTCA in patients with acute myocardial infarction. After administration of thrombolytic therapy, emergency PTCA is not indicated in the absence of ongoing pain, because of a higher incidence of complications than in patients not undergoing emergency PTCA. The controversy is now about whether intravenous thrombolytic therapy should be given versus emergency-direct PTCA. Intravenous thrombolysis may not be as effective (65%-70%) in opening arteries as PTCA (90%). However, this is counterbalanced by faster administration of intravenous thrombolysis and wider availability of the intravenous drug. Less than 10% of all hospitals have capability for emergency PTCA. Late patency (>24 hours) is 70%-80% for both methods. Thus, with the lack of available resources, intravenous thrombolytic therapy is still treatment of choice in patients with acute myocardial infarction. Emergency PTCA may be used in patients with 1) contraindication for intravenous thrombolysis, 2) cardiogenic shock, or 3) continued ischemia after thrombolytic therapy.

- Effectiveness of intravenous thrombolytic therapy versus emergency PTCA in patients with acute myocardial infarction is controversial.
- After giving thrombolytic therapy, emergency PTCA is not indicated in the absence of ongoing pain.
- Intravenous thrombolysis may not be as effective (65%-70%) in opening arteries as PTCA (90%).
- Less than 10% of hospitals have capability for emergency PTCA.
- Intravenous thrombolytic therapy is still treatment of choice in stable patients with acute myocardial infarction with no contraindications.

Indications for intravenous thrombolysis are a matter of controversy. Thrombolytic therapy definitely is indicated for patients presenting within 6 hours after the onset of pain who have ST-segment elevation and no contraindication. It should be considered for patients up to

12 hours after symptoms with continued pain. Whether thrombolytic therapy should be given to patients later than 6 hours after pain onset who have no evidence of continued ischemia is unclear. It should also be considered for patients presenting within 6 hours of pain onset and left bundle branch block. Thrombolytic therapy is not clearly indicated for patients with pain and other ECG abnormalities (ST-segment depression).

- Thrombolytic therapy definitely is indicated for patients presenting within 6 hours after the onset of pain who have ST-segment elevation and no contraindication.
- Whether thrombolytic therapy should be given to patients later than 6 hours after pain onset who have no evidence of continued ischemia is unclear.
- Thrombolytic therapy is not clearly indicated for patients with pain and other ECG abnormalities (ST-segment depression).

Contraindications to thrombolytic therapy include a history of bleeding, severe hypertension, recent stroke, diabetic hemorrhagic retinopathy, recent cardiopulmonary resuscitation, previous allergy to streptokinase, recent surgical procedure, suspected aortic dissection or pericarditis, and pregnancy. Major complications of intravenous thrombolysis include major bleeding (5%-6%), intracranial bleeding (0.5%), major allergic reaction (0.1%-1.7%), and hypotension (2%-10%). Higher incidence of myocardial rupture may occur in patients given thrombolytic therapy late (>12 hours after pain onset).

- Major complications of intravenous thrombolysis are major bleeding (5%-6%), intracranial bleeding (0.5%), major allergic reaction (0.1%-1.7%), and hypotension (2%-10%).
- Higher incidence of myocardial rupture may occur in patients given thrombolytic therapy late (>12 hours after pain onset).

Three agents are available for intravenous thrombolysis (Table 4-2). Streptokinase, a nonselective thrombolytic agent, combines with circulating plasminogen to split circulating and thrombus-bound plasminogen into plasmin, which splits fibrin. It lyses circulating

Table 4-2.--Thrombolytic Agents

	Clot specific	Half-life	Allergic reaction	Dosage	Cost
Streptokinase	+	++	++	1.5×10^6 U/hr	+
TPA (tissue plasminogen activator)	+++	+	-	10 mg i.v. bolus with 90 mg i.v. over 90 min	+++
APSAC (anisoylated plasminogen-streptokinase activator complex)	+	+++	+	30 U/5 min	++

-, none; +, some; ++, more; +++, most.

fibrinogen and thus has systemic effects. The dosage is a 250,000-U bolus and 1.5×10^6 U in 1 hour. TPA (tissue plasminogen activator) binds to preformed fibrin preferentially and lyses it without activating plasminogen in the general circulation. Thus, it has less effect on circulating fibrinogen and is "fibrin-specific." It has the fastest onset of action. The dosage is 100 mg over 90 minutes. Anistreplase (APSAC) is composed of anisolyated plasminogen and streptokinase bound together and inactivated by plasminogen. It requires spontaneous deacylation, which occurs in the plasma before the active streptokinase-plasminogen

complex is generated, splitting plasminogen to plasmin. Thus, anistreplase is a more stable agent and may be given as a single intravenous bolus. The dosage is 30 U over 5 minutes.

In the large European trials, there was no proven benefit of one thrombolytic therapy over the others. In the GUSTO trial, there was a lower mortality rate when an accelerated dose of TPA was given with intravenous heparin as compared with streptokinase. TPA is more costly than streptokinase and has a slightly increased risk of cerebral hemorrhage especially in the elderly. It is thus reasonable to preferentially give TPA in the younger patient who presents very early with a myocardial infarction.

After intravenous thrombolysis, a high-grade residual lesion is usually present. Reocclusion or ischemia occurs in 15%-20% of patients and reinfarction occurs in 2%-3%. In U.S., both heparin and aspirin are given after intravenous thrombolysis to prevent reinfarction. The benefit with aspirin is clear but is less clear with heparin. Indication for coronary angiography or PTCA after intravenous thrombolysis is continued pain or ischemia documented on functional testing. There is no benefit from routine intervention in all patients.

- After intravenous thrombolysis, reocclusion or ischemia occurs in 15%-20% of patients and reinfarction occurs in 2%-3%.
- Both aspirin and heparin are given after intravenous thrombolysis to prevent reinfarction.
- The benefit is clear with aspirin but not with heparin.
- Streptokinase is least expensive thrombolytic therapy.
- TPA is most clot-specific thrombolytic therapy.
- The least amount of antigenicity is with TPA.

Acute Mechanical Complications of Myocardial Infarction

Cardiogenic shock after myocardial infarction has a high mortality, approaching 90%. However, it is important to determine the cause of cardiogenic shock. Although most cases are due to extensive left ventricular dysfunction, there are other causes, e.g., right ventricular infarction and mechanical complications of myocardial infarction. Swan-Ganz catheterization and two-dimensional echocardiography may help in determining its cause (Table 4-3).

- Cardiogenic shock after myocardial infarction approaches 90% mortality.
- Most cases of cardiogenic shock are due to extensive left ventricular dysfunction.
- Swan-Ganz catheterization and two-dimensional echocardiography may help determine other causes of cardiogenic shock.

Right ventricular infarction occurs in up to 40% of patients with inferior myocardial infarction and is diag-

Table 4-3.--Diagnosis of Cause of Cardiogenic Shock

	Swan-Ganz catheterization				
	RA	PCWP	CO		2-Dimensional echocardiography
Left ventricular dysfunction	↑	↑↑	↓↓		Poor left ventricle
Right ventricular infarction	↑↑	↓	↓↓		Dilated right ventricle
Tamponade	↑↑	↑↑	↓↓	End-equalization	Pericardial tamponade
PM rupture	↑	↑↑	↓↓	Large "V"	Severe MR
VSD	↑	↑↑	↑	Step-up	Defect seen
PE	↑↑	=	↓	PADP > PCWP	Dilated right ventricle

CO, cardiac output; MR, mitral regurgitation; PADP, pulmonary artery diastolic pressure; PCWP, pulmonary capillary wedge pressure; PE, pulmonary emboli; RA, right atrial pressure; VSD, ventricular septal defect.

nosed by elevated jugular venous pressure in the presence of clear lung fields. In extreme circumstances, right ventricular infarction can cause cardiogenic shock, because the right ventricle is not able to pump effectively enough blood to fill the left ventricle. Treatment includes large amounts of fluids given intravenously and infusion of dobutamine.

- Right ventricular infarction occurs in up to 40% of patients with inferior myocardial infarction.

Myocardial free wall rupture may occur and cause

abrupt decompensation. Free wall rupture occurs in 85% of all ruptures. It occurs suddenly, usually 2-14 days after transmural myocardial infarction, most commonly in elderly hypertensive women. It presents as electromechanical dissociation or death. If rupture is contained in the pericardium, tamponade may occur. If the diagnosis can be made by emergency echocardiography, surgery should be performed. If the rupture is sealed off, pseudoaneurysm may occur; operation is required because of high incidence of further rupture.

- Free wall rupture occurs in 85% of all ruptures.

• It occurs suddenly, usually 2-14 days after transmural myocardial infarction.

Papillary muscle rupture occurs in 5% of all ruptures and usually 2-10 days after myocardial infarction. It is associated with inferior myocardial infarction, because of the single blood supply to the posteromedial papillary muscle. Papillary muscle rupture heralded by sudden onset of dyspnea and hypotension. Although a murmur may be present, it is not audible because of equalization of left atrial and left ventricular pressures. The diagnosis is made with echocardiography or Swan-Ganz catheterization, which demonstrates a large "V" wave on pulmonary capillary wedge pressure. The treatment is intra-aortic balloon pumping and emergency surgery.

• Papillary muscle rupture occurs in 5% of all ruptures.
• It usually occurs 2-10 days after myocardial infarction.
• It is associated with inferior myocardial infarction.
• It is heralded by sudden dyspnea and hypotension.
• It is diagnosed with echocardiography and Swan-Ganz catheterization.

Ventricular septal defects occur in 10% of all ruptures, usually 1-20 days after myocardial infarction. It is equally frequent in inferior and anterior myocardial infarctions. Ventricular septal defects associated with inferior myocardial infarctions have a poorer prognosis because of the serpiginous nature of the rupture and associated with ventricular infarction. They are indicated by sudden onset of dyspnea and hypotension. A loud murmur and systolic thrill are always present. The diagnosis is made with echocardiography or Swan-Ganz catheterization, which demonstrates a step-up in oxygen saturation from right atrium to pulmonary artery. Treatment is intra-aortic balloon pump and emergency surgery.

• Ventricular septal defects occur in 10% of all ruptures.
• They are equally frequent in inferior and anterior myocardial infarctions.
• They are indicated by sudden onset of dyspnea and hypotension.
• Ventricular septal defect almost always has a thrill and loud murmur.

Prehospital Dismissal Evaluation

To properly evaluate a patient with myocardial infarction before dismissal from the hospital, determine the predictors of mortality. These include status of the left ventricle, ventricular arrhythmias, and presence of continued myocardial ischemia.

Rehabilitation treadmill exertion testing should be performed in most patients after myocardial infarction to detect continued ischemia. It is a low-risk test in properly selected patients and is performed 8-10 days after the infarction. It is usually a limited workload to 5 metabolic equivalents (METs) or 70% of the maximum heart rate. High-risk patients identified by treadmill exertion testing have >1-mm ST-segment depression, decrease in blood pressure, or inability to achieve 4 METs on the exercise test. Imaging exercise tests may identify additional high-risk patients by demonstrating multiple areas of ischemia. Pharmacologic stress tests (dobutamine echocardiography, dipyridamole thallium scanning, or adenosine thallium scanning) may be useful in patients unable to exercise.

• After myocardial infarction, most patients should undergo rehabilitation treadmill testing.
• It is a low-risk test in properly selected patients and is performed 8-10 days after the infarction.

Coronary angiography is indicated after myocardial infarction if results of a rehabilitation treadmill exertion test are positive or postinfarction angina occurs. Whether it should be performed in all patients with non-Q-wave myocardial infarction is unclear.

• Coronary angiography is indicated if results of rehabilitation treadmill exertion test are positive or postinfarction angina occurs.

No randomized trials have examined the benefit of PTCA or bypass grafting after myocardial infarction. However, in high-risk patients (i.e., those with continued ischemia or positive results on treadmill exertion test), it is reasonable to proceed with intervention. PTCA can be undertaken if there is a single-vessel high-grade lesion amenable to the procedure. CABG should be performed if there is left main or proximal three-vessel disease or two- or three-vessel disease that supplies a large portion of the myocardium, especially when associated with moderate depression in left ventricular function.

The following apply to patients who survive acute myocardial infarction:

• Aspirin decreases recurrent myocardial infarction by 31% and late mortality by 15%, more so in cases of non-Q-wave myocardial infarction.

- Warfarin may cause a similar reduction in mortality and reinfarction, but it is not routinely used in the U.S.
- Diltiazem may be beneficial after non-Q-wave myocardial infarction to prevent reinfarction.
- β-Blockers improve survival after myocardial infarction.
- β-Blockers are most effective in high-risk patients (i.e., decreased left ventricular function and ventricular arrhythmias) and may not be required in low-risk patients.
- High dosages of β-blockers, equivalent to 200 mg of metoprolol per day, need to be administered.
- β-Blockers are also effective after thrombolytic therapy.
- Because antiarrhythmic agents are associated with increased mortality, they should not be used to suppress ventricular ectopy.
- ACE inhibitors reduce mortality after anterior myocardial infarction and depressed left ventricular function, presumably by inhibiting infarct remodeling.
- A rehabilitation program is essential for patient's well-being and cardiovascular fitness.

PART II
HEART FAILURE

DEFINITION

Heart failure is the inability of the heart to meet the metabolic demands of the body. Although the commonest cause is severe left ventricular dysfunction (as in dilated cardiomyopathy), other causes must be considered. To treat heart failure properly, the cause and precipitating factors must be identified. Backward heart failure is caused by elevated filling pressure, which affects the pulmonary circulation and causes shortness of breath and paroxysmal nocturnal dyspnea. Elevated filling pressure can also affect the systemic circulation and cause edema and ascites. Forward heart failure is caused by low cardiac output, which produces symptoms of fatigue and lethargy. Most patients will have a combination of the symptoms of backward and forward heart failure.

- Heart failure is the inability of heart to meet metabolic demands of the body.
- Its commonest cause is severe left ventricular dysfunction.
- Cause of backward heart failure is elevated filling pressure.
- Cause of forward heart failure is low cardiac output.

Myocardial dysfunction that causes heart failure may be due to systolic dysfunction, which is depression in contractile force of the myocardium leading to low stroke volume. The compensatory mechanism for improving stroke volume is ventricular dilatation. Ventricular dilatation results in increased end-diastolic pressures, which in turn cause symptoms of shortness of breath. Diastolic dysfunction is as important as systolic dysfunction in causing signs and symptoms of heart failure. As many as one-third of patients who present with heart failure have normal systolic function. Diastolic dysfunction is predominantly the cause of their heart failure. Diastolic dysfunction is an abnormality of filling of the left ventricle so that there is a greater rise in pressure per unit volume.

- Myocardial dysfunction that causes heart failure may be due to systolic dysfunction.
- Systolic dysfunction is depression in contractile force of the myocardium.
- Diastolic dysfunction is as important as systolic dysfunction in causing signs and symptoms of heart failure.
- One-third of patients with heart failure have normal systolic function.
- Diastolic dysfunction is an abnormality of filling of the left ventricle.

Diastolic function is a complex process. Three of its major components are relaxation, passive filling, and atrial contribution. Relaxation is an active process in which calcium is removed from the actin myosin filaments, causing contracted muscle to return to its original length. After relaxation, filling of the ventricle continues, with rise in pressure (passive filling). This is defined in terms of compliance, which is change in volume over change in pressure. Thus, abnormally low compliance produces high end-diastolic pressure. The contribution from atrial contraction further increases ventricular volume by as much as 15%-20% in normal subjects and 45%-50% in those with abnormality. In most disease states, a combination of systolic and diastolic abnormalities causes the signs and symptoms of heart failure.

- Three major components of diastolic function are relaxation, passive filling, and atrial contribution.
- In relaxation, calcium is removed from the actin myosin filaments.
- In most disease states, there is a combination of systolic and diastolic abnormalities.

ETIOLOGY

The cause of heart failure must be defined to properly define therapy. Several different types of categories can be used. A simple one is given in Table 4-4.

Clinically, the commonest cause of heart failure is a myocardial process in which there is severe left ventricular dysfunction. The treatment and prognosis are markedly different for other causes. Thus, the diagnosis is essen-

Table 4-4.--Causes of Heart Failure and Treatment

Cause	Treatment
Myocardial	
Dilated cardiomyopathy	Angiotension converting enzyme inhibitors, digoxin, diuretics, heart transplant
Hypertrophic cardiomyopathy	β-Blockers, calcium channel blockers, permanent pacing, surgery
Restrictive cardiomyopathy	Diuretics, heart transplant
Pericardial	
Tamponade	Pericardiocentesis
Constrictive pericarditis	Pericardiectomy
Valvular	Valve repair or replacement
Hypertension (increased afterload)	Afterload reduction
Pulmonary hypertension	Heart-lung transplant
High output	Correct underlying cause
Hyperthyroidism, Paget's disease	
Arteriovenous fistula	

tial and is made on the basis of physical examination and noninvasive testing, e.g., echocardiography and radionuclide angiography.

PRECIPITATING FACTORS

It is necessary to define an underlying cause in patients with heart failure. However, one or more precipitating factors are usually responsible for "tipping" a patient into congestive heart failure. If the precipitating factors are not identified and corrected, the severe symptoms of heart failure frequently return after initial therapy. In every patient, the following categories must be investigated to determine a precipitating factor (Table 4-5).

In evaluating each patient with heart failure, take the following steps: 1) medical history, delving into dietary history and history of medication compliance ("pill count"); 2) culture specimens of blood, urine, and sputum; 3) chest radiography and arterial blood gases should be performed to look for pneumonitis or pulmonary embolus; 4) ECG and creatine kinase-MB fraction blood test should be performed to rule out active ischemia. Other tests include hemoglobin, leukocyte count, sensitive thyroid-stimulating hormone, and creatinine. The heart rhythm should be documented.

- For different causes of heart failure, treatment and prognosis are different.
- For every patient with heart failure, precipitating factors must be identified and treated.

Table 4-5.--Precipitating Factors of Heart Failure

Diet (increased sodium intake)
Noncompliance of medication
Infection (infective endocarditis, urinary tract infection, upper respiratory tract infection)
Myocardial ischemia or infarction
Pulmonary embolus
Arrhythmia (atrial fibrillation, bradycardia)
Anemia
Metabolic (hyperthyroidism, chronic renal failure)

DEFINITION OF CARDIOMYOPATHIES

Cardiomyopathy is a disease of heart muscle without any known cause. Three major categories of cardiomyopathies are dilated, hypertrophic, and restrictive. Many other diseases have the same pathophysiology as true cardiomyopathies but have a known underlying cause. The different anatomical and pathophysiologic processes for each cardiomyopathy are listed in Table 4-6.

DILATED CARDIOMYOPATHY

The major abnormality in dilated cardiomyopathy is decreased systolic function (low ejection fraction). This results in compensatory enlargement of the left ventricular cavity, with increased left ventricular end-diastolic pressure due to diastolic dysfunction. These factors result in increased filling pressures and low cardiac output and produce symptoms of shortness of breath and fatigue.

- In dilated cardiomyopathy, the major abnormality is decreased systolic function (low ejection fraction).
- Low ejection fraction causes compensatory enlargement of left ventricular cavity, with increased left ventricular end-diastolic pressure due to diastolic dysfunction.

Table 4-6.--Anatomical and Pathophysiologic Processes for Each Cardiomyopathy

Type	Left ventricular cavity size	Left ventricular wall thickness	Systolic function	Diastolic function	Other
Dilated cardiomyopathy	↑↑↑	↑	↓↓↓	↓	
Hypertrophic cardiomyopathy	↓	↑↑↑	↑↑	↓↓	Left ventricular outflow obstruction
Restrictive cardiomyopathy	↑/↓	↑↑	↑/↓	↓↓↓	

↓, ↓↓, ↓↓↓, mild, moderate, severe decrease, respectively.
↑, ↑↑, ↑↑↑, mild, moderate, severe increase, respectively.

A true dilated cardiomyopathy is indicated by left ventricular dysfunction without any known cause. There appears to be a genetic link, with 20%-30% incidence of dilated cardiomyopathy in first-degree relatives. Some speculate there is a viral cause, perhaps starting out with a viral myocarditis. Other causes of severe left ventricular dysfunction include severe coronary artery disease ("hibernating myocardium"), multiple areas of previous infarctions, ethanol abuse, hyperthyroidism or hypothyroidism, postpartum cardiomyopathy, toxins and drugs, tachycardia-induced cardiomyopathy, and infiltrative cardiomyopathy (i.e., hemochromatosis or amyloidosis).

- Genetic link--20%-30% incidence of dilated cardiomyopathy in first-degree relatives.
- Other causes of severe left ventricular dysfunction: severe coronary artery disease ("hibernating myocardium"), multiple areas of previous infarction, ethanol abuse, hyperthyroidism or hypothyroidism, postpartum cardiomyopathy, toxins and drugs, tachycardia-induced cardiomyopathy, and infiltrative cardiomyopathy (i.e., hemochromatosis or amyloidosis).

Clinical Presentation of Dilated Cardiomyopathy

The presentation of dilated cardiomyopathy is highly variable. The patient may be asymptomatic, in which case the diagnosis is made on basis of chest radiography, ECG, or echocardiography. Patients may have symptoms of mild to severe heart failure (New York Heart Association functional class IV). Other patients may present with the sudden onset of a systemic embolus. Atrial and ventricular arrhythmias are common in dilated cardiomyopathy. If heart failure is present, the following are found on physical examination: jugular venous pressure is increased, up-stroke of carotid artery is low volume, left ventricular impulse is displaced with a rapid filling wave, third and fourth heart sounds are frequently audible, and apical systolic murmur of mitral regurgitation.

- Presentation of dilated cardiomyopathy is highly variable.
- Jugular venous pressure is increased and third and fourth heart sounds are often audible.

ECG frequently shows interventricular conduction delay or left bundle branch block and left ventricular hypertrophy. Premature atrial contractions or atrial fibrillation occurs. Premature ventricular contractions and short bursts of ventricular tachycardia are common. The chest radiography usually shows left ventricular enlargement. The diagnosis is made on the basis of reduced ejection fraction on analysis of left ventricular function (echocardiography, radionuclide angiography, or left ventriculography).

- ECG shows interventricular conduction delay or left bundle branch block and left ventricular hypertrophy.
- Premature ventricular contractions and short bursts of ventricular tachycardia are common.

Evaluation of Dilated Cardiomyopathy

After the diagnosis of depressed left ventricular function is made, rule out treatable secondary causes of left ventricular dysfunction. Sensitive thyroid-stimulating hormone level should be determined to exclude hyperthyroidism or hypothyroidism. Iron and iron-binding capacities should be measured (or ferritin level) to rule out hemochromatosis. Ethanol or drug abuse must be documented. Tachycardia-induced cardiomyopathy is a recently described entity. In patients with prolonged periods of tachycardia due to either atrial fibrillation or atrial tachycardia, left ventricular systolic function is frequently depressed. The mechanism of this is unknown but may be related to abnormalities of neurohumoral mechanisms. This is an important cause to establish because systolic dysfunction can be completely reversed after the tachycardia is treated. In severe coronary artery disease, reversible left ventricular dysfunction can be caused by hibernating myocardium. In these patients, long-standing diffuse ischemia depletes ATP stores in myocardial cells, which are thus functionally inactive. However, with revascularization, left ventricular function may gradually improve. A small percentage of patients with severe coronary artery disease probably have depressed left ventricular function because most of the patients have irreversible fibrosis. Differentiating between these two groups of patients is difficult. Currently, the standard method is PET scanning, which can demonstrate metabolic activity. Improvement in myocardial thickening after treatment with low doses of dobutamine or large areas of perfusion on thallium scanning may help diagnose hibernating myocardium.

- Rule out treatable secondary causes of left ventricular dysfunction.
- Sensitive thyroid-stimulating hormone test can exclude hyperthyroidism and hypothyroidism as causes.
- Tachycardia-induced cardiomyopathy is reversible.
- Hibernating myocardium is a reversible cause of left ventricular dysfunction.

A certain number of patients have left ventricular dysfunction caused by acute myocarditis. The natural history of these patients is unknown. Many patients continue to have progressive left ventricular dysfunction that eventually may lead to dilated cardiomyopathy. A small percentage of patients may undergo spontaneous improvement with time. Thus, it is necessary to measure left ventricular function 3-6 months after making the diagnosis. Endomyocardial biopsy may help in diagnosing myocarditis (but may not be practical because there is no proven therapy for myocarditis).

- Endomyocardial biopsy, usually performed at tertiary care centers, can diagnose myocarditis but may not be practical because there is no proven therapy for myocarditis.

Pathophysiology

To treat heart failure associated with dilated cardiomyopathy, the pathophysiology of heart failure must be understood. The relationship of stroke volume to preload and afterload and the neurohumoral response to decreased myocardial contractility are important.

The relationship of stroke volume to preload is shown on the Starling curve in Figure 4-4.

The relationship of stroke volume to afterload is shown in Figure 4-5.

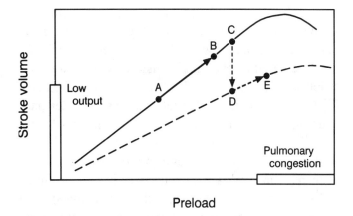

Fig. 4-4. Starling curve. Solid line is patient with normal contractility, and the dotted line is one with depressed systolic function. Normally, stroke volume depends on preload of the heart. Increasing preload increases stroke volume (A to B). Myocardial dysfunction causes a shift of the curve downward and to the right (C to D), causing a severe decrease in stroke volume, which leads to symptoms of fatigue and lethargy. The compensatory response to decrease in stroke volume is an increase in preload (D to E). Because the diastolic pressure-volume relationship is curvilinear, increased left ventricular volume produces increased left ventricular end-diastolic pressure, causing symptoms of pulmonary congestion. Note flat portion of the curve at its upper end; here, there is little increase in stroke volume for increase in preload.

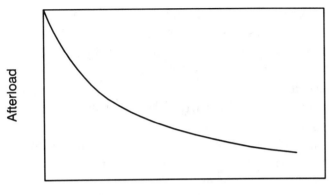

Fig. 4-5. As opposed to preload, increase in afterload produces a decrease in stroke volume. Therefore, a shift of the Starling curve up and to the left can be accomplished by either increase in myocardial contractility or decrease in afterload.

Figure 4-6 illustrates the neurohumoral response to decreased myocardial contractility. Decreased stroke volume produces compensatory increase in left ventricular end-diastolic volume and end-diastolic pressure (Starling curve mechansim); this results in symptoms of pulmonary congestion. Decreased stroke volume activates baroreceptors and the sympathetic nervous system. Sympathetic nervous system stimulation causes an increased heart rate and contractility. Alpha-stimulation of the arterioles causes increase in afterload. Renin-angiotensin system is activated by sympathetic stimulation, decreased renal blood flow, and decreased renal sodium. This system in turn activates aldosterone, causing increased renal retention of sodium and, thus, more pulmonary congestion. Low rate of renal blood flow results in renal retention of sodium. Increased level of angiotensin II causes vasoconstriction and increase in afterload. In congestive heart failure, there is inappropriate increase in afterload, causing further decrease in stroke volume.

- Increase in preload causes increase in stroke volume.
- Increase in afterload causes decrease in stroke volume.
- Either increase in afterload or decrease in myocardial contractility can shift the Starling curve downward and to the right.
- Inappropriate increase in afterload in patients with heart failure causes further decrease in stroke volume.

Treatment of Dilated Cardiomyopathy

In treating dilated cardiomyopathy, it is important to diagnose and remove precipitating factors, as mentioned above. Treatment of congestive heart failure in patients with dilated cardiomyopathy should be based on the pathophysiologic mechanisms described above (Fig. 4-7).

- In treating dilated cardiomyopathy, diagnose and remove precipitating factors.

Drugs that directly affect contractility include digoxin and phosphodiesterase inhibitors (milrinone and amrinone). Digoxin provides symptomatic relief if the ejection fraction is <40%, particularly in patients with a third heart sound or concomitant atrial fibrillation. Whether digoxin improves mortality is unknown. Because digoxin is excreted by the kidneys, its dosage needs to be decreased with increased levels of creatinine and for older patients. The normal dosage is 0.25 mg/day but should be decreased to 0.125 mg/day if creatinine clearance is <70. In patients with chronic renal failure, digoxin can be given at a dosage of 0.125 mg three times weekly. Because of drug-to-drug interaction, digoxin dosage should be decreased with concomitant administration of quinidine, verapamil, and amiodarone. Although newer inotropic agents (milrinone and amrinone) may improve symptoms short-term, their overall effect is to increase mortality. Therefore, they should not be used in most cases of congestive heart failure.

- Digoxin and phosphodiesterase inhibitors (milrinone and amrinone) directly affect contractility.
- Because digoxin is excreted by the kidneys, its dosage needs to be decreased with increased levels of creatinine and for older patients.
- Digoxin dosage should be decreased with concomitant administration of quinidine, verapamil, and amiodarone.

Diuretics and nitrates reduce pulmonary congestion. Diuretics are mainstay of therapy and should be used in most patients with symptoms of pulmonary congestion. The daily use of diuretics may cause neurohumoral and electrolyte imbalances, thus, a "pulsed" dosage of diuretics (three times weekly), if tolerated, may be more beneficial. Nitrates reduce preload through venodilatation. They should be given three times daily with a nitrate-free interval to prevent nitrate tolerance.

- Diuretics and nitrates reduce pulmonary congestion.
- If tolerated, "pulse" dosage of diuretics (three times weekly) may be more beneficial.
- Nitrates reduce preload through venodilatation.

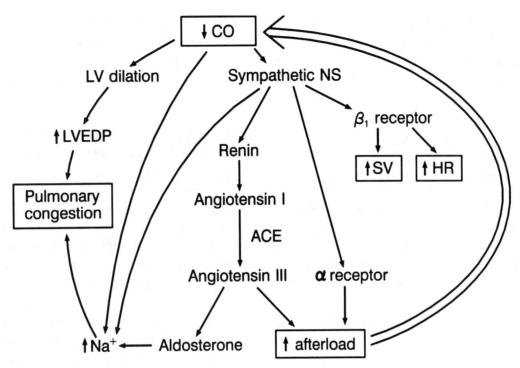

Fig. 4-6. Neurohumoral response to decreased myocardial contractility. ACE, angiotensin converting enzyme; CO, cardiac output ; HR, heart rate; LV, left ventricle; LVEDP, left ventricular end-diastolic pressure; NS, nervous system; SV< stroke volume.

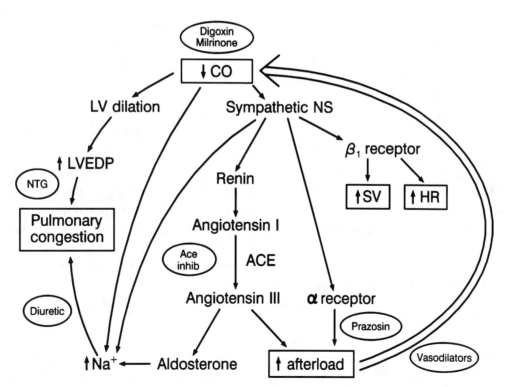

Fig. 4-7. The effect of various drugs used to treat heart failure on the neurohumoral responses in patients with dilated cardiomyopathy. NTG, nitroglycerin. Other abbreviations as in Figure 4-6.

With reduced afterload, stroke volume improves, as do symptoms. Prazosin, a selective α_1-blocker, has a high rate of tachyphylaxis and no effect on mortality. The combination of nitrates and hydralazine provides symptomatic improvement, probably to a greater degree than ACE inhibitors, in patients with heart failure. For severely symptomatic patients, the combination of nitrates and hydralazine also improves mortality. However, the rate of intolerance to these medications is high. When afterload reduction is used, diuretics should be given concomitantly to prevent the compensatory increase in sodium retention.

- Stroke volume improves with reduced afterload.
- Prazosin, selective α_1-blocker, has high rate of tachyphylaxis.
- Combination of nitrates and hydralazine improves mortality.

Mainstays of therapy in the 1990s are ACE inhibitors. By blocking conversion of angiotensin I to angiotensin II, ACE inhibitors decrease afterload by inhibition of angiotensin II and decrease sodium retention by inhibition of aldosterone. Also, ACE inhibitors may directly affect myocardial cells at the molecular level. This may explain how ACE inhibitors prevent ventricular dilatation and improve mortality. Overall, ACE inhibitors provide symptomatic improvement in patients with New York Heart Association functional class III or IV failure and improve mortality in patients with moderate and severe heart failure.

- ACE inhibitors are mainstays of therapy in the 1990s.
- ACE inhibitors decrease afterload by inhibition of angiotensin II and decrease sodium retention by inhibition of aldosterone.
- ACE inhibitors improve mortality in patients with moderate and severe heart failure.

In asymptomatic or mildly symptomatic patients, ACE inhibitors prevent onset of heart failure and reduce need for hospitalization. After anterior myocardial infarction, ACE inhibitors prevent progressive ventricular dilatation and reduce mortality. These agents need to be given initially as a small dose (comparable to 6.25 mg of captopril) because of a hypotensive effect. Dosage should be titrated up as tolerated, with a final dosage equivalent to 50 mg of captopril three times daily. To achieve this, diuretics should be withheld for several days before administering ACE inhibitors for equilibration of intravascular

volume. Side effects of ACE inhibitors include hypotension, proteinuria, dysgeusia, cough, acute renal failure (with bilateral renal artery stenosis or renal artery stenosis in a single kidney), granulocytopenia, and thrombocytopenia.

- In asymptomatic/mildly symptomatic patients, ACE inhibitors prevent onset of heart failure and reduce need for hospitalization.
- After anterior myocardial infarction, ACE inhibitors probably prevent progressive ventricular dilatation and reduce mortality.
- ACE inhibitor side effects: hypotension, proteinuria, dysgeusia, cough, acute renal failure, granulocytopenia, thrombocytopenia.

β-Blockers may be helpful in the treatment of selected patients with dilated cardiomyopathy. β-Blockers are most useful in patients with resting tachycardia but need to be given carefully to prevent left ventricular decompensation. The benefit of beta-blockade may be achieved through prevention of sympathetic-induced myocardial necrosis.

- β-Blockade is most useful in patients with resting tachycardia.
- β-Blockade may prevent sympathetic-induced myocardial necrosis.

A 48-hour infusion of dobutamine gives symptomatic relief, but the effect is temporary (1-2 months) and mortality is increased. The infusion must be given with continuous ECG monitoring to look for arrhythmia. The usual dosage is 10-25 µg/kg per minute to get resting heart rate 15-20 beats per minute above baseline. Dobutamine may replenish low catecholamine stores. This therapy is reserved for severely symptomatic patients who are unresponsive to other therapies.

- 48-Hour infusion of dobutamine gives symptomatic relief.
- Effect is for 1-2 months.
- Dobutamine may cause increased mortality.
- Dobutamine may replenish low cathecholamine stores.

Several investigational calcium channel blockers may be beneficial for patients with dilated cardiomyopathy. Their major effect appears to be by lowering afterload. Forty percent of patients with severe dilated cardiomyopathy have left ventricular thrombus with high embolic potential. Therefore, anticoagulation with warfarin is recommended if the ejection fraction is <30% (or <50% in patients in atrial fibrillation).

- Of patients with severe dilated cardiomyopathy, 40% have left ventricular thrombus with high embolic potential.
- Anticoagulation with warfarin is recommended if ejection fraction is <30% (or <50% in patients with atrial fibrillation).

Even with optimal medical therapy, prognosis for patients with dilated cardiomyopathy is poor, with a 2-year mortality of 50% after symptoms are severe. Heart transplantation is procedure of choice for patients with severe dilated cardiomyopathy and severe symptoms. With successful transplantation, 1-year survival is 90%. The major contraindication for transplantation in otherwise healthy patient is a high pulmonary arteriolar resistance (>4 Wood units/m^2). In the U.S., donor availability is the major limiting factor.

- After symptoms are severe, 2-year mortality is 50% for patients with dilated cardiomyopathy, even with optimal medical therapy.
- The procedure of choice for these patients is heart transplantation.
- With successful transplantation, 1-year survival is 90%.

Recapitulation of Drug Therapy of Heart Failure
- ACE inhibitors improve mortality in patients with severely symptomatic dilated cardiomyopathy.
- ACE inhibitors prevent deterioration and subsequent hospitalizations in patients with asymptomatic dilated cardiomyopathy.
- ACE inhibitors prevent ventricular dilatation and improve mortality in patients with anterior myocardial infarction.
- Combination of nitrates and hydralazines may improve symptoms to a greater degree than ACE inhibitors. These drugs improve mortality in severely symptomatic patients, but intolerance to these medications is high.
- Nitrates should be used on a three-times-a-day dosage with a nitrate-free interval to prevent nitrate tolerance.
- Diuretics should be given as a "pulsed dose" to prevent neurohumoral and electrolyte imbalances that occur with daily dosages.
- Digoxin is useful for symptomatic treatment of patients with dilated cardiomyopathy, particularly those in atri-

al fibrillation or with a third heart sound.
- Phosphodiesterase inhibitors and prolonged infusion of dobutamine directly increase contractility, may improve symptoms but probably increase mortality.

HYPERTROPHIC CARDIOMYOPATHY

Etiology
Hypertrophic cardiomyopathy is a disease in which massive hypertrophy of the myocardium occurs without any known cause. There is usually dynamic left ventricular outflow tract obstruction, but 20%-40% of patients have no obstruction. The diagnosis is based on echocardiographic finding of severe hypertrophy of the myocardium in the absence of a secondary cause, such as hypertension, chronic renal failure, or infiltrative disease.

- Hypertrophic cardiomyopathy--massive hypertrophy of myocardium without known cause.
- Dynamic left ventricular outflow tract obstruction occurs, but not in 20%-40% of patients.
- Diagnosis is based on echocardiographic finding of severe myocardial hypertrophy.

Primary abnormality of patients with hypertrophic cardiomyopathy appears to be abnormal calcium metabolism at cellular level. Hypertrophic cardiomyopathy is a hereditary disease (autosomal-dominant), although sporadic cases are frequent. All patients with hypertrophic cardiomyopathy should have screening of first-degree relatives. Genetic counseling is advised for potential parents. A gene mutation is highly prevalent in certain families with hypertrophic cardiomyopathy. Patients with this gene mutation have a high incidence of sudden death.

- The primary abnormality apparently is abnormal calcium metabolism at cellular level.
- It is hereditary disease (autosomal-dominant), but sporadic cases are frequent.
- Genetic counseling is advised.
- A gene mutation is highly prevalent in certain families with hypertrophic cardiomyopathy.
- Patients with this gene mutation have a high incidence of sudden death.

Symptoms
Hypertrophic cardiomyopathy has several different manifestations. There appears to be a bimodal age dis-

tribution of presentation. Young males (usually in teens or early 20s) have a high propensity for syncope and sudden death. Older patients (in 50s and 60s) present with symptoms of shortness of breath and angina and may have a better prognosis than young patients. The classic presentation of the younger group is a young male athlete undergoing a physical examination for participating in a sport who is found to have a heart murmur and left ventricular hypertrophy on ECG. The classic presentation of the older group is an elderly woman in whom pulmonary edema develops after noncardiac surgery and whose condition worsens, with diuresis, afterload reduction, and inotropic support (all of which worsen dynamic left ventricular outflow tract obstruction). The classic symptom triad is syncope, angina, and dyspnea. These symptoms are similar to those of patients with valvular aortic stenosis. Some patients have a small hyperdynamic left ventricle with hypertrophy due to hypertension and associated dynamic left ventricular outflow tract obstruction—"hypertensive-hypertrophic cardiomyopathy." Although they do not have true cardiomyopathy, the pathophysiology may be the same as for hypertrophic cardiomyopathy. These patients are not at increased risk for sudden death and ventricular fibrillation.

- The classic presentation of hypertrophic cardiomyopathy is the triad of angina, syncope, and dyspnea.
- Bimodal distribution of presentation: young males with high incidence of sudden death and older patients with dyspnea and angina.
- Prognosis for older patients may be better than for younger patients.
- Patients with hypertension may have hypertrophy and dynamic left ventricular outflow tract obstruction similar to those of patients with hypertrophic cardiomyopathy.

Pathophysiology

Signs and symptoms of patients with hypertrophic cardiomyopathy are caused by four major abnormalities: diastolic dysfunction, left ventricular outflow tract obstruction, mitral regurgitation, and ventricular arrhythmias.

Diastolic dysfunction is caused by many mechanisms. Severe hypertrophy and increased muscle mass produce decreased compliance so that there is increased pressure per given volume entering the left ventricle during diastole. Marked abnormality in calcium metabolism causes abnormal ventricular relaxation. High afterload due to left ventricular tract obstruction also delays ventricular relaxation.

All these events cause increased left ventricular diastolic pressure, which leads to angina and dyspnea.

In many patients, dynamic left ventricular tract obstruction is caused by the hypertrophied septum encroaching into the left ventricular outflow tract. This subsequently "sucks in" the anterior leaflet of the mitral valve (systolic anterior motion), thus the occurrence of left ventricular outflow tract obstruction. Because of this pathophysiologic process, a dynamic outflow tract obstruction increases dramatically with decreased preload or afterload or increased contractility.

Systolic anterior motion of the mitral valve distorts the mitral valve apparatus during systole and may cause significant mitral regurgitation. The degree of mitral regurgitation is also dynamic and depends on the degree of left ventricular outflow tract obstruction. Patients with severe mitral regurgitation usually have severe symptoms of dyspnea.

Because of cellular disarray in patients with hypertrophic cardiomyopathy, the electrical conduction system is dispersed, leading to a high propensity for ventricular arrhythmias. The frequent occurrence of ventricular arrhythmias may cause sudden death. Also, arrhythmias usually cause recurrent episodes of syncope.

- The major pathophysiologic abnormality in patients with hypertrophic cardiomyopathy is diastolic dysfunction.
- Left ventricular outflow tract obstruction and mitral regurgitation are caused by distortion of the mitral valve apparatus (systolic anterior motion).
- The propensity for ventricular arrhythmias causing syncope and sudden death is high.

Examination

Hypertrophic cardiomyopathy can be diagnosed with the combination of carotid artery upstroke and left ventricular impulse. The carotid artery upstroke is very rapid compared with that of patients with aortic stenosis. If left ventricular outflow tract obstruction is significant, carotid artery upstroke has a bifid quality. The left ventricular impulse is always very sustained, indicating significant left ventricular hypertrophy. It frequently has a palpable "A" wave. Patients with significant left ventricular outflow tract obstruction have a triple impulse. The first heart sound is normal, and the second heart sound is paradoxically split. A loud systolic ejection murmur indicates left ventricular outflow tract obstruction. The murmur changes in intensity with changes in loading conditions

(Table 4-7). A holosystolic murmur of mitral regurgitation may be present; it increases with increases in left ventricular outflow murmur. The changes in mitral regurgitation with different maneuvers are opposite the changes that occur with mitral regurgitation due to other causes. There is an increased intensity of the murmur on the beat after a premature ventricular contraction. Arterial pulse rate decreases because the obstruction is increased. This is due to increased contractility and decreased afterload and is called Brockenbrough's sign.

- Diagnosis of hypertrophic cardiomyopathy can be made by palpating sustained left ventricular impulse and rapid upstroke of the carotid artery.
- The murmur changes dramatically with changes in loading conditions of the heart.
- Mitral regurgitation murmur changes in same direction as that of left ventricular outflow tract obstruction under different loading conditions.
- First heart sound is normal, and the second heart sound is paradoxically split.

Diagnostic Testing in Patients With Hypertrophic Cardiomyopathy

Patients with hypertrophic cardiomyopathy almost always have abnormal ECG, which shows significant left ventricular hypertrophy. Apical hypertrophic cardiomyopathy is a variant of hypertrophic cardiomyopathy in which the hypertrophy is localized at the apex of the left ventricle. The ECG in these patients typically has large, diffuse, symmetrical T-wave inversions across the precordium.

Hypertrophic cardiomyopathy is diagnosed with echocardiography, which shows severe hypertrophy of myocardium (left ventricular wall thickness >16 mm in diastole) without any known cause. Although asymmetric septal hypertrophy was required for the diagnosis (septum-to-posterior-wall ratio >1.3), it is now recognized that hypertrophy can be in any part of the myocardium, e.g., lateral wall only or diffuse concentric hypertrophy. Therefore, the M-mode criterion of asymmetric septal hypertrophy is no longer valid. Doppler echocardiography is useful in diagnosing left ventricular outflow tract obstruction. If left ventricular outflow tract obstruction is present, velocity across the left ventricular outflow tract is increased. Severity of the outflow obstruction can be measured by applying modified Bernoulli equation (pressure gradient = $4 \times V^2$). Mitral regurgitation can be detected with Doppler echocardiography.

Table 4-7.--Dynamic Left Ventricular Outflow Tract Obstruction

Increased obstruction
Decreased afterload
Amyl nitrite
Vasodilators
Angiotensin converting enzyme inhibitors
Increased contractility
Postpremature ventricular contraction beat
Digoxin
Dopamine
Decreased preload
Squat-to-stand
Nitrates
Diuretics
Valsalva maneuver
Decreased obstruction
Increased afterload
Handgrip
Decreased contractility
β-Blockers
Calcium channel blockers
Increased preload
Fluids

Cardiac catheterization is no longer necessary for diagnosing dynamic left ventricular outflow tract obstruction because all diagnostic data can be obtained by two-dimensional and Doppler echocardiography. Because of strong association with ventricular arrhythmias and sudden death, 48- to 72-hour Holter monitoring is recommended for all patients with hypertrophic cardiomyopathy.

- ECG always shows evidence of left ventricular hypertrophy in cases of hypertrophic cardiomyopathy.
- Asymmetric septal hypertrophy is diagnosed by the presence of large inverted T-waves in precordial leads on ECG. It is confirmed by echocardiography, which demonstrates localized apical hypertrophy.
- Diagnosis of hypertrophic cardiomyopathy is made with echocardiography, which shows hypertrophy in absence of any known cause.
- Strong association with ventricular arrhythmias and sudden death.
- 48- to 72-Hour Holter monitoring recommended for all patients with hypertrophic cardiomyopathy.

Treatment

Treatment of Symptomatic Patients

For symptomatic patients with hypertrophic cardiomyopathy, treatment is with drugs that decrease contractility in attempt to decrease left ventricular outflow tract obstruction (Fig. 4-8). The most effective medication is a high dose of β-blockers (>240 mg equivalent of propranolol/day). Although calcium channel blockers may be used if β-blockade fails, they may cause sudden hemodynamic deterioration in patients with high resting left ventricular outflow tract gradients. Disopyramide may give symptomatic improvement by decreasing left ventricular outflow tract obstruction, but anticholinergic side effects limit its use. All drugs that reduce afterload or preload and those that increase contractility must be avoided in patients with hypertrophic cardiomyopathy.

Surgical myectomy is reserved for patients who are severely symptomatic despite optimal medical therapy and produces dramatic symptomatic relief. Mortality associated with this procedure is 5%-10%. Its complications include complete heart block, aortic regurgitation, and ventricular septal defect. Myectomy is a highly operator-dependent procedure and should be performed only at medical centers that specialize in this procedure.

Dual-chamber pacing may be an alternative to myectomy for patients with hypertrophic cardiomyopathy and severe left ventricular outflow tract obstruction. Its mechanism is unclear but may be due to altered electrical activation of the septum, decreasing movement of the septum into the outflow tract during systole. Dual chamber pacing can produce a modest improvement in gradient, and in the initial studies, symptomatic improvement may be achieved. More studies need to be completed before recommending dual chamber pacing for all patients with severely symptomatic hypertrophic obstructive cardiomyopathy.

Sudden death is a problem in patients with hypertrophic cardiomyopathy. Predictors of sudden death include a family history of sudden death, young male, history of syncope, and nonsustained ventricular tachycardia on Holter monitoring. Genetic markers may identify patients with strong propensity for sudden death. Whether to treat asymptomatic patients with nonsustained ventricular tachycardia is a controversial subject (Fig. 4-9). No conventional antiarrhythmic agent is effective and may make the arrhythmia worse. In selected patients with multiple risk factors for sudden death, a low dose of amiodarone or an automatic implantable cardiac defibrillator might

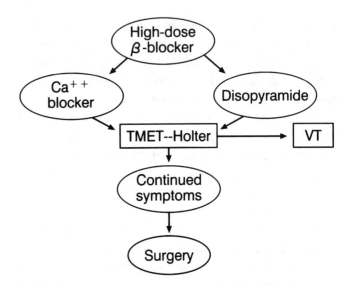

Fig. 4-8. Treatment of symptomatic patients. TMET, treadmill exertion test; VT, ventricular tachycardia.

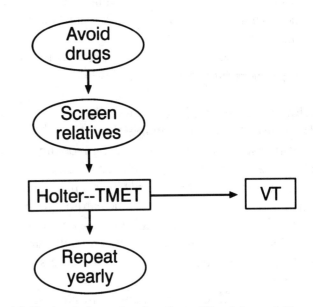

Fig. 4-9. Treatment of asymptomatic patients. Abbreviations as in Figure 4-8.

be chosen. In patients who have already had an out-of-hospital arrest, treatment of choice is automatic implantable cardiac defibrillator.

- β-Blockade is treatment of choice for patients with symptomatic hypertrophic cardiomyopathy.
- Surgical myectomy is reserved for severely symptomatic patients unresponsive to medical therapy.
- Calcium channel blockers may cause sudden hemodynamic deterioration in patients with high resting left ventricular outflow tract obstruction.
- Predictors of sudden death: family history of sudden death, nonsustained ventricular tachycardia, young

male, and history of syncope.

- No conventional antiarrhythmic agent is effective and may worsen the arrhythmia.
- Automatic implantable cardiac defibrillator is treatment of choice for patients with out-of-hospital arrest.

RESTRICTIVE CARDIOMYOPATHY

Definition

The primary abnormality in restrictive cardiomyopathy is diastolic dysfunction. As mentioned above, diastolic dysfunction causes abnormal left ventricular filling so that rise in pressure per unit volume is greater. This is reflected back to the pulmonary circulation, causing symptoms of shortness of breath and edema. Also, because the ventricle cannot fill to meet its preload requirements (Starling mechanism), cardiac output is low, causing fatigue and lethargy. Systolic function is maintained in many patients with restrictive cardiomyopathy. However, at the end stage of the disease, there is decompensation of systolic function as well.

- In restrictive cardiomyopathy, primary abnormality is diastolic dysfunction.
- Diastolic dysfunction causes abnormal left ventricular filling so that rise in pressure per unit volume is greater.
- Left ventricle cannot fill to meet its preload requirements.
- Low cardiac output causes fatigue and lethargy.

The cause of primary restrictive cardiomyopathy is unknown. There are two major categories: idiopathic restrictive cardiomyopathy and endomyocardial fibrosis. In idiopathic restrictive cardiomyopathy (seen mainly in the U.S.), there is progressive fibrosis of the myocardium. Endomyocardial fibrosis is probably an end stage of eosinophilic syndromes in which there is intracavitary thrombus filling of the left ventricle. This restricts filling and causes increased diastolic pressures. Secondary fibrosis may also involve the mitral valve, causing severe mitral regurgitation. There may be two different forms of endomyocardial fibrosis: active inflammatory eosinophilic myocarditis in temperate zones and chronic endomyocardial fibrosis in tropic zones. Diseases that cause infiltration of the myocardium have a presentation and pathophysiology similar to those of primary restrictive cardiomyopathy. These diseases include amyloidosis, sarcoidosis, hemochromatosis, and chronic renal failure. Patients after radiation therapy and following heart transplantation may also develop signs and symptoms similar to patients with restrictive cardiomyopathy.

- Endomyocardial fibrosis is probably an end stage of eosinophilic syndromes.
- Secondary fibrosis may involve mitral valve, causing severe mitral regurgitation.
- Diseases causing infiltration of myocardium: amyloidosis, sarcoidosis, hemochromatosis, chronic renal failure.

Signs and Symptoms

Patients with restrictive cardiomyopathy usually present with severe right-sided failure and low output symptoms. Thus, a major symptom is onset of ascites and edema. Atrial arrhythmias are frequently present, and the patient may present with atrial fibrillation. Jugular venous pressure is almost always elevated, with rapid X and Y descents. The precordium is quiet, and heart sounds are soft. There may be apical systolic murmur of mitral regurgitation and a left sternal border murmur of tricuspid regurgitation. A third heart sound may be present. Dullness at the bases of the lungs is consistent with bilateral pleural effusions. ECG is usually low voltage with atrial arrhythmias. Chest radiography shows pleural effusions with normal cardiac silhouette.

- Restrictive cardiomyopathy: severe right-sided failure and low output symptoms.
- Atrial arrhythmias are frequently present.
- Jugular venous pressure is elevated, with rapid X and Y descents.
- Heart sounds are soft.
- ECG is low voltage with atrial arrhythmias.

Diagnosis

Restrictive cardiomyopathy is diagnosed with echocardiography. Typical findings are normal left ventricular cavity size and function and marked enlargement of both atria. Echocardiography is usually nonspecific about the cause except in two instances. One, in endomyocardial fibrosis, the typical appearance of an echo density indicates thrombus in left ventricular apex. Two, amyloid heart disease has typical echocardiographic features of thickened myocardium with a scintillating appearance of the myocardium, pericardial effusion, and valvular regurgitation. Cardiac catheterization shows elevation and end-equalization of all end-diastolic pressures. A typical "square-root sign" and "dip and plateau" pattern consistent with early rapid filling is present. Endomyocardial biopsy usually is not helpful unless there is a systemic disease that has caused infiltration of the myocardium (i.e., amyloid, sarcoid).

- Restrictive cardiomyopathy is diagnosed with echocardiography.
- Typical findings: normal left ventricular cavity size and function and marked enlargement of both atria.
- Endomyocardial fibrosis: typical appearance of echo density indicating thrombus in left ventricular apex.
- Amyloid heart disease: typical echocardiographic features of thickened myocardium with scintillating appearance of myocardium, pericardial effusion, valvular regurgitation.

Treatment

There is no treatment for restrictive cardiomyopathy. Diuretics decrease filling pressures and give symptomatic relief, but this may be at the expense of further decreasing cardiac output. Although calcium channel blockers have been proposed for treating diastolic dysfunction, they may be harmful and cause elevation of end-diastolic pressures. Digoxin usually is not helpful, because systolic contractility is maintained. Heart transplantation is only proven therapy for patients with severe restrictive cardiomyopathy.

- There is no treatment for restrictive cardiomyopathy.
- Diuretics decrease filling pressures.
- Digoxin usually is not helpful.
- Heart transplantation is only proven therapy.

It is important to differentiate restrictive cardiomyopathy from constrictive pericarditis. Both have similar presentations and findings on clinical examination and diagnostic studies. However, in constrictive pericarditis, pericardiectomy produces symptomatic improvement and, frequently, prolongation of longevity. Therefore, exploratory thoracotomy is usually indicated in patients with normal left ventricular systolic function, large atria, and severe elevation of diastolic filling pressures.

- It is important to differentiate restrictive cardiomyopathy from constrictive pericarditis.
- In constrictive pericarditis, pericardiectomy produces symptomatic improvement and prolongation of longevity.

QUESTIONS
(See "Answers" section)

Part I
Multiple Choice

1. Which of the following is not useful in the treatment of a large anterior myocardial infarction?
   a. β-Blockers
   b. Calcium channel blockers
   c. Thrombolytic therapy
   d. Emergency percutaneous transluminal coronary angioplasty
   e. Aspirin

2. Which of the following agents can be given as an isolated intravenous bolus in the setting of an acute anterior myocardial infarction?
   a. Streptokinase
   b. Tissue-plasminogen activator
   c. Anisoylated plasminogen streptokinase activator complex
   d. Urokinase
   e. Nitroglycerin given intravenously

3. The four components of myocardial oxygen demand include all of the following except:
   a. Heart rate

b. Contractility
c. Coronary perfusion pressure
d. Afterload
e. Wall tension

4. For a 50-year-old man with an acute anterior myocardial infarction of 3 hours' duration, what is the optimal therapy?
   a. Streptokinase, 500,000 U; aspirin, 325 mg; and metoprolol, 5 mg intravenously times three
   b. Streptokinase, 1,500,000 U; diltiazem, 5 mg intravenously; and aspirin, 325 mg
   c. Streptokinase, 500,000 U; enalapril, 5 mg intravenously; and aspirin, 325 mg
   d. Streptokinase, 1,500,000 U; aspirin, 325 mg; and metoprolol, 5 mg intravenously times three
   e. Streptokinase, 500,000 U; metoprolol, 5 mg intravenously times three; and enalapril, 5 mg intravenously

5. A 60-year-old man with typical angina and a history of tobacco abuse and hypertension had a treadmill exercise test. He went 100% of his functional aerobic capacity without electrocardiographic changes. Which of the following is the best descriptor of his status?
   a. He does not have significant coronary heart disease
   b. He has coronary artery spasm
   c. He has coronary artery disease but a good prognosis
   d. He has significant left main coronary artery disease
   e. He has normal ventricular function

True/False
6. With regard to catheter-based interventions, indicate whether the following are true or false:
   a. Laser angioplasty produces a lower restenosis rate than percutaneous transluminal coronary angioplasty
   b. Percutaneous transluminal coronary angioplasty decreases the incidence of myocardial infarction in a 90% left anterior descending coronary artery lesion
   c. The immediate success rate of percutaneous transluminal coronary angioplasty approached 90% in 1993
   d. Percutaneous transluminal coronary angioplasty should be performed in all patients with high-grade

lesions after thrombolytic therapy for myocardial infarction
   e. Percutaneous transluminal coronary angioplasty reduces mortality in patients with a high-grade left anterior descending coronary artery lesion

7. With regard to coronary artery bypass grafting, indicate whether the following are true or false:
   a. It will prolong survival in patients with left main coronary artery disease
   b. It will prevent myocardial infarction in patients with left anterior descending coronary artery disease
   c. It will prolong survival in patients with three-vessel disease and an ejection fraction of 40%
   d. It will improve left ventricular function in patients with an ejection fraction <20%
   e. It is effective in the treatment of sustained ventricular tachycardia

Part II
Multiple Choice
8. Dilated cardiomyopathy frequently has all the following except:
   a. Systolic dysfunction
   b. Diastolic dysfunction
   c. Mitral regurgitation
   d. Dynamic left ventricular outflow tract obstruction
   e. Apical thrombus

9. Which of the following decreases mortality in severely symptomatic patients with dilated cardiomyopathy?
   a. Digoxin
   b. A 48-hour infusion of dobutamine
   c. Prazosin (a selective α_1-blocker)
   d. Enalapril (an angiotensin-converting enzyme inhibitor)
   e. Nitrates and diuretics

10. Which of the following should not be used in symptomatic patients with dilated cardiomyopathy?
   a. Warfarin (Coumadin)
   b. Digoxin
   c. Milrinone
   d. Angiotensin-converting enzyme inhibitors
   e. Nitrates/hydralazine

11. An increase in stroke volume can occur with all the

following except:
a. A selective α_1-blocker
b. A β_1-agonist
c. A long-acting nitrate
d. An angiotensin-converting enzyme inhibitor
e. Digoxin

12. Which of the following is the primary pathophysiologic mechanism in restrictive cardiomyopathy:
a. Systolic dysfunction
b. Dynamic left ventricular outflow tract obstruction
c. Apical thrombus formation
d. Atrial arrhythmias
e. Diastolic dysfunction

True/False
13. Angiotensin-converting enzyme inhibitors have been shown to do the following:
a. Prolong life in severely symptomatic patients with dilated cardiomyopathy
b. Prevent ventricular dilatation after anterior myocardial infarction
c. Decrease future hospitalization in asymptomatic patients with dilated cardiomyopathy
d. Be more effective than nitrates/hydralazine in decreasing symptoms in patients with dilated cardiomyopathy
e. Improve symptoms of low output in patients with symptomatic dilated cardiomyopathy
f. Prevent sudden death in patients with dilated cardiomyopathy

14. The following cardiac diseases have a hereditary component:
a. Hypertrophic cardiomyopathy
b. Dilated cardiomyopathy
c. Coronary artery disease
d. Bicuspid aortic stenosis
e. Mitral stenosis
f. Mitral valve prolapse

CHAPTER 5
CARDIOLOGY II

Stephen C. Hammill, M.D.

CARDIAC ARRHYTHMIAS

MYOCARDIAL CELLULAR CONDUCTION

Cells in the sinus and atrioventricular (AV) nodes are slow-conducting and activated by opening calcium channels and blocked by calcium channel blockers such as verapamil. Cells in the atrium, His-Purkinje system, and ventricle are fast-conducting and activated by opening sodium channels and blocked by sodium channel blockers such as class I antiarrhythmic drugs (quinidine, lidocaine, propafenone).

MECHANISMS OF TACHYCARDIA

Reentrant Rhythm

Three conditions are required for reentry to occur (Fig. 5-1 and 5-2): 1) two or more functionally distinct pathways connected proximally and distally to form a closed circuit, 2) unidirectional block in one pathway, and 3) slowed conduction in the other pathway.

Reentry is the most common mechanism responsible for cardiac arrhythmias and can occur in a micro-reentrant circuit within the sinus node, AV node, or small area of injured myocardium bordering a myocardial infarction. Large reentrant circuits involve the atrium (as in atrial flutter) or the atrium, AV conduction system, ventricle, and accessory pathway (as in patients with Wolff-Parkinson-White syndrome).

● Reentry is the most common mechanism for cardiac arrhythmias.

Automatic Rhythm

Automatic rhythms occur when accelerated phase IV depolarization results in enhanced automaticity. The sinus

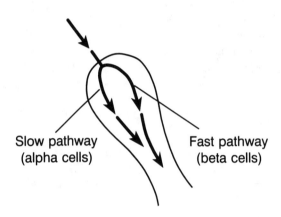

Fig. 5-1. Reentry within AV node demonstrates the two limbs of reentrant circuit.

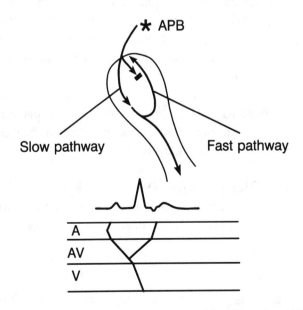

Fig. 5-2. AV nodal reentrant tachycardia. An atrial premature beat (APB) blocks in fast pathway but conducts over slow pathways to ventricle. Impulse then returns to atria over recovered fast pathway and can reenter slow pathway and initiate tachycardia. A, atrium; AV, atrioventricular node; V, ventricle.

node demonstrates normal physiologic automaticity. When other cells in the heart have increased automaticity, they may exceed the rate of sinus node automaticity and replace the sinus node as the cardiac pacemaker. The factors that enhance automaticity are listed in Table 5-1.

Table 5-1.--Factors That Enhance Automaticity

Autonomic changes
Increased sympathetic tone
Decreased parasympathetic tone
Metabolic changes
Increased carbon dioxide
Decreased oxygen
Increased acidity
Mechanical factors
Increased stretch
Drugs
Digitalis
Electrolyte alterations
Decreased potassium
Increased calcium

Automaticity is the mechanism responsible for multifocal atrial tachycardia in patients with decompensated lung disease and patients with ventricular ectopy early after myocardial infarction. In both cases, automaticity is enhanced by increased sympathetic tone, hypoxia, acid-base and electrolyte disturbances, and atrial or ventricular stretch.

- Automaticity is enhanced by increased sympathetic tone, hypoxia, acid-base and electrolyte disturbances, and atrial or ventricular stretch.

Early or Delayed After-Depolarization

This arrhythmia mechanism is identified in the cellular laboratory and may be one of the causes of torsades de pointes.

Parasystole

Parasystole occurs when an ectopic focus in the atrium or ventricle is isolated from the dominant rhythm because of conduction block into the focus. Cells within this area undergo automatic depolarization and, because of entrance block, are not constantly reset by the dominant rhythm. These cells capture the regional myocardium unless the myocardium is refractory from a previously conducted beat. This mechanism causes 3% of premature ventricular complexes (PVCs) noted during routine monitoring and, in general, is benign.

- Parasystole is caused by ectopic focus in atrium or ventricle.
- Parasystole causes 3% of PVCs during routine monitoring.
- Parasystole is benign.

DIAGNOSTIC TECHNIQUES

Ambulatory Monitoring and Transtelephonic Event Recording

Ambulatory (Holter) monitoring is used to document symptomatic and asymptomatic rhythm disturbances if they occur frequently enough to be recorded during the 24- or 48-hour recording period. It is also used to determine the effect of treatment, such as control of ectopic beats and managing heart rate response during atrial fibrillation. Patients may have adequate control of heart rate in response to atrial fibrillation at rest in the physician's office but inappropriately rapid heart rates in response to mild exercise. Such inappropriate rates can be shown by 24-hour monitoring or exercise testing.

Ambulatory monitoring can assess pacemaker function and determine the relationship of arrhythmia to daily activity (e.g., exercise). Finally, ambulatory monitoring is used to confirm episodes of myocardial ischemia, most of which are usually not associated with typical symptoms of angina.

- Ambulatory monitoring assesses pacemaker function, determines relationship of arrhythmia to daily activity, and confirms episodes of myocardial ischemia (most of which do not have typical symptoms of angina).

Transtelephonic event recording determines heart rate during symptoms that occur infrequently. Patients either wear a device continuously for several days or briefly attach themselves to it during symptoms. The device permanently stores the electrocardiogram (ECG) in memory when activation button is depressed, and this ECG is later transmitted over the telephone for evaluation. This device documents the rhythm when a patient experiences typical symptoms. About 20% of transmissions document abnormal heart rhythm, although often the transmissions are helpful for patient management even if normal rhythm is identified.

- Transtelephonic event recording determines heart rate during symptoms that occur infrequently.
- About 20% of transmissions document abnormal heart rhythm.
- Transtelephonic event recording is often helpful for patient management even if normal rhythm is identified.

Exercise Testing

Exercise testing is helpful when patients describe symptoms consistent with cardiac arrhythmia which occur during exercise. This allows for evaluation in a controlled setting with ECG monitoring to determine whether cardiac arrhythmia is causing the exercise-related symptoms. Exercise testing is also useful to determine whether the beneficial effect of a drug at rest is reversed with exercise. Patients with atrial fibrillation may have adequate control of heart rate at rest but poor control with moderate exercise. Those with ventricular tachycardia or complex ventricular ectopy may have adequate suppression of arrhythmia at rest in response to medical therapy only to have ventricular tachycardia with exercise.

- Exercise testing evaluates cardiac arrhythmia during exercise.
- Exercise testing determines whether effect of a drug is reversed with exercise.

PVCs occur during exercise testing in 10% of patients without and 60% of patients with coronary artery disease. Response of PVCs during exercise does not predict severity of coronary artery disease. Elimination of PVCs with exercise is not an indication that coronary artery disease is less severe.

- PVCs occur during exercise in 10% of patients without and 60% of patients with coronary artery disease.
- Response of PVCs during exercise does not predict severity of coronary artery disease.
- Elimination of PVCs with exercise does not indicate less severe coronary artery disease.

Exercise testing is useful for assessing sinus node function to determine whether there is chronotropic incompetence in a patient who complains of dyspnea on exertion. It is also used to assess AV block. AV block at the AV node is usually benign and does not require pacing. This type of block (Wenckebach or Mobitz I) improves with exercise when increased catecholamines enhance AV node conduction. AV node block due to failure of conduction in the His-Purkinje system (Mobitz II) has a worse prognosis; it has a high incidence of heart block and requires pacing. This type of block often worsens with exercise because the increase in catecholamines enhances AV node conduction and results in increased frequency of activation of the diseased His-Purkinje system with progressive block.

- Exercise testing assesses sinus node function in patients with dyspnea on exertion.
- Mobitz I block improves with exercise.
- Mobitz II block worsens with exercise.
- Mobitz II block has worse prognosis and requires pacing.

Signal-Averaged ECG

Signal-averaged ECG is a noninvasive test used to detect low-level signals, termed "late potentials," that result from delayed conduction through diseased myocardium. These signals usually arise in the border zone adjacent to a myocardial infarction, where conducting myocardial cells are mixed in among scar tissue. This disrupted architecture results in delayed conduction and is the substrate for myocardial reentry. Signal-averaged ECG amplifies this low-level signal by several thousandfold and averages multiple QRS complexes to eliminate random noise. The low-level activity is then measured to determine whether a late potential is present. Late potentials have independent prognostic value for identifying patients at risk for ventricular tachycardia after myocardial infarction and inducible ventricular tachycardia at the time of electrophysiologic testing. Signal-averaged ECG has a positive predictive accuracy of 25%-50% and a negative predictive accuracy of 90%-95% for identifying patients at risk for ventricular tachycardia.

- Signal-averaged ECG is noninvasive.
- Signal-averaged ECG identifies patients at risk for ventricular tachycardia.
- Positive predictive accuracy is 25%-50%; negative predictive accuracy is 90%-95%.

Electrophysiologic Testing

Electrophysiologic testing involves placement of electrode catheters in the heart to record and stimulate heart rhythm. In general, catheters are placed in high right atrium, across tricuspid valve in the region of the AV node and His bundle, in right ventricular apex, and, in selected patients, in coronary sinus to record from the left atrium and ventricle. This testing is indicated in patients with cardiogenic syncope of undetermined origin (Fig. 5-3), for evaluation of mechanism of supraventricular tachycardia, for assessing symptomatic patients with Wolff-Parkinson-White syndrome, and for evaluating patients with sustained ventricular tachycardia and survivors of out-of-hospital cardiac arrest. Complication rate of the test is 0.5%-1%.

- Electrophysiologic testing is invasive.
- Electrophysiologic testing is indicated for cardiogenic syncope of undetermined origin.
- Complication rate is 0.5%-1%.

THERAPY

Pacing

Pacing uses a four-letter classification system (Table 5-2). The first letter is the chamber paced; second letter, the chamber sensed; third letter, the mode of response; and fourth letter, the programmable capabilities. Common pacing modes are VVI, which is ventricular paced, ventricular sensed, and inhibited in response to a ventricular event; VVIR, in which rate responsiveness is added (R); and DDD, which is atrial and ventricular paced and sensed and also triggered and inhibited in response to a sensed atrial or ventricular event.

Physiologic pacing attempts to maintain heart rate with

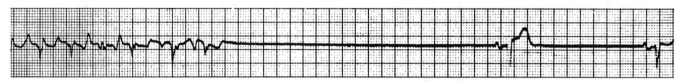

Fig. 5-3. Tachycardia-bradycardia with episode of atrial fibrillation terminating spontaneously; these are followed by a 4.5-second pause until sinus node recovers. (From MKSAP IX: Part C Book 1, 1992. American College of Physicians. By permission.)

normal AV synchrony and increase heart rate in response to physical activity. DDD pacing is used to track atrial activation in patients with normal sinus node activity but some type of AV block. As sinus activity increases in response to exercise or some other stress, the pacemaker tracks this response and paces the ventricle with normal AV conduction delay (P-R interval) at a rate following sinus rate. In patients whose sinus node does not work appropriately because of chronotropic incompetence or patients who have failure of sinus activity as a result of a rhythm such as atrial fibrillation, rate-modulated pacing (the "R" in VVIR) is used to increase heart rate in response to physical demand. An external sensor that

senses body motion, respiratory rate, and blood temperature, or some other sensor, is used to drive the pacemaker to keep up with increased metabolic demands. This type of pacemaker increases exercise endurance during treadmill testing.

- Physiologic pacing maintains heart rate with normal AV synchrony and increases rate during physical activity.
- Rate-modulated pacing increases exercise endurance during treadmill testing.

Pacemaker syndrome is a complication that occurs during ventricular pacing in patients who have intact ret-

Table 5-2.--Code of Permanent Pacing

Chamber(s) paced	Chamber(s) sensed	Mode(s) of response	Programmable capabilities
V = Ventricle	V = Ventricle	T = Triggered	P = Limited (rate or output, or both)
A = Atrium	A = Atrium	I = Inhibited	
D = Dual (atrium and ventricle)	D = Dual (atrium and ventricle)	D = Dual (triggered and inhibited)	M = Multiprogrammable
	O = None	O = None	R = Rate modulated
			O = None

rograde conduction between the ventricle and the atrium (Fig. 5-4). When the ventricle is paced, the impulse conducts retrogradely to the atrium, and simultaneous atrial and ventricular contractions result. The atria are then trying to contract against closed tricuspid and mitral valves, and as a result the atrial contribution to ventricular filling is eliminated and atria are distended. The increased atrial pressure distends the neck veins and can result in hypotension; symptoms include a full sensation in the neck, light-headedness, and fatigue. These are eliminated with dual-chamber pacing.

- Pacemaker syndrome is a complication of pacemakers.
- Atria contract against closed tricuspid and mitral valves.
- Increased atrial pressure distends neck veins and results in hypotension.
- Symptoms: full sensation in neck, light-headedness, fatigue.
- Dual-chamber pacing eliminates symptoms.

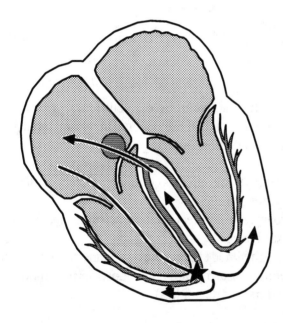

Fig. 5-4. Pacemaker syndrome with retrograde atrial activation during ventricular pacing (*star*), resulting in simultaneous atrial and ventricular contractions.

Pacemaker-mediated tachycardia occurs with DDD pacing when there is intact retrograde conduction between the ventricle and atrium. In this type of tachycardia, the pacemaker generator acts as one limb of the reentrant circuit. Typically, a PVC occurs that conducts retrogradely to the atrium. The retrograde atrial activity is sensed by the pacemaker, which awaits the normal AV delay and

then paces the ventricle. The ventricular activity then conducts retrogradely to the atrium, and the reentrant circuit is completed. This abnormality is corrected through programming changes of the pacemaker generator.

- Pacemaker-mediated tachycardia occurs with DDD pacing, when there is intact retrograde conduction between ventricle and atrium.
- Abnormality is corrected by programming changes of pacemaker generator.

Antiarrhythmic Drugs

Therapeutic range, half-life, and routes of metabolism of antiarrhythmic drugs are listed in Table 5-3. Table 5-4 lists the relative effectiveness of these drugs for treating PVCs, ventricular tachycardia, paroxysmal tachycardia utilizing the AV node as part of the reentrant circuit, and atrial fibrillation.

Half-life is an important concept for use of antiarrhythmic drugs. It is the time required for 50% of a dose to be eliminated. It takes 5 half-lives for a drug to reach steady state or be eliminated. If a drug has a half-life of 90 minutes (e.g., lidocaine), a steady state will be reached in 6 hours; therefore, a loading dose is given to achieve a therapeutic level more promptly. The newer antiarrhythmic drugs often have half-lives approaching 24 hours, and effectiveness is not achieved until 4 or 5 days after initiation of therapy. Therefore, a patient may have adequate suppression of arrhythmia after 2 days of therapy only to have intolerable side effects after 4 days (including proarrhythmia), when steady state is finally achieved.

- Half-life is important concept for use of antiarrhythmic drugs.
- Half-life is time required for 50% of a dose to be eliminated.

Proarrhythmic effect (Table 5-5), a common problem of all antiarrhythmic drugs, occurs when the drug creates an adverse rhythm disturbance (Fig. 5-5), including sinus node suppression and sinus bradycardia, AV block, or increased frequency of or new-onset atrial or ventricular arrhythmias. It was first described in association with quinidine and causes quinidine syncope, which occurs in 1% of patients who take this drug. In such patients, a rapid ventricular tachycardia with polymorphic morphology develops, termed "torsades de pointes." The frequency of proarrhythmia is higher in patients who have reduced ventricular function and a history of sustained

Table 5-3.--Properties of Antiarrhythmic Drugs

Drug	Therapeutic range, µg/mL	Half-life, hours	Route of metabolism	
			Hepatic, %	Renal, %
Class IA				
Quinidine	2-5	5-12	80	20
Procainamide	4-10	3-6	50	50
Disopyramide	2-8	6-8	50	50
Class IB				
Lidocaine	1.5-5	1-2	100	...
Mexiletine	1-2	10-13	100	...
Tocainide	5-12	9-20	60	40
Class IC				
Flecainide	0.2-1	12-27	75	25
Propafenone	Not helpful[*]	5-8	100	...
Class I				
Moricizine	Not helpful	2-3[†]	60	40
Class III				
Amiodarone	1-2	25-110 days	Unknown	...
Sotalol	...	7-18	...	100

[*]Therapeutic effects for propafenone are generally associated with a QRS width increase of 10% above baseline.
[†]Effects of moricizine persist for 14-24 hours; thus, an unmeasured metabolite is suggested.
From MKSAP IX: Part C Book 1, 1992. American College of Physicians. By permission.

Table 5-4.--Relative Effectiveness of Antiarrhythmic Drugs

Drug	Effectiveness[*]			
	PVCs	VT	PSVT	AF
Quinidine	2+	2+	2+	2+
Procainamide	2+	2+	2+	2+
Disopyramide	2+	2+	2+	2+
Lidocaine	2+	2+	0-1+	0
Mexiletine	2+	2+	0-1+	0
Tocainide	2+	2+	0-1+	0
Flecainide	4+	2+	3+	2-3+
Propafenone	4+	2+	3+	2-3+
Moricizine	2+	2+	0-1+	0
Amiodarone	4+	3+	3+	3+
Sotalol	4+	2-3+	3+	2-3+

[*]0, not effective; 1+, least effective; 4+, most effective.
AF, atrial fibrillation (prevention of paroxysmal AF); PSVT, paroxysmal tachycardia utilizing AV node as part of reentrant circuit; VT, ventricular tachycardia.

ventricular tachycardia or ventricular fibrillation. Unfortunately, it is these patients in whom antiarrhythmic drugs are most often required.

- Proarrhythmic effect is common problem of all antiarrhythmic drugs.
- Proarrhythmic effect occurs when drug creates rhythm disturbance.
- Proarrhythmic effect causes quinidine syncope: a rapid ventricular tachycardia with polymorphic morphology (torsades de pointes).

The Cardiac Arrhythmia Suppression Trial (CAST) study indicated that patients with asymptomatic or mildly symptomatic ventricular ectopy after myocardial infarction had decreased survival rate with drug therapy, even though the drugs suppressed the spontaneous ectopy. These patients had approximately a threefold increase in death rate compared with the rate in patients taking placebo. The CAST study evaluated flecainide, encainide, and moricizine; however, similar results have been demonstrated for class IA drugs (quinidine, procainamide, and disopyramide) and the class IB drug mexilitine.

- CAST study indicated decreased survival rate with drug therapy in patients with asymptomatic or mild ventricular ectopy after infarction.

Adenosine slows conduction in the AV node and is eliminated by uptake in endothelial cells and erythrocytes. Its half-life is 10 seconds. Adenosine is indicated in supraventricular reentrant tachycardia that utilizes the AV node as part of the reentrant circuit (i.e., AV nodal reentry or reentry utilizing an accessory pathway). The drug does not terminate atrial fibrillation, flutter, or tachycardia, and it slows the ventricular rate for only a few seconds because of its short half-life. Both adenosine and verapamil have equal efficacy at the highest recommended doses (adenosine, 12 mg; verapamil, 10 mg). Because of adenosine's short half-life, approximately 10% of patients have recurrent supraventricular tachycardia after its administration, whereas recurrent supraventricular tachycardia is rare after administration of verapamil. In patients with a wide QRS tachycardia (ventricular tachycardia) or atrial fibrillation and associated Wolff-Parkinson-White syndrome, hemodynamic collapse is common when they are given verapamil. This problem is not associated with adenosine. The cost of adenosine is approximately twice that of verapamil.

- Adenosine slows conduction in AV node.
- Adenosine is used for supraventricular reentrant tachycardia.
- Adenosine does not terminate atrial fibrillation, flutter, or tachycardia.
- Efficacy of 12 mg of adenosine is equal to that of 10 mg of verapamil.
- Adenosine causes recurrent supraventricular tachycardia in 10% of patients (short half-life).
- Cost of adenosine is twice that of verapamil.

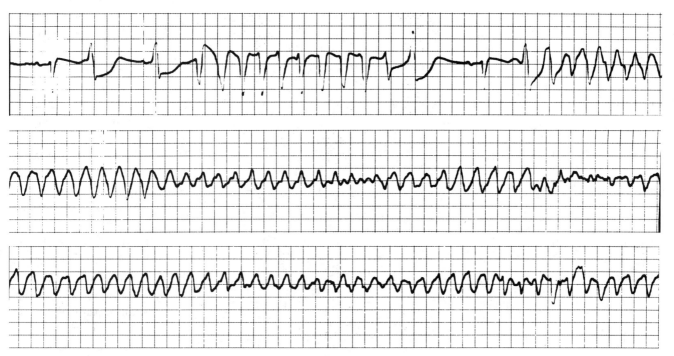

Fig. 5-5. Proarrhythmic response to quinidine. Quinidine resulted in prolongation of QT interval, and late-coupled PVC initiated polymorphic ventricular tachycardia, termed "torsades de pointes."

Electrophysiology-Guided Serial Drug Testing

This technique is used to identify an effective drug before dismissal from the hospital in patients who have life-threatening arrhythmias and for whom outpatient management is unsafe. Arrhythmia is induced in the baseline state, an antiarrhythmic drug is then administered orally, and the electrophysiology study is done. A drug that prevents induction of tachycardia is termed effective. In patients who have ventricular tachycardia occurring spontaneously, the chance of that tachycardia being induced in the laboratory is 95% if they have underlying coronary artery disease and 75% if they have dilated cardiomyopathy or valvular heart disease. In patients who present with out-of-hospital cardiac arrest and ventricular fibrillation, the chance of life-threatening ventricular arrhythmia being induced at testing is 70%. For

Table 5-5.--Toxicity and Side Effects of Antiarrhythmic Drugs

Drug	Frequency of side effects, %	Organ toxicity	% proarrhythmia at treatment for:		Risk of congestive heart failure[*]		Side effects
			PVC	VT	EF ≥ 30%	EF ≤ 30%	
Quinidine	30	Moderate	3	10	0	0	Nausea, abdominal pain, diarrhea, thrombo-cytopenia, hypo-tension, ↓ warfarin
Procainamide	30	High	3	10	0	1+	Lupus-like syndrome, rash, fever, headache, nausea, hallucinations, diarrhea
Disopyramide	30	Low	3	10	1+	4+	Dry mouth, urinary hesitancy, blurred vision, constipation, urinary retention
Lidocaine	40	Moderate	2	5	0	0	L-H, seizure, tremor, confusion, memory loss, nausea
Mexiletine	40	Low	2	5	0	0	L-H, tremor, ataxia, confusion, memory loss, altered liver function
Tocainide	40	High	2	5	0	0	L-H, tremor, ataxia, confusion, memory loss, blood dyscrasia
Flecainide	30	Low	2	5-15+	1+	3+	L-H, visual disturbance, headache, nausea
Propafenone	30	Low	2	5-10[†]	0-1+	2+	L-H, headache, nausea, constipation, metallic taste
Moricizine	30	Low	1	5	0	1+	L-H, nausea, headache, fatigue, dyspnea
Amiodarone	65	High	1	2	0	1+	Corneal deposits, photosensitivity, sleep disturbance, nausea, anorexia, tremor, ataxia, neuropathy, pulmonary toxicity, thyroid disorders, hepatotoxicity, ↓ warfarin
Sotalol	30	Low	2	5	1+	2-3+	L-H, fatigue, dyspnea, nausea

[*]Congestive heart failure risk: 0, no risk; 4+, high risk.
[†]Proarrhythmia risk increases in presence of reduced ventricular function.
EF, ejection fraction; L-H, light-headedness; PVC, premature ventricular complex; VT, sustained ventricular tachycardia.
From MKSAP IX: Part C Book 1, 1992. American College of Physicians. By permission.

patients with ventricular tachycardia, an effective drug is identified in approximately 40%, and each drug has a 25% chance of being effective with electrophysiology-guided serial drug testing. For patients who survive cardiac arrest and have inducible ventricular tachycardia, the survival rate at 1 year is 95% if an effective drug is identified. Alternatively, the 1-year survival rate is 65% if an effective drug cannot be identified and 85% if ventricular tachycardia is not inducible during baseline study and no therapy is given.

- Electrophysiology-guided serial drug testing identifies effective drug in patients with life-threatening arrhythmias before dismissal from hospital.
- With out-of-hospital cardiac arrest and ventricular fibrillation, chance of life-threatening arrhythmia during testing is 70%.
- Serial drug testing identifies effective drug in 40% of patients with ventricular tachycardia.

Implantable Antitachycardia Devices

Because serial drug testing identifies only 40% of patients with life-threatening ventricular arrhythmias, alternative therapy has been developed to treat recurrences of tachycardia. The most effective therapy has been the implantable cardioverter-defibrillator. This device monitors the rhythm and treats a ventricular arrhythmia with a 30-joule shock (first-generation device), a first shock that can be programmed to low energy followed by high-energy shocks if needed (second-generation device), or antitachycardia pacing as the initial therapy followed by low-energy cardioversion and high-energy defibrillation if needed (third-generation device). Current limitations of the device are a battery life of 4-5 years, requirement for thoracotomy, large and cumbersome size, and presence of uncomfortable and potentially dangerous shocks during sinus rhythm or atrial fibrillation.

Implantable cardioverters-defibrillators have improved mortality in patients surviving sudden cardiac death when compared with historical controls. Historically, such patients had a 70% survival rate at 1 year with either no treatment or empiric antiarrhythmic drug therapy. Use of the device has improved the overall 1-year survival rate to 90%; recurrent sudden cardiac death occurs in 2% of patients at 1 year and 4% of patients at 4 years.

- Limitations of implantable cardioverter-defibrillator: battery life of 4-5 years, requires thoracotomy, large,

uncomfortable and potentially dangerous shocks during sinus rhythm or atrial fibrillation.
- Overall 1-year survival rate with the device is 90%.

Transcatheter Ablation

This technique involves placing an electrode catheter within a heart chamber. It is placed adjacent to a critical portion of a reentrant circuit, which might include one of the pathways participating in AV nodal reentrant tachycardia or an accessory pathway in patients with Wolff-Parkinson-White syndrome, an automatic atrial focus, or a portion of the reentrant circuit adjacent to scar in the ventricle in patients with ventricular tachycardia. Previously, direct current was then passed through the catheter, exiting the catheter tip and resulting in a 1-cm scar that was 2-3 mm in depth. Most ablations are now performed with radiofrequency energy, which is passed through the catheter, heating its tip; the result is smaller scar with a lesion size that is easier to control.

- Catheter placement for ablation: pathway in AV nodal reentrant tachycardia, accessory pathway in Wolff-Parkinson-White syndrome, automatic atrial focus, or reentrant circuit.
- Catheter ablation is performed with radiofrequency energy passed through catheter.

Radiofrequency energy used to treat an accessory pathway (Wolff-Parkinson-White syndrome) or reentrant tachycardia within the AV node is successful in 90%-95% of cases. About 1%-2% of patients have complications, including vascular injury where the catheters are placed, cardiac perforation, and infection. In addition, if the accessory pathway is close to the normal conduction system or if AV nodal reentrant tachycardia is ablated, there is a 5% risk of creating complete heart block that requires permanent pacing. Compared with previous surgical approaches for treatment of similar tachycardias, the technique has reduced the hospital stay from 7 days to 2-3 days and the time to return to work or school from 6-8 weeks to 3-5 days. The cost is approximately 40% of the surgical cost.

- Catheter ablation is successful in 90%-95% of cases of accessory pathway or reentrant tachycardia in AV node.
- Complication rate is 1%-2%.
- Reduces hospital stay to 2-3 days.
- Cost is 40% of surgical cost.

Catheter ablation is also used to achieve complete heart block in patients with supraventricular tachycardias (usually atrial fibrillation or atrial flutter) that are refractory to medications and associated with rapid ventricular rates. Either direct-current or radiofrequency ablation results in heart block in approximately 80%-90% of patients, and permanent pacing is then required. Such patients have significant symptomatic improvement because the heart rate is regular and they respond normally to exercise because of rate-responsive pacing. This technique trades tachycardia-associated problems for problems associated with permanent pacemaker implantation and follow-up.

- Catheter ablation achieves complete heart block in supraventricular tachycardias that are refractory to medication and associated with rapid ventricular rates.
- Catheter ablation results in heart block in 80%-90% of patients; permanent pacing then required.
- Symptoms improve significantly.

Antitachycardia Surgery

Operation is a standard technique for treating ventricular tachycardia. The border zone adjacent to myocardial scar (including aneurysm) is generally the location for the reentrant circuit. This border zone is located with mapping systems at the time of operation and is then removed with a technique called subendocardial resection. The operative mortality rate is approximately 10%; arrhythmia is cured in 85% of survivors.

- Operation is standard for treating ventricular tachycardia.
- Operative mortality rate is 10%.
- Arrhythmia cured in 85% of survivors.

Operation is also a standard technique for treating an accessory pathway or AV nodal reentrant tachycardia. Either sharp dissection or cryoablation of the accessory pathway is used. Surgical success rates approach 95%. The surgical mortality rate is 1%, and the risk of heart block is 1%-2%. For the most part, surgical techniques have been replaced by transcatheter radiofrequency ablation.

- Operation is standard for treating accessory pathway or AV nodal reentrant tachycardia.
- Success rate is 95%.

SPECIFIC ARRHYTHMIA PROBLEMS

Sinus Node Dysfunction

Also called sick sinus syndrome, this includes sinus bradycardia, sinus pauses, tachycardia-bradycardia syndrome (Fig. 5-3), and sinus arrest. It is usually associated with conduction system disease and lack of an appropriate junctional escape focus during sinus pause or sinus bradycardia. The diagnosis is made from the history and results of ECG and Holter monitoring, which are the most useful diagnostic tests. Electrophysiologic testing is used to evaluate patients with a history consistent with sinus node disease but in whom ECG or Holter monitoring has not shown the mechanism because of infrequent spells. Electrophysiologic testing has low sensitivity because patients may be in an increased adrenergic state in the laboratory and catecholamines prevent the sinus bradycardia or sinus pauses from being apparent. Prolonged monitoring with an event recorder is also useful for diagnosis.

- Sinus node dysfunction includes sinus bradycardia, sinus pauses, tachycardia-bradycardia syndrome, sinus arrest.
- Associated with conduction system disease.
- Diagnosed from history and ECG and Holter monitoring.
- Electrophysiology testing used for patients in whom mechanism of dysfunction is not shown by ECG or Holter.

Asymptomatic patients with sinus node dysfunction are followed without specific therapy. Symptomatic patients are usually treated with pacemakers. Often, patients with tachycardia-bradycardia have atrial fibrillation that at times presents with rapid ventricular rates and at other times with inappropriate, symptomatic bradycardia. Pacemakers are used to prevent the bradycardia, and drugs are used to slow conduction through the AV node and prevent episodes of rapid ventricular rate.

- Asymptomatic patients with sinus node dysfunction: followed without specific therapy.
- Symptomatic patients with sinus node dysfunction: treated with pacemakers.

Conduction System Disorders

First-degree AV block results in a prolonged P-R interval and is usually due to conduction delay within the AV node. In patients with associated bundle-branch block, the conduction delay may be distal to the AV node in the His-Purkinje system. Patients with *second-degree AV block of the Mobitz I* or Wenckebach variety have a gradual prolongation of the P-R interval before the nonconducted P wave. The subsequent P-R interval is shorter than the P-R interval before the nonconducted P wave (Fig. 5-6 and 5-7). Also, the R-R interval that encompasses the nonconducted P wave is shorter than two R-R intervals between conducted beats. Wenckebach conduction often accompanies an inferior myocardial infarction, which results in ischemia of the AV node. This problem generally does not require pacing unless there are documented hemodynamic problems associated with the slow heart rate.

- First-degree AV block results in prolonged P-R interval.
- Second-degree AV block of Mobitz I type results in gradual prolongation of P-R interval before nonconducted P wave.
- Wenckebach conduction accompanies inferior myocardial infarction.
- Wenckebach conduction does not require pacing unless hemodynamic problems are associated with slow heart rate.

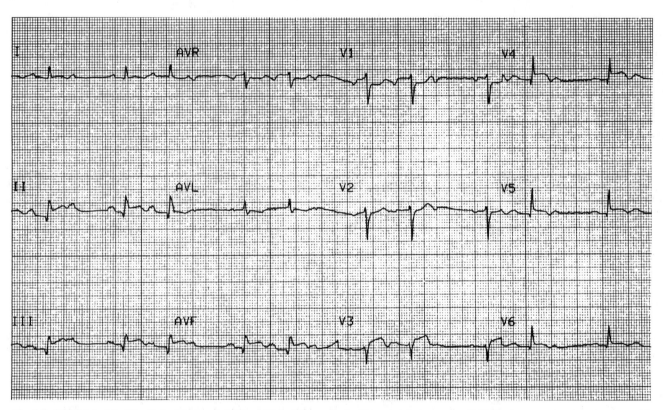

Fig. 5-6. 3:2 Mobitz I (or Wenckebach) second-degree AV block in a patient with acute inferior myocardial infarction.

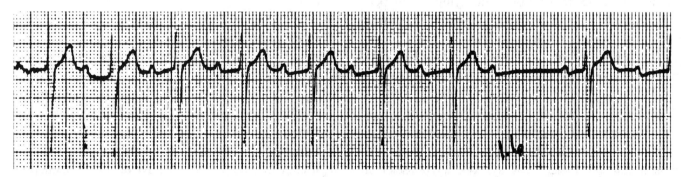

Fig. 5-7. Mobitz I second-degree AV block; note gradual P-R prolongation. P-R after nonconducted P wave is shorter than P-R preceding nonconducted P wave.

Second-degree AV block due to the Mobitz II mechanism is generally caused by conduction delay in the His-Purkinje system and is associated with bundle-branch block (Fig. 5-8). This conduction abnormality is shown on the ECG as a sudden failure of a P wave to conduct to the ventricle with no change in the P-R interval either before or after the nonconducted P wave. This problem often heralds complete heart block, and strong consideration should be given to permanent pacing. *Complete heart block* is diagnosed when there is no relationship between the atrial rhythm and the ventricular rhythm and the atrial rhythm is faster than the ventricular escape rhythm (Fig. 5-9). The ventricular escape rhythm is either

a junctional escape focus, with a conduction pattern similar to the conduction pattern seen during normal rhythm, or a ventricular escape focus, with a wide QRS conduction pattern. Complete heart block is treated with permanent pacing in most cases.

- Second-degree AV block of Mobitz II type is due to conduction delay in His-Purkinje system.
- Often heralds complete heart block; consider permanent pacing.
- Complete heart block: no relationship between atrial rhythm and ventricular rhythm and atrial rhythm is faster than ventricular escape rhythm.

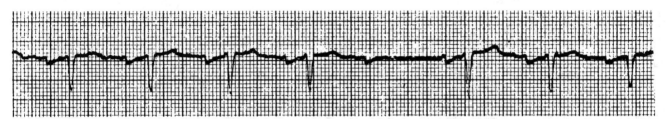

Fig. 5-8. Mobitz II second-degree AV block with no change in P-R interval before or after nonconducted P wave.

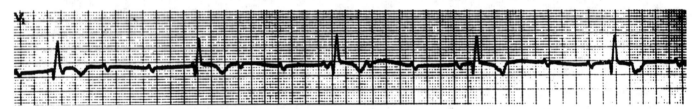

Fig. 5-9. Complete heart block with an atrial rate at 70 beats per minute and a ventricular escape rhythm at 30 beats per minute.

Bifascicular block refers to left bundle-branch block, right bundle-branch block with left anterior fascicular block (marked left-axis deviation), or right bundle-branch block with left posterior fascicular block (right-axis deviation). Bifascicular block is usually associated with underlying structural heart disease and has a 1% chance of progressing to complete heart block in asymptomatic persons. Patients presenting with syncope and bifascicular block may have intermittent complete heart block caused by their conduction system disease or ventricular tachycardia caused by the underlying myocardial disease. Permanent pacing can be used to treat syncope due to complete heart block, but syncope due to ventricular tachycardia requires antiarrhythmic medications, an implantable defibrillator, or surgery, depending on the clinical situation. Patients with syncope and bifascicular block should undergo electrophysiologic testing to determine whether they have ventricular tachycardia because

this rhythm occurs in 40% of such patients. If these patients receive only permanent pacing, the pacing, although it improves their syncope, does not decrease their risk of sudden death.

- Bifascicular block is associated with structural heart disease.
- Bifascicular block progresses to complete heart block in 1% of asymptomatic persons.
- Permanent pacing is used to treat syncope in complete heart block.
- Syncope due to ventricular tachycardia requires antiarrhythmic medications, implantable defibrillator, or surgery.
- Patients with syncope, bifascicular block, and ventricular tachycardia who receive only permanent pacing have improvement in syncope but no decrease in risk of sudden death.

High-degree AV block is diagnosed when there is 2:1 or higher AV conduction block (Fig. 5-10). It might be caused by a Wenckebach or a Mobitz II mechanism. A Wenckebach mechanism is more likely if the QRS conduction is normal, and a Mobitz II-type mechanism is more likely if the QRS complex demonstrates additional conduction disease, such as bundle-branch block.

During an electrophysiologic study, the *H-V interval* is measured. It is the conduction time after the impulse leaves the AV node to the time when the ventricles are activated (Fig. 5-11). The normal H-V interval is 35-55 ms. In asymptomatic persons, an H-V interval of 50-70 ms is associated with a 1% per year risk of complete heart block and does not require pacing, an H-V interval of 70-100 ms is associated with a 4% per year risk of complete heart block and treatment should be individualized, and an H-V interval >100 ms is associated with an 8% per year risk of complete heart block and should be treated with permanent pacing.

Indications for pacing include symptomatic Mobitz II heart block, complete heart block, and bifascicular block. Pacing should be considered in asymptomatic patients with Mobitz II and complete heart block.

- Indications for pacing: symptomatic Mobitz II, complete, bifascicular heart block.
- Pacing considered for asymptomatic persons with Mobitz II and complete heart block.

Carotid Sinus Syndrome

Carotid sinus massage is performed to identify carotid sinus hypersensitivity (Fig. 5-12). Approximately 40% of patients older than 65 years have hyperactive carotid sinus reflex (3-second pause or decrease in blood pressure of 50 mm Hg), although most of these patients have no spontaneous syncope. Carotid sinus massage should be performed over the carotid bifurcation at the angle of the jaw in patients without evidence of carotid bruit on carotid auscultation or a history of cerebrovascular disease. Carotid sinus massage is performed with moderate pressure over the carotid bifurcation for 5-10 seconds while monitoring heart rate and blood pressure. Approximately 35% of patients with hyperactive carotid sinus reflex have a pure cardioinhibitory component manifested only by a pause in ventricular activity exceeding 3 seconds. Fifteen percent of patients have a pure vasodepressor component with a normal heart rate maintained but a decrease in

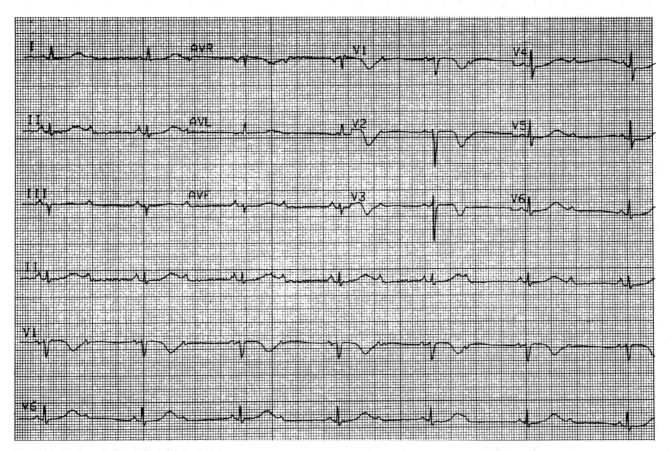

Fig. 5-10. High-grade 2:1 AV conduction block.

AVF

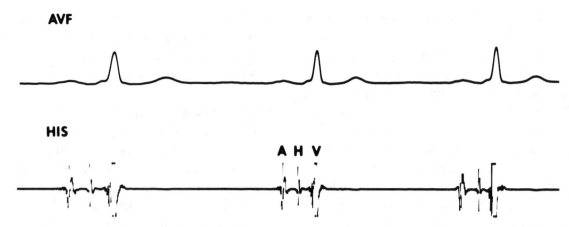

HIS

Fig. 5-11. Intracardiac recording of the AV node-His bundle area (HIS) with surface lead AVF. The A-H interval is conduction through AV node, and H-V interval is conduction through His-Purkinje system.

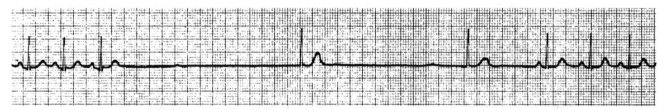

Fig. 5-12. Carotid sinus massage resulting in sinus pause with junctional escape beats before sinus rhythm returns.

blood pressure exceeding 50 mm Hg. Sixty percent of patients have a combined response with both cardioinhibitory and vasodepressor components. In such patients, permanent pacing may prevent the cardioinhibitory response, but the vasodepressor response continues to result in symptoms.

- Carotid sinus massage is used to identify carotid sinus hypersensitivity.
- About 40% of patients >65 years have carotid sinus reflex (3-second pause or decrease in blood pressure of 50 mm Hg).

Occasionally, associated neck abnormalities, including lymph node enlargement, previous neck surgery, and regional tumor, result in carotid sinus syndrome. Surgical techniques to treat this condition are usually unsuccessful, and the primary form of therapy is AV sequential pacing for the cardioinhibitory component and elastic stockings for the vasodepressor component. On occasion, patients respond to anticholinergic medications.

Atrial Flutter

Atrial flutter is identified by the characteristic saw-tooth pattern of atrial activity at a rate of 240-320 beats per minute. Patients with normal conduction systems maintain 2:1 AV conduction; thus, the ventricular rate is often

close to 150 beats per minute. Higher degrees of AV block (3:1 or higher) in the absence of drugs to slow AV node conduction (digoxin, β-adrenergic blocker, calcium antagonist) imply AV conduction disease (Fig. 5-13). Patients with 2:1 AV conduction and a heart rate of 150 beats per minute often have one of the flutter waves buried in the QRS complex. Carotid sinus massage results in increased AV block, revealing the flutter waves and establishing the diagnosis.

- Atrial flutter: atrial activity at 240-320 beats per minute.
- Ventricular rate is close to 150 beats per minute.

Treatment is aimed at preventing paroxysms and controlling the ventricular rate. Paroxysms of atrial flutter (or atrial fibrillation) can be prevented or decreased with class IA (quinidine, procainamide, disopyramide), class IC (propafenone, flecainide), and class III (amiodarone, sotalol) antiarrhythmic drugs. In general, these drugs control paroxysms of atrial flutter or atrial fibrillation in 50%-60% of cases during the first year of use. Side effects, including proarrhythmia, need to be weighed against symptoms during tachycardia to ensure that the potential benefits of therapy outweigh the risk.

- Antiarrhythmic drugs control atrial flutter (fibrillation) in 50%-60% of cases.

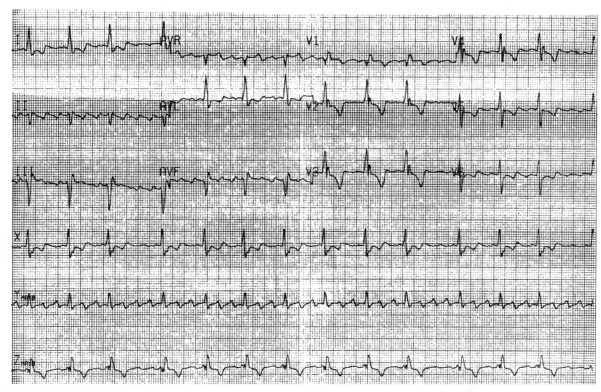

Fig. 5-13. Atrial flutter with 3:1 conduction in a patient with AV conduction disease.

Atrial Fibrillation

This rhythm is diagnosed by the characteristic irregular baseline without clear-cut P waves and irregularly irregular ventricular response. A slow ventricular response in the absence of drugs to block the AV node implies associated AV conduction disease. Patients with this slow response may have prolonged sinus node recovery and so should be electrically cardioverted with temporal external pacing standby because the combination of atrial fibrillation and a slow ventricular rate implies tachycardia-bradycardia syndrome or sinus node dysfunction.

Most patients with atrial fibrillation have sympathetically mediated arrhythmia that may be made worse with sympathetic stimulation that occurs with activity, stress, smoking, and consumption of alcohol and caffeine. In about 5%-10% of patients with atrial fibrillation, the rhythm is due to increased parasympathetic activity resulting in sinus bradycardia and dispersion of atrial refractoriness. An atrial premature complex then finds part of the atrium refractory, whereas other parts of the atrium are either partially refractory or fully recovered. This sets up the substrate for a reentrant arrhythmia and the development of atrial fibrillation. Typically, the arrhythmias occur during sleep or at rest. They are worse with drugs that slow sinus rate, such as digoxin and β-adrenergic blockers.

- Most patients with atrial fibrillation have sympathetically mediated arrhythmia that may be worse with activity, stress, smoking, alcohol and caffeine consumption.
- In 5%-10% of patients, rhythm is due to increased parasympathetic activity.

Acute atrial fibrillation or flutter should be treated with electrical cardioversion if there is hemodynamic compromise. In a patient who is adequately tolerating the new arrhythmia, initial therapy should be aimed at controlling the ventricular rate with digoxin, a β-adrenergic blocker, or a calcium antagonist. Attention should then be directed to reversing the underlying cause, which might include fever, anemia, thyrotoxicosis, myocardial infarction, pulmonary embolism, or worsening heart failure. A patient who has been in atrial fibrillation for >24-48 hours should undergo anticoagulation with warfarin for 3 weeks before and 4 weeks after elective cardioversion. After 3 weeks of anticoagulation, chemical cardioversion can be tried with a class IA or IC antiarrhythmic agent. These drugs should be initiated in the hospital during continuous monitoring to observe for proarrhythmia. If drugs are ineffective, electrical cardioversion can be performed; if sinus rhythm is obtained, the drug can be maintained for several weeks to help ensure maintenance of sinus rhythm. Continuation of drug therapy depends on the underlying heart disease and the propensity for relapse into atrial fibrillation or flutter. Use of the antiarrhythmic drug should be stopped if recurrent atrial fibrillation occurs, and it should not be used in patients with chronic atrial fibrillation.

- Acute atrial fibrillation or flutter is treated with electrical cardioversion if there is hemodynamic compromise.
- Initial therapy should be digoxin, β-adrenergic blocker, or calcium antagonist.
- Underlying cause should be reversed.
- If atrial fibrillation is present >24-48 hours, treat with warfarin for 3 weeks before elective cardioversion.
- If drugs are ineffective, perform electrical cardioversion.

Digoxin is not as effective as a β-adrenergic blocker or a calcium antagonist for controlling ventricular rate in response to exercise during atrial fibrillation. Patients with atrial fibrillation or flutter treated with digoxin may have adequate rate control at rest only to have inappropriately fast heart rates with exercise. Such patients benefit from the addition of either a β-adrenergic blocker or calcium antagonist to their drug regimen.

- Digoxin not as effective for controlling ventricular rate in response to exercise during atrial fibrillation.
- Patients treated with digoxin may have control at rest but fast heart rates with exercise; β-adrenergic blocker or calcium antagonist should be added.

Anticoagulation with warfarin is indicated in patients with atrial fibrillation if there is associated heart disease or congestive heart failure. Anticoagulation is not indicated for lone atrial fibrillation (patients younger than 60 years with no associated heart disease and no history of hypertension). Warfarin is better than aspirin, and both are better than placebo for preventing stroke or major systemic embolization in patients with either chronic or paroxysmal atrial fibrillation. The optimal prothrombin time is 1.3-1.5 times normal (INR 2-3); in this range, the benefit of reducing stroke outweighs the risk of bleeding complications. Aspirin has not been helpful in patients older than 75 years.

- Anticoagulation indicated if there is heart disease or congestive heart failure.
- Anticoagulation not indicated for lone atrial fibrillation (patients younger than 60 years, no heart disease, and no history of hypertension).
- Warfarin is better than aspirin.
- Aspirin not helpful in patients older than 75 years.

Supraventricular Tachycardia
Paroxysmal supraventricular tachycardia (PSVT) refers to cardiac arrhythmias of supraventricular origin using a reentrant mechanism with an abrupt onset and termination, a regular R-R interval, and a narrow QRS complex unless there is rate-related or preexisting bundle-branch block (Fig. 5-14). In patients with a normal QRS during sinus rhythm (lack of preexcitation), PSVT is due to reentry within the AV node in 60%, reentry utilizing a concealed accessory pathway in 30%, and reentry in the sinus node or atrium in the remaining 10% (Fig. 5-15). Episodes usually respond to vagal maneuvers; if these fail, intravenously administered adenosine or verapamil terminates the arrhythmia in 90% of patients.

- PSVT is arrhythmia with abrupt onset and termination.
- PSVT usually responds to vagal maneuvers; if not, adenosine or verapamil effective in 90% of cases.

PSVT is generally not a life-threatening arrhythmia and only occasionally is associated with near-syncope or syncope. The rhythm is more serious when it is associated with significant heart disease, and cardiac decompensation results with the sudden increase in heart rate. This can occur in patients with congenital heart disease, cardiomyopathy, or ischemic heart disease. Patients with AV nodal reentrant tachycardia usually have simultaneous activation of the atrium and ventricle, in which case the atria contract against closed tricuspid and mitral valves (similar to pacemaker syndrome) and produce symptoms associated with atrial distention, including a fullness in the neck, hypotension, and polyuria. Hypotension and polyuria are in part due to release of atrial natriuretic factor.

- PSVT is generally not a life-threatening arrhythmia.
- PSVT is more serious when associated with heart disease.

PSVT responds to most antiarrhythmic drugs, including drugs that suppress AV node conduction (digoxin, β-adrenergic blocker, and calcium antagonist), assuming

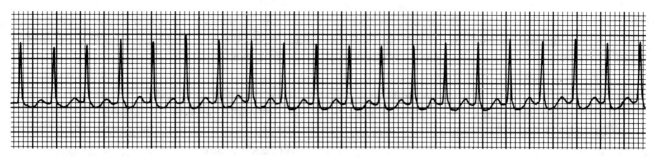

Fig. 5-14. Paroxysmal supraventricular tachycardia.

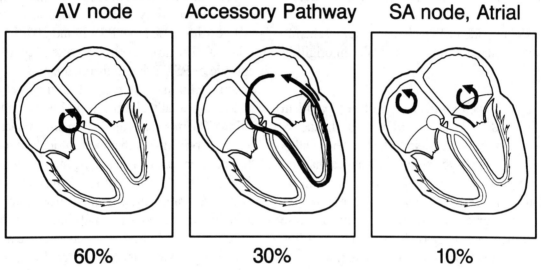

AV node   Accessory Pathway   SA node, Atrial

60%   30%   10%

Fig. 5-15. Mechanisms of paroxysmal supraventricular tachycardia in patients with a normal ECG during sinus rhythm. SA, sinoatrial.

part of the reentrant circuit utilizes the AV node, and drugs that slow conduction within the reentrant circuit, including class IA (quinidine, procainamide, disopyramide), IC (propafenone, flecainide), and III (amiodarone, sotalol) antiarrhythmic drugs.

• PSVT responds to most antiarrhythmic drugs.

Multifocal atrial tachycardia is an automatic atrial rhythm diagnosed when three or more distinct atrial foci (P waves of different morphology) are present and the rate exceeds 100 beats per minute (Fig. 5-16). The rhythm occurs primarily in patients with decompensated lung disease with associated hypoxia, increased catecholamines (exogenous and endogenous), atrial stretch, and local tissue acid-base and electrolyte disturbances. This rhythm is made worse by digoxin, which shortens atrial refractoriness but does respond to improved oxygenation and slow channel blockade with verapamil or diltiazem.

• Digoxin worsens multifocal atrial tachycardia.

Distinguishing Supraventricular Tachycardia With Aberrancy From Ventricular Tachycardia

A wide QRS tachycardia may be due to supraventricular tachycardia with aberrancy or to ventricular tachycardia. Useful findings to identify ventricular tachycardia are listed in Table 5-6.

Table 5-6.--Findings That Identify Ventricular Tachycardia

1.	Evidence of AV dissociation with P waves "marching through" the QRS complexes
2.	A QRS width >0.14 second if the tachycardia has a right bundle-branch block pattern and >0.16 second if the tachycardia has a left bundle-branch block pattern
3.	Northwest axis (axis between -90° and -180°)
4.	A different QRS morphology in patients with a preexisting bundle-branch block
5.	A history of ischemic heart disease

Approximately 85% of wide QRS tachycardias are ventricular in origin and are often well tolerated. The absence of hemodynamic compromise during tachycardia is not a clue that the tachycardia is supraventricular in origin. In patients with a wide QRS tachycardia and a history of ischemic heart disease (angina, myocardial infarction, Q wave on ECG), the tachycardia is ventricular in origin in 90%-95%. Therefore, the vast majority of wide QRS complex tachycardias are ventricular tachycardia (Fig. 5-17).

- About 85% of wide QRS tachycardias are ventricular in origin.
- In patients with wide QRS tachycardia and ischemic heart disease, tachycardia is ventricular in origin in 90%-95%.

Avoid intravenous administration of verapamil in patients with a wide QRS tachycardia unless the tachycardia is supraventricular in origin. Most patients with a wide QRS tachycardia have ventricular tachycardia, and verapamil causes hemodynamic deterioration requiring cardioversion in more than half of these patients. The verapamil results in peripheral vasodilatation, further increase in catecholamines, and decreased cardiac contractility, all of which contribute to adverse hemodynamics.

- Avoid intravenously administered verapamil for wide QRS tachycardia.
- Verapamil causes hemodynamic deterioration requiring cardioversion.

Wolff-Parkinson-White Syndrome

This abnormality is defined as 1) symptomatic tachycardia, 2) a short P-R interval (<0.12 second), 3) a delta wave, and 4) a prolonged QRS interval (>0.12 second).

In Wolff-Parkinson-White syndrome, normal activation of the ventricle is a fusion complex. Part of activation is due to conduction over accessory pathway, and remaining activation is due to conduction through the normal His-Purkinje conduction system. Not all patients with preexcitation have a short P-R interval. Normal P-R conduction may occur if the accessory pathway is far removed from the AV node. In patients with a far left lateral accessory pathway, the heart is activated through the AV node before atrial activation reaches the accessory pathway. The P-R interval thus may be normal before the onset of the delta wave.

Ventricular activation is abnormal in patients with Wolff-Parkinson-White syndrome. Infarction, ventricular hypertrophy, and ST-T wave changes should not be interpreted once the diagnosis is established because these changes are usually due to the abnormal pattern of ventricular activation.

- In Wolff-Parkinson-White syndrome, P-R interval may be normal before onset of delta wave.
- Ventricular activation is abnormal in Wolff-Parkinson-White syndrome.

Preexcitation occurs in about 2 of 1,000 patients; tachycardia subsequently develops in 70%. Of patients with tachycardia, 70% have PSVT, and 30% have atrial fibrillation. The atrial fibrillation often occurs after a short episode of PSVT due to disorganized conduction in the atrium. Elimination of PSVT after surgery or catheter ablation generally eliminates problems with atrial fibrillation. The most serious rhythm disturbance is the onset of atrial fibrillation with rapid ventricular conduction over the accessory pathway resulting in ventricular fibrillation (Fig. 5-18). Most asymptomatic patients do not benefit from risk stratification with electrophysiologic testing, including induction of atrial fibrillation, unless they have a high-risk occupation. Patients who are asymptomatic have a negligible chance of sudden death, and in patients who are symptomatic the incidence of sudden death is 0.0025 per patient-year.

- Preexcitation occurs in 2 of 1,000 patients; tachycardia develops in 70%.
- Of patients with tachycardia, 70% have PSVT and 30% have atrial fibrillation.
- Asymptomatic patients have negligible chance of sudden death.
- In symptomatic patients, incidence of sudden death is 0.0025 per patient-year.

Patients with Wolff-Parkinson-White syndrome may have either 1) a manifest accessory pathway resulting in preexcitation on the ECG (Fig. 5-19) due to antegrade conduction over the accessory pathway or 2) a concealed accessory pathway that is capable of conducting only in the retrograde direction, and therefore, the surface ECG in sinus rhythm is normal. Both manifest and concealed accessory pathways have the same mechanism of reentrant tachycardia, in which antegrade conduction over the normal conduction system results in a normal QRS complex (unless there is rate-related bundle-branch block) and conduction continues through the ventricle, returns retrogradely over the accessory pathway, and continues

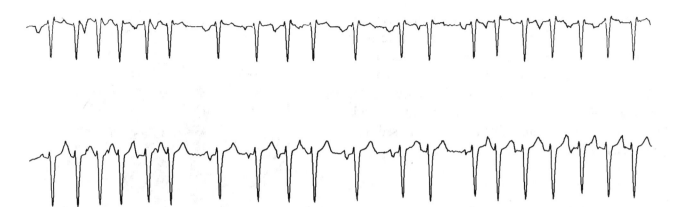

Fig. 5-16. Simultaneous recordings from patient with multifocal atrial tachycardia, showing three or more P waves of different morphology. (*Lower panel*, From MKSAP IX: Part C Book 1, 1992. American College of Physicians. By permission.)

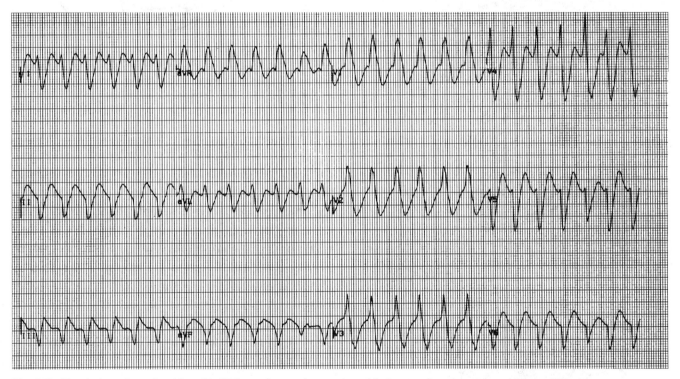

Fig. 5-17. Ventricular tachycardia with a wide QRS complex, northwest axis, and fusion complexes in a patient with normal blood pressure.

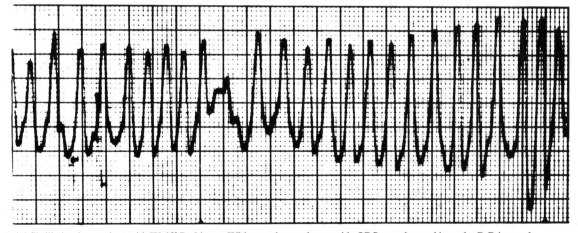

Fig. 5-18. Atrial fibrillation in a patient with Wolff-Parkinson-White syndrome shows wide QRS complex and irregular R-R intervals.

through the atrium to complete the reentrant circuit, termed "orthodromic AV reentry" (Fig. 5-20). Five percent of patients may have reentrant tachycardia that goes in the reverse direction (antidromic AV reentry), in which ventricular activation over the accessory pathway activates the ventricle from an ectopic location; the result is a wide QRS complex tachycardia that is often confused with ventricular tachycardia (Fig. 5-21).

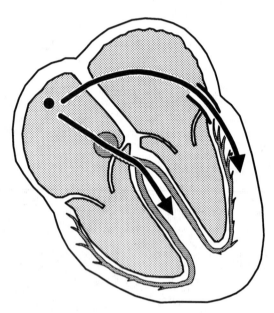

Fig. 5-19. Conduction of sinus impulse in Wolff-Parkinson-White syndrome. Ventricles are activated over normal AV node–His-Purkinje system and accessory pathway; result is a fusion complex (QRS and delta wave).

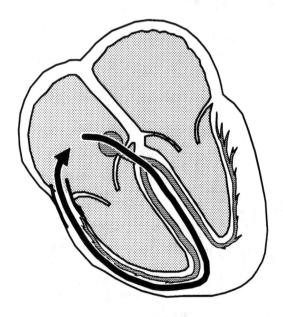

Fig. 5-20. Typical mechanism of supraventricular tachycardia in patients with Wolff-Parkinson-White syndrome; result is narrow QRS complex because ventricular activation is over the normal conduction system.

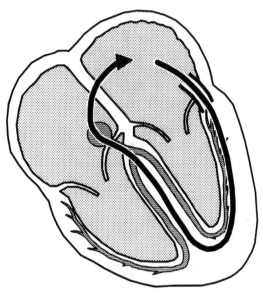

Fig. 5-21. Unusual mechanism of supraventricular tachycardia in patients with Wolff-Parkinson-White syndrome; result is a wide QRS complex because ventricular activation is over accessory pathway. This arrhythmia is difficult to distinguish from ventricular tachycardia.

Electrophysiologic testing should be done in patients with Wolff-Parkinson-White syndrome who have reentrant tachycardia with significant symptoms, have a heart rate >200 beats per minute, fail to respond to antiarrhythmic drugs, or need to avoid antiarrhythmic drugs, including young patients. In addition, patients who have had atrial fibrillation with a rapid ventricular rate or a history of syncope are candidates for electrophysiologic testing. This testing identifies the pathway location, confirms that the pathway is an integral part of the reentrant circuit and not an innocent bystander (i.e., the arrhythmia is AV nodal reentry), and evaluates for a second accessory pathway that occurs in approximately 15% of patients.

- Indications for electrophysiologic testing in Wolff-Parkinson-White syndrome: reentrant tachycardia with significant symptoms, heart rate >200 beats per minute, no response to antiarrhythmic drugs, need to avoid antiarrhythmic drugs.

During acute atrial fibrillation, intravenously administered digoxin and verapamil should be avoided because they accelerate the ventricular rate. Digoxin shortens the refractoriness of the accessory pathway, and verapamil results in vasodilatation with reflex increase in catecholamines and more rapid conduction over the accessory pathway. Both drugs have been associated with ventricular fibrillation when used to treat atrial fibrillation in the presence of Wolff-Parkinson-White syndrome. If the rate is rapid or there is hemodynamic compromise, cardioversion should be done. Intravenously administered procainamide can be used to slow conduction over the accessory pathway and attempt to convert the atrium to sinus rhythm if immediate cardioversion is not indicated.

- Avoid intravenously administered digoxin and verapamil during acute atrial fibrillation.
- If heart rate is rapid and there is hemodynamic compromise, perform cardioversion.
- Use intravenously administered procainamide to slow conduction and convert atrium to sinus rhythm.

PSVT in patients with an accessory pathway often ends with vagal maneuvers or intravenously administered adenosine or verapamil. Further episodes can be prevented with β-adrenergic blocker, calcium antagonist, and class IA (quinidine, procainamide, disopyramide), class IC (propafenone, flecainide), and class III (amiodarone, sotalol) antiarrhythmic drugs. Radiofrequency ablation is used to ablate the accessory pathway and cure the tachycardia and so eliminates need for medical therapy. This should be used in patients with tachycardias not responding to antiarrhythmic drugs, patients with demonstrated rapid conduction during tachycardia resulting in hemodynamic compromise or syncope, and patients in whom long-term drug therapy is not desired.

- Further PSVT is prevented with β-adrenergic blocker, calcium antagonist, and class IA, IC, and III antiarrhythmic drugs.
- Radiofrequency ablation used to cure tachycardia.
- Radiofrequency ablation used for tachycardias not responding to antiarrhythmic drugs, for rapid conduction during tachycardia, and when long-term drug therapy is not wanted.

Tachycardia-Mediated Cardiomyopathy

Supraventricular tachycardia, atrial fibrillation with a rapid ventricular rate, and ventricular tachycardia have been associated with cardiomyopathy. Treatment of the tachycardia has allowed cardiac performance to return to near normal. When patients present with heart failure and tachycardia is identified, determine whether the heart failure is causing the tachycardia or the tachycardia has caused the heart failure. Control of ventricular rate often improves ventricular function. In a patient with heart failure who has a rhythm with an abnormal P-wave axis, tachycardia-mediated cardiomyopathy should be suspected.

Premature Ventricular Complexes

Complex PVCs are defined as >10 per hour, multiform morphology, PVC pairs, or runs of nonsustained ventricular tachycardia. Patients who are asymptomatic with a normal heart and complex PVCs have an excellent long-term prognosis, and the PVCs in general are considered benign. Management includes reassurance and antiarrhythmic drugs only if necessary for intolerable palpitations.

In patients with asymptomatic complex ventricular ectopy and associated heart disease, the risk for syncope or sudden death is 10%-20%. However, antiarrhythmic agents for all such patients are not warranted because 80%-90% will not have syncope or sudden death, and these agents would expose them to the risks of drug toxicity and proarrhythmia. Studies are now under way to identify the best test to stratify patients at highest risk for sudden death. These tests include the signal-averaged ECG, measuring of ventricular function, and electrophysiologic testing.

- In patients with asymptomatic complex ventricular ectopy and heart disease, risk for syncope or sudden death is 10%-20%.
- Antiarrhythmic drugs not warranted because 80%-90% will not have syncope or sudden death.

Ventricular Tachycardia and Fibrillation

Patients who present with ventricular tachycardia or fibrillation or who survive sudden cardiac death have lethal ventricular arrhythmias and a significant risk of recurrence. Survivors of sudden cardiac death have a risk of death approaching 30% in 1 year after hospital dismissal. They should receive electrophysiology-guided therapy, which improves outcome. In about 40% of patients, an antiarrhythmic drug is identified that prevents induction of ventricular tachycardia or fibrillation, and these patients have approximately a 5% chance of death at 1 year if dismissed with that medication. Patients in whom the baseline electrophysiology study is negative or an antiarrhythmic drug cannot be identified to prevent tachycardia continue to have increased risk for sudden death and should be considered for antitachycardia surgery or an implantable cardioverter-defibrillator. This device has reduced the recurrence rate of sudden death to 2% at 1 year and to 4% at 4 years; the overall mortality rate is 10% at 1 year and 20% at 4 years.

- Patients with ventricular tachycardia or fibrillation who

survive sudden cardiac death have significant risk of recurrence.
- Survivors of sudden cardiac death have a risk of death of 30% at 1 year after hospital dismissal.
- Electrophysiology-guided therapy improves outcome.
- In 40% of patients, effective antiarrhythmic drug can be identified.

Torsades de Pointes

This is a form of ventricular tachycardia with a characteristic polymorphic morphology described as a twisting of the points (Fig. 5-5). The QT interval is prolonged, and the tachycardia is initiated by a late-coupled PVC. The arrhythmia is usually due to a medication (quinidine, procainamide, disopyramide, sotalol, tricyclic antidepressants), electrolyte disturbance (hypokalemia), and bradycardia (especially after myocardial infarction). Once the tachycardia has been converted to sinus rhythm (electrically or spontaneously), treatment should be aimed at shortening the QT interval until the offending drug can be metabolized or the electrolyte disturbance or bradycardia corrected. Treatment options include temporary overdrive pacing, isoproterenol infusion, or magnesium. Patients with QT prolongation in the absence of medications, electrolytes, or bradycardia have a congenital form of this problem and are usually treated with a β-adrenergic blocker.

- Torsades de pointes is a form of ventricular tachycardia involving prolonged QT interval.
- Torsades de pointes is usually due to a medication, electrolyte disturbance, and bradycardia.
- Treatment includes temporary overdrive pacing, isoproterenol, or magnesium.

Ventricular Arrhythmias During Acute Myocardial Infarction

Prevention of myocardial ischemia and the use of β-adrenergic blockers are essential after acute myocardial infarction to reduce the frequency of life-threatening ventricular arrhythmias. Asymptomatic complex ventricular ectopy, including nonsustained ventricular tachycardia, should not be treated empirically because the risk of proarrhythmia outweighs the potential benefit of therapy for reducing the incidence of sudden cardiac death after hospital dismissal. Studies are assessing the use of amiodarone or risk stratification with ejection fraction, signal-averaged ECG, and electrophysiology testing after myocardial infarction in an attempt to reduce the inci-

dence of sudden death.

Ventricular tachycardia and fibrillation occurring within 24 hours after myocardial infarction are independent risk factors for in-hospital mortality at the time of the acute myocardial infarction but are not risk factors for subsequent total mortality or mortality due to an arrhythmic event after hospital dismissal and do not require antiarrhythmic therapy.

Ventricular tachycardia and fibrillation occurring 24 hours or longer after an acute myocardial infarction in the absence of reinfarction are independent risk factors for increased total mortality and death due to an arrhythmic event after hospital dismissal. Patients should be assessed with electrophysiology testing, and treatment options include serial-guided antiarrhythmic drug testing, implantable cardioverter-defibrillator, and endocardial resection.

Episodes of refractory ventricular tachycardia and fibrillation during acute myocardial infarction should be treated with intravenously administered lidocaine, procainamide, or bretylium, and patients should have adequate oxygenation and normal electrolyte values. If these drugs are ineffective, alternative therapies to prevent recurrences of tachycardia include overdrive pacing if the tachycardia follows a bradycardia event, high-dose amiodarone, interaortic balloon pump, and coronary revascularization.

- Refractory ventricular tachycardia and fibrillation during acute myocardial infarction should be treated with intravenously administered lidocaine, procainamide, or bretylium.
- Alternative therapies are overdrive pacing, high-dose amiodarone, and coronary revascularization.

Role of Pacing in Acute Myocardial Infarction

Among patients with an acute inferior myocardial infarction, 5%-10% have Mobitz I second-degree or third-degree block in the absence of bundle-branch block, and the site is usually in the AV node. This is usually transient, tends not to recur, and requires pacing only if there are symptoms as a result of bradycardia.

Bundle-branch block occurs in 10%-20% of patients with acute myocardial infarction; in half of these patients, it is present at initial presentation, often representing pre-existing conduction system disease. Approximately 40% of patients with right bundle-branch block and either left-axis or right-axis deviation (fascicular block) will have transient complete heart block in the first few days after myocardial infarction. In 20% of patients with new left bundle-branch block or bundle-branch block of uncertain duration, complete heart block develops. The appearance of new bundle-branch block is an indication for prophylactic temporary pacing.

- Bundle-branch block occurs in 10%-20% of patients with acute myocardial infarction.
- In 20% of patients with new left bundle-branch block or bundle-branch block of uncertain duration, complete heart block develops.

Death in patients with myocardial infarction and bundle-branch block is usually due to advanced heart

failure and ventricular arrhythmias rather than to development of complete heart block. Patients in whom transient complete heart block develops in association with bundle-branch block are at risk for recurrent complete heart block and should undergo permanent pacing. New bundle-branch block that never progresses to complete heart block is not an indication for permanent pacing.

- Death in patients with myocardial infarction and bundle-branch block is due to advanced heart failure.
- New bundle-branch block that never progresses to complete heart block is not an indication for permanent pacing.

QUESTIONS
(See "Answers" section)

Multiple Choice
1. A 62-year-old black man has a cardiac arrest while golfing. The ambulance attendants initiate cardiopulmonary resuscitation, and ventricular fibrillation is converted to sinus rhythm with a single 200-joule countershock. After admission to the hospital, he improves rapidly. His pulse is 62 beats per minute and blood pressure 138/80 mm Hg. His electrocardiogram shows left bundle-branch block. He develops no further cardiac rhythm abnormalities or evidence of a myocardial infarction during the subsequent 48 hours of observation. During an exercise thallium test, he exercises 8.2 minutes using the Bruce protocol, increasing his heart rate from 52 to 163 beats per minute and blood pressure from 128/74 to 192/86 mm Hg. He has no electrocardiographic abnormalities, chest discomfort, or perfusion defects during the test. Which one of the following tests would you now perform?
   a. Coronary angiography
   b. Echocardiography
   c. Twenty-four-hour ambulatory electrocardiographic recording (Holter)
   d. Signal-averaged electrocardiography
   e. Electrophysiology study

2. A 72-year-old white man is admitted to the hospital after an episode of syncope. The following rhythm strip is recorded at a time when the patient is sleeping:

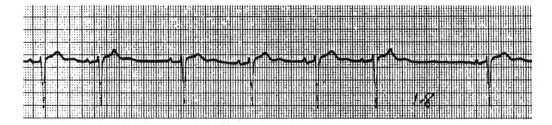

The 1.8-second pause is due to which of the following?

a. Sinoatrial exit block
b. Nonconducted atrial premature complex
c. Atrioventricular nodal Wenckebach
d. Mobitz II block at the level of the atrioventricular node
e. Carotid sinus hypersensitivity

3. A 47-year-old white man undergoing a treadmill exercise test develops chest pressure consistent with angina, 1.5 mm of horizontal ST depression involving the inferolateral electrocardiographic leads, and then the following arrhythmia:

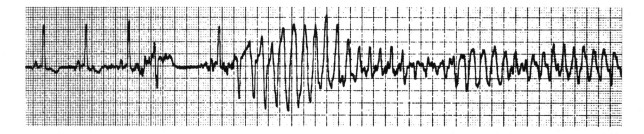

He is cardioverted to sinus rhythm and admitted to the hospital, and a myocardial infarction is ruled out. Which one of the following would be the best approach in this patient?

a. Signal-averaged electrocardiography
b. Exercise thallium test
c. Coronary angiography
d. Initiate β-adrenergic blocker therapy and dismiss from hospital
e. Amiodarone

4. A 54-year-old Hispanic woman presents with a wide QRS complex tachycardia. Which one of the following suggests supraventricular tachycardia?

a. Blood pressure of 120/80 mm Hg

b. QRS morphology similar to sinus rhythm
c. Atrioventricular dissociation
d. Prior history of myocardial infarction
e. QRS width of 0.18 second

5. A 72-year-old black woman with a history of hypertension complains of intermittent palpitations. Telephone transmission of her electrocardiogram at a time when she feels palpitations demonstrates atrial fibrillation. The best approach to antithrombotic therapy is:

a. Adequate control of hypertension
b. Observation
c. Warfarin
d. Aspirin, 81 mg daily
e. Aspirin, 5 g daily

6. A 26-year-old Hispanic man with Wolff-Parkinson-White syndrome presents to the emergency room in atrial fibrillation. Which one of the following intravenous medications could be used to slow the ventricular rate, the others being either not helpful or dangerous because of accelerating the ventricular rate?
   a. Adenosine
   b. Verapamil
   c. Lidocaine
   d. Procainamide
   e. Digoxin

7. Which of the following should not be considered when treating a patient who has survived sudden cardiac death?
   a. Administering quinidine to achieve a therapeutic level before dismissal
   b. Coronary angiography to assess for significant coronary artery disease
   c. Electrocardiography and cardiac enzyme tests to evaluate for acute myocardial infarction
   d. Electrophysiologic testing to guide management
   e. Use of an implantable defibrillator in patients who have no inducible arrhythmias during electrophysiologic testing

8. A 54-year-old woman presents with acute inferior myocardial infarction, and the following rhythm strip is recorded (AVF, atrioventricular fibrillation):

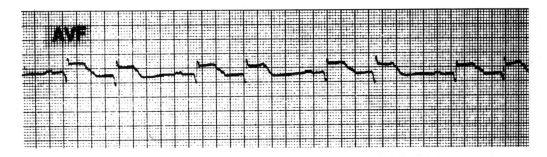

The best approach to managing this asymptomatic arrhythmia is:
   a. Observation
   b. Adenosine
   c. Atropine
   d. Temporary pacing
   e. β-Adrenergic blocker

9. A 73-year-old black woman presents with an acute myocardial infarction, and the following asymptomatic arrhythmia is recorded:

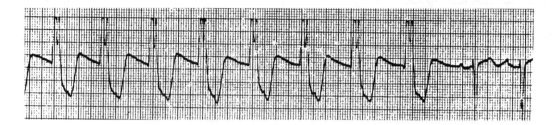

The best approach to management is:
a. Atropine
b. Observation
c. Lidocaine
d. Magnesium
e. Overdrive pacing

True/False

10. A 48-year-old white man presents with syncope that develops during church services, and an electrocardiographic rhythm strip in the emergency room demonstrates the following arrhythmia:

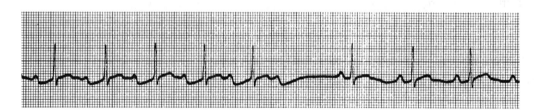

Are the following statements concerning this arrhythmia true or false?
a. The mechanism is Mobitz II second-degree atrioventricular block
b. This is the most likely cause of the patient's syncope
c. The arrhythmia does not require further evaluation or treatment
d. The mechanism is Mobitz I second-degree atrioventricular block
e. A permanent pacemaker should be placed
f. It can be due to an acute inferior myocardial infarction

11. The following medications are useful for preventing episodes of atrial fibrillation:

a. Quinidine
b. Mexiletine
c. Propafenone
d. Digoxin
e. Sotalol
f. Amiodarone

12. The following are complications of amiodarone therapy:
a. Hyperthyroidism
b. Skin photosensitivity
c. Hepatitis
d. Pulmonary toxicity
e. Ataxia
f. Hypothyroidism

13. This rhythm strip demonstrates the following findings of ventricular tachycardia:

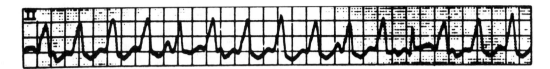

    a. Wide QRS complex (>0.16 second)
    b. Atrioventricular dissociation
    c. Fusion beat
    d. Retrograde conduction
    e. Northwest axis
    f. Concordance

14. A 26-year-old Native American woman with mitral valve prolapse and premature ventricular complexes was given quinidine. She had two episodes of syncope, and the following rhythm was recorded in the emergency room:

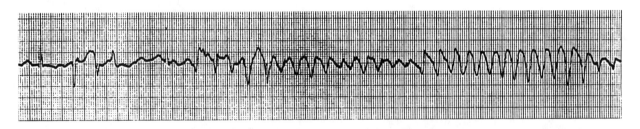

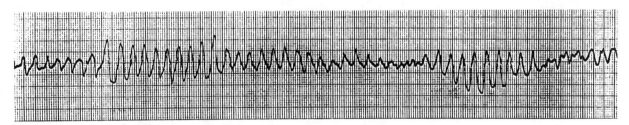

The following statements can be used to describe this arrhythmia:
    a. The mechanism is atrial fibrillation
    b. The mechanism is torsades de pointes
    c. This rhythm can occur after the first dose of quinidine
    d. Procainamide would be useful to prevent recurrence
    e. The arrhythmia is unrelated to quinidine
    f. Isoproterenol would be useful to prevent recurrence

NOTES

CHAPTER 6
CARDIOLOGY III

Carole A. Warnes, M.D.

PHYSICAL EXAMINATION, VALVULAR DISEASES, PERICARDIUM, MISCELLANEOUS

PHYSICAL EXAMINATION

Jugular Venous Pressure

This pressure is normally 6-8 cm H_2O. It will not be visible when the patient is sitting up. When it is elevated, consider not only biventricular failure but also constrictive pericarditis, pericardial tamponade, cor pulmonale (especially pulmonary embolus), and superior vena cava syndrome. The normal waves are *a*, which reflects atrial contraction; *c*, closure of tricuspid valve; and *v*, ventricular filling.

- Normal jugular venous pressure: 6-8 cm H_2O.
- Normal waves: *a*, atrial contraction; *c*, closure of tricuspid valve; *v*, ventricular filling.

Abnormalities of the waves indicate various conditions, as follows:

1) Large "a" wave: tricuspid stenosis, right ventricular hypertrophy, pulmonary hypertension
2) Cannon "a" wave: atria contracting against a closed atrioventricular valve (atrioventricular dissociation)
3) Large cv wave: tricuspid regurgitation
4) Rapid x + y descent: constrictive pericarditis
5) Kussmaul's sign: pericardial tamponade or constriction

- Abnormalities of waves:
    large "a" wave: tricuspid stenosis, right ventricular hypertrophy, pulmonary hypertension.

cannon "a" wave: atria contracting against closed atrioventricular valve (atrioventricular dissociation).
rapid x + y descent: constrictive pericarditis.

Arterial Pulse

Palpation of radial pulse is useful only for rate. Check brachial or carotid pulse for contour. "Tardus" describes the rate of rise of upstroke, and "parvus" describes the volume. In hypertension, look for radiofemoral delay (check radial and femoral pulses simultaneously) to determine whether coarctation is present.

Abnormalities of the arterial pulse and their indicated conditions are as follows:

1) parvus and tardus: aortic stenosis
2) parvus only: low output, cardiomyopathy
3) bounding: aortic regurgitation or atrioventricular fistulae
4) bifid: hypertrophic obstructive cardiomyopathy (from midsystolic obstruction)
5) bisferiens: aortic stenosis and regurgitation

- Abnormalities of arterial pulse:
    parvus and tardus: aortic stenosis.
    parvus only: low output, cardiomyopathy.
    bisferiens: aortic stenosis and regurgitation.

Apical Impulse

This is normally a discrete area of localized contraction. It is usually maximal at the fifth intercostal space, midclavicular line.

Abnormalities of the apical impulse and their indicated

conditions are as follows:
1) apex displaced, impulse poor and diffuse: cardiomyopathy
2) sustained: left ventricular hypertrophy, aortic stenosis, often with large "a" wave
3) trifid: hypertrophic cardiomyopathy
4) hyperdynamic and diffuse with rapid filling wave: mitral regurgitation
5) tapping quality, localized: mitral stenosis

● Abnormalities of apical impulse:
 apex displaced, impulse poor and diffuse: cardiomyopathy.
 trifid: hypertrophic cardiomyopathy.
 tapping quality, localized: mitral stenosis.

Thrills

These indicate turbulent flow (e.g., aortic stenosis, ventricular septal defect).

Heart Sounds

First

This consists of mitral valve closure followed shortly by tricuspid valve closure. A *loud* first heart sound occurs with a short P-R interval and mitral stenosis because the mitral valve is wide open when the left ventricle begins to contract and then slaps shut. The intensity of the first sound is *decreased* if mitral valve is heavily calcified (severe mitral stenosis) and also if P-R interval is long (occurs classically with acute rheumatic fever).

● Loud first heart sound: short P-R interval and mitral stenosis.
● Decreased intensity of first heart sound: mitral valve heavily calcified, long P-R interval.

Second

This consists of aortic closure followed by pulmonary closure. Intensity of both is increased by hypertension (loud P_2 with pulmonary hypertension, and P_2 is audible at apex). Intensity is decreased with heavily calcified valves (severe aortic stenosis). Normally, second sound widens on inspiration.

● Intensity of second heart sound increased by hypertension.

● Intensity decreased with heavily calcified valves.
 Abnormalities of splitting of the second heart sound and their indicated conditions are as follows:
1) fixed split: atrial septal defect
2) paradoxic split (caused by delay in aortic closure so it closes after pulmonary valve): left bundle-branch block, left ventricular hypertrophy

● Abnormalities of splitting of second heart sound:
 fixed split: atrial septal defect.
 paradoxic split: left bundle-branch block, left ventricular hypertrophy.

Third

This is probably caused by tensing of the chordae as the blood distends the left ventricle during diastole. It is heard normally in young people and in older adults and is associated with volume load on the left ventricle such as aortic regurgitation, mitral regurgitation, and cardiomyopathy.

● Third heart sound is heard in young people and older adults in association with volume load on left ventricle (e.g., aortic regurgitation, mitral regurgitation, cardiomyopathy).

Fourth

This occurs with the atrial kick as blood is forced into the left ventricle by atrial contraction. It occurs when the left ventricle is stiff and noncompliant, such as in aortic stenosis, systemic hypertension, hypertrophic cardiomyopathy, and ischemia.

● Fourth heart sound occurs in aortic stenosis, systemic hypertension, hypertrophic cardiomyopathy, and ischemia.

Opening Snap

This is virtually always caused by mitral stenosis, and the interval from the second heart sound to the opening snap helps determine the severity. With severe mitral stenosis, the left atrial pressure is very high and thus the valve opens earlier, and the interval is <60 m/second.

● Opening snap virtually always caused by mitral stenosis.

Murmurs

These are discussed with the individual valvular lesions

described later in this chapter, but some broad guidelines follow here.

A systolic ejection murmur occurs when blood is ejected from a ventricle into a vascular structure. It begins after the first heart sound and ends before the second sound. It may have a diamond-shaped quality with crescendo and decrescendo components, but in general the more severe the obstruction, the longer the murmur and there is less decrescendo quality. It may be preceded by an ejection click.

- Systolic ejection murmur: the more severe the obstruction, the longer the murmur.

A holosystolic murmur occurs when blood goes from a high-pressure to a low-pressure system (mitral regurgitation, ventricular septal defect). It engulfs the first and second heart sounds.

- Holosystolic murmur occurs with mitral regurgitation and ventricular septal defect and engulfs first and second heart sounds.

MANEUVERS THAT ALTER CARDIAC MURMURS

- *Inspiration* increases venous return and so increases right-sided murmurs of tricuspid regurgitation, pulmonary stenosis, pulmonary regurgitation.
- *Valsalva* increases intrathoracic pressure, inhibiting venous return to right side of heart.
- Most cardiac murmurs and sounds diminish in intensity during Valsalva maneuver because of decreased ventricular filling and decreased cardiac output (except hypertrophic obstructive cardiomyopathy and mitral valve prolapse).
- *Handgrip* increases cardiac output and systemic arterial pressure.
- A change in *posture* from supine to upright causes decrease in venous return; therefore, stroke volume falls, and this decrease causes a reflex rise in heart rate and peripheral resistance.
- *Squatting* and the *Valsalva maneuver* have opposite hemodynamic effects. Squatting increases peripheral resistance and increases venous return.

The effects of maneuvers are shown in Table 6-1.

Table 6-1.--Effects of Physical Maneuvers and Other Factors on Valvular Diseases

| Maneuver | Result | Effect on murmur | | |
		Mitral regurgitation	Aortic stenosis	HOCM
Amyl nitrite	↓ afterload	↓	↑	↑
Valsalva	↓ preload	↓	↓	↑
Handgrip	↑ afterload	↑	↓	↓
Post-PVC	↑ contractility ↓ afterload	=	↑	↑*

*Although the murmur ↑, the peripheral pulse ↓ because of the increase in outflow obstruction.
HOCM, hypertrophic obstructive cardiomyopathy; PVC, premature ventricular complex.

VALVULAR HEART DISEASE

Aortic Stenosis

Supravalvular

The two major types of supravalvular aortic stenosis are diaphragmatic and localized hourglass-shaped narrowing immediately above the aortic sinuses, often associated with hypoplasia of the ascending aorta.

Supravalvular aortic stenosis is associated with Williams' syndrome, which is characterized by so-called elfin facies, mental retardation, and hypercalcemia. Systemic hypertension is a common association. An important feature is large, dilated, thick-walled coronary arteries because the coronary ostia are proximal to the obstruction. This lesion also causes premature atherosclerosis.

Physical Examination

Findings include a prominent left ventricle, a thrill in

suprasternal notch and over carotid artery (thrill is often more marked in right carotid artery and pulse upstroke is often brisker on right side than left side), systolic murmur without click, and a loud A_2.

- Features of supravalvular aortic stenosis: thrill in suprasternal notch and over carotid artery, systolic murmur without click, loud A_2.

Subvalvular

The types of subvalvular stenosis are discrete ("membranous") and fibromuscular (fixed or dynamic). These two types can coexist.

Physical Examination

Findings include a prominent left ventricle, reduced pulse pressure, no click, and arterial thrill when the stenosis is severe. Subvalvular aortic stenosis is commonly associated with aortic regurgitation because there is a jet lesion on the aortic valve cusps.

- Features of subvalvular aortic stenosis: prominent left ventricle, reduced pulse pressure, no click, arterial thrill when the stenosis is severe.
- Commonly associated with aortic regurgitation.

Diagnosis

The diagnosis can usually be made with two-dimensional and Doppler echocardiography, often without the need for cardiac catheterization. Two-dimensional echocardiography can determine the severity of the stenosis and the site and presence or absence of additional valvular abnormality. In addition, it determines the presence or absence of left ventricular hypertrophy. If cardiac catheterization is performed, when the catheter is pulled back from the left ventricle toward the aorta there is a low subvalvular left ventricular pressure tracing before the aortic valve is crossed.

- Diagnosis of subvalvular aortic stenosis is made with two-dimensional and Doppler echocardiography.
- Echocardiography determines presence or absence of left ventricular hypertrophy.

Valvular

Types

The *congenital bicuspid* type occurs in 1% of the population. It may be associated with obstruction in infancy through early adulthood. It is the most common cause of aortic stenosis in adults <55 years old. Even in young adults the valve is frequently still pliable and auscultation is thus different from that of degenerative aortic valve disease. An ejection click often precedes the systolic murmur. The earlier the click (i.e., the closer to the first sound), the more severe the stenosis. A_2 becomes later with increasing stenosis, and when severe there may be paradoxic splitting of the second sound. The lesion may be associated with coarctation. The diagnosis can usually be made successfully with two-dimensional and Doppler echocardiography without the need for cardiac catheterization in young people.

- Congenital bicuspid valvular aortic stenosis occurs in 1% of population.
- It is most common cause of aortic stenosis in adults <55 years old.
- Ejection click often precedes systolic murmur.
- Earlier the click (closer to first heart sound), more severe the stenosis.
- A_2 becomes later with increasing stenosis; when severe, there may be paradoxic splitting of second sound.

Degenerative aortic valve disease is the most common cause of aortic stenosis in adults >55 years old. The valve is three-cuspid and calcified. When calcification is extensive, A_2 becomes inaudible.

- Degenerative aortic valve disease is most common cause of aortic stenosis in adults >55 years old.
- When calcification is extensive, A_2 becomes inaudible.

The *rheumatic* type is less common. It is associated with thickening and fusion of the aortic cusps at the commissures. It always occurs with a rheumatic mitral valve, although important mitral stenosis or regurgitation may not always be evident. It usually occurs in early adulthood (age 40-60 years).

- Rheumatic type is less common cause of valvular aortic stenosis.
- Usually occurs at 40-60 years of age.

Symptoms

The classic triad of symptoms includes exertional dyspnea, syncope, and angina; however, most patients are symptom-free. The presence of angina does not necessarily indicate coexisting coronary disease.

- Symptoms of valvular type of aortic stenosis: exertional dyspnea, syncope, angina.
- Angina does not necessarily indicate coexisting coronary disease.

Physical Examination

The pulse is parvus and tardus. The left ventricular impulse is localized and sustained. There may be a palpable fourth sound. Arterial thrills may be palpable in the carotid, suprasternal notch, second intercostal space, or left and right sternal borders. A fourth heart sound may be present. A_2 will be diminished or absent. Ejection systolic murmur becomes longer with increasing severity radiating to the carotid arteries and the apex.

- Pulse is parvus and tardus.
- Ejection systolic murmur becomes longer with increasing severity.

Diagnosis

Electrocardiography may show left ventricular hypertrophy (although it is not a sensitive index, and echocardiography is better). Electrocardiogram is often normal in young patients. Left bundle-branch block is common, and in later stages of the condition conduction abnormalities may develop (e.g., complete heart block) if the calcium impinges on the conducting system. On chest radiography, the heart size is usually normal, even when the stenosis is severe. The aortic root may show post-stenotic dilatation. In degenerative aortic valve disease, calcium in the valve leaflets may be seen, especially on a penetrated lateral view.

- Electrocardiogram often normal in young patients.
- Left bundle-branch block is common on electrocardiogram.
- Aortic root may show post-stenotic dilatation on chest radiograph.

Differential diagnoses include 1) hypertrophic cardiomyopathy (note different carotid upstroke and changing murmur with maneuvers) and 2) mitral regurgitation (murmur may radiate anteriorly and upward, particularly if there is rupture of a posterior mitral valve leaflet).
Aortic stenosis can be diagnosed with bedside physical

examination. The most important physical finding is the parvus and tardus pulse. However, the degree of aortic stenosis can be difficult to determine, particularly in older patients. Doppler echocardiography is particularly useful for assessing gradient and correlates well with cardiac catheterization. Severe aortic stenosis is present when the gradient is >50 mm Hg and the valve area is <0.75 cm². Patients being considered for operation should also have coronary angiography if they are older than 50 years.

- Aortic stenosis can be diagnosed with bedside physical examination.
- Most important physical finding: parvus and tardus pulse.
- Doppler echocardiography is useful for diagnosis.
- Severe aortic stenosis: gradient is >50 mm Hg, valve area is <0.75 cm².

Aortic Regurgitation

Etiology

Valvular

Causes of valvular aortic regurgitation include 1) congenital bicuspid valve, 2) rheumatic fever, 3) endocarditis, 4) degenerative aortic valve disease, 5) seronegative arthritis, 6) ankylosing spondylitis, and 7) rheumatoid arthritis.

Aortic Root Dilatation

Various conditions have been associated with aortic root dilatation. Marfan syndrome can be associated with progressive dilatation of the aortic root and sinuses (so-called cystic medial necrosis). Syphilis is an uncommon cause and usually causes aortic root dilatation above the sinuses (syphilis spares the sinuses). Remember that syphilis is associated with calcium in the aortic root on chest radiography. Age is also a related factor. With advancing age, the aorta dilates, and hypertension also tends to accelerate this process. Acute aortic regurgitation may be associated with an aortic dissection.

- Marfan syndrome can be associated with aortic root dilatation.
- Syphilis is uncommon cause.

Symptoms

The symptoms of aortic regurgitation include fatigue,

dyspnea, palpitations, and exertional angina.

Physical Examination

A bounding, collapsing Corrigan's pulse resulting from wide pulse pressure is found. Other findings are de Musset's head nodding, Durozier's sign over femoral artery, and Quincke's sign (pulsatile capillary nail bed). The left ventricular impulse is diffuse and hyperdynamic, and the apex beat is often displaced. A diastolic decrescendo murmur is heard at either the left or the right sternal border, and the second heart sound may be paradoxically split because of increased left ventricular volume. The loudness of the murmur does not correlate with the severity of aortic regurgitation, particularly in acute aortic regurgitation (e.g., with dissection). There may be little or no murmur when there is an abrupt rise in left ventricular end-diastolic pressure. Systolic flow murmur is common. It does not necessarily indicate coexistent aortic stenosis, and so the pulse should be checked.

- Findings indicative of aortic regurgitation: bounding, collapsing Corrigan's pulse, diastolic decrescendo murmur, second heart sound may be paradoxically split.

Diagnosis

On electrocardiography, features of left ventricular hypertrophy may be found. Ruptured sinus of Valsalva should be considered in the differential diagnosis. The diagnosis can be made at bedside clinical examination, but it can be missed if a patient with acute aortic regurgitation presents with little or no murmur. Doppler echocardiogram is useful and also helps evaluate left ventricular size and function. If dissection is suspected, transthoracic echocardiography may be insufficient, and computed tomography, transesophageal echocardiography, or even aortography may be needed.

- Electrocardiography may show left ventricular hypertrophy.
- Differential diagnosis: ruptured sinus of Valsalva.
- Doppler echocardiogram is useful.

Timing of Surgery

The timing of surgical management is still controversial. Despite a large volume load on the left ventricle and compensatory left ventricular enlargement, patients with aortic regurgitation may remain asymptomatic for several years. The development of symptoms, however, usu-

ally reflects left ventricular dysfunction, and survival is limited unless surgical intervention is prompt. Once left ventricular dysfunction is established, patients are less likely to have a return of normal function after aortic valve replacement. There is still controversy, however, regarding the timing of operation for patients who are asymptomatic or who have very mild symptoms. Certainly when the ejection fraction decreases below normal, operation is needed. Other factors that have been used include echocardiographic data: a systolic dimension >55 mm or a diastolic dimension >80 mm. Asymptomatic patients with large left ventricles need to be followed carefully; therefore, if there is evidence of resting left ventricular dysfunction or of rapidly progressive left ventricular dilatation, they should have operation.

- Timing of operation for aortic regurgitation is controversial.
- Patients can be asymptomatic for several years.
- If symptoms develop, survival is limited unless surgical intervention is prompt.
- If ejection fraction decreases below normal, operation is needed.

When the cause of aortic regurgitation is acute infective endocarditis, antibiotic therapy should always be instituted first. Surgery is indicated for uncontrolled infection, development of left ventricular dysfunction, or pulmonary congestion. Conduction abnormalities suggest an aortic root abscess.

- If cause of aortic regurgitation is acute infective endocarditis, antibiotic therapy should be given first.
- Indications for operation: uncontrolled infection, left ventricular dysfunction, pulmonary congestion.
- Conduction abnormalities suggest aortic root abscess.

Mitral Stenosis

Mitral stenosis is almost always due to rheumatic heart disease causing leaflet thickening with fusion of the commissures and later calcification. Symptoms do not usually develop for several years after mitral stenosis is apparent on physical examination. These symptoms are usually dyspnea and later orthopnea with paroxysmal nocturnal dyspnea. Atrial fibrillation usually causes significant deterioration of symptoms. Other symptoms include hemoptysis, and later pulmonary hypertension may cause signs of right-sided failure with ascites and peripheral edema.

Systemic emboli may also result from atrial fibrillation.

- Mitral stenosis is almost always due to rheumatic heart disease.
- Symptoms do not develop for several years after mitral stenosis is found on physical exam.
- Symptoms: dyspnea, orthopnea with paroxysmal nocturnal dyspnea.
- Atrial fibrillation causes significant deterioration of symptoms.

Physical Examination

The first heart sound is loud. The shorter the interval from the second heart sound (A_2) to the opening snap, the more severe the mitral stenosis. An opening snap occurs only with a pliable valve, and it disappears when the valve calcifies. The stenosis is mild if this interval is >90 ms, moderate if it is 80 ms, and severe if it is <60 ms. The diastolic murmur is a low-pitched apical rumble, and the longer it is, the more severe the stenosis. The murmur has presystolic accentuation. Right ventricular lift and increased P_2 are associated with pulmonary hypertension.

- Physical exam in mitral stenosis:
    loud first heart sound.
    shorter the interval from A_2 to opening snap, more severe stenosis.
    diastolic murmur is low-pitched apical rumble.
    longer the murmur, more severe stenosis.

Diagnosis

Electrocardiography shows P mitrale and later right ventricular hypertrophy. Chest radiography (Fig. 6-1) shows straightening of the left heart border with a large left atrial shadow and dilated upper lobe pulmonary veins. With pulmonary hypertension, the central pulmonary arteries become prominent. In severe stenosis, Kerley B lines may be present.

- Electrocardiography: P mitrale, later right ventricular hypertrophy.
- Chest radiography: straightening of left heart border, large left atrial shadow, dilated upper lobe pulmonary veins, Kerley B lines in severe stenosis.

Two-dimensional and Doppler echocardiography is the tool of choice to diagnose mitral stenosis and deter-

mine its severity. Information is gained about valve gradient and valve area (Table 6-2), and pulmonary artery pressures can be noninvasively assessed. Cardiac catheterization is usually unnecessary unless the coronary arteries need to be studied or the echocardiographic findings do not concur with the clinical situation. Severe stenosis usually correlates with a mean gradient >12 mm Hg.

- Two-dimensional and Doppler echocardiography: tools to diagnose mitral stenosis and determine severity.
- For diagnosis of mitral stenosis, cardiac catheterization usually unnecessary.
- Severe stenosis: mean gradient >12 mm Hg.

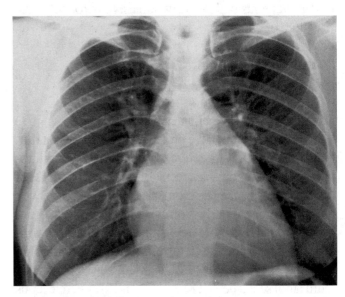

Fig. 6-1. Chest radiograph from a patient with severe mitral stenosis, showing a typical straight left heart border, prominent pulmonary artery, large left atrium, right ventricular contour, and pulmonary venous hypertension.

Table 6-2.--Severity of Mitral Stenosis, by Valve Area

Severity	Valve area, cm^2
Mild	1.5-2
Moderate	1-1.5
Severe	<1

Indications for Surgery

Because there is no concern about left ventricular dysfunction (left ventricle is small and underfilled) in mitral stenosis, operation is not needed until there are symptoms of exertional dyspnea or pulmonary edema. A trial fibrillation does not necessarily indicate the need for operation because it can often be controlled medically. With a pliable valve that is noncalcified and has no regurgitation, a commissurotomy can be performed without valve replacement, and this may preclude the need for valve replacement for at least 10 years. Another consideration is a percutaneous balloon valvuloplasty if the valve is pliable and there is no regurgitation. This is probably the procedure of choice.

- Operation for mitral stenosis indicated with exertional dyspnea or pulmonary edema.
- Atrial fibrillation not necessarily indicative of operation (can be controlled medically).
- Percutaneous balloon valvuloplasty is probably procedure of choice.

Mitral Regurgitation

Etiology

Causes of mitral regurgitation include the following: 1) rheumatic; 2) mitral valve prolapse (with or without ruptured chordae); 3) infective endocarditis; 4) papillary muscle dysfunction--as a result of ischemia, fibrosis, or rupture (note that the posteromedial papillary muscle with its single blood supply from the right coronary artery becomes infarcted more frequently than the anterior papillary muscle); 5) dilated left ventricle; 6) hypertrophic cardiomyopathy; 7) cleft mitral valve associated with primum atrial septal defect; 8) trauma; and 9) systemic lupus erythematosus. Mitral annular calcification, when severe, can also cause mitral regurgitation. This may be accelerated by systemic hypertension, diabetes, and hypercalcemic states (e.g., resulting from chronic renal failure).

- In mitral regurgitation, posteromedial papillary muscle becomes infarcted more often than anterior papillary muscle.
- Mitral annular calcification accelerated by systemic hypertension, diabetes, hypercalcemic states.

Symptoms

Fatigue, dyspnea (due to increased left atrial pressure), and pulmonary edema can be present. Symptoms worsen with atrial fibrillation.

Physical Examination

The findings include a diffuse and hyperdynamic left ventricular impulse, which may be visible, and a palpable rapid filling wave. The first heart sound is usually obliterated, and there is a holosystolic murmur. The second heart sound is widely split (early A_2), and there is a third heart sound. A low-pitched early diastolic rumble is significant for severe regurgitation, but does not mean there is coexistent mitral stenosis. In acute mitral regurgitation, the murmur may be short because of increased left atrial pressure. The left atrium may be palpable with systole, and the left ventricle with diastole; there may be both third and fourth heart sounds. If the cause is ruptured chordae, an anterior leaflet murmur radiates to the axilla and back, and a posterior leaflet murmur radiates to the base and carotids. Consider acute mitral regurgitation with a normal-sized heart and pulmonary edema.

- Physical exam in mitral regurgitation:
  first heart sound usually obliterated.
  holosystolic murmur.
  second heart sound widely split (early A_2).
  low-pitched early diastolic rumble significant for severe regurgitation, but does not mean coexistent mitral stenosis.

Diagnosis

Chest radiography may first show a dilated left atrium and then, as mitral regurgitation increases, dilatation of the left ventricle.

Pathophysiology

Mitral regurgitation "offloads" the left ventricle, so filling volume must increase to maintain adequate forward output. This results in a hyperdynamic ventricle, and thus many patients with significant mitral regurgitation remain asymptomatic for many years. A low or low-normal ejection fraction therefore suggests significant ventricular dysfunction. Left atrial compliance may determine the hemodynamic picture. The left atrium may enlarge slightly and the pressure will rise significantly within it; conversely, it may markedly enlarge and permit a near-normal pressure.

- Many patients remain asymptomatic for many years.
- Low or low-normal ejection fraction suggests significant ventricular dysfunction.

Timing of Surgery

Asymptomatic patients with an ejection fraction >50%

can continue to undergo regular observation. Operation should be considered for symptomatic patients (note that ventricular function significantly influences postoperative outcome), and because "afterload is removed" when the mitral valve is replaced, left ventricular function may actually deteriorate. Mildly symptomatic patients may be considered for operation, particularly if serial examinations reveal progressive cardiac enlargement. Earlier operation may be indicated in those who are obviously suitable for mitral valve repair rather than replacement.

- Symptomatic patients with mitral regurgitation should be considered for operation.
- Mildly symptomatic patients, particularly with progressive cardiac enlargement, may be considered for operation.

Tricuspid Stenosis

The cause of tricuspid stenosis is almost always rheumatic, and it is never an isolated lesion. Carcinoid syndrome may cause tricuspid stenosis, and in rare cases atrial tumors may be the cause.

- Cause of tricuspid stenosis: almost always rheumatic; rarely, carcinoid syndrome and atrial tumors.

Tricuspid Regurgitation

This is usually caused by dilatation of the right ventricle. When there is right ventricular hypertension, tricuspid regurgitation is also common. It often results from mitral valve disease, but it may be related to 1) biventricular infarction, 2) primary pulmonary hypertension, 3) congenital heart disease (e.g., Ebstein's anomaly), or 4) carcinoid syndrome--more commonly associated with tricuspid regurgitation than tricuspid stenosis.

- Tricuspid regurgitation is caused by dilatation of right ventricle.
- Often results from mitral valve disease.

Tricuspid Valve Prolapse

This may occur as an isolated entity or in association with other connective tissue abnormalities. The tricuspid valve may prolapse or become flail secondary to trauma or endocarditis (commonly fungal or staphylococcal in drug addicts).

Physical Examination

Findings on physical examination include jugular venous distention with a prominent v wave, a prominent right ventricular impulse, a pansystolic murmur at left sternal edge increasing with inspiration, possibly a right-sided third heart sound, and peripheral edema, ascites, and hepatomegaly.

Surgical Therapy

Tricuspid annuloplasty may be helpful if regurgitation is a result of right ventricular dilatation; however, if there is significant pulmonary hypertension, tricuspid valve replacement is usually required. This can be done with either a biologic or a mechanical valve. In patients with endocarditis, the tricuspid valve can be removed completely, and patients may tolerate this well for several years.

CONGENITAL HEART DISEASE

Atrial Septal Defect

Secundum

Patients with secundum atrial septal defect often survive to adulthood and may be asymptomatic. The condition is often detected on routine examination with the finding of a murmur. If the defect has gone undetected, patients frequently develop atrial fibrillation in their 50s with onset of symptoms, usually dyspnea with subsequent tricuspid regurgitation and right-sided heart failure. The condition may present with a neurologic event.

- Patients with secundum atrial septal defect often survive to adulthood and may be asymptomatic.
- Condition is found on routine examination with finding of murmur.
- Patients often develop atrial fibrillation in their 50s with onset of symptoms.
- Condition may present with neurologic event.

Physical Examination

Findings include a normal or slightly prominent jugular venous pressure, a right ventricular heave, an ejection systolic murmur in the pulmonary artery (never more than grade 3/6), a fixed splitting of the second sound, and a tricuspid diastolic flow rumble if the shunt is large.

- Findings of secundum atrial defect:
    ejection systolic murmur in pulmonary artery (never

more than grade 3/6).

fixed splitting of second sound.

tricuspid diastolic flow rumble if shunt is large.

Diagnosis

Electrocardiography usually shows right bundle-branch block. Chest radiography shows pulmonary plethora, a prominent pulmonary artery, and right ventricular enlargement (Fig. 6-2). Young patients (<40 years) with secundum atrial septal defect and sinus rhythm do not have left atrial enlargement. If the chest radiograph shows left atrial enlargement, consider another lesion, particularly primum atrial septal defect with mitral regurgitation.

- If chest radiograph shows left atrial enlargement, consider primum atrial septal defect with mitral regurgitation.

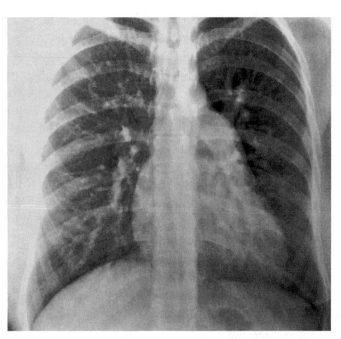

Fig. 6-2. Chest radiograph from a patient with a large left-to-right shunt due to a secundum atrial septal defect. Notice cardiac enlargement with right ventricular contour, very prominent pulmonary artery, and pulmonary plethora.

Two-dimensional and color Doppler echocardiography can usually demonstrate the defect and right ventricular enlargement with volume overload. If visualization is poor, transesophageal echocardiography can be performed. Cardiac catheterization is usually unnecessary, unless coexisting coronary disease is suspected.

Sinus Venosus

An uncommon condition, this occurs in the superior portion of the atrial septum. It is often associated with anomalous pulmonary veins, usually the right upper. If echocardiography shows right ventricular volume overload and no secundum defect, consider sinus venosus atrial septal defect or anomalous pulmonary veins.

Primum (Partial Atrioventricular Canal)

This is a defect in the lower portion of the septum. The mitral valve is usually cleft and produces various degrees of regurgitation.

Diagnosis

On electrocardiography, findings are different from those of secundum type with left-axis deviation and right bundle-branch block. More than 75% of patients have first-degree atrioventricular block. The chest radiographic findings are the same as those for secundum atrial septal defect, although there may be left atrial enlargement because of mitral regurgitation. Atrioventricular defects are the most common cardiac anomaly associated with Down's syndrome.

- Electrocardiography shows left-axis deviation with right bundle-branch block and, commonly, first-degree atrioventricular block.
- Atrioventricular defects are most common cardiac anomaly of Down's syndrome.

Ventricular Septal Defect

Ventricular septal defect occurs in different parts of the ventricular septum, most commonly either in the membranous septum or in the muscular septum. Small defects produce a loud noise, and patients are often asymptomatic. The size of the hole determines the degree of left-to-right shunting. Small defects may have a long holosystolic murmur, often with a thrill at the left sternal edge, usually around the fourth interspace. Large defects may produce a mitral diastolic flow rumble at the apex, especially when the shunt is more than 2.5:1.

- Ventricular septal defects are most common in membranous septum or muscular septum.
- Small defects produce loud noise.
- Size of hole determines degree of left-to-right shunting.

Patent Ductus Arteriosus

This condition is associated with maternal rubella. It produces essentially an "arteriovenous fistula." A small ductus is compatible with a normal lifespan. The ductus may calcify in adult life. A continuous "machinery" murmur envelops the second heart sound around the second interspace beneath the left clavicle. A large patent ductus arteriosus may produce ventricular failure. Surgical ligation is curative. Patients then do not need endocarditis prophylaxis.

All of the above-described shunt lesions, when large, may produce elevated pulmonary pressures and subsequently pulmonary vascular disease.

- Patent ductus arteriosus is associated with maternal rubella.
- Small ductus compatible with normal lifespan.
- Continuous "machinery" murmur is present.
- Surgical ligation is curative, and endocarditis prophylaxis then not needed.
- All described shunt lesions, when large, may produce elevated pulmonary pressures and subsequently pulmonary vascular disease.

Eisenmenger's Syndrome

This syndrome develops in the first few years of life when a large shunt produces pulmonary hypertension and irreversible pulmonary vascular disease. This condition causes the shunt to reverse so that blood flows from the right to left and subsequent cyanosis occurs. Patients are then inoperable. Death commonly occurs in the third or fourth decade of life as a result of exercise-induced syncope, arrhythmia, hemoptysis, and stroke. The cyanosis produces significant erythrocytosis, often with hemoglobin values in the teens or 20s. There is no need to phlebotomize patients with a hemoglobin value <20 g/dL or a hematocrit value <65%. Also, repeated phlebotomies frequently lead to iron deficiency, and iron-deficient erythrocytes are more rigid than ordinary ones, and the risk of stroke is thereby increased. Phlebotomy may be necessary in symptomatic patients with a hemoglobin value >20 g/dL. Always remember to replace fluid concomitantly in patients with Eisenmenger's syndrome because hypotension and syncope may be fatal.

- Eisenmenger's syndrome develops in first few years of life.
- Syndrome produces pulmonary hypertension and irreversible pulmonary vascular disease.
- Death common in third or fourth decade of life.
- Associated conditions: exercise-induced syncope, arrhythmia, hemoptysis, stroke.
- Cyanosis produces significant erythrocytosis.

Pulmonary Stenosis

This may occur as an isolated lesion or in association with a ventricular septal defect. Valvular pulmonary stenosis often causes few or no symptoms. The valve is frequently pliable, and it may be bicuspid. Thickened dysplastic valves, often stenotic, occur in association with Noonan's syndrome.

- Thickened dysplastic valves, often stenotic, occur with Noonan's syndrome.

Physical Examination

Findings include a prominent "a" wave in the jugular venous pulse; right ventricular heave; ejection click--the earlier the click, the more severe the stenosis (the click indicates that the valve is pliable and noncalcified); ejection systolic murmur--the longer the murmur and the later peaking, the more severe the stenosis; and soft and late P_2 (with severe stenosis P_2 becomes inaudible).

- Findings of pulmonary stenosis:
    prominent "a" wave in jugular venous pulse.
    ejection click (earlier the click, the more severe the stenosis).
    soft and late P_2.

Diagnosis

Electrocardiography shows right ventricular hypertrophy. On chest radiography, pulmonary oligemia is found only with *very severe* pulmonary stenosis. There is poststenotic pulmonary dilatation, especially of the left pulmonary artery (Fig. 6-3).

The diagnosis can be reliably made with two-dimensional echocardiography, and Doppler reliably predicts the gradient and estimates right ventricular pressure. In asymptomatic patients, no treatment is indicated unless the right ventricular pressure approaches two-thirds that of the systemic pressure. Later in life, the valve may become calcified when the ejection click disappears. The treatment of choice for a pliable valve is percutaneous balloon valvuloplasty. This has essentially replaced surgical valvotomy.

- Diagnosis of pulmonary stenosis is made with two-dimensional and Doppler echocardiography.

- Treatment for pliable valve is percutaneous balloon valvuloplasty.

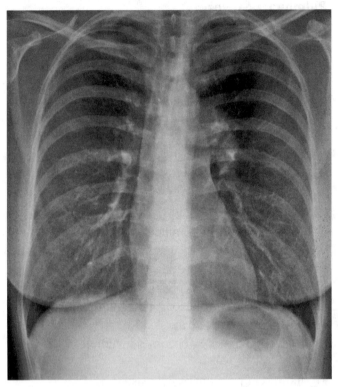

Fig. 6-3. Typical chest radiograph of valvar pulmonary stenosis, showing normal cardiac size and marked prominence of main and left pulmonary arteries, representing poststenotic dilatation. This does not occur with infundibular pulmonary stenosis. Lung fields appear mildly oligemic.

Coarctation of the Aorta

This is usually either a discrete or a long segment of narrowing adjacent to the left subclavian artery. It is more common in males and frequently is associated with a bicuspid aortic valve. Most cases of coarctation are diagnosed in childhood; only about 20% are diagnosed in adulthood. This is the most common cardiac anomaly associated with Turner's syndrome. Other associations include aneurysms of the circle of Willis and aortic dissection or rupture. There is an increased incidence of aortic dissection or rupture in Turner's syndrome even in the absence of coarctation. As a result of the coarctation, systemic collaterals develop from the subclavian and axillary arteries through the internal mammary, scapular, and intercostal arteries.

- Coarctation of aorta is more common in males.
- Condition is frequently associated with bicuspid aortic valve.

- Only 20% of cases are diagnosed in adulthood.
- Most common cardiac anomaly associated with Turner's syndrome.
- Increased incidence of aortic dissection or rupture in Turner's syndrome even in absence of coarctation.

There are five major complications of coarctation of the aorta: 1) cardiac failure, 2) aortic valve disease, 3) rupture or dissection, 4) endarteritis, and 5) rupture of an aneurysm of the circle of Willis--this is exacerbated by the presence of hypertension, which occurs in the upper limbs. Systemic hypertension may be the presenting feature in adults. Some patients complain of pain in the legs on exercise.

Physical Examination

Findings include an easily palpable brachial pulse; the femoral pulse is weak and delayed. There are differences in systolic pressure between the upper and lower extremities. Exercise may exaggerate the systemic hypertension. An ejection click is present when there is an associated bicuspid valve. A_2 may be loud as a result of hypertension. A fourth heart sound may be present with associated left ventricular hypertrophy and hypertension. Murmurs may originate from 1) the coarctation, which can produce a systolic murmur over the left sternal edge and over the spine in the mid-thoracic region, and it sometimes extends into diastole in the form of a continuous murmur; 2) arterial collaterals, which are spread widely over the thorax; and 3) the bicuspid aortic valve, which may generate a systolic murmur.

- Findings of coarctation of aorta: easily palpable brachial pulse, weak and delayed femoral pulse, differences in systolic pressure between upper and lower extremities.
- Coarctation can produce systolic murmur over left sternal edge and over spine in mid-thorax.
- Arterial collaterals are spread widely over thorax.

Diagnosis

Electrocardiography may be normal. With more severe coarctation or hypertension, left ventricular hypertrophy with or without repolarization changes is found. Chest radiography may show rib notching from the dilated and pulsatile intercostal arteries and a "3" configuration of the aortic knob, which represents the coarctation site with proximal and distal dilatations.

- Chest radiographic findings in coarctation of aorta are rib notching and a "3" configuration of aortic knob.

The condition may be demonstrated by echocardiography and Doppler, although imaging may be difficult in this area, and additional visualization may be necessary with digital subtraction angiography, magnetic resonance imaging, or computed tomography. Angiography can also be performed.

Treatment

Balloon angioplasty has been performed in some patients, although it is associated with aneurysm formation and re-coarctation. Surgical treatment has been an accepted approach since 1945. However, there is a significant rate of hypertension after coarctation repair. As many as 75% of patients are hypertensive at 30-year follow-up. Surgically treated patients still often die prematurely of coronary disease, heart failure, stroke, or ruptured aorta. Age at operation is important. The 20-year survival rate is 91% in patients who have operation when they are <14 years old and 79% in patients who have operation when they are >14 years old.

- Surgical repair of coarctation of aorta is associated with significant rate of hypertension; 75% of patients are hypertensive at 30-year follow-up.
- Surgically treated patients often die prematurely of coronary disease, heart failure, stroke, ruptured aorta.

Ebstein's Anomaly

This unusual congenital lesion is thought to be associated with maternal lithium ingestion during pregnancy. It has a variable spectrum. It involves an inferior displacement of the tricuspid valve ring into the right ventricular cavity. The degree of displacement is variable, as is the degree of abnormality of the tricuspid valve. The inferior displacement results in "atrialization" of the right ventricle, the small contractile chamber beneath.

- Ebstein's anomaly is thought to be associated with maternal lithium ingestion during pregnancy.
- Anomaly involves inferior displacement of tricuspid valve ring into right ventricular cavity.

Physical Examination

The extremities are usually cool, often with peripheral cyanosis (a reflection of low cardiac output). There

may be an "a" wave in the jugular venous pressure (although this is variable because the large right atrium may accommodate a large tricuspid regurgitant volume). A subtle right ventricular lift is noted. The first heart sound has a loud T_1 component. A holosystolic murmur increases on inspiration at the left sternal edge from tricuspid regurgitation. One or more systolic clicks are noted (may be multiple). Common associated conditions are secundum atrial septal defect and preexcitation syndrome. Patients with secundum atrial septal defects are often very cyanotic because of the right-to-left shunting. They may present with neurologic events.

- Findings of Ebstein's anomaly include cool extremities, often with peripheral cyanosis, and a holosystolic murmur that increases on inspiration.
- One or more systolic clicks are noted (may be multiple).
- Associated conditions: secundum atrial septal defect, preexcitation syndrome.
- Patients with secundum atrial septal defects are often very cyanotic.
- They may present with neurologic events.

Diagnosis

Chest radiography shows a narrow pedicle with enlarged globular silhouette and right atrial enlargement. The lung fields are normal or oligemic. On electrocardiography a tall P wave (Himalayan P waves) and right bundle-branch block are found.

Two-dimensional and Doppler echocardiography delineates the anatomy precisely, and cardiac catheterization is unnecessary. Electrophysiology study may be necessary to delineate the bypass tract, if present.

PREGNANCY AND CARDIAC DISEASE

Physiologic Changes of Pregnancy

Plasma volume starts to increase in the first trimester, peaking around the second trimester to almost 50% above normal. An increase in red cell mass also begins early and peaks in the second trimester, but not to the same degree as the plasma volume; thus, there is a relative anemia. The cardiac output increases, and peripheral resistance decreases. Increased venous pressure in the lower extremities leads to pedal edema in 80% of healthy pregnant women.

- Physiologic changes of pregnancy include increased

plasma volume, red cell mass, cardiac output.
- Peripheral resistance decreases.

Because of these changes, the physical examination may suggest cardiac abnormalities to the unwary. Normal results of physical examination in a healthy pregnant woman include elevation of the jugular venous pressure, bounding carotid pulses, and an ejection systolic murmur in the pulmonary area (never more than grade 3/6). The second heart sound is loud, and there is a third heart sound or diastolic filling sound. A fourth heart sound occasionally may be heard.

- Ejection systolic murmur (never more than grade 3/6) is a normal finding in pregnancy.

Although a third heart sound or diastolic filling sound is common, a long rumble should raise the possibility of mitral stenosis. Because of the decrease in peripheral resistance and increased output changes, stenotic lesions are less well tolerated than regurgitant ones; for example, a patient with aortic stenosis has exaggeration of the aortic valve gradient, whereas a patient with mitral regurgitation experiences "afterload reduction" with peripheral vasodilatation and so tolerates pregnancy better. Functional class of the patient is a consideration in terms of whether pregnancy is possible. Patients who are in functional class III or IV have a maternal mortality rate approaching 7%.

- Third heart sound or diastolic filling sound common in pregnancy, but long rumble should raise possibility of mitral stenosis.
- Functional class III or IV: maternal mortality rate approaches 7%.

Pregnancy is *absolutely contraindicated* in patients with the following conditions: 1) Marfan syndrome with a dilated aortic root--increased risk of dissection and rupture because hormonal changes soften the connective tissue (unpredictable risk of dissection and rupture in Marfan syndrome and pregnancy even when aortic root has normal size), 2) Eisenmenger's syndrome (maternal mortality rate is 50%), 3) primary pulmonary hypertension, 4) symptomatic severe aortic stenosis, 5) symptomatic severe mitral stenosis, 6) symptomatic dilated cardiomyopathy.

Although not absolute contraindications, the follow-ing conditions are also of concern in pregnancy: 1) atrial septal defect (deep venous thrombosis may lead to paradoxical embolus) and 2) coarctation (increased risk of dissection and rupture).

Patients at risk during pregnancy should minimize activity (decreases cardiac output), reduce sodium in the diet, and minimize anemia with iron and vitamin supplements.

If symptoms deteriorate and congestive heart failure supervenes, bed rest may need to be instituted. Arrhythmias such as atrial fibrillation need to be treated promptly in these situations. If necessary, cardioversion can be performed with apparently low risk to the fetus. Fetal cardiac monitoring should be performed at the same time. Occasionally patients need operative intervention. Operation during the first trimester is associated with a significantly increased rate of fetal loss. Percutaneous aortic and mitral balloon valvuloplasty have been performed during pregnancy and may obviate bypass. Careful lead shielding of the fetus is needed during these procedures.

Drugs
Many cardiac drugs cross the placenta into the fetus but yet can be used safely when necessary and are not absolutely contraindicated in pregnancy. These include digoxin, quinidine, procainamide, β-adrenergic blockers, and verapamil. The β-adrenergic blockers can be associated with growth retardation of the fetus, neonatal bradycardia, and hypoglycemia. They may need to be used, however, in large doses in patients with hypertrophic cardiomyopathy, and fetal growth must be monitored.

Drugs that should be avoided are captopril, which causes fetal renal dysgenesis; phenytoin, which causes hydantoin syndrome and teratogenicity; and warfarin, which causes teratogenicity and abortion.

- Drugs to avoid in pregnancy: captopril, phenytoin, warfarin.

Delivery
Delivery is a time of rapid hemodynamic swings. With each uterine contraction, about 500 mL of blood is released into the circulation. Cardiac output goes up with advancing labor. High-risk patients need careful monitoring with Swan-Ganz catheterization to maintain preload at an optimal level, maternal and fetal electrocardiography monitoring, careful analgesia and anesthesia to avoid hypotension, delivery in the left lateral position so the

fetus is not lying on the inferior vena cava (this position maintains venous return), and a short second stage (delivery may need to be facilitated if labor progresses slowly).

Vaginal delivery is safer for most women because the average blood loss is 500-800 mL; with cesarean section it is 800 mL. Usually, cesarean section is performed only for obstetric indications. The new guidelines of the American Heart Association state there is no need for antibiotic prophylaxis in an uncomplicated vaginal delivery.

- With each uterine contraction, 500 mL of blood is released into circulation.
- No need for antibiotic prophylaxis in uncomplicated vaginal delivery.

Prosthetic Valves and Pregnancy

Most women of childbearing age who need a valve replacement will receive a biologic valve, and if they are in sinus rhythm they will usually not be receiving anticoagulants. Women with mechanical valves will be taking warfarin, and this poses a problem with teratogenicity and increased risk of abortion. In general, diagnose pregnancy as soon as possible and switch the therapy to subcutaneous heparin, monitoring the activated partial thromboplastin time, and continue this approach throughout pregnancy. This agent is also associated with increased fetal loss, however.

- In pregnant patients with mechanical valves, switch therapy from warfarin to subcutaneous heparin.
- Heparin is associated with increased fetal loss.

PERICARDIAL DISEASE

The pericardium has an inner layer, the visceral pericardium, and an outer layer, the parietal pericardium. Space between the two layers contains approximately 15-25 mL of clear fluid. The pericardium has three main functions: prevent cardiac distention, limit cardiac displacement because of its attachment to neighboring structures, and protect the heart from nearby inflammation.

Acute or Subacute Inflammatory Pericarditis

Presenting Symptoms

The chest pain of pericarditis is often aggravated by movement of the trunk, by inspiration, and by coughing.

The pain is often relieved by sitting up. *Low-grade fever* and malaise are other findings.

Diagnosis

Pericardial friction rub may be variable. Chest radiography is usually normal. It may show globular enlargement if pericardial effusion is significant (at least 250 mL). Occasionally, pulmonary infiltrate or small pleural effusion is noted. Left pleural effusion predominates, and the cause is unknown. Electrocardiography shows acute concave ST elevation in all ventricular leads. The PR segment is also depressed in the early stages. Echocardiography allows easy diagnosis of pericardial effusion.

- Chest pain is presenting symptom of pericarditis.
- Electrocardiography shows concave ST elevation and depressed PR segment.

Causes

The causes of pericarditis include viral pericarditis, idiopathic pericarditis, autoimmune and collagen diseases (systemic lupus erythematosus, rheumatoid arthritis, scleroderma), and postmyocardial infarction. The postcardiotomy syndrome follows open heart procedures. It presents with pyrexia, increased sedimentation rate, and pleural or pericardial chest pain. It occurs weeks to months after operation. Its incidence decreases with age, and it usually responds to anti-inflammatory agents. Pericarditis is also associated with radiation and neoplasm, namely, Hodgkin's disease, leukemia, and lymphoma. Breast, thyroid, and lung tumors can metastasize to the pericardium and cause pericarditis or pericardial effusion. Melanoma also metastasizes to the heart. Uremia and tuberculosis can also cause pericarditis. If no cause can be documented, idiopathic viral pericarditis is the most likely diagnosis, and treatment with nonsteroidal anti-inflammatory agents or high-dose aspirin usually resolves the condition.

- Causes of pericarditis: autoimmune and collagen diseases; postmyocardial infarction; radiation; neoplasm; breast, thyroid, and lung tumors; uremia; tuberculosis.

Pericardial Effusion

The response of the pericardium to inflammation is to exude fluid, fibrin, and blood cells, causing a pericardial effusion. The amount of effusion needed before it shows on the chest radiograph is 250 mL. If fluid accumulates slowly, the pericardial sac distends slowly with no cardiac compression. If fluid accumulates rapidly, such as with bleeding, tamponade can occur with relatively small amounts of fluid. Tamponade restricts the blood entering the ventricles and causes a decrease in ventricular volume. The raised intrapericardial pressure increases the ventricular end-diastolic pressure and mean atrial pressure, and the increased atrial pressure increases the venous pressure. The decreased ventricular volume and filling diminish cardiac output. Any of the previously listed causes of pericarditis can cause tamponade, but other acute causes of hemopericardium should be considered, such as ruptured myocardium after infarction, aortic dissection, ruptured aortic aneurysm, and sequelae of cardiac operation.

- Amount of effusion needed to be seen on chest radiograph is 250 mL.
- Tamponade can occur with small amounts of fluid.
- Tamponade restricts blood entering ventricles and decreases ventricular volume.

Clinical Features

Tamponade produces a continuum of features, depending on its severity. The blood pressure is low, the heart is small and quiet, jugular venous pressure is increased, and pulsus paradoxus develops (increased flow of blood into the right heart during inspiration, decreased flow into the left heart). An increase in inspiratory distention of neck veins (Kussmaul's sign) is infrequent unless there is underlying constriction.

Treatment

Emergency pericardiocentesis is performed with echocardiography-directed guidance.

Constrictive Pericarditis

Diastolic filling of both ventricles is prevented by the pericardium. The smaller the ventricular volume, the higher is the end-diastolic pressure. The most common causes are recurrent viral pericarditis, irradiation, previous open heart operation, tuberculosis, and neoplastic disease.

Symptoms

Dominantly right-sided failure, peripheral edema, ascites, and often dyspnea and fatigue are present.

- Symptoms of constrictive pericarditis: peripheral edema, ascites, dyspnea, fatigue.

Physical Examination

The jugular venous pressure is elevated (remember to look at the patient when he or she is sitting or standing), and inspiratory distention of neck veins (Kussmaul's sign) is present. The jugular venous pressure may show rapid descents, and pericardial knock is present in fewer than 50% of cases (sound is probably due to sudden cessation of ventricular filling). Ascites and peripheral edema may be present. Chest radiography may show pericardial calcification, but no specific changes are found on electrocardiography.

- Signs of constrictive pericarditis: elevated jugular venous pressure, inspiratory distention of neck veins, rapid descents of jugular venous pressure, pericardial knock in <50%.
- Chest radiograph may show pericardial calcification.
- No specific changes on electrocardiogram.

Diagnosis

Echocardiography and Doppler may be helpful, particularly Doppler, which shows respiratory changes in mitral and tricuspid inflow velocities. Other methods such as computed tomography and magnetic resonance imaging help to delineate the thickness of the pericardium, although they do not prove physiologic significance. The major confounding diagnosis is restrictive cardiomyopathy, and the distinction can be very difficult. Diastolic expansion of both ventricles is affected equally; therefore, diastolic pressure is elevated and equal in all four chambers. Ventricular pressure curve shows characteristic "√" from rapid ventricular filling and equalization of pressures (also may be seen in restrictive cardiomyopathy). The "a" and v waves are usually equal and x and y descents are rapid. If pulmonary artery systolic pressure is >50 mm Hg, myocardial disease is likely. If the end-diastolic pulmonary artery pressure is <30% of systolic pressure, myocardial disease is likely. Both of these findings are nonspecific, however. The treatment of choice for constrictive pericarditis is exploratory operation to remove the pericardium.

- Constrictive pericarditis diagnosed from respiratory changes in mitral and tricuspid inflow velocities.
- Major confounding diagnosis is restrictive cardiomyopathy.

● Diastolic pressure is elevated and equal in all four chambers.

EVALUATION OF THE PATIENT WITH CARDIAC DISEASE BEFORE NONCARDIAC SURGERY

Risks

The major risk for most patients with cardiac disease who undergo noncardiac operations arises from the presence of coronary artery disease. In patients without previous evidence of heart disease, the risk of perioperative myocardial infarction during noncardiac procedure is 0.15%. In patients who have had myocardial infarction, the frequency of reinfarction during a major noncardiac operation is about 6%. The risk of perioperative reinfarction is inversely related to the interval between preoperative infarction and noncardiac operation (Table 6-3). With aggressive perioperative management and invasive hemodynamic monitoring, these rates may be significantly reduced. The mortality rate from a perioperative myocardial infarction is approximately 50%.

● Patients without previous heart disease: risk of perioperative myocardial infarction during noncardiac operation is 0.15%.
● Patients with previous myocardial infarction: risk of reinfarction during major noncardiac operation is 6%.
● Risk of perioperative infarction inversely related to time from previous infarction to noncardiac operation.
● Mortality rate from perioperative myocardial infarction is 50%.

Table 6-3.--Risk of Perioperative Reinfarction, by Time From Initial Infarction

Time from MI to noncardiac operation, mo	Risk of perioperative MI, %
<3	27-37
3-6	11-16
>6	4-5

MI, myocardial infarction.

Certain surgical procedures are associated with a threefold greater chance of myocardial infarction: major intrathoracic, upper abdominal, and great vessel surgical procedures. Other preoperative cardiac risks include age >70 years, S_3 gallop, jugular venous pressure >12 cm H_2O, and significant aortic stenosis. Electrocardiographic risk factors are a rhythm other than sinus, atrial ectopy, or >5 premature ventricular contractions per minute. Other factors to consider are general medical status (e.g., PaO_2 <60 or $PaCO_2$ >50 mm Hg, potassium <3 mEq/L, bicarbonate <20 mEq/L), blood urea nitrogen value >50 or creatinine value >3 mg/dL, chronic liver disease, general debilitation, and type of operation (e.g., emergency procedure or intraperitoneal, thoracic, or aortic procedure).

● Risk of myocardial infarction is threefold more with major intrathoracic, upper abdominal, great vessel operations.

Because of a strong association between coronary disease and peripheral vascular disease, patients who are to undergo a peripheral vascular operation are at high risk of having important coronary disease. In patients having routine coronary angiography before a vascular operation, approximately 60% with clinically suspected ischemic heart disease have severe multivessel or even inoperable coronary artery disease. Approximately 20% of patients with no prior history to suggest coronary disease have diffuse, severe coronary artery disease.

● At routine angiography before vascular operation, 60% of patients with clinically suspected ischemic heart disease have severe multivessel or inoperable coronary artery disease.
● Of patients without history of coronary artery disease, 20% have diffuse, severe coronary artery disease.

Therefore, use of a cardiac risk index (e.g., Goldman) has limitations. Obviously, the risks are much higher, for example, in patients undergoing a vascular operation. Risk indices thus depend on referral patient population, nature of the operation, expertise of the surgeon and anesthesiologist, and uncommon problems or events (e.g., emergency procedure).

● Strong association between coronary disease and peripheral vascular disease.

A low risk score index does not exclude a patient from having a perioperative event but rather indicates a low probability of a cardiac event. Preoperative cardiovascular assessment with a thorough cardiac history is important, corroborated by examination, chest radiography, and electrocardiography. The presence or absence and severity of angina pectoris and the efficacy of current medical therapy need to be considered. The history and time of the previous myocardial infarction are important. If operation is not urgent, waiting more than 6 months after myocardial infarction is probably appropriate.

- Low risk score index does not exclude a perioperative event but does indicate low probability of cardiac event.
- Preoperative cardiovascular assessment important.
- History and time of previous infarction are important.

Mild Angina

Most patients who can perform vigorous activity of daily living and are functional class I or II tolerate the stress of most noncardiac operations. However, if they are to undergo one of the more risky procedures (intrathoracic, upper abdominal, or vascular), preoperative stress testing should be considered. If functional limitation is not clear from the history, stress testing should be performed, if possible.

Class III or IV Angina

Significant limitation because of symptoms suggests the need for direct coronary angiography.

- Patients limited by class III or IV angina need direct coronary angiography.

Exercise Testing

Different end points have been used in stress testing. If during routine exercise treadmill testing the patient has no ischemic changes and achieves >75% of maximal predicted heart rate, the risk of a perioperative myocardial infarction is low. If ischemia develops on electrocardiogram during treadmill exercise testing and the patient can only exercise <5 METs, the risk is twice that with a normal exercise electrocardiogram and exercise >5 METs. For various reasons, some patients are unable to exercise, and for them dipyridamole thallium scanning may be useful. This has a high sensitivity (particularly when used before vascular operation) but not a very high specificity. The negative predictive value, however, is high. In other words, a negative dipyridamole thallium scan suggests a low risk of operation.

- Dipyridamole thallium scanning has high sensitivity but not specificity.
- Negative dipyridamole thallium scan suggests low risk of operation.

Before a series of tests are done, the risks and benefits of coronary revascularization before a major noncardiac operation should be considered. For example, the Coronary Artery Surgery Study (CASS) found that the operative mortality rate was 2.3% with coronary artery bypass grafting, 2.9% when the left ventricular ejection fraction was <50%, and 7.9% in patients >70 years old. Thus, the risk of bypass may be higher than the potential risk of noncardiac surgery. Each case needs to be considered individually. Angina therapy needs to be optimized. If left ventricular dysfunction is present, noninvasive assessment of left ventricular ejection fraction may be indicated and treatment optimized. If left ventricular dysfunction is severe, hemodynamic monitoring should be performed perioperatively, especially when optimization of cardiac status is not possible preoperatively. Antianginal therapy should be maintained perioperatively.

- Risk of coronary artery bypass grafting may be higher than potential risk of noncardiac operation.
- Therapy for angina needs to be optimized.
- Antianginal therapy should be maintained perioperatively.

Aortic or Mitral Stenosis

Assess stenosis with two-dimensional and Doppler echocardiography. If it is severe, patients should have cardiac operation before a noncardiac procedure. Percutaneous balloon valvuloplasty can occasionally be used to "get patients through" the operation. Asymptomatic patients with significant aortic stenosis can often tolerate a noncardiac operation safely with careful anesthesia and hemodynamic monitoring.

- If aortic or mitral stenosis is severe, cardiac operation should be done before noncardiac procedure.
- Asymptomatic patients with significant aortic stenosis can often tolerate noncardiac operation safely.

Mechanical Valvular Prostheses

Management depends on the degree of operation being undertaken. Depending on the risk and degree of the procedure, anticoagulant therapy can be discontinued 1 to 3 days preoperatively and restarted 2 to 5 days postoperatively with a low risk of a thromboembolic event. The risk of bleeding complications may be higher, depending on the extent of the operation. For patients needing more extensive procedures, oral anticoagulation may be changed to heparin, continued 6 hours before operation with resumption 24 hours postoperatively, or days later if necessary.

THE HEART IN SYSTEMIC DISEASE

Hyperthyroidism

Effects

The cardiovascular effects include increased heart rate, stroke volume, and cardiac output, decreased peripheral resistance, and widened pulse pressure. All of these lead to increased myocardial work and may precipitate angina. Symptoms include palpitations, tachycardia, and exertional dyspnea.

- Cardiovascular effects of hyperthyroidism: increased heart rate, stroke volume, cardiac output; decreased peripheral resistance; widened pulse pressure.
- Effects lead to increased myocardial work and perhaps angina.

Physical Examination

Common findings are tachycardia, bounding pulse, forceful apical impulse, systolic ejection murmur, and scratchy systolic murmur at the left sternal border resembling a pericardial friction rub. Cardiac arrhythmias are common, particularly supraventricular tachycardia or atrial fibrillation. Atrial fibrillation occurs in 10%-20% of patients. Always suspect thyrotoxicosis in a patient with unexplained atrial fibrillation. Arterial embolization is rare.

- Findings: tachycardia, bounding pulse, forceful apical impulse, systolic ejection murmur.
- Cardiac arrhythmias are common (supraventricular tachycardia, atrial fibrillation).
- Suspect thyrotoxicosis in patient with atrial fibrillation.

Hypothyroidism

This disorder causes a decrease in metabolic rate and circulatory demand, bradycardia, decreased myocardial contractility and stroke volume, and increased peripheral resistance.

Physical Examination

There may be cardiac enlargement due to either intrinsic myocardial disease or pericardial effusion. Myocardial contractility is reduced. These changes usually resolve with thyroid hormone therapy. Pericardial effusion occurs in approximately one-third of patients with hypothyroidism. Heart failure is rare in the absence of associated cardiac disease. Coronary atherosclerosis occurs twice as often in patients with hypothyroidism as in age- and sex-matched controls.

- Physical findings in hypothyroidism: cardiac enlargement, reduced myocardial contractility, pericardial effusion in one-third.
- Heart failure rare in absence of associated cardiac disease.
- Coronary atherosclerosis occurs twice as often as in controls.

Diabetes Mellitus

This condition is frequently associated with premature coronary atherosclerosis, and the prevalence is increased among females. Fatal myocardial infarctions occur at least twice as often in diabetic men and three times as often in diabetic women as in the nondiabetic population. The cause is uncertain. The prevalence of hypertension is increased among diabetic patients. Hyperlipidemia is common. Angina and myocardial infarction are often manifested by atypical symptoms. The incidence of silent myocardial infarction is high. Congestive heart failure may be the first manifestation of coronary disease.

- Fatal myocardial infarction occurs twice as often in diabetic men and three times as often in diabetic women as in nondiabetics.
- Prevalence of hypertension increased in diabetics.
- Angina and myocardial infarction manifested by atypical symptoms.
- Incidence of silent myocardial infarction is high.

There is some evidence that diabetes may also be associated with cardiomyopathy unassociated with coronary artery disease. Some studies suggest that this may be due to small vessel disease, similar to that in the kidney.

Amyloidosis

Primary amyloidosis is characterized by accumulation

of protein ground substance in many organs, typically the kidneys and the heart but also the tongue, skin, nerves, and liver. Secondary amyloidosis occurs in association with chronic disease (rheumatoid arthritis, tuberculosis, chronic infection, neoplasia). Cardiac abnormality is not a prominent feature. In senile systemic amyloidosis the heart is the most involved organ. Prevalence increases from age 60 on. Familial amyloidosis is autosomal dominant. The characteristic amyloid protein is prealbumin. It can involve the heart.

- Primary amyloidosis: protein ground substance in many organs.
- Secondary amyloidosis: cardiac abnormality not prominent.
- Senile systemic amyloidosis: heart is most involved organ.
- Familial amyloidosis: autosomal dominant, can involve heart.

Primary Amyloidosis

About 90% of patients with primary amyloidosis have clinical evidence of cardiac dysfunction. The heart is often enlarged, due mostly to thickened ventricular myocardium caused by the infiltration, and the atria tend to enlarge. Abnormalities of conduction may occur. Amyloid also deposits in the cardiac valves, and there is a high frequency of atrioventricular valve regurgitation.

- In primary amyloidosis, 90% of patients have cardiac dysfunction.
- Abnormalities of conduction may occur.
- Amyloid deposits in cardiac valves.

Clinical Features

The following can occur: congestive heart failure, arrhythmias, sudden death, angina-like chest pain, pericardial effusion, and murmurs of atrioventricular valve regurgitation. Natural history is usually intractable biventricular cardiac failure. Diastolic abnormalities are common, particularly features of "restrictive cardiomyopathy." Most patients have evidence of renal disease associated with serum and urine protein abnormalities.

- Clinical features of primary amyloidosis: arrhythmias, sudden death, "restrictive cardiomyopathy," evidence of renal disease.

Diagnosis

Electrocardiography shows classic low-voltage QRS complex, which is nonspecific. In addition to the systemic abnormalities described, echocardiography is particularly useful. This typically demonstrates the increased ventricular wall thickness without cavity dilatation and a granular appearance of the ventricular myocardium. Atria are usually dilated. The cardiac valves may also show some thickening and reduction in motion associated with atrioventricular valve regurgitation. Various hemodynamic features have been shown in amyloidosis, and Doppler techniques have recently been useful for characterizing these. An early-stage finding is prolonged relaxation with an important contribution to filling from atrial contraction. In later stages, rapid early filling suggestive of restrictive cardiomyopathy may be found.

- Echocardiographic findings in primary amyloidosis: increased ventricular wall thickness, granular appearance of ventricular myocardium, dilated atria.
- Early stage: prolonged relaxation.
- Later stages: rapid, early filling.

Hemochromatosis

This is an iron-storage disease, either a primary form or a secondary form related to exogenous iron (usually from repeated blood transfusions). Iron deposits within the cardiac cells. Cardiac hemochromatosis never occurs alone and is always accompanied by involvement of other organs. Clue to diagnosis is tetrad of diabetes, liver disease, brown skin pigmentation, and heart disease. The condition may present with cardiomegaly and congestive failure or cardiac arrhythmias. It may have features of dilated or restrictive cardiomyopathy. Therefore, it can present with abnormalities of either systolic or diastolic dysfunction. Once clinical symptoms of heart failure or arrhythmias develop, most patients will be dead within 1 year unless treatment is initiated either with phlebotomy or iron chelation.

- In hemochromatosis, iron deposits within cardiac cells.
- Cardiac hemochromatosis never occurs alone.
- Tetrad: diabetes, liver disease, brown skin pigmentation, heart disease.

Carcinoid Heart Disease

Metastatic malignant carcinoid tumors produce serotonin-like substance that causes systemic flushing. In patients with hepatic metastases, right-sided valves are involved. Therefore, changes occur in the tricuspid and pulmonary valves. The tricuspid leaflets become thickened with deposition on the underside of the valve. Leaflets become thickened, stiff, and relatively immobile, and the chordae may also be involved. The dominant lesion is tricuspid regurgitation. There may be some element of stenosis. Pulmonary valve is also involved, and the leaflets become thickened and rigid. Pulmonary regurgitation is common, and the valve is also often stenotic. Surgical therapy includes tricuspid valve replacement (with a mechanical valve because carcinoid may also affect bioprostheses). Pulmonary valve resection may be necessary.

- Carcinoid tumors produce serotonin-like substance that causes systemic flushing.
- Changes occur in tricuspid and pulmonary valves.
- Dominant lesion is tricuspid regurgitation.
- Pulmonary regurgitation is common.
- Pulmonary valve is often stenotic.

PROSTHETIC VALVES

Bioprostheses

These are made of animal or human tissue, which may be unmounted or mounted in a frame. Different types include 1) homograft (human tissue), either aortic or pulmonary; 2) heterograft (porcine valve), e.g., Hancock or Carpentier-Edwards; and 3) pericardial (bovine valve), e.g., Ionescu-Shiley. Tissue valves have the advantage that they are not as thrombogenic as mechanical valves, thus most patients in sinus rhythm do not require anticoagulation. There is a risk of systemic embolism, however, with biologic prostheses in patients with atrial fibrillation, particularly with a mitral prosthesis. The disadvantage is that tissue valves degenerate and calcify and thus patients will need reoperation. Approximately 50% of patients will need valve replacement at 10 years. Tissue valves last a little longer in the tricuspid position than in positions on the left side of the heart. Aortic valves have a slightly better durability than mitral valves. Prosthesis failure can be detected by clinical evaluation and two-dimensional and Doppler echocardiography.

- Tissue valves are not as thrombogenic as mechanical valves.

- Most patients with tissue valves who are in sinus rhythm do not require anticoagulation.
- Risk of systemic embolism with biologic prostheses in patients with atrial fibrillation, particularly with a mitral prosthesis.
- Tissue valves degenerate and calcify.
- About 50% of patients will need valve replacement.

Mechanical Valves

An example of a *ball valve* is the Starr-Edwards. It has excellent longevity and is a so-called high-profile valve. A small size may be associated with a higher transvalvular pressure gradient. Types of *tilting disc valves* are the Björk-Shiley and St. Jude. All mechanical valves have a risk of thromboembolism. Reported rates vary. For example, in a Mayo Clinic series of patients with a Starr-Edwards prosthesis, 81% were free of embolism at 5 years when the valve was in the aortic position, and 93% were free of embolism when it was in the mitral position. Hemolysis often occurs with mechanical prostheses, especially with perivalvular leak. Anticoagulation can also be associated with hemorrhage and thrombosis. Rate of minor hemorrhages is approximately 2%-4% per year, and that of major hemorrhages is 1%-2% per year.

- All mechanical valves have a risk of thromboembolism.
- Hemolysis often occurs with mechanical prostheses, especially with perivalvular leak.
- Anticoagulation can be associated with hemorrhage and thrombosis.

TUMORS OF THE HEART

Most cardiac tumors are metastatic. Most common primary cardiac tumor is myxoma.

Cardiac Myxoma

Most cardiac myxomas are sporadic, but there have been some reports of familial occurrence. A syndrome of cardiac myxomas with lentiginosis (spotty pigmentation) and recurrent myxomas has been recognized. About 75% are in the left atrium, 18% are in the right atrium, and the rest are in the ventricles. Most of the atrial tumors arise from the atrial septum, usually adjacent to the fossa ovalis. About 95% are single. Most myxomas have a short stalk, are often gelatinous and friable, and tend to embolize. They occasionally calcify, so they may be visible on a chest radiograph.

The main clinical features are obstruction to blood flow, embolization, and systemic effects. Left atrial tumors prolapse into the mitral valve orifice and produce mitral stenosis. They mimic mitral valvular stenosis with symptoms of dyspnea, orthopnea, cough, pulmonary edema, and hemoptysis. Classically, symptoms occur with a change in body position. Physical findings suggest mitral stenosis. Pulmonary hypertension may also occur. An early diastolic sound, the tumor "plop," may be heard. This has a lower frequency than an opening snap.

- Most cardiac tumors are metastatic.
- Most common primary cardiac tumor is myxoma.
- 75% of cardiac myxomas are in left atrium, 18% in right atrium.
- Clinical features: obstruction to blood flow, embolization, systemic effects.
- Symptoms occur with change in body position.
- Early diastolic sound, tumor "plop," may be heard.

Embolization

Systemic emboli may occur in 30%-60% of patients with left-sided myxoma, frequently to brain and lower extremities. Histologic examination of embolized material is important. Coronary embolization is rare, but it should be considered in a young patient with no known previous cardiac disease. Systemic effects are fatigue, fever, weight loss, and arthralgia. Systemic effects may be associated with an elevated sedimentation rate, leukocytosis, hypergammaglobulinemia, and anemia. Elevated immunoglobulins are usually of IgG class.

Echocardiography is the preferred approach to diagnosis. Transesophageal echocardiography helps delineate the precise site of origin and accurately assesses tumor size and degree of mobility. Operation is indicated when the diagnosis is made.

- Systemic emboli occur in 30%-60% of cases of left-sided myxoma, frequently to brain and lower extremities.
- Coronary embolization is rare.
- Systemic effects: fatigue, fever, weight loss, arthralgia.
- Systemic effects may be associated with elevated sedimentation rate, leukocytosis, hypergammaglobulinemia, anemia.
- Elevated immunoglobulins are usually IgG.
- Echocardiography preferred for diagnosis.
- Operation indicated.

Primary Cardiac Neoplasm

Rhabdomyoma is most common in women and children. It can produce obstruction of cardiac valves simulating other abnormalities and can cause cardiac arrhythmias. Other tumors, such as Kaposi's sarcoma associated with acquired immunodeficiency syndrome (AIDS), do not usually cause cardiac symptoms.

Secondary tumors most often originate from bone, breast, lymphoma, leukemia, and thyroid. More than half of patients with malignant melanoma have metastases to the heart.

- Rhabdomyoma is most common in women and children.
- More than half of patients with malignant melanoma have metastases to heart.

DIAGNOSTIC TESTS

Echocardiography

Echocardiography uses an ultrasonic beam (frequency, >20,000 cps) produced by electric excitation of a piezoelectric crystal. The properties of this beam include linear transmission through a homogeneous medium, poor transmission through air, and reflective/refractive phenomena when the directed waves traverse an interface between two media of differing density (acoustic impedances). The greatest reflection of ultrasound occurs when the acoustic impedances of the neighboring structures are dissimilar and when the beam strikes this interface at a perpendicular angle. The reflected waves return to the ultrasound generator (transducer) with a time delay proportional to the distance of the interface from the transducer. Knowledge of the velocity of the ultrasound beam allows relative distances (and dimensions) of various structures to be determined. This forms the basis of M-mode echocardiography, which displays the distances as continuous lines of varying intensities on a moving strip of paper. This technique gives a "one-dimensional" look at a small portion of the heart. If instead of a single crystal a linear array of crystals is excited sequentially, a plane of ultrasound is generated, which when reflected and appropriately analyzed produces a tomographic or two-dimensional image of cardiac structure. An infinite variety of planes transecting the heart is possible; the examiner orients the ultrasound plane appropriately to transect desired structures.

Doppler Echocardiography

Doppler echocardiography is able to detect and measure abnormal blood velocities in the cardiac chambers and great vessels. It uses the Doppler principle, which states that a sound beam reflected off a moving object will change its frequency. This change in frequency, known as the Doppler shift, is proportional to the velocity of the moving object. Thus, by reflecting the Doppler beam off moving erythrocytes, one can measure blood velocities. From this information, it is possible to calculate gradients across stenotic valves, intracardiac pressures, and cardiac output. A semiquantitative estimate of the severity of valvular regurgitation and intracardiac shunts may also be obtained. Color flow imaging allows a real-time visualization of blood flow by superimposing different color maps (indicating direction and velocity of blood flow) on top of a moving two-dimensional echocardiogram.

- Doppler echocardiography detects and measures abnormal blood velocities in cardiac chambers and great vessels.
- Allows calculation of gradients across stenotic valves, intracardiac pressures, cardiac output.
- Color flow imaging allows real-time visualization of blood flow.

Practical Applications of Echocardiography

Chamber Size and Function

Echocardiography is an excellent method for determination of the size of all four cardiac chambers. In addition, left ventricular function (ejection fraction) can be easily and accurately determined in most patients. Based on left ventricular dimensions in systole and diastole measured on M-mode echocardiography, the equation for ejection fraction is

$$[(\text{diastolic dimension})^2 - (\text{systolic dimension})^2]$$
$$- (\text{diastolic dimension})^2$$

This has been well validated when compared with ejection fractions obtained by cardiac catheterization or radionuclide angiography.

- Echocardiography is excellent method for determination of size of all four cardiac chambers.
- Left ventricular function (ejection fraction) can be easily and accurately determined.

Regional Wall Abnormalities

Because of its ability to determine endocardial motion, as well as myocardial thickening, echocardiography is an ideal method for evaluation of regional wall abnormalities. This is a sensitive marker for either ongoing ischemia or myocardial infarction. Currently, a subjective visual analysis is used to determine wall motion abnormalities.

- Echocardiography is ideal for evaluation of regional wall abnormalities.
- Sensitive marker for ongoing ischemia or myocardial infarction.

Valvular Abnormalities

M-mode and two-dimensional echocardiography are sensitive methods for analysis of structural valvular lesions. Calcified stenotic valves are easily identified. Prolapsed and flail valves as a cause of valvular regurgitation may be detected. Doppler echocardiography adds hemodynamic information to allow an accurate estimate of the severity of stenosis and regurgitation.

- M-mode and two-dimensional echocardiography are sensitive for analysis of structural valvular lesions.

Intracardiac Shunts

Both atrial septal defects and ventricular septal defects can be visualized on two-dimensional echocardiography if they are more than 2-3 mm in diameter. Color flow imaging has allowed the detection of even smaller shunts.

Cardiac Output

Knowledge of 1) the cross-sectional area of a valvular orifice or great vessel utilizing M-mode and two-dimensional echocardiography and 2) the velocity of blood flow through the area of Doppler echocardiography allows a volumetric flow rate to be calculated. This provides a noninvasive instantaneous measurement of cardiac output which is accurate and reproducible.

Miscellaneous

Two-dimensional echocardiography is the method of choice in the evaluation of pericardial effusion. It has greatly enhanced the safety and feasibility of pericardiocentesis by directing the placement and angle of the puncture needle. Intracardiac masses (tumors, thrombus) are well visualized with two-dimensional echocardiography. Valvular vegetations are also able to be detected.

Because echocardiography is totally noninvasive and risk-free, sequential examinations are facilitated. Because transmission of ultrasound through the chest wall to the heart requires an "ultrasonic window" (i.e., an area without overlying lung and resultant air dispersion of sound waves), not all patients can have adequate imaging with this technique, and a 10%-20% failure rate is the largest single drawback. Transesophageal echocardiography overcomes several of these drawbacks and is especially useful for examining 1) valve pathology (ruptured chord, vegetations), 2) atrial septum (? patent foramen ovale/atrial septal defect), 3) anomalous pulmonary veins, and 4) left atrial appendage, in a search for thrombus.

QUESTIONS
(See "Answers" section)

Multiple Choice

1. Which one physical sign might be expected with this chest radiograph?

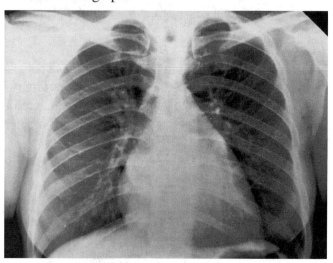

   a. Systolic ejection murmur
   b. Diastolic decrescendo murmur
   c. Soft first heart sound
   d. Diastolic rumble
   e. Holosystolic murmur

2. Which of the following occurs with hypertrophic cardiomyopathy?
   a. Increase in outflow murmur with handgrip
   b. Decreased murmur on standing
   c. Decreased murmur with amyl nitrite
   d. Decreased murmur with Valsalva
   e. Increased murmur after a premature ventricular complex

3. Which one of the following is true about mitral stenosis?
   a. Once a patient reaches 30 years of age, the valve is usually calcified
   b. The longer the interval from the second heart sound to opening snap, the more severe the stenosis
   c. Percutaneous valvotomy may relieve the stenosis if the valve is pliable
   d. It is more common in males than females
   e. The first heart sound is usually soft

4. Which of the following need antibiotic prophylaxis?
   a. An 18-year-old with a ventricular septal defect having a vaginal delivery
   b. A 24-year-old with an atrial septal defect having a dental extraction
   c. A 40-year-old with a ligated patent ductus arteriosus having a cystoscopy
   d. A 20-year-old with a bicuspid aortic valve without stenosis or regurgitation having a dental extraction
   e. A 40-year-old with a ventricular septal defect having a cardiac catheterization

5. A 60-year-old man, 2 months after resection of lung carcinoma, presents with rapidly increasing dyspnea and fatigue. On examination, he has a systolic blood

pressure of 80 mm Hg and an elevated jugular venous pressure. The echocardiogram shows a normal left ventricle with a large pericardial effusion and a swing heart. Which of the following would *not* be expected to be present?

a. Electrical alternans
b. Kussmaul's sign
c. Pulsus alternans
d. Pulsus paradoxus >20 mm Hg
e. Narrow pulse pressure

6. The following physical signs are commonly expected in a normal pregnant woman except:

a. Loud third heart sound
b. Holodiastolic murmur
c. Peripheral edema
d. Bounding pulses
e. Systolic ejection murmur

7. Which of the following physical signs would *not* be expected in a patient with the congenital lesion associated with this chest radiograph?

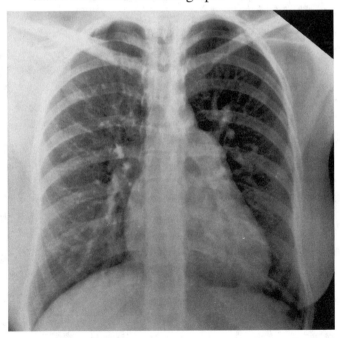

a. Pansystolic murmur
b. Ejection systolic murmur
c. Right ventricular lift
d. Diastolic rumble

8. Which of the following is true of coarctation of the aorta?

a. It is associated with mitral valve prolapse
b. It is more common in men

c. It usually is not detected until adulthood
d. It usually occurs proximal to the left subclavian artery
e. After good surgical repair, normal longevity can be anticipated

9. The following tumors commonly metastasize to the heart except:

a. Thyroid carcinoma
b. Colon carcinoma
c. Breast carcinoma
d. Melanoma
e. Lymphoma

10. An 80-year-old woman presents with acute abdominal pain and needs emergency resection of an infarcted bowel. She had an anterior myocardial infarction 1 year previously and has had poorly controlled congestive heart failure since. Examination reveals an increased jugular venous pulse and bibasilar rales. Chest radiography shows cardiomegaly and pulmonary venous redistribution. Which of the following is the most appropriate?

a. Urgent coronary arteriography
b. Dipyridamole thallium scanning
c. Echocardiography
d. Proceed with surgery with hemodynamic monitoring and optimize medical treatment
e. Defer surgery until her congestive heart failure has improved

True/False

11. Auscultation when the patient rises from squatting to standing results in which of the following changes?

a. A click and murmur of mitral valve prolapse occur earlier after first heart sound
b. The murmur of hypertrophic obstructive cardiomyopathy gets softer
c. The jugular venous pressure increases if the patient has an impediment to right ventricular filling
d. The timing of an early diastolic sound changes, allowing distinction to be made between atrial myxoma and pericardial knock
e. A pulmonary flow murmur gets louder
f. The murmur of mitral regurgitation gets louder

12. The following conditions elevate the jugular venous pressure:

a. Right ventricular infarct

b. Septic shock
c. Constrictive pericarditis
d. Pericardial tamponade
e. Superior vena cava obstruction
f. Severe tricuspid regurgitation

13. The following drugs should be avoided during pregnancy:
    a. Verapamil
    b. Propranolol
    c. Digoxin
    d. Captopril

e. Warfarin (Coumadin)
f. Quinidine

14. These physical signs are often associated with Eisenmenger ventricular septal defect:
    a. Loud systolic murmur
    b. Ejection click
    c. Thrill at left sternal edge
    d. Right ventricular lift
    e. Decrescendo diastolic murmur
    f. Loud P2

CHAPTER 7
CHEST X-RAYS

Edward C. Rosenow III, M.D.

INTRODUCTION

Internists should read every chest x-ray (CXR) of their patients. The only way to learn to read CXRs is to look at hundreds of them, including normal ones. By doing this, you will be able to recognize an abnormality, although you may not know what it is. The important thing is to recognize that something is different. Do not read the radiologist's report before interpreting the CXR. This is a way of testing yourself in learning to read CXRs.

Radiologists miss 10%-15% of the abnormalities on CXRs. For this reason, internists (generalists or subspecialists) must also read CXRs, just as they read electrocardiograms. Radiologists read a "normal" in less than 20 seconds, and at least 70% of the abnormalities seen on a CXR are noted in less than the first one-half second!

Experienced chest radiographers miss 90% of early (<1 cm) peripheral solitary pulmonary lung cancers. With overall 5-year survivorship of lung cancer still at about 10%, as it has been for over 40 years, it is only through early detection of peripheral nodules that this overall average can be raised, because 5-year survival of peripheral nodules is 50%-80% (only 50%-80%, not 100%, but better than 10%). Thus, every smoker's or former smoker's CXR must be carefully scrutinized. Any subtle change should be compared with previous CXRs. If no previous CXRs are available and tomography or computed tomography (CT) is not indicated, perform a follow-up CXR in 6-12 weeks and compare with the current one. Keep in mind that 15% of lung cancers occur in never-smokers.

Never accept the reading of a "normal CXR." The most difficult CXR to read is a "normal" one. How do you know it is normal? You might find something in a "normal CXR" that explains why you are examining the patient

in the first place--and it might be for a nonthoracic problem.

What you see on CXR is usually not diagnostic of a single entity. You need the benefit of the medical history, physical findings, and, sometimes, laboratory and tissue findings. What you are doing is narrowing the differential diagnosis to a few options.

PROCEDURE

It cannot be emphasized enough that previous CXRs are extremely important for comparison. It costs nothing and is painless. A subtle abnormality may be present and unchanged on previous CXRs but was overlooked, possibly because the radiologist missed it or because the technique was not sufficient for projecting this newly discovered "change." At the Mayo Clinic, the last CXR is available to compare with the current one. When something subtle shows up and you are uncertain whether it is normal variation or a new, possibly significant, abnormality, comparison with the old CXR usually settles the question quickly.

In comparing two CXRs, how do you know they are of the same patient? Could the labeling be a mistake? Comparing two CXRs is not as easy as it might seem, especially if the CXR is of a patient of the same sex, size, and build. An area to compare to see whether the CXR is of the same person is the first rib costochondral junction, which calcifies earlier than other rib functions. Of course, comparing calcified Ghon complex on two CXRs is easy. Aortic arch calcification is another way to compare two CXRs. Also, other anomalies (distortion, eventration of the diaphragm) help with the comparison.

Begin by looking at CXRs from a distance of 6-8 feet.

If too close, you miss abnormalities. Be sure to note "left" and "right" on the film. Are there physical findings of the thorax that you can relate to what is shown in the CXR (giving you an advantage over radiologists)?

About 15% of lung parenchyma is hidden by cardiovascular structures and the diaphragm. Thus, lateral CXR helps visualize these areas, but still you need specifically to look behind the heart and through the diaphragm for any abnormality. Whether a CXR is a right or left lateral is unimportant except lesions in the lateral part of the lung are more distinct on a lateral CXR of that side because the lesions are closer to the film and scatter is less. However, a lateral CXR definitely helps localize lesions, including mediastinal ones.

In reviewing an abnormal CXR, do not become fixed on the first abnormality noted, because there may be others. Compare the two lung fields for asymmetry. Look carefully behind heart, under clavicles, and under ribs. Form your own approach to viewing all areas on the CXR, and follow the same pattern so no area is overlooked. One way of remembering to look at all areas is to divide the CXR into chest wall, lung parenchyma and airways, and mediastinum.

Chest Wall

Chest wall refers to the pleura, ribs, spine, clavicles, diaphragm, and all extrathoracic structures, including infradiaphragmatic area. The following should be noted:

1. Pleural thickening or calcification.
2. Costophrenic angles--are they blunted? It takes at least 200-400 mL of pleural effusion before the angle is blunted. In some individuals, for unknown reasons, there is no meniscus fluid and all the fluid is infrapulmonary, mimicking elevated hemidiaphragm. Therefore, be suspicious of unexplained elevated hemidiaphragm, which would be clarified with a decubitus film.
3. Diaphragm--normally, right hemidiaphragm is higher than the left. Elevated hemidiaphragm is one of most common abnormalities on CXR in pulmonary embolism. Compare CXR with one made before pulmonary embolus.
4. Check inferior margin of ribs for notching (coarctation).
5. Look at bones for metastasis.
6. Are any unusual infradiaphragmatic abnormalities noted? Gastric bubble is absent in 80% of achalasics and 10%-15% of normals. Splenomegaly displaces the colon or gastric bubble medially.
7. Are any unusual extra-rib abnormalities seen?

Check the extrathoracic trachea, neck, soft tissues, shoulder, and clavicles.
8. Is there arm pain? Look for asymmetry in apex for Pancoast lesion.

Lung Parenchyma

Lung parenchyma includes all lung tissue. Points to consider include:

1. About 15% of the lung is hidden behind diaphragm and mediastinal structures.
2. Look behind the heart. With proper technique, you should be able to see rib and lung detail through the heart.
3. Carefully scan apices under clavicle and first rib. Many lesions can be hidden here.
4. Because lungs are paired organs, they are ideal for comparing right and left areas for asymmetry representing subtle change.
5. Overreading interstitial markings is common. Correlate findings with medical history, physical findings, pulmonary function, and, most important, earlier CXRs.
6. Look carefully for Kerley's B lines if interstitial changes are present.
7. Distribution of lung parenchymal changes between the upper and lower halves can also be important in narrowing differential diagnosis (see below).

Mediastinum

Be comfortable with the normal silhouette of this structure.

1. Right paratracheal area--subtle lymphadenopathy here may be only CXR evidence of sarcoidosis, metastasis, or lymphadenopathy of many causes; compare with previous CXRs.
2. There should be a notch between inferior margin of aortic knob and left pulmonary artery. A small bronchogenic carcinoma or lymphadenopathy can occur here and fill the space.
3. Esophageal disease is seldom detected on CXR except for large diaphragmatic hernia, leiomyoma, enterogenous cyst, and, occasionally, dilated fluid-filled achalasic esophagus.
4. On lateral CXR, the right ventricle should occupy no more than lower 1/3 of substernal space. If higher, it may indicate right ventricular hypertrophy.
5. About 10% of neurogenic tumors in posterior mediastinum are associated with intraspinal component (dumbbell tumor). Spine CT or magnetic resonance imaging (MRI) is indicated.

The most difficult areas to read on CXRs are the hila and whether there are increased interstitial markings. There are no good rules to follow here except experience and old CXRs. In 95% of people, the left hilus is normally higher than the right but never by more than 3 cm. The right is almost never higher than the left. This is important in detecting loss of volume not otherwise evident on that side. At this point, it is helpful to consult with a radiologist about which procedure might help delineate whether there is abnormality. Tomograms and/or special techniques in CT may be sufficient, or if there is no suspicion of abnormality, if it is possible that the area seen is within normal variation, and if no old CXRs are available, follow-up CXR in 6-8 weeks may be best alternative. MRI (expensive!) is effective in distinguishing large pulmonary artery from hilar mass.

With few exceptions, "emphysema" should not be read into a CXR. You can say "low-lying flattened diaphragm, increased AP diameter consistent with emphysema." This only describes hyperinflation. This and the uncommon finding of decreased peripheral vascular markings are characteristic of emphysema. A patient with severe asthma or an asthmatic in status has severely hyperinflated lungs, which mimics emphysema but is reversible. Panlobular emphysema, as in α_1-antitrypsin-deficient emphysema, involves mainly the bases and is one of the exceptions in describing emphysema on CXR.

Instead of describing the "disease" or disorder you see, describe the abnormality to define it anatomically, i.e., describe what you see and not what you think it is. If you do this, the disorder or at least a narrower differential diagnosis may come to mind. Trying to list conditions or diseases may cause confusion, especially when learning to interpret CXRs.

A silhouette sign is a poor man's lateral CXR. A positive sign is when a process (infiltration, lesion of any kind, collapsed lobe) obliterates cardiac diaphragm or aortic border; this occurs when the density is in direct continuity with the border. It is a localizing sign on the PA CXR and is usually confirmed with a lateral CXR.

Bronchogenic carcinoma can have many different appearances on CXR, including solitary pulmonary nodule (SPN), mass lesion (>3.5 cm), collapsed lobe, inflammatory-appearing infiltrate, pleural effusion, mediastinal adenopathy, and "pneumonia." "Pneumonia" in patients especially over 45 years should be followed up until complete resolution to be sure it is not obstructive pneumonitis (I have never seen complete resolution with antibiotics in this setting). It is important to remember that an unexplained shadow in a smoker or former smoker is bronchogenic carcinoma until proved otherwise. This does not mean it is necessary to bronchoscope or operate on every unexplained infiltrate, but there are appropriate ways of evaluating these.

Loss of volume is seen most commonly in obstruction of a bronchus. In adults, the commonest cause is bronchogenic carcinoma. Radiographic signs include 1) displacement of interlobar septa bounding the affected lobe (most direct and reliable sign of lobar collapse), 2) elevation of hemidiaphragm, 3) shift of mediastinum toward obstructed side, 4) narrowing of rib margins, 5) compensatory "emphysema" (hyperinflation) of remaining lobe and/or contralateral lung, and 6) hilar displacement. However few or none of these may be present in some cases.

Bronchography is of little value, with rare exception, for detecting any condition other than suspected bronchiectasis. High-resolution chest CT is as sensitive as bronchography and is more tolerable procedure for patients.

Indications for pulmonary tomography are 1) reveal calcium in "coin lesion"; 2) reveal cavities; 3) examine areas obscured by dense shadows, especially apical and hilar areas; and 4) demonstrate vessels in suspected arteriovenous fistulas.

Tomography costs about 1/3 that of CT, and chest MRI is 2-3 times as expensive as CT. Tomography clarifies the nature of an SPN in two-thirds of cases.

Chest fluoroscopy may be helpful in evaluating mid-mediastinal lesions adjacent to or involving esophagus, but demonstration of pulsation is usually meaningless: many aortic aneurysms do not pulsate, but any structure adjacent to the heart or aorta does. Up-and-down motion with swallowing occurs in substernal goiter, leiomyoma, and enterogenous cyst of foregut.

Cavitary lesions include abscess, neoplasms (usually squamous cell carcinoma), tuberculosis, coccidioidomycosis, cryptococcus, Wegener's granulomatosis.

Kerley's B lines represent passive congestion and lymphangitic carcinoma. When present, they help narrow differential diagnosis to two likely conditions: left heart failure and lymphangitic carcinoma. Kerley's B lines are not distended lymphatics (as originally thought) but are either tumor or fluid in the septa of secondary lobules. As isolated descriptive events, Kerley's A, C, and D lines are not as specific as B lines.

Air bronchograms in localized lesions are best seen with tomography and/or chest CT and, until proved otherwise, should be considered to represent bronchioalveolar cell carcinoma, lymphoma, or pseudolymphoma.

Occasionally, it is difficult to localize a small lesion or infiltrate on a lateral CXR. The best way to do this is to locate it in distance from the top of the aortic arch, with either the thumb or long finger on the lesion. With these two fingers fixed in same position, run them along same lines on the lateral CXR.

CXRS FOR THE BOARD EXAMINATION

It is unlikely that the examination will include a normal CXR. Look for a missing breast (radical mastectomy); metastatic disease may explain what is going on. Coarctation is a favorite, so look for rib notching; internists are supposed to be expert on secondary causes of hypertension. Look for "left" and "right" markers to be sure you are not dealing with dextrocardia. It is unlikely you will need to interpret a CT unless the finding is so obvious "anybody" could see it. With rare exception, there is almost no abnormality on CXR that is diagnostic for a single disease entity (you do not need to know the exceptions). You do need to know the differential diagnosis and the potential meaning of what the differential consists of and then be able to relate it to the information given in the stem, at which point you can probably come up with a single diagnosis. For any unexplained "shadow," think of bronchogenic carcinoma until proved otherwise, especially in a smoker or former smoker.

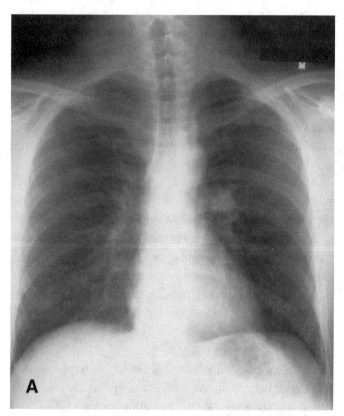 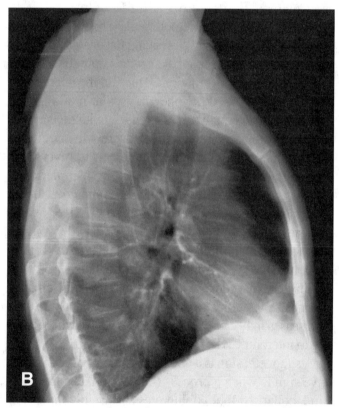

Fig. 7-1. Normal CXR. *A*, Posteroanterior (PA) and *B*, lateral. Look at the whole CXR first, without honing in on any perceived abnormality. Beginning with the chest wall, carefully look at all ribs for abnormalities, including notching. Assess the infradiaphragmatic portion for any abnormality, such as a mass displacing the colon or gastric bubble, or any calcifications. Look carefully at the neck for any variation of normal. Next, look at the mediastinal silhouette, including the heart. There should be a notch below the aortic knob on the left just above the left pulmonary artery. This can be filled with a neoplasm or lymphadenopathy. The right paramediastinal area can also contain subtle adenopathy. Look for this. The vascular shadow of the superior vena cava is subtle, without any discrete markings associated with it. Look carefully at the superior paramediastinal area for a thoracic outlet or Pancoast tumor. The hila are among the more difficult areas to interpret because they can be prominent but normal in some people. Normally, the left hilus is equal to or higher than the right one; if this is not the case, it may be evidence of loss of volume that is not otherwise apparent. Finally, look carefully at lung parenchyma and be careful not to overinterpret increased interstitial lung markings. Comparison with previous films is extremely important in interpreting the hila and interstitial markings. Look behind heart and diaphragm where at least 15% of lung is present. You should be able to see lung markings and rib detail behind the heart if the technique is proper. Are the costophrenic angles blunted (it takes 200-400 mL of fluid before a meniscus is produced)? Are there any subtle changes for bronchiectasis, meaning two parallel lines with widened bronchi, particularly in the lower lobes? You should always look at the trachea and mainstem bronchi for narrowing or a tumor process. This is not always easy, depending on technique of CXR, but should be done. On the lateral view, the right ventricle should come up only as far as the lower third of the retrosternal space; otherwise, there could be a mass there or right ventricular hypertrophy that is not evident on the PA view. The density overlying the vertebrae decreases as you go down to the lower thoracic vertebrae, because of less overlying muscle mass.

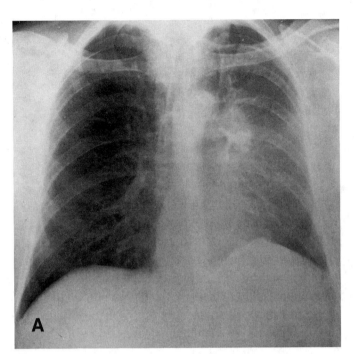

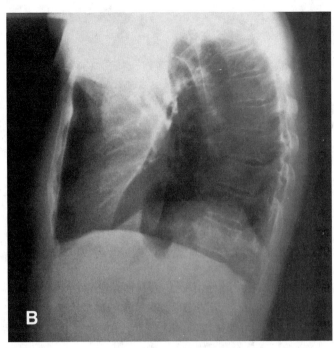

Fig. 7-2. Collapsed left upper lobe. *A*, PA CXR and *B*, lateral CXR. The ground glass haze over left hemithorax is typical of partially collapsed left upper lobe. In a little over one-half of patients with collapsed lobes, there is evidence of loss of volume. In this situation, left hemidiaphragm is elevated, medi-astinum is shifted to left, and left hilus is pulled cranially. Also, left mainstem bronchus deviates cranially. The calcification in left hilar mass represents unre-lated old granulomatous infection. In *B*, the density from left hilus down toward anterior portion of chest represents the partially collapsed left upper lobe. The radiolucency substernally is right lung.

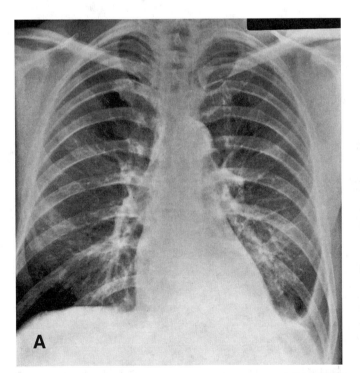

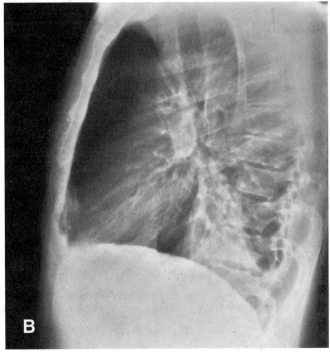

Fig. 7-3. Collapsed left lower lobe. *A*, PA CXR and *B*, lateral CXR. This is example of no evidence of loss of volume despite almost complete collapse of a large lobe. Note that rib detail and lung markings cannot be seen behind the heart due to the collapsed left lower lobe, with the border paralleling left bor-der of heart. Lateral CXR shows wedge-shaped density of collapsed left lower lobe, but in a moderate number of cases the only evidence may be seeming-ly increased density over the vertebrae without wedge-shaped infiltrate being so obvious.

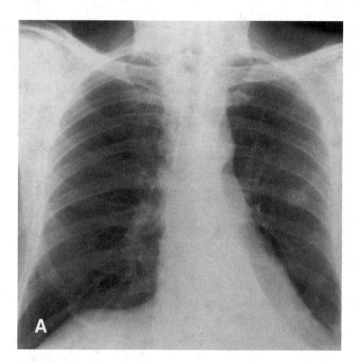

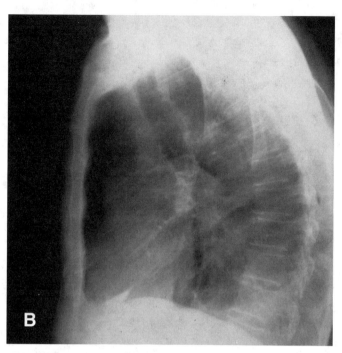

Fig. 7-4. Collapsed left lower lobe. *A*, PA CXR and *B*, lateral CXR. Nodule in left mid-lung field plus collapsed left lower lobe, as can be seen with a density behind the heart. This entity represents two separate primary lung cancers, viz., synchronous bronchogenic carcinomas. Do not stop with the first evident abnormality, such as nodule in mid-lung field, without carefully looking at all other areas. *B* demonstrates finding of increased density over lower thoracic vertebrae without any obvious wedge-shaped infiltrate, as in Figure 7-3. Over anterior portion of hemidiaphragm, the small wedge-shaped infiltrate is not fluid in left major fissure, because left major fissure is pulled away posteriorly. Instead, it is an incidental normal variant of fat pushed up into right major fissure.

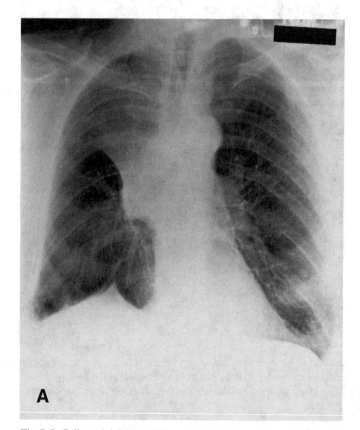

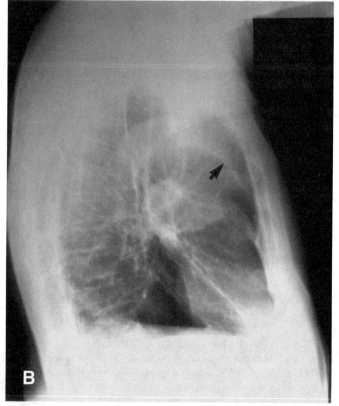

Fig. 7-5. Collapsed right upper lobe. *A*, PA CXR and *B*, lateral CXR. *A*, This is classic "reversed S" of mass in right hilus with partial collapse of right upper lobe. Loss of volume is evident with the elevation of the right hemidiaphragm. In *B*, the partially collapsed right upper lobe can be faintly seen in the upper anterior portion of hemithorax (*arrow*).

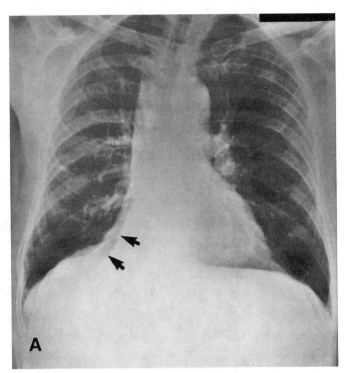

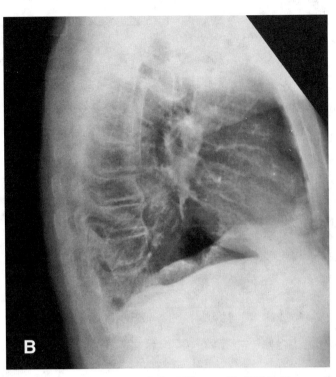

Fig. 7-6. Collapsed right lower lobe. *A*, PA CXR and *B*, lateral CXR. *A*, This 75-year-old smoker had hemoptysis for 1 1/2 years; his CXR had been read as "normal" on several occasions. Note linear density (*arrows*) projecting downward and laterally along right border of heart. It projects below diaphragm and is not a normal line. Also, right hilus is not evident; it has been pulled centrally and downward because of carcinoma obstructing bronchus of right lower lobe. Note very slight shift in mediastinum to the right, indicative of some loss of volume. In spite of significant collapse of right lower lobe, only subtle increased density over lower thoracic vertebrae represents this collapse.

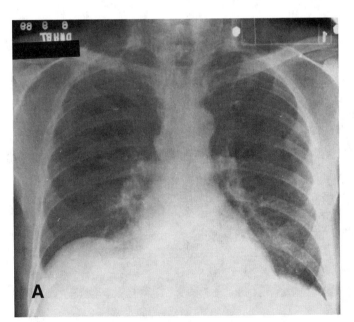

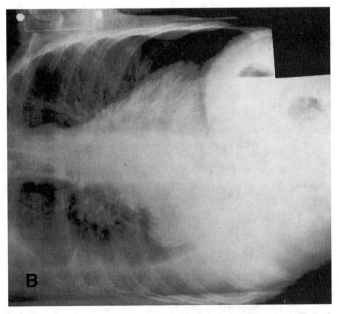

Fig. 7-7. *A*, "Elevated right hemidiaphragm" that is really infrapulmonic effusion, as seen on decubitus film, *B*. For reasons unknown, a meniscus is not formed in some people with infrapulmonic pleural effusion. Thus, any seemingly elevated hemidiaphragm should be examined with suspicion it could be infrapulmonic effusion. Decubitus CXR or ultrasonography would disclose the free fluid.

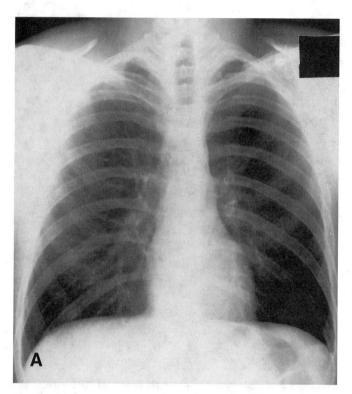

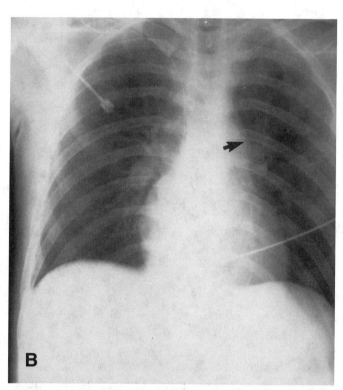

Fig. 7-8. *A*, Normal, pre-pulmonary embolism on PA CXR; *B*, pulmonary embolism. CXR is read as normal in 20%-30% of patients with angiographically proved pulmonary embolism. In comparison with *A*, *B* shows subtle elevation of right hemidiaphragm. In *A*, right and left hemidiaphragms are equal. Elevated hemidiaphragm is the most common finding with acute pulmonary embolism in some series. Also, note plumpness of right pulmonary artery, prominent pulmonary outflow tract on left (*arrow*), and subtle change in cardiac diameter. This 28-year-old man was in shock at the time of CXR from massive pulmonary emboli as result of major soft tissue trauma produced by a motorcycle accident 7 days earlier.

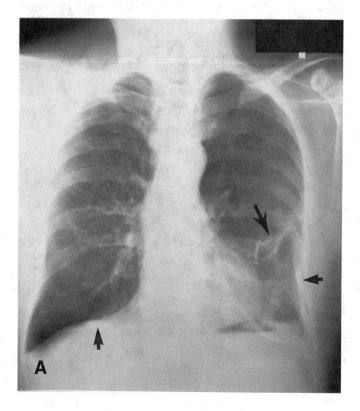

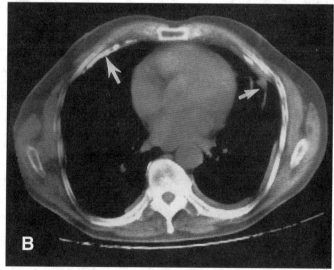

Fig. 7-9. Abnormal CXR, *A*, in 68-year-old asymptomatic man. *Small arrows* outline areas of pleural calcification, particularly on right hemidiaphragm. This is tip-off to prior asbestos exposure. The process in left mid-lung was worrisome (*large arrow*), perhaps indicating a new process such as bronchogenic carcinoma in this smoker. However, CT, *B*, disclosed rounded atelectasis (*small arrow*). The comma extending from this mass is characteristic of rounded atelectasis, which is result of subacute-to-chronic pleural effusion resolving and trapping some lung as it heals. Also note pleural calcification in *B* (*large arrow*).

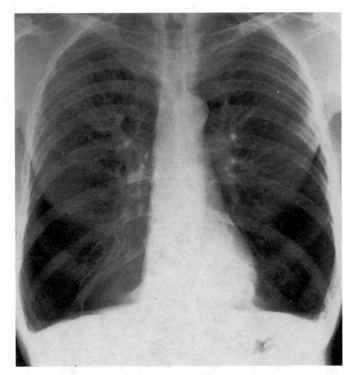

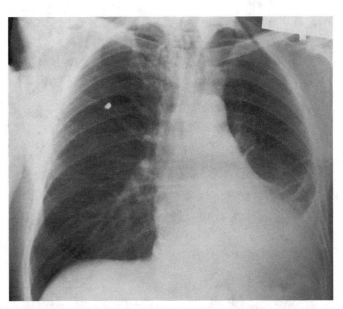

Fig. 7-11. Left pleural effusion, with loss of volume toward instead of away from effusion. This implies loss of volume on the left side for unexplained reasons, because there was no previous injury or surgical procedure in left hemithorax. The cause of left pleural effusion is collapsed left lower lobe from bronchogenic carcinoma (effusion was exudate with negative findings on cytology). Lateral CXR did not help show collapsed left lower lobe. Radiodensity over right hemithorax is shrapnel.

Fig. 7-10. Panlobular emphysema at the bases consistent with diagnosis of α_1-antitrypsin-deficiency emphysema. Emphysema should not be read into CXR, because all it usually represents is hyperinflation that can occur with severe asthma as well. However, in this setting there are markedly diminished interstitial markings at the bases, with radiolucency. Also, there is increased blood flow to the upper lobes because that is where most of the viable lung tissue is. Note flattening of hemidiaphragms from hyperinflation. In early stages, this is a treatable disease.

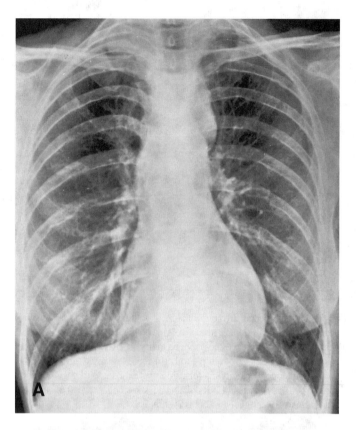

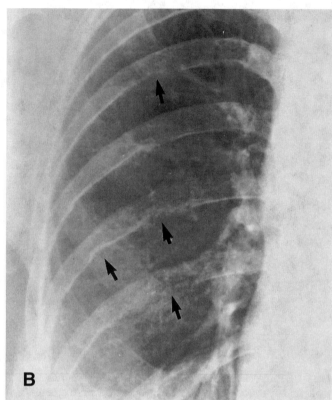

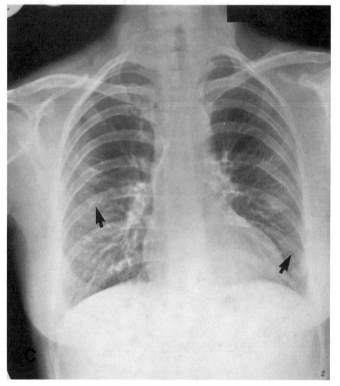

Fig. 7-12. *A*, *B*, and *C*, PA CXR. *A* and *B*, Coarctation with tortuous aorta, mimicking mediastinal mass. This occurs in about 1/3 of patients with coarctation. *C*, Coarctation without mediastinal abnormality. Most important is the rib notching that is very evident on the inferior borders of only a few of the ribs (*arrows* in *B* and *C*).

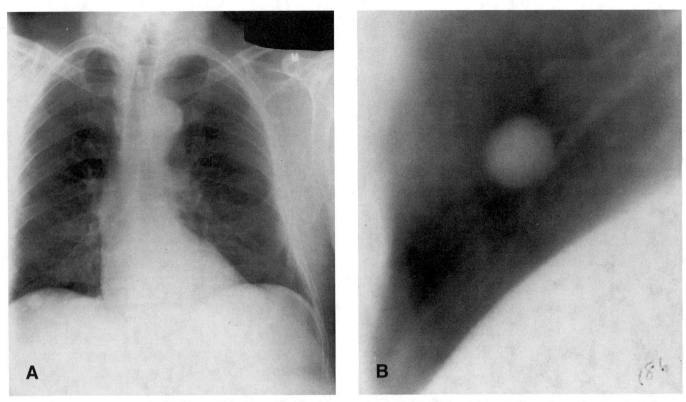

Fig. 7-13. *A*, Solitary pulmonary nodule evident below right hemidiaphragm, where at least 15% of lung is obscured. *B*, Tomography shows nodule has discrete border but is noncalcified. It was not present 18 months earlier. This is an adenocarcinoma.

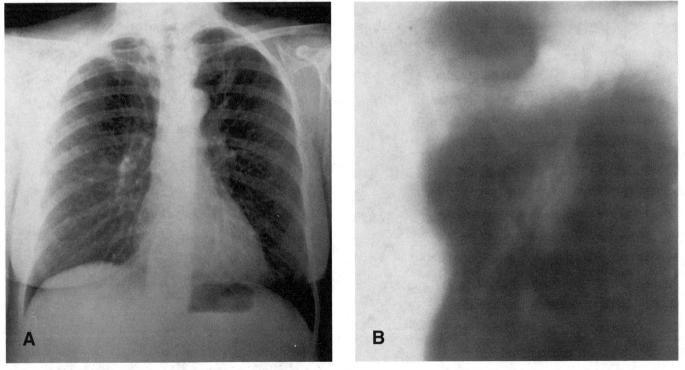

Fig. 7-14. *A*, Solitary infiltrate in left upper lobe with air bronchogram, as evident on tomography or CT. *B*, Air bronchogram should be considered sign of bronchioalveolar cell carcinoma or lymphoma until proved otherwise.

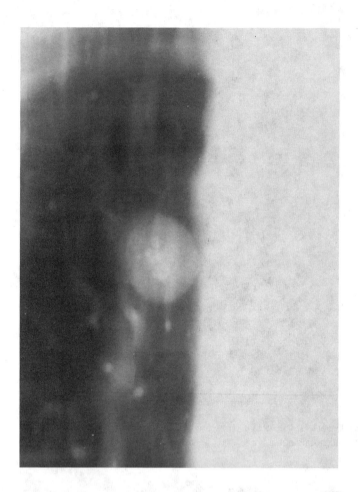

Fig. 7-15. Popcorn calcification of hamartoma. This can also be seen in granuloma and represents a benign process.

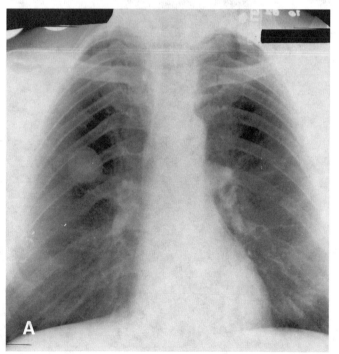

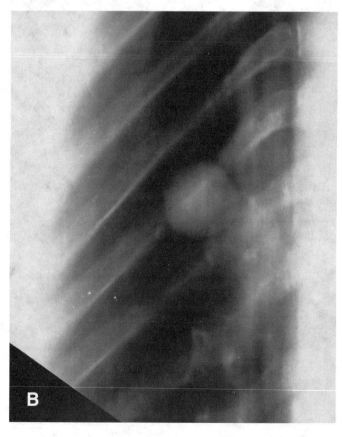

Fig. 7-16. *A* and *B*, Bull's-eye calcification characteristic of granuloma in solitary pulmonary nodule. They occasionally enlarge but even then almost never warrant removal.

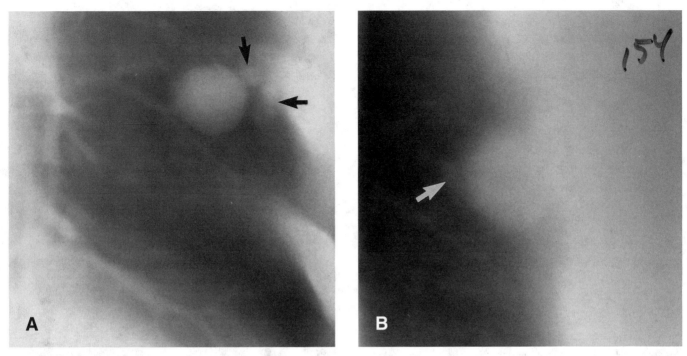

Fig. 7-17. *A* and *B*, Tomography of solitary pulmonary nodules showing satellite nodules (*arrows*). This is characteristic of granulomas.

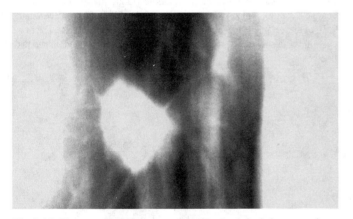

Fig. 7-18. Tomography of solitary nodule showing spiculation, or sunburst effect, characteristic of primary bronchogenic carcinoma. Spicules represent extension of tumor into septa. CT shows similar appearance.

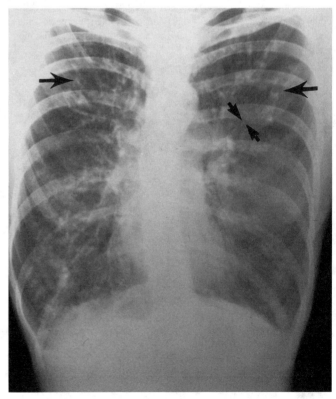

Fig. 7-19. Advanced cystic fibrosis, showing hyperinflation with low-lying hemidiaphragms, bronchiectasis (*small arrows* on parallel lines), and microabscesses (*large arrows*) representing small areas of pneumonitis distal to mucous plug that has been coughed out. For reasons unknown, cystic fibrosis almost always begins in upper lobes.

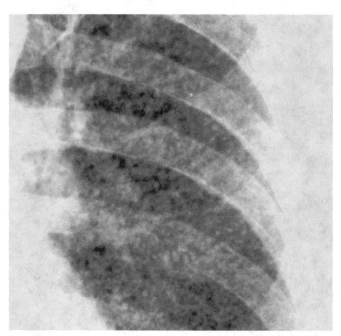

Fig. 7-20. Miliary tuberculosis. CXR shows miliary pattern of relatively discrete micronodules, with little interstitial (linear or reticular) markings. Disseminated fungal disease has similar appearance, as does bronchioalveolar cell carcinoma; however, these patients do not usually have the systemic manifestations of miliary tuberculosis. Other, less common differential diagnoses include lymphoma, lymphocytic interstitial pneumonitis, and pulmonary edema. *Pneumocystis carinii* pneumonia usually has more interstitial reaction.

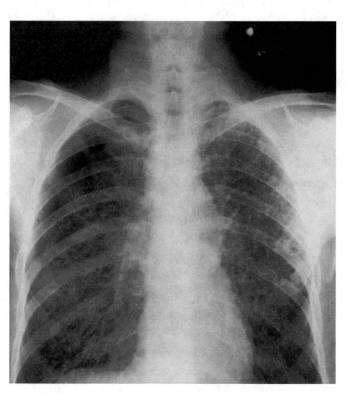

Fig. 7-21. Histiocytosis X, or eosinophilic granuloma, shows extensive change but predominantly in upper two-thirds of lung fields. Eventually 25% of these patients have pneumothorax, as seen on this CXR. The honeycombing, also described as microcysts, is characteristic of advanced histiocytosis X.

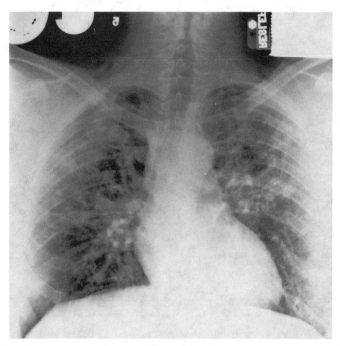

Fig. 7-22. Sarcoidosis in 35-year-old patient. This CXR shows the predominant upper 2/3 parenchymal pattern seen in many patients with stage II or III sarcoidosis. The pattern can be interstitial, alveolar (which this one predominantly is), or a combination. There probably is some residual adenopathy in hila and right paratracheal area.

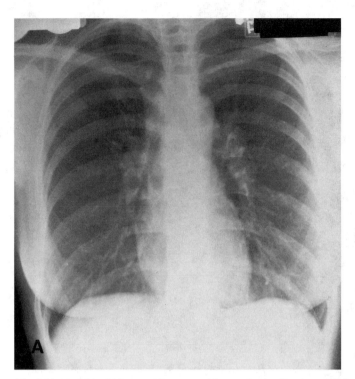
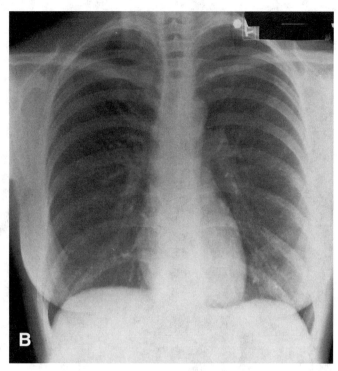

Fig. 7-23. *A*, CXR of 30-year-old woman with stage I pulmonary sarcoidosis with subtle bilateral hilar and mediastinal adenopathy, particularly right para-tracheal and left infra-aortic adenopathy. *B*, CXR 1 year later, after spontaneous regression of sarcoidosis.

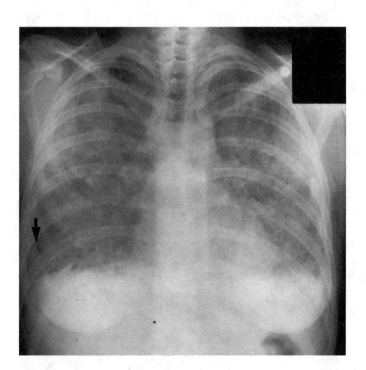

Fig. 7-24. Lymphangitic carcinoma in 27-year-old woman with 6-week history of progressive dyspnea and weight loss. Because of her young age, neoplasm was not considered. Yet, features present on this CXR should have suggested it, viz., bilateral pleural effusions, Kerley's B lines as evident in right base (*arrow*), and mediastinal and hilar lymphadenopathy in addition to diffuse parenchymal infiltrate.

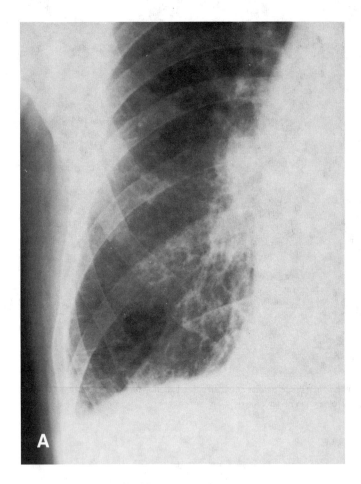

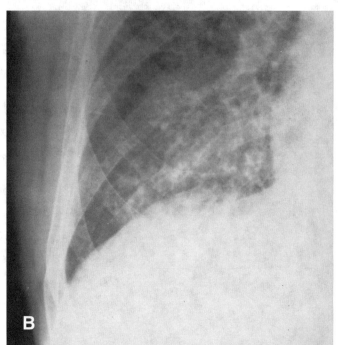

Fig. 7-25. *A* and *B*, Two examples of Kerley's B lines that can be helpful in interpreting CXRs. *A*, Kerley's B lines in a 75-year-old man with colon cancer. *B*, Kerley's B lines are from metastatic adenocarcinoma of the colon and were tip-off that parenchymal process in this patient was due to metastatic carcinoma and not to primary pulmonary process such as pulmonary fibrosis, which was the working diagnosis.

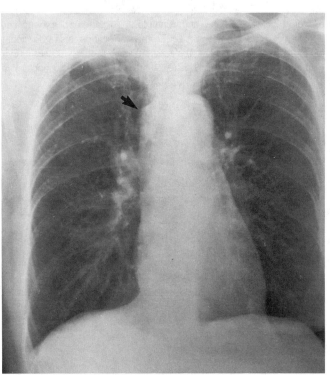

Fig. 7-26. CXR of 55-year-old woman who had had right mastectomy for breast carcinoma now shows subtle but definite right paratracheal (*arrow*) and right hilar adenopathy from metastatic carcinoma of breast.

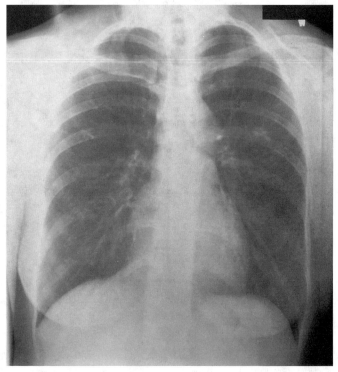

Fig. 7-27. Nodule in left mid-lung field is technically not "solitary pulmonary nodule" because of another abnormality in thorax that might be related to it, viz., left infra-aortic adenopathy. The differential would be bronchogenic carcinoma with hilar nodal metastasis or, as in this case, acute primary pulmonary histoplasmosis. Had this patient been in an area with coccidioidomycosis, that would also be in differential diagnosis.

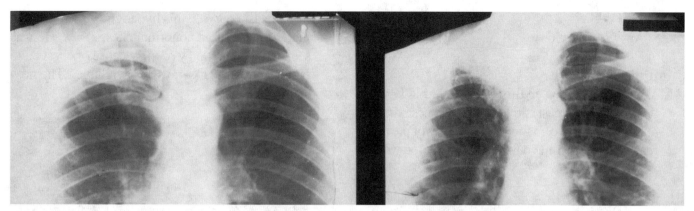

Fig. 7-28. Pancoast tumor. Subtle asymmetry at apex of the right lung was more obvious 3 1/2 years later, at which time the diagnosis of Pancoast lesion (primary bronchogenic carcinoma) was made. The patient was symptomatic at time of initial CXR, with symptoms attributed to cervical disk.

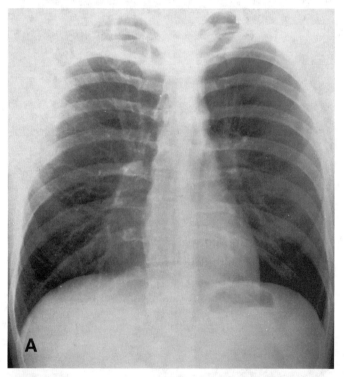

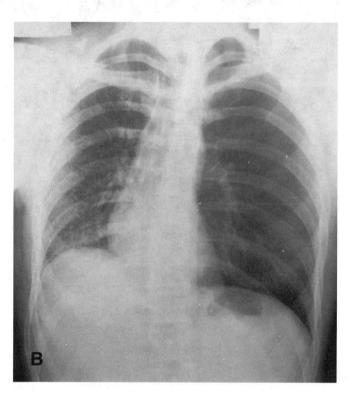

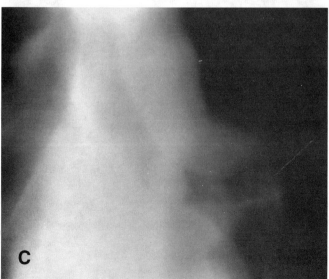

Fig. 7-29. The adage that "not all that wheezes is asthma" should be remembered every time you encounter an asthmatic whose condition does not seem to improve. In the case shown here, A, wheezes were predominant over the left hemithorax. A forced expiration film, B, showed air trapping in left lung. Tomography, C, confirmed a lesion in left mainstem bronchus that was a bronchial carcinoid at bronchoscopy.

Multiple Choice

1. You are asked to see this 59-year-old lady with previous right breast carcinoma. The chest x-ray is read as normal except for "hyperlucency of previous mastectomy." From your interpretation, you would:

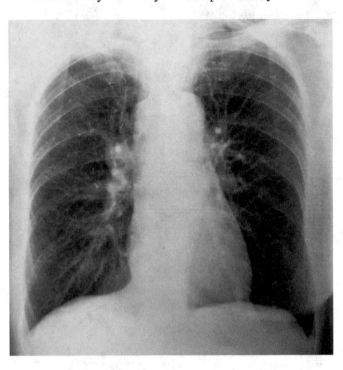

   a. Perform bronchoscopy
   b. Do nothing; repeat chest x-ray in 1 year
   c. Compare with old chest x-rays
   d. Repeat the chest x-ray in 3 months
   e. Order a chest CT

2. You are asked to see this hypertensive 48-year-old man because of an abnormal chest x-ray. He was seen in the emergency room because of chest pain. No previous chest x-rays are available. The next step would be:

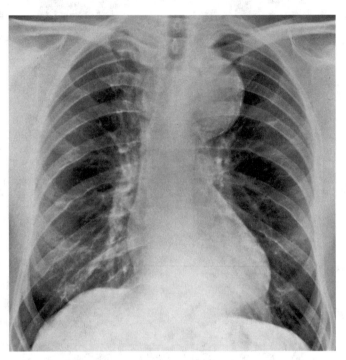

   a. Chest CT
   b. Mediastinoscopy
   c. Barium examination of esophagus
   d. Chest MR
   e. Complete the physical examination

3. The chest x-ray on this 64-year-old woman with a previous carcinoma of the breast was read as within normal limits. On your review you have some concern and order the following:

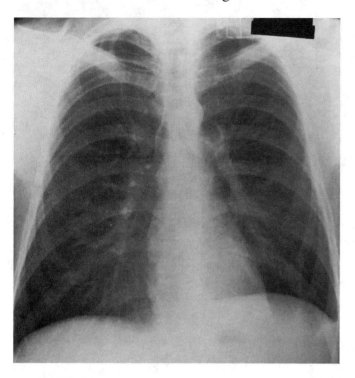

a. CT
b. Right and left decubitus views
c. Bronchoscopy
d. Pulmonary function studies
e. An antibiotic, and suggest follow-up chest x-ray in 3-4 weeks

4. A discrete lesion was found in this chest x-ray (*A*) of an asymptomatic 60-year-old man. The tomogram (*B*) and CT (*C*) are shown. No previous chest x-rays are available. Which of the following is appropriate?

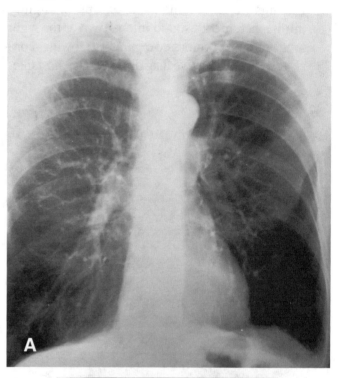

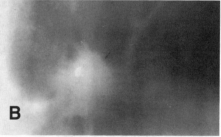

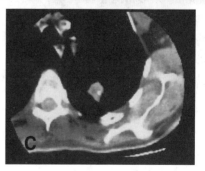

a. Consider thoracotomy
b. A course of broad-spectrum antibiotics and repeat the chest x-ray in 4-6 weeks
c. Repeat chest x-ray in 1 year
d. Bronchoscopy
e. Reassure the patient, because no further follow-up is needed

5. A 42-year-old man who is an office worker presents to you with acute onset of dyspnea. He has smoked 1 1/2 packs per day for 25 years and had been relatively asymptomatic except for a smoker's cough and mild dyspnea on exertion. Physical examination findings were not remarkable except for slightly diminished breath sound intensity over the right lung and some prolonged expiratory slowing, consistent with obstructive lung disease. The most likely diagnosis is:

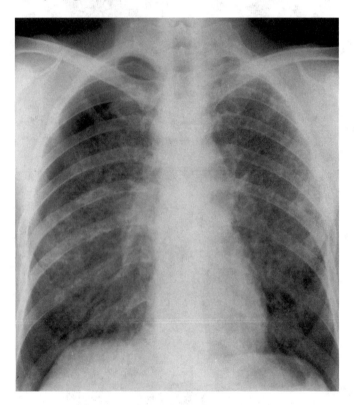

a. Alveolar proteinosis
b. Silicosis
c. Sarcoidosis
d. Idiopathic pulmonary fibrosis
e. Histiocytosis X (eosinophilic granuloma)

6. Which will be the most important question to ask this 56-year-old man whose chest x-ray is shown?

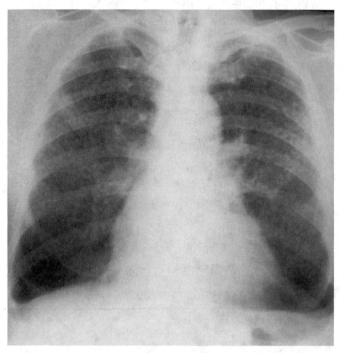

a. Occupational history
b. Smoking history
c. Family history
d. Drug ingestion history
e. History of exposure to tuberculosis

7. A 60-year-old man who is a salesman smoked two packs a day for 40 years. His routine chest x-ray shows that the lesion that has been observed for 2 years is slightly but definitely larger now. He denies all pulmonary complaints. Physical examination findings are normal. Sputum cytology is negative. At this point, you should:
a. Suggest only a repeat chest x-ray yearly
b. Repeat chest x-ray in 3-4 months
c. See if there are any chest x-rays available from more than 2 years ago
d. Reassure the patient and make no recommendations
e. None of the above

True/False

8. The cause of this chest x-ray abnormality is almost always infectious

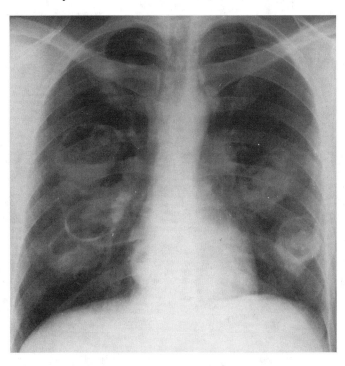

9. The least invasive test to evaluate the mid-lung infiltrate in this patient entails the use of high-resolution CT

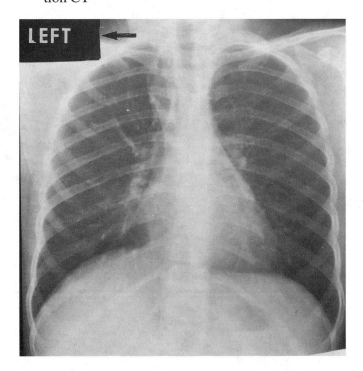

10. The treatment of this pulmonary condition is surgical

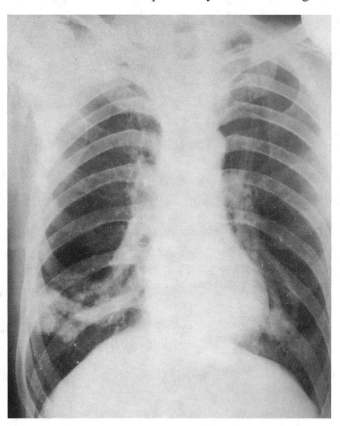

NOTES

CHAPTER 8
CLINICAL PHARMACOLOGY AND TOXICOLOGY

Thomas F. Bugliosi, M.D.

EPIDEMIOLOGY

Most exposures to poison (71%) reported to the American Association of Poison Control Centers in 1991 occurred in persons younger than 19 years. Overall, accidental poisoning outnumbers intentional poisoning in all age groups. However, if only fatal cases are considered (764 in 1991), most occurred in adults, and suicide was the cause in 53%. It is important to remember that the vast majority of all poisonings are not deadly, and most patients do well with good supportive care (Am. J. Emerg. Med. 10:452-491, 1992).

- Most exposures to poison are in persons younger than 19 years.
- Accidental poisoning outnumbers intentional poisoning.
- Vast majority of poisonings are not deadly.

DIAGNOSIS

Clinical

Any patient who presents with an altered mental status should be considered to have taken an overdose. The history provided by the patient is often unreliable, and every effort should be made to interrogate family, friends, paramedics, and law enforcement officers present at the scene. Ask them to bring in pill remnants and containers.

- Patient with altered mental status should be considered to have taken overdose.
- History given by patient is often unreliable.

The next most important step is a thorough general examination. Many frequently encountered poisonings produce classic physical signs and symptoms, and you should be familiar with these. The findings associated with various agents are listed below.

- Many poisonings produce classic physical signs.

Anticholinergic syndrome (atropine, belladonna alkaloid, tricyclic antidepressants, antipsychotics, medications for Parkinson's disease, and antihistamines):

    Dry skin and mucous membranes
    Hyperthermia
    Flushing
    Tachycardia
    Hypertension
    Mydriasis
    ↓ Salivation
    ↓ Sweating
    Ileus
    Urinary retention
    Anxiety/confusion
    Seizures

Pneumonic: "Red as a beet, hot as a hare, dry as a bone, blind as a bat, and mad as a hatter"

Cholinergic syndrome (organophosphate poisoning):

    Sweating
    Salivation
    Lacrimation
    Miosis
    Bradycardia
    Vomiting
    Diarrhea
    Wheezing
    Muscle cramps/fasciculations
    Altered mental status

Acronym is "SLUDGE":
*Salivation, Lacrimation, Urination, Defecation,
Gastrointestinal upset, Emesis*
Opiates (e.g., morphine, codeine, heroin, methadone):
Miosis
Respiratory depression
Drowsiness
Nausea/vomiting
Pulmonary edema
Seizures

Classic triad is depressed mental status, depressed
respiration, miosis.
Barbiturates (e.g., pentobarbital, phenobarbital):
Central nervous system depression
Respiratory depression
Bradycardia
Hypotension
Hypothermia
Areflexia
Pulmonary edema
Blisters
Pupils variable
Stimulants (amphetamines, cocaine, aminophylline):
Central nervous system excitation/agitation
Seizures
Hypertension
Tachycardia
Hallucinations
Arrhythmias/cardiovascular collapse
Mydriasis
Substance withdrawal:
Agitation
Confusion
Mydriasis
Tachycardia
Hypertension
Nausea
Vomiting
Abdominal pain
Seizures

Laboratory Evaluation

Toxicologic Screening

Many misconceptions exist regarding the utility of the standard drug screen. Many commonly encountered drugs cannot be easily detected. The predictive value of a negative toxicologic test is only 40%. Of the drugs that can be detected, quantitative results can be obtained in only 5%-10% of cases. When quantitative results can be measured, they often correlate poorly with clinical signs and symptoms. Most qualitative tests require urine samples, and most quantitative tests require serum samples.

- Predictive value of negative toxicologic test is only 40%.
- Quantitative results reliable in only 5%-10% of cases.
- Most qualitative tests require urine samples; most quantitative tests require serum samples.
- Treat the patient, not the toxicologic screen.

Quantitative drug levels have important therapeutic implications in only a handful of cases:
Acetaminophen
Salicylates
Theophylline
Methanol
Ethylene glycol
Iron
Lithium
Seizure medications (for seizure prophylaxis)
Carbon monoxide
Methemoglobin

Arterial Blood Gases

Perhaps the most useful ancillary blood test that can be performed is the arterial blood gas analysis. This not only will give critical acid-base information but also can diagnose specific poisonings such as carbon monoxide and methemoglobin.

- Arterial blood gas analysis is very useful test.

Osmolar Gap

This is calculated as the difference between the osmolarity as measured by freezing point depression and the calculated osmolarity.

- Calculated osmolarity $= 2\,[Na^+] + \dfrac{BUN}{2.8} + \dfrac{Glucose}{18}$
  (BUN, blood urea nitrogen)
- Osmolar gap = measured osmolarity - calculated osmolarity.
- If osmolar gap >10, consider acetone, ethanol, methanol, ethylene glycol, isopropanol, and diuretics (mannitol, glycerol, or sorbitol).

Anion Gap

The anion gap can be extremely useful in patients with

suspected overdose.

Anion gap = $Na^+ - (Cl^- + HCO_3^-)$; normal gap is 8-12 mEq.

A decreased anion gap can occur in patients with hypermagnesemia, bromide or lithium ingestion, or hypoalbuminemia. An increased anion gap can occur in patients who have ingested methanol, ethylene glycol, propylene glycol, salicylates, strychnine, isoniazid, paraldehyde, phenformin, carbon monoxide, cyanide, or iron. Nontoxicologic causes of an increased anion gap include uremia, diabetic ketoacidosis, and lactic acidosis.

- Iron ingestion is a cause of increased anion gap that is often forgotten.
- Acetaminophen, narcotics, hallucinogens, and stimulants generally do not cause an increased anion gap.

ESSENTIALS OF CARE

Care of the poisoned patient can be divided into 1) supportive care, 2) prevention of further absorption, 3) enhancement of excretion, and 4) administration of a specific antidote.

Supportive Care

Any patient who presents with an altered mental status or confusing symptom complex should be evaluated for drug overdose. Secure airway, breathing, and circulation (ABCs). Most patients will do well with careful attention to the ABCs, including endotracheal intubation if necessary. Intravenous access and cardiac monitoring should be initiated. Confused, agitated, or violent patients require close observation and possibly physical restraints.

- Any patient with altered mental status should be evaluated for drug overdose.
- Secure airway, breathing, circulation (ABCs).
- Establish intravenous access and cardiac monitoring.

Dextrose (D_{50}) was once considered "standard" care of patients with altered mental status. A growing body of evidence, however, suggests that elevated glucose concentrations during cerebral ischemia worsen brain injury and decrease functional recovery. Therefore, every patient with altered mental status should have a quick fingerstick blood glucose determination. Dextrose should be admin-

istered to patients with documented hypoglycemia. In addition, administer 100 mg thiamine intramuscularly to alcoholic patients.

- Elevated glucose concentrations during cerebral ischemia may worsen brain injury and decrease functional recovery.
- Every patient with altered mental status should have quick fingerstick blood glucose determination.
- Alcoholic patients should be treated with 100 mg thiamine intramuscularly.

Naloxone (Narcan) was also considered standard care of patients with altered mental status. Naloxone has been reported to cause pulmonary edema in a few anecdotal case reports. Patients with hypoventilation, miosis, or other signs of narcotic abuse who present with altered mental status should be given 2 mg naloxone by intravenous push. Naloxone can also be given subcutaneously or intramuscularly or by endotracheal tube. Remember that many narcotics have longer half-lives than naloxone, so all patients require prolonged monitoring for resedation.

- Naloxone has been reported to rarely cause pulmonary edema.
- Naloxone 2 mg intravenously should be given in patients with hypoventilation, miosis, or signs of narcotic abuse.
- All patients require prolonged monitoring for resedation.

Prevention of Further Absorption

Many toxins can be absorbed through the skin, and decontamination of the skin is mandatory in such cases. Gastric emptying can be accomplished with induced emesis or gastric lavage utilizing a large-bore (32- to 40-French) tube. In general, there has been a significant trend away from these treatments for several reasons.

- No studies prove that these efforts positively influence outcome.
- Recent studies have shown that activated charcoal alone may be superior to either induced emesis or gastric lavage, and it seems to cause fewer complications.
- Gastric emptying is time-consuming in a busy emergency department.
- Either method of gastric emptying removes only about 30% of ingested material.

Induced Emesis

Syrup of ipecac is the only acceptable emetic. It acts centrally (medulla) and peripherally. Vomiting usually occurs within 20 minutes. The usual adult dose is 30 mL, which may be given again in 30 minutes if vomiting has not occurred.

An indication for ipecac is ingestion of a potentially toxic substance in the home setting in persons older than 6 months. Contraindications are nontoxic ingestions, caustic ingestions, hydrocarbon ingestions, age younger than 6 months, altered mental status, poor gag reflex, seizures, and substance likely to alter mental status rapidly (e.g,. tricyclics). Complications are prolonged vomiting, Mallory-Weiss tear, aspiration pneumonia, intracranial hemorrhage, and delayed charcoal administration.

- Ipecac is the only acceptable emetic.
- Usual adult dose is 30 mL; may be repeated in 30 minutes.
- Aspiration is major concern with ipecac.
- Patient must be alert and likely to stay that way.

Gastric Lavage

This is accomplished with the patient in the left lateral decubitus position; a large-bore orogastric tube is used. A cuffed endotracheal tube should be placed before procedure if patient has altered mental status, depressed gag reflex, or seizures. Indications are recent (<1 hour) ingestion of a potentially toxic substance, substances not well bound by charcoal, or toxic substances that delay gastric emptying. Contraindications are nontoxic ingestions, caustic ingestions, and patients who present >1 hour after ingestion, except in cases of potentially delayed gastric emptying. Complications are aspiration pneumonia, perforation of esophagus or stomach, and inadvertent tracheal intubation.

- Before gastric lavage, cuffed endotracheal tube should be placed if patient has altered mental status, depressed gag reflex, or seizures.

Activated Charcoal

Activated charcoal is emerging as the treatment of choice for most poisonings. It is an inert compound that binds to most substances. The dose is generally 1 g/kg body weight. This may be given as a slurry down an orogastric tube or nasogastric tube, or the patient can drink it. Charcoal is generally ineffective for absorbing small ionic compounds such as lithium, magnesium, arsenic,

and alcohols. In addition, charcoal should not be given in cases of caustic ingestions because the caustic substances are poorly bound by activated charcoal, and the subsequent endoscopic view will be obscured. Pulse charcoal in which 50 g of charcoal is given every 2 to 4 hours has theoretical value in overdoses involving drugs that undergo enterohepatic circulation (e.g., barbiturates, meprobamate, carbamazepine, theophylline, phenytoin, tricyclics). Data are not conclusive, however, and the complication rate may be increased. Administration of cathartics after charcoal administration has not been proved to be effective.

- Activated charcoal emerging as treatment of choice for most poisonings.
- Dose is 1 g/kg body weight.
- Charcoal generally ineffective for absorbing small ionic compounds such as lithium, magnesium, arsenic, alcohols.
- Charcoal should not be given for caustic ingestion.

Enhancement of Excretion

Several methods may enhance excretion: forced diuresis, alkaline or acid diuresis, hemodialysis, and hemoperfusion. A brief review of volume of distribution is necessary to understand the limited role enhancement of excretion plays in most overdoses.

The volume of distribution (V_d) is defined as that volume of fluid into which a drug seems to distribute with the concentration equal to that in plasma. It is a hypothetical volume only. It does not refer to any physiologic space. When V_d is large (>1 liter/kg), the tissue concentration is large (and vice versa).

$$V_d = \frac{A \text{ (amount ingested)}}{C \text{ (plasma concentration)}}$$

The V_d can be used to predict the serum level of a drug if the amount ingested is known. For example, if a 70-kg patient ingested 50 100-mg tablets of phenytoin ($V_d = 0.75$ liter/kg), the plasma level can be predicted:

$$V_d = \frac{A}{C} \qquad V_d = 0.75 \text{ liter/kg x 70 kg} = 52.5 \text{ liters}$$

$$52.5 \text{ liters} = \frac{5,000 \text{ mg}}{C} = 95 \text{ mg/liter}$$

Drugs are eliminated by first order, zero order, or combination kinetics. First-order elimination is how the kidney handles toxins. A constant fraction of the drug is eliminated per unit time. The higher the plasma concentration, the greater the amount of drug excreted per unit time. Zero-order elimination is how the liver handles toxins. This type of elimination involves saturable enzymes that, when saturated, allow only for a constant amount of drug to be eliminated. Once enzymes are saturated, serum levels can increase dramatically. Examples include phenytoin, salicylates, and ethanol. Combination elimination occurs with salicylates, phenytoin, and ethanol. These drugs switch their elimination from first-order to zero-order elimination.

- First-order elimination is how kidney handles toxins.
- Zero-order elimination is how liver handles toxins.
- Combination elimination occurs with salicylates, phenytoin, ethanol in the therapeutic range.

Forced Diuresis

Most attempts at increasing drug elimination by forced diuresis (thereby increasing urine flow) are not successful. In general, for many drugs, elimination by renal excretion is not dependent on urine flow rates. In addition, drugs that are highly protein-bound or have a large volume of distribution (V_d) are not affected by forced diuresis.

- Most attempts at forced diuresis are not successful.
- Drugs that are highly protein-bound are not affected by forced diuresis.

Urine Alkalinization

Weak acids such as salicylates, phenobarbital, and isoniazid are ionized in a more alkaline medium. Promoting an alkaline urine by alkalinizing a patient slows reabsorption of weakly acidic compounds because they will exist as anions that do not readily cross lipid membranes. As a result, urinary clearance is increased. An alkaline diuresis is accomplished by adding 1 ampule of $NaHCO_3$ to 1 liter of 0.45 normal saline and monitoring urine pH.

Urine Acidification

Although several drugs (e.g., amphetamines and phencyclidine) may have their elimination enhanced by acidifying the urine, this is not recommended because of the possibility of acute tubular necrosis caused by rhabdomyolysis.

- Urine acidification not recommended because of possibility of acute renal tubular necrosis.

Hemodialysis

Hemodialysis has very limited application in drug overdoses. Suitable substances should be of small molecular weight and soluble, have limited protein and lipid binding, and have a small volume of distribution (V_d). The driving force is the concentration gradient of unbound, ultrafiltrable solute.

Hemodialysis is indicated in some cases of the following overdoses (depending on patient's condition): ethylene glycol, methanol, lithium, salicylates, bromide. Hemodialysis is not indicated for overdoses of tricyclic antidepressants, antihistamines, benzodiazepines, digitalis, phenothiazines, opiates, ethchlorvynol.

Hemoperfusion

Hemoperfusion is accomplished by pumping a patient's blood through an extracorporeal cartridge containing adsorbent particles (activated charcoal, carbon, or polystyrene resin). The factors that limit toxin removal in hemodialysis are not as important in hemoperfusion.

Hemoperfusion is indicated in some cases of ingestions of phenobarbital, other barbiturates, diphenylhydantoin, and theophylline. The major rate-limiting factors are the affinity of the absorbent for the toxin and the rate of blood flow through the circuit. Complications include thrombocytopenia, leukopenia, hypoglycemia, and hypocalcemia. Most overdoses can be managed without hemodialysis or hemoperfusion. Applications must be considered on an individual basis.

- In hemoperfusion, major rate-limiting factors are affinity of absorbent for toxin and rate of blood flow through circuit.
- Complications include thrombocytopenia, leukopenia, hypoglycemia, hypocalcemia.
- Most overdoses can be managed without hemodialysis or hemoperfusion.

Administration of an Antidote

There are specific antidotes for only a few agents involved in overdoses. Even when a specific antidote is available, it is often not needed, and supportive care is all that is necessary. A partial list of antidotes is included in Table 8-1.

CYCLIC ANTIDEPRESSANTS

Overdose with cyclic antidepressants (e.g., imipramine, amitriptyline, desipramine, doxepin) is one of the most

Table 8-1.--Antidotes for Agents Associated With Overdose

Drug/toxin	Antidote
Acetaminophen	*N*-acetylcysteine
Anticholinergics	Physostigmine
Benzodiazepines	Flumazenil
Carbon monoxide	Oxygen
Cyanide	Amyl nitrite, sodium nitrite, sodium thiosulfate
Ethylene glycol	Ethanol
Iron	Deferoxamine
Isoniazid	Pyridoxine
Methanol	Ethanol
Narcotics	Naloxone
Nitrites	Methylene blue
Organophosphates	Atropine
	Pralidoxime
Tricyclics	Sodium bicarbonate

From Bryson PD: Comprehensive Review in Toxicology. Second edition. New York, Raven Press, 1989, p 11. By permission of publisher.

serious types of overdose; it causes approximately 25% of all deaths due to poisoning. They are rapidly absorbed and readily distribute to body tissues and fat. In fact, tissue levels may be much higher than plasma levels. Cyclic antidepressants have a high degree of protein binding (85%-99%) and a huge volume of distribution (V_d) (i.e., not removed by hemodialysis or hemoperfusion). Increasing pH increases protein binding; thus, less free drug is available to exert its effect.

- Overdose with cyclic antidepressants one of most serious types of overdose.
- Causes about 25% of all deaths due to poisoning.
- Cyclic antidepressants are rapidly absorbed and readily distribute to body tissues and fat.
- They have high degree of protein binding.

Tricyclics (most cyclic antidepressants have three rings) have four main actions (Table 8-2):
1. Block reuptake of norepinephrine in central nervous system
2. Class IA antiarrhythmic effects (quinidine-like)
3. Antihistamine (H_1 and H_2 antagonist)
4. Anticholinergic activity

Table 8-2.--Effects of Tricyclic Antidepressants

Action	Clinical findings
1. Quinidine-like effect	↓ Myocardial contractility
	↑ Myocardial conduction
	Increased P-R and Q-T intervals
	Widened QRS
	Ventricular arrhythmia
	Hypotension
2. Anticholinergic	Supraventricular tachycardia, hyperthermia, mydriasis, anxiety, hallucinations, seizures, coma, death
3. Block reuptake of norepinephrine	↓ Myocardial contractility
	Hypotension
	Bradycardia
4. Antihistamine	

Toxic effects vary, but rapid deterioration is common. Ventricular arrhythmias, seizures, hypotension, and respiratory depression are some of the more dangerous side effects to anticipate. Maprotiline (Ludiomil) is a tetracyclic antidepressant that demonstrates more seizures but fewer cardiovascular side effects. Remember, cardiotoxicity is the main cause of death associated with cyclic antidepressants.

- Toxic effects vary, but rapid deterioration is common with overdose of cyclic antidepressants.

Treatment of patients who have overdosed on cyclic antidepressants first includes securing the ABCs. Because seizures or rapid deterioration is common, many patients require endotracheal intubation. Do not induce vomiting. After ABCs are secured, gastric lavage is indicated even if several hours have elapsed since ingestion because the anticholinergic effects cause delayed gastric emptying. Activated charcoal is recommended and, because of enterohepatic circulation, pulse charcoal may be of benefit. Cardiac monitoring is needed for all patients for a minimum of 24 hours.

- Seizures or rapid deterioration is common with overdose of cyclic antidepressants.
- Do not induce vomiting.
- Activated charcoal is recommended.

Treatment of specific complications is outlined below:

1) Cardiotoxicity: Alkalinization causes more cyclic antidepressant to be protein-bound, leaving less free drug to exert its effect. It may be the best treatment of most forms of cardiovascular toxicity and can narrow widened QRS complexes, abolish arrhythmias, and improve perfusion. The goal is a serum pH of about 7.5. Dysrhythmias should be treated with alkalinization. Lidocaine and phenytoin are both reasonable choices for ventricular arrhythmias. Bretylium has an effect similar to that of the tricyclics and should be avoided. Class IA agents (quinidine, procainamide, and disopyramide) should be avoided.

2) Seizures: After alkalinization, diazepam and phenytoin are used, as for other patients with seizures. Refractory seizures should be treated with phenobarbital or general anesthesia.

3) Hypotension: After fluid challenge and alkalinization, you may need catecholamine pressors such as epinephrine, norepinephrine, or phenylephrine. Isoproterenol, dobutamine, and low-dose dopamine should be avoided because they may worsen hypotension through unopposed β-adrenergic effect. (Cyclic antidepressants produce strong α-adrenergic blockade.)

4) Anticholinergic toxicity: Physostigmine can reverse the anticholinergic effects of cyclic antidepressants, but its use is controversial. It has a low therapeutic:toxic ratio and can produce cholinergic crises. Its use should be limited to patients with severe hypertension, seizures, or dysrhythmias not responsive to other forms of therapy.

- Lidocaine and phenytoin are reasonable choices for ventricular arrhythmias.
- Refractory seizures should be treated with phenobarbital or general anesthesia.
- For hypotension, avoid isoproterenol, dobutamine, and low-dose dopamine.

- Physostigmine can reverse anticholinergic effects of cyclic antidepressants; it has low therapeutic:toxic ratio and can produce cholinergic crises.

ACETAMINOPHEN

Acetaminophen is the active metabolite of phenacetin and is a common over-the-counter antipyretic analgesic available in many forms. It is rapidly absorbed. Toxicity is from a minor metabolite formed via the cytochrome P450 system. Actually, most of an acetaminophen dose is conjugated with glucuronic acid and sulfate and then excreted by the kidneys. Only a very small amount is metabolized by the cytochrome P450 system. In cases of overdose, however, the sulfate and glucuronide conjugating systems are saturated, so more metabolism occurs through the cytochrome P450 system. Under normal circumstances, the metabolite of this system is conjugated with hepatic glutathione and excreted. In the case of overdose, however, hepatic glutathione is rapidly depleted and the metabolite binds to hepatocytes, producing cell death.

- Acetaminophen is active metabolite of phenacetin.
- It is rapidly absorbed.
- In acetaminophen overdose, sulfate and glucuronide conjugating systems are saturated, so more metabolism occurs through cytochrome P450 system.
- In overdose, metabolite binds to hepatocytes, producing cell death.

Hepatotoxicity, the main complication of acetaminophen overdose, can be predicted accurately with a nomogram (Fig. 8-1). This is based on the estimate that 15 g of acetaminophen in a single ingestion causes hepatotoxicity in an adult. For safety, and because patients with chronic liver disease have less glutathione stores, 7.5 g is used for the nomogram. Remember that patients taking phenobarbital and alcohol have stimulated cytochrome P450 systems and are more likely to experience toxicity at any given dose.

- Hepatotoxicity is main complication of acetaminophen overdose.

Treatment of acetaminophen overdose requires precise determination of the time of ingestion and quantified serum levels of acetaminophen. For patients who are in the "toxic" range on the nomogram, treatment with

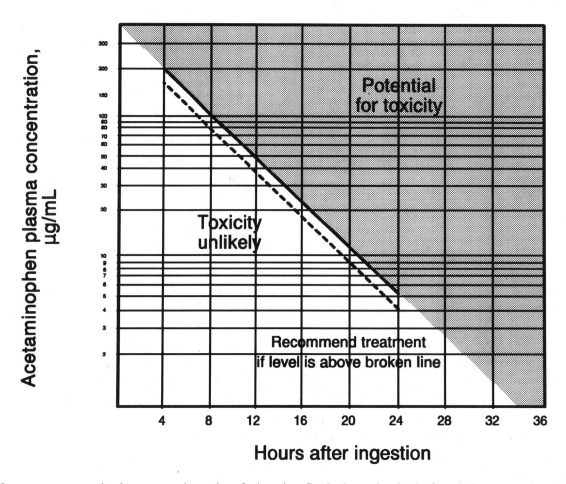

Fig. 8-1. Plasma or serum acetaminophen concentration vs. time after ingestion. Graph relates only to levels after a single acute overdose. Broken line represents 25% allowance below solid line; it is included to allow for possible errors in acetaminophen assays and estimated time from ingestion of overdose. (From Chiang WK, Wang RY: Evaluation and management of acute acetaminophen toxicity. Emerg Med Reports 14:83-90, 1993 and from McNeil Consumer Products Co., as adapted from Rumack BH, Matthews H. Acetaminophen poisoning and toxicity. Pediatrics 55:871-876, 1975. By permission of American Health Consultants, McNeil Conumer Products Co., and Pediatrics.)

N-acetylcysteine is indicated. *N*-Acetylcysteine provides a -SH group for the toxic intermediary to bind to, thus sparing the hepatocytes. *N*-Acetylcysteine is given orally in the United States, but it has been used intravenously in other countries for years, and it should be given within 24 hours of ingestion. The loading dose of 140 mg/kg is followed by 70 mg/kg every 4 hours for 17 doses. The odor is offensive, and it may be best to give it through a nasogastric tube.

- For patients in toxic range of acetaminophen overdose, treatment with *N*-acetylcysteine is indicated.
- Treatment should be given within 24 hours of ingestion.

There is some debate regarding the initial treatment of acetaminophen overdose. There is theoretical concern that if you give activated charcoal initially, it may also bind the antidote (*N*-acetylcysteine). In practice, however, this is not a major concern, and because activated charcoal binds acetaminophen well, most investigators recommend it. Induced emesis should be avoided because prolonged vomiting may delay giving *N*-acetylcysteine if it is found to be indicated.

SALICYLATES

Salicylates are weak acids that are rapidly absorbed and have a small volume of distribution (V_d, 0.2 liter/kg). Although the half-life is short (15 minutes) under normal conditions, in case of overdose the half-life may be prolonged to 20 hours. Overall, the number of accidental ingestions has decreased, and most toxicity is now related to chronic salicylate use. A 50% increase in the daily dose of aspirin can result in a 300% increase in plasma level. As salicylate levels increase, a typical pattern of acid-base disturbances occurs:

Respiratory → Respiratory → Metabolic acidosis
alkalosis   alkalosis   (anion gap)
                        +
             Metabolic acidosis
                (anion gap)

This pattern may be accelerated in children. About the only abnormality that does not occur is metabolic alkalosis.

- In salicylate overdose, half-life may be prolonged to 20 hours.
- Most toxicity related to chronic salicylate use.
- 50% increase in daily dose of aspirin can result in 300% increase in plasma level.

Other symptoms and signs of salicylate overdose are listed in Table 8-3.

Table 8-3.--Clinical and Laboratory Abnormalities in Salicylate Overdose

Central nervous system	Gastrointestinal	Pulmonary	Renal	Miscellaneous
Tinnitus	Nausea	Tachypnea	Tubular	Hyperpyrexia
Delirium	Vomiting	Noncardiogenic	necrosis	Hypokalemia
Stupor	Gastritis	pulmonary edema		Hypoglycemia
Coma				Platelet dysfunction
Seizures				Acid-base
				disturbances

An elderly patient who is confused and has a high anion gap metabolic acidosis or unexplained respiratory alkalosis may have salicylate toxicity. This is a common presentation. Salicylate intoxication can cause noncardiogenic pulmonary edema.

Treatment includes usual supportive care and activated charcoal. Consider gastric lavage if the duration since ingestion is <1 hour. Fluids should be given to correct losses and to promote diuresis. Potassium levels need to be monitored carefully. Alkalinization increases urinary excretion of salicylates dramatically and may prevent salicylates from crossing the blood-brain barrier (ion trapping). Hemodialysis is used in certain cases, such as renal failure, noncardiogenic pulmonary edema, persistent or progressive central nervous system manifestations, and deterioration despite adequate supportive care and alkaline diuresis.

- Treatment of salicylate overdose: activated charcoal, fluids to correct losses and promote diuresis, monitoring of potassium levels, alkalinization to increase urinary excretion, hemodialysis in some cases.

THEOPHYLLINE

Theophylline is approximately 50% protein-bound, and about 90% of excretion occurs through liver metabolism. Metabolism is increased with cigarette smoking and use of phenobarbital or phenytoin. Metabolism is decreased with erythromycin, cimetidine, propranolol, ciprofloxacin, and heart failure or liver disease. The clinical presentation of theophylline toxicity depends not only on the amount of drug ingested but also on whether the patient is chronically maintained on theophylline. Patients who chronically take theophylline have more toxicity, in general, than their counterparts at the same serum level.

- Theophylline is 50% protein-bound; 90% of excretion is through liver metabolism.
- Patients who chronically take theophylline have more toxicity than their counterparts at same serum level.

Symptoms of theophylline toxicity are nausea and vomiting, agitation, tachypnea, cardiac arrhythmia (atrial fibrillation, multifocal atrial tachycardia, ventricular tachycardia, ventricular fibrillation), and seizures. Seizures increase mortality and may be first manifestation. Hypokalemia, hypophosphatemia, and hyperglycemia are also seen.

Treatment includes routine supportive decontamination procedures. Pulse charcoal may be beneficial. Hemoperfusion is indicated for patients with rising serum levels or seizures from sustained-release products and for patients whose condition is deteriorating despite appropriate initial management. Although levels do not correlate well with toxicity, if the plasma level is >40 µg/mL in chronic overdose or >80 μg/mL in acute overdose, consider hemoperfusion.

IRON

Iron poisoning is a common cause of pediatric ingestion emergencies. It is much less common in adults. Toxicity may occur at doses of 20-60 mg/kg. Lethal dose is 60-80 mg/kg of elemental iron.

Clinically, several phases are encountered in overdose: *Phase I* (gastrointestinal symptoms 1/2 to 6 hours)-- nausea, vomiting, hematemesis, abdominal pain, diarrhea
Phase II (6-24 hours): latent period, patient seems to improve. Anion gap metabolic acidosis
Phase III (systemic toxicity): altered mental status, seizures, hepatic/renal failure, coagulopathy, death
Phase IV (late complications): gastrointestinal obstruction

Initial treatment includes standard supportive care and gastric emptying. Some authors recommend gastric lavage be performed with $NaHCO_3$, which converts iron to a less absorbable salt. This practice is controversial and not thoroughly investigated. Activated charcoal may be given but is of questionable value. Overall, iron is fairly resistant to various stomach decontamination regimes.

Patients suffering from significant iron overdose should have adequate crystalloid fluid resuscitation. Deferoxamine is a chelating agent that enhances iron elimination by producing a water-soluble substance (ferrioxamine) that can be excreted by the kidneys. It is administered intravenously at a rate of 15 mg/kg per hour. Deferoxamine should be given in any moderately or severely symptomatic patient regardless of iron levels, if serum iron level is >350 μg/dL, or in any patient whose serum iron level is greater than total iron-binding capacity.

A word of caution is in order in regard to treating patients for iron overdose. First, although iron tablets often show up on abdominal radiograph, their absence is not a guarantee that a significant iron overdose has not occurred. Second, a patient who presents to the emergency department in phase II (latent period) may appear well despite having taken a serious overdose. Finally, do not withhold chelation therapy in moderately or severely symptomatic patients while waiting for determination of serum iron levels.

- Deferoxamine is a specific chelating agent for iron.

- Serum iron levels should not be solely relied on in determining need for deferoxamine therapy.
- A normal abdominal radiograph does not exclude severe iron overdose.

LITHIUM

In general, lithium has a low therapeutic index. In acute intoxication, serum levels may not accurately reflect the severity of overdose. Early signs of toxicity are nausea and vomiting, dysarthria, and hand tremor. Later signs are ataxia, fasciculations, hyperreflexia, confusion, seizures, coma, and cardiotoxicity (rare).

Charcoal is not used for treatment because it does not absorb lithium. Rehydration with normal saline is helpful (lithium can cause nephrogenic diabetes insipidus). Alkalinization of the urine can increase renal excretion of lithium. Hemodialysis should be considered for patients with renal failure, patients with deterioration after appropriate treatment, or if serum lithium levels exceed 4 mEq/L.

β-ADRENERGIC BLOCKERS

Extremely small doses of β-blockers can produce life-threatening reactions. Blood levels are not helpful. Clinical findings include bradycardia (many rhythm types), hypotension, peripheral cyanosis, pulmonary edema, altered mental status, and many electrocardiographic abnormalities.

The treatment of β-adrenergic blocker overdose includes gastric lavage rather than emesis induction because β-adrenergic blockers taken in large quantity exert their effects quickly. Activated charcoal should also be administered. The hypotension and bradycardia are often refractory to usual therapies, including dopamine, epinephrine, and atropine. Intravenous glucagon seems to be the most consistent agent for reversing the toxic effects of β-adrenergic blocker overdose. Glucagon is given as an intravenous bolus (0.05-0.15 mg/kg) followed by a continuous infusion at 2-5 mg/hour.

- Glucagon is most consistent agent for reversing β-adrenergic blocker toxicity.

DIGITALIS

Clinical manifestations of digitalis toxicity include both cardiac and noncardiac symptoms. Toxic effects of digitalis in patients receiving chronic therapy can occur at any serum level. Acute overdoses of digitalis are rare but usually severe.

Noncardiac signs and symptoms are nausea, vomiting, abdominal pain, confusion, hallucinations, occasionally seizures, visual disturbances (many), and hyperkalemia. Cardiac symptoms are junctional tachycardia, ventricular premature contractions, ventricular tachycardia, ventricular fibrillation, atrial flutter, atrial fibrillation, and all types of atrioventricular block. Although hypokalemia increases the risk of toxicity in patients chronically taking digitalis, hyperkalemia is a complication of acute digitalis overdose.

Treatment includes supportive care with cardiac monitoring, and gastric emptying if ingestion was recent. Treat dangerous hyperkalemia with intravenous glucose, insulin, and bicarbonate. AVOID calcium in cases of digitalis toxicity. Atropine may be effective for bradycardias, as may external pacemakers. Treat stable ventricular arrhythmias with lidocaine or phenytoin. Magnesium sulfate may be beneficial. Digoxin immune Fab (ovine) (Digibind) is digoxin-specific antibody fragments that have been induced in sheep. It acts by binding digoxin molecules, making them incapable of binding at their receptor, the Na^+K^+-ATPase. Its use should be reserved for severe intoxication. It is given intravenously, and its dose is titrated to clinical effect. Many vials are often required. Because serum digoxin levels reflect both bound and unbound drug, they may actually increase over several hours.

- Avoid calcium in digitalis toxicity.
- Atropine may be effective for bradycardias.
- Lidocaine or phenytoin is preferred agent for ventricular irritability.
- Digoxin-specific Fab fragments reserved for severe intoxication.

CYANIDE

Cyanide binds to iron in cytochrome oxidase, and the result is cellular hypoxia. It does not combine with the iron in hemoglobin. Cyanide is used in many industries, and the natural environment contains various cyanogenic glycosides that, when broken down and ingested, can release cyanide.

- Cyanide binds to iron in cytochrome oxidase.
- It does not combine with the iron in hemoglobin.

Clinical symptoms with inhalation (symptoms within seconds) are dry, burning throat, air hunger, hyperpnea, apnea, seizures, and death. Symptoms with ingestion (symptoms delayed) are nausea, vomiting, confusion, vertigo, giddiness, seizures, and cardiac dysrhythmias.

The diagnosis of cyanide overdose must initially be made clinically because rapid deterioration leading to death can occur well before any laboratory confirmation can be obtained. The history may provide clues to occupational cyanide exposure (electroplating, metallurgy, etc.), intentional cyanide exposure (suicide attempt), or accidental ingestion (apricot, plum, or peach pits). The odor of bitter almonds or peach pits is diagnostic of cyanide poisoning. Finally, a patient with altered mental status and tachypnea but no cyanosis suggests cyanide overdose.

Treatment includes supplemental high-flow 100% oxygen. If cyanide is ingested, consider gastric lavage and charcoal. Nitrite-thiosulfate therapy is the therapy of choice in cyanide overdose. The nitrite causes creation of methemoglobin, which allows cyanide to bind to this rather than the cytochromic system. Thiosulfate then converts this to thiocyanate, which can be excreted by the kidney.

OPIOIDS

Opioids include many drugs that often are abused in society (e.g., morphine, heroin, methadone, codeine, propoxyphene, opium, fentanyl, meperidine). Morphine, opium, and codeine are the only natural (opium-derived) opioids. All other opioids require minor or major chemical alterations to produce.

Clinical features of opioid overdose are drowsiness, lethargy, respiratory depression, coma, nausea, vomiting, miosis, ileus, urinary retention, and pulmonary edema.

- Morphine, opium, and codeine are natural opioids.
- Heroin and methadone cause pulmonary edema.
- Classic opioid triad: respiratory depression, pinpoint pupils, coma.

Opioid ingestions are associated with other drugs in 90% of cases, and 95% of all emergency room visits by opioid abusers are for infections or trauma (not overdose). Thiamine, 100 mg intramuscularly, is given. If the blood glucose level is <80 mg/dL, 50 mL of dextrose (D_{50}, push) is given. Naloxone (Narcan), 2 mg by intravenous bolus, is given and repeated as necessary. A continuous infusion is occasionally required. Naloxone can be given intravenously, intramuscularly, or subcutaneously or by endotracheal tube. Many opioids have a longer half-life than naloxone, so prolonged monitoring for resedation is necessary.

- 90% of opioid ingestions are associated with other drugs.
- Patients successfully treated with naloxone require prolonged monitoring.

COCAINE

Although legally classified as a narcotic, cocaine is the only naturally occurring local anesthetic. When abused, it may be injected intravenously or subcutaneously, swallowed, smoked, or applied to oral or genital mucous membranes. Cocaine is cut with many substances, some of which have toxicity of their own.

Clinical features of cocaine use are excitement, euphoria, restlessness, nausea, vomiting, headache, seizures, tachycardia or hypertension, hypoventilation, psychosis, and mydriasis. Serious effects are malignant hyperthermia, seizures, and ventricular tachycardia.

The treatment of cocaine overdose is generally supportive. Seizures may be treated with diazepam and phenytoin. Propranolol can be used for severe hypertension or tachycardia, although some authors prefer labetalol (an α- and β-adrenergic blocker), which would not cause unopposed α-stimulation. Haloperidol can be used for hallucinations, although some authors prefer benzodiazepines.

In an attempt to smuggle cocaine, some patients have swallowed balloons or condoms filled with it ("body packers"). If an abdominal radiograph demonstrates this, consideration should be given to endoscopic or surgical removal.

AMPHETAMINES

Amphetamines are noncatechol sympathomimetic adrenergic agents that have more central nervous system stimulant activity than catecholamines. Symptoms of intoxication include tachycardia, headache, hypertension, euphoria, mydriasis, anxiety, hypothermia, seizures, diaphoresis, hallucinations, and arrhythmias. The hypertension and cardiac arrhythmias may be severe.

In general, emesis or lavage is not helpful for treatment. Phentolamine (α-adrenergic blocker) can be used

to treat hypertensive crisis. Haloperidol is used for psychosis and agitation.

BENZODIAZEPINES

Most drug overdoses in persons older than 17 are caused by benzodiazepines. The morbidity and mortality are directly related to respiratory depression. Flumazenil (1,4-imidazobenzodiazepine), a new antagonist, has recently become available in the United States.

Flumazenil (Romazicon) is a relative pure antagonist with limited agonist or inverse agonist properties. It effectively antagonizes the neurologic, behavioral, and respiratory depressant effects of benzodiazepines. The initial dosage is 0.2 mg intravenously over 30 seconds. Subsequent dosages of 0.3-0.5 mg intravenously over 30 seconds can be given until desired effects are achieved or cumulative dose of 3-5 mg is given. Adverse reactions, including nausea, vomiting, dizziness, and, rarely, seizures, can occur, especially if cyclic antidepressants were also ingested. Two other problems can occur: 1) the precipitation of a withdrawal-type syndrome if the patient chronically uses benzodiazepines, and 2) resedation is very common, so prolonged monitoring is required.

Endotracheal intubation and ventilation is the treatment of choice for hypoventilatory patients. The exact role of flumazenil in benzodiazepine overdose has yet to be determined.

- For benzodiazepine overdose, endotracheal intubation and ventilation is used in hypoventilatory patients.
- Flumazenil can effectively reverse benzodiazepine-induced central nervous system and respiratory depression, but its role in overdose situations is unclear.

ALCOHOLS AND GLYCOLS

Ethanol, isopropyl alcohol (rubbing alcohol), methanol (wood alcohol), and ethylene glycol all produce an osmolar gap (see page 146). Methanol and ethylene glycol produce a large anion gap metabolic acidosis (serum bicarbonate level usually <10 mEq/L). Ethylene glycol produces calcium oxalate crystalluria. Isopropyl alcohol produces ketones but no acidosis.

Ethanol

Ethanol is the most abused drug. It is metabolized by liver alcohol dehydrogenase through zero-order kinetics (i.e., enzymes that are saturable). Blood alcohol levels are a poor predictor of level of impairment and anticipated morbidity. Clinical findings are slurred speech, ataxia, nystagmus, dulled sensory perception, tachycardia, hypoventilation, hypothermia, and coma.

Because alcoholics also experience trauma, hypoglycemia, and life-threatening infections, part of treatment is to be vigilant. Observation until the patient is sober is a good general rule. Thiamine, 100 mg intramuscularly, can be given. If blood glucose value is <80 mg/dL, 50 mL of dextrose is given. Naloxone, 2 mg intravenously, should be given if any signs of narcotic overdose are present. Severe intoxication occasionally requires endotracheal intubation and gastric lavage (especially if multiple drugs are ingested).

- Alcoholics also experience trauma, hypoglycemia, life-threatening infection.
- General rule, observe patient until he or she is sober.
- If blood glucose value <80 mg/dL, give 50 mL dextrose.

Isopropyl Alcohol

Isopropyl alcohol is rubbing alcohol. It can cause toxicity by ingestion or inhalation, but it is not absorbed through the skin. On an equal-dose basis, it is more toxic than ethyl alcohol, causing more central nervous system depression. It is also metabolized by alcohol dehydrogenase, the end products being acetone, CO_2, and H_2O. Thus, it produces an osmolar gap and ketosis without significant metabolic acidosis.

- Isopropyl alcohol is rubbing alcohol.
- More toxic than ethyl alcohol.
- Produces osmolar gap and ketosis without significant metabolic acidosis.

Clinical effects are the same as those of ethanol; other effects are hemorrhagic gastritis, hypotension, rhabdomyolysis, hepatocellular toxicity, and breath with a sweet odor.

Treatment is generally supportive, as for ethanol. Only in extremely rare cases is hemodialysis considered (e.g., severe coma or isopropyl alcohol level >400 mg/dL).

Methanol

Methanol (wood alcohol) is metabolized by liver alcohol dehydrogenase to formaldehyde and formic acid (toxicity). Thus, it produces an osmolar gap and an impressively elevated anion gap metabolic acidosis. In fact, serum bicarbonate levels may reach 3 mEq/L. There is a latent period of 8-72 hours, and then visual symptoms (blurred vision, photophobia, papilledema), central nervous system effects (confusion, lethargy, coma), abdominal pain, nausea, and vomiting develop.

- Methanol produces osmolar gap and elevated anion gap metabolic acidosis.

Gastric lavage and activated charcoal are used for treatment. Ethanol has a greater affinity for alcohol dehydrogenase and, thus, helps prevent the formation of toxic metabolites. The goal is to achieve an ethanol level of 100 mg/dL. There are many dosing regimens. Hemodialysis works well and should be considered if methanol level is >50 mg/dL or if patient has deteriorated on ethanol therapy. Thiamine, other vitamins, magnesium, and glucose are given as needed. Bicarbonate therapy is controversial and should be guided by blood gas values.

- For methanol intoxication, gastric lavage and activated charcoal are used for treatment.
- Hemodialysis works well.
- Bicarbonate therapy controversial.

Ethylene Glycol

Ethylene glycol is commonly found in antifreeze and many other products. It is also metabolized by liver alcohol dehydrogenase to its toxic metabolites. Clinically, ethylene glycol overdose affects the central nervous system (ataxia, nystagmus, seizures, coma, papilledema), kidney (calcium oxalate crystals, acute tubular necrosis), and gastrointestinal tract (abdominal pain, nausea, vomiting). Late effects are pulmonary edema and cardiac failure. Similar to methanol, ethylene glycol produces an osmolar gap and an impressive anion gap metabolic acidosis.

- Ethylene glycol found in antifreeze.
- Produces an osmolar gap and impressive anion gap metabolic acidosis.
- Produces calcium oxalate crystalluria.

Treatment is similar to that for methanol toxicity, i.e., ethanol and hemodialysis if the ethylene glycol level is >50 mg/dL or there is clinical deterioration on ethanol therapy.

ORGANOPHOSPHATES

The inhibition of acetylcholinesterase by organophosphates results in increased cholinergic activity. Carbamates are also inhibitors of acetylcholinesterase, but they cause less toxicity because their binding is reversible. Clinical findings of pesticide overdose are bradycardia, lacrimation, salivation, sweating, urinary incontinence, wheezing, fecal incontinence, and miosis. Delayed effects are fasciculations, tachycardia, mydriasis, and hypertension.

Evaluation of patients includes determination of both serum (easier) and red blood cell (more accurate) cholinesterase levels.

● Organophosphates inhibit acetylcholinesterase.

Treatment includes establishment of an airway. Atropine, 2-4 mg, is given as needed. The stabilized patient is fully decontaminated by removing clothing and irrigating. Charcoal is used depending on route of contamination. Pralidoxime (Protopam, 2-PAM) reactivates cholinesterase and reverses cholinergic and nicotine effects. Dosage in adults is 1 g over 15 minutes.

● Treatment of pesticide toxicity includes atropine, 2-4 mg as needed.
● Pralidoxime also used.

CARBON MONOXIDE POISONING

Carbon monoxide is the leading cause of toxin-related death. It is a colorless, odorless, nonirritating gas that reversibly displaces oxygen in hemoglobin to produce carboxyhemoglobin (COHb). Symptoms are often vague and misdiagnosed.

Although at time of exposure COHb level can correlate with symptoms, the COHb level after initiation of treatment with 100% oxygen can be deceptively low (Table 8-4). Diagnosis is established from the history (especially if 100% oxygen administered) and from COHb levels.

● In carbon monoxide poisoning, carboxyhemoglobin level at exposure can correlate with symptoms, but after treatment with 100% oxygen, level can be deceptively low.

Table 8-4.--Relationship of Carboxyhemoglobin Levels to Clinical Presentation

COHb, %	Signs and symptoms
0	None
10	Headache
20	Headache, dyspnea
30	Nausea, dizziness, impaired judgment
40	Confusion, syncope
50	Coma, seizures
60	Hypotension, respiratory failure
70	Death

Treatment is administration of 100% oxygen ($\downarrow$ half-life COHb by 400%). The use of hyperbaric oxygen is very controversial. It may prevent delayed neurologic sequelae, but controlled studies are lacking. Consider it for patients in coma, those with neurologic deficits, chest pain, or acidosis, or in pregnant patients. COHb value >30% may also be an indication, but the decision should be based on the clinical picture.

METHEMOGLOBINEMIA

Methemoglobinemia is an abnormal, nonfunctioning ferric hemoglobin ($HbFe^{3}+$) that cannot bind oxygen. It is caused by hereditary diseases (rare) but also by drugs of abuse such as amyl nitrite and isobutyl nitrite. These are used for short-term "rush" effect and as orgasm enhancers.

Diagnosis is based on the finding of chocolate-brown cyanosis unrelieved by oxygenation and arterial blood gases with low saturation but normal arterial oxygen partial pressure.

Treatment includes supplemental oxygen. Methylene blue acts as a cofactor in methemoglobinemia reductase system. Its use is reserved for patients with hypoxic symptoms or methemoglobin levels >30%. It may cause hemolysis in high doses.

QUESTIONS
(See "Answers" section)

Multiple Choice

1. Which of the following signs or symptoms is *not* associated with the anticholinergic syndrome?
   a. Tachycardia
   b. Mydriasis
   c. Miosis
   d. Hyperthermia
   e. Hypertension

2. Which of the following would produce an osmolar gap, an elevated anion gap metabolic acidosis, and calcium oxalate crystalluria?
   a. Ethylene glycol
   b. Methanol
   c. Isopropyl alcohol
   d. Paraldehyde
   e. Ethanol

3. What is the metabolic abnormality generally noted first in acute aspirin overdose?
   a. Respiratory acidosis
   b. Metabolic acidosis
   c. Metabolic alkalosis
   d. Metabolic acidosis with respiratory acidosis
   e. Respiratory alkalosis

4. A 37-year-old previously healthy man is admitted to the intensive care unit after an ingestion of aspirin. He was treated initially with gastric lavage, charcoal, and intravenous alkalinization. Six hours later, however, he is in florid pulmonary edema and his urine output has dropped to zero. You would:
   a. Order emergency ultrasonography of the kidneys
   b. Arrange for emergency hemodialysis
   c. Arrange for emergency hemoperfusion
   d. Continue to force fluids and intravenous alkalinization
   e. Pass a nasogastric tube and give pulse charcoal therapy

5. A 16-year-old boy arrives in the emergency department by ambulance, 30 minutes after ingesting a large amount of tricyclic antidepressants. He is tachycardic, hypertensive, and deeply comatose. You should:
   a. Intubate the patient with a cuffed endotracheal tube and then perform gastric lavage
   b. Perform gastric lavage immediately
   c. Pass a nasogastric tube and administer 50 g of activated charcoal
   d. Intubate the patient and prepare for emergency hemodialysis
   e. Do nothing until confirming drug overdose via drug levels

True/False

6. Hemodialysis may be required in some ingestions of:
   a. Ethanol
   b. Ethylene glycol
   c. Methanol
   d. Digoxin
   e. Tricyclic antidepressants
   f. Aspirin

7. Activated charcoal binds the following well:
   a. Acetaminophen
   b. Theophylline
   c. Barbiturates
   d. Ethanol
   e. Lithium
   f. Isopropyl alcohol

NOTES

CHAPTER 9
CRITICAL CARE MEDICINE

Steve G. Peters, M.D.

Critical Care Medicine encompasses multidisciplinary aspects of the management of severely ill patients. All areas of medicine may have relevance for critically ill patients, but this review focuses on aspects of cardiopulmonary monitoring and life support, technological interventions, and disease states typically managed in the intensive care unit (ICU).

A few general tips for preparing for the broad examination: 1) Stress the acute care of common life-threatening conditions. Review a general manual or text of medical therapeutics. 2) Try to identify important areas with which you are less familiar or experienced. Also, review situations encountered in major hospitals of large U.S. cities, e.g., complications of alcohol, drug overdose, and trauma. 3) Common things are commonly tested, but be aware of unusual causes or features of common conditions, e.g., adult respiratory distress syndrome (ARDS) secondary to thrombotic thrombocytopenic purpura. 4) In reviewing drugs, stress common agents having serious toxicity, e.g., antihypertensive agents, theophylline, antibiotics, immunosuppressive agents, and antidepressants. 5) Know the indications for (and complications of) common invasive procedures, e.g., pulmonary angiography, cardiac catheterization, and hemodialysis.

- Stress acute care of common life-threatening conditions.
- Identify important areas with which you are less familiar or experienced.
- Be aware of unusual causes or features of common conditions.
- Know indications for (and complications of) invasive procedures.

RESPIRATORY FAILURE

Effective functioning of the respiratory system requires normal central nervous system control, neuromuscular transmission and bellows function, and gas exchange at the alveolar-capillary level. Respiratory failure may result from disease at any of these levels.

Physiologic Definitions and Relationships

Lung Volumes

TLC = total lung capacity--total volume of gas in the chest at the end of a maximal inspiration. VC = vital capacity--volume of a maximal breath (expired or inspired). V_T = tidal volume--volume of a normal breath. FRC = functional residual capacity--lung volume at the end of a normal expiration. It reflects the relaxation point of the respiratory system or the point at which outward recoil of the chest wall is balanced by inward recoil of the lungs. Compliance of the lungs or respiratory system is defined by the change in volume (ΔV) for a given change in pressure (ΔP).

$$C_{STATIC} = \frac{\Delta V}{\Delta P}$$

where ΔV is measured in L and ΔP in cm H_2O. Emphysema causes loss of recoil and, thus, increased compliance. Most other disease states, particularly interstitial diseases, fibrosis, pulmonary edema, and ARDS, cause decreased compliance (i.e., "stiff" lungs, or increased transpulmonary pressure for given volume change).

- Normal compliance = 0.2 L/cm H_2O.

- Emphysema causes loss of recoil and increased compliance.
- Interstitial diseases, fibrosis, pulmonary edema, ARDS cause decreased compliance.

Resistance (R) to air flow is defined by the change in pressure (ΔP) for a given change in flow ($\Delta \dot{V}$)

$$R = \frac{\Delta P}{\Delta \dot{V}}$$

where ΔP is measured in cm H_2O and $\Delta \dot{V}$ in L/sec. Common causes of increased airway resistance include bronchospasm and airway secretions.

- Causes of increased airway resistance: bronchospasm and airway secretions.

The total pressure required to inflate the respiratory system (spontaneously or by mechanical ventilator) is the pressure required to overcome elastic recoil plus the pressure to overcome flow resistance:

$$P_{inflation} = \frac{\Delta V}{C_{ST}} + R \times \Delta \dot{V}$$
$$\text{(Elastic)} \qquad \text{(Resistive)}$$

Gas exchange requires alveolar ventilation for elimination of carbon dioxide, oxygen uptake across alveolar-capillary membrane, and delivery of O_2 to tissues. Hypoxemia may result from a decrease in the inspired fraction of O_2 (FIO_2) (e.g., high altitude), hypoventilation, ventilation-perfusion ($\dot{V}$/Q) mismatch, shunting, or diffusion barrier. Estimation of the alveolar-arterial gradient for oxygen (A-aO_2 difference) is essential in analyzing the cause of hypoxemia. Important relationships include the following:

The partial pressure of carbon dioxide ($PaCO_2$) in the blood is directly proportional to amount of CO_2 produced ($\dot{V}CO_2$), and inversely proportional to alveolar ventilation ($\dot{V}A$):

$$PaCO_2 = k \frac{\dot{V}CO_2}{\dot{V}A}$$

Alveolar ventilation is equal to total ventilation ($\dot{V}E$) minus dead space ventilation (VD). Thus, physiologic dead space is defined by the portion of a breath which does not participate in gas exchange. Dead space may be anatomical (conducting airways) or alveolar (areas of ventilation which receive no perfusion):

$$\dot{V}A = \dot{V}E - VD \times f$$

where f = breaths/min.

$\frac{VD}{VT}$ normally is <0.25 - 0.30

$$\frac{VD}{VT} = \frac{PaCO_2 - P_ECO_2}{PaCO_2}$$

where P_ECO_2 is the partial pressure of expired CO_2. The dead space to tidal volume ratio is calculated by measuring the partial pressure of carbon dioxide in an arterial blood ($PaCO_2$) gas sample and an expired gas sample (P_ECO_2). The greater the dead space, the greater the difference between $PaCO_2$ and P_ECO_2.

- Physiologic dead space is defined by the portion of breath not participating in gas exchange.
- Dead space may be anatomical or alveolar.

Alveolar gas consists of inspired gases saturated with water vapor. The alveolus also contains CO_2 delivered from the blood. The sum of the partial pressures of all gases present equals the ambient barometric pressure. The alveolar air equation defines this relationship:

$$PaO_2 = FIO_2 (PB - PH_2O) - \frac{PaCO_2}{R}$$

where PB is barometric pressure, PH_2O is water-vapor pressure (47 mm Hg), and R is the respiratory quotient. The simplified equation is:

$$R = \frac{\dot{V}CO_2}{\dot{V}O_2} \quad nl \quad 0.8$$

The alveolar-arterial O_2 difference is defined by PAO_2 minus PaO_2, which is normally <10-20 mm Hg when breathing room air. The A-a gradient normally increases to approximately 50-100 mm Hg as the FIO_2 increases from 0.21 to 1.0. Hypoxemia due to hypoventilation is characterized by increased $PaCO_2$ and decreased PaO_2 but a relatively normal A-a gradient. Hypoxemia due to ventilation-perfusion mismatch shows an elevated A-a gradient. A shunt is defined by perfusion in the absence of ventilation (i.e., V/Q = 0). With a pure shunt, PaO_2 does not increase even though FIO_2 is increased to 100%. Normal shunt fraction is <3%-5% of total cardiac output. The shunt fraction (simplified on FIO_2 1.0):

$$\frac{Qs}{Qt} = \frac{Cc'O_2 - CaO_2}{Cc'O_2 - C\bar{v}O_2} = \frac{P(A-a)O_2 \times 0.003}{P(A-a)O_2 \times 0.003 + (Ca-C\bar{v})O_2}$$

The content of O_2 in the blood is the total amount of O_2 bound to hemoglobin plus the amount dissolved.

$$O_2 \text{ content: } C_xO_2 = 1.34 \times Hgb \times S_xO_2 + 0.003 \times P_xO_2$$
$$\text{(Bound)} \qquad \text{(Dissolved)}$$

where x may equal arterial, venous, capillary, etc.

Under steady state conditions, the amount of O_2 used by the tissues equals the amount taken up by the lungs. The O_2 uptake, $\dot{V}O_2$, can be defined by amount of O_2 leaving the lungs in pulmonary venous blood minus the amount of O_2 coming into the lungs in the pulmonary arteries. This should be familiar as the Fick equation:

$$\dot{V}O_2 = Q (Ca-C\bar{v})O_2$$

where Q is cardiac output.

- Hypoxemia due to hypoventilation: increased $PaCO_2$, decreased PaO_2, relatively normal A-a gradient.
- Shunt is defined by perfusion in absence of ventilation, i.e., V/Q = O.
- Normal shunt fraction is <3%-5% of total cardiac output.

Many applications of the Fick equation are important in managing critically ill patients. One application involves continuous monitoring of mixed venous O_2 saturation by recently developed pulmonary artery catheters. Expressing O_2 content in terms of saturation and rearranging the Fick equation to solve the $S\bar{v}O_2$ yields the following:

$$S\bar{v}O_2 = SaO_2 - \frac{\dot{V}O_2}{Q \times Hgb \times 1.34}$$

Note that decreased mixed venous O_2 saturation may be due to decreased arterial saturation, increased O_2 consumption, decreased cardiac output, or decreased hemoglobin. Certain disease states, particularly early sepsis, may be characterized by normal or increased mixed venous O_2 saturation, because cardiac output initially increases, along with impaired O_2 uptake by the tissues. Later in sepsis, mixed venous $S\bar{v}O_2$ typically decreases due to decreased O_2 delivery.

- Decreased mixed venous O_2 may be due to: decreased arterial saturation, increased O_2 consumption, decreased cardiac output, or decreased hemoglobin.
- Early sepsis: normal or increased mixed venous O_2 saturation.

Under normal circumstances, O_2 demand by the tissues is met by the supply. O_2 delivery is defined by cardiac output times arterial O_2 content, i.e.,

$$O_2 \text{ delivery} = Q \times CaO_2$$

Although cardiac output may decrease, $\dot{V}O_2$ of the tissues may be maintained by increased O_2 extraction. Supply dependence of O_2 consumption refers to disease states in which O_2 delivery falls below a certain point where O_2 extraction cannot maintain the required $\dot{V}O_2$. Below such a threshold of O_2 delivery, O_2 consumption varies directly with the available supply. Such conditions usually imply coexisting anaerobic metabolism and accumulation of lactic acid.

- O_2 delivery = cardiac output x arterial O_2 content.

ACID-BASE BALANCE AND ARTERIAL BLOOD GASES

The production of acid byproducts is the normal result of cellular metabolism. An acid is defined as a hydrogen ion, $[H^+]$, or proton donor. A base accepts protons. The dissociation constant (K) for an acid (HA) may be defined as

$$K = \frac{[H^+][A^-]}{[HA]}$$

Buffer systems minimize the changes in pH associated with the addition of acid or base. For carbonic acid:

$$H_2O + CO_2 \overset{K}{\leftrightarrow} H_2CO_3 \leftrightarrow H^+ + HCO_3^-$$

$$\text{and } K = \frac{[H^+][HCO_3^-]}{[H_2CO_3]}$$

The Henderson-Hasselbalch equation:

$$pH = pK + \log \frac{[HCO_3^-]}{[H_2CO_3]}$$

where $pH = -\log[H^+]$ and $pK = -\log K$. The pK for carbonic acid is 6.1. $[H_2CO_3]$ is often measured by taking $0.03 \times Paco_2$ (i.e., dissolved CO_2). So the Henderson-Hasselbalch equation can be rewritten,

$$pH = 6.1 + \log \frac{[HCO_3^-]}{0.03 \times Paco_2}$$

Hydrogen ions are buffered by several mechanisms in different body fluid compartments. In plasma and interstitial fluid, bicarbonate is the major buffer, with proteins and phosphate compounds contributing to a lesser extent. In erythrocytes, hemoglobin is the major buffer, but bicarbonate contributes approximately 30% and phosphate 10% of the buffering capacity. The kidney eliminates organic acid and also contributes by 1) reabsorption of bicarbonate from tubular fluids, 2) formation of titratable acid, and 3) elimination of $[H^+]$ as ammonium ions.

- Bicarbonate is the major buffer in plasma and interstitial fluid.
- In erythrocytes, hemoglobin is the major buffer.
- Kidney eliminates organic acid and reabsorbs bicarbonate from tubular fluids.

Given the importance of the carbonic acid-bicarbonate system, most acid-base problems involve some method for solving variables of the Henderson-Hasselbalch equation. Because pK is constant, given two of the three values for pH, Pco_2, and $[HCO_3^-]$, the missing variable can be calculated. Graphic displays are commonly used; two of the variables are plotted at constant values (isopleths) for the third variable (the Davenport diagram is an example).

Pattern of Acid-Base Disorder

Acute respiratory acidosis is defined by rapid development of CO_2 retention with a concomitant decrease in pH. Common causes include respiratory depression by drugs such as narcotics, central nervous system injury, acute diaphragm or neuromuscular weakness, and severe parenchymal respiratory failure or cardiac failure. Chronic respiratory acidosis is typically seen in patients with severe chronic obstructive lung disease (particularly chronic bron-

chitis or bronchiectasis) and in other states associated with chronic alveolar hypoventilation. Respiratory acidosis may be partly compensated by renal mechanisms, i.e., increased reabsorption of bicarbonate and excretion of acid in the urine. Acute respiratory alkalosis is the result of rapid decrease in $Paco_2$ due to hyperventilation. Hyperventilation is usually associated with anxiety or pain. Other important causes are early shock states, pulmonary embolism, other causes of hypoxemia, hyperthermia, salicylate intoxication, liver failure, and central nervous system disorders. Patients with unexplained hypocapnia should be evaluated for these disorders.

- Acute respiratory acidosis: rapid development of CO_2 retention with a concomitant decrease in pH.
- Chronic respiratory acidosis is typically seen in patients with severe chronic obstructive lung disease and other states associated with chronic alveolar hypoventilation.
- Respiratory acidosis may be partly compensated by renal mechanisms.
- Acute respiratory alkalosis: result of rapid decrease in $Paco_2$ due to hyperventilation.

Metabolic acidosis results from accumulation of organic acids such as lactate, pyruvate, or keto acids. Acidosis may develop by increased acid production or decreased renal excretion of acid. Conditions causing metabolic acidosis are further characterized by the anion gap, i.e.:

$$[Na^+] - ([Cl^-] + [HCO_3^-])$$

with a normal value of 8-14 mEq/L.

A normal anion gap or non-anion gap acidosis is characterized by an increase in chloride balancing the loss of bicarbonate. Causes include gastrointestinal losses of bicarbonate, i.e., diarrhea, urinary diversion procedures, or intestinal fistulas. Renal losses of bicarbonate (renal tubular acidosis) are also associated with a normal anion gap. Causes of acidosis associated with other anions--increased anion gap disorders--are diabetic ketoacidosis, lactic acidosis, uremia, and toxins (ethylene glycol, methanol, paraldehyde, and salicylate).

- Metabolic acidosis: result of accumulation of organic acids, e.g., lactate, pyruvate, keto acids.
- Normal anion gap or non-anion gap acidosis is characterized by increase in chloride balancing loss of bicarbonate.

- Increased anion gap disorders: diabetic ketoacidosis, lactic acidosis, uremia, toxins (ethylene glycol, methanol, paraldehyde, salicylate).

Metabolic alkalosis is characterized by increased bicarbonate and pH. Hypokalemia and hypochloremia are commonly associated and further perpetuate the alkalosis. Common causes are volume contraction states, particularly those associated with further loss of chloride and hydrogen ion (vomiting and nasogastric suctioning). Diuretic therapy and mineralocorticoids are also common contributing factors. Although respiratory compensation (hypoventilation) for metabolic alkalosis might seem counterproductive, it can occur and may contribute to hypoxemia. As with other acid-base disorders, therapy is directed at the underlying cause, but support with volume and potassium and chloride replacement are important.

- Metabolic alkalosis is characterized by increased bicarbonate and pH.
- Hypokalemia and hypochloremia are commonly associated and further perpetuate alkalosis.
- Common causes are volume contraction states, particularly those associated with further loss of chloride and hydrogen ion (vomiting, nasogastric suctioning).

CLINICAL APPROACH TO ARTERIAL BLOOD GASES

There are many ways to assess problems of acid-base balance and gas exchange. When interpreting arterial blood gases, the following approach is useful:

1. Consider the pH. Are conditions normal (pH 7.35-7.45), acidemic (<7.35), or alkalemic (>7.45)?
2. Assess $Paco_2$. Does the $Paco_2$ change (from 40 mm Hg) account for the pH change (from 7.40)? Evaluation of this relationship requires calculation, graphic display, or a rule of thumb, such as: an acute change in $Paco_2$ of 10 mm Hg should be associated with a pH change in the opposite direction of approximately 0.08 unit. If an abnormal pH can be accounted for by the change in $Paco_2$, a simple respiratory disturbance is present. If not, a mixed acid-base disorder is defined.
3. The change in bicarbonate, i.e., base deficit or excess, should confirm the conditions already defined by pH and $Paco_2$.

4. Consider Pao_2. If hypoxemia is present, estimate the alveolar-arterial gradient. If this is normal and $Paco_2$ is increased, hypoventilation alone should account for the hypoxemia. The alveolar-arterial gradient should be increased in conditions of ventilation-perfusion mismatching, shunting, or diffusion barrier.

- Consider the pH.
- Assess $Paco_2$.
- Change in bicarbonate should confirm the conditions already defined by pH and $Paco_2$.
- Consider Pao_2.

Airway Management

Endotracheal intubation allows control of the airway, ability to deliver specific inspired O_2 and positive pressure ventilation, and protection from aspiration. Indications for intubation include: airway protection in cases of obstruction or loss of normal gag and cough reflexes, central nervous system injury or sedation with loss of normal controls of ventilation, and any cause of respiratory failure requiring positive pressure-assisted ventilation. Oral-tracheal intubation is usually achieved via direct visualization with a laryngoscope. In experienced hands, this procedure should be relatively quick and safe. Complications may include vomiting and aspiration, hypoxemia during the procedure, and inadvertent intubation of the esophagus. The major contraindication for laryngoscopic intubation is an unstable cervical spine (due to trauma or degenerative conditions such as rheumatoid arthritis). In such cases, fiberoptic intubation (passing a tube over a bronchoscope) or tracheostomy may be necessary. In semiconscious and spontaneously breathing patients, nasotracheal intubation may be accomplished "blindly" and may be more comfortable for patients. Complications include bleeding, obstruction of sinus drainage with sinusitis, and damage to nasal structures.

- Endotracheal intubation allows control of the airway.
- Contraindication: unstable cervical spine (trauma or rheumatoid arthritis).
- In semiconscious, spontaneously breathing patients, nasotracheal intubation may be accomplished blindly.

In emergency situations where airway control is required, cricothyrotomy may be lifesaving. This procedure involves identification and puncture of the cricothyroid membrane. In patients requiring prolonged mechanical ventilation or airway support, the timing of tracheostomy is controversial. Newer high-volume low-pressure endotracheal tube cuffs have decreased the frequency of tracheal injury and stenosis caused by prolonged intubation. Tracheostomy has the advantages of decreased laryngeal injury, increased patient comfort, ease of suctioning, and, in certain patients, allowance for oral ingestion and speech. Complications may include tracheal injury and stenosis, bleeding, tracheoesophageal fistula, and possibly increased bronchial or pulmonary infections. Tracheostomy is commonly considered in patients who have needed or are expected to need intubation and mechanical ventilation for >2-4 weeks.

- In emergency situations, cricothyrotomy may be life-saving.
- High-volume low-pressure endotracheal tube cuffs have decreased frequency of tracheal injury and stenosis.
- Tracheostomy is for patients who have needed or are expected to need intubation and mechanical ventilation for >2-4 weeks.

Mechanical Ventilation

Mechanical ventilation may be valuable in various conditions of respiratory failure, including loss of respiratory controls, neuromuscular or respiratory pump failure, and disorders of gas exchange. Many specific variables have been suggested as criteria for ventilator support and are listed in Table 9-1.

Table 9-1.--Criteria for Ventilator Support

Respiratory rate >30/min
Minute ventilation >10 L/min
Maximal inspiratory pressure <-20 cm H_2O
Vital capacity <10 mL/kg
PaO_2 <60 mm Hg with FIO_2 >0.60
PaO_2/FIO_2 <100-150
$P(A-a)O_2$ >300 mm Hg on FIO_2 1.0
VD/VT >0.60
$PaCO_2$ >50 mm Hg

Complications of Mechanical Ventilation

Complications of mechanical ventilation may relate to airway access, physiologic responses to positive pressure, and complications related to other organ systems. Examples are given in Table 9-2.

Table 9-2.--Complications of Mechanical Ventilation

Airway injury, bleeding, infection
Ventilator malfunction--leaks, power loss, incorrect settings, or alarm failures
Barotrauma; pneumothorax; interstitial, subcutaneous, or mediastinal air
Decreased right ventricular filling, increased right ventricular afterload, decreased cardiac output, hypotension
Gastrointestinal bleeding, stress gastritis, ulceration
Decreased urine output
Alteration in intracranial pressure

Other complications, such as pulmonary embolism or malnutrition, may also reflect the underlying disease state. Management of these complications requires ongoing surveillance and recognition. Diagnosis of pneumonia may be difficult in patients receiving mechanical ventilation, because pulmonary infiltrates are frequently present, tracheal secretions may be colonized by bacteria, and signs such as fever and leukocytosis are frequently blunted. Prophylaxis is commonly given to reduce stress-related gastritis and ulceration. H_2-Blockers may increase colonization of the respiratory tract by gram-negative bacteria. Sucralfate or frequent use of antacids are alternatives. The hemodynamic complications of increased intrathoracic pressure may be overcome by fluid administration; however, there is often a coexisting condition of capillary leak and pulmonary edema which may worsen.

- Diagnosis of pneumonia may be difficult in patients receiving mechanical ventilation.
- Prophylaxis is commonly given to reduce stress-related gastritis and ulceration.
- H_2-Blockers may increase colonization of respiratory tract by gram-negative bacteria.
- Sucralfate or frequent use of antacids are alternatives.

An important and occasionally subtle complication of positive pressure ventilation is called intrinsic positive end-expiratory pressure (PEEP), auto-PEEP, breath stacking, or dynamic hyperinflation. This refers to a phenomenon of inadequate time during the expiratory phase of the respiratory cycle, so that a mechanically assisted breath is delivered before passive expiration of the lungs is complete. Thus, a new machine breath is delivered before the previous breath is completely exhaled. This may worsen hyperinflation, increase intrathoracic pressure, and worsen the associated complications, especially in patients with airway obstruction. Intrinsic PEEP may exist in spontaneously breathing patients with obstructive airway disease, but the effect is most significant in mechanically ventilated patients. Treatment typically involves optimizing bronchodilator therapy and altering the ventilator cycle to allow maximal expiratory time.

- Complication of positive pressure ventilation is called intrinsic PEEP, auto-PEEP, breath stacking, or dynamic hyperinflation.
- It is inadequate time during the expiratory phase of the respiratory cycle.
- It may worsen hyperinflation, increase intrathoracic pressure, and worsen associated complications, especially in patients with airway obstruction.

"Modes of mechanical ventilation" refers to the pattern of cycling of the machine breath and its relation to the spontaneous breaths of the patient. Assist-control mode is defined by a machine-assisted breath for every inspiratory effort by the patient. If no spontaneous breaths occur during a preset time interval, a controlled breath of predetermined tidal volume will be delivered by the ventilator. The backup rate should determine the minimum minute ventilation the patient will receive. The advantage of the assist-control mode is that it should allow maximal rest for the patient and maximal control of ventilation. The disadvantage is that hyperventilation and/or air trapping can occur in patients making rapid inspiratory efforts. Intermittent mandatory ventilation (IMV) allows a preset number of machine-assisted breaths of a given tidal volume. Between machine breaths, patients may breathe spontaneously. The advantage of IMV is that the number of machine breaths can be decreased gradually during weaning efforts, providing that the patient is able to maintain satisfactory spontaneous ventilation. This is common clinical practice but it has not been proved superior to other weaning techniques, e.g., T-piece trials alternated with full ventilator support.

- Assist-control mode: machine-assisted breath for every inspiratory effort by the patient.
- Assist-control mode advantage: allows maximal rest for patient and maximal control of ventilation.
- Assist-control mode disadvantage: hyperventilation and/or air trapping in patients making rapid inspiratory efforts.

- IMV: allows preset number of machine-assisted breaths of a given tidal volume.
- Between machine breaths, patients may breathe spontaneously.
- IMV advantage: number of machine breaths can be decreased gradually during weaning efforts.
- IMV not proved superior to other weaning techniques (T-piece trials).

Pressure support may be used to assist spontaneously breathing patients, with or without IMV breaths. In this technique, for each inspiratory effort of the patient, the ventilator delivers a high rate of flow of inspired gas, up to a preset pressure limit. This pressure support lasts only during the spontaneous inspiratory effort, so that the rate and pattern of respiration are determined by the patient. Initial ventilator settings require specification of the mode of ventilation, tidal volume, respiratory rate, inspiratory and expiratory ratio (I:E) for the respiratory cycle, F_{IO_2}, level of pressure support, and PEEP.

- For each inspiratory effort of the patient, the ventilator delivers a high flow of inspired gas, up to preset pressure limit.

PEEP is intended to increase functional residual capacity, recruit partially collapsed alveoli, improve lung compliance, and to improve $\dot{V}/Q$ matching. An adverse effect of PEEP is an excessive increase in intrathoracic pressure with decreased cardiac output. Overdistention of lung units may also worsen $\dot{V}/Q$ mismatch. At levels of PEEP >10-15 cm H_2O, barotrauma is of particular concern. Optimal, or best, PEEP may be defined as lowest level of PEEP needed to achieve satisfactory oxygenation at a nontoxic F_{IO_2}.

- PEEP: to increase functional residual capacity, recruit partially collapsed alveoli, improve lung compliance, improve $\dot{V}/Q$ matching.
- Adverse effect of PEEP: excessive increase in intrathoracic pressure with decreased cardiac output.
- Overdistention of lung units may also worsen $\dot{V}/Q$ mismatch.
- Optimal, or best, PEEP: lowest level of PEEP needed to achieve satisfactory oxygenation at a nontoxic F_{IO_2}.

Pulmonary O_2 toxicity appears to be the result of direct exposure to high tensions of inspired O_2 or alveolar O_2. For adults, O_2 toxicity is not believed to be a major clinical concern below an FIO_2 of 0.40-0.50. Higher levels of inspired O_2 may be associated with acute tracheobronchitis (most likely an irritant effect). After several days of exposure, a syndrome of diffuse alveolar damage and lung injury may develop. The pathologic picture may resemble that of ARDS.

- Pulmonary O_2 toxicity: result of direct exposure to high tensions of inspired O_2 or alveolar O_2.
- Syndrome of diffuse alveolar damage and lung injury may develop.
- The pathologic picture may resemble that of ARDS.

ADULT RESPIRATORY DISTRESS SYNDROME

Diffuse lung injury with acute hypoxic respiratory failure may result from various injuries. Acute lung injury is a frequent primary cause of critical illness and may occur as a complication or coexisting feature of multisystem disease. Mortality from all causes averages about 50%. Existing therapies do not significantly alter overall mortality in established ARDS. Recent emphasis is on identification of patients at high risk for acute lung injury and on possible early interventions. ARDS is commonly defined as diffuse acute lung injury that has the following major features: diffuse pulmonary infiltrates, severe hypoxemia due to shunting and ventilation-perfusion mismatch, and normal or low pulmonary capillary wedge pressure (i.e., noncardiogenic pulmonary edema). Criteria for the diagnosis of ARDS are listed in Table 9-3.

- Diffuse lung injury with hypoxic respiratory failure may result from various injuries.
- Mortality from all causes averages about 50%.
- Existing therapies do not significantly alter overall mortality in established ARDS.

ARDS was initially described as a post-traumatic or shock-induced injury, but it occurs with various states, as outlined in Table 9-4.

Relative risks of developing ARDS have been estimated from studies of predisposed groups. The greatest frequency is among patients with sepsis (approximately 40%), gastric aspiration (30%), multiple transfusions (25%), pulmonary contusion (20%), disseminated intravascular coagulation (20%), pneumonia requiring ICU management (12%), and trauma with long-bone or

Table 9-3.--Criteria for Diagnosis of Adult Respiratory Distress Syndrome

Appropriate setting
Pulmonary injury, shock, trauma
Acute event
Clinical respiratory distress, tachypnea
Diffuse pulmonary infiltrates on chest radiograph
Interstitial and/or alveolar pattern
Hypoxemia
PaO_2/FIO_2 ratio <150
Decreased compliance of respiratory system
<50 mL/cm H_2O
Exclude
Chronic pulmonary disease accounting for clinical picture
Left ventricular failure (most series require pulmonary artery wedge measurement <18 mm Hg)

Table 9-4.--Disorders Associated With Adult Respiratory Distress Syndrome

Shock	Any cause
Sepsis	Lung infections, other bacteremic or endotoxic states
Trauma	Head injury, lung contusion, fat embolism
Aspiration	Gastric, near-drowning, tube feedings
Hematologic	Transfusions, leukoagglutinin, intravascular coagulation, thrombotic thrombocytopenic purpura
Metabolic	Pancreatitis, uremia
Drugs	Narcotics, barbiturates, aspirin
Toxic	Inhaled--O_2, smoke
	Irritant gases--NO_2, Cl_2, SO_2, NH_3
	Chemicals--paraquat
Miscellaneous	Radiation, air embolism, altitude

pelvic fractures (5%).

The pathophysiology of ARDS depends on damage to the alveolar-capillary unit. The earliest histologic changes are endothelial swelling followed by edema and inflammation. Mononuclear inflammation, loss of alveolar type I cells, and protein deposition in the form of hyaline membranes may occur within 2-3 days. Fibrosis may develop after days or weeks of the process. Damage to type II alveolar epithelial cells leads to loss of surfactant. The surfactant that is produced may also be inactivated by proteins present in the airways. Alveolar filling and collapse cause intrapulmonary shunting and $\dot{V}/Q$ mismatch with hypoxemia.

Death from ARDS usually is not due to isolated hypoxemic respiratory failure. The most frequent causes of mortality are complications of infection, sepsis syndrome, or failure of other organ systems. In addition to clinical risk factors listed above, specific variables associated with mortality include <10% band forms on peripheral blood smear, persistent acidemia, bicarbonate <20 mEq/L, and blood urea nitrogen >65 mg/dL. Therefore, the systemic effects associated with ARDS may be important to outcome.

- Death from ARDS is not usually due to isolated hypoxemic respiratory failure.
- Infection, sepsis syndrome, or failure of other organ systems are usual causes of mortality.
- Variables associated with mortality: <10% band forms on peripheral blood smear, persistent acidemia, bicarbonate <20 mEq/L, blood urea nitrogen >65 mg/dL.

Traditional therapy of ARDS involves optimization of physiologic variables and supportive management of associated complications. Measures include optimization of gas exchange and hemodynamics, nutrition, ambulation, and control of infections. Hypoxemia is typically corrected with positive pressure ventilation with supplemental O_2 and PEEP. PEEP provides potential benefits of increased lung volume and lung compliance and improvement in ventilation-perfusion relationships. Beyond an optimal level of PEEP, increase in intrathoracic pressure may be associated with decreased venous return, increased pulmonary vascular resistance, decreased left ventricular filling, and corresponding decrease in cardiac output. Supportive management of associated complications includes screening for underlying infections and early antibiotic therapy. Selective bowel decontamination by oral or nasogastric administration of a combination of nonabsorbable antibiotics may decrease colonization of airway by gram-negative organisms (reported to decrease the incidence of pneumonia in patients receiving mechanical ventilation).

- Hypoxemia is typically corrected with positive pressure ventilation with supplemental O_2 and PEEP.
- Screen for underlying infections and early antibiotic therapy.
- Selective bowel decontamination may decrease colonization of airway by gram-negative organisms.

Because increased capillary permeability allows greater intravascular fluid leak at any given hydrostatic pressure, attempt to limit intravascular volume to that necessary for systemic perfusion. However, associated shock states may demand volume expansion or increased inotropic support. Crystalloids can provide adequate filling pressures in patients with shock states, but large volumes may be required. Specific applications for colloids in ARDS include blood products (e.g., for coagulopathies or anemia). Supplemental nutrition is typically provided throughout the course of critical illness. Many patients with ARDS have associated multiorgan injury and may have ileus and/or gastrointestinal dysfunction precluding enteral feedings. Such feedings are recommended if tolerated. Consequences of malnutrition may include impairment of respiratory muscle function, depressed ventilatory drive, and limitation of host defenses. Mobilization, ambulation, and ventilator weaning are carried out as early as practical.

- Crystalloids can provide adequate filling pressures in patients with shock states.
- Many patients with ARDS have associated multiorgan injury.

Pharmacologic therapies have been directed against proposed biochemical and cellular mechanisms of ARDS. Presumed pathogenesis of acute lung injury is centered on role of polymorphonuclear leukocytes. Activation of complement by many stimuli associated with lung injury may lead to recruitment and activation of neutrophils, which may injure endothelium by releasing proteolytic enzymes and liberating toxic O_2 species (e.g., hydrogen peroxide, hydroxyl radical, singlet oxygen, superoxide). Bronchoalveolar lavage fluid from patients with established ARDS and from high-risk patients may show increased numbers of cells, predominantly neutrophils. (Normal lavage fluid contains about 93% alveolar macrophages, with 5%-7% lymphocytes and few neutrophils.) Percentage of neutrophils is correlated with abnormalities of gas exchange and alveolar protein content. However, experimental lung injury may occur in the absence of neutrophils, and typical ARDS is seen in severely neutropenic patients. Thus, other mechanisms presumably have a role. Arachidonic acid metabolites are implicated in many biochemical events associated with acute lung injury. Arachidonic acid is released from cell membranes by phospholipases. Arachidonate may then be metabolized via lipoxygenase pathway to leukotriene compounds or via cyclooxygenase pathway to prostaglandins or thromboxane. These compounds are potentially crucial in pathogenesis of acute lung injury. Thromboxane A_2, a potent vasoconstrictor, induces platelet aggregation. Prostacyclin, or PGI_2, has the opposite effects on smooth muscle and platelet aggregation and is a potential therapeutic agent for ARDS. PGE_1, a prostaglandin, relaxes vascular and bronchial smooth muscle and inhibits neutrophil chemotaxis.

- Acute lung injury: presumed pathogenesis centers on polymorphonuclear leukocytes.
- Neutrophils may injure endothelium by releasing proteolytic enzymes and liberating toxic O_2 species.
- Experimental lung injury may occur in absence of neutrophils.
- Arachidonic acid metabolites are implicated in many biochemical events associated with acute lung injury.
- Thromboxane A_2: potent vasoconstrictor, induces platelet aggregation.
- PGE_1: relaxes vascular and bronchial smooth muscle, inhibits neutrophil chemotaxis.

Potential therapeutic and prophylactic agents have been directed against steps in arachidonate pathways. Corticosteroids decrease cell membrane disruption and have other anti-inflammatory properties. However, in ARDS and sepsis syndrome, steroids are potentially harmful and have no known benefit. Specifically, no differences in mortality have been observed in prospective, randomized studies of ARDS patients receiving methylprednisolone or placebo. Trials of corticosteroids in sepsis have also shown no difference in overall mortality. Steroids may delay resolution of secondary infections; a greater number of deaths related to secondary infection after steroids has been observed.

- Corticosteroids decrease cell membrane disruption and have other anti-inflammatory properties.
- In ARDS and sepsis syndrome, steroids are potentially harmful and have no known benefit.
- In sepsis, no difference in overall mortality with corticosteroids.

Nonsteroidal anti-inflammatory drugs (NSAIDs), e.g., ibuprofen and indomethacin, block cyclooxygenase and thromboxane formation. In animal models of acute lung injury and septic shock, NSAIDs have beneficial effects if used prophylactically. However, no benefit is known for established ARDS. Other mediators, particularly those associated with sepsis, may be important factors in pathogenesis of acute lung injury. Endotoxin, a complex lipopolysaccharide, may activate complement; it has been associated with neutrophilic alveolitis. Monoclonal antiendotoxin antibodies are reported to have beneficial effects in some septic patients.

The prognosis for patients who survive ARDS is good. Studies of survivors have shown nearly normal lung volumes and airflow 6-12 months after the illness, with mild impairment in gas exchange--decreased diffusing capacity, desaturation with exercise, or widened A-a gradient. Therefore, the incentive is strong to continue aggressive measures in those patients with otherwise reversible organ dysfunction.

- Prognosis for patients surviving ARDS is good.

CARDIOPULMONARY RESUSCITATION

General clinical algorithms for standardized responses to cardiac dysrhythmias or arrest should be reviewed. Ideally, in ICUs, cardiorespiratory problems should be prevented or anticipated and recognized quickly.

Basic Life Support

Airway Control

Relieve obstruction. Remove any foreign bodies. If not dislodged or obstructing, dentures may improve the seal of a face mask. However, dentures are usually removed before endotracheal intubation.

Suction (saliva, emesis, blood). A rigid suction catheter is most useful. Use head-tilt, chin-lift, or forward thrust of the jaw to open posterior pharynx. Oropharyngeal or nasopharyngeal airway may help maintain patency and facilitate suctioning and mask ventilation.

Supply a high rate of flow of supplemental O_2. Ventilation is usually begun with a bag-valve-mask technique. Because a combined respiratory and metabolic acidosis is common, hyperventilation should be carried out to the extent possible.

Endotracheal intubation provides better control of the airway for ventilation, oxygenation, and suctioning and should be performed as soon as practical during resuscitation effort. However, the best possible ventilation and oxygenation should be provided before any attempt at intubation, and efforts should be limited to 15-30 seconds before resuming mask ventilation.

For chest compressions, a 5:1 compression-to-ventilation ratio is recommended for two-person resuscitation. Check femoral pulse for effectiveness of compressions. Monitoring of expired CO_2 (capnometry) by various devices is used to assess adequacy of ventilation and confirm endotracheal (versus esophageal) intubation. Under conditions of controlled ventilation and cardiac resuscitation, expired CO_2 may be an indicator of effective chest compressions (i.e., by Fick equation for CO_2--$\dot{V}CO_2 = Q$ x ($C\overline{V}$-Ca) CO_2--and CO_2 delivery to lungs depends on adequate cardiac output).

- Relieve obstruction.
- Oropharyngeal or nasopharyngeal airway may help maintain patency.
- Supply a high rate of flow of supplemental O_2.
- Endotracheal intubation: better control of the airway for ventilation.

Electrical Therapy

Ventricular fibrillation is commonest rhythm in sudden cardiac arrest. The time to defibrillation is the most important factor determining successful resuscitation. In monitored patients in ICUs, defibrillation should typically be the first treatment, with other life support efforts initiated only after immediate attempts at electrical conversion. Electrical pacing may be useful in some cases of bradycardia and heart block.

- Ventricular fibrillation is commonest rhythm in sudden cardiac arrest.
- Time to defibrillation is most important factor determining successful resuscitation.
- In monitored patients in ICUs, defibrillation should typically be first treatment.

Drug Therapy

Several recent trends and changes in recommendations about drug use are noteworthy. Electrical defibrillation is the treatment of choice for ventricular fibrillation. As additional therapy, lidocaine and bretylium have similar results in clinical outcome. Because bretylium may have adverse hemodynamic effects (hypotension), lidocaine is the recommended first-line therapy.

Sodium bicarbonate is still often used despite potential adverse effects and lack of documented efficacy. A rapid bolus of sodium bicarbonate may induce osmotic and ionic shifts and, by generating CO_2, may transiently worsen intracellular acidosis. Currently, bicarbonate is recommended only after another initial treatment has been established and if persistent metabolic acidosis and/or hyperkalemia is documented.

- Bicarbonate is recommended only after another initial treatment has been established.

Calcium may provide positive inotropic effects and vasoconstriction, but benefits in cardiac arrest have not been confirmed. Current indications for calcium include calcium channel blocker toxicity, acute hyperkalemia, or hypocalcemia.

- Indications for calcium: calcium channel blocker toxicity, acute hyperkalemia, hypocalcemia.

Epinephrine is administered during resuscitation from cardiac arrest for documented effects of peripheral vasoconstriction and improved coronary artery and cerebral blood flow during cardiopulmonary resuscitation. Epinephrine should also increase contractility in the beating heart. However, myocardial O_2 consumption may also increase, and automaticity and arrhythmias may be promoted. The optimal dose of epinephrine is debated. Blood flow may increase to a greater extent at doses higher than the standard 1 mg recommended for adult humans. High dose of epinephrine (about 0.2 mg/kg) increases coronary artery perfusion in humans. Outcome and complications between standard and high doses of epinephrine: no additional toxicity but no improvement in survival. Standard doses and interval should remain the routine.

- High dose of epinephrine (about 0.2 mg/kg) increases coronary artery perfusion in humans.

VASCULAR ACCESS AND HEMODYNAMIC MONITORING

Central Venous Catheterization

The first choice for access in stable patients requiring intravenous therapy is peripheral veins. However, in ICUs, central venous catheterization is often necessary for the following indications: lack of adequate peripheral veins, need for hypertonic or phlebitic medications or solutions, need for long-term access, measurement of central pressures, and access for procedures (hemodialysis, cardiac pacing). Relative contraindications include inexperience of practitioner, coagulopathy, inability to identify landmarks, infection or burn at entry site, and thrombosis of proposed central venous site. Central venous catheters are usually placed over a guide wire (modified Seldinger technique). Complications of central venous catheterization include infections, cardiac arrhythmias, pneumothorax, air embolism, catheter or guide wire embolism, catheter knotting, bleeding, and other potential complications of needle or catheter misplacement.

- Central venous catheterization is often necessary.
- Contraindications: inexperienced practitioner, coagulopathy, inability to identify landmarks, infection or burn at entry site, thrombosis of proposed central venous site.
- Complications: infections, cardiac arrhythmias, pneumothorax, air embolism, catheter or guide wire embolism, catheter knotting, bleeding.

Catheter-related infections are usually attributed to migration of bacteria from skin along catheter tract. Catheter-related infection is usually defined by >15 colonies (CFU/mL) on semiquantitative culture of catheter tip. Catheter-related bacteremia is defined by similar growth and blood cultures positive for the same organism. Risk factors include infected catheter site or cutaneous breakdown, multiple manipulations, number of catheter lumens, and duration of use of the same site (particularly after 3-4 days). Treatment should include catheter removal and replacement at another site if necessary.

- Catheter-related infections usually are attributed to migration of bacteria from skin along catheter tract.
- Risk factors: infected catheter site or cutaneous breakdown, multiple manipulations, number of catheter lumens, duration of use of same site.

Pulmonary Artery Catheterization

Although common use (or overuse) of pulmonary artery catheterization is criticized, data from pulmonary artery catheterization may aid diagnosis and therapy in many disorders encountered in ICUs. Physiologic data that may be obtained are listed in Table 9-5.

Table 9-5.--Hemodynamic Data Obtained With Pulmonary Artery Catheterization

Variable	Normal value
Right atrial pressure (RAP)	2-8 mm Hg
Pulmonary arterial pressure (PAP)	16-24/5-12 mm Hg
Pulmonary capillary wedge pressure (PCWP)	5-12 mm Hg
Cardiac output (Q)	4-6 L/min
Cardiac index (CI = Q/body surface area)	2.5-3 L/min per m^2
Stroke volume (SV = Q/heart rate)	50-100 mL/beat
Stroke volume index (SVI = SV/body surface area)	35-50 mL/m^2
Systemic vascular resistance [SVR = (blood pressure - RAP)/Q]	10-15 mm Hg/L per min (x80 to convert to 800-1,200 dyne $\cdot$ s/cm^5)
Pulmonary vascular resistance [PVR = (PAP - PCWP)/Q]	1.5-2.5 mm Hg/L per min (100-200 dyne $\cdot$ s/cm^5)

Clinical conditions for which hemodynamic data may be useful include shock states, pulmonary edema, oliguric renal failure, indeterminate pulmonary hypertension, and myocardial and valvular disorders. Intravascular volume may be assessed more accurately, and effects of therapeutic interventions (volume, vasodilator therapy, or inotropes) may be evaluated. Mixed venous oxygen saturation may also be measured, as indicated above. This may be particularly useful in assessing the effects of PEEP on O_2 delivery (i.e., improving arterial saturation but potentially decreasing cardiac output).

Complications of pulmonary artery catheterization include arrhythmias, right bundle-branch block, complete heart block in patients with preexisting left bundle-branch block, vascular or right ventricular perforation, thrombosis and embolism, catheter knotting, infection, and pulmonary infarction or rupture due to persistent wedging or overdistention of the balloon.

- Complications of pulmonary artery catheterization: arrhythmias, right bundle-branch block, complete heart block in patients with preexisting left bundle-branch block, vascular or right ventricular perforation, thrombosis and embolism, catheter knotting, infection, pulmonary infarction or rupture due to persistent wedging or overdistention of balloon.

Use of pulmonary capillary wedge pressure (PCWP) as indicator of left ventricular end-diastolic pressure assumes a continuous hydrostatic column from pulmonary capillary to left atrium. Although digital displays of PCWP are usually available, the pressure wave should be examined for potential artifacts and for degree of respiratory variation. Because varying intrathoracic pressure may be sensed by the pulmonary artery catheter, recorded PCWP should be obtained at end expiration. Even with these measures, PCWP may be influenced by airway pressure--thus, not accurately reflecting ventricular filling pressure--especially with high levels of PEEP.

- PCWP is indicator of left ventricular end-diastolic pressure.
- PCWP may be influenced by airway pressure, especially with high levels of PEEP.

SHOCK STATES

Shock is defined by evidence of end-organ hypoperfusion, usually (but not necessarily) associated with hypotension. Common classification is cardiogenic (decreased cardiac output), hypovolemic (decreased blood volume), and septic (variable cardiac output, decreased systemic vascular resistance). All forms of shock may be characterized by hypotension, tachycardia, tachypnea, altered mental status, decreased urine output, and lactic acidosis. The clinical history often helps determine the diagnosis, e.g., blood loss, trauma, myocardial infarction, systemic infection. Compared with other causes, septic shock is often characterized by relatively warm extremities and normal or elevated cardiac output.

- Shock is defined by evidence of end-organ hypoperfusion, usually associated with hypotension.
- Common classification: cardiogenic, hypovolemic, septic.
- Shock is characterized by hypotension, tachycardia, tachypnea, altered mental status, decreased urine output, lactic acidosis.
- Septic shock is often characterized by relatively warm extremities and normal or elevated cardiac output.

Sepsis syndrome is typically defined by a known or presumed source of infection associated with fever (or hypothermia) and leukocytosis (or leukopenia) *and* evidence of systemic effects, including hypotension, decreased urine output, or metabolic acidosis. After rapid initial assessment, treatment is directed at the presumed source, e.g., volume (blood loss, hypovolemia), vasodilator, or inotropic therapy (cardiogenic) or fluids, antibiotics, and drainage of any infected space (sepsis). If response to initial therapy is inadequate, and especially if intravascular volume status is uncertain clinically, pulmonary artery catheterization may be useful. For example, if the wedge pressure remains <12-15 mm Hg, further volume support and/or erythrocytes should be administered. If the wedge pressure is >18-20 mm Hg and there is evidence of cardiac dysfunction, a vasodilator (nitroprusside) and diuretic therapy might be considered. If "hyperdynamic" indices are observed, i.e., increased cardiac output and low peripheral resistance, fluids should first be given to achieve a high-normal wedge pressure. Low doses of dopamine, 2-5 µg/kg per minute, may improve renal perfusion. *After* volume support has been given and tissue perfusion is still inadequate, careful administration of vasoconstrictors (norepinephrine) may improve organ perfusion. Septic shock is commonly associated with multiorgan injury. Multisystem organ failure is typically defined as acute dysfunction of two or more organ systems lasting >2 days. Sepsis is the commonest cause. The pathogenesis is attributed to hemodynamic and immunologic effects of endotoxin, cytokines (tumor necrosis factor [TNF-α]), interleukins (IL-1, IL-2, IL-6), platelet activating factor, arachidonic acid metabolites, polymorphonuclear leukocyte-derived toxic products, and myocardial depressant factors. Corticosteroids have no known benefit and potential adverse effects in patients with sepsis syndrome, with or without ARDS.

- Sepsis syndrome is typically defined by known or presumed source of infection associated with fever (or hypothermia) and leukocytosis (or leukopenia) and evidence of systemic effects (hypotension, decreased urine output, metabolic acidosis).
- Treatment is directed at the presumed source.
- Septic shock is commonly associated with multiorgan injury.
- Multisystem organ failure: acute dysfunction of two or more organ systems lasting >2 days.
- Pathogenesis is attributed to hemodynamic and immunologic effects of endotoxin, cytokines (TNF-α),

IL-1, IL-2, IL-6, platelet activating factor, arachidonic acid metabolites, polymorphonuclear leukocyte-derived toxic products, and myocardial depressant factors.
- Corticosteroids have no known benefit.

Mortality in patients with sepsis and multiorgan failure may be >70%-90%. Adverse risk factors include age >65 years, continued systemic signs of sepsis, persistent deficit in O_2 delivery, and preexisting renal or liver failure. Physiologic scoring systems (e.g., APACHE) may predict outcome more accurately for patient subgroups.

- Mortality in patients with sepsis and multiorgan failure may be >70%-90%.

ETHICS IN THE ICU

The principles listed in Table 9-6 provide a framework for assessing ethical issues in the ICU. However, the potential for conflict frequently arises because patients are often unable to participate in their own care, multiple family members may be involved, and medical staff may disagree about prognosis and proposed interventions.

Recent legal opinions have supported the concept that a competent person may refuse life-sustaining therapy. Decision making for incompetent patients is more controversial, and living-will legislation has been designed partly to address such conflicts.

- A competent person may refuse life-sustaining therapy.
- Decision making for incompetent patients is more controversial; living-will legislation has been designed partly to address such conflicts.

Do Not Resuscitate orders have become increasingly common and important in recent years. Guidelines of the American Medical Association include:
1. Consent to cardiopulmonary resuscitation is presumed unless the patient (or patient's surrogate) has expressed in advance the wish not to be resuscitated or if, in the judgment of the treating physician, an attempt to resuscitate the patient would be futile. Resuscitation efforts should be considered futile if they cannot be expected either to restore cardiac or respiratory function or to achieve the expressed goals of the patient.
2. The appropriateness of cardiopulmonary resuscitation should be discussed with those patients at risk of cardiopulmonary arrest, preferably in the outpa-

Table 9-6.--Principles for Assessing Ethical Issues in Intensive Care Units

Beneficence--acting in the patient's benefit by sustaining life, treating illness, and relieving pain

Nonmaleficence--do no harm

Autonomy--fundamental right to self-determination

Informed consent--providing factual and adequate information for competent patients to make decisions about their care

Substituted judgment--ability of a family member, guardian, or other surrogate to make decisions on behalf of the patient on the basis of what he or she believes the patient would have chosen if competent

Social justice--allocation of medical resources according to need (note that this concept implies overt health care rationing and may conflict with perceived individual rights)

Advance directives--living will: designed for persons to express their wishes regarding life-sustaining treatment at such time when they are deemed terminally ill and no longer able to participate in such decisions; typically there is provision or request for denial of specific life-support measures and designation of a surrogate decision maker.

tient setting or early during hospitalization, and resuscitation status should be reassessed periodically.
3. The physician is ethically obligated to honor resuscitation preferences of the patient or surrogate except when this would mandate use of futile therapeutic efforts (potential conflicts may arise in the application of this principle).
4. "Do Not Resuscitate" orders should be entered in the medical record.
5. "Do Not Resuscitate" orders affect administration of cardiopulmonary resuscitation only; other therapeutic interventions should not be influenced by the order.

Withholding Life Support Versus Withdrawal of Existing Support

Recent deliberations and court rulings have supported the concept that withholding and withdrawing of life support are essentially equivalent. In general, an irreversible or terminal illness is considered a prerequisite for withdrawal of support, but interpretation may vary widely.

- Withholding and withdrawing of life support are essentially equivalent.

QUESTIONS
(See "Answers" section)

Multiple Choice
1. Which of the following variables would most likely indicate need for mechanical ventilation:
    a. V_D/V_T of 0.30
    b. Shunt fraction of $Q_S/Q_T = 0.08$
    c. Maximal inspiratory pressure, -15 cm H_2O
    d. Minute ventilation, 8 L
    e. Alveolar-arterial gradient, 50 mm Hg on 50% O_2

2. A 30-year-old asthmatic man is admitted in acute respiratory distress. $Paco_2$ is 50 mm Hg. Mechanical ventilation is begun with assist-control mode; tidal volume, 1 L; rate, 20 breaths/minute. Progressive hypotension develops over 15 minutes. Which of the following is the least appropriate admission order:
    a. Decrease respiratory rate
    b. Corticosteroids
    c. Bronchodilators
    d. Dopamine infusion
    e. Saline given intravenously

3. A 40-year-old woman survived a 3-month hospitalization for ruptured gallbladder with sepsis and adult respiratory distress syndrome. One year later, pulmonary function studies would most likely show which one of the following:
    a. Pao_2, 55 mm Hg on room air
    b. CO diffusing capacity, 80% predicted
    c. Total lung capacity, 60% predicted
    d. FEV_1, 50% predicted
    e. Lung compliance, 60% predicted

4. A pulmonary artery catheter yields the following values in a hypotensive 50-year-old man: pulmonary artery pressure, 25/5 mm Hg; pulmonary artery wedge, 4 mm Hg; Svo_2, 75%; cardiac output, 8 L/min. Which of the following is most likely:
    a. Cardiac tamponade
    b. Pulmonary embolism
    c. Adult respiratory distress syndrome
    d. Sepsis
    e. Mitral regurgitation

5. Which of the following is most often associated with multiorgan failure?
    a. Long-bone fracture
    b. Gastric aspiration
    c. Multiple transfusions
    d. Closed head injury
    e. Sepsis

True/False
6. A 19-year-old man was admitted after a drug overdose suicide attempt. Arterial blood gas values on room air show Pao_2, 30 mm Hg; $Paco_2$, 80 mm Hg; and pH 7.10. Indicate whether the following are true or false:
    a. Aspiration pneumonia is likely
    b. Hypoventilation is the main cause of hypoxemia
    c. Supplemental O_2 should increase the $Paco_2$
    d. Assisted ventilation should increase the Pao_2
    e. $NaHCO_3$ should be given
    f. Anion gap is most likely normal

7. Indicate whether or not the following are characteristic of adult respiratory distress syndrome:
    a. Evidence of intrapulmonary shunting
    b. Increased lung compliance
    c. Neutrophilic alveolitis
    d. Overall survival less than 20%
    e. Loss of type II pneumocytes
    f. Improved survival with high doses of steroids

NOTES

CHAPTER 10
DERMATOLOGY

Marian T. McEvoy, M.D.
Margot S. Peters, M.D.

CUTANEOUS SIGNS OF UNDERLYING MALIGNANCY

Cutaneous metastasis occurs in 1%-5% of patients with metastatic neoplasms. The types of malignancy metastatic to the skin reflect the most common types of visceral carcinoma, in particular, lung, breast, kidney, gastrointestinal, melanoma, and ovary. Lesions usually present on the scalp, face, or trunk.

- Cutaneous metastasis occurs in 1%-5% of patients with metastatic neoplasms.
- Lesions usually present on scalp, face, trunk.

Paget's disease of the nipple is an erythematous, scaly, or weepy eczematous eruption of the areola. Virtually all patients with Paget's disease have an underlying ductal carcinoma of the breast. In contrast, *extramammary Paget's disease*, a morphologically similar eruption that usually occurs in the anogenital region, is associated with underlying carcinoma in only about 50% of cases. Extramammary Paget's disease may be associated with underlying cutaneous adnexal carcinoma or with underlying visceral carcinoma (particularly of the genitourinary or distal gastrointestinal tracts).

- Patients with Paget's disease have underlying ductal carcinoma of breast.
- Extramammary Paget's disease is associated with underlying carcinoma in only 50% of cases.

Acanthosis nigricans (color plate 10-1) consists of velvety hyperpigmentation of the intertriginous regions, particularly the axillae and groin. It has been associated with adenocarcinoma of the gastrointestinal tract, particularly the stomach, and insulin-resistant diabetes. Acanthosis nigricans may also be associated with obesity or certain medications (such as prednisone and nicotinic acid) or have an autosomal-dominant variant.

- Acanthosis nigricans associated with adenocarcinoma of gastrointestinal tract, particularly stomach, and insulin-resistant diabetes.
- May also be associated with obesity and certain medications.

Pyoderma gangrenosum (color plate 10-2) consists of ulcers with irregular, undermined, inflammatory, violaceous borders that heal with cribriform scarring. The lesions are most commonly associated with inflammatory bowel disease or rheumatoid arthritis. The bullous form of pyoderma gangrenosum is associated with malignancy of the hematopoietic system, particularly leukemia.

- Pyoderma gangrenosum most commonly associated with inflammatory bowel disease or rheumatoid arthritis.
- Bullous form is associated with leukemia.

The skin lesions of *glucagonoma syndrome (necrolytic migratory erythema)* (color plate 10-3) consist of erosions, crusting, and peeling, particularly involving the perineum and perioral areas, but may be generalized. The syndrome also includes stomatitis, glossitis (beefy tongue), anemia, diarrhea, and weight loss. It is associated with an islet cell (α) tumor of the pancreas.

- Glucagonoma syndrome consists of erosions, crusting, and peeling involving perineum and perioral areas.

- Associated with islet cell tumor of pancreas.

Leser-Trélat syndrome consists of sudden onset of numerous seborrheic keratoses, and it may be associated with underlying malignancy.

Torre's (Muir-Torre) syndrome consists of multiple sebaceous tumors of the skin associated with visceral carcinomas. These tumors are sebaceous adenomas, sebaceous epitheliomas, or sebaceous carcinomas. Patients may have one or numerous lesions. In addition, keratoacanthomas of the skin are also part of this syndrome. Of the underlying malignancies, carcinoma of the colon is the most common, although breast, hematologic, and other malignancies have been observed. There is a genetic predisposition and, in some cases, an association with the "cancer family syndrome."

- Torre's syndrome consists of multiple sebaceous tumors of skin associated with visceral carcinomas.
- Carcinoma of colon is most common underlying malignancy.

Cowden's syndrome has autosomal dominant inheritance. Cutaneous abnormalities include trichilemmomas, verrucous papules, and oral fibromas. The syndrome is associated with thyroid and breast carcinoma. There is an increased incidence of fibrocystic disease of breast and thyroid adenoma.

- Cowden's syndrome has autosomal-dominant inheritance.
- Cutaneous abnormalities: trichilemmomas, verrucous papules, oral fibromas.

Gardner's syndrome is a hereditary (autosomal dominant) form of colonic polyposis. Clinical features include adenomatous polyps of the colon, osteomas of the skull and face, scoliosis, soft tissue tumors (including dermoids, lipomas, and fibromas), and sebaceous (epidermal inclusion) cysts of the face and scalp. There is a high incidence of colonic carcinoma. Approximately 60% of patients develop adenocarcinoma of the colon by age 40 years, and malignancies of other sites have been associated with this syndrome, including adrenal, ovarian, and thyroid.

- Gardner's syndrome is a hereditary (autosomal-dominant) form of colonic polyposis.
- Clinical features: soft tissue tumors, sebaceous cysts of face.

- There is a high incidence of colonic carcinoma.

Acquired ichthyosis has most often been associated with Hodgkin's disease, but it has been reported with other types of lymphoma, multiple myeloma, and various carcinomas.

- Acquired ichthyosis associated with Hodgkin's disease.

Paraneoplastic acrokeratosis of Bazex consists of psoriasiform lesions of the hands, feet, ears, and nose, onychodystrophy, and carcinoma of the upper respiratory system, pharynx, or esophagus.

- Paraneoplastic acrokeratosis of Bazex consists of psoriasiform lesions and carcinoma of the upper respiratory system.

Hirsutism may reflect androgen excess due to an adrenal or ovarian tumor.

Hypertrichosis represents increase in hair unrelated to androgen excess, such as hypertrichosis lanuginosa acquisita (growth of soft downy hairs). It has been associated with carcinoid tumor, adenocarcinoma of the breast, lymphoma, gastrointestinal malignancy, and other types of neoplasms.

Erythema gyratum repens presents with a striking pattern of concentric erythematous bands in a "wood grain" pattern almost universally associated with underlying malignancy. The classic association is with breast carcinoma, but other types of malignancies have been reported.

- Erythema gyratum repens classically associated with breast carcinoma.

Sweet's syndrome (acute febrile neutrophilic dermatosis) has skin lesions that consist of erythematous plaques and nodules, most commonly located on the extremities and face. The association is with leukemia, particularly acute myelocytic or acute myelomonocytic leukemia.

- Sweet's syndrome is associated with leukemia.

Generalized pruritus is the presentation for many cutaneous and systemic disorders. Pruritus may be the presenting symptom in lymphoma.

- Pruritus may be presenting symptom in lymphoma.

In *dermatomyositis*, the pathognomonic skin lesions are Gottron's papules (color plate 10-4) involving the skin over the joints of the fingers, elbows, and knees. Poikilodermatous lesions or erythematous macular-papular eruptions may diffusely involve the face, particularly the periorbital area ("heliotrope rash" [color plate 10-5]), and the trunk and extremities. The cutaneous lesions are photosensitive. The disease is characterized by proximal myositis. Although creatine phosphokinase levels are usually elevated in patients with myositis, it is important to verify the diagnosis by obtaining a muscle biopsy specimen. Dermatomyositis is associated with an increased incidence of underlying malignancy.

- Dermatomyositis may involve periorbital area ("heliotrope rash") or dorsal aspect of hands (Gottron's papules).
- Lesions are photosensitive.
- Characterized by proximal myositis.

Multiple mucosal neuromas syndrome is associated with autosomal dominant inheritance. The main features include neuromas of the skin or mucosa (anterior tongue, lips, eyelids, conjunctiva), medullary carcinoma of the thyroid, pheochromocytoma, and parathyroid adenoma.

- Multiple mucosal neuromas syndrome: medullary carcinoma of thyroid, pheochromocytoma, parathyroid adenoma.

Cutaneous *amyloidosis* may present clinically as macroglossia (color plate 10-6), waxy papules on the eyelids or nasolabial folds, pinch-purpura, and postproctoscopic purpura (color plate 10-7). Multiple myeloma may be associated with amyloid.

- Amyloidosis may be associated with multiple myeloma.

Tylosis is a rare disorder characterized by palmar-plantar keratoderma associated with esophageal carcinoma. It has autosomal dominant inheritance.

- Tylosis is associated with esophageal carcinoma.

The *autoimmune bullous diseases* are a heterogeneous group of disorders characterized by antibody deposition at the basement membrane zone or epidermis. An association with malignancy has been demonstrated in several of these disorders.

- Pemphigus is associated with thymoma with or without myasthenia gravis.
- Paraneoplastic pemphigus that presents with clinical and histologic features of pemphigus and erythema multiforme is associated with lymphomas and leukemia.
- Patients with dermatitis herpetiformis rarely develop intestinal lymphoma.
- Epidermolysis bullosa acquisita is associated with amyloidosis and multiple myeloma.
- Bullous pemphigoid has not been associated with an increased risk of underlying malignancy.

DERMATOLOGY: AN INTERNIST'S PERSPECTIVE

Respiratory

The skin is involved in 15%-35% of patients with *sarcoidosis*. Lesions may present as 1) lupus pernio (erythematous swelling of the nose), 2) translucent papules around the eyes and nasolabial folds, 3) annular lesions with central atrophy, 4) nodules on the trunk and extremities, and 5) scar sarcoid. Acute sarcoidosis may present with a combination of erythema nodosum, bilateral hilar lymphadenopathy, fever, and arthralgias (Löfgren's syndrome).

- Skin involved in 15%-35% of patients with sarcoidosis.
- Lesions may present as lupus pernio (erythematous swelling of nose).

Erythema nodosum (color plate 10-8) is a reactive condition that may be associated with acute sarcoidosis. Erythema nodosum typically presents as tender, erythematous, subcutaneous nodules localized to pretibial areas. The lesions may be acute and self-limited or chronic, lasting for months up to years.

- Erythema nodosum is caused by many conditions.
- May be associated with acute sarcoidosis.

In *Wegener's granulomatosis*, cutaneous involvement

occurs in >50% of patients and is manifested by cutaneous infarction, ulceration, hemorrhagic bullae, purpuric papules, or urticaria. A skin biopsy may show hypersensitivity vasculitis or granulomatous vasculitis.

- In Wegener's granulomatosis, cutaneous involvement in >50% of patients.
- Manifestations: ulceration, hemorrhagic bullae, purpuric papules, urticaria.

Churg-Strauss granulomatosis/allergic granulomatosis syndrome is characterized by combination of adult-onset asthma, peripheral eosinophilia, and pulmonary involvement with recurrent pneumonia or transient infiltrates. Skin lesions have been reported in up to 60% of patients and consist of palpable purpura, cutaneous infarcts, and subcutaneous nodules.

- Skin lesions of Churg-Strauss granulomatosis occur in up to 60% of patients.
- Skin lesions include palpable purpura, cutaneous infarct, subcutaneous nodules.

In *relapsing polychondritis*, there is episodic destructive inflammation of cartilage of the ears, nose , and upper airways. There may be associated arthritis and ocular involvement. In the acute stage, the ears may be red, swollen, and tender. Later, they become soft and flabby. Nasal chondritis may lead to saddle-nose deformities. Relapsing polychondritis is mediated by antibodies to type II collagen.

- Relapsing polychondritis: episodic destructive inflammation of cartilage of ears, nose, upper airways.
- Nasal chondritis may lead to saddle-nose deformities.

Cardiovascular

In several syndromes, lentigines have been associated with cardiac abnormalities. These include the *LEOPARD*, *NAME*, and *LAMB* syndromes.

- LEOPARD syndrome (Moynahan's syndrome): *l*entigines, *e*lectrocardiographic changes, *o*cular hypertelorism, *p*ulmonary stenosis, *a*bnormal genitalia, *r*etardation of growth, *d*eafness.
- NAME syndrome: *n*evi, *a*trial myxoma, *m*yxoid neurofibromas, *e*philides.
- LAMB syndrome: *l*entigines, *a*trial myxoma, *m*ucocutaneous myxomas, *b*lue nevi.

Pseudoxanthoma elasticum may be transmitted by autosomal dominant or autosomal recessive inheritance. Yellow xanthoma-like papules are seen on the neck (plucked-chicken skin), axillae, groin, and abdomen. Angioid streaks may be seen in the fundus. Skin biopsy shows degeneration of elastic fibers. Systemic associations include stroke, myocardial infarction, and peripheral vascular disease.

- Pseudoxanthoma elasticum associated with stroke, myocardial infarction, peripheral vascular disease.

Ehlers-Danlos syndrome includes 10 subgroups that vary in severity and systemic associations. Cutaneous findings are skin hyperextensibility with hypermobile joints and fish-mouth scars. Angina, peripheral vascular disease, and gastrointestinal bleeding may be associated.

- Ehlers-Danlos syndrome associated with angina, peripheral vascular disease, gastrointestinal bleeding.

Erythema marginatum is one of the diagnostic criteria for acute rheumatic fever. This uncommon eruption occurs on the trunk and is characterized by erythematous plaques with rapidly mobile serpiginous borders.

- Erythema marginatum is one of diagnostic criteria for acute rheumatic fever.

Gastrointestinal

Osler-Weber-Rendu syndrome (hereditary hemorrhagic telangiectasia), with autosomal dominant inheritance, is manifested by cutaneous and mucosal telangiectasias. Frequent nosebleeds and gastrointestinal bleeds may be a presenting feature. Pulmonary arteriovenous malformations and central nervous system angiomas are also features of this syndrome.

- Osler-Weber-Rendu syndrome has autosomal dominant inheritance.
- Features: nosebleeds, gastrointestinal bleeds, pulmonary arteriovenous malformations, central nervous system angiomas.

Acrodermatitis enteropathica is an inherited (autosomal recessive) or acquired disease characterized by zinc deficiency (failure of absorption or failure to supplement). The clinical features include angular cheilitis, a seborrheic dermatitis-like eruption, erosions, blisters, and pustules, with skin lesions particularly involving the face, hands, feet, and perineum. Alopecia and diarrhea are other features of this syndrome.

- Acrodermatitis enteropathica: inherited (autosomal recessive) or acquired disease.
- Characterized by zinc deficiency (failure of absorption or failure to supplement).
- Alopecia and diarrhea are other features.

Peutz-Jeghers syndrome is an inherited (autosomal dominant) syndrome of intestinal polyposis. Patients have hamartomas, mostly involving the small bowel, without an increased risk of developing carcinoma. Cutaneous lesions include macular pigmentation (freckles) of the lips, periungual skin, fingers, and toes and pigmentation of the oral mucosa.

- Peutz-Jeghers syndrome is inherited (autosomal dominant) syndrome of intestinal polyposis.
- No increase in risk of developing carcinoma.

Dermatitis herpetiformis (color plate 10-9) is an immune-mediated bullous disease that presents with intensely itchy vesicles on extensor surfaces (elbows, knees, buttocks, scapula). Gluten-sensitive enteropathy occurs in up to 70% of patients.

- Dermatitis herpetiformis is immune-mediated bullous disease.
- Gluten-sensitive enteropathy occurs in up to 70% of patients.

Extensive *aphthous ulceration* may be associated with Crohn's disease or gluten-sensitive enteropathy.

- Aphthous ulceration may be associated with Crohn's disease or gluten-sensitive enteropathy.

Pyoderma gangrenosum (color plate 10-2) presents with ulceration, predominantly on the lower extremities, with inflammatory undermined borders. The lesions heal with cribriform scarring. The phenomenon whereby lesions occur at sites of trauma is known as pathery-- the occurrence of the disease at sites of trauma is classic. Systemic disease associations include inflammatory bowel disease (ulcerative colitis more commonly than Crohn's disease), rheumatoid arthritis, and paraproteinemia.

- Pyoderma gangrenosum occurs at sites of trauma.
- Associated diseases are inflammatory bowel disease (ulcerative colitis more than Crohn's disease), rheumatoid arthritis, paraproteinemia.

Cutaneous Crohn's disease may present as skin nodules with granulomatous histology. Other manifestations include pyostomatitis vegetans (granulomatous inflammation of the gingivae), granulomatous cheilitis, oral aphthous ulceration, perianal skin tags, and perianal fistulae.

- Manifestation of Crohn's disease: pyostomatitis vegetans (granulomatous inflammation of gingivae).

Bowel bypass syndrome presents with a flu-like illness with fever, malaise, arthralgias, myalgias, and inflammatory papules and pustules on the extremities and upper trunk. The disease is recurrent and episodic and occurs in up to 20% of patients after jejunoileal bypass. The condition responds to antibiotics or to reversal of the bypass procedure.

- Bowel bypass syndrome: flu-like illness, inflammatory papules and pustules.
- Occurs in up to 20% of patients after jejunoileal bypass.

Gardner's syndrome is described on page 178, and *glucagonoma syndrome* is described on page 177.

Nephrology
Partial lipodystrophy is associated with C3 deficiency and the nephrotic syndrome.

Neurocutaneous
Fabry's disease is an X-linked recessive disorder due to deficiency of the enzyme α-galactosidase A. The skin changes consist of numerous vascular tumors (angiokeratomas) that develop during childhood and adolescence. Corneal opacities are present in 90% of patients. Systemic manifestations include paresthesias and pain due to involved peripheral nerves, renal insufficiency, and vascular insufficiency of the coronary and central nervous system.

- Fabry's disease is recessive disorder due to deficiency of α-galactosidase A.
- Systemic manifestations: paresthesias, renal insufficiency, vascular insufficiency.

The clinical features of *ataxia-telangiectasia* include

cutaneous and ocular telangiectasia, cerebellar ataxia, choreoathetosis, IgA deficiency, and recurrent pulmonary infections.

Tuberous sclerosis may be inherited in an autosomal dominant pattern (25%) or may occur sporadically (new mutation). Predominant cutaneous lesions include hypopigmented macules, adenoma sebaceum, subungual or periungual fibromas, and shagreen patch (connective tissue nevus) (color plate 10-10). This syndrome is associated with epilepsy (80%) and mental retardation (60%). Rhabdomyomas may occur in the heart in childhood. Angiomyolipomas occur in the kidneys in up to 80% of adults with this syndrome.

- Tuberous sclerosis may be inherited in autosomal dominant pattern or be sporadic.
- Associated with epilepsy (80%) and mental retardation (60%).
- Angiomyolipomas occur in kidneys in up to 80% of affected adults.

Neurofibromatosis (von Recklinghausen's disease) (color plate 10-11) occurs in 1 in 3,000 births. Inheritance is autosomal dominant, and approximately 50% of cases are new mutations. The major signs of the disease are café-au-lait spots, axillary freckling (Crowe's sign), neurofibromas, and Lisch nodules of the iris.

- Neurofibromatosis is autosomal dominant.
- Major signs: café-au-lait spots, axillary freckling, neurofibromas.

Neurofibromatosis has various clinical manifestations, as reflected in Ricardi's classification:

1. Classic: Neurofibromas, café-au-lait spots, Lisch nodules of iris, chromosome 17, positive family history.
2. Central: Bilateral acoustic neuromas, few neurofibromas, few café-au-lait spots, *no Lisch nodules*, chromosome 22, positive family history.
3. Mixed: Features of no. 1 and no. 2, central nervous system tumors, positive family history.
4. Variant: Variable family history, diffuse café-au-lait spots, neurofibromas, with or without central nervous system tumors.
5. Segmental or dermatomal: Neurofibromas or café-au-lait spots, skin involvement only, negative family history.
6. Multiple café-au-lait spots: Skin involvement only, negative family history, no neurofibromas.

7. Late onset: Cutaneous disease for >30 years.
8. Other: Clinical syndromes not fitting the above classifications.

The associated central nervous system tumors include acoustic neuromas, optic gliomas, and meningiomas. Other associated tumors include pheochromocytoma, neuroblastoma, and Wilms' tumor. Café-au-lait spots and neurofibromas frequently occur in the absence of neurofibromatosis. The diagnostic criteria for neurofibromatosis include two or more of the following:

1. Six or more café-au-lait macules > 0.5 cm in greatest diameter in prepubertal patients, or >1.5 cm in diameter in adults.
2. Two or more neurofibromas of any type, or one plexiform neurofibroma.
3. Freckling of skin in axillary or inguinal regions.
4. Optic gliomas.
5. Lisch nodules.
6. An osseous lesion such as sphenoid dysplasia or thinning of long bone cortex with or without pseudarthrosis.
7. A first-degree relative with neurofibromatosis that meets the above diagnostic criteria.

Sturge-Weber-Dimitri syndrome is characterized by capillary angioma (port-wine stain) in the distribution of the upper or middle branch of the trigeminal nerve. There may be associated meningeal angioma in the same distribution. Intracranial tramline calcification, mental retardation, epilepsy, contralateral hemiparesis, and visual impairment may be associated.

- Sturge-Weber-Dimitri syndrome characterized by capillary angioma in distribution of upper or middle branch of trigeminal nerve.
- Associated features: intracranial calcification, mental retardation, epilepsy, contralateral hemiparesis, visual impairment.

Klippel-Trenaunay-Weber syndrome is the constellation of hemangiomas in a dermatomal distribution with associated arteriovenous malformation.

Cobb's syndrome is a noninherited disorder in which port-wine stain or angiokeratoma occurs in a dermatomal distribution associated with spinal cord angioma within one to two segments of the cutaneous lesions.

Sneddon's syndrome involves extensive livedo reticularis and cerebrovascular accidents, possibly as manifestation of the antiphospholipid syndrome.

Cerebral granulomatous angiitis is a sequela of ophthalmic herpes zoster and is responsible for the combination of ophthalmic zoster followed by a delayed contralateral hemiplegia (weeks to months; average, 8 weeks).

Rheumatology: Cutaneous Associations of Arthritis

Psoriasis has a frequency of approximately 1% in the United States. Onset of lesions is usually in the third decade of life, and about one-third of patients have a family history of psoriasis. The cutaneous disease is usually chronic, and the most common presentation is with papules or plaques covered with silvery scales. Removal of the scale results in pinpoint bleeding, a phenomenon referred to as Auspitz sign. Approximately 50% of patients have nail abnormalities, most commonly onycholysis, pitting, and oil spots. Psoriatic lesions are characterized by "koebnerization" (induction of lesions at sites of trauma).

- Onset of psoriasis lesions is in third decade of life.
- One-third of patients have family history.
- 50% of patients have nail abnormalities.

Psoriatic arthritis occurs in 4%-5% of patients with psoriasis. It is characterized by involvement of the distal interphalangeal joints, but also with involvement of the proximal interphalangeal joints. Most patients have asymmetric involvement of few joints of the fingers or toes. A small percentage of patients have symmetric polyarthritis resembling rheumatoid arthritis. The most severe form of psoriatic arthritis, arthritis mutilans, is associated with osteolysis resulting in "telescoping" of digits and dissolution of distal phalanges. Approximately 5% of patients with psoriatic arthritis have ankylosing spondylitis.

- Psoriatic arthritis occurs in 4%-5% of patients with psoriasis.
- Characterized by involvement of distal interphalangeal joints.
- 5% of patients have ankylosing spondylitis.

Reiter's syndrome consists of the triad of urethritis, conjunctivitis, and arthritis. The disease usually affects young men. Two-thirds of patients have skin lesions, namely, circinate balinitis, consisting of erythematous plaques of the penis, and keratoderma blennorrhagicum, a pustular psoriasiform eruption of the palms and soles. Most patients are HLA-B27 positive.

- Reiter's syndrome triad: urethritis, conjunctivitis, arthritis.
- Most patients are HLA-B27 positive.

Multicentric reticulohistiocytosis may affect the skin, mucosa, joints, bones, and viscera. Most patients have skin lesions and arthritis. Skin lesions consist of red-brown papules and nodules, most commonly located on the dorsal aspects of hands and face. Approximately half of all patients have mucosal lesions, particularly of the lips, buccal mucosa, tongue, gingiva, or nose. The arthritis consists of severely destructive and mutilating involvement, particularly of the interphalangeal joints of the hands ("opera glass hand" or "telescope fingers"), knees, wrists, hips, ankles, feet, elbows, and spine. Multicentric reticulohistiocytosis has also been associated with underlying malignancy.

- Multicentric reticulohistiocytosis involves skin lesions and arthritis.
- May be associated with underlying malignancy.

Erythema chronicum migrans is an annular, sometimes urticarial, erythematous lesion presenting as a manifestation of Lyme disease. The lesion develops subsequent to, and surrounding the site of, a tick bite. Lesions are single in 75% of patients and multiple in 25%. Other acute features of Lyme disease include fever, headaches, myalgias, arthralgias, and lymphadenopathy. The tick, *Ixodes dammini*, contains a spirochete, *Borrelia burgdorferi*, that is thought to be responsible for the syndrome. Arthritis is a late complication of Lyme disease. Weeks or months after the initial illness, patients may develop meningoencephalitis, peripheral neuropathy, myocarditis, atrioventricular node block, or destructive erosive arthritis.

- Erythema chronicum migrans presents as manifestation of Lyme disease.
- Lesion develops subsequent to and surrounding site of tick bite.
- Lesions are single in 75% of patients and multiple in 25%.

In *rheumatoid arthritis,* nodules occur over the extensor surfaces of joints, most commonly on the dorsal hands and elbows. Rheumatoid vasculitis with ulceration may occur in the setting of rheumatoid arthritis with a high circulating rheumatoid factor.

During the late stages of *gout*, tophi (urate deposits with surrounding inflammation) occur in the subcutaneous tissues. Improved methods of treatment account for the decrease in the incidence of tophaceous gout in recent years.

- With gout, tophi occur in subcutaneous tissues.

In *lupus erythematosus* (LE), cutaneous abnormalities occur in approximately 80% of patients. LE has been classified into chronic cutaneous LE (localized discoid LE and generalized discoid LE), subacute cutaneous LE, and acute cutaneous LE (malar rash, generalized macular-papular erythema, or bullous LE).

- In LE, cutaneous abnormalities occur in 80% of patients.

Discoid LE (color plate 10-12) is characterized by erythematous papules and plaques with follicular hyperkeratosis and scaling. Localized discoid LE is usually not associated with systemic LE. Generalized discoid LE or disseminated discoid LE refers to lesions involving the head and neck area or the trunk and extremities. Discoid LE most commonly affects the face, scalp, and ears. Although most patients with discoid LE lack manifestations of systemic LE, approximately 25% of patients with systemic LE have had cutaneous lesions of discoid LE at some point during the course of their illness.

- Discoid LE characterized by erythematous papules and plaques with follicular hyperkeratosis and scaling.
- Discoid LE most commonly affects face, scalp, ears.
- 25% of patients with systemic LE have had cutaneous manifestations of discoid LE.

Subacute cutaneous LE (color plate 10-13) usually presents with generalized annular or polycyclic papules and plaques. The lesions may appear papulosquamous or vesiculobullous. Subacute cutaneous LE is characterized by the presence of anti-Ro (anti-SSA) antibodies in serum and photosensitivity.

- Subacute cutaneous LE presents with annular or polycyclic papules and plaques.
- Characterized by presence of anti-Ro (anti-SSA) antibodies and photosensitivity.

The "lupus band test" consists of the finding of immunoglobulin and complement at the basement membrane zone of skin biopsy tissue as determined by direct immunofluorescence testing. In biopsy of lesional tissue from discoid LE or systemic LE, immunoglobulin and complement are demonstrable at the basement membrane zone in >90% of patients. Only 50%-60% of patients with subacute cutaneous LE have a positive lupus band test of lesional skin. The lupus band test is positive in nonlesional skin (normal-appearing, non-sun-exposed skin, typically buttock) from 50% of patients with systemic LE and in nonlesional sun-exposed skin of the forearm from 75% of patients with systemic LE, and it is generally negative in nonlesional skin of patients with discoid LE. Therefore, direct immunofluorescence testing of nonlesional, non-sun-exposed skin is specific, but not highly sensitive, for LE.

- Only 50%-60% of patients with subacute cutaneous LE have positive lupus band test of lesional skin.
- Direct immunofluorescence testing of nonlesional, non-sun-exposed skin is specific, but not sensitive, for LE.

Circulating antinuclear antibodies are demonstrable in most patients with systemic LE and subacute cutaneous erythematosus, but they are present in only a small percentage of patients with discoid LE. A homogeneous antinuclear antibody pattern tends to correlate with the diagnosis of systemic LE, peripheral (rim) pattern correlates with lupus nephritis, speckled anticentromere pattern is associated with the CREST variant of scleroderma (CREST: *c*alcinosis cutis, *R*aynaud's phenomenon, *e*sophageal dysmotility, *s*clerodactyly, and *t*elangiectasia), nucleolar pattern usually correlates with the diagnosis of scleroderma and uncommonly with lupus, and the particulate pattern is associated with various connective tissue diseases, including LE. In addition to association with subacute cutaneous LE, anti-Ro (anti-SSA) antibodies are associated with Sjögren's syndrome, LE with C2 deficiency, and neonatal LE.

Scleroderma encompasses a spectrum of diseases, including progressive systemic sclerosis, localized scleroderma, localized morphea, generalized morphea, linear scleroderma (including en coup de sabre), facial hemiatrophy, CREST syndrome, and eosinophilic fasciitis.

Morphea manifests as discrete sclerotic plaques with white shiny center and erythematous or violaceous periphery. Localized or linear scleroderma may have various presentations depending on extent, location, and depth of sclerosis. Most lesions are characterized by sclerosis and atrophy associated with depression or "delling" of the soft tissue; underlying bone may be affected.

- Morphea manifests as discrete sclerotic plaques with white shiny center.
- Underlying bone may be affected.

Systemic scleroderma consists of diffuse sclerosis associated with smoothness and hardening of the skin, with masklike face and microstomia. Sclerodactyly, periungual telangiectasia, hyperpigmentation, and cutaneous calcification may be observed. Esophageal, pulmonary, renal, and cardiac involvement may be associated with systemic scleroderma. The CREST syndrome (color plate 10-14) is associated with circulating anticentromere antibodies.

- Systemic scleroderma may include sclerodactyly, periungual telangiectasia, hyperpigmentation, and cutaneous calcification.

Eosinophilic fasciitis manifests as tightly bound thickening of the skin and underlying soft tissue of the extremities. Other features include arthralgias, hypergammaglobulinemia, and peripheral blood eosinophilia.

- Eosinophilic fasciitis manifests as tightly bound thickening of skin and underlying soft tissue of extremities.

Hematologic

Graft-versus-host disease (GVHD) most commonly occurs after bone marrow transplantation and represents the constellation of skin lesions, diarrhea, and liver function abnormalities. GVHD occurs in 60%-80% of patients who undergo allogeneic bone marrow transplantation.

- GVHD commonly occurs after bone marrow transplantation.
- Includes skin lesions, diarrhea, liver function abnormalities.

GVHD generally occurs in two phases. Acute GVHD begins 7-21 days after transplantation, and chronic GVHD begins within months to 1 year after transplantation. One or both phases may occur in the same patient. Acute GVHD results from attack of donor immunocompetent T lymphocytes and null lymphocytes against host histocompatibility antigens. Chronic GVHD results from immunocompetent lymphocytes that develop in the recipient.

The cutaneous abnormalities of acute GVHD include pruritus, numbness or pain of the palms and soles, an erythematous macular-papular eruption of the trunk, palms, and soles, and blisters that, when extensive, resemble toxic epidermal necrolysis. Acute GVHD also includes intestinal abnormalities resulting in diarrhea and liver function changes.

- Cutaneous abnormalities of GVHD: pruritus, numbness or pain of palms and soles, erythematous macular-papular eruption of trunk, palms, and soles.

Chronic GVHD mainly affects skin and liver. Early chronic GVHD is characterized by a lichenoid reaction consisting of cutaneous and oral lesions that resemble lichen planus, with coalescing violaceous papules, but also pigmentary changes. Late chronic GVHD is characterized by cutaneous sclerosis, poikilodermatous-reticulated lesions, and scarring alopecia. The histologic pattern of GVHD includes lymphocytes in proximity to dyskeratotic keratinocytes, so-called satellite cell necrosis. The cutaneous infiltrate is composed predominantly of suppressor/cytotoxic T cells.

- Chronic GVHD: lichenoid reaction consisting of cutaneous and oral lesions.

Mastocytosis (mast cell disease) can be divided into four groups, depending on the age at onset and the presence or absence of systemic involvement: 1) urticaria pigmentosa arising in infancy or adolescence without significant systemic involvement, 2) urticaria pigmentosa in adults without significant systemic involvement, 3) systemic mast cell disease, and 4) mast cell leukemia.

The cutaneous lesions may be brown to red macules, papules, nodules, or plaques that urticate on stroking. Less commonly, the lesions may be bullous, erythrodermic, or telangiectatic. The systemic manifestations are due to histamine release and consist of flushing, tachycardia, and diarrhea.

- Cutaneous lesions of mastocytosis: brown to red macules, papules, nodules, or plaques that urticate on stroking.
- Systemic manifestations--flushing, tachycardia, diarrhea--due to histamine release.

Necrobiotic xanthogranuloma--indurated plaques with associated atrophy and telangiectasia with or without ulceration--may occur on the trunk or periorbital areas. Serum electrophoresis shows an IgG κ paraproteinemia or multiple myeloma.

Endocrine

Diabetes Mellitus

Several dermatologic disorders have been described in diabetics.

Necrobiosis lipoidica diabeticorum (color plate 10-15) classically occurs on the shins and presents as yellow-brown atrophic telangiectatic plaques that occasionally ulcerate. Two-thirds of patients have diabetes.

- Necrobiosis lipoidica diabeticorum occurs on shins.
- Two-thirds of patients have diabetes.

Granuloma annulare is an asymptomatic eruption consisting of small, firm, flesh-colored or red papules in an annular configuration (color plate 10-16) (less commonly nodular or generalized). The association with diabetes is disputed.

- Granuloma annulare consists of small, firm, flesh-colored or red papules in annular configuration.

Rarely, patients with poorly controlled diabetes present with spontaneously occurring *subepidermal blisters* (bullosa diabeticorum) on the dorsal aspects of the hands and feet.

The *stiff hand syndrome* has been reported in juvenile-onset insulin-dependent diabetes. Patients have limited joint mobility and tight waxy skin on the hands. There is an increased risk of subsequent renal and retinal microvascular disease.

- Stiff hand syndrome: increased risk of subsequent renal and retinal microvascular disease.

In *scleredema*, there is an insidious onset of thickening and stiffness of the skin on the upper back and posterior neck. The condition is more common in middle-aged men with diabetes. The diabetes is often long-standing and poorly controlled.

- Scleredema is more common in middle-aged men with diabetes.

- Diabetes is often long-standing and poorly controlled.

Thyroid

Pretibial myxedema and thyroid acropachy are cutaneous associations of Graves' disease.

Metabolic

The *porphyrias* are a group of inherited or acquired abnormalities of heme synthesis. Each type is associated with deficient activity of a particular enzyme. The porphyrias are usually divided into three types: erythropoietic, hepatic, and mixed.

Erythropoietic porphyria (Günther's disease) is a hereditary form (autosomal recessive) characterized by marked photosensitivity, blisters, scarring alopecia, hirsutism, red-stained teeth, hemolytic anemia, and splenomegaly. The skin lesions are severely mutilating. Onset is in infancy or early childhood.

- Erythropoietic porphyria is autosomal recessive.
- Skin lesions are severely mutilating.

Erythropoietic protoporphyria is an autosomal dominant syndrome that usually begins during childhood. It is characterized by variable degrees of photosensitivity and a marked itching, burning, or stinging sensation that occurs within minutes after sun exposure. It is associated with deficiency of ferrochelatase.

- Erythropoietic protoporphyria is autosomal dominant.
- It is associated with deficiency of ferrochelatase.

Porphyria cutanea tarda, one of the hepatic porphyrias, is an acquired or hereditary (autosomal dominant) disease associated with a defect in uroporphyrinogen decarboxylase. The disease may be precipitated by exposure to toxins (such as chlorinated phenols or hexachlorobenzene), alcohol, estrogens, iron overload, and infection with hepatitis C. Porphyria cutanea tarda usually presents in the third or fourth decade of life. Clinical manifestations include photosensitivity, skin fragility, erosions and blisters (particularly on dorsal surfaces of the hands) (color plate 10-17), hyperpigmentation, milia, hypertrichosis, and facial suffusion. Some patients develop sclerodermoid skin changes. The diagnosis is confirmed by the finding of elevated porphyrin levels in the urine. Treatment includes phlebotomy and low-dose chloroquine.

- Porphyria cutanea tarda is acquired or hereditary (autosomal dominant).
- Associated with defect in uroporphyrinogen decarboxylase.
- May be precipitated by exposure to toxins or infection with hepatitis C.

Pseudoporphyria is a porphyria cutanea tarda-like clinical syndrome induced by drugs, including tetracycline, furosemide, and nalidixic acid, or by hemodialysis. The clinical features resemble those of porphyria cutanea tarda, but there is usually no demonstrable biochemical abnormality of porphyrin metabolism.

- Pseudoporphyria is induced by drugs (tetracycline, furosemide, nalidixic acid) or by hemodialysis.

Acute intermittent porphyria ("Swedish porphyria") lacks skin lesions and is characterized by acute attacks of abdominal pain or neurologic symptoms.

- Acute intermittent porphyria lacks skin lesions.
- Involves acute attacks of abdominal pain or neurologic symptoms.

Variegate porphyria (mixed porphyria) also follows autosomal dominant inheritance. Variegate porphyria is characterized by cutaneous abnormalities that are similar to those of porphyria cutanea tarda and by acute abdominal episodes, as in acute intermittent porphyria. Variegate porphyria tends to be precipitated by drugs, such as barbiturates and sulfonamides.

- Variegate porphyria is autosomal dominant.
- Tends to be precipitated by drugs, such as barbiturates and sulfonamides.

NAIL CLUES TO SYSTEMIC DISEASE

Onycholysis consists of distal and lateral separation of the nail plate from the nail bed. Onycholysis may be due to psoriasis, infection (such as *Candida* or *Pseudomonas*), a reaction to nail cosmetics, or a drug reaction. Drugs that have been noted to induce onycholysis include tetracycline and chlorpromazine. Association with thyroid disease (hyperthyroidism more than hypothyroidism) has also been observed.

- Onycholysis may be due to psoriasis, infection

(*Candida* or *Pseudomonas*), nail cosmetics, or drug reaction.

Pitting is a common feature of psoriatic nails. Pits have also been associated with alopecia areata.

Twenty-nail dystrophy is most often associated with lichen planus or alopecia areata.

Terry's nails consist of whitening of the proximal or entire nail as a result of changes in the nail bed. This abnormality is associated with cirrhosis.

- Terry's nail associated with cirrhosis.

Muehrcke's lines consist of white parallel bands associated with hypoalbuminemia.

- Muehrcke's lines associated with hypoalbuminemia.

"Half-and-half" nails (Lindsay's nails) are nails in which the proximal half is white and the distal half is red. This abnormality may be associated with renal failure.

- "Half-and-half" nails may be associated with renal failure.

Yellow nails are associated with chronic edema, pulmonary disease, pleural effusion, chronic bronchitis, bronchiectasis, and lung carcinoma.

Beau's lines are transverse grooves in the nail associated with high fever, systemic disease, and drugs.

Koilonychia (spoon nails) is associated with iron-deficiency anemia, but it may also be idiopathic, familial, or related to trauma.

- Koilonychia associated with iron-deficiency anemia.

Blue-colored lunula is associated with hepatolenticular degeneration (Wilson's disease) and argyria.

Mees' lines are white bands associated with arsenic.

- Mees' lines associated with arsenic.

CUTANEOUS MANIFESTATIONS OF AIDS

Epidemic Kaposi's sarcoma usually presents as oval papules or plaques oriented along skin lines of the trunk, extremities, face, and mucosa. This presentation is in contrast to that of classic Kaposi's sarcoma seen in elderly patients, which occurs predominantly on the distal lower extremities. Although epidemic Kaposi's sarcoma is most commonly associated with human immunodeficiency virus (HIV) infection, the finding of a small percentage of homosexual men with Kaposi's sarcoma who are HIV negative has suggested that Kaposi's sarcoma may be related to another sexually transmitted infectious disease.

- Epidemic Kaposi's sarcoma: oval papules or plaques along skin lines of trunk, extremities, face, mucosa.
- Most commonly associated with HIV infection.

Severe herpes simplex virus infection, manifested as chronic progressive erosions or ulcers, has been associated with HIV infection.

Herpes zoster infection is considered a sign of underlying HIV infection and occurs 7 times more often in homosexual men with HIV than in HIV-negative controls.

Oral hairy leukoplakia is caused by Epstein-Barr virus infection of the oral mucosa and usually occurs in patients with advanced HIV infection.

Molluscum contagiosum, a common viral infection of otherwise healthy children, has been observed in 10%-20% of patients with HIV infection.

- Molluscum contagiosum observed in 10%-20% of patients with HIV infection.

Bacillary angiomatosis consists of one or more vascular papules or nodules caused by a *Rickettsia*-like organism related to *Rochalimaea quintana*.

Syphilis, which is severe and often resistant to therapy, is commonly associated with HIV disease.

There is a marked increase in the incidence of *Reiter's syndrome* in HIV infection.

Eosinophilic pustular folliculitis is associated with HIV disease.

SELECTED DERMATOLOGY TOPICS

Melanoma and Skin Cancer

More than 500,000 new cases of skin cancer were documented in the United States in 1991. The incidence of malignant melanoma has almost tripled in the past 40 years, and there were approximately 32,000 new cases in 1991. Squamous cell carcinoma and basal cell carcinoma occur predominantly on sun-exposed sites, where-

as most malignant melanomas occur on nonexposed areas. Although various factors may contribute to the occurrence and increased incidence of skin cancers, ultraviolet light seems to be the main etiologic factor.

- Squamous cell carcinoma and basal cell carcinoma occur on sun-exposed sites.
- Malignant melanoma occurs on nonexposed areas.
- Ultraviolet light seems to be main etiologic agent.

Dermatologists encourage regular use of sunscreens with a sun protection factor (SPF) of at least 15. It has been estimated that sun exposure during the first 18 years of life accounts for up to 80% of cumulative lifetime sunlight exposure. Therefore, sunscreen use is particularly important in children and adolescents. People with skin types I and II and those with outdoor occupations have an increased risk of developing basal cell and squamous cell carcinoma. Risk factors for development of malignant melanoma include fair skin, family history of malignant melanoma, personal or family history of dysplastic nevus syndrome, certain congenital nevi, and history of severe (blistering) sunburns during childhood.

- Risk factors for malignant melanoma: fair skin, family history of malignant melanoma, personal or family history of dysplastic nevus syndrome, certain congenital nevi, history of severe (blistering) sunburns during childhood.

During the past decade, there has been emphasis on the subject of dysplastic nevus as a precursor of malignant melanoma. The clinical features of dysplastic nevus include irregularity of border and color, size >6 mm, occurrence predominantly on the trunk, and numerous nevi (sometimes hundreds). Data suggest that even large numbers of nondysplastic nevi may be associated with increased risk of malignant melanoma. The risk of developing a malignant melanoma in a small congenital nevus (usually defined as <2 cm in diameter) is not well established. The lifetime risk of malignant melanoma arising in a giant congenital nevus is generally considered to be 6%.

- Dysplastic nevus as precursor of malignant melanoma.
- Risk of malignant melanoma in small congenital nevus is not well established.

The key to improved survival rate with malignant melanoma has been early diagnosis. The most important prognostic feature of malignant melanoma is tumor thickness; this is defined as the measurement from the stratum granulosum to the deepest tumor cell in the histologic section and is referred to as Breslow's thickness. The 5-year survival rate approaches 100% in patients with lesions <0.75 mm thick, approximately 94% for lesions 0.76-1.50 mm, 84% for lesions 1.5-2.25 mm, 77% for lesions 2.26-3.00 mm, and 46% for lesions >3 mm. The 5-year survival rate is approximately 36% in patients with lymph node metastases and 5% in patients with extranodal metastases. Clark's levels of invasion (level 1, intraepidermal tumor only; level 2, tumor extending into papillary dermis; level 3, tumor pushing on papillary dermal-reticular dermal junction; level 4, lesion has invaded reticular dermis; level 5, invasion into subcutaneous fat) are not used for prognostic classification. Other factors such as sex and anatomic site have sometimes been cited as criteria of independent prognostic significance.

- Key to improved survival rate with malignant melanoma is early diagnosis.
- Most important prognostic feature is tumor thickness (Breslow level).

Stage I malignant melanoma consists of the cutaneous lesion without lymph node involvement, stage II consists of the primary skin lesion plus lymph node involvement, and stage III represents distant metastases. The recommended management of stage I malignant melanoma is surgical. The previous recommendation of a 5-cm margin of excision for all types of malignant melanoma has been revised. Although "wide" excision of malignant melanoma is still the standard of treatment, excision margins >3 cm are no longer advocated. For excision of a thin melanoma (<1 mm thick), a 1-cm margin is generally recommended, and a 3-cm margin is advised for thicker lesions. Elective lymph node dissection does not improve outcome in patients with stage I disease. For stage II disease, excision of the primary skin lesion and regional lymph node dissection are usually recommended. Again, early diagnosis is the key to management, as no form of adjuvant therapy has been shown to improve survival in patients with advanced disease.

- Surgical management of stage I malignant melanoma consists of excision with tumor-free margins of 1-3 cm.

Forms of *cutaneous T-cell lymphoma* are mycosis fun-

goides and Sézary syndrome. Mycosis fungoides generally manifests as discrete or coalescing patches, plaques, or nodules of the skin. Mycosis fungoides may progress to involve lymph nodes and viscera. From the time of extracutaneous involvement, the median duration of survival has been estimated at 2.5 years. The course of patients with patch- or plaque-stage cutaneous lesions, without extracutaneous disease, is less predictable, but the median duration of survival is approximately 12 years. Sézary syndrome is characterized by generalized erythroderma, keratoderma of the palms and soles, and a Sézary cell count of >1,000/mm^3 in the peripheral blood. Most patients have severe pruritus.

- Mycosis fungoides and Sézary syndrome are forms of cutaneous T-cell lymphoma.
- Mycosis fungoides may progress to involve lymph nodes and viscera.
- Median survival for patients with mycosis fungoides is 12 years, 2.5 years from time of extracutaneous involvement.

Both mycosis fungoides and Sézary syndrome are characterized by the presence of Sézary cells (lymphocytes with hyperchromatic and convoluted nuclei) involving the epidermis (epidermotrophism) and dermis. Immunostains of cutaneous lesions demonstrate that these neoplastic T cells usually express CD3 and CD4 antigens, and molecular genetic studies reveal clonal rearrangement of the T-cell receptor gene in lymphocyte populations from skin biopsy, lymph node, and peripheral blood specimens of patients with cutaneous T-cell lymphoma.

- Mycosis fungoides and Sézary syndrome are T-cell lymphomas characterized by presence of Sézary cells in skin and peripheral blood.

Treatment of cutaneous T-cell lymphoma includes topical nitrogen mustard, psoralen with ultraviolet-A light (PUVA), radiotherapy (electron beam, orthovoltage), and systemic chemotherapy. Interferon, retinoids, and other agents have also been used. Most recently, extracorporeal photopheresis has become popular in the treatment of cutaneous T-cell lymphoma. After ingestion of methoxsalen, the patient's leukocytes are exposed to ultraviolet light A and then reinfused.

Autoimmune Bullous Diseases

Bullous pemphigoid is the most common autoimmune

bullous disease. The disease predominantly occurs in elderly patients and usually presents with large, tense bullae on erythematous bases with predilection for flexural areas (color plate 10-18). Lesions are often generalized but may be localized. The most common histologic pattern is a subepidermal bulla with eosinophils, although there is a subset of patients with neutrophil-rich lesions, noninflammatory lesions, or eosinophilic spongiosis without evidence of blisters histologically.

- Bullous pemphigoid is most common autoimmune bullous disease.
- Occurs predominantly in elderly patients.
- Presents as large, tense bullae with predilection for flexural areas.

Immunofluorescence testing is important for diagnosis of bullous pemphigoid. Direct immunofluorescence testing of perilesional skin shows deposition of C3 in a linear pattern at the basement membrane zone in almost all cases and of IgG in >90%. A minority (usually <20%) of biopsy specimens also have IgA or IgM in a linear pattern at the basement membrane zone. Indirect immunofluorescence testing of serum demonstrates IgG anti-basement-membrane zone antibodies in approximately 70% of cases. Routine indirect immunofluorescence testing of serum in patients suspected to have autoimmune bullous diseases is usually performed with monkey esophagus as substrate. The sensitivity of detection of anti-basement- membrane zone antibodies is increased by use of sodium chloride (NaCl)-split human skin as substrate. In addition, use of NaCl-split skin as substrate for indirect immunofluorescence testing is useful in distinguishing between bullous pemphigoid and epidermolysis bullosa acquisita. On NaCl-split skin substrate, basement membrane zone antibodies from patients with bullous pemphigoid localize to the epidermal side (roof) of the substrate, or occasionally to both the roof and the floor of the substrate, whereas basement membrane zone antibodies from patients with epidermolysis bullosa acquisita localize to the dermal side (floor) of the substrate. This procedure often obviates immunoelectron microscopy to distinguish between bullous pemphigoid and epidermolysis bullosa acquisita.

- Immunofluorescence testing important for diagnosis of bullous pemphigoid.
- Almost all cases have deposition of C3 in linear pattern at basement membrane zone.

Immunoelectron microscopy of bullous pemphigoid lesions demonstrates deposition of IgG at the lamina lucida and hemidesmosomes. Immunoblotting and immunoprecipitation studies have demonstrated that bullous pemphigoid antigens are a heterogeneous group of noncollagenous glycoproteins, predominantly consisting of two proteins of 230 kd and 180 kd.

Treatment of bullous pemphigoid includes systemic corticosteroids, dapsone, azathioprine, and cyclophosphamide. In general, bullous pemphigoid requires less immunosuppressive therapy than does pemphigus. Also in contrast to pemphigus, the titer of circulating antibodies does not correlate with disease activity.

Epidermolysis bullosa acquisita is another subepidermal bullous disease. It is characterized clinically by blisters or erosions induced by trauma, which predominantly occur on acral locations. A small subset of patients have generalized lesions, which clinically may be difficult to distinguish from bullous pemphigoid. The histologic pattern is a subepidermal bulla, with or without eosinophils or neutrophils.

- Epidermolysis bullosa acquisita characterized by blisters or erosions induced by trauma.
- Occurs predominantly on acral sites.

Direct immunofluorescence testing reveals a pattern similar to that in bullous pemphigoid, namely, deposition of IgG and C3 in a linear pattern at the basement membrane zone. In contrast to bullous pemphigoid, C3 may be absent or IgG may be the dominant immunoreactant. Indirect immunofluorescence testing of serum on monkey esophagus substrate demonstrates IgG anti-basement-membrane zone antibodies in 25%-50% of patients; these antibodies localize to the dermal side (floor) of NaCl-separated human skin substrate. In patients who lack circulating antibodies, the NaCl-split skin technique may be applied to skin biopsy tissue from the patient. Immunoelectron microscopy demonstrates IgG deposits below and at the lamina densa. The epidermolysis bullosa acquisita antigen is a 290-kd collagenous glycoprotein, representing the globular carboxyl terminus of type VII procollagen. Epidermolysis bullosa acquisita tends to be resistant to immunosuppressive therapy.

- On direct immunofluorescence, epidermolysis bullosa acquisita shows deposition of IgG and C3 in linear pattern at basement membrane zone.
- Tends to be resistant to immunosuppressive therapy.

Cicatricial pemphigoid is characterized by mucosal lesions, with limited or no cutaneous lesions. The disease predominantly affects oral and ocular mucous membranes, and less frequently the genital, pharyngeal, or upper respiratory mucosa. This disease is also known as benign mucous membrane pemphigoid, which is often a misnomer because untreated ocular involvement may lead to blindness. Patients may present with oral erosions or diffuse gingivitis.

- Cicatricial pemphigoid affects oral and ocular mucous membranes, and less frequently genital, pharyngeal, or upper respiratory mucosa.

Direct immunofluorescence testing of mucosal tissue shows deposition of C3 and IgG in a linear pattern at the basement membrane zone, as in bullous pemphigoid. There may be IgA deposition, in addition to IgG and C3, in approximately 20% of patients. The diagnostic yield of oral mucosal tissue is better than that of conjunctiva. Serum rarely contains IgG anti-basement-membrane zone antibodies demonstrable on monkey esophagus substrate. Use of NaCl-split human skin or oral mucosa as substrate increases the sensitivity of detection of circulating anti-basement-membrane zone antibodies. Immunoelectron microscopy demonstrates deposition of IgG somewhat lower in the lamina lucida in cicatricial pemphigoid than in bullous pemphigoid. Immunoblotting and immunoprecipitation studies demonstrate that cicatricial pemphigoid antigens appear to be similar to bullous pemphigoid antigens by molecular weight, suggesting that the different disease expression is related to a different location of target antigens.

- In cicatricial pemphigoid, direct immunofluorescence shows deposition of C3 and IgG in linear pattern at basement membrane zone.

Treatment of cicatricial pemphigoid is similar to that of bullous pemphigoid, with systemic corticosteroids, dapsone, azathioprine, or cyclophosphamide. Cyclophosphamide has been used particularly in patients with ocular involvement.

Herpes gestationis, also referred to as pemphigoid gestationis, consists of intensely pruritic urticarial papules, plaques, or blisters usually occurring in last half of pregnancy. The lesions are histologically characterized by a subepidermal bulla with eosinophils.

- Herpes gestationis consists of intensely pruritic urticarial papules, plaques, or blisters.

Direct immunofluorescence testing of perilesional skin demonstrates deposition of C3 in a linear pattern at the basement membrane zone. In contrast to bullous pemphigoid, IgG is deposited at the basement membrane zone in only 30%-40% of cases. Direct immunofluorescence testing is particularly useful because the other dermatoses of pregnancy (such as pruritic urticarial papules and plaques of pregnancy, PUPP) are negative by immunofluorescence testing. The serum from approximately half of patients with herpes gestationis contains the "HG factor," which is a complement-fixing IgG anti-basement-membrane zone antibody. IgG1 is the major subclass in serum and tissue from patients with herpes gestationis, whereas it is IgG4 in patients with bullous pemphigoid. Immunoelectron microscopy of a skin lesion from herpes gestationis demonstrates deposition of C3 throughout the lamina lucida. The herpes gestationis antigen appears to be a 180-kd molecule, although a higher -molecular-weight antigen may also exist.

- In herpes gestationis, direct immunofluorescence shows deposition of C3 in linear pattern at basement membrane zone.

Dermatitis herpetiformis (color plate 10-9) is characterized by extremely pruritic, grouped vesicles occurring predominantly over the elbows, knees, buttocks, back of the neck and scalp, and low back, usually beginning in the third or fourth decade of life. The characteristic histologic pattern in skin biopsy tissue consists of papillary stuffing with neutrophils underlying a microvesicle. Virtually all patients have some degree of gluten-sensitive enteropathy, although it is usually low-grade and subclinical. This association is important in terms of management of dermatitis herpetiformis. Dermatitis herpetiformis is also associated with thyroid disease.

- In dermatitis herpetiformis, virtually all patients have some degree of gluten-sensitive enteropathy.

The hallmark of the diagnosis of dermatitis herpetiformis is the direct immunofluorescence finding of IgA deposits in a stippled, granular, or clumped pattern, concentrated in papillary bodies and along the basement membrane zone. It is recommended that skin biopsy specimens be obtained from an area 0.5 to 1 cm away from an active lesion. IgA deposits tend to persist in the skin over time. A small percentage of patients who strictly adhere to a gluten-free diet may show diminution in IgA deposits after many years, but IgA deposits in the skin are unaffected by pharmacologic therapy. The serum of patients with dermatitis herpetiformis may contain IgA anti-reticulin and IgA anti-endomysial antibodies. IgA anti-endomysial antibodies and IgA anti-reticulin antibodies are found in approximately 70% of patients with dermatitis herpetiformis or celiac disease and in close to 100% of such patients who have grade III or IV gluten-sensitive enteropathy. Testing for IgA anti-endomysial antibodies is useful for both diagnosis and management of dermatitis herpetiformis, although these antibodies correlate with the degree of gluten-sensitive enteropathy rather than the skin lesion per se.

- In dermatitis herpetiformis, direct immunofluorescence shows IgA deposits in stippled, granular, or clumped pattern.
- Testing for IgA anti-endomysial antibodies useful for diagnosis and management.

The mainstay of treatment of dermatitis herpetiformis consists of dapsone and a gluten-free diet. Patients who strictly adhere to a gluten-free diet may have a decreased need for dapsone. Patients must adhere to the diet for at least 8 months before its efficacy is assessed. The titer of IgA anti-endomysial antibodies decreases during strict adherence to a gluten-free diet. Systemic corticosteroids are generally not helpful in the treatment of dermatitis herpetiformis.

- Treatment of dermatitis herpetiformis: dapsone and gluten-free diet.

Linear IgA bullous dermatosis is immunologically distinct from dermatitis herpetiformis. It is characterized by vesicles or blisters on erythematous bases in a more generalized distribution than dermatitis herpetiformis, a high rate of mucosal involvement, and absence of gluten-sensitive enteropathy. *Chronic bullous disease of childhood* seems to be immunologically identical to linear IgA bullous dermatosis of adults. Both diseases have clinical and histologic features in common with dermatitis herpetiformis and bullous pemphigoid. The histologic pattern is a subepidermal bulla with features of dermatitis herpetiformis or pemphigoid.

The diseases are characterized by the direct immunofluorescence finding of IgA deposition in a linear pattern at the basement membrane zone, with or without C3 or IgG deposition. Circulating IgA anti-basement-membrane zone antibodies, usually in low titer, are better demonstrated with use of NaCl-split skin as substrate than with monkey esophagus as substrate. Immunoelectron microscopy demonstrates deposits of IgA in the lamina lucida, sublamina densa, or both locations. Treatment of linear IgA bullous dermatosis and chronic bullous disease of childhood includes systemic corticosteroids, dapsone, and sulfapyridine.

- In linear IgA bullous dermatosis and chronic bullous disease of childhood, direct immunofluorescence shows IgA deposition in linear pattern at basement membrane zone.

Bullous eruption of systemic lupus erythematosus shares clinical and histologic features with dermatitis herpetiformis. The blisters were therefore originally thought to represent the coexistence of dermatitis herpetiformis and lupus erythematosus, but they are now established as a distinct subset of lupus.

Direct immunofluorescence testing demonstrates deposition of IgG, IgM, IgA, or C3 in a linear or granular pattern at the basement membrane zone, similar to the classic "lupus band." Indirect immunofluorescence testing of serum may show IgG anti-basement-membrane zone antibodies; testing on NaCl-split skin substrate reveals a pattern identical to that with serum from patients with epidermolysis bullosa acquisita--staining of the floor (dermal side) of separated skin. The antigen of bullous lupus erythematosus appears to be the same as the epidermolysis bullosa acquisita antigen (a 290-kd glycoprotein).

- In bullous eruption of systemic lupus erythematosus, direct immunofluorescence shows deposition of IgG, IgM, IgA, or C3 in a linear or granular pattern at basement membrane zone.
- Antigen is same as that of epidermolysis bullosa acquisita.

The clinical variants of *pemphigus* include pemphigus vulgaris and pemphigus foliaceus (with subsets pemphigus erythematosus and fogo selvagem, the latter being an endemic form of pemphigus that occurs in South America). There is also a drug-induced variant of pemphigus, particularly associated with D-penicillamine, captopril, or other thiol-containing medications.

- A drug-induced variant of pemphigus is associated with D-penicillamine.

More than 50% of patients with pemphigus vulgaris present with oral lesions, and >90% have oral mucosal involvement at some point in the course of the disease. Pemphigus vulgaris is characterized by coalescing blisters and erosions, often with generalized involvement. In contrast, pemphigus foliaceus, considered to represent the "superficial" variant of pemphigus, may present with superficial scaling-crusting lesions of the head and neck area (in a seborrheic dermatitis-like pattern) or generalized distribution (color plate 10-19).

The histologic hallmark of pemphigus is the presence of acantholysis (detachment of intercellular adhesion resulting in rounded keratinocytes). Pemphigus vulgaris is characterized by an intraepidermal bulla in a suprabasilar location. Pemphigus foliaceus involves acantholysis at the granular layer.

- Histologic hallmark of pemphigus is presence of acantholysis.

All types of pemphigus are characterized by the deposition of IgG and C3 at the intercellular space (epidural cell surface) on direct immunofluorescence testing (intercellular substance antibody, ICS). Indirect immunofluorescence testing demonstrates IgG anti-ICS antibodies in approximately 90% of cases. The titer of IgG anti-ICS antibodies is useful in both diagnosis and management of pemphigus. IgG in pemphigus is predominantly IgG4.

- All types of pemphigus are characterized by direct immunofluorescence finding of IgG and C3 deposition at the epidural cell surface.
- Titer of IgG anti-ICS antibodies is useful in diagnosis and management.

Pemphigus antibodies are pathogenic in that they have been demonstrated to induce acantholysis in vitro and in animal models. Immunoelectron microscopy shows that IgG and C3 are localized to cell membranes, not intracellularly. The pemphigus vulgaris antigen complex consists of a 130-kd glycoprotein (the binding site for pemphigus vulgaris antibodies) linked to plakoglobin. The pemphigus foliaceus antigen complex is composed of a 160-kd protein

(which is desmoglein 1--the binding site for pemphigus foliaceus antibodies) linked to plakoglobin.

- Pemphigus antibodies induce acantholysis.

High-dose corticosteroids are generally required to control pemphigus. Various "steroid-sparing" immunosuppressive agents have been used, including azathioprine, cyclophosphamide, gold, and dapsone.

- High-dose corticosteroids generally required to control pemphigus.

Erythema Multiforme

This is an acute, usually self-limited eruption of maculopapular, urticarial, occasionally bullous lesions characterized by "iris" or "target" morphology (color plate 10-20). A subset of patients with erythema multiforme may have recurrent lesions. When erythema multiforme presents with extensive cutaneous and mucosal lesions, it is referred to as Stevens-Johnson syndrome. Various etiologic factors have been implicated in erythema multiforme. The most commonly cited precipitating factor is viral infection, particularly herpes simplex virus. This is responsible for a significant percentage of recurrent erythema multiforme. Other infectious agents that have been noted to cause erythema multiforme include *Mycoplasma pneumoniae* and *Yersinia enterocolitica*. Drugs have been reported to induce erythema multiforme, particularly sulfonamides, but also barbiturates and anticonvulsants. Erythema multiforme may be associated with underlying connective tissue disease or malignancy. A small subset of patients with erythema multiforme have disease of the oral mucosa. Erythema multiforme tends to involve the lips, buccal mucosa, and tongue, in contrast to pemphigus vulgaris, which typically involves the pharynx, buccal mucosa, and tongue, and pemphigoid, which most often involves gingivae. Neither pemphigus nor pemphigoid tends to involve the lips.

- Erythema multiforme presents with extensive cutaneous and mucosal lesions (referred to as Stevens-Johnson syndrome).
- Most commonly cited precipitating factor is viral infection, particularly herpes simplex.
- Other agents: *Mycoplasma pneumoniae* and *Yersinia enterocolitica*.
- Drugs are reported to induce erythema multiforme: sulfonamides, barbiturates, anticonvulsants.

Urticaria

Urticaria is a type I, IgE-dependent hypersensitivity reaction. It has numerous causes, including hypersensitivity to foods, drugs, pollens, animal danders, and insect venom. The physical urticarias include dermographism, pressure urticaria, vibratory angioedema, cold-induced urticaria, solar urticaria, and cholinergic urticaria.

- Urticaria is type I, IgE-dependent hypersensitivity reaction.
- It has numerous causes.

Erythema Nodosum

Erythema nodosum typically presents as tender, erythematous, subcutaneous nodules localized to the pretibial areas. The lesions may be acute and self-limited or chronic, lasting for months up to years. The most common cause is streptococcal pharyngitis. Other infectious agents that have been implicated in the development of erythema multiforme include *Yersinia enterocolitica*, *Coccidioides*, and *Histoplasmosis*. Drug-induced erythema nodosum is most often associated with oral contraceptives and sulfonamides. Other associations with erythema nodosum include sarcoidosis, inflammatory bowel disease, and Behçet's syndrome.

- Most common cause of erythema nodosum is streptococcal pharyngitis.
- Drug-induced erythema nodosum most often associated with oral contraceptives and sulfonamides.
- Other associations: sarcoidosis, inflammatory bowel disease, Behçet's syndrome.

Drug Reactions

The morphologic spectrum of reactions that may be induced by medications is broad, and hundreds of drugs may produce a cutaneous reaction. Types of cutaneous lesions induced by drugs include morbilliform maculopapular eruptions, acne-folliculitis, necrotizing vasculitis, vesiculobullous lesions, erythema multiforme, erythema nodosum, fixed drug eruptions, lichenoid reactions, photosensitivity reactions, and hair loss.

It has been estimated that approximately 2% of hospitalized patients have cutaneous drug reactions and that penicillin, sulfonamides, and blood products are responsible for approximately two-thirds of such reactions. The most common types of clinical presentations (in descending order of frequency) are exanthematous or morbilliform eruptions, urticaria or angioedema, fixed drug erup-

tion, and erythema multiforme. Stevens-Johnson syndrome, exfoliative erythroderma, and photosensitive eruptions are less common. Urticarial drug reactions are most often related to aspirin, penicillin, or blood products. Photoallergic reactions are most often associated with sulfonamides, thiazides, griseofulvin, or phenothiazines. Phototoxic (sunburn-like, nonimmunologic) reactions may be induced by tetracyclines. Chronic use of chlorpromazine may be associated with slate-gray discoloration of sun-exposed skin, and amiodarone has been associated with slate-blue discoloration of sun-exposed areas, particularly the face. Antimalarial drugs induce yellow pigmentation.

- 2% of hospitalized patients have cutaneous drug reactions.
- Penicillin, sulfonamides, blood products responsible for about two-thirds of drug reactions.
- Urticarial drug reactions most often related to aspirin, penicillin, blood products.
- Photoallergic reactions most often associated with sulfonamides, thiazides, griseofulvin, phenothiazines.
- Phototoxic reactions may be induced by tetracyclines.

Exanthematous or morbilliform eruptions are the most common type of cutaneous drug reaction. This type of eruption usually begins within a week of onset of therapy, but it may occur >2 weeks after initiation of the drug or up to 2 weeks after use of the drug has been discontinued. Ampicillin, penicillin, and cephalosporins are commonly associated with morbilliform eruptions. A fixed drug eruption is one or several lesions that recur at the same anatomic location on rechallenge with the medication. The genital and facial areas are common sites of involvement. Phenolphthalein, barbiturates, salicylates, and oral contraceptives have been implicated in the cause of fixed drug eruptions.

- Exanthematous or morbilliform eruptions are most common cutaneous drug reaction.
- Fixed drug eruption is one or several lesions that recur at same location on rechallenge.
- Phenolphthalein, barbiturates, salicylates, oral contraceptives implicated in fixed drug eruptions.

Lichenoid drug eruptions are morphologically similar to lichen planus (with violaceous papules of the skin and lacelike white plaques of the oral mucosa) and have most often been associated with gold and antimalarial drugs, although various medications may induce this type of reaction.

Allergic Contact Dermatitis

This is a type IV hypersensitivity reaction (delayed, cell-mediated). Recognition of antigens by T-lymphocytes requires participation of Langerhans cells, which are the "antigen-presenting" cells of the epidermis. Langerhans cells are dendritic cells of the epidermis, which express CD1 (OKT6) antigen and contain Birbeck granules. During investigation of the cause of allergic contact dermatitis, one must consider the anatomic location of the cutaneous lesions and environmental exposure to allergens, including occupational, household, and recreational contactants.

- Allergic contact dermatitis is type IV hypersensitivity reaction (delayed, cell-mediated).
- Langerhans cells are "antigen-presenting" cells of epidermis.

Patch testing consists of application of various substances to the patient's back; each substance is under a small aluminum disk covered with adhesive tape. These are left on the patient's back for 48 hours, and the results are interpreted at 48 and 96 hours. According to the North American Contact Dermatitis Group, the most common allergens include nickel sulfate, paraphenylenediamine, potassium dichromate, thimerosal, ethylenediamine, neomycin sulfate, ammoniated mercury, mercaptobenzothiazole, benzocaine, thiuram, formalin, and paraben mixture.

Nickel sulfate allergies are mainly associated with jewelry. Paraphenylenediamine is present in hair dyes and other cosmetics; *para*-aminobenzoic acid (PABA) in sunscreens is immunologically related to paraphenylenediamine. Potassium dichromate sensitivity is one of the most common types of occupational allergic contact dermatitis and occurs in construction workers exposed to cement, leathers, and certain paints. Formaldehyde is a common preservative in cosmetics and shampoos. Parabens are also commonly found in cosmetics. Neomycin sulfate is a component of many topical antimicrobial preparations. Thiuram is a rubber accelerator and fungicide and therefore may correlate with occupational dermatitis or dermatitis related to wearing shoes containing rubber.

- Nickel sulfate allergies associated with jewelry.

- Potassium dichromate sensitivity occurs in construction workers exposed to cement, leathers, certain paints.
- Formaldehyde is common preservative in cosmetics and shampoos.

Miscellaneous Therapies

Systemic Retinoids

Isotretinoin (13-*cis*-retinoic acid) is a synthetic vitamin A derivative used primarily for the treatment of severe nodulocystic acne vulgaris. The mechanism of action of 13-*cis*-retinoic acid in acne is probably multifactorial, including improvement in keratinization, decrease in sebum production, and decrease in inflammation. A 4- to 5-month course of 13-*cis*-retinoic acid at a dosage of approximately 1 mg/kg per day is the standard regimen.

- Isotretinoin used for treatment of severe acne vulgaris.

Etretinate has been used effectively for treatment of pustular psoriasis, erythrodermic psoriasis, and generalized chronic plaque-type psoriasis. It has been used successfully as a single agent or in combination with PUVA therapy.

The greatest risk associated with use of systemic retinoids is teratogenicity. Before isotretinoin is prescribed, female patients must be counseled on this side effect and follow contraception during therapy and for at least 1 month after use of the drug is discontinued. Because of its long half-life (at least 3 months) and deposition in subcutaneous fat, etretinate is not recommended for treatment of females of childbearing potential.

- Greatest risk with use of systemic retinoids is teratogenicity.

The systemic retinoids are associated with various side effects, including xerosis, dermatitis, cheilitis, sticky skin, peeling skin, epistaxis, conjunctivitis, hair loss, and nail dystrophy. Symptoms of arthralgias and myalgias may also occur. Most patients develop some degree of hyperlipidemia, including hypertriglyceridemia and hypercholesterolemia. Other laboratory abnormalities include elevation of liver function measurements and leukopenia. Skeletal hyperostosis occurs particularly in association with long-term use.

- Side effects of systemic retinoids include xerosis, dermatitis, cheilitis, sticky skin, peeling skin, epistaxis, conjunctivitis, hair loss, nail dystrophy.

Ultraviolet Light

Natural sunlight may be divided into ultraviolet B (UVB, 280-320 nm), ultraviolet A (320-400 nm), and visible light. UVB radiation is responsible for the sunburn reaction. In treating inflammatory dermatoses, UVB has been used most commonly in combination with tar, as in the Goeckerman therapy of psoriasis. UVB may also benefit atopic dermatitis, lichen planus, and certain other inflammatory dermatoses.

PUVA

PUVA consists of ingestion of psoralen followed by exposure of the skin to ultraviolet-A light. PUVA has most commonly been used for therapy of generalized psoriasis, but it is also effective in treatment of various other dermatoses, including lichen planus, mycosis fungoides, and urticaria pigmentosa. PUVA therapy is associated with minimal or no systemic side effects. The main side effect of PUVA therapy is an increased risk (>12 times) of cutaneous squamous cell carcinoma in patients who have received long-term therapy.

- PUVA commonly used for therapy of generalized psoriasis.
- Associated with minimal or no systemic side effects.
- Main side effect is increased risk of cutaneous squamous cell carcinoma.

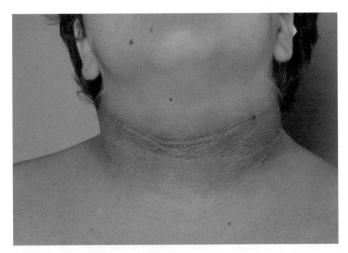

Color plate 10-1. Acanthosis nigricans.

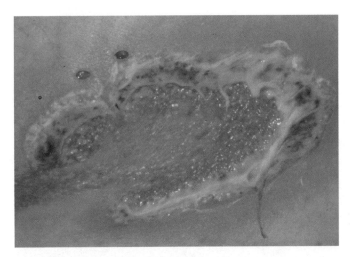

Color plate 10-2. Pyoderma gangrenosum.

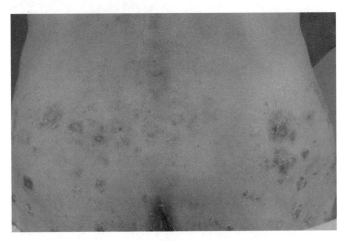

Color plate 10-3. Glucagonoma syndrome (necrolytic migratory erythema).

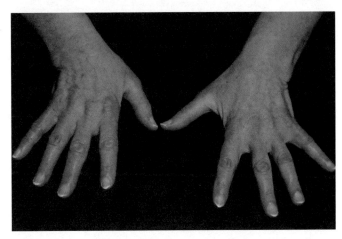

Color plate 10-4. Dermatomyositis: Gottron's papules.

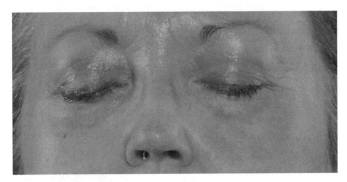

Color plate 10-5. Dermatomyositis: heliotrope discoloration.

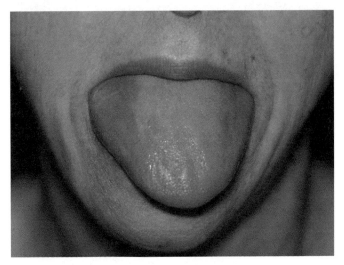

Color plate 10-6. Amyloidosis: macroglossia.

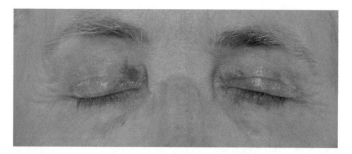

Color plate 10-7. Amyloidosis: postproctoscopic purpura.

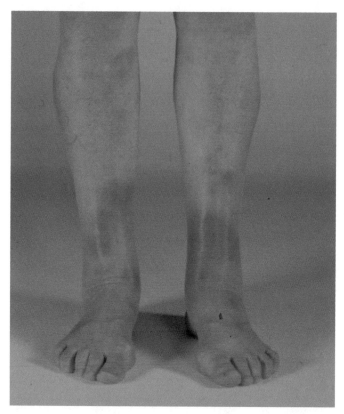

Color plate 10-8. Erythema nodosum.

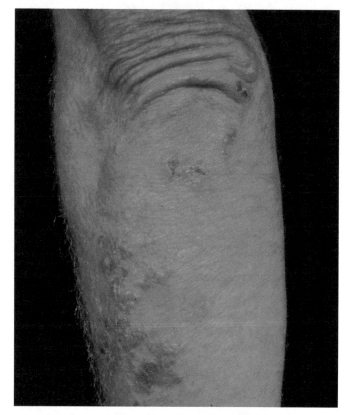

Color plate 10-9. Dermatitis herpetiformis.

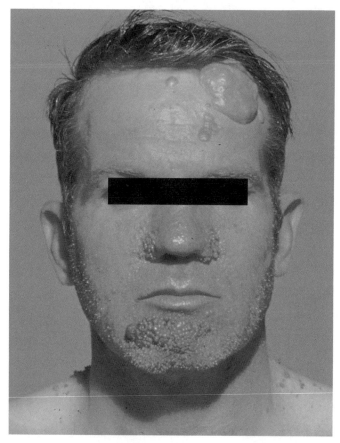

Color plate 10-10. Tuberous sclerosis: adenoma sebaceum and forehead plaque.

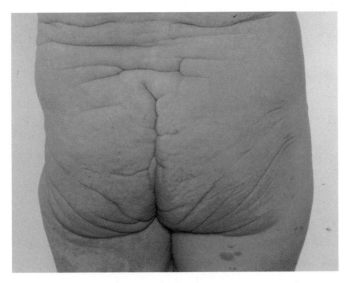

Color plate 10-11. Neurofibromatosis: plexiform neurofibroma.

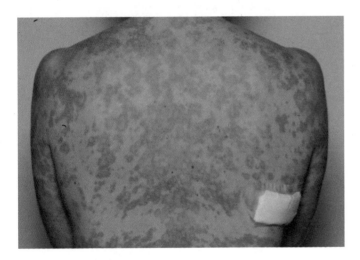

Color plate 10-13. Subacute cutaneous lupus erythematosus.

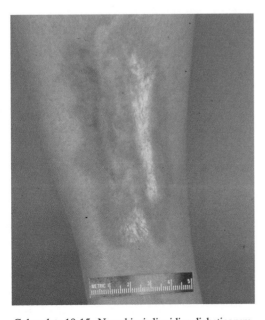

Color plate 10-15. Necrobiosis lipoidica diabeticorum.

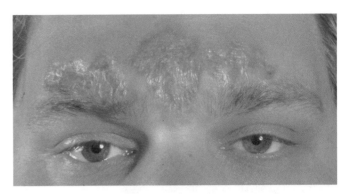

Color plate 10-12. Discoid lupus erythematosus.

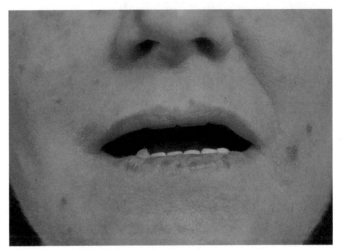

Color plate 10-14. Scleroderma: CREST syndrome.

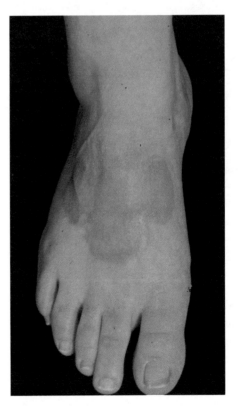

Color plate 10-16. Granuloma annulare.

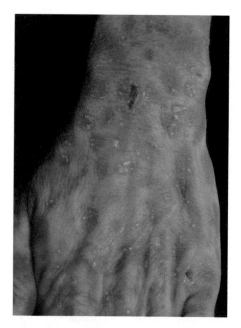

Color plate 10-17. Porphyria cutanea tarda.

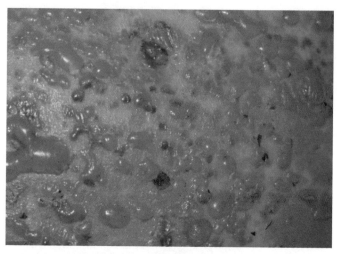

Color plate 10-18. Bullous pemphigoid.

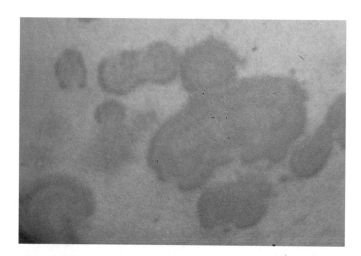

Color plate 10-20. Erythema multiforme.

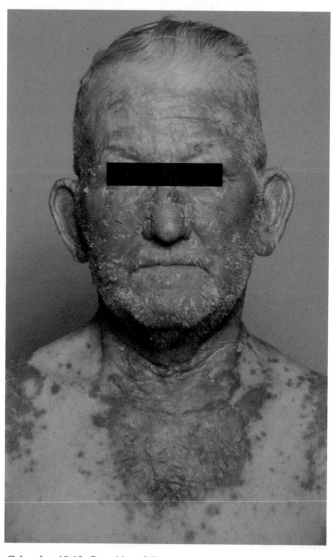

Color plate 10-19. Pemphigus foliaceus.

QUESTIONS
(See "Answers" section)

Multiple Choice

1. Acrodermatitis enteropathica has the following features except:
   a. Autosomal dominant inheritance
   b. Angular cheilitis
   c. Alopecia
   d. Zinc deficiency
   e. Periorificial dermatitis

2. All the porphyrias have cutaneous abnormalities except:
   a. Porphyria cutanea tarda
   b. Erythropoietic porphyria
   c. Variegate porphyria
   d. Acute intermittent porphyria
   e. Erythropoietic protoporphyria

3. Pseudoporphyria is most often associated with:
   a. Captopril
   b. Cirrhosis
   c. Hemodialysis
   d. Corticosteroids
   e. Penicillin

4. Skin diseases typically associated with the following underlying malignancies include:
   a. Pemphigus erythematosus and thymoma
   b. Ichthyosis and leukemia
   c. Acute febrile neutrophilic dermatosis and breast carcinoma
   d. Erythema gyratum repens and leukemia
   e. Dermatitis herpetiformis and adenocarcinoma of the stomach

5. Photosensitivity, annular skin lesions, circulating anti-Ro antibodies, and negative "lupus band" are most characteristic of:
   a. Disseminated discoid lupus erythematosus
   b. Systemic lupus erythematosus
   c. Progressive systemic sclerosis
   d. Dermatomyositis
   e. Subacute cutaneous lupus erythematosus

6. Sézary syndrome
   a. Is characterized by neoplastic proliferation of B cells
   b. Usually spares the palms
   c. Is histologically similar to mycosis fungoides in the skin
   d. Lacks circulating neoplastic lymphocytes
   e. Is usually asymptomatic

7. The following are subepidermal autoimmune bullous diseases except:
   a. Herpes gestationis
   b. Cicatricial pemphigoid
   c. Linear IgA dermatosis
   d. Pemphigus foliaceus
   e. Bullous lupus erythematosus

8. Dermatitis herpetiformis
   a. Is characterized by deposition of IgM at the basement membrane zone
   b. Is associated with gluten-sensitive enteropathy
   c. Does not respond to treatment with gluten-free diet
   d. Improves with systemic corticosteroids
   e. Is asymptomatic

9. The most common association with erythema nodosum is:
   a. *Yersinia enterocolitica*
   b. Streptococcal pharyngitis
   c. Sarcoidosis
   d. Ulcerative colitis
   e. Behçet's syndrome

10. The following are true of allergic contact dermatitis except:
    a. Allergic contact dermatitis is mediated by mast cells
    b. Paraphenylenediamine is present in hair cosmetics
    c. Thiuram sensitivity should be suspected in patients with dermatitis of the feet
    d. Chromate sensitivity should be considered in a construction worker with hand dermatitis
    e. Allergic contact dermatitis is mediated by Langerhans cells

True/False

11. The following are recognized associations:
    a. Angiokeratomas and renal insufficiency
    b. Acanthosis nigricans and hypernephroma
    c. Paget's disease and lung carcinoma
    d. Pyoderma gangrenosum and leukemia
    e. Sebaceous adenomas and colonic carcinoma

f. Bullous pemphigoid and breast carcinoma

12. The following lesions as a component of specific syndromes are recognized associations:
   a. Osteomas and adenocarcinoma of the colon
   b. Macular pigmentation of the lips and intestinal
       polyposis
   c. Trichilemmomas and breast carcinoma
   d. Palmar keratoderma and thyroid carcinoma
   e. Café-au-lait spots and acoustic neuromas
   f. Zinc deficiency and perineal dermatitis

13. Side effects of 13-cis-retinoic acid include:
   a. Hypertriglyceridemia
   b. Sticky skin
   c. Leukocytosis

   d. Osteopenia
   e. Teratogenicity
   f. Conjunctivitis

14. Dermatologic manifestations of human immunodeficiency virus (HIV) infection include:
   a. Kaposi's sarcoma typically presenting on the lower
       extremities
   b. Herpes simplex infection with cutaneous ulcers
   c. Oral hairy leukoplakia caused by Epstein-Barr
       virus
   d. Bacillary angiomatosis lesions resembling heman-
       giomas
   e. Syphilis responds to intramuscular benzathine peni-
       cillin
   f. Disseminated molluscum contagiosum

CHAPTER 11
ENDOCRINOLOGY

Charles F. Abboud, M.D.

HYPOTHALAMIC-PITUITARY DISORDERS

The Pituitary Gland

The pituitary gland has two distinct parts: the adeno-hypophysis (or anterior pituitary) and the neurohypophysis (or posterior pituitary). The adenohypophysis is composed of the anterior lobe, intermediate lobe, and pars tuberalis. It is an endocrine gland with at least five types of cells that produce at least eight hormones (Table 11-1). The neurohypophysis is composed of the supraoptic and paraventricular hypothalamic nuclei, their axons, the pituitary stalk, and the posterior lobe. The posterior lobe is not an endocrine gland; it is a storehouse for hormones of the supraoptic and paraventricular nuclei, i.e., arginine vasopressin (AVP) and oxytocin. You should know the anatomical relationships of the pituitary gland (Fig. 11-1). Blood supply--The adenohypophysis does not have a direct arterial supply; the long portal venous system from superior hypophyseal arteries and the short portal system from inferior hypophyseal arteries form its blood supply.

- Adenohypophysis: endocrine gland with at least five types of cells producing at least eight hormones.
- Posterior lobe: not an endocrine gland but a storehouse for hormones (AVP and oxytocin), of supraoptic and paraventricular nuclei.

Table 11-1.--Anterior Pituitary Hormones and Their Hypothalamic Regulators

Anterior pituitary cell type	Pituitary hormone	Hypothalamic regulatory hormone
Somatotrope	Somatotropin or growth hormone (GH)	(-) Growth hormone release-inhibiting hormone (somatostatin)
		(+) Growth hormone-releasing hormone (GHRH), dominant
Lactotrope	Lactotropin or prolactin (PRL)	(-) Prolactin-inhibiting hormone (dopamine), dominant
		(+) Vasoactive intestinal peptide (VIP)
Thyrotrope	Thyrotropin or thyroid-stimulating hormone (TSH)	(+) Thyrotropin-releasing hormone (TRH), dominant
		(-) Somatostatin
Gonadotrope	Follicle-stimulating hormone (FSH)	(+) Gonadotropin-releasing hormone (GnRH)
	Luteinizing hormone (LH)	
Corticotrope	Corticotropin or adrenocorticotropic hormone (ACTH)	(+) Corticotropin-releasing hormone (CRH)
	Lipotropin (β-LPH)	
	Endorphin (β-END)	

(+), stimulatory effect; (-), inhibitory effect.

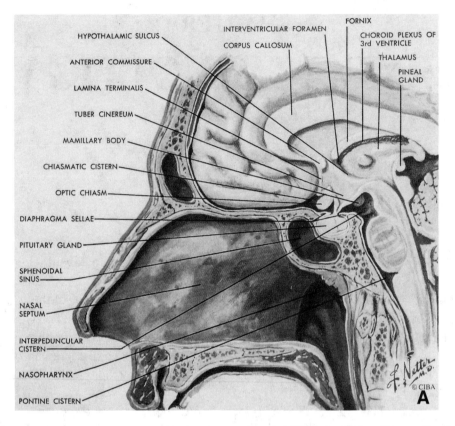

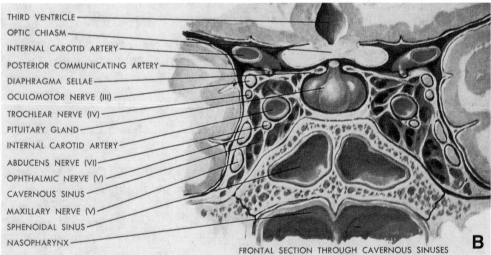

Fig. 11-1. Anatomical relationships of the pituitary gland. A, sagittal and, B, frontal views. (From Netter FH: The CIBA Collection of Medical Illustrations. Vol 4. Endocrine System and Selected Metabolic Diseases. Summit, New Jersey, CIBA, 1965, pp 6-7. By permission of CIBA Pharmaceutical Company.)

Anterior Pituitary Gland

Tropic Hormones

Gonadotropins (LH, FSH), corticotropin (ACTH), and thyrotropin (TSH) are discussed in the sections dealing with their respective target glands.

Growth Hormone

Growth hormone (GH) is secreted in bursts. Its bio-logical effects are 1) generalized protein anabolic effect, 2) generation of insulin-like growth factors (IGF) by peripheral tissues (IGFs mediate the growth-promoting effect), and 3) control of intermediary metabolism. IGF-I (somatomedin-C [SM-C]) is a peptide that resembles proinsulin and is produced by GH-responsive peripher-al tissues. It acts in an autocrine, paracrine, and endocrine manner. Cell differentiation and growth require both GH and IGF-I. GH secretion is under the control of neural influences, is sleep-entrained, and is subject to feedback by IGF-I and intermediary metabolites such as glucose, amino acids, and fatty acids (Fig. 11-2). Growth hormone-releasing hormone (GHRH) is the dominant hypothalamic control and is stimulatory.

- Biologic effects of GH: anabolic effect, generation of IGF by peripheral tissues, control of intermediary metabolism.
- IGFs mediate growth-promoting effect.
- IGF-I acts in autocrine, paracrine, and endocrine manner.
- Cell differentiation and growth require both GH and IGF-I.
- GH secretion is under control of feedback by IGF-I and intermediary metabolites.
- GHRH is the dominant hypothalamic control and is stimulatory.

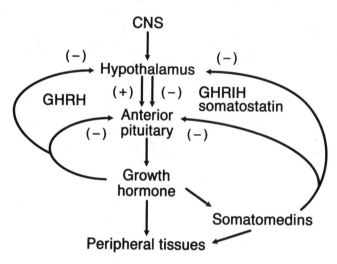

Fig. 11-2. Hypothalamic-pituitary-growth hormone axis. CNS, central nervous system. GHRH, growth hormone-releasing hormone.

Prolactin

Prolactin is also secreted in bursts. Its main biologic effects are on breast development and lactogenesis. Its physiologic role in the fetus, children, and adult males is not known. Prolactin levels start to increase early in pregnancy and continue to rise through the third trimester, reaching a level about 10x normal. Levels are high in the postpartum state and decrease to normal within a few weeks in nonlactating females. Prolactin secretion is under neural influence and is sleep-entrained; it is stimulated by suckling and stress and inhibited by prolactin itself (Fig. 11-3). Dopamine (DA) is the dominant hypothalamic control and is inhibitory.

- Prolactin: main biologic effects are on breast development and lactogenesis.
- Prolactin levels increase early in pregnancy and continue to rise through third trimester.
- DA is the dominant hypothalamic control and is inhibitory.

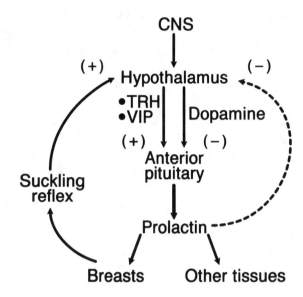

Fig. 11-3. Hypothalamic-pituitary-prolactin axis. CNS, central nervous system. TRH, thyrotropin-releasing hormone; VIP, vasoactive intestinal peptide.

Manifestations of Hypothalamic Disease

Anatomical effects are produced by mass lesions and include obstructive hydrocephalus and chiasmal syndrome.

- Anatomical effects are produced by mass lesions.

Functional effects are related to disordered hypothalamic vegetative or endocrine functions. These include 1) vegetative dysfunction such as disorders of thirst, appetite, or temperature regulation, and 2) endocrine disorders affecting AVP and/or hypophysiotropic functions, including diabetes insipidus, syndrome of inappropriate antidiuretic hormone (ADH), hypopituitarism, or hyperpituitarism.

- Functional effects are related to disordered hypothalamic vegetative or endocrine functions.

Hypopituitarism

Disorders of the anterior pituitary gland can affect one, more than one, or all of its hormones. When more than one hormone is affected, the disorder can affect them concurrently or in succession. In multitropic failure, the usual sequence of hormone loss is GH, LH/FSH, TSH, ACTH, and, last, PRL. However, failure can occur in any sequence.

● Disorders of the anterior pituitary gland can affect one, more than one, or all of its hormones.

The causes of hypopituitarism are outlined in Table 11-2, and the usual presentations of hypopituitarism are described in Table 11-3. However, hypopituitarism can present acutely: 1) acute adrenocortical crisis may be precipitated by acute medical/surgical illness or by thyroid hormone replacement in a patient with associated unrecognized ACTH deficiency, 2) hypoglycemia (ACTH and GH lack), 3) hyponatremia (ACTH and TSH lack), and 4) sedative/anesthetic "sensitivity" (ACTH and TSH lack).

● Hypopituitarism can present acutely: acute adrenocortical crisis, hypoglycemia, hyponatremia, sedative/anesthetic "sensitivity."

Table 11-2.--Causes of Hypopituitarism

Primary pituitary disease
   Congenital--idiopathic
   Traumatic--neurosurgical (pituitary tumors, breast carcinoma, diabetic retinopathy); radiotherapeutic (to sella, nasopharynx,
     or intracranial contents)
   Inflammatory or infiltrative--infections (tuberculosis, syphilis, fungal), sarcoidosis, hemochromatosis, autoimmune
    hypophysitis
   Vascular
     Ischemic necrosis--postpartum pituitary necrosis (Sheehan's syndrome), diabetes mellitus, temporal arteritis, sickle-cell
       disease and trait, eclampsia
     Pituitary apoplexy
   Neoplastic
     Primary--pituitary tumors, craniopharyngioma
     Metastatic
   Miscellaneous--primary empty sella syndrome, idiopathic
Secondary pituitary disease: hypothalamic
   Destruction of pituitary stalk--trauma, neurosurgical, compression by tumor or aneurysm
   Hypothalamic or other central nervous system disease
     Functional
       Stress--psychogenic
       Nutritional--starvation, obesity
       Anorexia nervosa/bulimia syndrome
       Systemic disease--renal, hepatic failure, uncontrolled diabetes mellitus
       Drugs--vincristine
       Hormones--glucocorticoids, gonadal steroids, thyroid hormones
     Organic
       Traumatic--neurosurgery, irradiation
       Inflammatory/infiltrative--sarcoidosis, histiocytosis X
       Neoplastic
         Primary--gliomas, ectopic pinealoma, craniopharyngioma
         Metastatic
         Lymphoma and leukemia
       Idiopathic
Extrasellar disease
   Parasellar--meningioma, optic nerve glioma, chordoma
   Cysts--arachnoid
   Nasopharyngeal carcinoma
   Sphenoid sinus mucocele
   Aneurysm of internal carotid artery
   Cavernous sinus thrombosis

Table 11-3.--Manifestations of Hypopituitarism

Hormone lack	Childhood-adolescence	Adulthood
Growth hormone	Shortness of stature Hypoglycemia	Hypoglycemia(?) Asthenia
Prolactin	None	Failure of postpartum lactation in women None in men
Gonadotropin	Failure of sexual maturation in adolescents	Failure of gametogenesis in both sexes and of maintenance of secondary sex characteristics and of other sex steroid hormone-dependent functions
Thyrotropin	Impairment of central nervous system development in newborn infants Slowing of emotional, mental, and physical functions Failure of sexual maturation in adolescents	Slowing of emotional, mental, and physical functions
Corticotropin	Ill health, anorexia, weight loss, gastrointestinal disturbances, weakness, orthostatic hypotension, hypoglycemia, inability to excrete a water load, pallor, inability to tan, and propensity to adrenocortical crises	Same as in childhood and adolescence

Diagnostic Approach

"Function" Evaluation

Growth hormone. Low serum level of GH is unresponsive to stimulation. Definitive provocative options: insulin-hypoglycemia, L-dopa, arginine, propranolol-glucagon, or clonidine. Screening provocative options: sleep or exercise. GH provocative tests are not needed in adults until future delineation of need and availability of GH therapy.

Prolactin. Low serum level of prolactin is unresponsive to stimulation. Options: TRH, chlorpromazine, metoclopramide, or insulin-hypoglycemia. Provocative tests for prolactin are rarely needed in clinical practice.

Gonadotropins. Male: low sperm count, low serum level of testosterone, and inappropriately low serum levels of LH and FSH. Female: low serum levels of estradiol and inappropriately low serum levels of LH and FSH. Provocative tests for LH and FSH are not clinically indicated.

ACTH. Low serum levels of cortisol and inappropriately low serum level of ACTH. Cosyntropin (Cortrosyn) test usually shows no response unless ACTH lack is partial or of recent onset. Prolonged exogenous ACTH tests show a stepwise response. Other provocative tests, including insulin-hypoglycemia and metyrapone tests, document pituitary ACTH-adrenal unresponsiveness.

TSH. Low serum levels of T_4 and free T_4 (or free thyroxine index [FTI]) and inappropriately low serum level of TSH.

- Low serum level of GH unresponsive to stimulation.
- GH provocative tests not needed in adults.
- Low serum level of prolactin unresponsive to stimulation.
- Males: low sperm count, low serum level of testosterone, inappropriately low serum levels of LH and FSH.
- Females: low serum level of estradiol and inappropriately low serum levels of LH and FSH.
- Low serum level of cortisol and inappropriately low serum level of ACTH.
- Cosyntropin test usually shows no response.
- Prolonged exogenous ACTH tests show stepwise response.
- Low serum levels of T_4 and free T_4 or FTI and inappropriately low serum level of TSH.

"Anatomical" Evaluation

Computed tomography (CT) or magnetic resonance (MR) imaging and ophthalmic evaluation to assess visual fields, visual acuity, and optic disks.

- Anatomical evaluation: CT or MR imaging and ophthalmic evaluation.

In diagnosing hypopituitarism, the physician must document the presence of hypopituitarism and delineate its cause. For tropic hormone deficiencies, the diagnosis rests on the evaluation of the function of the target gland. If target gland failure is present, additional studies are required to distinguish between primary target gland failure and target gland failure secondary to hypothalamic-pituitary disease.

- In diagnosing hypopituitarism, the presence of hypopituitarism must be documented and its cause delineated.
- Diagnosis of tropic hormone deficiencies rests on evaluation of target gland function.
- For target gland failure, additional studies need to distinguish between primary target gland failure and failure due to hypothalamic-pituitary disease.

In hypothyroid patients, a high serum level of TSH or presence of goiter points to primary hypothyroidism, and an inappropriately low serum level of TSH confirms the diagnosis of TSH deficiency.

- In hypothyroid patients, inappropriately low serum level of TSH confirms diagnosis of TSH deficiency.

In suspected hypogonadism, high serum levels of LH and FSH point to primary gonadal failure. In hypogonadism due to hypothalamic-pituitary disease, serum LH and FSH levels are inappropriately low. Presence of anosmia or hyposmia strongly suggests Kallmann's syndrome.

- In hypogonadism due to hypothalamic-pituitary disease, serum LH and FSH levels are inappropriately low.
- Presence of anosmia or hyposmia strongly suggests Kallmann's syndrome.

If a hypocortisol state is present, a diagnosis of primary adrenocortical failure is supported by the presence of hyperpigmentation and low aldosterone and low sex steroid levels. It is documented by increased serum levels of ACTH or lack of adrenocortical responsiveness to exogenous ACTH stimulation. In adrenocortical failure due to hypothalamic-pituitary disease, there is pallor, loss of tanning ability, no mineralocorticoid deficiency, inappropriately low serum ACTH levels, and adrenal responsiveness to prolonged exogenous ACTH stimulation.

- Adrenocortical failure due to hypothalamic-pituitary disease: pallor, loss of tanning ability, no mineralocorticoid deficiency, inappropriately low serum levels of ACTH, adrenal responsiveness to prolonged exogenous ACTH stimulation.

For the nontropic hormones, GH and PRL, a basal high-normal or high value excludes deficiency; otherwise, a provocative test is needed to assess hormone reserve. Clinically, such provocative tests are needed to document GH deficiency only in children with hypopituitarism.

- GH and PRL (nontropic hormones): basal high-normal or high value excludes deficiency.
- Otherwise, a provocative test is needed to assess hormone reserve.

In determining the cause of hypopituitarism, suspected functional causes must be removed or corrected. Normalization of pituitary function lends support to functional hypopituitarism. If functional causes are excluded or if hypopituitarism persists despite removal or correction of a functional cause, then evaluate for organic hypothalamic-pituitary disease. This evaluation is based on the clinical setting and appropriate laboratory and radiologic studies.

- In determining cause of hypopituitarism, suspected functional causes must be removed or corrected.
- Next, evaluate for organic hypothalamic-pituitary disease based on clinical setting and appropriate laboratory and radiologic studies.

Diagnostic Pitfalls

1) Failure to determine the extent and degree of hypopituitarism. It is important to evaluate all pituitary functions in patients with suspected hypopituitarism. 2) Failure to rule out functional causes. These are important causes of hypopituitarism because they are common and potentially reversible. 3) Failure to look for an organic cause and to follow up closely those patients with hypopituitarism in whom no organic cause is found. Hypopituitarism may precede the clinical appearance of its cause by a long time.

- Do not fail to determine extent and degree of hypopituitarism.
- Do not fail to rule out functional causes.

- Do not fail to look for organic cause and follow up those patients with hypopituitarism in whom no organic cause is found.

Therapy of Hypopituitarism

Therapy includes treating the cause and, when applicable, administering pituitary hormones or hormones of the target gland.

- Therapy: treat cause and, if needed, administer pituitary hormones or those of target gland.

Glucocorticoids. Hydrocortisone, 20 mg in early a.m. and 10 mg in early p.m. for adults (or equivalent dosage of prednisone). Instruct patients in dose modification during acute illness. In patients with combined ACTH-TSH lack, initiate glucocorticoid therapy before thyroid hormone therapy to avoid thyroid hormone-induced increased need for cortisol and precipitation of acute adrenocortical crisis.

- Instruct patients in dose modification during acute illness.
- In patients with combined ACTH-TSH lack, initiate glucocorticoid therapy before thyroid hormone therapy.

Thyroid hormones. T_4 is the drug of choice. Initiate therapy with a low dose and gradually increase it over a period of weeks. Assess adequacy of therapy by feeling of well-being and serum levels of T_4. Do not use sTSH levels to monitor adequacy of T_4 dosage, because they are characteristically low in untreated persons.

- T_4 is drug of choice.
- Initiate therapy with low dose and gradually increase it over weeks.
- Do not use sTSH to monitor adequacy of therapy.

Gonadal hormone replacement. 1) In females, conjugated estrogens, 0.6-1.25 mg (or equivalent) daily. Use progestational agents for women with a uterus: medroxyprogesterone acetate, 10 mg daily for days 1-12 of each month. 2) In males, long-acting testosterone parenteral preparation (T enanthate or cypionate), 100-200 mg every 2-3 weeks. The goal is to restore full androgenicity.

For restoration of fertility, FSH/LH or GnRH therapy may be indicated. Delay therapy in puberty to avoid premature closure of epiphyses and to allow maximal linear growth. Evaluate psychosexual needs and patient's lifestyle to assess the impact of the therapy. Assess prostate and prostate-specific antigen (PSA) in middle-aged men before therapy and follow annually.

- Conjugated estrogens; supplemental progestational agents for women with a uterus.
- Long-acting parenteral testosterone esters are drugs of choice in men.
- In adolescents, delay sex hormone therapy as long as possible to avoid premature closure of epiphyses.

Growth hormone. In children, GH is used to treat impaired linear growth due to GH deficiency. Recombinant GH is given parenterally until an acceptable height is attained (goal, 5'4"). Careful attention is given to concomitant thyroid and cortisol replacement in order to avoid under- or overtreatment. Delay using sex steroid therapy to avoid premature closure of the epiphyses.

- GH: used in children to treat impaired linear growth due to GH deficiency.

Pituitary Tumors

Pituitary tumors are "microadenomas" (<10 mm) or "macroadenomas" (>10 mm) in size, "sellar" or "sellar/extrasellar" in extent, and "functioning" or "nonfunctioning." In functioning tumors, the incidence is: PRL, 50%; GH, 15%; ACTH, 15%; LH/FSH, 5%; TSH, α-glycoprotein subunit, 5%; and "nonfunctioning," 10%. Pituitary tumors can be "isolated" or part of multiple endocrine neoplasia type I (MEN I) (see below).

- Tumor size: microadenoma (<10 mm) or macroadenoma (>10 mm).
- Tumor extent: sellar or sellar/extrasellar.
- Functioning or nonfunctioning tumor.
- Pituitary tumors: isolated or part of MEN I.

Clinical Manifestations

Chronic

Mass effects include headaches and evidence of tumor extension beyond the confines of the sella. Superior extension of the tumor may cause 1) chiasmal syndrome with impaired visual acuity and visual field defects; 2) hypothalamic syndrome with vegetative disturbance in thirst, appetite, satiety, sleep, and temperature regulation and with endocrine disorder of diabetes insipidus or syndrome of ADH; 3) obstructive hydrocephalus; and 4) frontal lobe dysfunction. Lateral extension of the tumor may cause impairment of cranial nerves III, IV, VI, V, with diplopia, facial pain, and temporal lobe dysfunction. Inferior extension of the tumor may lead to a nasopharyngeal mass or cerebrospinal fluid (CSF) rhinorrhea.

- Mass effects: headaches and evidence that tumor extends beyond the sella.

Endocrine effects result from either hypersecretory states or hypopituitarism caused by destruction of the pituitary gland by tumor growth. Hyperpituitarism can cause gigantism/acromegaly (GH excess), hyperprolactinemic syndrome (PRL excess), Cushing's disease and Nelson/Salassa syndrome (ACTH excess), and thyrotoxicosis (TSH excess). Generally, LH/FSH and α-subunit excess are clinically silent. Hypopituitarism can be expressed in several ways (see above). Endocrine associations of pituitary tumors include MEN I, i.e., parathyroid tumor or hyperplasia (primary hyperparathyroidism), endocrine pancreas tumor or hyperplasia (various endocrine syndromes), and other endocrine gland tumors (thyroid, adrenal) and lipomas.

- Endocrine effects: due to hypersecretory states or to hypopituitarism caused by destruction of pituitary gland by tumor growth.
- Endocrine associations of pituitary tumors: MEN I.

Acute

Pituitary apoplexy (see below) may occur in patients with known pituitary tumor. Occasionally, it may be the first indication of an underlying tumor.

- Pituitary apoplexy may occur in patients with known pituitary tumor.
- It may be first indication of underlying tumor.

Diagnosis

The presence of a pituitary tumor is suggested by clinical assessment and by CT or MR imaging. Ophthalmic evaluation, including assessing visual acuity, visual fields, and optic disks, is critical. Hormonal evaluation includes evaluating hormonal excess (see below) or hormonal lack (see below) and for presence of any associated MEN I.

- Pituitary tumor: presence suggested by clinical assess-

ment and CT and MR imaging.

The differential diagnosis includes 1) other hypothalamic or pituitary masses (outlined below); and 2) pituitary hyperplasia of pregnancy, target gland primary failure (e.g., primary hypothyroidism), and hypothalamic regulatory hormone disorder (eutopic or ectopic excess production).

Treatment

Pituitary tumors usually are treated with ablation or irradiation. Drug therapy is available for PRL-, GH-, or TSH-producing tumors; it can be a useful adjunct to ablative therapy. Treat associated hypopituitarism.

- Treatment: ablation or irradiation.
- Drug therapy for PRL-, GH-, TSH-producing tumors.
- Drug therapy: can be useful adjunct to ablation.

Surgery--Transsphenoidal surgery is the operation of choice for most tumors; transfrontal operation is reserved for tumors with large suprasellar extensions. Surgical morbidity and mortality as well as neurosurgical expertise should be considered. Radiotherapy--Issues to be considered are 1) long latent period (few months to years), 2) postradiation hypopituitarism (30%-40% of cases), and 3) potential for central nervous system (CNS) damage (rare) or development of CNS tumors (very rare). Drug therapy--Dopamine agonists (bromocriptine in U.S.) for management of prolactinoma or GH-producing tumors. Somatostatin analog (octreotide) for GH- or TSH-producing tumors. Consider the efficacy, long-term safety, and cost. "No therapy" can be an option if the tumor is small and has no effect on quality/quantity of life. Follow-up is essential for all therapeutic options to monitor for persistence, recurrence, and development of other aspects of MEN I.

- Follow-up essential to monitor for persistence, recurrence, development of other aspects of MEN I.

Hyperprolactinemic Syndrome and Prolactinomas

Pituitary tumors associated with hyperprolactinemia may be prolactinomas, "mixed" tumors (e.g., GH- and PRL-producing tumors), or any tumor or mass lesion with suprasellar extension and "stalk effect." (In the "stalk effect" type, the serum level of PRL is usually <200 ng/mL; bromocriptine can control the hyperprolactinemia but does not cause regression of tumor size.) The causes of hyperprolactinemia are outlined in Table 11-4.

● Pituitary tumors associated with hyperprolactinemia: prolactinomas, mixed tumors, or any tumor/mass lesion with suprasellar extension and stalk effect.

Table 11-4.--Causes of Hyperprolactinemia

Physiologic
Newborn, pregnancy, lactation, stress
Pathologic
Eutopic pituitary disorder
Primary pituitary disease
Pituitary tumors
Hypophysitis
Empty sella syndrome
Secondary pituitary disorder
Hypothalamic/stalk disease
Functional
Drugs
Primary hypothyroidism
Chest wall disease
Chronic renal or hepatic failure
Organic
Traumatic
Inflammatory/infiltrative
Vascular
Neoplastic, primary or secondary
Ectopic tumors--lung, kidney, ovary

Clinical Manifestations

Prolactinomas usually present with manifestations of hyperprolactinemia and, occasionally, mass effects. The characteristic presentation is amenorrhea/galactorrhea in women; decreased libido and potency in men; and delayed sexual maturation in adolescents.

● Prolactinomas: usually present with manifestations of hyperprolactinemia and, occasionally, mass effects.
● Characteristic presentation: amenorrhea/galactorrhea in women, decreased libido and potency in men, delayed sexual maturation in adolescents.

Endocrine effects include disorders caused by hyperprolactinemia: 1) in women, galactorrhea, ovulatory and menstrual dysfunction (short luteal phase or anovulation) leading to infertility, oligo/amenorrhea and hypogonadism, hyperandrogenic manifestations (hirsutism or acne), and decreased libido; 2) in men, libido and potency impairment, oligospermia (infertility), and galactorrhea and gynecomastia (very rare); and 3) in adolescents, delayed puberty. Endocrine effects also include associated pituitary dysfunction (hypopituitarism) and associated MEN I (see above).

● Endocrine effects: hyperprolactinemia, associated pituitary dysfunction, associated MEN I.

Neurologic effects are caused by mass effects of pituitary tumors (see above).

● Neurologic effects: mass effects.

In men, recognition of hyperprolactinemia is frequently delayed because decreased libido and impaired potency may be dismissed by the patient and physician as a result of psychiatric factors. In those harboring a pituitary tumor, marked hyperprolactinemia and a macroprolactinoma are usual at the time of presentation.

● In males, recognition of hyperprolactinemia is frequently delayed; a macroprolactinoma is usually present at diagnosis.

Diagnostic Approach

Rule out physiologic causes. A pregnancy test is an essential part of the work-up of any female of reproductive age.

● Rule out physiologic cause: pregnancy test is essential.

Check serum PRL. If the level is >10x normal (>250 ng/mL), it establishes the diagnosis of prolactinoma. However, prolactinomas may be associated with lower levels. Thus, check CT or MR imaging and visual fields if extrasellar tumor extension is present, and evaluate other pituitary functions.

If the serum level of PRL is <10x normal (<250 ng/mL), rule out functional causes, e.g., exclude drugs, irritative lesion of the chest wall, primary hypothyroidism, and chronic renal failure. If a functional cause is present, remove or treat if possible. If hyperprolactinemia does not resolve in about 3 months, then evaluate for hypothalamic-pituitary disease. If no functional cause is present, rule out hypothalamic-pituitary disease by CT or MR imaging and by evaluating other pituitary functions and the visual fields if necessary.

- Check serum level of PRL.
- Level >250 ng/mL: establishes the diagnosis (but prolactinomas may be associated with lower levels).
- Level <250 ng/mL: rule out functional cause, e.g., exclude drugs, irritative lesion of the chest wall, primary hypothyroidism, chronic renal failure.
- If no functional cause, rule out hypothalamic-pituitary disease by CT or MR imaging.

Diagnostic possibilities include pituitary tumor, other organic hypothalamic-pituitary disease, or "idiopathic" hyperprolactinemia.

In evaluating hyperprolactinemia and galactorrhea, rule out pregnancy and obtain a careful drug history. If the patient is taking a drug that can cause hyperprolactinemia, decide whether use of the drug can be discontinued. If use of the drug is discontinued, the serum level of PRL is checked again in a few weeks. If the repeat serum level of PRL is normal, the diagnosis is drug-related hyperprolactinemia. If use of the drug cannot be discontinued or if the hyperprolactinemia persists despite discontinued use, the work-up is continued to rule out organic disease.

A careful history and physical examination and appropriate laboratory and radiologic studies are usually sufficient to rule out a chest wall lesion, renal or hepatic failure, systemic disease, or metastatic disease. The next step is to rule out primary hypothyroidism. Thyroid function tests should be performed in all hyperprolactinemia patients because many patients with primary hypothyroidism are asymptomatic and the findings may be subtle (total and free T_4 [or FTI] and serum TSH).

The next step is to rule out a pituitary tumor or other hypothalamic-pituitary mass lesion. The diagnosis of pituitary tumor is based on considering the serum level of PRL and CT or MR findings on scans of the pituitary area. Most patients with a serum PRL level >100 ng/mL and almost all patients with PRL levels >250 ng/mL harbor a pituitary tumor. A substantial portion of patients with serum PRL levels between 25 and 100 ng/mL have pituitary tumors; therefore, marginally increased values do not rule out a tumor. Radiologic studies, especially CT or MR imaging, are crucial for the diagnosis. A mass lesion supports the diagnosis of tumor, but definitive proof may come only with surgery.

If no discernible cause is found after a thorough evaluation, the hyperprolactinemia is considered to be of indeterminate origin. Follow-up evaluation is critical in these patients because some of them may harbor microadenomas or other hypothalamic-pituitary space-occupying lesions that are below the limit of radiologic detection, and follow-up examinations may show evidence of a mass. The serum level of PRL should be checked every 6-12 months and a CT or MR scan repeated in 1-2 years or earlier if deemed necessary by the development of new symptoms.

Treatment of Microprolactinoma or Idiopathic Hyperprolactinemia

Treatment is indicated for management of infertility, hypogonadism, significant galactorrhea, and hirsutism or to meet the patient's desire. Treatment options include bromocriptine or transsphenoidal surgery for microprolactinoma. Otherwise, observe, check serum PRL level annually, and perform CT or MR imaging every 2-3 years.

Treatment of Macroprolactinoma

Surgical excision is usually incomplete; for persistent disease, the options are radiotherapy with or without interim bromocriptine or bromocriptine. Radiotherapeutic ablation with 1) interim bromocriptine while awaiting the effects of radiotherapy or 2) surgical excision for persistent or progressive disease. Pharmacologic--The dopamine agonist bromocriptine is the mainstay of medical treatment; surgical excision or radiotherapy are then reserved for persistent or progressive disease or for drug intolerance.

Bromocriptine

Bromocriptine is a dopamine agonist. It suppresses hyperprolactinemia and restores gonadal function (80%-90% of cases), and it may decrease tumor size (<50%). Its effect may be dramatic. The drug is not antimitotic. It is costly and can have side effects that are usually minimal and include nausea, fatigue, nasal stuffiness, and postural hypotension. Its long-term safety is unknown. The usual dose in cases of prolactinoma is 5.0-7.5 mg/day. Bromocriptine is a temporizing therapy and discontinuation of its use leads to resumption of tumor growth and endocrine dysfunction.

- Bromocriptine is a dopamine agonist.
- It suppresses hyperprolactinemia and restores gonadal function.
- It may decrease tumor size.
- Discontinuation of its use: resumption of tumor growth and endocrine dysfunction.

Bromocriptine and Pregnancy

Restoration of gonadal function and fertility is the major goal of drug therapy. The use of bromocriptine should be stopped at the earliest sign of pregnancy. In pregnancy, the risk of tumor growth for microprolactinoma is <5% and for macroprolactinoma, 20%-40%. Observe patients closely, especially if they have macroprolactinomas, and periodically perform clinical and visual field evaluations. If significant tumor growth complicates pregnancy, consider surgical excision or reinstituting bromocriptine therapy.

- Use of bromocriptine should be stopped at earliest sign of pregnancy.
- In pregnancy, risk of tumor growth for microprolactinoma is <5% and for macroprolactinoma, 20%-40%.
- If significant tumor growth complicates pregnancy, consider surgical excision or reinstituting bromocriptine therapy.

Surgical Treatment for Prolactinomas

The surgical cure rates for microadenomas and macroadenomas are 60%-80% and 0%-30%, respectively. The recurrence rate for hyperprolactinemia is 10%-50% and for pituitary tumors, 5%-10%. Morbidity is <1%-5% and mortality, 0%-1%.

Growth Hormone-Producing Tumors

Etiology

1. Pituitary disorder: primary cause, >99% are GH-producing tumors. Secondary causes are eutopic GHRH-tumors and ectopic GHRH-tumors.
2. Ectopic GH-producing tumors.

Clinical Features

The clinical presentations are related to GH/IGF-I excess, the pituitary tumor, and the associations of acromegaly. 1) Excess GH/IGF-I leads to acromegalic features/gigantism, hyperhidrosis, heat intolerance, increased skin porosity and oiliness, carbohydrate intolerance (20%; frank diabetes mellitus is rare), hypercalciuria, hyperphosphatemia, acroparesthesias, nerve entrapment syndromes, myopathy, hypertension or cardiomyopathy, Raynaud's phenomenon, fibromas or acanthosis nigricans, and sleep apnea or narcolepsy. 2) Pituitary tumor manifestations include hypopituitarism, hyperprolactinemia (which may be caused by mixed tumor or stalk effect of extrasellar extension), and anatomical effects related to extrasellar extension. 3) The associations of acromegaly include diffuse or nodular goiter, thyrotoxicosis (which may be related to mixed GH/TSH tumor, associated Graves' disease, or multinodular toxic goiter), MEN I (see above), or colon polyps/cancer.

- Clinical presentation: related to GH/IGF-I excess, pituitary tumor, associations of acromegaly.

Diagnostic Approach

Assess the clinical features. A random serum level of GH may be helpful. Values <2 ng/mL exclude acromegaly, and those >50 ng/mL confirm acromegaly. Values in the range of 2-50 ng/mL are nondiagnostic. Measure the serum IGF-I, increased levels (Som C) are diagnostic of acromegaly if one excludes physiologic elevations of pregnancy and adolescence. Perform oral glucose tolerance test with GH responses; nonsuppressible GH during an oral glucose tolerance test is the standard test. GH levels will not suppress to <2 ng/mL in active acromegaly. If the results are borderline, check for paradoxical GH responses to TRH or L-dopa.

- Assess clinical features.
- Random serum level of GH may be helpful.
- Measure serum level of IGH-I: increased serum level is diagnostic of acromegaly.
- Perform oral glucose tolerance test with GH responses.
- Reference standard test: nonsuppressible GH during an oral glucose tolerance test.
- If borderline results, check for paradoxical GH responses to TRH or L-dopa.

Usually, there is no problem in the diagnosis of flagrant cases. The challenge is to make the diagnosis early, because untreated chronic disease can cause irreversible physical changes, increase patients' morbidity (by the effects of tumor, GH hypersecretion, and other endocrine dysfunctions), and increase mortality (from hypertension, diabetes, and cardiovascular effects). The syndrome should be considered in the differential diagnosis of increased perspiration, oiliness of the skin, hyperpigmentation, menstrual irregularities, galactorrhea, hypertension, diabetes, premature and significant degenerative joint disease, carpal tunnel and other entrapment neuropathies, peripheral neuropathy, sellar enlargement, and chiasmal syndrome and in the setting of MEN I.

Treatment

Pituitary tumor. Surgical excision is the treatment of choice. Transsphenoidal surgery is the usual approach; the transfrontal operation is reserved for tumors with a large suprasellar extension. For persistent disease, consider radiotherapy plus interim pharmacologic therapy (either bromocriptine or somatostatin analogue or both) (see below). Radiotherapy--Interim pharmacologic therapy (see above) can be considered. For persistent or progressive disease proceed with surgical therapy.

- Therapy of choice: surgical excision.
- Transsphenoidal approach is the usual one.
- For persistent disease: radiotherapy plus interim pharmacologic therapy.

Ectopic GH or GHRH tumor. Surgical resection is the therapy of choice. For persistent disease, consider somatostatin analogue.

The transsphenoidal operation has a cure rate of 60%-80%; hypopituitarism, 5%-10%; diabetes insipidus, 2%-3%; and mortality, 0%-1%. Radiation therapy has a cure rate of 70% after 10 years; hypopituitarism, 50%; other morbidity, rare. Bromocriptine therapy, usual dose, 5-20 mg/day or higher; normal GH/Som C, <10%; tumor shrinkage, <10%. This is a temporizing therapy. Somatostatin analogue (octreotide) is an investigational treatment. The average dose, 100-200 mg/8 hours given subcutaneously; normal GH/Som C, 80%; tumor shrinkage, 30%-50%. The side effects include nausea, flatulence, mild malabsorption, cholelithiasis (10% of cases), and impairment of glucose tolerance. This, too, is a temporizing therapy.

Gonadotropin-Producing Tumors

Gonadotropin-producing tumors are rare, accounting for 3%-4% of all pituitary tumors. They usually are macroadenomas. These tumors may be selective for gonadotropins or be plurihormonal. Usually there is hypersecretion of FSH, occasionally of FSH and LH, and rarely of LH only. Also, these tumors may secrete α-glycoprotein subunit. Clinically, the tumor may present at any age but usually in middle-aged or elderly persons, predominantly males. Extrasellar effects dominate the clinical picture, and some degree of hypopituitarism is usually present. Rarely, in children, sexual precocity may be the presenting feature. Laboratory findings are high levels of FSH (85%), high levels of LH and FSH (10%-15%), or high levels of LH only (rarely). In males, serum levels of testosterone are variable and semen analysis is normal or oligospermic. CT or MR imaging reveals the sellar mass with extrasellar extension. Chiasmal syndrome may be present. The treatment is usually surgical with or without postoperative irradiation. Endocrine replacement therapy is given for management of hypopituitarism. Drug therapy for these tumors is ineffective.

- Gonadotropin-producing tumors: are rare; 3%-4% of all pituitary tumors.
- Are usually macroadenomas.
- Usually hypersecretion of FSH.
- Usually in middle-aged or elderly persons, predominantly males.
- "Extrasellar" effects dominate the clinical picture.
- High FSH level (85% of cases); high LH and FSH levels (10%-15%).
- Treatment: surgical with or without postoperative irradiation.

Thyrotropin-Producing Tumors

The clinical presentations of primary TSH tumors include diffuse goiter and hyperthyroidism. The major differential diagnosis is Graves' disease. In TSH-producing tumors, one finds equal sex incidence, absence of ophthalmopathy/dermopathy, normal or high sTSH values in patients with hyperthyroidism, and absence of thyroid-stimulating immunoglobulins. Other presentations include extrasellar mass effects and hypopituitarism. Laboratory evaluation reveals that in thyrotoxic patients sTSH value is normal or high, α-glycoprotein subunit levels are high, and TSH responsiveness to TRH is absent. CT or MR imaging shows sellar mass with or without extrasellar extension. Treatment options include ablation (either surgically or with irradiation), pharmacologic therapy with somatostatin analogue, and ancillary measures for the management of thyrotoxicosis.

- Clinical presentation of primary TSH tumors: diffuse goiter, hyperthyroidism.
- Major differential diagnosis: Graves' disease.
- In patients with hyperthyroidism, normal or high sTSH values.
- Other presentations: mass effects, hypopituitarism.
- Treatment: ablative, pharmacologic (somatostatin analogue).

α-Glycoprotein Subunit-Producing Tumors

These rare tumors may also be unihormonal, with selective hypersecretion of the α-subunit, or plurihormonal, with cosecretion of GH, PRL, LH/FSH, or TSH. The dominant clinical presentations are mass effects with extrasellar manifestations and hypopituitarism. α-Subunit excess is clinically silent. Also, there may be associated cosecreted hormone excess, such as acromegaly, hyperprolactinemia, or thyrotoxicosis. Laboratory evaluation documents the high serum level of the α-subunit. Radiologic imaging reveals a sellar mass with or without extrasellar extension. Therapy for selective α-subunit tumors is either surgical excision or irradiation. Radiotherapy is also indicated as a secondary treatment for surgical patients with postoperative persistence or recurrence.

- Dominant clinical presentations: mass effects and hypopituitarism.
- High serum levels of α-subunit.
- Therapy for selective α-subunit tumors: surgical excision or radiation.

ACTH-Producing Tumors
These are discussed below in the section on the adrenal gland.

Empty Sella Syndrome
Primary empty sella syndrome is usually a normal variant commonly seen in obese females who are evaluated for headache. Visual changes are absent (unless primary empty sella is associated with increased intracranial pressure). Clinical hypopituitarism is rare, although decreased pituitary reserve by laboratory testing is seen in up to 40% of patients. Primary empty sella syndrome can occur in association with other pituitary disorders, e.g., pituitary microadenomas.

- Primary empty sella syndrome: usually a normal variant commonly found in obese females.
- Visual changes are absent.
- Clinical hypopituitarism is rare.
- Primary empty sella syndrome can occur in association with other pituitary disorders.

Secondary empty sella syndrome occurs in the setting of previous pituitary surgery/irradiation or apoplexy, Sheehan's syndrome, hypophysitis, or in idiopathic hypopituitarism. Its presentations include headaches and visual defects due to traction on the optic pathways. The major diagnostic challenge is to differentiate it from recurrent pituitary tumor.

- Secondary empty sella syndrome: occurs in setting of previous pituitary surgery/irradiation or apoplexy, Sheehan's syndrome, hypophysitis, or in idiopathic hypopituitarism.
- Presentation: headaches, visual defects.
- Major diagnostic challenge: differentiation from recurrent pituitary tumor.

Radiology of empty sella. A lateral skull film may show the characteristic ballooned or cupped enlarged sella. A radiographic clue may be the presence of myelographic dye in the sella in patients who have had previous myelographic studies. CT or MR imaging reveals a sella filled with CSF; the stalk is midline and extends down to the compressed pituitary gland in the floor of the sella (Fig. 11-4). The major radiologic diagnostic feature in the differentiation from a cystic pituitary tumor is that in cystic tumors the pituitary stalk is displaced or obscured.

- CT/MR imaging: sella filled with CSF; stalk is in midline and extends down to compressed pituitary gland in floor of sella.

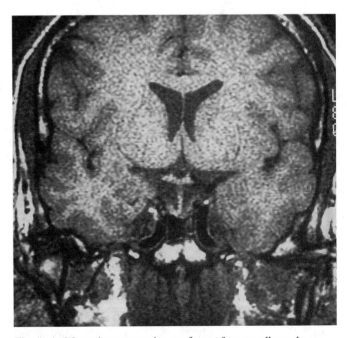

Fig. 11-4.--Magnetic resonance image of case of empty sella syndrome.

Craniopharyngioma
Craniopharyngioma is a slow-growing encapsulated squamous cell tumor originating from remnants of

Rathke's pouch. It is the commonest pituitary region tumor in childhood but can occur at any age. Two-thirds of the tumors are suprasellar, and one-third originate in or extend into the sella. Most are cystic, and some are solid or mixed. These tumors have a propensity to calcification. The clinical presentation includes obstructive hydrocephalus, hypothalamic syndrome (diabetes insipidus/ hyperprolactinemia), chiasmal defects, hypopituitarism, or calcification in or around the sella, as seen incidentally on radiography. Radiography shows calcification in intrasellar or suprasellar regions (75% of children; 25% of adults). CT or MR imaging reveals a mass or cysts, calcification on CT, and low attenuation values (cholesterol content). Treatment--Surgical, biopsy for diagnosis; excision is possible for only small craniopharyngiomas. Decompression for large craniopharyngiomas includes cyst puncture and evacuation or subtotal solid mass excision. A VP shunt is used for obstructive hydrocephalus. Other treatments include postoperative radiotherapy and management of endocrine dysfunction.

- Craniopharyngioma: slow-growing encapsulated squamous cell tumor.
- Commonest pituitary region tumor in children but can occur at any age.
- Propensity to calcification.
- Clinical presentation: obstructive hydrocephalus, hypothalamic syndrome, chiasmal defects, hypopituitarism, or calcification in or around sella.
- Treatment: surgical, postoperative radiotherapy, management of endocrine dysfunction.

Pituitary Apoplexy

Pituitary apoplexy refers to hemorrhagic infarction of the pituitary gland with or without underlying disease. The usual clinical setting is that of a pituitary tumor, irradiated pituitary tumor, pregnancy, anticoagulation, increased intracranial pressure, vascular disease (e.g., diabetes), or vasculitis (e.g., temporal arteritis). Presentations: 1) asymptomatic if small or gradual bleeding; 2) acute if sudden or large hemorrhage--severe headache, ophthalmoplegia, visual defects, meningismus, depressed sensorium, and acute adrenocortical crisis. Death may occur. The diagnosis is made by the characteristic clinical, radiologic, and surgical findings. Treatment includes neurosurgical decompression and hormonal support. Late sequelae may include hypopituitarism, secondary empty sella, or regression of hypersecretory syndrome in infarcted functioning pituitary tumor.

- Pituitary apoplexy: hemorrhagic infarction of pituitary gland with or without underlying disease.
- Acute if sudden or large hemorrhage.
- Severe headache, ophthalmoplegia, visual defects, meningismus, depressed sensorium, acute adrenocortical crisis.
- Death may occur.
- Characteristic clinical, radiologic, surgical findings.
- Treatment: neurosurgical decompression, hormonal support.

Lymphocytic Hypophysitis

Lymphocytic hypophysitis is presumed to be of autoimmune origin. It usually occurs in association with other autoimmune endocrinopathies and it affects adults, predominantly women, especially during pregnancy and the postpartum state. The clinical presentation may include hypopituitarism or the presence of a sellar mass associated with hyperprolactinemia. The major differential diagnoses are prolactinoma and Sheehan's syndrome. The diagnosis depends on the associations and the results of surgical exploration. No specific therapy is available. Hormonal replacement is given as needed.

- Lymphocytic hypophysitis: autoimmune origin.
- Affects adults, predominantly women, especially during pregnancy and postpartum state.
- Clinical presentation: hypopituitarism; sellar mass associated with hyperprolactinemia.

THE NEUROHYPOPHYSIS

The biologic effects of arginine vasopressin (AVP or antidiuretic hormone [ADH]) and its regulatory influences are outlined in Fig. 11-5 and 11-6.

Control of water balance. The input and output of water are regulated by changes in the volume of the liquid ingested, which is controlled by thirst, and in urine volume, which is controlled by AVP. Thirst and AVP secretion are regulated primarily by hypothalamic neurons in response to changes in plasma osmolality and volume. Increased plasma osmolality causes shrinkage and stimulation of the hypothalamic osmoreceptors, leading to increased AVP secretion and increased thirst. Osmoreceptors are extremely sensitive to changes in plasma osmolality, even to changes <1%. In extreme circumstances, decreased plasma volume sensed by volume

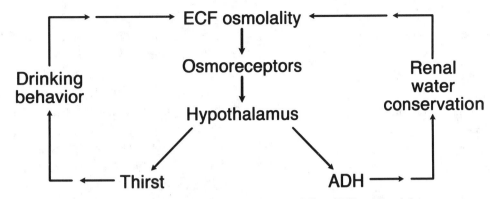

Fig. 11-5. Homeostatic control of extracellular fluid (ECF) osmolality. ADH, antidiuretic hormone.

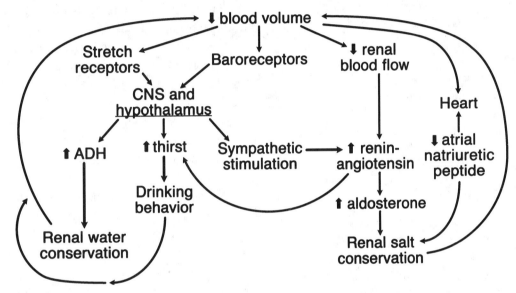

Fig. 11-6. Homeostatic control of blood volume. ADH, antidiuretic hormone; CNS, central nervous system.

receptors in the atria or pulmonary vessels, carotid sinuses, and aortic arch can also produce increased thirst and AVP secretion. Volume stimuli can override the effects of osmolality stimuli.

- Thirst and AVP secretion: regulated primarily by hypothalamic neurons in response to changes in plasma osmolality and volume.
- Osmoreceptors: extremely sensitive to changes in plasma osmolality, even changes <1%.
- Volume stimuli can override effects of osmolality stimuli.

Vasopressin Deficiency: Diabetes Insipidus

Etiology

Diabetes insipidus can result from decreased production of AVP ("central diabetes insipidus"), unresponsiveness of renal tissue to AVP ("nephrogenic diabetes insipidus"), or functional suppression of AVP ("primary polydipsia"). The causes of diabetes insipidus are outlined in Table 11-5.

Polyuria (3-15 L/day) and polydipsia, often with preference for ice-cold water, are characteristic. Both of them are almost always accompanied by nocturia, except in psychogenic primary polydipsia. The abrupt onset of symptoms usually points to central diabetes insipidus. No other ill effects are seen unless patients do not have access to water. When access to water is restricted, hypertonic encephalopathy and circulatory collapse may ensue. In childhood, dilatation of the bladder, ureters, and renal pelvis may occur. In hypertonic encephalopathy, loss of cellular water leads to brain shrinkage and disturbances of consciousness, ranging from lethargy to coma. If it develops acutely, mortality is considerable. Those who survive may have permanent neurologic sequelae. If hyperosmolarity develops gradually, the brain adapts by accumulation of idiogenic osmoles, and the incidence of encephalopathy is decreased.

Table 11-5.--Causes of Vasopressin Deficiency
(Diabetes Insipidus)

AVP-deficient (neurogenic, hypothalamic, or central)
  Idiopathic
    Familial--autosomal dominant
    Sporadic--30%-40% of all cases
  Secondary
    Congenital
    Trauma--surgical, accident
    Inflammation
      Infections--meningitis, encephalitis, etc.
      Granulomatous--sarcoidosis, histiocytosis
    Vascular--Sheehan's syndrome, aneurysms, vasculitis,
      etc.
    Neoplasia
      Primary hypothalamic
      Extrahypothalamic--craniopharyngioma
      Metastatic
AVP-resistant (nephrogenic)
  Idiopathic
    Familial--X-linked recessive
    Sporadic
  Secondary
    Metabolic--hypercalcemia, hypokalemia
    Toxic--lithium, demeclocycline, methoxyflurane,
      colchicine
    Vascular--sickle cell disease or trait
    Inflammatory--pyelonephritis, sarcoidosis, Sjögren's
      syndrome
    Degenerative--amyloidosis
    Postobstructive
    Polycystic disease
Primary polydipsia
  Psychogenic
  Dipsogenic
    Idiopathic
    Secondary--sarcoidosis, vasculitis, etc.
    Drug-induced--thioridazine, chlorpromazine
AVP-resistant diabetes insipidus of pregnancy
  Presence of vasopressinase (rare)

- Diabetes insipidus characteristics: polyuria (3-15 L/day) and polydipsia, with preference for ice-cold water.
- Abrupt onset of symptoms usually points to central diabetes insipidus.
- When access to water is restricted, hypertonic encephalopathy and circulatory collapse may ensue.

Diagnostic Approach

Does the patient have diabetes insipidus? If so, what type? The diagnosis depends on a careful and complete clinical evaluation. Rule out solute diuresis (e.g., diabetes mellitus), electrolyte abnormalities (hypercalcemia, hypokalemia), associated diseases (e.g., sickle cell disease), and drugs. Consider compulsive water drinking if urine volume is >18 L/24 hours, random plasma osmolality is <285 mOsm/kg, or if symptoms are intermittent or have varying intensity.

Check random plasma and urine osmolality values and, if necessary, perform the water deprivation/exogenous AVP test. Plasma and urine osmolality in different types of diabetes insipidus is shown in Table 11-6.

The responses of patients with different types of diabetes insipidus to water deprivation/exogenous AVP test are shown in Table 11-7.

- When to start the water deprivation test: begin the night before the test in patients with mild polyuria, and start the morning of the test in patients with severe symptoms.
- When to give exogenous AVP: when two sequential urine osmolalities vary by <30 mOsm/kg or when 3%-5% body weight is lost.
- A >10% increase in urine osmolality constitutes a normal AVP response.
- The usefulness of AVP assays is not clearly defined.

Table 11-6.--Plasma and Urine Osmolality in
Different Types of Diabetes Insipidus

Osmolality		
Plasma	Urine	Diagnosis
Decreased	Decreased	Primary polydipsia
Increased	Decreased	Central or nephrogenic diabetes insipidus
Normal	Decreased	Any type of diabetes insipidus

Etiology

After diabetes insipidus and its type have been diagnosed, appropriate studies are needed to define the cause. In cases of central diabetes insipidus, perform CT or MR imaging, examine the visual fields, and assess anterior pituitary function. Diagnostic pitfalls include differentiating partial central diabetes insipidus, partial nephrogenic diabetes insipidus, and primary polydipsia with

Table 11-7.--Water Deprivation/Exogenous
Vasopressin Test

Water conservation	Response to vasopressin	Diagnosis
Normal	Absent	Primary polydipsia
Impaired	Present	Central diabetes insipidus
Impaired	Absent	Nephrogenic diabetes insipidus

renal medullary washout. These are best differentiated by plotting plasma osmolality against plasma AVP values obtained during the water deprivation test.

- After diagnosing diabetes insipidus and its type, determine the cause.
- In central diabetes insipidus, perform CT or MR imaging, examine the visual fields, assess anterior pituitary function.

Therapy

There is no need for drug therapy for patients with mild diabetes insipidus (urine output, 2-5 L/day) and free access to water. For central diabetes insipidus, desmopressin acetate (DDAVP) is currently the drug of choice. It is administered by nasal instillation or spray in a dose of 5-10 μg once or twice daily. For patients with partial central diabetes insipidus, AVP agonists such as chlorpropamide (250-500 mg/day; carbamazepine is less desirable) or thiazides such as hydrochlorothiazide (50-100 mg daily) can be used. Note that the effect of thiazide is diminished by ample salt intake. For nephrogenic diabetes insipidus, thiazides are the only available treatment.

- No need for drug therapy in patients with mild diabetes insipidus and free access to water.
- For central diabetes insipidus, desmopressin acetate is drug of choice.
- For partial central diabetes insipidus, use AVP agonists such as chlorpropamide, 250-500 mg/day.
- For nephrogenic diabetes insipidus, thiazides are the only available treatment.

The treatment of hypertonic encephalopathy includes the gradual replenishment of body water which should be administered at a rate to decrease the serum concentration of sodium by 1 mEq/L every 2 hours. Caution: rapid repletion leads to translocation of water into brain cells and cerebral edema. If volume contraction is mild, use hypotonic saline. If volume contraction is significant, treat initially with normal saline to restore volume; 5% dextrose in water can be used in the absence of circulatory insufficiency; the rate should be less than that which induces glycosuria.

Vasopressin Hypersecretion: Syndrome of Inappropriate ADH

Pathophysiology

AVP excess and continued water intake are the basic events. Renal retention of water leads to hypo-osmolality of extracellular body fluids and hyponatremia, relative hyperosmolality of urine (usually >300 mOsm/kg) and increased extracellular fluid volume. Extracellular fluid volume expansion produces increased glomerular filtration rate, atrial natriuretic peptide, and suppression of the renin-aldosterone system. Natriuresis follows. Syndrome of inappropriate ADH is also characterized by the absence of edema and low serum levels of creatinine and uric acid. This syndrome is often asymptomatic, particularly if the hyponatremia is mild or has developed gradually over a few weeks to months. Otherwise, frequent symptoms are anorexia, nausea, or vomiting. If hyponatremia is severe or develops acutely, CNS dysfunction occurs, with symptoms of cerebral edema, irritability, confusion, or convulsions. Coma may occur.

- Syndrome of inappropriate ADH: basic events are AVP excess and continued water intake.
- Relative hypo-osmolality of body fluids, relative hyperosmolality of urine, increased extracellular fluid volume.
- Natriuresis; absence of edema.
- Often asymptomatic, particularly if hyponatremia is mild or has developed gradually.
- Anorexia, nausea, or vomiting are frequent symptoms.
- In severe or acute hyponatremia, CNS dysfunction.

The causes of hypersecretion of AVP are outlined in Table 11-8.

Diagnostic Approach

1) Check serum concentration of sodium. If it is normal, consider water loading. Is it true hyponatremia? 2) Check serum osmolality. Rule out factitial (hyperlipidemia, hyperproteinemia, hyperglycemia) and hyperosmolar states (e.g., hyperglycemia). Is it due to syndrome

Table 11-8.--Causes of Hypersecretion of
Vasopressin

Vasopressin hypersecretion
    Physiologic or appropriate ADH secretion
        Hyperosmolar states
        Decreased effective blood volume/pressure
            States with generalized edema
            States with volume depletion
    Pathologic or inappropriate ADH secretion
        Exogenous
            AVP or its analogs
            Oxytocin
        Ectopic
            Malignancy
                Cancer--bronchus, pancreas, ureter, prostate,
                    bladder
                Lymphoma, leukemia
                Thymoma, mesothelioma
            Benign pulmonary disorders
                Pneumonia, lung abscess, empyema,
                    pneumothorax
                Tuberculosis, cystic fibrosis
                Asthma, positive pressure breathing
        Eutopic
            Central nervous system/hypothalamic disease of
              diverse causes
                Traumatic
                Inflammatory/degenerative
                Vascular
                Neoplastic
            Drugs that stimulate AVP secretion and/or
              action--vincristine, vinblastine, cyclophospha-
              mide, phenothiazines, monoamine oxidase
              inhibitors, tricyclic antidepressant agents,
              chlorpropamide, clofibrate, carbamazepine,
               nicotine
        Postoperative period
        Old age

- What is the cause of syndrome of inappropriate ADH? Look for eutopic or ectopic disorder.

The major diagnostic challenge is to differentiate syndrome of inappropriate ADH from subclinical hypovolemia. Consider urine concentration of sodium, serum levels of creatinine and uric acid, and plasma renin activity.

- Major challenge: distinguishing syndrome of inappropriate ADH from subclinical hypovolemia.

Treatment

The treatment of syndrome of inappropriate ADH includes 1) water restriction to 800-1,000 mL daily. Follow patient's weight and serum concentration of sodium. 2) Use AVP antagonists if necessary: demeclocycline, 900-1,200 mg/day. Lithium is not recommended because of its potential serious side effects. 3) If acute neurologic sequelae are present, give hypertonic saline intravenously, 200-300 mL of 5% NaC1 over 3-4 hours. Rapid correction of hyponatremia can lead to central pontine myelinolysis, which is often fatal. 4) Identify and correct the cause.

- Water restriction.
- AVP antagonists, if necessary.
- For acute neurologic sequelae, hypertonic saline.
- Rapid correction of hyponatremia can lead to central pontine myelinolysis.
- Identify and correct cause.

THYROID DISORDERS

Physiology

The normal hypothalamic-pituitary-thyroid axis is shown in Fig. 11-7. Euthyroidism is maintained by a negative feedback system. TRH is the dominant hypothalamic regulator of TSH secretion. Thyroid hormones feed back principally at the pituitary level: triiodothyronine (T_3) directly and T_4 mainly by its intracellular monodeiodination to T_3. T_4 is produced exclusively by the thyroid gland. T_3 has two sources: 20% from the thyroid and 80% from peripheral deiodination of T_4. Peripheral deiodination of T_4 by deiodinase can lead to the formation of T_3, the bioactive hormone, or reverse T_3, which is bioinert. Thyroid hormones circulate in two forms: bound to binding proteins (TBG, TBPA, albumin) and free. (99.95% of T_4 and 99.50% of T_3 are bound,

of inappropriate ADH? 3) Rule out appropriate AVP excess, and exclude generalized edema, volume depletion, cortisol deficiency, and thyroid deficiency. What is the cause of the syndrome? 4) Look for a eutopic or ectopic disorder.

- Check serum concentration of sodium; if normal, consider water loading.
- Is it true hyponatremia? Check serum osmolality.
- Is it due to syndrome of inappropriate ADH? Rule out appropriate AVP excess.

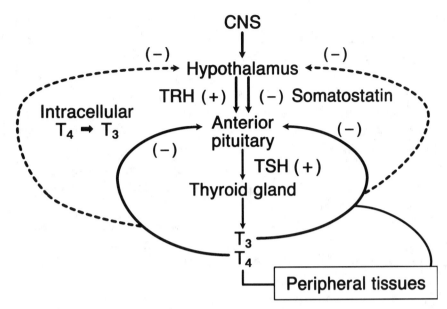

Fig. 11-7. The hypothalamic-pituitary-thyroid axis. CNS, central nervous system; TRH, thyrotropin-releasing hormone; TSH, thyroid-stimulating hormone. T_3, triiodothyronine; T_4, thyroxine.

and 0.05% of T_4 and 0.50% of T_3 are free.) The free hormone is the physiologically active component responsible for thyroid function. The bound hormone is bioinert; its quantity depends on availability and affinity of binding proteins.

- Euthyroidism is maintained by a negative feedback system.
- TRH is the dominant hypothalamic regulator of TSH secretion.
- T_4 is produced exclusively by the thyroid gland.
- T_3 has two sources: 20% from the thyroid and 80% from peripheral deiodination of T_4.
- Thyroid hormones circulate in 2 forms: bound and free.
- T_4, 99.95% bound and 0.05% free.
- T_3, 99.50% bound and 0.50% free.

Assessment of the Thyroid Axis

Serum T_4. Two determinants are thyroid function and the quantity and quality of binding proteins. Decreased: hypothyroidism; euthyroid patients with low concentration of binding proteins in serum (androgen and anabolic steroid therapy, glucocorticoid excess, chronic liver disease, acromegaly, genetic TBG deficiency); euthyroid sick syndrome. Increased: thyrotoxicosis; euthyroid patients with increased TBG (estrogen use, pregnancy, acute hepatitis, acute intermittent porphyria, perphenazine use, and familial TBG excess); patients with genetic excess in albumin or prealbumin-binding protein; peripheral resistance to thyroid hormones; euthyroid sick syndrome.

Serum T_3. Determinants: thyroid function, conversion of T_4 to T_3 in peripheral tissues, and binding proteins. Decreased: hypothyroidism; euthyroid state in the neonate, elderly, euthyroid sick syndrome, and patients with caloric deprivation; use of drugs such as propranolol, glucocorticoids, certain iodinated contrast agents, and amiodarone that block T_4 to T_3 conversion; states with decreased TBG levels (see above). Increased: thyrotoxicosis (including the T_3 toxicosis variety); euthyroid patients with TBG excess (see above); peripheral hormone resistance.

Free T_4. Determinant is thyroid function. Decreased: hypothyroidism, euthyroid sick syndrome. Increased: hyperthyroidism, euthyroid patients with euthyroid sick syndrome or peripheral hormone resistance.

FTI. Determinants: total T_4, resin T_3 uptake (an indirect measure of TBG). FTI is equivalent to the free T_4. Decreased: hypothyroidism, euthyroid sick syndrome. Increased: hyperthyroidism; euthyroid patients with euthyroid sick syndrome; peripheral hormone resistance; genetic albumin and prealbumin-binding protein excess; anti-T_4 antibodies.

Serum sensitive TSH (sTSH). Sensitivity is >10x the sensitivity of the previously available standard TSH assays. It clearly delineates low-normal from low values. Its major impact: 1) diagnosis of hyperthyroidism;

sTSH is low or undetectable in all types of thyrotoxicosis except that due to TSH-producing tumor, and 2) monitoring replacement or suppressive thyroid hormone therapy. Serum sTSH can be used alone as a thyroid function screening test in outpatients. Normal sTSH value implies absence of thyroid dysfunction and no further studies are indicated. If sTSH is increased, determine FTI: primary hypothyroidism, decreased FTI; TSH-producing tumor, increased FTI. If sTSH is decreased, determine FTI: thyrotoxicosis (except that induced by TSH-producing tumor), increased FTI; central hypothyroidism, decreased FTI.

- sTSH clearly delineates low-normal from low values.
- sTSH major impact: diagnosis of hyperthyroidism and monitoring replacement or suppressive thyroid hormone therapy.
- Serum sTSH: can be used alone as thyroid function screening test in outpatients.

Thyroid scanning--The main indications are for documentation of thyroid agenesis or dysgenesis and ectopic thyroid and for evaluation of nodular goiter, fine needle aspiration "suspicious" single nodule, retrosternal goiter, struma ovarii, or metastatic functioning thyroid tumor.

Radioactive iodine (^{131}I) uptake--A 24-hour ^{131}I uptake is indicated for differential diagnosis of thyrotoxicosis with diffuse goiter (Graves' disease [high] from silent thyroiditis [low]); diagnosis of silent or subacute thyroiditis (low); diagnosis of exogenous or ectopic hyperthyroidism (low); pre-^{131}I treatment of thyrotoxicosis; and management and follow-up of differentiated thyroid malignancy postoperatively.

Serum thyroglobulin--Although thyroglobulin levels can be increased in many benign or malignant thyroid disorders, its main clinical usefulness is as a tumor marker for follow-up of differentiated thyroid carcinoma and in distinguishing between silent thyroiditis (high) and exogenous hyperthyroidism (low).

TSH receptor-stimulating immunoglobulins--These are markers for Graves' disease and are helpful in diagnosing euthyroid endocrine ophthalmopathy, predicting relapse of drug-treated Graves' disease, and predicting neonatal thyrotoxicosis.

Antithyroglobulin and antimicrosomal antibodies-- These usually are used to assess the presence of autoimmune thyroid disorder. The antimicrosomal antibodies are more specific as indicators of such a disorder. Highest titers occur in Hashimoto's thyroiditis (95%). Lower titers are found in primary atrophic hypothyroidism and Graves' disease, and modest or low titers can be found in other autoimmune disorders (e.g., systemic lupus erythematosus, rheumatoid arthritis). Negative test results do not exclude the presence of autoimmune thyroid disease.

Thyroid ultrasonography--Potential indications include assessing thyroid size and configuration, assessing nodular goiter size and consistency of the nodule, and following up thyroid malignancy to demonstrate preclinical cervical metastatic nodes.

Hypothyroidism

The causes of hypothyroidism are outlined in Table 11-9.

Table 11-9.--Causes of Hypothyroidism

Primary thyroid failure (95% of cases)
    Permanent--Hashimoto's thyroiditis, primary atrophic, postablative (surgery, radioiodide, radiation), others
    Reversible--hypothyroid phase of subacute or silent thyroiditis, iodide deficiency, goitrogens (iodides, antithyroid agents, lithium)
Secondary/tertiary failure or central hypothyroidism (5% of cases)
    Permanent--organic hypothalamic-pituitary disease, postpartum necrosis, tumors, others
    Reversible--withdrawal of thyroid hormone therapy in euthyroid person
Tissue resistance to thyroid hormone (rare)

Atypical Presentations: The Great Mimicker

- Neuropsychiatric: dementia, dysarthria, deafness, cerebellar ataxia, carpal tunnel syndrome, peripheral neuropathy, or psychoneurosis/psychoses.
- Cardiopulmonary: hypertension, cardiomegaly/failure, pericardial/pleural effusions, or respiratory depression.
- Gastrointestinal: constipation, ileus, or ascites.
- Genitourinary: potency impairment in males and menorrhagia, dysmenorrhea, or amenorrhea/galactorrhea in females.
- Musculoskeletal: arthritis or cramps/stiffness.
- Hematologic: normocytic anemia, macrocytic anemia, pernicious anemia, or microcytic anemia (iron deficiency).
- Endocrine: growth retardation, abnormalities of sex-

ual maturation, galactorrhea, associated autoimmune endocrinopathies, or syndrome of inappropriate ADH.
- Metabolic/laboratory findings: hyperlipidemia, hypercalcemia, hyperuricemia, or increased SGOT-LDH-CPK.

Diagnostic Approach

The diagnosis of hypothyroidism is based on the assessment of clinical features and evaluation of the results of FTI and sTSH. The diagnostic process should delineate the presence of hypothyroidism, its type (whether primary or central), its cause, and whether it is reversible.

- Diagnosis of hypothyroidism: assessment of clinical features and results of FTI and sTSH.

FTI (or equivalent) and sTSH are the critical tests. Diagnostic clues: 1) normal FTI and sTSH exclude hypothyroidism; 2) normal FTI and high sTSH point to subclinical hypothyroidism; 3) low FTI and high sTSH point to primary hypothyroidism (rule out reversible causes and associated autoimmune disease); 4) low FTI and low sTSH point to hypothalamic-pituitary disease (check other pituitary functions and perform radiologic studies); 5) high FTI and high sTSH point to peripheral resistance to thyroid hormone.

- Normal FTI, high sTSH: subclinical hypothyroidism.
- Low FTI, high sTSH: primary hypothyroidism.
- Low FTI, low sTSH: hypothalamic-pituitary disease.
- High FTI, high sTSH: peripheral resistance to thyroid hormone.

Therapy

Synthetic T_4 is the drug of choice. The usual replacement dose is 1.5 µg T_4/kg; the average dose is 0.1 mg/day. Start low and increase slowly (except in young patients or if hypothyroidism is of recent onset). Monitor clinical response and serum level of T_4 in central hypothyroidism. Monitor TSH and clinical response in primary hypothyroidism. In patients with primary hypothyroidism receiving previously documented adequate therapy, an increase in sTSH may indicate substandard medication, poor compliance, malabsorption (e.g., bile acid sequestrant therapy), ongoing progressive thyroid disease, increased binding proteins (pregnancy and estrogen therapy), or increased hormone clearance (phenytoin, rifampin). A decrease in sTSH may indicate reduced requirements of aging, patient's self-induced overmed-

ication, regeneration of autonomous thyroid remnant, decreased binding protein, or decreased clearance.

- Synthetic T_4 is the drug of choice.
- Start low and increase slowly (except in young patients or if hypothyroidism is of recent onset).
- Monitor clinical response and serum level of T_4 in central hypothyroidism.
- Monitor TSH and clinical response in primary hypothyroidism.

Chronic Autoimmune Thyroiditis: Hashimoto's Thyroiditis

Chronic autoimmune thyroiditis disorder is the commonest form of thyroiditis. It can affect any age or sex, predominantly older women. Autoimmune disorder; association with other autoimmune disorders. Two types: goitrous and atrophic. Incidence: antimicrosomal antibodies occur in 10% of women and 3% of men; 10%-20% have subclinical hypothyroidism.

- Affects predominantly older women.
- Autoimmune disorder; association with other autoimmune disorders.
- Familial.
- 10%-20% have subclinical hypothyroidism.

Clinical Presentations

The size of the goiter is variable, and the texture is rubbery to firm. It is usually diffuse but may be nodular. Euthyroid or hypothyroid; hypothyroidism may be overt or subclinical. Occasionally, Hashimoto's thyroiditis may present with thyrotoxicosis, indistinguishable from Graves' disease. It may also present with postpartum thyroid dysfunction: transient hyperthyroidism followed by transient hypothyroidism, usually appears within 6 months after delivery, may occur in as many as 5%-10% of women, often recurs in subsequent pregnancies, increased risk of permanent hypothyroidism.

- Goiter: variable size, rubbery to firm, usually diffuse (may be nodular).
- Euthyroid or hypothyroid.
- May present with postpartum thyroid dysfunction.

Laboratory Findings

Antimicrosomal antibodies (antigen is thyroid peroxidase), 95%; antithyroglobulin antibodies, 50%-60%. FTI and sTSH may reveal euthyroidism, subclinical primary hypothyroidism, or overt primary hypothyroidism. Radioiodide uptake is variable, and isotopic scan usually shows heterogeneous uptake; these tests are not indicated. Fine needle aspiration may be needed in the evaluation of "nodular goiter"; in Hashimoto's thyroiditis, it shows the characteristic lymphocytic infiltration.

- Antimicrosomal antibodies (antigen in thyroid peroxidase), 95%; antithyroglobulin antibodies, 50%-60%.
- FTI and sTSH may show: euthyroidism, subclinical primary hypothyroidism, overt primary hypothyroidism.

Treatment

For euthyroid goiter, T_4 therapy to decrease goiter size (successful in 50% of cases) and to preempt development of hypothyroidism (5%-10%/year). For subclinical or overt hypothyroidism, T_4 therapy. For obstructive goiter, surgical excision if no response to T_4 treatment. For thyrotoxicosis: treat as for Graves' disease.

Hyperthyroidism

The causes of hyperthyroidism are outlined in Table 11-10.

Table 11-10.--Causes of Hyperthyroidism

Exogenous
    Thyroid hormones
    Iodides
Endogenous
    Eutopic
        Primary thyroid disease
            Nodular goiter--single, multiple
            Thyroiditis--silent, subacute
            Follicular carcinoma
        Abnormal thyroid regulation
            Autoimmune
                Antibody-mediated--Graves' disease
            TSH--pituitary tumor
            hCG--hydatidiform mole
    Ectopic
        Struma ovarii

Graves' Disease

Graves' disease is an autoimmune, multisystem disease characterized by the triad of hyperthyroidism, diffuse goiter, and mesenchymal extrathyroidal manifestations of ophthalmopathy and dermopathy. These manifestations can occur singly or in combination. Graves' disease is the commonest cause of hyperthyroidism. Although it is seen most often in young females, it can occur at any age and in either sex. There is a strong familial predisposition. The immediate cause of the hyperthyroidism is the production of thyroid-stimulating autoantibodies that bind to the TSH receptor, activating it and causing cellular growth and increased hormonogenesis. Spontaneous remissions can occur. The goiter is usually 2x-3x normal size, diffuse, smooth, and somewhat firm. Twenty percent of the patients, especially the elderly, may not have goiter. The two types of ocular findings are infiltrative and noninfiltrative. The infiltrative findings (lid puffiness, chemosis, proptosis, extraocular muscle dysfunction, optic neuritis, or atrophy) are specific for Graves' disease. The noninfiltrative findings (lid lag and lid retraction) can occur with any type of thyrotoxicosis. Localized pretibial myxedema occurs in patients who either have or have had Graves' thyroid disease (raised thickened peau d'orange changes usually affecting the dorsum of the feet and legs). Thyroid acropachy may accompany the dermal changes.

- Graves' disease: autoimmune multisystem disease.
- Characteristic triad: hyperthyroidism, diffuse goiter, mesenchymal extrathyroidal effects (ophthalmopathy and dermopathy).
- Commonest cause of hyperthyroidism.
- Strong familial predisposition.
- Immediate cause of hyperthyroidism: production of thyroid-stimulating antibodies.
- 20% of patients, especially elderly, may not have goiter.
- Two types of ocular findings: infiltrative, noninfiltrative.
- Infiltrative findings: specific for Graves' disease.
- Noninfiltrative findings: can occur with any type of thyrotoxicosis.

Toxic Multinodular Goiter

Toxic multinodular goiter is a disease of the elderly and occurs in patients who have had a long-standing simple nodular goiter with autonomy in one or more nodules. The hyperthyroidism is usually less severe than that of Graves' disease and may be characterized by the dominance of organ-specific manifestations. Cardiovascular effects (arrhythmias, congestive heart failure), weakness (and frequently wasting), loss of appetite, and listlessness may dominate the picture--the so-called apathetic hyperthyroidism. The goiter is usually large, nodular, and asymmetrical; it may be difficult to palpate in some patients because of either a short neck or a substernal extension.

- Toxic multinodular goiter: disease of the elderly.
- Occur in patients with long-standing simple nodular goiter with autonomy in one or more nodules.
- Hyperthyroidism may be characterized by dominance of organ-specific manifestations.
- Goiter may be difficult to palpate because of short neck or substernal extension.

Toxic Adenoma

Toxic adenoma is caused by a hyperfunctioning autonomous follicular adenoma and is seen most often in middle-aged women. The solitary nodule is >3 cm in diameter, easily palpable, and firm. Radioisotopic scan shows intense uptake in the nodule, with no uptake in the rest of the gland.

- Solitary nodule: >3-cm diameter, easily palpable, firm.
- Radioisotopic scan: intense uptake in nodule, none elsewhere.

Thyroiditis

Thyrotoxicosis can occur in thyroiditis because of release of stored hormone from the inflamed, damaged thyroid follicles. It is transient and lasts a few weeks, until the hormone stores are depleted. A short period of hypothyroidism may ensue until the thyroid recovers. Thyroiditis-induced thyrotoxicosis can be caused by subacute thyroiditis (see below) and by painless lymphocytic thyroiditis (see below).

- Thyrotoxicosis can occur in thyroiditis through release of stored hormone from damaged thyroid follicles.
- It is transient, lasting a few weeks.
- Short period of hypothyroidism may occur until thyroid recovers.
- Can be caused by subacute thyroiditis or painless lymphocytic thyroiditis.

Painless Lymphocytic Thyroiditis

Painless lymphocytic thyroiditis is probably a variant of Hashimoto's thyroiditis. It occurs most commonly in females, especially in the postpartum period. This type of hyperthyroidism may account for 5%-20% of all patients with hyperthyroidism. It is usually mild and transient, lasting for several weeks, and, in about one-third of patients, may be followed by transient hypothyroidism lasting several weeks. The small diffuse, painless, nontender goiter may be firm. Painless lymphocytic thyroiditis has a tendency to recur, especially in subsequent pregnancies. FTI and sTSH indicate hyperthyroidism: FTI is increased and sTSH is suppressed; low uptake of ^{131}I. Antithyroid antibodies are normal or modestly increased; leukocyte count is normal, and erythrocyte sedimentation rate is normal or slightly increased. There is no associated ophthalmopathy or dermopathy. The differential diagnosis includes Graves' disease and factitial hyperthyroidism. Graves' disease with iodide exposure and low uptake of ^{131}I: history of iodide exposure and high urinary iodide. Factitial hyperthyroidism: no goiter, ^{131}I uptake is low, and the serum thyroglobulin level is low (in contrast to painless thyroiditis, in which the serum thyroglobulin level is high). Painless lymphocytic thyroiditis is self-limiting, and the thyroid dysfunction is transient. No treatment is required for most patients. Use β-blockers if hyperthyroidism is symptomatic. Symptomatic hypothyroidism may have to be treated with T_4 for a few months. If recurrences are significant, the gland may have to be ablated with ^{131}I in the euthyroid state to prevent recurrences. Annual follow-up of thyroid function is needed because of the increased risk of permanent hypothyroidism.

- Painless lymphocytic thyroiditis: most commonly in females, especially in postpartum period.
- This type of hyperthyroidism may account for 5%-20% of all patients with hyperthyroidism.
- Usually mild and transient.
- May be followed by transient hypothyroidism in about a third of patients.
- Tendency to recur.
- FTI increased, sTSH suppressed, low uptake ^{131}I, antithyroid antibodies normal or modestly increased.
- No associated ophthalmopathy or dermopathy.
- Disease is self-limiting.
- No treatment is required in most patients.

Exogenous Hyperthyroidism

Exogenous hyperthyroidism can be caused by prescribed or factitiously ingested thyroid hormone(s), ingestion of iodides in susceptible persons (see below), or ingestion of ground meat contaminated with thyroid tissue. Factitial thyrotoxicosis should be suspected in thyrotoxic patients with no palpable goiter who have suppressed ^{131}I uptake and low serum levels of thyroglobulin.

- Causes: prescribed or factitiously ingested thyroid hormone(s), ingestion of iodides, ingestion of ground meat contaminated with thyroid tissue.
- Factitial thyrotoxicosis suspected in thyrotoxic patients with: no palpable goiter, suppressed ^{131}I uptake, low serum levels of thyroglobulin.

Atypical Presentations

Cardiac: tachyarrhythmias, congestive heart failure, or systolic hypertension. Gastrointestinal: hyperdefecation, chronic diarrhea, or increased alkaline phosphatase and other liver enzymes. Reproductive: oligomenorrhea/amenorrhea or gynecomastia in men. Neurologic: myopathy or hypokalemic periodic paralyses, particularly in Oriental males. Metabolic bone disease: osteoporosis.

Diagnostic Approach

- FTI and sTSH are the cornerstones of laboratory diagnoses.
- Serum T_3 assay may be needed in the 10%-20% of patients who present with T_3 toxicosis.
- TRH test is needed rarely and has been replaced by the sTSH assay.
- Mesenchymal manifestations = Graves' disease.
- Diffuse goiter; no mesenchymal manifestations: decreased sTSH and increased ^{131}I uptake = Graves' disease. Decreased sTSH and decreased ^{131}I uptake = silent thyroiditis. Normal or increased sTSH = TSH-producing tumor.
- Nodular goiter: single = toxic nodule; many = toxic multinodular goiter; and metastasis = follicular carcinoma.
- Painful tender goiter = subacute thyroiditis (increased erythrocyte sedimentation rate and decreased radioiodine uptake).
- No goiter and presence of pelvic mass = struma ovarii; otherwise, exogenous or factitial thyrotoxicosis.
- Normal FTI and normal sTSH exclude hyperthyroidism.
- High FTI and low sTSH indicate thyrotoxicosis of any type except TSH tumor or euthyroid sick syndrome.
- Low FTI and low sTSH indicate need for serum T_3 assay. Increased T_3 points to T_3 toxicosis; if T_3 is low, think of euthyroid sick syndrome or hypothalamic-

pituitary disease.
- High FTI and high sTSH point to TSH tumor or peripheral hormone resistance.

T_3 toxicosis: serum level of T_4 is low without deficiency of binding proteins and serum level of T_3 is increased. It occurs in about 20% of patients with thyrotoxicosis and may develop in any type of thyrotoxicosis. It may be the first manifestation of hyperthyroidism and may herald relapses and recurrences of the disease. It may also be caused by exogenous supraphysiologic T_3 therapy.

- T_3 toxicosis: low serum level of T_4 without deficiency of binding proteins and increased serum level of T_3.
- T_3 toxicosis: occurs in about 20% of patients with thyrotoxicosis.
- May be first manifestation of hyperthyroidism.
- May herald relapses and recurrences.

T_4 toxicosis: serum level of T_4 is increased, with a normal or low serum level of T_3. This may occur in the thyrotoxic elderly or sick. It usually is seen in the hospital setting. T_4 toxicosis due to decrease in the conversion of T_4 to T_3.

- T_4 toxicosis: serum level of T_4 is increased, with a normal or low serum level of T_3.
- May occur in the thyrotoxic elderly or sick and is usually seen in the hospital setting.

Management

Available modalities include symptomatic (rest, β-blockers), ablative (surgery, radioiodide), and temporizing (block thyroid hormone formation, antithyroid drugs; block release of thyroid hormones, iodides [days]) therapies.

Antithyroid Drugs

Methimazole and propylthiouracil block thyroid hormone formation and may decrease the production of thyroid-stimulating immunoglobulins. In addition, propylthiouracil decreases T_4 to T_3 conversion. The effect of these drugs is temporary and lasts only while the drugs are being given. They do not damage the thyroid and are given to control hyperthyroidism and, in Graves' disease, with the hope that the disease will enter a spontaneous remission during their use (<50% chance). Therapy is initiated with either methimazole, 20 mg daily as a single dose, or with propylthiouracil, 300-450 mg/day in divided doses. Improvement is evident in 1-2 weeks, and euthyroidism is usually achieved in 6-8 weeks. Maintenance doses are then given to maintain euthyroidism. In Graves' disease, therapy is continued for 6-12 months; the use of the drug is then discontinued and the patient is assessed periodically. Most recurrences develop in the first few months after discontinuing use of the drug. Side effects are uncommon (<5%). Remember the serious side effects of agranulocytosis, vasculitis, hepatitis, and aplastic anemia (<0.2%). Agranulocytosis can develop abruptly within a few hours.

- Methimazole and propylthiouracil block thyroid hormone formation and may decrease the production of thyroid-stimulating immunoglobulins.
- Propylthiouracil: decreases T_4 to T_3 conversion.
- Drug given to control hyperthyroidism (in Graves' disease, with hope of spontaneous remission--<50% chance).
- In Graves' disease, treat for 6-12 months; discontinue therapy and assess patient periodically.
- Serious side effects: agranulocytosis, vasculitis, hepatitis, and aplastic anemia (<0.2%).
- Agranulocytosis can develop abruptly within a few hours.

Radioiodine

Radioiodine therapy is safe and effective. Its major drawback is the almost certain eventual development of ^{131}I-induced hypothyroidism. It does not carry the risk of thyroid carcinogenesis or leukemogenic potential. [131]I can be given to the young and old, with the only absolute contraindication being pregnancy. However, in practice, most physicians avoid its use in very young patients. The usual dose is 150-200 μCi/g (estimated weight). Lower doses are less likely to relieve hyperthyroidism and do not obviate eventual hypothyroidism. The maximal effect from a given dose of ^{131}I is obtained in 2-3 months. Doses can be repeated if necessary. Radiation thyroiditis may appear in 7-10 days and rarely is severe. It is most likely to occur in the elderly; because of the risk of aggravating thyrocardiac disease, it is best to render these patients euthyroid with antithyroid drug therapy before administering [131]I.

- [131]I: safe and effective.
- Major drawback is the eventual development of [131]I-

induced hypothyroidism.
- Only absolute contraindication: pregnancy.
- In practice, most physicians avoid using it in very young patients.
- Maximal effect is obtained in 2-3 months.
- Radiation thyroiditis may appear in 7-10 days and is most likely in the elderly.

Surgery

As a therapeutic option, subtotal thyroidectomy is reserved for the management of toxic nodular goiter and/or patients with Graves' disease who are young, pregnant, or with large obstructive-compressive goiters. It is customary to render the patient euthyroid and to give iodides for 7-10 days preoperatively to prevent thyrotoxic crisis and excessive bleeding from the overactive friable gland. Damage to the recurrent laryngeal nerves or parathyroid glands should be a rare occurrence for experienced surgeons.

- Subtotal thyroidectomy: reserved for toxic nodular goiter and/or patients with Graves' disease who are young, pregnant, or with large obstructive-compressive goiters.
- It is customary to render the patient euthyroid and to give iodides 7-10 days preoperatively.

Special Considerations

Inorganic iodides have a transient inhibitory effect on hormone release (7-10 days). Iodides can be used as adjunctive agents in patients being prepared for surgery, with severe thyrocardiac disease, or with an actual or impending crisis. Iodides are also a temporary expedient while awaiting the full effect in those patients given radioiodine treatment.

- Iodides: for patients being prepared for surgery or with actual or impending crisis.
- Temporary expedient while awaiting full effect of radioiodine therapy.

β-Blockers should be used only as adjunctive therapy. Propranolol is used most commonly in a dose of 40-120 mg/day. Such therapy only controls the adrenergic manifestations of hyperthyroidism and may also decrease the conversion of T_4 to T_3. The major uses of these drugs are in thyrotoxic crisis and while awaiting the effects of more definitive therapy. These drugs should not be used alone in the preoperative preparation of thyrotoxic patients, because they do not prevent thyrotoxic crisis.

- β-Blockers: use only as adjunctive therapy.
- Major uses: in thyrotoxic crisis; while awaiting effects of more definitive therapy.
- Should not be used alone in preoperative preparation of thyrotoxic patients.

Summary of Management

Graves' disease: radioiodine therapy (unless pregnant or very young, in which case use surgical excision or antithyroid drugs).

"Too sick": antithyroid drugs until euthyroid, then ^{131}I or surgical excision.

Toxic single nodule: surgical excision or ^{131}I.

Toxic multinodular: surgical excision or ^{131}I plus temporizing antithyroid drug therapy.

Silent thyroiditis: symptomatic supportive.

Subacute thyroiditis: symptomatic supportive plus steroids.

Tumor-induced, e.g., struma, hydatidiform, or pituitary: surgical excision.

Goiter

Diffuse Euthyroid Goiter

Causes: simple goiter, Hashimoto's thyroiditis, euthyroid Graves' disease, goitrogens, lymphoma, or Riedel's thyroiditis.

Diagnostic approach: the two most important issues in the clinical evaluation of diffuse goiter in a euthyroid patient are an assessment of the onset and course of development of the goiter and an inquiry into the use of or exposure to goitrogens.

1. Goitrogen: history, removal of goitrogen leads to resolution of goiter.
2. If gradual onset and slow progression: consider Hashimoto's thyroiditis (bosselated goiter, high antibody titer, presence of other autoimmune diseases), Graves' disease (ophthalmopathy/dermopathy and presence of thyroid-stimulating immunoglobulins), simple goiter (adolescence, spontaneous resolution in 1-2 years).
3. If rapid onset and progression: consider Hashimoto's thyroiditis or lymphoma. Check thyroid antibodies. Tissue diagnosis is critical.

Multinodular Euthyroid Goiter

Causes--If benign multinodular goiter: Hashimoto's

thyroiditis. If malignancy: primary carcinoma, metastatic carcinoma, or lymphoma.

Diagnostic approach--If any nodule is dominant: manage as single nodule (see below). If any features suggest malignancy: tissue diagnosis, fine needle aspiration, and surgical therapy. If gradual onset and slow progression: differential diagnosis is benign multinodular goiter versus Hashimoto's thyroiditis; check for other autoimmune disorders and thyroid antibodies.

Single or Dominant Thyroid Nodule

Etiology. Benign: adenoma, cyst, focal thyroiditis, benign multinodular goiter with dominant nodule, or remnant hyperplasia (postsurgical ablation). Malignant: 1) primary (thyroid follicle--differentiated [papillary or follicular] or undifferentiated [anaplastic]--or parafollicular C cell [medullary carcinoma]); 2) secondary (metastatic or lymphoma).

Diagnostic approach. Identify any factors that increase suspicion of malignancy: young age, male, rapid growth, invasive characteristics, history of irradiation, family history of thyroid cancer, or appearance while patient is receiving suppressive doses of thyroid hormone.

- Identify any factors that increase suspicion of malignancy.

Fine needle aspiration is an integral part of the evaluation of a single or dominant thyroid nodule. Interpretation of the aspirated tissue by an experienced cytopathologist is critical to the usefulness of the procedure.

- "Benign aspirate": observe.
- "Suspicious" aspirate: scan. "Hot nodule," observe or ablate; "cold nodule," surgical excision.
- "Malignant" aspirate: surgical excision.
- "Nondiagnostic" aspirate (10%): repeat fine needle aspiration or make decisions based on clinical assessment.

Thyroid Cancer

Thyroid cancer may arise from the thyroid follicle or parafollicular C cells. Also, the thyroid gland may be affected by lymphoma or metastatic disease. Thyroid carcinoma may be differentiated (papillary or follicular) or undifferentiated (anaplastic). Medullary thyroid cancer arises from the parafollicular C cells.

- Thyroid cancer: may arise from thyroid follicle or

parafollicular C cells.

- Thyroid may also be affected by lymphoma or metastatic disease.

Papillary cancer is the commonest type (50%-60% of patients). Its incidence peaks in early and late adulthood. Papillary cancer spreads typically to lymph nodes and usually has the best prognosis. It can present with a thyroid mass or cervical lymphadenopathy or it can be found incidentally in surgically excised thyroid glands. Follicular carcinoma (20%) spreads preferentially by the hematogenous route. Its follicles can form thyroid hormones. Its presentations are with a thyroid mass or metastatic deposits (can be stained with antithyroglobulin stains). Rarely, if the tumor burden is large, follicular carcinoma can lead to thyrotoxicosis. Anaplastic carcinoma usually presents in the elderly with a rapidly progressive thyroid mass. It has a poor prognosis and longevity is <6-9 months.

- Papillary cancer: the most common (50%-60%). It spreads to lymph nodes and has the best prognosis. Presentation: thyroid mass, cervical lymphadenopathy, found incidentally in excised thyroid glands.
- Follicular carcinoma (20%): spreads preferentially by hematogenous route. Presentation: thyroid mass, metastatic deposits. It can lead to thyrotoxicosis (rare).
- Anaplastic carcinoma: usually presents in the elderly with rapidly progressive thyroid mass. Prognosis is very poor.

Treatment of Differentiated Thyroid Cancer

Surgical excision is the definitive therapy: either lobectomy with or without subtotal contralateral lobectomy or near total thyroidectomy. The affected lymph nodes are selectively excised, and postoperatively, the thyroid remnant is ablated with ^{131}I. Suppressive doses of T_4 are used (monitored by sTSH). Follow-up on regular basis with physical examination, chest radiography, serum thyroglobulin, high resolution ultrasonography of the thyroid and neck, and radioiodide study. Radioiodine therapy is given for functioning metastases. Radiotherapy is given for local bony painful metastasis. The treatment of anaplastic carcinoma is palliative.

- Surgical excision is the definitive therapy.
- Suppressive doses of T_4 are used (monitored by sTSH).
- Radioiodine therapy is given for functioning metastases.

Medullary Carcinoma of the Thyroid

Medullary carcinoma of the thyroid arises from C cells and has the distinctive pathologic feature of amyloid deposits among sheets of cells. It secretes calcitonin and can occur sporadically or be familial. Familial medullary carcinoma of the thyroid may be isolated or part of an endocrine complex. In MEN IIA, it may be associated with primary hyperparathyroidism and pheochromocytoma, and in MEN IIB, it occurs in association with pheochromocytoma, mucosal neuroma syndrome, and a distinctive marfanoid habitus. Medullary cell hyperplasia may precede the medullary carcinoma in some of the affected families. Medullary carcinoma of the thyroid can present with a thyroid nodule, cervical lymphadenopathy, or metastatic disease. It may be detected in an asymptomatic relative during a family screen. In addition, the tumor may secrete other hormones such as ACTH, AVP, serotonin, and histamine and present with "ectopic" humoral syndromes. A search for associated pheochromocytoma and hyperparathyroidism should be conducted in all patients. The diagnosis is confirmed by an increased serum level of calcitonin or an abnormal calcitonin response to a calcium and/or pentagastrin stimulation test. Treatment is surgical (after the exclusion of pheochromocytoma). Currently, no effective chemotherapy is available.

- Medullary carcinoma of thyroid: arises from C cells. Calcitonin is the tumor marker.
- Feature: amyloid deposits.
- It can occur sporadically or be familial.
- Familial form may be isolated or part of an endocrine complex, e.g., MEN IIA and MEN IIB.
- In some families, medullary cell hyperplasia may precede medullary carcinoma of thyroid.
- Presentation: thyroid nodule, cervical lymphadenopathy, metastatic disease.
- Search for associated pheochromocytoma and hyperparathyroidism in all patients.
- Medullary carcinoma of thyroid may secrete other hormones and present with "ectopic" humoral syndromes.
- Diagnosis confirmed by an increased serum level of calcitonin or abnormal calcitonin response to a calcium and/or pentagastrin stimulation test.
- Treatment: surgical.

"Painful" Goiter

Cause: inflammatory (subacute thyroiditis, acute suppurative thyroiditis, and, rarely, Hashimoto's thyroiditis), hemorrhage into cyst or adenoma, or neoplastic (anaplastic carcinoma or lymphoma). Diagnostic approach: clinical (onset, course, duration, systemic features, e.g., recent viral disease, pyogenic source), characteristics of goiter, and search for cervical lymphadenopathy. Laboratory studies: leukocyte count and differential, erythrocyte sedimentation rate, FTI, sTSH, ^{131}I uptake, other thyroid antibodies, and, when needed, fine needle aspiration.

Subacute Painful Thyroiditis (Granulomatous or de Quervain's)

Subacute painful thyroiditis, probably a viral illness, is the commonest cause of painful, tender thyroid. It occurs mostly in women in the 3rd-5th decades. The onset is gradual or abrupt, and the dominant symptom is a painful, tender thyroid area. Pain may radiate to the upper neck, jaws, throat, or ears. Many patients may have fever, malaise, myalgia, and a history of upper respiratory tract infection. The thyroid is tender and enlarged: involvement is usually diffuse but may be unilateral and involve the two lobes sequentially. Hyperthyroidism of a few weeks' duration may be present in 50% of patients; almost all patients have biochemical hyperthyroidism related to follicular destruction. It may be followed by transient hypothyroidism. The illness is self-limiting, usually subsiding in weeks to months. The disease is characterized by remissions and relapses, but it eventually resolves completely. Restoration of function is the rule, but permanent hypothyroidism occurs in <5% of patients. Marked increase in the erythrocyte sedimentation rate is characteristic. The leukocyte count is mildly increased. FTI is increased and sTSH is suppressed in the hyperthyroid phase; ^{131}I uptake is suppressed. In the ensuing hypothyroid phase, the FTI is decreased, but the sTSH may still be suppressed (it may take 8 weeks to recover). The antibody titers are low or minimally increased. The major differential diagnosis is with hemorrhage into a thyroid nodule. In hemorrhage into a thyroid nodule, there are no systemic features; erythrocyte sedimentation rate is normal; ^{131}I uptake is normal; resolution occurs in a few days. Other differential diagnoses include radiation thyroiditis and pyogenic thyroiditis. Therapy--The disease is self-limited. For mild disease, no treatment is needed. For moderate disease, use nonsteroidal anti-inflammatory drugs; for severe disease, prednisone 20-40 mg/day; prompt response (a therapeutic test), treat for 2-3 weeks and withdraw over 3 weeks. For the hyperthyroid phase, use β-blockers. For the hypothyroid phase, T_4 treatment for a few months may be needed.

- Subacute painful thyroiditis: probably a viral illness.
- Onset: gradual or abrupt.
- Many patients: fever, malaise, myalgia, history of upper respiratory tract infection.
- Involvement: usually diffuse, may be unilateral.
- Hyperthyroidism of few weeks' duration may be present in 50% of patients.
- May be followed by transient hypothyroidism.
- Illness is self-limiting.
- Disease characterized by remissions and relapses.
- Restoration of function is the rule.
- Marked increase in erythrocyte sedimentation rate is characteristic.
- FTI is increased and sTSH is suppressed in hyperthyroid phase; ^{131}I uptake is suppressed.
- Major differential diagnosis is with hemorrhage into thyroid nodule.
- For moderate disease, use nonsteroidal anti-inflammatory drugs.
- For severe disease, prednisone 20-40 mg/day; prompt response (therapeutic test).

Euthyroid Sick Syndrome: "Adaptive Hypothyroidism"

In acute and chronically sick hospitalized patients:

- Decrease peripheral T_3 production = decreased serum level of T_3.
- Decrease serum T_4 and T_3 binding = decreased serum levels of T_4 and T_3.
- Change in hormone clearance = increased serum level of T_4.
- Central effects = decreased sTSH.

Note that the thyroid parameter abnormalities in the euthyroid sick syndrome can mimic 1) central hypothyroidism: decreased T_4 and T_3, normal or decreased sTSH; and 2) thyrotoxicosis: increased T_4 and decreased sTSH.

- In euthyroid sick syndrome, thyroid parameter abnormalities can mimic central hypothyroidism and thyrotoxicosis.

With recovery from the illness, thyroid function parameters return to normal within a few days.

Suppressed sTSH in the euthyroid sick syndrome: medical/surgical illness, 20%; psychiatric illness, 20%. Drugs: glucocorticoids, dopamine.

Increased sTSH in the euthyroid sick syndrome: during recovery from illness. Therefore, sTSH cannot be used alone as thyroid function screening test in hospitalized patients.

- sTSH cannot be used alone as thyroid function screening test in hospitalized patients.

Iodide-Induced Thyroid Dysfunction

Common causes of iodide-induced thyroid dysfunction are contrast agents, inorganic iodides, and amiodarone. Iodide-induced hypothyroidism: Hashimoto's thyroiditis, Graves' disease after radioiodine therapy or surgery, fetal and neonatal thyroid, others. Iodide-induced hyperthyroidism: autonomous thyroid (jodbasedow) Graves' disease, multinodular thyroid, others.

Pregnancy and the Thyroid

In patients with primary hypothyroidism, optimize the therapy before pregnancy is contemplated. Untreated hypothyroidism may lead to early loss of pregnancy. Also, closely follow TSH levels during pregnancy, because the dose of thyroid hormone may need to be increased. The dosage is returned to prepregnancy dosage after delivery.

- In patients with hypothyroidism, optimize therapy before pregnancy is contemplated.
- Closely follow TSH levels during pregnancy.
- Dose of thyroid hormone may need to be increased.
- After delivery, dosage is returned to prepregnancy dosage.

In patients with diffuse euthyroid goiter early in pregnancy, check antithyroid antibodies. Positive antimicrosomal antibodies may identify patients at increased risk for developing postpartum thyroid disease.

- If diffuse euthyroid goiter occurs early in pregnancy, check antithyroid antibodies.
- Positive antibodies: may identify patients at increased risk for postpartum thyroid disease.

Thyrotoxicosis in pregnancy--In normal pregnancy, T_4 and T_3 levels increase because of estrogen-induced increase in TBG. The resin T_3 uptake is decreased, and the FTI is normal. sTSH may be decreased modestly, as low as 0.1 µU/mL (normal, 0.4-5 µU/mL). The thyroid may be slightly enlarged. An increase in FTI and an sTSH <0.1 µU/mL point to thyrotoxicosis. Obviously, a [131]I

uptake test is absolutely contraindicated.

- In normal pregnancy, T_4 and T_3 levels increase.
- Resin T_3 uptake is decreased; FTI is normal.
- sTSH may be decreased modestly.
- Increase in ^{131}I and sTSH <0.1 µU/mL indicates thyrotoxicosis.
- [131]I uptake test is absolutely contraindicated.

For management of Graves' thyrotoxicosis in pregnancy, most physicians rely on antithyroid drug therapy. Surgical excision may be an option after the first trimester. Antithyroid drugs cross the placenta and have an effect on the fetal thyroid; however, maternal T_4 and T_3 do not cross the placenta. Therefore, antithyroid drugs should be given in the smallest doses necessary to control the disease, usually <200 mg/day of propylthiouracil. Radioiodine therapy is absolutely contraindicated. Also, β-blockers should not be given, because of fetal growth retardation and neonatal respiratory depression. Inorganic iodides should be avoided; they can cross the placenta and cause fetal goiter and hypothyroidism.

- For Graves' thyrotoxicosis in pregnancy, most physicians rely on antithyroid drug therapy.
- Surgical excision may be an option after first trimester.
- Antithyroid drugs cross the placenta.
- Maternal T_4 and T_3 do not cross the placenta.
- Antithyroid drugs: give in smallest dose necessary to control disease.
- Radioiodine therapy is absolutely contraindicated.
- β-Blockers should not be given.

Thyrotoxic Crisis

Thyrotoxic crisis is a rare disorder seen in untreated or inadequately treated hyperthyroid patients undergoing surgical treatment or who have an acute nonthyroidal illness. It may be seen postoperatively in poorly prepared patients with thyrotoxicosis undergoing subtotal thyroidectomy. It is characterized by extreme irritability, delirium, hyperpyrexia, tachycardia, hypotension, vomiting, diarrhea, prostration, and coma. If untreated, it is fatal. Perform the appropriate diagnostic blood tests promptly, and start treatment without waiting for confirmation of the diagnosis. Give propylthiouracil to block thyroid hormone synthesis (150-250 mg/2-6 hr) followed 1 hour later by sodium iodide to inhibit release of thyroid hormones (1 g in slow intravenous infusion). Propranolol is given as a β-blocker and to decrease T_4 conversion to

T_3 (20-60 mg/6 hour orally or 0.5-2 mg/4 hour intravenously). Support the patient with fluids given intravenously, vitamin B complex, dexamethasone (2 mg/6 hour), and with symptomatic therapy. After recovery, plan for definitive therapy.

- Thyrotoxic crisis: seen in untreated or inadequately treated hyperthyroid patients undergoing surgical treatment or who have acute nonthyroidal illness.
- Characteristics: extreme irritability, delirium, hyperpyrexia, tachycardia, hypotension, vomiting, diarrhea, prostration, coma.
- Untreated, it is fatal.
- Start treatment without waiting for confirmation of diagnosis.
- Propylthiouracil to block thyroid hormone synthesis.
- Sodium iodide to inhibit release of thyroid hormones.
- Propranolol is given as a β-blocker and to decrease T_4 conversion to T_3.
- Support patient.
- After recovery, plan for definitive therapy.

Myxedema Crisis

Myxedema crisis occurs in patients with severe hypothyroidism and is either spontaneous or precipitated by acute illness, exposure to cold, or use of sedatives or opiates. It carries a high mortality (20%-50%). The onset is gradual, with progressive stupor culminating in coma. Seizures may occur, and hypothermia, hypotension, hypoventilation, hyponatremia, and hypoglycemia may be present. Most often, the patients are elderly and have overt hypothyroidism. Treatment--Perform confirmatory blood tests and start treatment promptly. Do not wait for confirmatory results. Institute supportive therapy and give aggressive thyroid hormone therapy. Conserve body heat; do not warm externally. Conserve vital functions; consider tracheal intubation and ventilatory support if respiratory depression occurs. Cautiously maintain hydration and hemodynamic functions and watch out for hyponatremia (syndrome of inappropriate ADH). Give T_4 2 μg/kg intravenously over 5-10 minutes; and 100 μg/24 hour intravenously thereafter. Support the patient with glucocorticoids in high doses (hypothyroidism may have slowed down adrenal responsiveness and there may be associated Addison's disease).

- Myxedema crisis: occurs in severe hypothyroidism, either spontaneously or precipitated by acute illness, exposure to cold, or use of sedatives or opiates.

- It carries a high mortality (20%-50%).
- Onset is gradual, with progressive stupor culminating in coma.
- Hypothermia, hypotension, hypoventilation, hyponatremia, hypoglycemia may occur.
- Perform confirmatory blood tests; start treatment promptly.
- Institute supportive therapy and give aggressive thyroid hormone therapy.
- Support patient with glucocorticoids in high doses.

THE PARATHYROID GLANDS AND METABOLIC BONE DISEASE

Physiology

Parathyroid Hormone

Parathyroid hormone (PTH) is critical for maintenance of eucalcemia. It acts on bone to mobilize calcium and phosphate (osteolytic osteolysis and osteoclastic bone resorption), an effect that needs the permissive action of calcitriol, $1\text{-}25(OH)_2D$. Its renal effects include stimulation of calcium reabsorption by distal tubule of the nephron, inhibition of phosphate reabsorption by proximal tubule of the nephron, and stimulation of 1-hydroxylation of $25(OH)D$ to $1\text{-}25(OH)_2D$. PTH stimulates the absorption of calcium and phosphate from the gut indirectly via $1\text{-}25(OH)_2D$. PTH acts via cell membrane receptors and activates adenylate cyclase; cyclic AMP is the second messenger. The serum level of calcium is the major determinant of PTH secretion: low serum levels of calcium stimulate and high serum levels suppress PTH secretion. Magnesium is necessary for the secretion and action of PTH. PTH is a single-chain polypeptide of 84 amino acids; its N-terminal (1-34) is biologically active and has a short half-life. The C-terminal is biologically inert, has a long half-life, and is excreted by the kidney. Standard assays use C-terminal, N-terminal, or mid-region antisera. C-terminal assays are falsely elevated in renal failure. New immunoradiometric assays measure the intact PTH molecule with high sensitivity and specificity and are the immunoassays of choice.

- PTH: critical for maintenance of eucalcemia.
- Bone effects: mobilization of calcium and phosphate.
- Renal effects: stimulation of calcium reabsorption by distal tubule of the nephron, inhibition of phosphate reabsorption by proximal tubule of the nephron, stim-

ulation of 1-hydroxylation of 25(OH)D to 1-25(OH)₂D.

- Intestinal effect: stimulation of absorption of calcium and phosphate indirectly via 1-25(OH)₂D.
- Serum calcium is the major determinant of PTH secretion.
- Magnesium is necessary for PTH secretion and action.
- PTH: single-chain polypeptide of 84 amino acids.
- N-terminal (1-34) is biologically active.
- C-terminal is biologically inert.
- New immunoradiometric assays: measure PTH molecule assays with high sensitivity and specificity and are the immunoassays of choice.

Vitamin D

The sources of vitamin D are the diet and the irradiation of vitamin D precursors in the skin. The bioactivation of vitamin D is shown in Fig. 11-8.

1-25(OH)₂D, or calcitriol, is the active hormone. It stimulates active absorption of calcium and phosphate from the gut, has a permissive role in the PTH effect on bone, and optimizes calcium-phosphate product in the extracellular fluids to allow mineralization of new osteoid. It has other effects on the skin and immune system. 1-25(OH)₂D is a steroid and acts through specific intracellular cytoplasmic or nuclear receptors.

- Sources of vitamin D: diet and irradiation of vitamin D precursors in the skin.
- 1-25(OH)₂D is the active hormone.
- Stimulates active absorption of calcium and phosphate from gut.
- Permissive role in PTH effect on bone.
- Optimizes calcium-phosphate product in extracellular fluids to allow mineralization of new osteoid.

Calcium

Total body calcium is 1,000-1,200 g. Bone and teeth contain about 99%; cells, 1%; and extracellular fluid, 0.1% (about 1 g). The total serum calcium is ionized (50%); complexed to citrate, phosphate, and other anions (5%-10%); and bound to protein (40%), especially albumin. Ionized calcium is the biologically active component and the major determinant of PTH secretion. The average intake of calcium is 400-1,000 mg/day. Absorption occurs in the proximal small intestine and is enhanced by 1-25(OH)₂D. Calcium is filtered by the glomeruli; 98%-99% of filtered calcium is reabsorbed by the renal tubules, mostly in the proximal tubule; distal tubular reabsorption is enhanced by PTH. In men, 24-hour urine excretion is <275 mg and in women, <250 mg.

- Total serum calcium: ionized (50%); complexed to citrate, phosphate, other anions (5%-10%); bound to protein (40%), especially albumin.
- Ionized calcium is the biologically active component and major determinant of PTH secretion.
- Gut absorption occurs in proximal small intestine and is enhanced by 1-25(OH)₂D.
- Distal tubular reabsorption is enhanced by PTH.

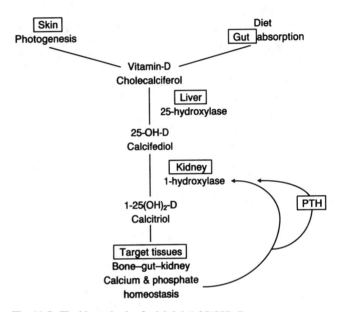

Fig. 11-8. The biosynthesis of calcitriol, 1-25(OH)₂D.

Syndrome of Hypercalcemia

Clinical Presentation

Hypercalcemia may be asymptomatic or present with a single or multisystem disorder. Renal: polyuria, polydipsia due to nephrogenic diabetes insipidus; renal colic, nephrolithiasis; and chronic renal failure. Neuropsychiatric: fatigue, weakness, impairment of consciousness, confusion, depression, and hyporeflexia. Gastrointestinal: anorexia, nausea, vomiting, and constipation; hypercalcemia may be associated with peptic ulcer and pancreatitis. Cardiovascular: hypertension and arrhythmias; hypercalcemia potentiates the cardiac effects of digitalis; ECG may show shortened QT intervals. Metastatic calcification: band keratopathy or nephrocalcinosis.

- Hypercalcemia: may be asymptomatic or present with single or multisystem disorder.

Etiology

The causes of hypercalcemia are outlined in Table 11-11. Fundamentally, hypercalcemia can result from

Table 11-11.--Causes of Hypercalcemia

Parathyroid hormone-dependent
    Hyperparathyroidism--primary or tertiary
    Familial benign hypocalciuric hypercalcemia
    Drug-induced--thiazides, lithium
    Ectopic hyperparathyroidism (rare)
Parathyroid hormone-independent
    Malignancy
        With bone metastasis
        Hematologic--multiple myeloma, leukemia, lymphoma
        Humoral hypercalcemia
    Endocrine disorders
        Thyroid dysfunction
        Pheochromocytoma
        Adrenal insufficiency
        Acromegaly
    Hypervitaminosis D
        Exogenous vitamin D
        Endogenous--granulomatous disorders, some
          lymphomas
    Immobilization, especially in patients with high turnover
      of bone as in Paget's disease
    Milk-alkali syndrome

increased bone resorption, increased intestinal absorption, or decreased urinary excretion of calcium. More than one mechanism may be involved in any given disorder. The causes can most usefully be categorized as either PTH-dependent or PTH-independent.

Parathyroid-Dependent Hypercalcemia

Primary hyperparathyroidism--Adenoma is the commonest cause. It can be single (80% of patients) or multiple (3%); hyperplasia of all four glands occurs in 15% of patients; carcinoma is rare (2%). Adenoma may be ectopic in 6%-10% of cases and be found in the thyroid, thymus, or mediastinum. Primary hyperparathyroidism may be isolated or familial. The familial form may be a part of MEN I (in association with tumors of the anterior pituitary and endocrine pancreas) or MEN IIA (in association with medullary carcinoma of the thyroid and pheochromocytoma). The usual parathyroid lesion in familial hyperparathyroidism is hyperplasia. Most patients with primary hyperparathyroidism are asymptomatic and identified by random blood screening; others may present with features of hypercalcemia (see above). Characteristic skeletal lesions include osteopenia, subperiosteal bone resorption, salt and pepper lesions in the

skull, and ostitis fibrosis cystica. Primary hyperparathyroidism has known associations with chondrocalcinosis and pseudogout. Hypercalcemia may be mild and intermittent; serum levels of phosphate are usually low but may be normal; chloride is often increased and bicarbonate often decreased. Urine calcium is usually normal or modestly increased, which helps to differentiate it from familial hypocalciuric hypercalcemia. ECG may show short QT interval or arrhythmia. The serum level of PTH is increased (90% of patients); it may be "normal" in 10% of patients but is always inappropriately increased for the degree of hypercalcemia. Immunoradiometric assay of PTH is most reliable and in most patients distinguishes primary hyperparathyroidism from humoral hypercalcemia of malignancy. Preoperative localization is not required except in the surgical management of postoperative persistent or recurrent disease (high-resolution ultrasonography for cervical adenomas and CT scan, thallium/technetium subtraction scan, or angiography for mediastinal tumors). Conservative therapy may be indicated in cases of mild uncomplicated disease, especially in the elderly; otherwise, adenomectomy for adenoma and subtotal parathyroidectomy (leaving 50 mg of parathyroid tissue) for hyperplasia. Medical therapy for chronic hypercalcemia is usually not effective; options include phosphate and estrogen given orally.

- Primary hyperparathyroidism: adenoma is commonest cause.
- It can be single (80%) or multiple (3%).
- Hyperplasia of all four glands in 15% of patients.
- Carcinoma is rare (2%).
- It may be isolated or familial.
- Familial hyperparathyroidism: may be part of MEN I or IIA.
- Usual parathyroid lesion in familial hyperparathyroidism: hyperplasia.
- Most patients with hyperparathyroidism are asymptomatic.
- Characteristic skeletal lesions: osteopenia, periosteal bone resorption, salt and pepper lesions in skull, ostitis fibrosis cystica.
- Primary hyperparathyroidism: known associations with chondrocalcinosis and pseudogout.
- Urine calcium: usually normal or moderately increased (helps distinguish from familial hypocalciuric hypercalcemia).
- Serum PTH is increased (90%), may be "normal" in 10%, but is always inappropriately increased for the

degree of hypercalcemia.

- Immunoradiometric PTH is most reliable and in most patients distinguishes primary hyperparathyroidism from humoral hypercalcemia of malignancy.
- Preoperative localization not necessary except in surgical management of preoperative persistent or recurrent disease.
- Conservative therapy may be indicated in mild uncomplicated disease (especially in elderly).
- Adenomectomy for adenoma.
- Subtotal parathyroidectomy for hyperplasia.

Familial hypocalciuric hypercalcemia is characterized by hypercalcemia in a relatively young patient, normal or slightly elevated PTH, low-to-normal phosphate, and decreased fractional excretion of calcium and magnesium. The measured calcium clearance to creatinine clearance ratio is <0.1. The parathyroid glands show chief cell hyperplasia. Familial hypocalciuric hypercalcemia is familial and autosomal dominant; the hypercalcemia may be detected in affected family members before age 10. Screening of family members is important. Hypercalcemia is usually asymptomatic and uncomplicated. No medical or surgical therapy is indicated. Surgical therapy does not relieve hypercalcemia unless all parathyroid tissue is removed.

- Familial hypocalciuric hypercalcemia: hypercalcemia in a relatively young patient.
- Normal or slightly elevated PTH.
- Decreased fractional excretion of calcium and magnesium.
- Autosomal dominant.
- Hypercalcemia may be detected in affected family members before age 10.
- Hypercalcemia is usually asymptomatic and uncomplicated.

Thiazides may potentiate the effects of PTH on bone and kidney and may cause mild hypercalcemia. Unlike other diuretics, thiazides decrease urine calcium. The mild hypercalcemia should resolve within a few weeks after discontinuing use of the drug. Many patients have underlying mild primary hyperparathyroidism. Use thiazides with caution in patients with increased bone turnover and hypercalciuria, e.g., Paget's disease and thyrotoxicosis.

- Thiazides: may potentiate effects of PTH on bone and

kidney.
- Mild hypercalcemia should resolve in few weeks after use of drug is discontinued.
- Use thiazides with caution in patients with increased bone turnover and hypercalciuria.

Lithium--Hypercalcemia occurs in 10% of patients who take lithium. Lithium increases the set-point of parathyroid secretion. The hypercalcemia is reversible if the use of lithium is discontinued.

- Hypercalcemia occurs in 10% of patients who take lithium.
- Lithium increases set-point of parathyroid secretion.

Parathyroid-Independent Hypercalcemia

Hypercalcemia of malignancy is common, often develops acutely, and may be quite severe. It is the commonest cause of hypercalcemia in hospitalized patients. Its causes include local bone destruction by metastasis or myeloma, increased synthesis of 1-25(OH)$_2$D by lymphoma, and elaboration of other mediators of bone resorption (e.g., PTH-related protein, tumor necrosis factor, transforming growth factor, cytokines) by such tumors of the lung, kidney, squamous cell carcinoma, etc. Ectopic PTH is very uncommon. PTH-related protein (PTH-RP) shares with PTH its renal and bone effects; levels are increased in most patients with humoral hypercalcemia of malignancy and are low or normal in patients with primary hyperparathyroidism. Most PTH antisera do not cross react with PTH-related protein. Most patients with humoral hypercalcemia of malignancy show suppressed PTH by radioimmunoassay.

- Hypercalcemia of malignancy: common, often develops acutely, may be severe.
- Commonest cause of hypercalcemia in hospitalized patients.
- Cause: local bone destruction by metastasis or myeloma; increased synthesis of 1-25(OH)$_2$D by lymphoma; elaboration of other mediators of bone resorption.
- Increased levels of PTH-RP in majority of patients.
- Most patients show suppressed PTH on radioimmunoassay.

Vitamin D intoxication--Hypercalcemia, hypercalciuria, renal insufficiency, and soft tissue calcification follow prolonged ingestion of vitamin D in high dosages.

The condition may persist for months after discontinuing use of vitamin D, because of fat storage of the vitamin. Levels of 1-25(OH)$_2$D are increased. Response to glucocorticoids is prompt.

- Vitamin D intoxication: may persist for months after discontinued use of the vitamin.
- Prompt response to glucocorticoids.

Sarcoidosis and other granulomatous disorders-- Hypercalcemia occurs in 15% of patients (hypercalciuria is more common) and is caused by increased gut absorption and increased bone resorption. It is vitamin D-mediated. Levels of 25(OH)D are normal; the serum level of 1-25(OH)$_2$D is increased because granulomas have 1-hydroxylase and can generate 1-25(OH)$_2$D from circulating 25(OH)D. The condition is responsive to glucocorticoids.

- Hypercalcemia is vitamin D-mediated.
- Serum levels of 1-25(OH)$_2$D increase because granulomas have 1-hydroxylase.
- Glucocorticoid responsive.

In Addison's disease, hypercalcemia is frequent and related to an increase in the protein-bound fraction; it is reversible with glucocorticoid therapy.

In thyrotoxicosis, enhanced bone resorption is greater than bone formation. Hypercalcemia occurs in 25% of patients; hypercalciuria, in 50%. Hypercalcemia resolves with treatment of thyrotoxicosis.

Immobilization may result in hypercalcemia in patients with rapid bone turnover, such as adolescents and patients with Paget's disease.

Milk-alkali syndrome is a combination of high calcium intake and absorbable alkali. Features: hypercalcemia, low urine calcium, alkalosis, renal failure, and soft tissue calcification. It is preventable.

Diagnostic Approach

Rule out laboratory error and factitial causes. Confirm the hypercalcemia with repeated measurements. If serum albumin abnormalities are present, correct for serum albumin levels or measure ionized calcium. A change of 1.0 g/dL in serum albumin changes serum calcium by about 0.8 mg/dL, in the same direction.

- Rule out laboratory error and factitial causes.
- Correct for serum albumin or obtain ionized calcium.

If drug-induced hypercalcemia is suspected, stop use of the drug and reassess the serum concentration of calcium in a few weeks (few months in case of vitamin D). If hypercalcemia persists, proceed with evaluation.

- If drug-induced, stop use of the drug.
- Reassess serum concentration of calcium.

Determine serum level of PTH. The best assay is the two-site immunometric assay that measures intact PTH and is unaffected by renal function.

- Determine serum level of PTH.
- Best assay: two-site immunometric assay.

A suppressed PTH points to parathyroid-independent hypercalcemia. Proceed with careful clinical, biochemical, and radiologic assessment to identify the cause. Increased PTH-related protein points to humoral hypercalcemia of malignancy, and an increased 1-25(OH)$_2$D suggests a granulomatous disorder or some type of lymphoma.

- Suppressed PTH: parathyroid-independent hypercalcemia.
- Increased PTH-related protein: humoral hypercalcemia of malignancy.
- Increased 1-25(OH)$_2$D: granulomatous disorder or some type of lymphoma.

A high serum level of PTH points to primary hyperparathyroidism. A "normal" or "minimally elevated" serum level of PTH may be due to thiazides, lithium, familial hypocalciuric hypercalcemia, or primary hyperparathyroidism. A family history, benign clinical course, and low urinary concentration of calcium point to familial hypocalciuric hypercalcemia. Note that the serum concentration of phosphate may be low in any hypercalcemic state. High serum concentration of phosphate points to renal insufficiency or to non-PTH-dependent hypercalcemia. Low urinary level of calcium is seen in familial hypocalciuric hypercalcemia and with the use of thiazides. Significant hypercalciuria (>400 mg/24 hour) usually points to nonparathyroid cause.

- High serum PTH level: primary hyperparathyroidism.
- "Normal" or "minimally elevated" serum level of PTH: thiazides, lithium, familial hypocalciuric hypercalcemia, primary hyperparathyroidism.

- Family history, benign clinical course, low urinary concentration of calcium: familial hypocalciuric hypercalcemia.

Treatment

Specific--Treatment of the primary cause, if feasible, is the most important therapeutic option. For example, parathyroid adenomectomy for primary hyperparathyroidism and medical management of thyrotoxicosis. Glucocorticoids are the drugs of choice for the hypercalcemia seen in Addison's disease and in vitamin D excess, either of exogenous or endogenous origin (sarcoidosis and other granulomatous disorders). They are also effective for specific antitumor effects in some malignancies, such as multiple myeloma, some lymphomas, and breast cancer with metastasis. Indomethacin or aspirin as antiprostaglandins is usually ineffective.

- Most important therapeutic option: treatment of primary cause.
- Glucocorticoids: drugs of choice for hypercalcemia in Addison's disease and in vitamin D excess (exogenous or endogenous origin).
- Glucocorticoids may be effective in some malignancies: multiple myeloma, some lymphomas, breast cancer with metastasis.

Nonspecific--Consider the rapidity of the onset, severity of the hypercalcemia, coexisting illness, and age of patient. Nonspecific therapy is designed to decrease bone resorption and increase renal excretion.

- Nonspecific therapy: to decrease bone resorption and increase renal excretion.

Severe hypercalcemia leads to a decrease in renal concentrating ability, dehydration, decreased renal blood flow and glomerular filtration rate, and enhanced renal tubular absorption of calcium along with sodium. Rehydration is an essential first step in the treatment in order to correct these abnormalities. Forced saline diuresis can increase calcium urinary losses and reduce serum calcium level in 1-3 mg/dL. Furosemide, given intravenously, 40 mg/1-2 hours. Replace volume and electrolytes. Do not initiate forced saline diuresis until volume repletion is achieved. Often, central venous pressure monitoring and bladder catheterization are necessary. Treatment is temporizing. The dangers include cardiac decompensation, life-threatening hypokalemia, hypomagnesemia, and hypophosphatemia.

- Rehydration is an essential first step in the treatment.
- Do not initiate forced saline diuresis until volume repletion is achieved. Watch for volume or electrolyte abnormalities.

Calcitonin has a direct antiresorptive effect on osteoclasts; also, it is hypercalciuric. Calcitonin is nontoxic and has a rapid onset of action (few hours). Give in a dose of 2-8 IU/kg intravenously, intramuscularly, or subcutaneously every 6 hours. Unfortunately, the effect is modest and variable, and tachyphylaxis often develops (concomitant administration of glucocorticoids may prolong its effect). Side effects include nausea, flushing, and skin rash.

- Calcitonin has direct antiresorptive effect on the osteoclasts; also, it is hypercalciuric.
- It has rapid onset of action.
- Effect is modest and variable.
- Tachyphylaxis often develops.

Bisphosphonates are analogues of pyrophosphate, with a high affinity to hydroxyapatite of bone. They are taken up by osteoclasts and inhibit bone resorption. In addition, bisphosphonates inhibit differentiation of progenitor cells to osteoclasts. Etidronate is a first-generation bisphosphonate. It is poorly absorbed when given orally; so to be effective in managing hypercalcemia, it has to be given intravenously. The dose is 7.5 mg/kg daily in 5% dextrose in water over 2 hours for 3 successive days. It causes a dramatic decrease in the serum concentration of calcium, but normalizes calcium in only 30%-40% of patients. The improvement may last 5-7 days. The side effects include nausea, vomiting, and abdominal pain.

- Bisphosphonates: analogues of pyrophosphate.
- Inhibit bone resorption.
- Etidronate: first-generation bisphosphonate.
- It has to be given intravenously.
- Causes a dramatic decrease in serum calcium.
- Normalizes calcium in 30%-40% of patients.
- Improvement may last 5-7 days.

Pamidronate, a new generation bisphosphonate, is an extremely potent antiresorptive agent that recently has been approved by the FDA for management of hypercalcemia. It is given as a single intravenous dose of 60-

90 mg. Pamidronate is effective in 24-48 hours (in 70% to >90% of patients) and normalizes the serum concentration of calcium for weeks or months. The drug given orally is also effective. Unlike etidronate, chronic administration is not associated with mineralization defect. Side effects include low-grade fever (20% of patients), hypocalcemia (10%), hypophosphatemia, hypomagnesemia, and reversible hepatic injury.

- Pamidronate: a new generation bisphosphonate.
- It is an extremely potent antiresorptive agent.
- Given as a single intravenous dose of 60-90 mg.
- Effective in 24-48 hours in majority of patients.
- Normalizes serum concentration of calcium for weeks or months.
- Unlike etidronate, chronic administration is not associated with mineralization defect.

Plicamycin (mithramycin) inhibits osteoclastic resorption. A dose of 15-25 μg/kg is given over a period of 4-24 hours. The effect is rapid (24-48 hours); it normalizes calcium in 40%-60% of patients. The effect may last for 5-7 days. Side effects include thrombocytopenia and qualitative platelet defects, renal insufficiency, and liver abnormalities. Bisphosphonates have replaced plicamycin as "first-line" therapy.

- Plicamycin: inhibits osteoclastic resorption.
- Rapid effect.
- Normalizes calcium in 40%-60% of patients.
- Effect may last for 5-7 days.
- Bisphosphonates have replaced plicamycin as "first-line" therapy.

Gallium nitrate also inhibits osteoclastic bone resorption. A dose of 200 mg per square meter of body surface area in 1 L of fluid daily for 5 days. Therapy achieves eucalcemia in 75% of patients. This effect may last 7-10 days. Side effects include nausea, hypotension, and renal insufficiency.

- Gallium nitrate: inhibits osteoclastic bone resorption.
- Achieves eucalcemia in 75% of patients.
- Effect may last 7-10 days.

Phosphate given intravenously can have a dramatic effect in lowering the serum level of calcium by precipitating calcium phosphate in the skeleton and in soft tissues, including the kidneys and the heart. It is hazardous and can precipitate acute renal failure and hypotension. This treatment has been superseded by the other agents described above. Phosphate given orally is minimally effective, if at all. Dialysis, either peritoneal or hemodialysis, is reserved for patients with renal failure.

- Phosphate given intravenously: hazardous; can precipitate renal failure and hypotension.
- Dialysis (peritoneal or hemodialysis): reserved for patients with renal failure.

Syndrome of Hypocalcemia

Clinical Presentation

Hypocalcemia may be asymptomatic and detected only by biochemical screening. The symptoms of hypocalcemia reflect not only the degree but also the rate of its development. Neuromuscular: paresthesias and muscle spasms, such as carpopedal spasms, laryngeal stridor, and convulsions. Apathy, lethargy, and depression may occur. Specific neurologic sequelae include basal ganglia calcification, extrapyramidal manifestations, and benign intracranial hypertension. Gastrointestinal: abdominal pain, nausea, vomiting, and malabsorption. Cardiovascular: prolonged QT interval and congestive heart failure resistant to standard therapy but responsive to normalization of serum level of calcium. Other effects include premature cataracts, alopecia, and mucocutaneous candidiasis. Children may have enamel hypoplasia and failure of secondary dentition. The signs of Chvostek and Trousseau are characteristic of hypocalcemia, although they rarely can be elicited in normal persons.

- Symptoms of hypocalcemia reflect not only the degree but also the rate of its development.
- Carpopedal spasms, laryngeal stridor, and convulsions.
- Basal ganglia calcification, extrapyramidal manifestations, benign intracranial hypertension.
- Cardiovascular effects: prolonged QT; congestive heart failure resistant to standard therapy but responsive to normalization of serum level of calcium.
- Chvostek's and Trousseau's signs: characteristic of hypocalcemia.

Etiology

The causes of hypocalcemia are outlined in Table 11-12. Basically, hypocalcemia may result from decreased secretion of PTH or PTH resistance, from decreased pro-

Table 11-12.--Causes of Hypocalcemia

Decreased secretion of parathyroid hormone
    Hypoparathyroidism
        Functional--hypomagnesemia
        Organic--postoperative
        Autoimmune
        Hypomagnesemia
Decreased action of parathyroid hormone
    Pseudohypoparathyroidism
Vitamin D deficiency
    Nutritional
    Malabsorption
    Chronic liver disease
    Anticonvulsant agents
    Renal failure
Vitamin D resistance--types I and II
Other
    Phosphate excess
    Increased bone avidity for calcium
    Miscellaneous, e.g., acute pancreatitis

---

duction of vitamin D or vitamin D resistance, and from other, miscellaneous disorders that decrease the mobilization of calcium from bone or increase calcium deposition in tissues.

Hypoparathyroidism may result from inadvertent surgical damage to the parathyroid glands during thyroidectomy, radical neck dissection, or surgical management of primary hyperparathyroidism. It may be transient or permanent, and it may appear shortly or in few months or years after the surgical insult. Occasionally, hypoparathyroidism may result from other organic disorders: autoimmune, infiltrative (hemochromatosis or Wilson's disease), or congenital (DiGeorge syndrome). Idiopathic hypoparathyroidism often appears as a familial disorder, and may have an autoimmune basis. It occasionally accompanies other endocrine deficiency states. Hypomagnesemia is a cause of functional hypoparathyroidism; it decreases the secretion and action of PTH.

- Surgical hypoparathyroidism: may result from inadvertent damage to parathyroid glands and may be transient or permanent.
- May occasionally result from organic disorders: autoimmune, infiltrative, congenital.
- Idiopathic hypoparathyroidism: often appears as a familial disorder; may have an autoimmune basis.

- Hypomagnesemia: an important cause of hypoparathyroidism.
- Hypomagnesemia: decreases secretion and action of PTH.

Pseudohypoparathyroidism is an inherited disorder characterized by end-organ resistance to PTH action. The resistance may affect bone and kidney differentially; thus, clinical manifestations may vary. In type IA pseudohypoparathyroidism, there is a 50% decrease in the activity of Gs, the stimulatory guanyl nucleotide-binding protein coupled to adenylate cyclase; other hormone actions, e.g., TSH, gonadotropins, may be affected. In type IB, there may be a problem with the PTH receptor. In type II, there is a postreceptor defect. The characteristic features of type IA are short stature, round face, obesity, short neck, short metacarpals and metatarsals, subcutaneous calcification, and mild mental retardation. A variant disorder called "pseudopseudohypoparathyroidism" presents with the same characteristic physical features but without the biochemical abnormalities.

- Pseudohypoparathyroidism: inherited; characterized by end-organ resistance to PTH action.
- Type IA: Characteristic features are short stature, round face, obesity, short neck, short metacarpals and metatarsals, subcutaneous calcification, mild mental retardation.
- Pseudopseudohypoparathyroidism: variant disorder with same characteristic physical features but without the biochemical abnormalities.

In both hypoparathyroidism and pseudohypoparathyroidism, hypocalcemia of variable degree and hyperphosphatemia are present. The serum level of PTH is low in hypoparathyroidism and high in pseudohypoparathyroidism. Basal ganglia calcification may occur in either disorder.

- Hypoparathyroidism and pseudohypoparathyroidism: hypocalcemia (variable degree) and hyperphosphatemia.
- Serum level of PTH: low in hypoparathyroidism, high in pseudohypoparathyroidism.
- Basal ganglia calcification may occur in either disorder.

For vitamin D deficiency and resistance, see section on osteomalacia.

Diagnostic Approach

Rule out laboratory error and factitial hypocalcemia. Adjust for serum albumin abnormalities (if present): for every 1-g change in albumin, serum calcium changes by 0.8 mg/dL in the same direction, or measure serum concentration of ionized calcium. Confirm by repeated measurements. Rule out hypomagnesemia and renal insufficiency. If hypomagnesemia is present, treat; if hypocalcemia persists, proceed with evaluation. Check serum level of PTH. A low or undetectable level of PTH points to hypoparathyroidism; a high level may be related to pseudohypoparathyroidism, vitamin D deficiency, or renal failure. The diagnosis of pseudohypoparathyroidism is based on clinical stigmata, family history, and unresponsiveness to exogenous PTH. Vitamin D deficiency is suggested by the clinical setting and is confirmed by assays of 25(OH)D or 1-25(OH)$_2$D.

- Rule out laboratory error and factitial hypocalcemia.
- Adjust for serum albumin abnormalities (if present).
- Rule out hypomagnesemia and renal insufficiency.
- Low/undetectable serum level of PTH: hypoparathyroidism.
- High serum level of PTH: pseudohypoparathyroidism, vitamin D deficiency, or renal failure.

Treatment

The treatment of hypocalcemia includes treating the cause when identifiable and feasible, e.g., replacement of magnesium. Calcium supplementation and/or vitamin D therapy are the mainstays of therapy. Overreplacement leads to hypercalcemia, hypercalciuria, nephrolithiasis, or nephrocalcinosis. Therefore, it is important to monitor the efficacy of the therapy and to maintain the serum concentration of calcium in the range of 8.0 to 8.5 mg/dL and the 24-hour urine concentration of calcium to <300 mg/24 hours.

- Hypocalcemia: treat cause when identifiable and feasible.
- Mainstays of therapy: calcium supplementation, vitamin D therapy.
- Important to monitor efficacy of therapy.
- Serum level of calcium: maintain at 8.0-8.5 mg/dL.
- 24-hour urine concentration of calcium: maintain at <300 mg/24 hours.

If hypocalcemia is life-threatening, give calcium intravenously: calcium gluconate is administered slowly over a period of 5-10 minutes (10-20 mL; 93 mg of elemental calcium per 10 mL); it can be repeated if symptoms persist. Frequently monitor the serum level of calcium. Remember that calcium given intravenously may be hazardous in patients taking digitalis. For chronic therapy, give calcium orally. Vitamin D is usually needed in addition. Calcium carbonate (40% elemental calcium) is preferred, up to 2 g of elemental calcium daily. Ergocalciferol is started in a dose of 25,000 U/day (or dihydrotachysterol in a dose of 0.125 mg/day or calcitriol in a dose of 0.25 µg/day). Useful adjuncts in some patients include thiazides (to decrease urinary calcium excretion) and oral phosphate binders.

- If hypocalcemia is life-threatening, give calcium intravenously.
- Useful adjuncts in some patients: thiazides (to decrease urinary calcium excretion) and oral phosphate binders.

Osteoporosis

By definition, "osteoporosis" refers to a decrease in bone mass that compromises the mechanical support function of the skeleton. The remaining bone is morphologically normal. Calcium homeostasis is not affected.

Clinical Presentation

Fracture after minimal trauma (especially of the vertebrae, distal radius, femoral neck), loss of height, dorsal kyphosis, and drooping of the rib cage should suggest osteoporosis.

Etiology

The causes of osteoporosis are outlined in Table 11-13.

Diagnostic Approach

Document osteopenia. Radiography of the spine or other affected bones is a relatively insensitive diagnostic test. On spine films, the vertebral bodies may show loss of transverse trabeculations, thinning and sharpening of cortical margins, wedging, or collapse. In radiologic studies, it is important to look for specific signs of other disorders, such as subperiosteal resorption of primary hyperparathyroidism or Looser's zones of osteomalacia. Bone densitometry is the diagnostic procedure of choice: single-photon absorptiometry of the forearm, dual-photon absorptiometry of the spine, or dual energy x-ray absorptiometry of the spine and hip.

Table 11-13.--Causes of Osteoporosis

Primary (idiopathic)
  Postmenopausal
  Senile
  Juvenile
Secondary
  Endocrine
    Cushing's syndrome
    Thyrotoxicosis
    Hyperparathyroidism
    Hypogonadism
    Diabetes mellitus
  Malignancy
    Multiple myeloma
    Leukemia
    Lymphoma
    Systemic mastocytosis
  Immobilization
    Generalized
    Localized
  Genetic abnormalities in bone collagen synthesis
    Homocystinuria
    Ehlers-Danlos syndrome
    Osteogenesis imperfecta
  Drugs
    Corticosteroids
    Heparin therapy
    Methotrexate
  Nutritional
    Protein malnutrition
    Ascorbic acid deficiency
    Alcoholism
  Gastrointestinal
    Malabsorption
    Gastric surgery

- Document osteopenia.
- Radiography of spine or other affected bones is relatively insensitive diagnostic test.
- In radiologic studies, look for specific signs of other disorders, e.g., subperiosteal resorption of primary hyperparathyroidism and Looser's zones of osteomalacia.
- Bone densitometry is diagnostic procedure of choice.
- Single-photon absorptiometry of forearm, dual-photon absorptiometry of spine, dual energy x-ray absorptiometry of spine and hip.

In identifying the cause, rule out secondary causes of osteoporosis by history, physical examination, and appropriate laboratory and radiologic tests. The endocrine tests that are required include serum level of calcium (and, if necessary, PTH), FTI and sTSH, screen for Cushing's syndrome with 1-mg overnight dexamethasone suppression test or 24-hour urinary free cortisol. Assess gonadal status (serum level of sex steroids, LH and FSH) to rule out hypogonadism. Tests to rule out myeloma and malabsorption are important. In idiopathic osteoporosis, serum levels of calcium and phosphate are normal, and urine concentration of calcium is variable; alkaline phosphatase is normal unless there has been a recent fracture. Bone scans identify recent fractures but are otherwise negative. Localized increased uptake otherwise may indicate Paget's disease or neoplasm. Bone biopsy is indicated in osteopenia in all men, black women, and premenopausal white women when the cause is undetermined.

- To identify cause: first rule out secondary causes of osteoporosis.
- Required endocrine tests: serum level of calcium (and PTH if necessary), FTI, sTSH, screen for Cushing's syndrome, and assessment of gonadal status.
- Tests to rule out myeloma and malabsorption are important.
- Bone scan in idiopathic osteoporosis: identifies recent fractures, otherwise negative.
- Localized increased uptake, on bone scan, otherwise may indicate Paget's disease or neoplasm.
- Bone biopsy is indicated in osteopenia in all men, black women, and premenopausal white women when the cause is undetermined.

Differential Diagnosis

Osteomalacia: presence of biochemical abnormalities (low serum levels of calcium and phosphate and increased serum level of alkaline phosphatase). Pseudofractures are almost pathognomonic. The diagnosis is confirmed by bone biopsy. Remember that osteoporosis and osteomalacia can coexist.

- Presence of biochemical abnormalities, pseudofractures, or characteristic bone biopsy findings: point to osteomalacia.
- Osteoporosis and osteomalacia can coexist.

Metastatic bone disease: strongly suspected if vertebral collapse occurs above vertebra T-9, presence of primary tumor, if the lesion affects the posterior arches of the vertebra, or if hypercalcemia or hypercalciuria is present. Bone scan is positive.

- Strongly suspect metastatic bone disease if: vertebral collapse is above T-9, lesion affects posterior arches of vertebrae, or hypercalcemia or hypercalciuria is present.
- Bone scan is positive.

Management of Postmenopausal Osteoporosis

Prevention: adequate calcium intake, 1,000 mg/day in premenopausal women and up to 1,500 mg/day in postmenopausal women. Calcium carbonate is 40% elemental calcium and is the most inexpensive preparation. Also, adequate vitamin D of 400-800 U/day; adequate weight-bearing exercise program; and effective and rapid treatment of secondary causes of osteoporosis. If there are no known contraindications, initiate estrogen therapy as early as possible after the development of menopause and continue the therapy for life. A minimum dose of 0.625 mg of conjugated estrogens is necessary (or its equivalent). The concomitant administration of progesterone is only necessary in women with intact uterus to prevent endometrial hyperplasia and cancer.

- Adequate calcium intake.
- Adequate vitamin D.
- Adequate weight-bearing exercise program.
- Effective and rapid treatment of secondary causes of osteoporosis.
- If no known contraindications, initiate estrogen therapy as soon as possible after menopause develops.
- Minimum dose necessary: 0.625 mg conjugated estrogens.
- Concomitant administration of progesterone: only if uterus is intact.

Treatment: decrease bone resorption and/or enhance bone formation. Estrogen, calcium, and calcitonin are the only drugs approved for reduction of bone resorption. Fluoride can increase bone formation, but it is associated with inadequate mineralization and increased incidence of appendicular fractures; therefore, it is not recommended. Androgens in females may have unacceptable androgenic side effects. Bisphosphonates, e.g., etidronate, reduce bone resorption but have to be administered cyclically (2 weeks every 3 months) and are experimental.

- Decrease bone resorption and/or enhance bone formation.
- Only drugs approved for reduction of bone resorption: estrogen, calcium, calcitonin.
- Bisphosphonates (etidronate): reduce bone resorption, have to be given cyclically (2 weeks every 3 months), are experimental.

Osteomalacia

Definition, Clinical Presentation, and Etiology

Osteomalacia refers to failure of mineralization of bone osteoid resulting in an excess of unmineralized osteoid and deficiency of mature mineralized bone. In children, the disorder is known as "rickets" and is associated with failure of maturation of the growth plate and gross skeletal deformities. Features: bone pain and tenderness, fractures, deformity, proximal weakness, and waddling gait. The causes of osteomalacia are outlined in Table 11-14. Basically, osteomalacia can result from vitamin D deficiency or resistance; phosphate deficiency; or abnormal bone cell, matrix, or crystal.

- Osteomalacia: failure of mineralization of bone osteoid.
- Result: excess of unmineralized osteoid.
- Bone pain and tenderness, fractures, deformity, proximal weakness, waddling gait.

Renal osteodystrophy is related to phosphate retention, decreased $1-25(OH)_2D$, and acidosis. Three major disorders are a part of the syndrome: predominant hyperparathyroid bone disease (osteitis fibrosa), predominant impaired mineralization of bone (osteomalacia), and mixed hyperparathyroid/osteomalacic disorder. Another form of bone disease, amyloid arthropathy, is recognized with increasing frequency in patients receiving long-term hemodialysis and is attributable to an increased plasma level of β_2-microglobulin, a microglobulin deposited in tissues as amyloid fibrils.

- Renal osteodystrophy: related to phosphate retention, decreased $1-25(OH)_2D$, and acidosis.
- Three major disorders are part of syndrome: hyperparathyroid bone disease, predominant impaired mineralization of bone, mixed hyperparathyroid/osteomalacic disorder.

Diagnostic Approach

Clinical diagnosis depends on 1) the clinical picture; 2)

Table 11-14.--Causes of Osteomalacia

Disorders of vitamin D metabolism
    Vitamin D deficiency
        Nutritional
        Malabsorption syndromes
    Defects of 25(OH)D generation
        Anticonvulsant agents
        Severe hepatic disease
    Defects of 1-25(OH)$_2$D generation
        Renal failure
        Hyperphosphatemia
    Hereditary disorders
        Vitamin D-resistant rickets, types I and II
Phosphate deficiency
    X-linked hypophosphatemic rickets
    Phosphate-binding antacids
    Renal phosphate loss
        Proximal tubular defects
            Isolated
            Generalized (Fanconi)
        Renal tubular acidosis
    Nonfamilial adulthood hypophosphatemia
    Neoplasms
Abnormal bone cell, matrix, crystal
    Familial hypophosphatasia
    Fibrogenesis imperfecta ossium
    Axial osteomalacia
    Fluoride toxicity
    Aluminum toxicity
    Bisphosphonates

biochemical abnormalities of serum levels of calcium, phosphate, creatinine, and alkaline phosphatase; and 3) radiologic osteopenia and characteristic Looser's zone or pseudofractures. Pseudofractures are areas of linear decalcification that are perpendicular to the periosteal surface and along the course of blood vessels. Usually, they are bilateral and symmetrical; occur in the scapula, pelvis, proximal long bones; and represent stress fractures. In children, the epiphyses are wide, cupped, and irregular. Occasionally, the skeletal findings of secondary hyperparathyroidism may be seen. Bone scan may identify pseudofractures before skeletal radiographs show positive findings. Definitive diagnosis of osteomalacia rests on bone biopsy after tetracycline labeling.

- Clinical diagnosis depends on: clinical picture; biochemical abnormalities of serum levels of calcium, phosphate, creatinine, alkaline phosphatase; radiolog-

ic osteopenia and characteristic Looser's zone or pseudofractures.
- Bone scan may identify pseudofractures before skeletal radiographs show positive findings.
- Definitive diagnosis of osteomalacia rests on bone biopsy after tetracycline labeling.

Check serum levels of calcium, phosphate, creatinine, alkaline phosphatase, and PTH. Normal serum levels of calcium and PTH: 1) low phosphate = phosphate depletion; 2) normal phosphate, low alkaline phosphatase = hypophosphatasia; and 3) normal phosphate, normal alkaline phosphatase = primary disorder of bone with abnormal matrix, bone cell, or bone crystal.

Decreased or normal serum levels of calcium and high levels of PTH: 1) high phosphorus and creatinine = renal osteodystrophy; 2) if phosphorus is low, check 25(OH)D; 3) if phosphorus and 25(OH)D are low = vitamin D deficiency, liver disease, or use of anticonvulsant agents; and 4) if phosphorus, creatinine, and 25(OH)D are normal, check serum levels of 1-25(OH)$_2$D. If 1-25(OH)$_2$D is low = vitamin D-dependent rickets; if 1-25(OH)$_2$D is high = vitamin D-resistant rickets.

Treatment

Correct the underlying disorder if possible. Also, replenish the necessary minerals. Vitamin D is the mainstay of therapy; doses may be as low as 2,000-4,000 U/day in nutritional deficiency and up to 25,000-100,000 U/day in severe malabsorption. Equivalent doses of more potent analogues may be reasonable alternatives in some forms of osteomalacia, e.g., 1-hydroxylated derivatives in osteomalacia of renal failure. Supplemental calcium is given in a dose of 1-3 g of elemental calcium per day. Oral phosphate is added in hypophosphatemic states. Bone disease may take several months to heal. Be careful to avoid the complications of vitamin D therapy, i.e., hypercalciuria, hypercalcemia, nephrolithiasis, or nephrocalcinosis.

- Correct underlying disorder.
- Replenish necessary minerals.
- Mainstay of therapy: vitamin D.
- Doses from 2,000-4,000 U/day (in nutritional deficiency) to 25,000-100,000 U/day (in severe malabsorption).
- Supplemental elemental calcium is given in a dose of 1-3 g/day.
- Add oral phosphate in hypophosphatemic states.

- Be careful to avoid the complications of vitamin D therapy.

Paget's Disease

Paget's disease, a disorder of unknown cause, is characterized by disorganized bone remodeling, structurally weakened bone, skeletal pain, and deformities. Genetic factors and "slow virus" infection may have a role in its pathogenesis. Although this disease is rare in persons <40 years, it affects 3% of the population >45. Pagetoid bone is enlarged and characteristically evolves through three phases--the early "lytic phase" is followed by excessive bone formation and the "mosaic pattern" and finally the "sclerotic phase." Paget's disease may be monostotic or polyostotic; it affects the axial more than the appendicular skeleton. Sites of predilection are the sacrum, spine, femur, tibia, skull, and pelvis.

- Paget's disease characterized by: disorganized bone remodeling, structurally weakened bone, skeletal pain, and deformities.
- Affects 3% of the population >45 years old.
- Pagetoid bone is enlarged and evolves through three phases: early lytic phase, mosaic pattern, sclerotic phase.
- May be monostotic or polyostotic.
- Sites of predilection: sacrum, spine, femur, tibia, skull, pelvis.

Clinical presentation: asymptomatic to crippling disease. Pain, deformity, or fracture. Deformity and bowing of long bones, enlargement of the skull, erythema and warmth of overlying skin and dorsal kyphosis. Complications include compressive neurologic manifestations, high-output cardiac failure, malignant transformation (especially of lesions in the femur or humerus), and hypercalcemia with immobilization. Angioid streaks are seen in the optic fundus in 15% of patients.

- Pain, deformity, or fractures.
- Complications: compressive neurologic manifestations, high-output cardiac failure, malignant transformation (especially of tumors in femur or humerus), hypercalcemia with immobilization.

Laboratory evaluation--Increased serum level of alkaline phosphatase, which reflects increased osteoblastic activity, correlates with disease activity. It may be normal in monostotic disease. Serum levels of calcium are usually normal except with immobilization or coexistent primary hyperparathyroidism. Increased urinary hydroxyproline correlates with increased bone matrix resorption.

- Increased serum level of alkaline phosphatase correlates with disease activity.
- It may be normal in monostotic disease.
- Serum levels of calcium are usually normal except with immobilization or coexistent primary hyperparathyroidism.

Radiologic evaluation may show an early lytic lesion in the skull (osteoporosis circumscripta), in the ends of long bones (sharply defined V shape), or in the vertebra (picture frame). There may be mixed lesions in the skull (honeycomb or cotton wool), pelvis, and long bones or sclerotic lesions in the patella or vertebrae. Radioisotopic scans are more sensitive than radiography for detecting the lesions of Paget's disease. Active lesions appear hot. CT of the spine may be helpful in delineating arthritic from spinal compressive manifestations.

- Lytic lesion in the skull (osteoporosis circumscripta) and ends of long bone (sharply defined V shape).
- Mixed lesions in skull, pelvis, long bones.
- Radioisotopic scans: more sensitive than radiography for lesions of Paget's disease.
- CT: may help distinguish arthritic from spinal compressive manifestations.

Diagnostic Approach

Diagnosis is based on the clinical picture, increased serum level of alkaline phosphatase, and characteristic radiologic findings. Look for arthritic, neurologic, or cardiac complications, and keep in mind the possibility of malignant transformation. Note the differentiation from osteoblastic metastasis, especially in the pelvis: in Paget's disease, the external dimensions of the bone are increased. There is thickening of the pelvic brim and iliopectineal line (brim sign) and enlargement of the pubic and ischial bones.

- Diagnosis based on: clinical picture, increased serum level of alkaline phosphatase, characteristic radiologic findings.

- Look for arthritic, neurologic, or cardiac complications.
- Keep in mind: possibility of malignant transformation.
- Differentiate from osteoblastic metastasis, especially in pelvis.

Treatment

The objectives of medical treatment are to decrease bone pain, to prevent or reverse complications in the CNS, heart, or weight-bearing joints, and to prepare patients for orthopedic surgery (to minimize surgical bleeding and prevent hypercalcemia of immobilization). Medical treatment is monitored with serial alkaline phosphatase determinations every 2-3 months and serial annual radiographs of lytic lesions. Calcitonin is the mainstay of treatment. Currently, it is given parenterally as salmon calcitonin, 50-100 MRC units/day subcutaneously. The effects are usually seen in 2-4 weeks. Maintenance doses are 50 MRC units 3 times weekly. Calcitonin can be given in courses of 6-12 months. Side effects include nausea, facial flushing, and rash. The beneficial effects may be limited by antibody formation (such patients may respond to human calcitonin). Bisphosphonates--Etidronate is the only bisphosphonate approved for such use in the U.S. at this time. It is given orally in a dose of 5-10 mg/kg daily for 6 months. Higher doses or more prolonged administration may lead to osteomalacia. Supplemental calcium is given. More potent bisphosphonates, with lesser risk of osteomalacia, are being tested. Plicamycin is an effective alternate therapy in refractory progressive cases. It is not approved by the FDA. Platelet, renal, and hepatic toxicity may be associated with its use. Surgical therapy is indicated for decompression of neurologic sequelae or to enable ambulation (total hip arthroplasty, tibial osteotomy).

- Objectives of medical treatment: to reduce bone pain; to prevent or reverse complications in CNS, heart, or weight-bearing joints; to prepare patients for orthopedic surgery.
- Calcitonin: mainstay of treatment.
- Calcitonin can be given in courses of 6-12 months.
- Beneficial effects may be limited by antibody formation.
- Etidronate is only bisphosphonate approved for such use in the U.S.
- Plicamycin: effective alternative therapy in refractory progressive cases.
- Surgical therapy: for decompression of neurologic sequelae; to enable ambulation.

PANCREAS

Diabetes Mellitus

Diabetes mellitus is a metabolic disorder in which the basic defect is an absolute or relative lack of insulin. In its complete form, it is manifested by hyperglycemia, accelerated atherosclerosis, microvascular disease (retina and kidney), and neuropathy. It affects about 5% of the population in the U.S.

- Diabetes mellitus: metabolic disorder in which basic defect is absolute or relative lack of insulin.
- Complete form manifested by: hyperglycemia, accelerated atherosclerosis, microvascular disease (retina, kidney), neuropathy.

Type I, insulin-dependent, ketosis-prone diabetes mellitus (juvenile-onset diabetes mellitus) is characterized by severe absolute insulin deficiency, the patient's dependence on exogenous insulin therapy, and a high predisposition to ketosis. It affects 10%-20% of the diabetic population, usually appearing in patients <20 years old, but it can occur at any age. Both genetic and environmental factors are involved in its pathogenesis. There is concordance in twins in about 50% of cases, frequent association with certain histocompatibility antigen HLA types, and association with abnormal immune responses, including islet-cell antibodies. Some patients may show a remission of up to several months after initial insulin therapy restores the metabolic balance. This "honeymoon" is transient and followed by recurrence of insulin deficiency and symptomatic diabetes mellitus.

- Characterized by: severe absolute insulin deficiency, patient's dependence on exogenous insulin therapy, high predisposition to ketosis.
- Affects 10%-20% of the diabetic population.
- Genetic and environmental factors are involved in pathogenesis.
- Concordance in twins: about 50% of cases.
- Frequent association with certain histocompatibility antigen HLA types.
- Association with abnormal immune responses.
- Some patients may have remission of up to several months after initial insulin therapy restores metabolic balance. This "honeymoon" is transient.

Type II, non-insulin-dependent, ketosis-resistant diabetes mellitus is characterized by partial absolute or relative insulin deficiency, resistance to development of ketosis, and, in most patients, insulin resistance at target tissues. It affects 80%-90% of the diabetic population and can occur at any age but usually appears in older obese patients. Genetic susceptibility is strong, and twin concordance is almost 100%. Environmental factors such as obesity have a definite role in development of the disease.

- Characterized by: partial absolute or relative insulin deficiency, resistance to development of ketosis, and (in most patients) insulin resistance at target tissues.
- Affects 80%-90% of diabetic population.
- Usually appears in older obese patients.
- Genetic susceptibility is strong.
- Twin concordance is almost 100%.
- Environmental factors such as obesity have a definite role.

Clinical Presentation

Type I diabetes mellitus usually has a dramatic onset related to abrupt severe insulin deficiency. It usually presents with polyuria, polydipsia, polyphagia with associated weight loss, severe dehydration, ketoacidosis, and, eventually, coma. In very young children, nocturnal enuresis may signal the onset of disease.

- Type I diabetes mellitus: usually dramatic onset related to abrupt severe insulin deficiency.
- Presentation: polyuria, polydipsia, polyphagia with associated weight loss, severe dehydration, ketoacidosis.

Type II diabetes mellitus usually has an insidious onset. Initially, the patient may be asymptomatic, and the diagnosis is suggested by the presence of glycosuria or is made by the finding of fasting hyperglycemia. Patients may complain of blurring of vision and myopia, generalized pruritus, and episodes of recurrent infections, carbuncles, furuncles, urinary tract infections, monilial vaginitis in females, and balanitis in males. Occasionally, patients may present with evidence of chronic diabetic complications (neuropathy, nephropathy, or retinopathy) without symptoms relating to the glucose intolerance. Patients may develop polyuria, polydipsia, and polyphagia under certain conditions when the insulin output is stressed, e.g., in pregnancy, with infection, and with the use of certain drugs. Occasionally, patients can present with hyperosmolar nonketotic coma.

Some patients may present with transient postprandial hypoglycemia. The diagnosis should be suspected in women who have delivered large babies (>9 pounds) or who have a history of hydramnios, preeclampsia, and unexplained fetal losses.

- Type II diabetes mellitus: usually insidious onset.
- Initially, patient may be asymptomatic.
- Episodes of recurrent infections, carbuncles, furuncles, urinary tract infections, monilial vaginitis, or balanitis.
- Evidence of chronic diabetic complications.
- Under certain conditions when insulin output is stressed, polyuria, polydipsia, polyphagia may develop.
- Patients occasionally present with hyperosmolar nonketotic coma.
- Suspect diagnosis in women who deliver large babies (>9 pounds) or who have history of hydramnios, preeclampsia, unexplained fetal losses.

Diagnosis

Confirm the Presence of Diabetes

1. Fasting plasma glucose. The normal fasting plasma glucose is <115 mg/dL. In adults (but not pregnant women), values ≥140 mg/dL on two or more separate occasions confirm the diagnosis of diabetes.
2. Oral glucose tolerance test. The main usefulness of this test is to establish or refute the diagnosis of diabetes mellitus in the following circumstances: when the fasting plasma glucose values are borderline (between 115 and 139 mg/dL); when the patient presents with symptoms related to diabetes mellitus or its known chronic complications and fasting plasma glucose is normal or borderline; and when a diagnosis of diabetes mellitus must be made during pregnancy.

- In adults (not pregnant women): values ≥140 mg/dL on two or more separate occasions confirm diagnosis of diabetes.
- Main usefulness of oral glucose tolerance test: establish or refute diagnosis of diabetes mellitus. When fasting glucose values are borderline. When patient presents with symptoms related to diabetes mellitus or its known chronic complications and fasting plasma glucose is normal or borderline. When diagnosis of diabetes mellitus must be made during pregnancy.

3. A diagnosis of diabetes mellitus is made if on two separate occasions the fasting plasma glucose is >140 mg/dL and the 2-hour value and 1 additional value between 0.5 and 1.5 hour are ≥200 mg/dL. A 2-hour plasma glucose value <140 mg/dL effectively rules out the diagnosis of diabetes.

4. A diagnosis of impaired glucose tolerance is made if the fasting plasma glucose is <140 mg/dL, the 2-hour value is 140-200 mg/dL, and the intervening values are ≥200 mg/dL. Over time, patients with impaired glucose tolerance may decompensate to frank diabetes, may revert to normal glucose tolerance, or may remain unchanged. They should be reevaluated periodically or if clinical indications develop.

- Over time, patients with impaired glucose tolerance may: decompensate to frank diabetes, revert to normal glucose tolerance, or remain unchanged.
- They should be reevaluated periodically.

5. Patients with previous abnormality of glucose tolerance who have a history of documented hyperglycemia and have subsequently returned to normal glucose homeostasis. They include those with gestational diabetes and those who developed hyperglycemia during the acute phase of myocardial infarction, during serious trauma or sepsis, or during ingestion of diabetogenic drugs.

- Have a history of documented hyperglycemia and have subsequently returned to normal glucose homeostasis.

6. Patients with potential abnormality of glucose tolerance have normal glucose tolerance but are at increased risk for developing diabetes compared with the general population. They include monozygotic twins or other first-degree relatives of diabetic patients, obese persons, women who have delivered babies of >9 pounds, and certain racial/ethnic groups such as Native Americans and African and Hispanic Americans.

- Have normal glucose tolerance but are at increased risk for developing diabetes.
- They include: monozygotic twins or other first-degree relatives of diabetic patients, obese persons, women who delivered babies >9 pounds, certain racial/ethnic groups.

7. Pregnancy--Early detection and optimal management of diabetes during pregnancy can prevent congenital malformations and decrease neonatal morbidity and mortality. Screening for glucose intolerance is advisable in all pregnancies. Give 50 g of glucose orally at 24-26 weeks of gestation. Measure plasma level of glucose 1 hour later; if value is >140 mg/dL, perform the oral glucose tolerance test. In the oral glucose tolerance test during pregnancy, 100 g of glucose is given orally. The diagnostic criteria are those of O'Sullivan and Maher. Two or more of the following plasma glucose values must be met or exceeded: fasting, 105 mg/dL; 1 hour, 190 mg/dL; 2 hours, 165 mg/dL; and 3 hours, 145 mg/dL. By these criteria, 2%-3% of all pregnancies in the U.S. are attended by gestational diabetes. The status of the carbohydrate intolerance should be reclassified in the postpartum period. Reclassification can fall into three categories: diabetes mellitus, impaired glucose tolerance, and normal with previous abnormality of glucose tolerance.

- Early detection and optimal management of diabetes during pregnancy can prevent congenital malformations and decrease neonatal morbidity and mortality.
- Screening for glucose intolerance is advisable in all pregnancies and is usually done at 24-26 weeks of gestation.
- Oral glucose tolerance test during pregnancy: give 100 g of glucose orally. Diagnostic criteria of O'Sullivan and Maher.
- Reclassify status of carbohydrate intolerance in postpartum period.

Rule Out Secondary Diabetes

Diabetes mellitus may develop secondarily to destructive lesions or surgical removal of the pancreas or to hypersecretion of hormones with actions that are antagonistic to insulin or that interfere with insulin secretion.

- Diabetes mellitus may develop secondarily to: destructive lesions/surgical removal of pancreas and hypersecretion of hormones antagonistic to insulin or that interfere with insulin secretion.

1. Pancreatic diabetes may be caused by surgical removal of more than two-thirds of the pancreas or to chronic relapsing pancreatitis. Pancreatic dia-

betes differs from spontaneous insulin-dependent diabetes by requiring (in most cases) no more than 20-40 units of insulin per day, by a greater tendency to insulin-induced hypoglycemia, by a lesser tendency to ketosis, and by usual association with exocrine pancreatic insufficiency. Hemochromatosis is often associated with "bronze diabetes." Diabetes can be explained by increased insulin resistance resulting from cirrhosis, insulin deficiency caused by the effects of iron deposits in the pancreas, or associated genetic predisposition to diabetes. Pancreatic carcinoma should be considered in new onset of diabetes in elderly patients, particularly if associated with abdominal pain, weight loss, depression, etc.

- Pancreatic diabetes (unlike insulin-dependent diabetes): requires no more than 20-40 units of insulin per day.
- Greater tendency to insulin-induced hypoglycemia.
- Lesser tendency to ketosis.
- Usually associated with exocrine pancreatic insufficiency.

2. Features common to virtually all forms of endocrinopathy-associated diabetes mellitus include reversibility of the hyperglycemia after the underlying endocrine disorder is cured and, in most patients, absence of ketosis, because of the ongoing availability of endogenous insulin. In acromegaly, the prevalence of glucose intolerance is as high as 60%, fasting hyperglycemia is observed in only 15%-30% of patients, and <10% of patients require insulin. In Cushing's syndrome, whether of an exogenous or endogenous cause, there is insulin antagonism and increased neoglucogenesis. Fasting hyperglycemia is present in 20%-25% of patients. In pheochromocytoma, excess catecholamines interfere with either insulin secretion or its action. The degree of hyperglycemia is usually mild. Carbohydrate intolerance and, rarely, frank diabetes may accompany the hypokalemia of primary aldosteronism and is due to reversible inhibition of insulin secretion. Glucagon and somatostatin-secreting tumors of the pancreas (glucagonoma and somatostatinoma) are rare causes of the diabetic syndrome. In glucagonoma, there is weight loss, diarrhea, erythematous bullous skin eruption (necrolytic migratory erythema), anemia, hypokalemia, pancreatic tumor, and increased plas-

ma levels of glucagon. In somatostatinoma, there is weight loss, abdominal discomfort, diarrhea, steatorrhea, hypochlorhydria, increased incidence of cholelithiasis, pancreatic tumor, and high plasma levels of somatostatin. Isolated growth hormone deficiency is associated fairly commonly with glucose intolerance. Diabetes mellitus may coexist with multiple autoimmune endocrine deficiency syndromes (Addison's disease, Hashimoto's thyroiditis, Graves' disease, hypoparathyroidism, primary gonadal failure, pernicious anemia, etc.).

- Features common to virtually all forms of endocrinopathy-associated diabetes mellitus: reversibility of hyperglycemia after correction of underlying endocrine disorder and absence of ketosis.

3. Stress hyperglycemia occurs in association with acute illness (e.g., sepsis, myocardial infarction, burns, stroke, and severe trauma) and results from increased catecholamines and glucagon and decreased insulin release. It may unmask previous mild carbohydrate intolerance. Patients may not have evidence of diabetes before or after the episode. The tests of glucose intolerance should not be performed until several weeks or months after recovery and restoration of adequate nutrition and physical activity. Uremia and liver cirrhosis, particularly when accompanied by portal hypertension, may be associated commonly with glucose intolerance caused by insulin resistance and hyperglucagonemia.

In all these circumstances associated with secondary diabetes mellitus, the diagnosis is based on the clinical suspicion, clinical setting, appropriate laboratory studies, and hormonal studies.

Chronic Complications

Diabetic Eye Disease

In insulin-dependent diabetes, the prevalence of diabetic retinopathy is 50% by 10-15 years and 80% by 20 years. It is rare in those who have had diabetes mellitus for <5 years. In non-insulin-dependent diabetes, the prevalence is 50% by 15 years.

Simple background nonproliferative retinopathy can be manifested early with increased capillary permeability (detected by fluorescein angiography), occlusion and dilatation of capillaries (microaneurysms), and dilated veins. Intraretinal hemorrhages--"dot" in the deep retinal layers and "blot" in the superficial layers--may occur. Exudates may develop--"cotton wool" from microinfarcts and "hard" from leakage of protein and lipids from the damaged capillaries. Retinal ischemia can lead to retinal and macular edema, which is the commonest cause of decreased vision in simple retinopathy. In most patients, simple retinopathy tends to remain stable. In 10 years, 10%-15% of patients progress to proliferative retinopathy.

- Increased capillary permeability, microaneurysms, dilated veins.
- Intraretinal hemorrhages: dot and blot.
- Exudates: cotton wool and hard.
- In simple retinopathy, commonest cause of decreased vision: retinal and macular edema.
- In 10 years, 10%-15% of patients progress to proliferative retinopathy.

Proliferative retinopathy results from new vessel formation that occurs in response to the underlying retinal ischemia. New vessels may develop over any portion of the retina but mostly around the optic disk. They penetrate into the vitreous. Two complications may occur: 1) preretinal and vitreous hemorrhage and 2) retinal detachment due to the growth of fibrous tissue into the vitreous and the subsequent contraction of the fibrous tissue. This type of retinopathy can present with sudden loss of vision in one eye. It is the leading cause of blindness in the 20- to 64-year-old age group in the U.S. Proliferative retinopathy may also be caused by sickle cell anemia, retinal vein obstruction, and retrolental fibroplasia.

- Proliferative retinopathy: due to new vessel formation that occurs in response to underlying retinal ischemia.
- Two complications: preretinal and vitreous hemorrhage and retinal detachment.
- It can present with sudden loss of vision in one eye.
- It is leading cause of blindness in 20-64-year-old persons in U.S.

Other ophthalmic problems in diabetic patients include 1) temporary changes in the shape of the lens and marked fluctuation of visual acuity because of hyperglycemia; 2) increased frequency of cataract and glaucoma; 3) neoproliferation of vessels in the iris; and, occasionally, 4) isolated primary pupillary abnormalities such as anisocoria and Argyll Robertson pupil (i.e., decreased reactivity to light but normal reactivity in accommodation).

- Temporary changes in shape of lens.
- Increased frequency of cataract and glaucoma.
- Isolated primary pupillary abnormalities.

Ophthalmic evaluation is critical for all diabetic patients, at least annually. In all cases, the severity of diabetic retinopathy is worsened by increasing duration of the diabetes, poor control, and hypertension. Diabetes and hypertension should be controlled early and adequately. Caution: rapid tight control of diabetes, such as with intensive insulin therapy, may exacerbate the retinopathy. Photocoagulation is used for the management of macular edema and proliferative retinopathy. Vitrectomy and repair of retinal tears are considered in the appropriate setting.

- Ophthalmic evaluation: critical for all diabetic patients, at least annually.
- In all cases, severity of diabetic retinopathy is worsened by duration of diabetes, poor control, hypertension.

Diabetic Renal Disease

Diabetic nephropathy is present in 15% of patients with insulin-dependent diabetes after 15 years and in 40% after 30 years. Early lesions are those of microvascular glomerular disease, with glomerular hypertrophy, hyperfiltration, and microalbuminuria. As the disease progresses, diffuse thickening of the basement membrane and increased mesangial volume occur. This increased mesangial volume may lead to glomerular occlusion and diffuse or nodular (Kimmelstiel-Wilson) lesions. Glomerular hypertrophy and hyperfiltration can be reversed by optimizing control of the diabetes. Microalbuminuria (30-250 mg/24 hours) precedes overt proteinuria and can identify patients at risk for nephropathy. It can be reversed with adequate control of the diabetes and blood pressure. The development of persistent proteinuria in insulin-dependent diabetes (>0.5 g/24 hours) heralds a relentless progression to end-stage renal disease. In patients with non-insulin-dependent diabetes, proteinuria occurs earlier, and its occurrence does not necessarily indicate such progression. Persistent proteinuria of >3.5 g/day may progress to classic nephrotic syndrome and usually means that renal failure will occur within 3-5 years. The rate of progression of late phases can be affected by several factors: hypertension, infection, obstruction, or use of contrast agents. Glycemic control is of no benefit; protein restriction is under study. Hypertension is volume-dependent and can be treated with salt restriction, thiazide or loop diuretics, angiotensin-converting enzyme (ACE) inhibitors, or calcium channel blockers. Studies suggest that the use of ACE inhibitors in the microalbuminuria stage and before the development of hypertension may decrease the risk of the development of nephropathy. (Management of renal failure is discussed in Chapter 21.)

- Diabetic nephropathy: occurs in 15% of patients with insulin-dependent diabetes after 15 years and in 40% after 30 years.
- Early lesions: glomerular hypertrophy, hyperfiltration, microalbuminuria.
- With disease progression: diffuse thickening of basement membrane. May lead to glomerular occlusion and diffuse or nodular (Kimmelstiel-Wilson) lesions.
- Microalbuminuria (30-250 mg/24 hours) precedes overt proteinuria and can identify patients at risk for nephropathy.
- Can be reversed with adequate control of diabetes and blood pressure.
- Persistent proteinuria in insulin-dependent diabetes (>0.5 g/24 hours) heralds relentless progression to end-stage renal disease.
- Persistent proteinuria of >3.5 g/day may progress to classic nephrotic syndrome. It usually means renal failure within 3-5 years.
- Rate of progression of late phases affected by: hypertension, infection, obstruction, use of contrast agents.
- Use of ACE inhibitors in microalbuminuria stage before hypertension develops: may decrease risk of developing nephropathy.

The use of contrast dyes in diabetes mellitus may induce rapid deterioration of renal function and acute renal failure. This deterioration is manifested as oliguria and increasing serum levels of creatinine (which peaks in 2-4 days and resolves in 1-4 weeks) or as acute renal failure. Predisposing factors include old age, dehydration, preexisting renal impairment, and liver disease. Do not perform contrast studies unless they are clearly indicated and the benefits of the study outweigh the risks. Before and after the study, hydrate the patient well; monitor fluid balance, and check serum creatinine every 12 hours until a pattern is established.

- Contrast dyes: may induce rapid deterioration of renal function and acute renal failure.
- Deterioration manifested as oliguria and increased serum level of creatinine or as acute renal failure.

Other manifestations of diabetic kidney disease include syndrome of hyporeninemic hypoaldosteronism (see below), renal tubular acidosis after diabetic ketoacidosis, necrotizing papillitis, and acute/chronic pyelonephritis.

- Syndrome of hyporeninemic hypoaldosteronism.
- Acute renal tubular acidosis after diabetic ketoacidosis.
- Necrotizing papillitis.
- Acute/chronic pyelonephritis.

Diabetes and the Nervous System

Neuropathy may occur early in diabetes, but the frequency and severity increase in proportion to the duration and severity of the hyperglycemia. Neuropathy is clinically evident in about 30% of patients with diabetes of >10 years' duration.

- Neuropathy may occur early in diabetes.
- Frequency and severity increase proportional to duration and severity of hyperglycemia.
- Neuropathy is clinically evident in about 30% of patients with diabetes of more than 10 years' duration.

Peripheral polyneuropathy is the most commonly encountered type. It is usually bilateral and symmetrical and affects the lower extremities more commonly than the upper extremities. It presents with numbness, paresthesias, or hyperesthesia or with deep-seated moderate-to-severe pain that is worse at night. The onset may be insidious or acute, often occurring during the loss of diabetic control secondary to infection or other stresses. Peripheral polyneuropathy also presents with abnormalities of proprioceptive fibers, leading to gait abnormalities and development of Charcot's joints (painless progressive destruction of articular cartilage and joint architecture and function; radiography commonly reveals loss of arch and multiple fractures of the tarsal bones). Neurotrophic ulcers may develop, particularly on the plantar aspect of the feet, and may be complicated by osteomyelitis. Examination shows absence of deep tendon reflexes and decreased vibration sense. Therapy--Optimize control of diabetes; use amitriptyline with or without fluphenazine or local capsaicin cream for pain relief.

- Peripheral polyneuropathy: commonest type encountered.

Mononeuropathy, probably of vascular origin, can affect any single nerve trunk and characteristically can present with sudden wristdrop, footdrop, or painful diplopia resulting from cranial nerve III, IV, or VI dysfunction. There is a high degree of spontaneous reversibility, usually over several weeks. In cranial nerve mononeuropathy, pain precedes the development of paralysis by 5-10 days. When cranial nerve III is involved, there is a characteristic sparing of the pupillary fibers in >80% of patients. Aneurysms or intracranial mass lesions generally involve both the pupillary fibers and the fibers to the extraocular muscles.

- Mononeuropathy: probably of vascular origin.
- Characteristic presentation: sudden wristdrop, footdrop, or painful diplopia resulting from cranial nerve III, IV, or VI dysfunction.
- High degree of spontaneous reversibility.
- When cranial nerve III is involved, characteristic sparing of pupillary fibers in >80% of patients.

Radiculopathy is a sensory syndrome that can present with pain in the distribution of one or more spinal nerves, usually in the chest wall, abdomen, and lower extremities. It is also usually self-limited.

- Radiculopathy: sensory syndrome with pain in distribution of one or more spinal nerves.
- It is usually self-limited.

Autonomic neuropathy can involve virtually every organ system, but the gastrointestinal tract is the primary target. Although constipation is the commonest manifestation of this autonomic neuropathy, it tends to be overshadowed by the common, distressing diabetic diarrhea, which consists of intermittent explosive diarrhea that is not preceded by cramps and is seemingly worse at night. Radiologic studies may demonstrate characteristic patterns of disordered small-bowel motility. Steatorrhea suggests coexisting celiac disease or other causes of malabsorption. Diabetic gastroparesis may present with early satiety and nausea or vomiting. Radiologic or electrophysiologic studies may reveal impaired peristalsis and delayed gastric emptying. This complication is important because, as a result of the inconsistency of food absorption, there may be unpredictable swings in plasma levels of glucose and in levels of diabetic control. Esophageal dysfunction and dysphagia may also occur. Treatment is with metoclopramide, 10 mg four times daily.

- Autonomic neuropathy: can involve virtually every organ system.
- Gastrointestinal tract is the primary target.
- Commonest manifestation: constipation.
- Diabetic diarrhea.
- Steatorrhea suggests coexisting celiac disease or other diseases of malabsorption.
- Diabetic gastroparesis: important because, as a result of inconsistency of food absorption, there may be unpredictable swings in plasma level of glucose and in levels of diabetic control.

Genitourinary involvement includes urinary bladder dysfunction, which occurs in >50% of patients with diabetes of >20 years' duration. It can present as hesitancy, delayed and incomplete emptying, and residual urine. A voiding cystometrogram may reveal decreased propulsive efforts and increased residual urine. Urinary bladder dysfunction may be complicated initially by bacteriuria and later by overt urinary tract infection. Therapy is bladder drainage, antibacterial therapy for infections, and encouraging voiding every 3 hours by manual pressure. Potency impairment occurs in >50% of men with long-standing diabetes and may be the initial presentation of the diabetic syndrome. Another cause of potency impairment in diabetic patients is penile vascular insufficiency caused by aortoiliac occlusive disease (Leriche's syndrome). Diabetic male patients may also have retrograde ejaculation.

- Urinary bladder dysfunction is common and may be complicated by bacteriuria and overt urinary tract infection.

Potency impairment in diabetic males may be due to (among other causes) autonomic neuropathy or penile vascular insufficiency.

Features of cardiovascular autonomic neuropathy may include manifestations of persistent resting tachycardia, orthostatic hypotension, and neuropathic edema. Encourage slow change in position, Jobst leg compression, and use of fludrocortisone for orthostatic hypotension. Irregularity of sweating and partial and total anhidrosis may be observed; a patchy distribution of sweating may be particularly evident in the face. An unusual variant of autonomic instability may be manifested in some diabetic patients by gustatory sweating after eating.

Diabetic neuromuscular disease presents with symmetrical painless atrophy and weakness of the intrinsic hand muscles that may be associated with sensory impairment. It occurs more commonly in elderly patients and in males. Diabetic amyotrophy refers to a progressive weakness and wasting that involves the muscles of the pelvic girdle and anterior thigh compartments, most commonly the quadriceps femoris. It is usually accompanied by severe pain and may be distributed asymmetrically. It characteristically occurs in elderly men and generally resolves in 6-12 months after the time of diagnosis. A similar but less painful variant occurs in the upper extremities.

- Diabetic amyotrophy: progressive weakness and wasting of muscles of pelvic girdle and anterior thigh compartment.
- Is usually accompanied by severe pain.
- May be distributed asymetrically.
- Occurs characteristically in elderly men.
- Resolves in 6-12 months after diagnosis.

In diabetic neuropathy, electromyography may show a decrease in motor and sensory nerve conduction velocity, evidence of denervation and fasciculation, and characteristic distribution of nerve dysfunction. Examination of the CSF may show a slight increase in protein content.

Diabetic foot ulcers result from the effects of neuropathy and vascular disease. Abnormal pressure distribution results in callus formation; ill-fitting shoes cause blisters; and foreign bodies lead to abrasions and punctures. The ulcers are painless and frequently complicated by infection and osteomyelitis. Therapy consists of prevention or relief of maldistribution of pressure, prompt treatment of infections, and documentation and correction of vascular insufficiency.

- Diabetic foot ulcers: painless; frequently complicated by infection and osteomyelitis.

Macrovascular Disease

Arteriosclerosis, which appears earlier and is more extensive in diabetic patients than in the general popula-

tion, can present clinically as peripheral vascular disease (with intermittent claudication, gangrene, and impotence), coronary artery disease (with angina and myocardial infarction), and cerebrovascular disease (e.g., stroke). Coronary artery disease accounts for 70% of deaths in the diabetic population. It tends to involve the proximal and distal vessels in the right and left coronary arterial systems. Atypical manifestations may occur. Angina may present with epigastric distress, heartburn, and neck or jaw pain. Myocardial infarction may be silent (in 15% of cases) because of autonomic neuropathy. It should be suspected in those patients with sudden onset of left ventricular failure. Diabetes mellitus may also be associated with cardiomyopathy and heart failure (in 17% of cases) in the absence of other identifiable causes and with a normal coronary arterial system by angiography. Peripheral vascular disease has a higher frequency of distal involvement, particularly in the lower extremities. Arteriography should be used with caution if the patient has diminished renal function, because acute tubular necrosis may develop. Arteriography should be reserved for patients who are candidates for vascular surgery.

- Arteriosclerosis can present as: peripheral vascular disease, coronary artery disease, cerebrovascular disease.
- Atypical manifestations may occur.
- Myocardial infarction may be silent.
- Suspect myocardial infarction in patients with sudden onset left ventricular failure.
- Peripheral vascular disease: higher frequency of distal involvement, particularly lower extremities.
- Arteriography: use cautiously; reserve for candidates for vascular surgery.

Hypertension

ACE inhibitors are the first line of therapy in hypertensive diabetic patients with normal renal function. ACE inhibitors normalize intraglomerular pressure, reduce proteinuria, and have no adverse effects on glucose and lipid levels. Calcium channel blockers are reasonable alternatives, especially for patients with coexistent coronary artery disease. They may induce minimal impairment in glucose tolerance but have no adverse effects on lipids. Thiazides are no longer a first-line therapy, especially in non-insulin-dependent diabetes, because of their metabolic side effects. They impair glucose tolerance, partly due to hypokalemia, and increase low-density lipoprotein cholesterol and triglycerides.

- ACE inhibitors: first line of therapy in hypertensive diabetic patients with normal renal function.
- Calcium channel blockers: reasonable alternatives, especially for patients with coexistent coronary artery disease.
- Thiazides: no longer first-line therapy, especially in non-insulin-dependent diabetes, because of their metabolic side effects.

Infections

Although infections may not occur more frequently in diabetic than in nondiabetic patients, they tend to be more severe because of the presence of hyperglycemia (which impairs leukocyte function) and because of associated macro- and microvascular disease, which decreases regional blood flow. In diabetic patients, there is an increased frequency of cutaneous infections (*Staphylococcus* infections, furuncles, pyoderma, and carbuncles), urinary tract infections (cystitis, pyelonephritis, papillary necrosis), lung infections (pneumonia), extremity infections (gram-negative and anaerobic infections), and genital tract infections (vulvovaginitis and balanitis). Three unusual conditions appear to have specific relationships to the diabetic syndrome: malignant external otitis, rhinocerebral mucormycosis, and emphysematous cholecystitis.

- Increased frequency of: cutaneous, urinary tract, lung, extremity, and genital tract infections.
- Three unusual conditions having specific relationships to diabetic syndrome: malignant external otitis, rhinocerebral mucormycosis, emphysematous cholecystitis.

Dermatologic Complications

Various cutaneous lesions may occur in diabetic patients. Necrobiosis lipoidica diabeticorum consists of plaque-like lesions with central yellowish areas surrounded by a brownish border, usually occurring over the anterior surfaces of the legs. Ulceration may occur. Diabetic dermopathy consists of small rounded plaques with a raised border that occur over the anterior tibial surfaces. They may ulcerate centrally and crust at the edges. As these lesions heal, there is a depressed scar and diffuse brown discoloration. Dupuytren's contractures occur in 5%-20% of patients. Diabetic cheirarthropathy occurs in insulin-dependent diabetes and presents with finger stiffness, periarticular swelling, and waxy thickened skin, resembling scleroderma. Eruptive xanthomas caused by

significant hypertriglyceridemia may occur in uncontrolled diabetes.

Management of Diabetes Mellitus

Goals of Therapy

"Practical" goals--These apply to all patients and include 1) the elimination of ketosis and symptomatic hyper- and hypoglycemia, 2) preservation of well-being in adults and normal growth and development in children, 3) achieving and maintaining ideal body weight, and 4) provision of accessible care that encourages self-care and periodic surveillance. Currently, the available, standard therapeutic regimens can achieve these goals in most patients. Unfortunately, such regimens do not normalize the metabolic derangements in many patients and are associated with a high incidence of micro- and macrovascular complications, which develop with increasing duration of the disease.

Restoration of euglycemia--This goal, which is based on the assumption that normalization of hyperglycemia will prevent/delay the micro- and macrovascular complications of the disease, is difficult to achieve. In pregnancy-associated diabetes, current evidence mandates attempts at achieving and maintaining euglycemia before and certainly during pregnancy. The Diabetes Control and Complications Trial has shown that restoration of euglycemia in insulin-dependent diabetes prevents or reverses early manifestations of microvascular complications.

- In pregnancy-associated diabetes: achieving and maintaining euglycemia before and during pregnancy is mandated.
- Restoration of euglycemia in insulin-dependent diabetes prevents or reverses early manifestations of microvascular complications.

The generally accepted biochemical indices of metabolic control are listed in Table 11-15.

The modalities currently available in the U.S. are diet, exercise, oral antidiabetic agents, insulin, and combination therapy. Diet therapy is the first step. Its objective is to restore and maintain normal weight. In many patients with non-insulin-dependent diabetes, this can decrease insulin resistance, improve insulin secretion, and restore euglycemia. An optimal diet plan should address caloric content, distribution of nutrients, and, in diabetic patients receiving insulin therapy, timing of meals and snacks.

Table 11-15.--Biochemical Indices of Metabolic Control

	Ideal	Acceptable	Poor
Fasting plasma glucose, mg/dL	<115	116-140	>200
Postprandial plasma glucose, mg/dL	<140	141-200	>235
Glycosylated hemoglobin, %	<8	8-10	>12
Hemoglobin A_{1c}, %	<6	6-8	<10
Serum cholesterol, mg/dL	<200	200-239	>240
Serum triglycerides, mg/dL	<150	150-249	>250
Serum HDL cholesterol, mg/dL	>40	---	---

Nutrient distribution should be roughly 50%-60% complex carbohydrates (restrict glucose and sucrose and increase dietary fiber), 15%-20% proteins, and 20%-30% fats (<10% saturated fat and <300 mg cholesterol). Exercise--A regular exercise program is encouraged. Its benefits include reduction in cardiovascular risk factors, weight reduction, increased insulin sensitivity, and improved sense of well-being. The risks of exercise include hypoglycemia, arrhythmia, myocardial infarction or sudden death, increased blood pressure, vitreous hemorrhage, and injuries. If initial diabetic control is poor, exercise worsens glycemic control. The major problem with diet/exercise therapy is patient noncompliance.

- Modalities available in U.S.: diet, exercise, oral antidiabetic agents, insulin, combination therapy.
- Diet therapy is first step.
- Objective: restore and maintain normal weight.
- Optimal diet plan should address: caloric content, distribution of nutrients, timing of meals and snacks (for patients receiving insulin therapy).
- Regular exercise program is encouraged.
- Major problem with diet/exercise therapy: patient noncompliance.

When patients fail to meet the above outlined goals by diet and exercise, the therapeutic program should be advanced. The patient's age, weight, duration of diabetes, environment, and general health are among the factors that need to be considered in selecting the appropriate therapy.

Oral Sulfonylureas (Oral Antidiabetic Agents)

Oral sulfonylureas act primarily by increasing the ability of the pancreatic islets to secrete insulin and, indirectly, by improving tissue response to insulin. The dose, effectiveness, and duration of action of these drugs are listed in Table 11-16.

- Oral sulfonylureas: act primarily by increasing ability of pancreatic islets to secrete insulin and, indirectly, by improving tissue response to insulin.

Indications--Fasting plasma level of glucose <250 mg/dL, age at onset of non-insulin-dependent diabetes >40 years, duration of diabetes <5 years, normal or excessive weight, and no previous therapy with insulin or insulin dose <40 U/day. Contraindications--Insulin-dependent diabetes, pregnant or lactating diabetic women, hepatic/renal insufficiency, and sulfa allergy. Efficacy--The primary failure rate is 20%. Secondary failure is about 5%-10% a year and is probably caused by continued deterioration of islet reserve and/or progression of insulin resistance. Remember that transient failures may be due to intercurrent acute medical/surgical illness, failure to adhere to the diet, and weight gain. Complications--There are few serious adverse effects. The most serious one is hypoglycemia, especially in elderly patients who are ill-nourished and have renal/hepatic failure. Other side effects are gastrointestinal, dermatologic, and hematopoietic. Side effects with chlorpropamide use: antabuse-like effect and syndrome of inappropriate ADH. Selection of agent--Consider potency, duration of action, dosage range, metabolism, side effects, cost, convenience, and potential drug interactions. Also consider the known contraindications. Prescribe the lowest effective dose and increase it weekly until satisfactory control or the highest recommended dose is reached. Those patients who respond to oral antidiabetic agents should undergo periodic reassessment to find the lowest effective dose and to assess for secondary failure.

- Indications: fasting plasma glucose <250 mg/dL, age at disease onset >40 years, duration of disease <5 years, normal or excessive weight, no previous insulin therapy or insulin dose <40 U/day.
- Contraindications: insulin-dependent diabetes, pregnant or lactating diabetics, hepatic/renal insufficiency, sulfa allergy.
- Efficacy: primary failure rate, 28%; secondary failure, 5%-10% a year.

Table 11-16.--Oral Sulfonylureas

Name		Daily	Relative	Duration of
Generic	Brand	dose, mg	effectiveness	action, hr
Tolbutamide	Orinase	500-3,000	1	6-12
Chlorpropamide	Diabinese	100-500	5	60
Acetohexamide	Dymelor	250-1,500	2.5	12-18
Tolazamide	Tolinase	100-1,000	5	12-24
Glipizide	Glucotrol	5-40	20	12-24
Glyburide	DiaBeta, Micronase	2.5-20	40	16-24

● Transient failure due to: intercurrent acute medical/surgical illness, failure to adhere to diet, weight gain.

● Most serious complication: hypoglycemia, especially in the elderly who are ill-nourished and have hepatic/renal failure.

● Side effects include: antabuse-like effect, syndrome of inappropriate ADH.

Second-generation agents (glyburide, glipizide) are analogues of first-generation drugs and are considerably more potent (50x-100x). There is no difference in mechanism of action, efficacy, contraindications, or complications. Secondary failures may be less common. These drugs are nonionically bound to plasma proteins and so are not displaced by other ionically charged drugs such as warfarin and phenylbutazone. Concurrent use of the latter medications does not lead to variation in bioavailability of the second-generation oral antidiabetic agents.

● Second-generation agents: glyburide, glipizide.
● Nonionically bound to plasma proteins.
● Thus, not displaced by other ionically charged drugs, e.g., warfarin, phenylbutazone.

Treatment of oral antidiabetic agent failure--When patients fail to meet treatment goals, therapy should be escalated. Various approaches have been evaluated, and it is clear that any treatment that improves glycemic control can potentially improve the response to oral antidiabetic agents. The options are 1) stress treatment with diet; this may correct postreceptor defect and improve endogenous insulin response. 2) Try another oral agent; 10%-15% of patients failing to respond to one agent may respond to another. 3) Discontinue use of oral agent and start insulin. 4) Add insulin to the oral agent if patient continues to show some response to the drug; combination therapy may lead to better control than with an oral antidiabetic agent alone. Similar control can be achieved with insulin alone, although generally larger doses are required. Administration of insulin at bedtime to control fasting hyperglycemia has some merit and may require lower doses and cause less perturbation of patient's lifestyle.

● Stress treatment with diet.
● Try another oral agent.
● Discontinue using oral agent and start insulin.
● Add insulin to oral agent.

Insulin Therapy

Selection--The only demonstrable clinical advantage to using highly purified or human insulin is a decline in the incidence of local reactions, insulin allergy/immune resistance, and lipoatrophy. The peak effect of crystalline zinc insulin may be delayed (5-7 hours) and the duration may be prolonged (10-12 hours) in patients who have developed antibodies. Human crystalline zinc insulin and NPH insulins tend to have a more rapid onset and shorter duration of action than animal insulins; this may not be true of human Lente. The mixing of Lente and regular insulins may blunt the usual rapid peak of the regular component; premixing is not advisable.

● Only demonstrated clinical advantage to using highly purified or human insulin: decline in incidence of local reactions, insulin allergy/immune resistance, lipoatrophy.

Conventional Insulin Therapy

Conventional insulin therapy uses predominantly intermediate-acting insulins (NPH/Lente).

1. Single morning NPH/Lente. Three responses are

observed in well-controlled patients: a) 70% are adequately controlled on a single a.m. dose (type B). b) 15% have a delayed response with the nadir of plasma glucose occurring between 10 p.m. and 5 a.m. (late responders or type C); reduce the dose of NPH/Lente insulin and add a short-acting insulin before breakfast. c) 15% have an early response, with nadir of plasma glucose occurring at or shortly after noon (early responders of type A); split the dose of NPH/Lente giving 2/3 of the dose before breakfast and 1/3 before supper. Additional short-acting insulin may also be needed with one or both of the intermediate doses.

2. Difficult to control situations. Consider increased caloric intake, inadequate dose, failure to take insulin properly, infection/acute illness, emotional stress, use of thiazides or corticosteroids, dawn and Somogyi phenomena, and insulin resistance.

- In difficult to control situations, consider: increased caloric intake, inadequate dose, failure to take insulin properly, infection/acute illness, emotional stress, use of thiazides or corticosteroids, dawn and Somogyi phenomena, insulin resistance.

3. Poorly controlled patients brought under good control with insulin frequently experience a significant decrease in insulin requirements after several days or weeks (hyperglycemia aggravates insulin resistance).

Intensive Insulin Therapy

Simply stated, the goals of intensive insulin therapy are to achieve euglycemia and to avoid hypoglycemia. It attempts to duplicate the physiologic pattern of insulin release in nondiabetic persons and uses either an insulin pump or a multiple-dose insulin (MDI) program. It provides:

1. Basal rate of insulin. Pump--Constant delivery of 0.6 U/hour of CZI in a 50-kg patient. An increase in basal rate sometimes may be required between 4 a.m. and 8 a.m. to meet increased insulin needs (dawn phenomenon). MDI--Usually a single dose of Ultralente (at times a split dose is required). The basal rate is about half of the total daily dose and must be individually adjusted.

2. Preprandial boluses of CZI are superimposed to control postprandial glucose excursions. The bolus is delivered 15-60 minutes before a meal.

- Intensive insulin therapy: to achieve euglycemia and to avoid hypoglycemia.
- Attempts to duplicate physiologic pattern of insulin release.
- Uses either an insulin pump or MDI program.

In addition, various schemes that use intermediate insulin have been proposed. They include: 1) regimen with mixed crystalline zinc insulin and intermediate-acting insulin at breakfast, crystalline zinc insulin at dinner, and intermediate-acting insulin at bedtime. 2) Regimen with premeal crystalline zinc insulin and bedtime intermediate-acting insulin. In general, these regimens are less preferable for the following reasons: 1) the peak of intermediate insulin may vary from patient to patient and in any individual patient; 2) in the attempt to suppress overnight hepatic neoglucogenesis, the patient may be exposed to the risk of hypoglycemia during peak activity of the intermediate-acting insulin.

- Various schemes that use intermediate-acting insulin have been proposed.

Complications of intensive insulin therapy include:
1. Hypoglycemia. This is the major complication of intensive insulin therapy; the risk is twofold to threefold. The goal of euglycemia brings patients closer to hypoglycemic levels. Insulin pumps do not turn themselves off when blood glucose levels are low. Intensive therapy lowers the threshold for hypoglycemia awareness and for release of counterregulatory hormones. Many diabetic patients have impaired glucagon and epinephrine response to hypoglycemia.
2. Diabetic ketoacidosis. Pump-treated patients are more prone to diabetic ketoacidosis, because of limited insulin depot and frequent transient interruption of flow.
3. Catheter abscess. This occurs in about 10%-15% of patients. Skin care at insertion sites is important.

- Hypoglycemia: the major complication of intensive insulin therapy.
- Intensive therapy: lowers threshold for hypoglycemia awareness and for release of counterregulatory hormones. Many diabetic patients have impaired glucagon and epinephrine response to hypoglycemia.
- Diabetic ketoacidosis: pump-treated patients.
- Catheter abscess.

Indications--The only firm indications for intensive insulin therapy are pregnancy and patients with insulin-dependent diabetes, particularly early in the disease. All other indications remain unproved. Requirements-- Careful patient selection, i.e., sophisticated, motivated patients. Avoid intensive therapy in patients with established diabetic complications and those at greater risk for hypoglycemia; formal education and training program; intensive dietary and physical activity instruction; self-monitoring of blood glucose 4 times/day and at 3 a.m. at least once weekly; and frequent outpatient visits to review data and make adjustments.

- Only firm indications for therapy: pregnancy and patients with insulin-dependent diabetes, particularly early in the disease.

Insulin Therapy in Non-Insulin-Dependent Diabetes

Indications include 1) temporary use during pregnancy, major surgery, or serious infection. 2) Newly diagnosed non-insulin-dependent diabetes in a patient <40 years old of normal or below-normal weight and who has evidence of insulin lack, i.e., hyperglycemia >250 mg/dL, glycosuria, ketosis, and weight loss greater than can be accounted for by dehydration. Insulin therapy leads to rapid control of metabolic abnormalities. In these patients, oral antidiabetic agents are less likely to succeed and may take many weeks to achieve control. 3) Diet/exercise/oral agent failure: about 40% of patients with non-insulin-dependent diabetes require insulin therapy to achieve acceptable metabolic control.

- Temporary use during pregnancy, major surgery, serious infection.
- Newly diagnosed non-insulin-dependent diabetes in patient: <40 years old, normal/below-normal weight, evidence of insulin lack (hypoglycemia >250 mg/dL, ketosis, weight loss greater than accounted for by dehydration).
- Diet/exercise/oral agent failure.

Acute Complications of Diabetes Mellitus

Diabetic Ketoacidosis

Diabetic ketoacidosis is characterized by severe insulin deficiency, significant hyperglycemia, hypertonic dehydration, and ketonemia. Its pathophysiology includes insulin deficiency and counterregulatory hormone excess;

hyperglycemia, osmotic diuresis, dehydration, hyperosmolar state; and lipolysis, ketogenesis, ketonemia, and metabolic acidosis.

- Diabetic ketoacidosis: severe insulin deficiency, significant hyperglycemia, hypertonic dehydration, ketonemia.

Clinical presentation--The patient usually has insulin-dependent diabetes; in fact, diabetic ketoacidosis may be the initial presentation of the disorder. The features include gradual or abrupt onset of polyps, dehydration, anorexia, nausea and vomiting, abdominal pain, tachypnea, obtundation, and coma. Note that abdominal pain usually is not due to diabetic ketoacidosis if the patient is >40 years old or, if <40 years, the bicarbonate level is >10 mEq/L. It is important to know the precipitating factors: failure to take insulin, infection, other intercurrent illness such as myocardial infarction, pancreatitis, stroke, trauma, or emotional stress.

- Diabetic ketoacidosis: patient usually has insulin-dependent diabetes.
- May be initial presentation of the disease.
- Abdominal pain not due to diabetic ketoacidosis if patient is >40 years or (if <40 years) bicarbonate level is >10 mEq/L.
- Know precipitating factors: failure to take insulin, infection, other intercurrent illness (myocardial infarction), pancreatitis, stroke, trauma, emotional stress.

Diagnosis is based on demonstrating significant hyperglycemia, ketonemia, and metabolic acidosis. Pitfalls: hyperglycemia may be only of moderate degree (plasma glucose level <500 mg/dL), particularly with pregnancy or alcohol use. Ketoacidosis may be present with negative findings on nitroprusside tests (Ketostix, Acetest). Such tests react mainly with acetoacetate, less so with acetone, and none at all with β-hydroxybutyrate. The ratio of β-hydroxybutyrate to acetoacetate is usually 3:1. At pH 7.1, it increases to 6:1 and may be >30:1 in the presence of alcohol excess or lactic acidosis (altered redox state). The diagnostic process is not complete without a thorough search for precipitating factors and assessment of complications.

- Diagnosis based on demonstrating: significant hyperglycemia, ketonemia, metabolic acidosis.
- Ketoacidosis may be present with negative finding on

nitroprusside tests (Ketostix, Acetest).

- Diagnostic process not complete without thorough search for precipitating factors and assessment of complications.

Management--The goals of therapy are to correct the hyperglycemia, hyperketonemia and acidosis, hyperosmolar dehydration, and electrolyte depletion. These goals are achieved by insulin administration, replacement of fluid and electrolytes, treatment of precipitating factors, and avoidance of complications. Metabolic and volume correction have to be initiated rapidly. After improvement is established, one can proceed more cautiously.

- Goals: correct hyperglycemia, hyperketonemia and acidosis, hyperosmolar dehydration, electrolyte depletion.
- Achieve by: insulin administration, replacement of fluid and electrolytes, treatment of precipitating factors, avoidance of complications.

1. Insulin. Regular insulin is the mainstay of therapy. Initially, give a priming dose of 10-20 U intravenously and then set up an insulin infusion at the rate of 10 U/hour. This provides a plasma level of about 200 μU/mL, adequate to inhibit lipolysis and hepatic glucose production and maximize glucose uptake. Insulin infusion is preferred over subcutaneous or intramuscular insulin regimens because it provides smoother control with less risk of hypoglycemia.

- Regular insulin: mainstay of therapy.
- Insulin infusion preferred over subcutaneous or intramuscular insulin regimens.

2. Fluids. The aim is to restore volume and correct electrolyte and fluid losses and hyperosmolarity. The average fluid deficit in the adult is 5-8 L. Give 2 L of normal saline in the first hour; 1 L/hour in the second and third hours; then 250-500 mL/hour until vital signs stabilize. Then, switch to 0.45% saline and adjust as needed. As plasma glucose values approach 300 mg/dL, change to 0.45% saline in 5% dextrose in water. Maintain plasma glucose value between 200-250 mg/dL during the first 12-24 hours to reverse ketosis, to avoid rapid decrease in osmolarity and cerebral edema, and to avoid hypoglycemia.

3. Electrolytes. Potassium deficit is about 300-500 mEq. Regardless of the initial serum level of potassium, the total body stores of potassium are low. With therapy and correction of acidosis and hyperglycemia, the serum level of potassium decreases. Potassium should be added to the intravenous fluids as soon as renal perfusion and urine flow are assured. Add 40 mEq of potassium to each liter of intravenous fluid as potassium chloride. In controlled trials, potassium-phosphate is of no benefit. Phosphate repletion is indicated in the presence of phosphate levels <1 mg/dL. Give phosphate in the dose of 0.08 mM/kg intravenously over 6 hours. (Neutral potassium phosphate, 1 ampule contains 3 mM phosphate and 15 mEq of potassium.) Monitor serum level of phosphate carefully because of the risk of hypocalcemia, seizures, and death. Bicarbonate: if pH is <7.1, give bicarbonate (44 mEq/L) until pH increases to about 7.1. Avoid excessive bicarbonate, because it exacerbates hypokalemia and may result in paradoxical CSF fluid acidosis.

- With therapy and correction of acidosis and hyperglycemia, serum level of potassium decreases.
- Add potassium to intravenous fluids as soon as renal perfusion and urine flow are assured.
- If pH is <7.1, give bicarbonate (44 mEq/L) until pH is about 7.1.

The major complications of diabetic ketoacidosis mostly result from therapy failures. In most patients, persistent ketosis/acidosis, hypoglycemia, hypokalemia, paradoxical CSF acidosis, cerebral edema, metabolic alkalosis can be prevented.

Prognosis: 5%-15% mortality; higher rate among the elderly. With myocardial infarction, mortality is 50%. After successful therapy, the goal is to avoid recurrence by properly managing the diabetic state and by patient education.

- Prognosis: 5%-15% mortality; higher rate among elderly.
- After successful therapy, goal is to avoid recurrence by properly managing diabetic state and patient education.

Hyperglycemic Hyperosmolar Nonketotic Coma
Hyperglycemic hyperosmolar nonketotic coma is char-

acterized by significant hyperglycemia and dehydration without ketoacidosis. Its pathophysiology includes insulin deficiency, osmotic diuresis, dehydration, and decreased renal function; however, enough insulin is available to inhibit ketogenesis. It occurs predominantly in patients with non-insulin-dependent diabetes. It is often precipitated by acute illness such as myocardial infarction, pancreatitis, pneumonia, or other infections, surgical stress, dialysis, hyperalimentation, and the use of such drugs as glucocorticoids, thiazides, or phenytoin. Hyperglycemic hyperosmolar nonketotic coma may be the first presentation of non-insulin-dependent diabetes.

- Characteristics: significant hyperglycemia and dehydration without ketoacidosis.
- Pathophysiology: insulin deficiency, osmotic diuresis, dehydration, decreased renal function.
- Enough insulin is available to inhibit ketogenesis.
- Occurs predominantly in patients with non-insulin-dependent diabetes.
- Often precipitated by acute illness.
- Precipitated by use of: glucocorticoids, thiazides, phenytoin.
- May be first presentation of non-insulin-dependent diabetes.

Diagnostic approach--The disorder should be suspected in any diabetic patient presenting with altered sensorium, obtundation or coma, and severe dehydration. Laboratory evaluation reveals significant hyperglycemia (plasma glucose level is often >600 mg/dL), absence of significant ketonemia, and plasma hyperosmolarity (>320 mOsm/L). Associated findings may include renal insufficiency and lactic acidosis. After the diagnosis is made, prompt management is indicated; at the same time, search for complications and the precipitating disorder.

- Suspect disorder in any diabetic patient with: altered sensorium, obtundation/coma, severe dehydration.
- Laboratory evaluation shows: significant hyperglycemia (plasma glucose level is often >600 mg/dL), no significant ketonemia, plasma hyperosmolarity (>320 mOsm/L).
- Associated findings: renal insufficiency, lactic acidosis.
- Prompt management is indicated.
- Search for complications and precipitating disorder.

Management--The objectives are to restore volume and osmolarity and to manage the hyperglycemia. Supportive measures are initiated to manage shock, coma, and, in patients who have been or are receiving steroids, to provide increased dosages appropriate for an acute illness. Initial fluid therapy should be with normal saline to correct the volume deficit: 1 L normal saline per hour for 2-4 hours or more, followed by 0.45% saline to correct the hyperosmolarity. As the level of blood glucose decreases, with appropriate insulin therapy, 5% dextrose in water can be added. A dose of 20 U of regular insulin is given intravenously if the plasma glucose level is >600 mg/dL, then insulin infusion is begun. It is important to decrease the PG gradually to a level around 200 mg/dL. Then, stop the infusion, and start giving insulin subcutaneously. Potassium, phosphate, and magnesium replacements are as outlined above for diabetic ketoacidosis. Lactic acidosis usually responds to volume replacement; if pH is <7.1, bicarbonate can be given. The patient's condition has to be monitored closely. Repeated neurologic evaluation is needed because focal deficits or seizures may become apparent during therapy.

- Objectives: restore volume and osmolarity, manage hyperglycemia.
- Initial fluid therapy: normal saline to correct volume deficit.
- Next, 0.45% saline to correct hyperosmolarity.
- Regular insulin.
- Lactic acidosis: responds to volume replacement.
- If pH is <7.1, can give bicarbonate.
- Patient must be monitored closely.

Complications include vascular events such as myocardial infarction or cerebrovascular accident, hypoglycemia, cerebral edema, and hypokalemia. Mortality is 50%.

- Complications: vascular events (myocardial infarction, cerebrovascular event), hypoglycemia, cerebral edema, hypokalemia.
- Mortality: 50%.

Diabetes and Pregnancy

Diabetes may be newly diagnosed in pregnancy ("gestational diabetes") or antedate pregnancy. The well-being of the fetus dictates tight glucose control. Inadequate control early in pregnancy increases the risk of congenital malformations, and inadequate control in the latter part of pregnancy increases the risk of macrosomia, neonatal hypoglycemia, hypocalcemia, polycythemia, hyperbilirubinemia, and respiratory distress. The normal gestational changes in fuel metabolism include 1) fetal siphoning of glucose and neoglucogenic precursors, resulting in a tendency to fasting maternal hypoglycemia and to starvation ketosis; and 2) anti-insulin action of placental hormones (HPL, estrogen, progesterone) and increased cortisol secretion. Because of these stresses, gestational diabetes may develop in those with reduced B-cell reserve. In those with established diabetes, there is worsening of control.

- Well-being of fetus dictates tight glucose control.
- Inadequate control in early pregnancy: increased risk of congenital malformations.
- Inadequate control in latter part of pregnancy: increased risk of macrosomia, neonatal hypoglycemia, hypocalcemia, polycythemia, hyperbilirubinemia, respiratory distress.

Gestational diabetes complicates 2%-3% of all pregnancies. Increased risk is seen in patients with diabetes in a first-degree relative, previous abnormality of glucose tolerance, obesity, advanced maternal age, and abnormal obstetric history, i.e., large babies, unexplained stillbirths, congenital anomalies, and polyhydramnios. All pregnant women should be screened at 24-28 weeks or, if at high risk, at the first visit. A 50-g oral glucose load is given and plasma glucose is obtained 1 hour later. A plasma glucose level >140 mg/dL indicates the need for a complete oral glucose tolerance test (see above).

- Gestational diabetes complicates 2%-3% of all pregnancies.
- Increased risk in patients with: diabetes in first-degree relative, previous abnormality of glucose tolerance, obesity, advanced maternal age, abnormal obstetric history.
- Screen all pregnant women at 24-28 weeks; if at high risk, at first visit.
- 50-g oral glucose load; 1 hour later, plasma glucose level >140 mg/dL indicates need for complete oral glucose tolerance test.

The goals of therapy are 1) to ensure tight control of diabetes, with avoidance of hypoglycemia and fasting ketonemia (fasting and preprandial values of 70-100 mg/dL; 1 hour postprandial, <140 mg/dL; 2 hours postprandial, <120 mg/dL; normal glycohemoglobin; 2) to ensure ade-

quate nutrition and optimal weight gain; and 3) home monitoring for blood glucose and urine ketones. Insulin therapy is essential for achieving these goals, and dosage should be adjusted appropriately. Regular office visits and monthly glycohemoglobin values are required. In patients with prenatal diabetes, insulin requirements may decrease early in pregnancy, but after mid pregnancy, requirements increase progressively. Immediately post partum, insulin requirements usually return to prepregnancy levels. Timing of the delivery is based on tests of fetal maturity. An uncomplicated pregnancy should be allowed to progress to at least 37 weeks.

- Goals of therapy: ensure tight control of diabetes (avoiding hypoglycemia and fasting ketonemia), ensure adequate nutrition and optimal weight gain, home monitoring for blood glucose and urine ketones.
- Insulin therapy is essential.
- In patients with prenatal diabetes, insulin requirements may decrease early in pregnancy and increase progressively after mid pregnancy.
- Immediately post partum, insulin requirements usually return to prepregnancy levels.
- Timing of delivery: based on tests of fetal maturity.

In women with insulin-dependent diabetes and significant chronic diabetic complications, pregnancy may exacerbate retinopathy. Nephropathy may lead to toxemia, and borderline cardiac status may be decompensated. The well-controlled patient with mild and early chronic complications has a very good chance for a normal pregnancy, without harm to mother or fetus. The risk of diabetes in the offspring of a diabetic mother is 1%-5% and no greater than if the father is a diabetic.

Those with gestational diabetes who become euglycemic in the postpartum state should be followed up periodically; the risk of developing non-insulin-dependent diabetes approaches 60% in 15 years.

- Periodic follow-up of patients with gestational diabetes who become euglycemic post partum.
- Risk of developing non-insulin-dependent diabetes is almost 60% at 15 years.

Hypoglycemic Syndrome

Etiology

The maintenance of euglycemia involves a balance between glucose production and glucose utilization.

Hypoglycemia can result from decreased production and/or increased utilization of glucose. Factors involved in glucose production include glucose input from the gastrointestinal tract and from hepatic glycogenolysis and neoglucogenesis. Insulin and the counterregulatory hormones glucagon, epinephrine, cortisol, and GH exert major influences on glucose production and utilization. The causes of hypoglycemia are outlined in Table 11-17.

Table 11-17.--Causes of Hypoglycemia

Postprandial or reactive hypoglycemia
    Reactive, functional, or idiopathic
    "Diabetic"
    Alimentary
Fasting hypoglycemia
    Hepatic
        Extensive surgical resection
        Acute fulminant hepatic necrosis--viral, toxic
        Cirrhosis
        Hereditary enzyme deficiencies
            Glycogen storage diseases
            Galactosemia
            Hereditary fructose intolerance
    Endocrine
        Insulin excess
            Insulinoma
            Insulin and oral hypoglycemia agents--therapeutic
              error, factitial
            Autoimmune
        Hypopituitarism
        Cortisol deficiency
    Alcohol
    Severe medical illness
        Chronic renal failure
        Severe malnutrition
        Infection and sepsis
    Extrapancreatic islet tumors
        Mesenchymal tumors
        Hepatoma
        Adrenocortical carcinoma
        Gastrointestinal tract, bronchial, or pancreatic
            carcinoma
    Drugs and poisons
        β-Blockers
        Salicylates
        Mushroom poisoning
        Akee fruit
        Hepatotoxins

Postprandial hypoglycemia is due to asynchronous or excessive insulin secretion relative to prandial plasma glucose levels. It is characterized by symptomatic hypoglycemia occurring 1-5 hours after food ingestion. Postprandial hypoglycemia can occur as a rare hereditary abnormality in children. In these patients, hypoglycemia may follow the ingestion of fructose, galactose, or leucine. Postprandial hypoglycemia does not occur in patients with frank diabetes mellitus. However, in some patients who have impaired glucose tolerance with normal fasting plasma levels of glucose, symptomatic hypoglycemia, or "diabetic" hypoglycemia, may develop 4-6 hours after glucose ingestion. It is attributed to excessive and delayed insulin response to a glucose load.

- Postprandial hypoglycemia: due to asynchronous or excessive insulin secretion relative to prandial plasma glucose levels.
- Characteristic: symptomatic hypoglycemia occurring 1-5 hours after food ingestion.

"Alimentary" hypoglycemia most often follows gastrectomy, jejunostomy, or vagotomy and pyloroplasty. Symptomatic hypoglycemia in alimentary hypoglycemia occurs earlier (1-2 hours after a glucose meal) than in other forms of postprandial hypoglycemia. The mechanism is believed to be due to the rapid entry of large amounts of glucose into the small bowel, causing a precipitous increase in the plasma glucose level and dramatic secretion of insulin. Alimentary hypoglycemia may also occur in patients with thyrotoxicosis or rapid gastric emptying of unknown cause.

Contrary to popular belief, idiopathic postprandial syndrome (reactive or functional) is distinctly rare. Normal subjects may have low circulating level of glucose after an oral glucose load. Those who have hypoglycemia after oral glucose frequently have normal glucose levels after a mixed meal. Symptoms do not correlate with glucose levels. Also, patients frequently have psychiatric disorders.

- Contrary to popular belief, idiopathic postprandial syndrome (reactive or functional) is distinctly rare.

Fasting hypoglycemia--Symptomatic hypoglycemia occurs infrequently in liver disease, such as severe cirrhosis or acute fulminant hepatic necrosis of viral or toxic origin, or after extensive surgical resection. Inborn defects of hepatic enzymes required for normal carbohydrate metabolism are rare and include glycogen storage diseases, galactosemia, and hereditary fructose intolerance.

Insulinomas are rare islet-cell pancreatic tumors that can occur in all ages, but they occur most frequently in patients in the 4th-7th decades, with a slight preponderance in females. Of the affected patients, 80% have a single benign tumor; 10% of the insulinomas are multiple, and another 10% are malignant. Of insulinomas, 10% occur in the setting of MEN I.

- 80% have a single benign tumor.
- 10% of the insulinomas are multiple.
- 10% are malignant.
- 10% occur in setting of MEN I.

Autoimmune hypoglycemia is a rare entity that can occur in patients who have antibodies to insulin (without previous exposure to insulin) or in patients with autoantibodies to insulin receptors of indeterminate cause.

Drug-related hormonal causes are the most common causes of hypoglycemia. Insulin administration in a known diabetic can cause hypoglycemia. The causes of insulin-induced hypoglycemia include: excessive insulin dose because of erroneous prescription or inability to measure the correct dose; failure to reduce insulin dose, e.g., during weight reduction; associated hypopituitarism or adrenocortical insufficiency or renal or hepatic failure; at the termination of pregnancy in an insulin-requiring woman; or after recovery from a stressful situation. Surreptitious administration of insulin may also cause hypoglycemia, as may excessive dosage in oral antidiabetic therapy related to decreased degradation or excretion (e.g., in kidney failure), potentiation by other drugs (e.g., barbiturates, warfarin, phenylbutazone, salicylates, sulfonamides, thiazide, or monoamine oxidase inhibitors), or surreptitious administration.

Glucocorticoid deficiency, whether related to primary adrenal disease or secondary to hypothalamic-pituitary disease, can cause fasting or late postprandial hypoglycemia because of impaired hepatic neoglucogenesis. This deficiency can be corrected completely by adequate steroid replacement. In children, GH deficiency can cause clinical hypoglycemia because of enhanced peripheral glucose utilization related to unopposed insulin effects.

Hypoglycemia associated with severe medical illness can occur in chronic renal failure, in severely malnourished children or adults, and in infection and sepsis. Certain extrapancreatic tumors may be associated with hypoglycemia. It can occur in patients with tumors of any histologic type but most frequently in those who have mesenchymal tumors, massive fibroma or sarcoma (e.g., retroperitoneal or intrathoracic), hepatomas, adrenocortical carcinomas, and gastrointestinal, bronchial, and exocrine pancreatic carcinoma. The cause of the hypoglycemia is likely related to insulin-like growth factors. Hypoglycemia can be caused by other drugs and poisons: β-adrenergic blockers, salicylates, and, most commonly in children, drugs that interfere with glucose metabolism in the liver. Ingestion of certain poisonous plants, e.g., mushrooms and akee fruit, and hepatotoxins can cause fatal hypoglycemia. Alcohol-induced hypoglycemia is a common cause of fasting hypoglycemia. It occurs most commonly in chronically malnourished alcoholics who stopped food and alcohol intake 10-20 hours earlier. It can also occur in healthy adults or children after a short drinking spree. Hypoglycemia results mainly from inhibition of gluconeogenesis by the products of ethanol metabolism; NADH accumulates in the liver and prevents entry of substrates into the gluconeogenic pathway.

- Hypoglycemia associated with severe medical illness: most frequently in those with mesenchymal tumors.
- Cause: likely related to insulin-like growth factors.
- Hypoglycemia can be caused by other drugs and poisons.
- Alcohol-induced hypoglycemia is a common cause of fasting hypoglycemia.

Clinical Manifestations

Clinical manifestations are related to hypoglycemia and its cause. The degree of hypoglycemia required to produce symptoms and the clinical manifestations reported by different patients vary widely. However, a similar pattern of symptoms generally recurs in any one person. Hypoglycemic symptoms may be hyperepinephrinemic, resulting from sympathetic activation, or neuroglycopenic, resulting from impaired central nervous system function. Hyperepinephrinemic symptoms usually occur when the plasma glucose levels decrease rapidly. These symptoms include sweating, palpitation, tremor, nervousness, hunger, faintness, weakness, and acral and perioral numbness. They may be blunted or absent in patients receiving β-adrenergic blocking agents, e.g., propranolol. Neuroglycopenic symptoms usually predominate when the plasma glucose levels decline slowly and reach lower levels (≤40 mg/dL). These symptoms include headache, diplopia, confusion, inappropriate affect, motor incoordination, and, when hypoglycemia is severe, seizures, coma, and (ultimately) death. Hypoglycemic manifestations can mimic many neurologic and psychiatric abnormalities. In patients with cerebrovascular disease, hypoglycemic manifestations may occur at higher plasma glucose levels, and the localized neurologic findings may correlate with the underperfused regions of the brain. The manifestations of hypoglycemia are generally reversible, but permanent brain damage can result from a prolonged severe episode.

- Clinical manifestations are related to hypoglycemia and its cause.
- Hypoglycemic symptoms may be hyperepinephrinemic or neuroglycopenic.
- Hyperepinephrinemic symptoms occur when the plasma glucose levels decrease rapidly. Symptoms may be blunted or absent in patients receiving β-adrenergic blocking agents.
- Neuroglycopenic symptoms usually predominate when the plasma glucose levels decline slowly and reach lower levels (≤40 mg/dL).
- Hypoglycemic manifestations can mimic many neurologic and psychiatric abnormalities.
- Manifestations of hypoglycemia: usually reversible, but permanent brain damage can result from a prolonged severe episode.

Diagnostic Approach

Evaluation of patients for possible hypoglycemia has two diagnostic objectives: to demonstrate that the clinical manifestations are due to hypoglycemia and to identify the underlying cause. The most important step in the diagnostic approach to hypoglycemia is to document Whipple's triad, i.e., to show that typical symptoms and hypoglycemia occur during a spontaneous attack or a provocative test and that the symptoms are relieved promptly by the ingestion or infusion of glucose. The actual level of plasma glucose that defines hypoglycemia is a matter of controversy. A reasonable diagnostic criterion is a glucose level, <50 mg/dL in males and <40 mg/dL in females, that is associated with clinical symptoms. It is important to rule out artifactual hypoglycemia. Whole-blood glucose values may be spuriously low in polycythemia vera and in leukemia, but measurement of plasma glucose in these conditions should provide an accurate result. The possibility of laboratory error should be excluded by repeated measurements.

- Two diagnostic objectives in evaluating hypoglycemia: demonstrate that clinical manifestations are due to hypoglycemia and identify underlying cause.
- Most important step in diagnostic approach to hypoglycemia: documenting Whipple's triad.
- Actual level of plasma glucose that defines hypoglycemia: controversial matter.
- Reasonable diagnostic criterion is a glucose level (<50 mg/dL in males and <40 mg/dL in females) that is associated with clinical symptoms.
- Exclude possibility of laboratory error by repeating measurements in cases of spuriously low levels of blood glucose.

Fasting Hypoglycemia

In evaluating fasting hypoglycemia, the two critical laboratory determinations are measurement of plasma glucose (to document hypoglycemia) and serum insulin (to categorize its cause). They can be measured during a spontaneous attack, after an overnight fast, or after a provoked attack (during a 72-hour fast). When fasting glucose levels are <50 mg/dL, normal insulin production by the beta pancreatic cells is suppressed and serum insulin levels decrease to <10 µU/mL. When plasma glucose values are <40 mg/dL, insulin values should be <5 µU/mL. During continued fasting in normal persons, plasma glucose and serum insulin levels decline together. As a result, the ratio of insulin to plasma glucose remains constant and <0.3.

- Two critical laboratory determinations in evaluating fasting hypoglycemia: measuring plasma glucose (to document hypoglycemia) and serum insulin (to categorize cause).
- Measurements performed: during spontaneous attack, after overnight fast, after provoked attack (during 72-hour fast).

Hyperinsulinism is identified by plasma insulin levels >6 µU/mL in association with plasma glucose of <50 mg/dL in males and <40 mg/dL in females. In most patients with hyperinsulinism, the ratio of insulin to plasma glucose is >0.3. If hyperinsulinism is present, the diagnostic considerations are insulinoma or the surreptitious administration of insulin or oral antidiabetic agents.

- Hyperinsulinism: plasma insulin levels >6 µU/mL in association with plasma glucose of <50 mg/dL in males and <40 mg/dL in females.

● If hyperinsulinism, diagnostic considerations are: insulinoma or surreptitious administration of insulin or oral antidiabetic agents.

Surreptitious administration of insulin or oral antidiabetic agents occurs most commonly in family members of insulin-dependent diabetics or in hospital personnel who have ready access to insulin, syringes, and oral agents. All patients should be examined carefully for injection marks, and if surreptitious administration of insulin is suspected, the hospital room should be searched for hidden insulin and syringes. Detection of insulin antibodies in the plasma of a nondiabetic patient supports the diagnosis (remember: insulin autoantibodies also occur in some persons who have not received exogenous insulin). The diagnosis is confirmed by the measurement of serum C peptide. In patients with hyperinsulinism, a high C-peptide level implies endogenous insulin secretion, whereas a low C-peptide level suggests an exogenous source. The diagnosis of surreptitious ingestion of oral antidiabetic agents as a cause of the hypoglycemic syndrome is confirmed by the measurement of either plasma drug levels or urinary metabolites.

● Measurement of C peptide is critical in evaluating hyperinsulinemic states.
● In hyperinsulinism: high C-peptide levels imply endogenous insulin secretion and can result from insulinoma or the ingestion of sulfonylureas.
● Confirm diagnosis of sulfonylurea-induced hypoglycemia by measuring plasma sulfonylurea levels or urinary metabolites.
● Low C-peptide levels suggest exogenous source.

The exclusion of surreptitious administration of drugs points to insulinoma as the cause of the hyperinsulinemic state. The diagnosis can further be supported by high serum proinsulin levels. In >85% of patients with insulinoma, the percentage of proinsulin is >25%, and the more undifferentiated the tumor, the higher the percentage of proinsulin. The use of an exogenous insulin suppression test can help distinguish physiologically controlled pancreatic beta cell islet from autonomous nonsuppressible insulin production in insulinoma. Suppression is assessed by measuring serum C peptide after administering insulin to produce hypoglycemia. Provocative agents such as tolbutamide, glucagon, leucine, or calcium elicit more insulin secretion from insulinomas than from normal beta cells. These provocative tests can be helpful in selected patients.

● In hyperinsulinemic states, the exclusion of surreptitious administration of drugs points to insulinoma as the cause of the hyperinsulinemic state.

After the diagnosis of insulinoma is made, attempt to anatomically delineate the tumor. Ultrasonography or a CT scan of the pancreas can delineate tumors >2 cm. Angiography may be needed to detect smaller tumors. Intraoperative ultrasonography may be helpful in identifying small tumors. Serum levels of human chorionic gonadotropin (hCG) or its α or β subunits are increased in two-thirds of patients with malignant insulinomas but not in those with benign disease.

● After making the diagnosis of insulinoma: anatomically delineate the tumor.

If hyperinsulinism is absent in patients with documented hypoglycemia, the differential diagnosis includes hypopituitarism, hypoadrenalism, liver disease, drug-induced hypoglycemia, and extrapancreatic tumor. If the clinical evidence suggests hypopituitarism or hypoadrenalism, appropriate endocrine tests are in order. Severe liver disease or ingestion of alcohol, drugs, or toxins can generally be distinguished by the history, physical examination, and liver function tests. In inborn hepatic enzyme defects, symptoms usually begin in infancy, and the diagnosis depends on the clinical setting and appropriate enzyme assays. The diagnosis of primary liver disease is usually obvious, but physicians should remember that if hypoglycemia is noted in the course of cirrhosis, the presence of hepatoma needs to be excluded. The presence of an extrapancreatic tumor that causes hypoglycemia is likely if the clinical findings and specific laboratory tests do not support one of the above conditions, especially if significant wasting or an abdominal mass is present.

● If hyperinsulinism is absent in patients with documented hypoglycemia, the differential diagnosis includes hypopituitarism, hypoadrenalism, liver disease, drug-induced hypoglycemia, extrapancreatic tumor.
● For hypoglycemia noted in course of cirrhosis, exclude hepatoma.
● The presence of extrapancreatic tumor causing hypoglycemia is likely if the clinical findings and specific laboratory tests do not support one of the above conditions, especially in presence of wasting or abdomi-

nal mass.

Remember that alcohol-induced hypoglycemia is a frequent cause of fasting hypoglycemia. Its manifestations are often mistakenly attributed to drunkenness. The plasma glucose level should be determined in all symptomatic patients with a history of significant alcohol intake. Diabetic patients taking insulin or oral agents are especially susceptible to ethanol-induced hypoglycemia. Also, bear in mind that blood alcohol levels may not be increased when a patient with hypoglycemia is examined.

- Remember: alcohol-induced hypoglycemia is a frequent cause of fasting hypoglycemia.
- Its manifestations are often mistakenly attributed to drunkenness.
- Diabetic patients taking insulin or oral agents are especially susceptible to ethanol-induced hypoglycemia.
- When patient with alcohol-induced hypoglycemia is examined, blood alcohol levels may not be increased.

Postprandial Hypoglycemia

It is important to remember that 1) postprandial hypoglycemia is uncommon; 2) patients are inclined to attribute many types of symptoms to hypoglycemia; 3) lack of energy, chronic anxiety, lethargy, mental dullness, and similar complaints rarely result from hypoglycemia, and 4) physician's responsibility is to demonstrate that these symptoms have been incorrectly attributed to hypoglycemia. The patient is instructed in the use of glucose oxidase strip reagents (e.g., Chemstrip BG) and asked to measure the plasma glucose at the time of the symptoms. If the levels are >80 mg/dL, the diagnosis of hypoglycemia is ruled out. If the levels are <80 mg/dL, a glucose or mixed meal tolerance test is indicated. The patient should avoid drugs known to influence glucose tolerance and ingest at least 150 g of complex carbohydrates for 3 days before the test.

- Postprandial hypoglycemia is uncommon.
- Patients are inclined to attribute many symptoms to hypoglycemia.
- Physician's responsibility: demonstrate that symptoms have been incorrectly attributed to hypoglycemia.
- Measure plasma glucose at time of symptoms.
- If the levels are <80 mg/dL, a glucose or mixed meal tolerance test is indicated.

ADRENAL CORTEX

Physiology (Fig. 11-9)

The hypothalamic-pituitary-adrenal axis is shown in Fig. 11-10. Its three regulatory influences are diurnal rhythm, negative feedback, and stress. ACTH and cortisol are secreted episodically. ACTH is produced by the anterior pituitary corticotroph cell and is under the regulation of CRH. Cortisol circulates in bound (96%-98%) and free (2%) forms. It is bound to transcortin, a specific binding protein, and to albumin. The free form is biologically active. Cortisol enters the target cells freely and is recognized by a specific cytoplasmic and nuclear receptor. It has a critical permissive role in intermediary metabolism, in optimizing cardiovascular function, in the ability of the kidney to excrete a water load, and in central nervous system activity. It also has a role in the checks and balances of the inflammatory response and immune reaction.

- Three regulatory influences: diurnal rhythm, negative feedback, stress.
- ACTH is produced by the anterior pituitary corticotroph cell under the regulation of CRH.
- Cortisol circulates in bound (96%-98%) and free (2%) forms.
- The free form is biologically active.
- Cortisol: critical permissive role in intermediary metabolism, optimizing cardiovascular function, kidney's ability to excrete water load, central nervous system activity.
- Cortisol: role in checks and balances of inflammatory response and immune reaction.

The renin-angiotensin-aldosterone system and its control are shown in Fig. 11-11. The dominant physiologic effect of aldosterone is at the distal renal tubule, where it enhances sodium reabsorption and potassium excretion. Aldosterone has a crucial role in maintaining sodium balance, extracellular fluid volume, and potassium balance. Its major regulatory influences are blood volume (through its effects on renal perfusion, renin secretion, and atrial natriuretic hormone production), β-adrenergic influences, and serum potassium level. Decreased blood volume, increased β-adrenergic stimulation, and increased serum potassium levels stimulate aldosterone secretion. Increased blood volume, atrial natriuretic hormone, and hypokalemia suppress its secretion. ACTH has a minor, permissive role in aldosterone secretion.

- Dominant physiologic effect of aldosterone: at distal renal tubule.
- It enhances sodium reabsorption and potassium excretion.
- Aldosterone: crucial role in maintaining sodium balance, extracellular fluid volume, potassium balance.
- Its major regulatory influences: blood volume, β-adrenergic influences, serum potassium level.
- ACTH: minor, permissive role in aldosterone secretion.

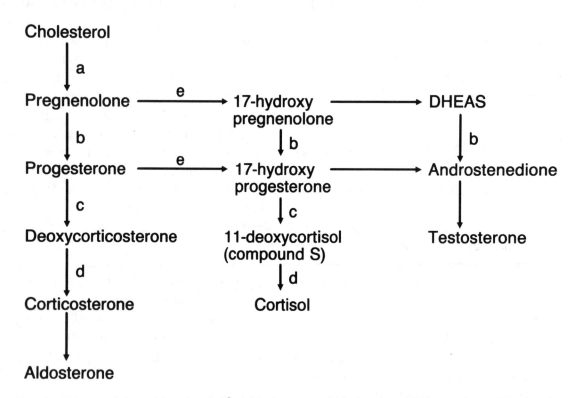

Fig. 11-9. Steroidogenic pathway. a, cholesterol desmolase; b, 3β-ol-dehydrogenase; c, 21-hydroxylase; d, 11-hydroxylase; e, 17-hydroxylase.

Adrenocortical Failure

Clinical Features

Weakness, fatigue, poor appetite, nausea, vomiting, weight loss, diarrhea, abdominal pain, salt craving, muscle cramps, hypotension with orthostatism; small heart seen on chest radiography; hypoglycemia, hyponatremia, hyperkalemia, and amenorrhea and loss of sexual hair in women. Pigmentary disorder (hyperpigmentation or vitiligo), neutropenia, lymphocytosis, eosinophilia, and adrenal calcification seen on abdominal radiography. About 25% of patients present with adrenocortical crisis.

- Features: weakness, fatigue, poor appetite, hypotension with orthostatism, hypoglycemia, hyponatremia, hyperkalemia.
- Pigmentary disorder.
- About 25% of patients present with adrenocortical crisis.

Etiology

Primary adrenocortical failure--Addison's disease is rare. It can be caused by autoimmune disease (>80% of patients), tuberculosis, hemorrhage into the adrenals (caused by sepsis, trauma, use of anticoagulant agents, bilateral infarction due to vasculitis), fungal disorders, malignancy (lymphoma or metastatic disease), bilateral adrenalectomy, and some forms of congenital adrenal hyperplasia (21- and 11-hydroxylase deficiency).

Secondary adrenocortical failure (see Hypopituitarism above)--Organic: hypothalamic-pituitary disease; functional: previous glucocorticoid therapy.

Peripheral resistance to ACTH or glucocorticoids (exceedingly rare).

Primary Adrenocortical Failure

Autoimmune Addison's disease is the commonest cause of adrenocortical failure in the U.S. (>80% of patients). Patients have circulating anti-adrenal antibodies (70%) with or without antibodies directed against other endocrine

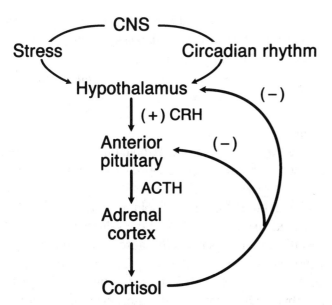

Fig. 11-10. Hypothalamic-pituitary-adrenal axis. ACTH, adrenocorticotropic hormone; CNS, central nervous system; CRH, corticotropin-releasing hormone.

glands, e.g., antithyroid (80%). It may occur in association with other autoimmune endocrine disorders such as Graves' disease, Hashimoto's thyroiditis, hypoparathyroidism, type I diabetes mellitus, hypogonadism, pernicious anemia, and vitiligo. Forty percent of patients have a family history of associated endocrinopathies.

- Autoimmune Addison's disease: commonest cause of adrenocortical failure in U.S. (>80%).
- May occur in association with other autoimmune endocrine disorders.
- 40% of patients have a family history of associated endocrinopathies.

Tuberculous Addison's disease is not associated with other endocrinopathies. Evidence of hematogenous dissemination and of adrenal calcification occurs in 50% of patients. Bilateral adrenal hemorrhage is probably the second most common cause in the U.S. It may be the result of systemic infections (e.g., meningococcemia), trauma, or use of anticoagulant agents. AIDS may cause adrenocortical failure in two ways: adrenalitis due to viral, bacterial, or fungal infections and hyporeninemic-hypoaldosteronism and hyperkalemia.

- Bilateral adrenal hemorrhage: is probably second most common cause in U.S. May result from: systemic infections, trauma, anticoagulant agents.

Secondary Adrenocortical Failure

In organic disease of the hypothalamic-pituitary unit, ACTH deficiency may be isolated or be part of hypopituitarism. The commonest cause of ACTH deficiency is functional suppression by prolonged exogenous steroid therapy. It may also follow from removal of tumor causing Cushing's syndrome. From 6 to 12 months may be needed for axis to recover after cessation of therapy, hence the need for interim steroid coverage. In ACTH lack, there is pallor but not hyperpigmentation. Aldosterone

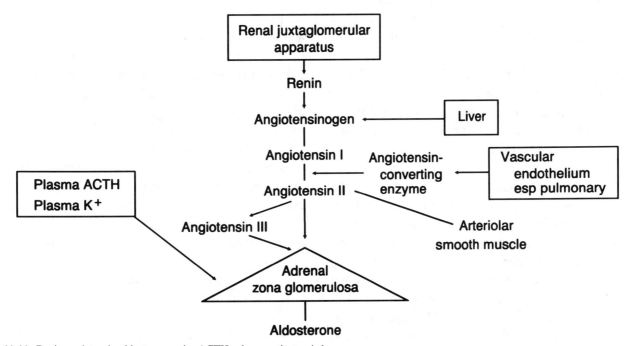

Fig. 11-11. Renin-angiotensin-aldosterone axis. ACTH, adrenocorticotropic hormone.

secretion is usually normal. Although serum levels of sodium may be low because of inability to excrete a water load due to cortisol or thyroid lack, the serum level of potassium is normal. Other features of hypothalamic-pituitary disease are usually present.

- Commonest cause of ACTH deficiency: functional suppression by prolonged exogenous steroid therapy.
- May occur after removal of tumor causing Cushing's syndrome.
- 6-12 months may be needed for axis to recover after cessation of therapy.

Aldosterone Deficiency

Aldosterone deficiency can result from decreased production or decreased tissue effect. Decreased production may be the result of:

1. Primary adrenocortical failure (decreased plasma aldosterone; increased plasma renin activity). This results from aldosterone and cortisol lack (from congenital adrenal hyperplasia or acquired adrenocortical failure, as in Addison's disease) or from isolated aldosterone lack due to 18-hydroxylase deficiency.
2. Abnormal regulation due to decreased renin (decreased PRA, decreased plasma aldosterone). This may result from acquired chronic renal disease or the use of drugs such as β-blockers and prostaglandin synthesis inhibitors. Abnormal regulation is also caused by decreased angiotensin II (decreased plasma aldosterone, increased PRA) due to use of drugs such as ACE inhibitors.

- Aldosterone deficiency: results from decreased production or decreased tissue effect.
- Decreased production results from: primary adrenocortical failure, abnormal regulation due to decreased renin or decreased angiotensin II.

Hyporeninemic hypoaldosteronism can occur in the elderly, especially those with diabetes mellitus and mild-to-moderate renal impairment. In the usual case, one can find hyperkalemia, mild metabolic acidosis, and hypertension related to associated renal disease. In such patients, drugs that can suppress the renin-angiotensin-aldosterone axis must be used with caution. These drugs include nonsteroidal anti-inflammatory agents, ACE inhibitors, β-blockers, calcium channel blockers, and chronic heparin therapy.

- Hyporeninemic hypoaldosteronism can occur in elderly, especially those with diabetes mellitus and mild-to-moderate renal impairment.
- In such patients, drugs that suppress renin-angiotensin-aldosterone axis must be used with caution.

Diagnostic Approach

Plasma cortisol level and 24-hour urinary levels of free cortisol, 17-hydroxysteroids, 17-ketogenic steroids, and 17-ketosteroids are not usually helpful in diagnosing adrenocortical failure. Plasma cortisol levels can be normal in partial adrenocortical failure. Low values can be seen in eucortisol normal patients (because of the timing of the sampling relative to the diurnal rhythm or episodic secretion) and in patients with decreased cortisol-binding globulin (hypothyroidism, liver disease, nephrotic syndrome, multiple myeloma). It is important to remember that "normal" values of plasma cortisol in a patient who is acutely sick are strong indications of adrenocortical failure.

- Not helpful in diagnosing adrenocortical failure: plasma cortisol level and 24-hour urinary levels of free cortisol, 17-hydroxysteroids, 17-ketogenic steroids, 17-ketosteroids.
- "Normal" values of plasma cortisol in a patient who is acutely sick are strong indications of adrenocortical failure.

Assays for urinary free cortisol are not sensitive enough to differentiate between low-normal and low values. The urinary levels of cortisol metabolites are usually low in adrenocortical failure (except that due to some types of congenital adrenal hyperplasia); however, they can be low in eucortisol persons because of inadequate 24-hour collections, starvation, liver disease, use of drugs that alter cortisol degradation (e.g., phenytoin, phenobarbital), hypothyroidism, and renal failure.

For the diagnosis of adrenocortical failure, adrenocortical provocative tests are critical; the cosyntropin test, overnight metyrapone test, or insulin hypoglycemia test can be used singly or in combination.

- Diagnosis of adrenocortical failure: adrenocortical provocative tests are essential.
- Cosyntropin test, overnight metyrapone test, insulin hypoglycemia test: use singly or in combination.

Is Adrenocortical Failure Present?

A cosyntropin test is done. The normal response is a

plasma cortisol increment >7 µg/dL with peak cortisol >18 µg/dL. Subnormal cortisol responses establish the diagnosis of adrenocortical failure but cannot differentiate Addison's disease from secondary failure due to hypothalamic-pituitary disease. A normal cortisol response excludes Addison's disease but does not rule out secondary adrenocortical failure that is partial or of recent onset.

- Do cosyntropin test.
- Subnormal cortisol response: establishes diagnosis of adrenocortical failure. Cannot differentiate Addison's disease from failure due to hypothalamic-pituitary disease.
- Normal cortisol response: excludes Addison's disease. Does not rule out secondary adrenocortical failure that is partial or of recent onset.

One can elect to proceed initially with overnight metyrapone test or insulin hypoglycemia test. A normal response to the metyrapone test is a serum level of 11-deoxycortisol (immediate precursor of cortisol) >7 µg/dL. A normal response to insulin hypoglycemia is a cortisol level >18 µg/dL. A normal response to either test indicates a normal hypothalamic-pituitary-adrenal axis. An impaired response documents adrenocortical failure but does not localize the level of axis impairment.

- One may initially proceed with overnight metyrapone test or insulin hypoglycemia test.
- Normal response (either test) indicates normal hypothalamic-pituitary-adrenal axis.
- Impaired response documents adrenocortical failure but does not localize level of axis impairment.

What Is the Cause of the Adrenocortical Failure?

The serum level of ACTH is critical in distinguishing between Addison's disease (high levels, >200 pg/mL) and secondary adrenocortical failure (low values, <50 pg/mL). If ACTH assays are not available, perform the 3-day prolonged ACTH stimulation test. In Addison's disease, the adrenal glands remain unresponsive; however, a stepwise response is seen in patients with secondary failure. In patients who have normal cosyntropin responsiveness and who are still suspected to have partial or recent secondary failure, an impaired response to the metyrapone test or insulin hypoglycemia test confirms the diagnosis.

- Serum level of ACTH: critical for distinguishing between Addison's disease and secondary adrenocortical failure.
- If ACTH assays are not available, perform 3-day prolonged ACTH stimulation test.
- In patients who have normal Cortrosyn responsiveness and still suspected to have partial or recent secondary failure, impaired response to metyrapone or insulin hypoglycemia test confirms the diagnosis.

After the diagnosis is established, search for the cause. In secondary failure, proceed with work-up as outlined in the section on hypopituitarism. In Addison's disease, a search for the cause includes clinical assessment, search for other autoimmune disorders, infections, neoplasms, etc.

- After diagnosis is established, search for the cause.

Treatment

Chronic--Primary adrenocortical failure requires glucocorticoid therapy and usually mineralocorticoid therapy. In most patients, secondary failure requires only glucocorticoid therapy. The patient needs to be educated about the disease, its replacement therapy, how to handle dosage during acute illness, and how to inject steroids when needed. Therapy in primary adrenocortical failure usually consists of 1) hydrocortisone, 20 mg in a.m. and 10 mg in early p.m., or prednisone, 5 mg in a.m. and 2.5 mg in early p.m. Monitor clinical symptoms; ACTH levels are not reliable for monitoring the adequacy of therapy, because they do not always decrease and are not widely available or reliable. 2) Mineralocorticoid therapy in the form of fludrocortisone, 0.05-0.2 mg orally; liberal salt intake. Monitor supine and standing blood pressure, presence of edema, serum potassium level, and, if needed, plasma renin activity.

- Primary adrenocortical failure requires glucocorticoid and usually mineralocorticoid therapy.
- Secondary failure (in most patients) requires only glucocorticoid therapy.
- Therapy for primary adrenocortical failure: hydrocortisone, 20 mg in a.m. and 10 mg in early p.m. or equivalent.
- Mineralocorticoid therapy: fludrocortisone, 0.05-0.2 mg orally; liberal salt intake.

Acute illness coverage: in mild-to-moderate acute illness, increase the glucocorticoid dosage x3 for the duration of the illness. In the presence of severe illness or if vomiting is present, the patient needs to use parenteral dexamethasone (4 mg intramuscularly) and seek prompt medical help. For minor procedures performed under local anesthesia and most radiologic procedures, no special preparation is required. For moderately stressful procedures such as endoscopy, hydrocortisone (100 mg intravenously) should be given just before the procedure. For major surgery, give 100 mg hydrocortisone intravenously before induction of anesthesia, and continue with 100 mg every 6-8 hours for the first 24 hours and taper dose rapidly (decrease by 50% per day) to maintenance level.

Management of adrenal crisis: Suspect a crisis in the presence of dehydration, hypotension or shock out of proportion to severity of current illness, nausea, vomiting with a history of anorexia and weight loss, abdominal pain (may mimic acute abdomen), unexplained fever, hyponatremia, hyperkalemia, azotemia, hypercalcemia, eosinophilia, and hypoglycemia.

Prompt management is critical. Establish intravenous access: draw blood for measuring electrolytes, glucose, plasma cortisol level, and serum ACTH level. Do not wait for the results, but institute management as soon as the diagnosis is suspected. Promptly infuse saline/dextrose to restore blood and extracellular fluid volume; give dexamethasone, 4 mg intravenously (hydrocortisone, 100 mg every 6 hours, may be used but will interfere with measurements of cortisol during the cosyntropin test). Mineralocorticoids are not necessary at this time. Use other supportive measures as needed.

- Prompt management is critical.
- Draw blood for measuring electrolytes, glucose, plasma cortisol level, serum ACTH level.
- Do not wait for results.
- Institute management as soon as diagnosis is suspected.

After patient's condition is stabilized, continue infusions but at a lower rate. Search for and treat possible infections and precipitating causes. Perform cosyntropin stimulation test and determine type and cause of adrenocortical failure. Taper glucocorticoids to maintenance, and begin mineralocorticoid replacement, if needed, after saline infusion is stopped.

- After stabilization, continue infusions at lower rate.
- Search for and treat possible infections and precipitating causes.
- Perform cosyntropin stimulation test.

Cushing's Syndrome

Clinical Features

1) Obesity with cushingoid characteristics. 2) Evidence of protein wasting such as thin skin, easy bruising, striae, muscle weakness and atrophy, or osteoporosis. 3) Diabetes mellitus. 4) Hypertension with or without hypokalemia. 5) Hyperandrogenicity with acne/hirsutism, menstrual disorders, and, rarely, virilization. 6) Psychiatric problems with depression or psychosis. 7) Hyperpigmentation (related to excess ACTH). 8) Growth failure in children. 9) Discovery of a pituitary, ectopic, or adrenal mass.

- Obesity with cushingoid characteristics.
- Evidence of protein wasting.
- Diabetes mellitus.
- Hypertension with or without hypokalemia.
- Hyperandrogenicity
- Psychiatric problems.
- Growth failure in children.
- Pituitary, ectopic, or adrenal mass.

Etiology

Exogenous causes are iatrogenic or factitial. Endogenous causes: 1) ACTH-dependent, including Cushing's disease (70%), ectopic ACTH-producing tumors (20%), eutopic or ectopic CRH-producing tumor (rare). 2) Non-ACTH-dependent, primary, adrenal; adrenal tumor (10%), either adenoma or carcinoma and the rare micronodular hyperplasia.

Cushing's disease is caused by an ACTH-producing pituitary tumor (>90% of patients) or hyperplasia (<10%). It usually presents with the classic clinical picture of gradual onset and slow progression and affects predominantly women between 20 and 40 years old. Hyperpigmentation and hypokalemic metabolic alkalosis are rare. Laboratory evaluation shows normal-to-modestly increased serum level of ACTH (40-200 pg/mL), mild-to-moderate cortisol excess, and mild proportionate increase in adrenal androgen production. The hypothalamic-pituitary-ACTH axis is impaired but responsive (cortisol hypersecretion is high-dose dexamethasone suppressible in >70% of patients). An ACTH-producing tumor is shown radiologically in about 50% of patients. MR imaging is currently the procedure of choice.

- Cushing's disease is caused by an ACTH-producing pituitary tumor (>90% of patients) or hyperplasia (<10%).

- Usual presentation: classic clinical picture of gradual onset and slow progression.
- Affects predominantly women 20-40 years old.

Most ectopic ACTH-producing tumors occur in men between 50 and 70 years old. The ectopic tumor is evident, such as lung carcinoma, thymoma, pancreatic carcinoma, medullary carcinoma of the thyroid, pheochromocytoma, and others. The hypercortisol state has a rapid onset and progression and is severe. The presentation includes weakness, debility, weight loss, hypertension, hypokalemic alkalosis, edema, diabetes mellitus, and hyperpigmentation. Cushingoid features are absent because of the short duration of the illness. There is an associated proportionate increase in mineralocorticoid and androgen production; ACTH is moderately to significantly increased, with 65% of patients having ACTH levels >200 pg/mL. The ACTH ectopic tumor is autonomous, and the hypothalamic-pituitary-ACTH axis is suppressed. Thus, cortisol secretion is non-high-dose dexamethasone-suppressible. (For bronchial carcinoid, see below.)

- Most ectopic ACTH-producing tumors occur in men 50-70 years old.
- Ectopic tumor is usually evident, such as lung carcinoma, thymoma, pancreatic carcinoma, medullary carcinoma of thyroid, pheochromocytoma, others.
- The hypercortisol state has a rapid onset and progression and is severe.
- Cushingoid features are absent because of short duration of illness.

Iatrogenic Cushing's syndrome is the commonest cause of the syndrome. It is more likely to be associated with benign intracranial hypertension, glaucoma, cataracts, pancreatitis, or avascular necrosis of the femur head. Cessation of therapy may be followed by clinical evidence of hypothalamic-pituitary-adrenal axis suppression and may need glucocorticoid replacement until recovery of the axis. To assess recovery of the axis, use the cosyntropin test; a basal serum cortisol level >11 μg/dL and a post-ACTH level >20 μg/dL indicate recovery.

- Iatrogenic Cushing's syndrome is commonest cause of the syndrome.
- More likely associated with: benign intracranial hypertension, glaucoma, cataracts, pancreatitis, avascular necrosis of femur head.

- Cessation of therapy may be followed by clinical evidence of hypothalamic-pituitary-adrenal axis suppression.
- Glucocorticoid replacement may be needed until axis recovers.

Diagnostic Approach

Is Cushing's Syndrome Present?
Diagnosis depends on the clinical picture and the biochemical demonstration of a pituitary-adrenal axis that does not suppress normally. The best screening tests are the 1-mg overnight dexamethasone suppression test or the 24-hour urinary free cortisol. The definitive test is the low-dose (2 mg/day for 2 days) dexamethasone suppression test. The demonstration of abnormal dexamethasone suppressibility or increased urinary free cortisol point to a diagnosis of Cushing's syndrome, but only after alcoholism, depression, and acute illness have been excluded.

- Diagnosis depends on clinical picture and biochemical demonstration of pituitary-adrenal axis that does not suppress normally.
- Best screening test: 1-mg overnight dexamethasone suppression test or 24-hour urinary free cortisol.
- Definitive test: low-dose (2 mg/day for 2 days) dexamethasone suppression test.
- Exclude alcoholism, depression, acute illness.

The 1-mg dexamethasone suppression test is a reliable screening test. The normal response is a plasma cortisol value of <5 μg/dL. Patients with Cushing's syndrome usually have values >10 μg/dL. False-positive test results occur in 13% of patients with simple obesity and in 25% of chronically ill patients. Other causes of false-positive responses include acute illness, depression, estrogen use, pregnancy, and the use of drugs that can accelerate dexamethasone metabolism (phenytoin, barbiturates).

Urinary free cortisol is increased in >97% of patients with Cushing's syndrome. However, it can also be increased in acute illness, trauma, surgery, alcoholism, and depression. Importantly, it can be modestly increased in simple obesity.

The 2-mg low-dose dexamethasone suppression test is the standard test for the diagnosis of Cushing's syndrome. False-positive results can be seen in patients with acute illness, severe stress, alcoholism, or depression and with the use of drugs known to accelerate dexamethasone metabolism (phenytoin, barbiturates).

What is the Cause of Cushing's Syndrome?

In searching for the cause, the most important diagnostic tools are serum ACTH level, high-dose (8 mg) dexamethasone suppression test, and radiologic studies for pituitary, ectopic, or adrenal tumors.

● In searching for cause, most important diagnostic tools: serum ACTH level, high-dose (8 mg) dexamethasone suppression test, radiologic studies for pituitary, ectopic, adrenal tumors.

If Cushing's syndrome is caused by an adrenal tumor, one will find a low or undetectable level of ACTH, nonsuppressible hypercortisol state, and an adrenal mass found on abdominal CT. Adrenal adenomas show "pure" glucocorticoid excess of gradual progressive nature, and the tumor is usually <3 cm in size. However, in adrenal carcinoma, the hypercortisol state develops rapidly and is "mixed" with mineralocorticoid and androgen overproduction; the tumor is usually >6 cm in size.

● Cushing's syndrome caused by adrenal tumor: low/undetectable ACTH level, nonsuppressible hypercortisol state, adrenal mass found on abdominal CT.

Cushing's syndrome caused by an ectopic ACTH tumor is characterized in most patients by an evident ectopic tumor, rapid clinical course, very high ACTH levels (>200 pg/mL), and nonsuppressibility.

● Cushing's syndrome caused by ectopic ACTH tumor: evident ectopic tumor, rapid clinical course, very high ACTH levels (>200 pg/mL), nonsuppressibility.

In Cushing's disease, ACTH values are "normal" or moderately increased (<200 pg/mL), the hypercortisol state is dexamethasone-suppressible in >66% of patients, and CT or MR imaging of the sella may show a pituitary tumor. However, about 50% of patients have normal sellar radiographic features, and 33% have nonsuppressibility. Also, patients with bronchial carcinoids may be clinically and biochemically indistinguishable from patients with Cushing's disease. If CT or MR imaging of the sella and CT of the chest do not show abnormality, resort to petrosal sinus selective venous sampling with CRH provocative testing. A central-to-peripheral ACTH gradient ≥2:1 points to Cushing's disease.

● Cushing's disease: ACTH values are normal/moderately increased (<200 pg/mL), hypercortisol state is dexamethasone suppressible in >66% of patients, CT/MR imaging of sella may show pituitary tumor.
● About 50% of patients have normal sellar radiographic features; about 33% have nonsuppressibility.
● Patients with bronchial carcinoids: clinically and biochemically may be indistinguishable from patients with Cushing's disease.
● If CT/MR of sella and CT of chest show no abnormality, resort to petrosal sinus selective venous sampling with CRH provocative testing.

Differential Diagnosis

False-positive biochemical evaluation. 1) Simple obesity: urinary free cortisol, urinary ketogenic and ketosteroids, and other urinary steroids may be mildly increased. Overnight dexamethasone suppression may be abnormal in 10%-20% of obese patients, but the low-dose 2-mg dexamethasone suppression test shows normal suppressibility. 2) Estrogen, oral contraceptives, and pregnancy: high cortisol-binding globulin and increase in plasma cortisol. Overnight 1-mg dexamethasone suppression test may give abnormal results, but urinary free cortisol is normal. Results of low-dose 2-mg dexamethasone suppression test are normal. 3) Pseudo-Cushing's syndrome in alcoholics: exclude this in every patient with suspected Cushing's syndrome. Clinical and biochemical similarities to Cushing's syndrome. Increased cortisol production, nonsuppressible low-dose 2-mg dexamethasone suppression test. Abnormalities return to normal in a few weeks to a few months after abstention from alcohol. 4) Depression: biochemical similarities to Cushing's syndrome include increased cortisol production and nonsuppressible low-dose dexamethasone test. Typical features of Cushing's syndrome are absent. These patients maintain normal cortisol responses to insulin provocative test (patients with true Cushing's syndrome have blunted cortisol responses to hypoglycemia). The hypercortisol state is reversible with recovery from depression. 5) Acute and chronic illness in hospital setting: steroid values may be increased and dexamethasone suppression may be impaired. Repeat the steroid evaluation after the illness resolves.

● False-positive evaluation with: simple obesity; estrogen, oral contraceptives, pregnancy; pseudo-Cushing's in alcoholics; depression; acute and chronic illness in hospital setting.

False-negative evaluation. This occurs in patients with delayed dexamethasone clearance or with periodic hormonogenesis. Periodic hormonogenesis can occur with any cause of endogenous Cushing's syndrome. The hypercortisol state is periodic or cyclic, lasting a few weeks to a few months; between cycles of activity, cortisol secretion and dexamethasone suppressibility are normal. Repeated evaluations at intervals of a few weeks to a few months are required to establish the cyclic nature of the disorder.

● False-negative evaluation occurs in patients with delayed dexamethasone clearance or with periodic hormonogenesis.

Treatment

1. Cushing's disease--Transsphenoidal adenomectomy is the treatment of choice. The tumor can be identified in >90% of patients, surgical cure can be achieved in >80%, and for experienced surgeons, mortality and morbidity should be <1%. Alternatively, heavy particle irradiation or conventional radiotherapy can be given (only one medical center in the U.S. can deliver heavy particle irradiation). Radiotherapy, although effective in children with Cushing's disease, is effective in only 15%-25% of adults. If therapy fails, consider bilateral adrenalectomy and, in addition, for those who failed transsphenoidal surgery, postoperative pituitary irradiation. Drug therapy, such as cyproheptadine or valproic acid, to inhibit ACTH secretion is rarely successful. However, drugs that inhibit cortisol secretion, such as ketoconazole, metyrapone, aminoglutethimide, or the antimitotic op'DDD, can be used as adjunctive therapy or when therapy has failed. These drugs are expensive, have frequent side effects, and may produce a hypocortisol state.

● Cushing's disease: transsphenoidal adenomectomy is treatment of choice.
● Radiotherapy: effective in children but in only 15%-25% of adults.
● If therapy fails: bilateral adrenalectomy plus (for those failing transsphenoidal surgery) postoperative pituitary irradiation.

2. Ectopic ACTH--Unfortunately, surgical excision of the tumor is possible only in a small number of patients. If cortisol excess (rather than the primary tumor) is life-threatening, consider bilateral adrenalectomy. Otherwise, drug therapy is used (see above).

3. Adrenal tumor--For adrenal adenoma, surgical excision is curative. In adrenal carcinoma, surgical excision or debulking is undertaken with generally poor results; op'DDD and/or other drug therapy is given for residual disease.

In Cushing's syndrome of whatever cause, the normal hypothalamic-pituitary-adrenal axis is suppressed. After tumor ablation, the axis may take up to 1-2 years to recover. During this time, glucocorticoid replacement therapy should be given.

Aldosteronism

Clinical Features

The most important clinical clues are hypertension and hypokalemia. Symptoms related to potassium deficiency include fatigue, muscle weakness, polyuria/polydipsia (due to either nephrogenic diabetes insipidus or diabetes mellitus), orthostatic hypotension, and paresthesias/tetany.

● Most important clinical clues: hypertension and hypokalemia.

Etiology

Primary causes: adenoma, 70% of patients; hyperplasia, 30%; carcinoma (rare); and glucocorticoid-remediable aldosteronism (very rare). Secondary causes: 1) with hypertension--increased renin, renal artery stenosis, malignant hypertension, primary renin-tumor, hypertension, and diuretics; also, increased angiotensinogen, estrogen therapy. 2) Without hypertension--increased renin, decreased renal perfusion of any cause; pregnancy; and Bartter's syndrome.

Diagnostic Approach

Document hypokalemia--If unprovoked hypokalemia is present, continue with the work-up. If the patient has a normal serum level of potassium and has been taking a potassium-sparing diuretic, discontinue use of the drug and reassess in a few weeks. If the patient has a normal serum level of potassium and has been on a low salt diet, salt load and measure the serum level of potassium in a few days. Otherwise, normokalemia excludes primary aldosteronism.

- Document hypokalemia.
- If patient has normal serum level of potassium and takes potassium-sparing diuretic, discontinue use of drug and reassess in a few weeks.
- If patient has normal serum level of potassium and has been on low sodium diet, salt load and measure serum level of potassium in a few weeks.
- Otherwise, normokalemia excludes aldosteronism.

If the patient has hypokalemia and has been taking a potassium-wasting diuretic, you could stop use of the diuretic, replenish the potassium, and repeat serum level of potassium in about 2 weeks. If hypokalemia persists, proceed with study. Alternatively, you could check plasma renin activity: if suppressed in a patient receiving diuretic therapy, it points to mineralocorticoid excess. Then proceed with the study.

- If patient has hypokalemia and has been taking a potassium-wasting diuretic, stop use of diuretic, replenish potassium, repeat serum level of potassium in about 2 weeks.

Document kaliuresis--Check urinary potassium level. In mineralocorticoid excess, urinary potassium in hypokalemic patients is >30 mEq/L.

- Document kaliuresis. Check urinary potassium level.

Document aldosterone overproduction--Check plasma or urinary aldosterone level. Note that because potassium is an aldosterone secretagogue and because significant hypokalemia may decrease aldosterone secretion in primary aldosteronism, potassium should be replenished before aldosterone measurements are made. If aldosterone levels are high, proceed with work-up. If aldosterone levels are low, consider other causes of hypertension and hypokalemia (see above).

- Document aldosterone overproduction. Check plasma or urinary aldosterone levels.
- Replenish potassium before measuring aldosterone.

Document the type of aldosterone overproduction-- Check plasma renin activity. If low, it points to primary aldosteronism; high values imply that the aldosteronism is secondary.

- Document type of aldosterone overproduction. Check

plasma renin activity.

Identify the cause of primary aldosteronism-- Distinguishing between adenoma and hyperplasia in most patients is impossible on clinical and biochemical grounds and is best achieved by radiographic study. Abdominal CT is the imaging procedure of choice. If findings are negative, proceed with selective bilateral adrenal venous sampling. Aldosterone levels are 2x-3x higher on the side harboring the adenoma. The selective sampling procedure is technically difficult and laborious. Alternatively, one may elect to proceed with medical treatment for hyperaldosteronism and repeat the CT study in 1-2 years.

- Identify cause of primary aldosteronism.
- Distinguishing adenoma and hyperplasia in most patients is impossible on clinical and biochemical grounds.
- Distinguishing between the two is achieved with radiography.
- Abdominal CT is imaging procedure of choice.

Many patients with adenoma have anomalous postural decrease in plasma level of aldosterone and increased 18-hydroxycorticosterone levels; unfortunately, in individual patients, these tests usually are of limited value.

Differential diagnosis--1) Hypertension, hypokalemia, low aldosterone level, and suppressed renin: other mineralocorticoid excess such as deoxycorticosterone-secreting tumor, 11- and 17-hydroxylase deficiency, licorice ingestion, and 11-β-hydroxysteroid dehydrogenase deficiency. 2) Hypertension, hypokalemia, high aldosterone level, suppressed renin: familial glucocorticoid-remediable aldosteronism; correction of clinical abnormalities occurs after few weeks of dexamethasone therapy at 1-2 mg/day.

Special Considerations

Syndrome of apparent mineralocorticoid excess is characterized by hypertension, hypokalemia, suppressed renin, and suppressed aldosterone. The defect is in 11-β-hydroxysteroid dehydrogenase, which catalyzes the conversion of the active cortisol to the inactive cortisone in the peripheral tissues. Thus, tissue cortisol levels increase and the cortisol binds to the mineralocorticoid receptor. The diagnosis is made by measuring metabolites of cortisol and cortisone in the urine. Licorice-induced mineralocorticoid excess syndrome occurs because licorice inhibits 11-β-hydroxysteroid dehydrogenase.

- Syndrome of apparent mineralocorticoid excess: hypertension, hypokalemia, suppressed renin, suppressed aldosterone.
- Defect: 11-β-hydroxysteroid dehydrogenase.
- Diagnosis: measuring metabolites of cortisol and cortisone in urine.
- Licorice-induced mineralocorticoid excess syndrome: due to licorice inhibition of 11-β-hydroxysteroid dehydrogenase.

Glucocorticoid-remediable aldosteronism is a rare syndrome, familial and autosomal dominant, that primarily affects young males. Hyperaldosteronism is dexamethasone suppressible; cortisol and ACTH secretion are normal.

Treatment

Surgical excision is the treatment of choice for aldosteronoma unless the patient is a poor surgical risk. For such patients and those with hyperplasia, medical treatment is indicated. This consists of dietary salt restriction and the use of potassium-sparing diuretics. Spironolactone, an aldosterone antagonist, is given in a dose of 25-100 mg/8 hours. It restores normokalemia and normalizes blood pressure in most patients. In men, it is associated with gynecomastia and impaired libido and potency. For such patients, use amiloride or triamterene. Surgical treatment in hyperplasia requires bilateral adrenalectomy; it normalizes potassium but rarely restores blood pressure to normal levels. For this reason, surgical treatment is not indicated in the management of hyperplasia. In glucocorticoid-remediable hyperaldosteronism, one may give dexamethasone in the dose of 1 mg/day.

- Surgical excision: treatment of choice for aldosteronoma (unless patient is poor surgical risk).
- For patients who are poor surgical risks and those with hyperplasia, medical treatment.
- Medical treatment: dietary salt restriction and potassium-sparing diuretics.
- In glucocorticoid-remediable hyperaldosteronism: dexamethasone at 1 mg/day.

THE ADRENAL MEDULLA

The sympathochromaffin system consists of the sympathetic nervous system and the chromaffin tissues of the adrenal medulla. The catecholamines norepinephrine, epinephrine, and dopamine are the hormones and neurotransmitters of this system. The biosynthesis and biodegradation of these hormones are outlined in Fig. 11-12. Tyrosine hydroxylase is the rate-limiting enzyme. Epinephrine is a hormone of the adrenal medulla. Norepinephrine is the neurotransmitter of sympathetic ganglionic neurons. Dopamine is principally a neurotransmitter in the CNS. The catecholamines exert their biologic actions by binding to cell membrane α and β receptors in the target tissues. Their principal endocrine role is to provide an integrated homeostatic stress response.

- Sympathochromaffin system: sympathetic nervous system plus chromaffin tissues of adrenal medulla.
- Catecholamines: norepinephrine, epinephrine, and dopamine.
- They are hormones and neurotransmitters of sympathochromaffin system.
- Epinephrine: hormone of adrenal medulla.
- Norepinephrine: neurotransmitter of sympathetic ganglionic neurons.
- Principal endocrine role of catecholamines: integrated homeostatic stress response.

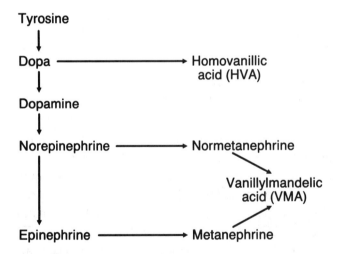

Fig. 11-12. Catecholamine synthesis and degradation.

Pheochromocytoma

Pheochromocytomas are rare chromaffin tumors. They are important because they 1) may be potentially malignant; 2) present with a distinctive hypertensive syndrome (although rare--<1% of all hypertensive disorders--it can be cured, and if untreated, it can be potentially lethal); and 3) they may be familial. Over 90% of tumors are sporadic, adrenal, unilateral, and benign. Familial pheochromocytomas are more likely to be intra-adrenal, bilateral, and malignant. Extra-adrenal tumors are usually located in the abdomen. Less than 1% of pheochromocytomas are in the chest or neck. Pheochromocytomas generally secrete both epinephrine and norepinephrine. Epinephrine-secreting tumors are either located in the adrenals or in the organs of Zuckerkandl. Pheochromocytomas can secrete catecholamines persistently or episodically.

- Pheochromocytomas are important because they are potentially malignant and may present with a distinctive hypertensive syndrome.
- May be familial.
- Over 90% of tumors are sporadic, adrenal, unilateral, benign.
- Extra-adrenal tumors are usually in the abdomen.
- Less than 1% are in chest or neck.
- They generally secrete epinephrine and norepinephrine.
- Epinephrine-secreting tumors: either in adrenals or organs of Zuckerkandl.
- Pheochromocytomas can secrete catecholamines persistently or episodically.

Clinical Presentations

Pheochromocytomas are great mimickers. They can be asymptomatic and discovered incidentally on abdominal imaging. More commonly, they are suspected because of the presence of: 1) hypertension, particularly if it is labile, intermittent, or refractory to treatment; 2) paroxysmal symptoms of headaches, palpitations, sweating, anxiety and a feeling of impending doom, and pallor; 3) heat intolerance, sweating, and weight loss; 4) unexplained abdominal or chest pain; 5) orthostatic hypotension, unexplained shock after trauma, surgery or parturition; and 6) family history of pheochromocytoma, MEN IIA (Sipple's syndrome) or MEN IIB (mucosal neuroma syndrome), or von Hippel-Lindau disease or neurofibromatosis. In most patients, the paroxysmal symptoms are stereotyped and vary only in severity or frequency. The common symptoms are headaches, palpitations, and sweating; absence of all three in a hypertensive patient strongly points away from pheochromocytoma.

- Pheochromocytomas: great mimickers.
- They can be asymptomatic; discovered incidentally on abdominal imaging.
- More commonly, are suspected because of hypertension.

- Paroxysmal symptoms.
- Heat intolerance, sweating, weight loss.
- Unexplained abdominal or chest pain.
- Orthostatic hypotension.
- Unexplained shock.
- Family history of pheochromocytoma, MEN IIA, or MEN IIB.
- In most patients, paroxysmal symptoms are stereotyped, vary only in severity or frequency.
- Common symptoms: headache, palpitations, sweating.
- Absence of all three symptoms in hypertensive patient: strongly points away from pheochromocytoma.

Diagnostic Approach

Document Catecholamine Hypersecretion

1. Check the levels of urinary catecholamines or metabolites. Diagnosis is based principally on urinary measurements of free catecholamines and their urinary metabolites, metanephrines and vanillylmandelic acid. No one measurement is clearly superior to the others, and in practice, the three measurements are made on the same 24-hour urine collection. Demonstration of increased values in hypertensive patients establishes the diagnosis if such conditions as severe stress, intercurrent illness, and acute myocardial ischemia are excluded. Normal values in hypertensive or otherwise symptomatic patients are adequate to exclude the diagnosis. In borderline cases, the urinary studies can be repeated. In patients who have paroxysmal symptoms, the diagnostic yield can be significantly increased by initiating collection during or shortly after a paroxysm. In all urine collections, assay for creatinine to ensure the adequacy of the sample. Among the drugs that can interfere with the usefulness of the assay are α-methyldopa, labetalol, MAO-inhibitors, and β-adrenergic blockers.

- Document catecholamine hypersecretion.
- Check urinary catecholamines or metabolites.
- Increased values in hypertensive patients establish diagnosis (if severe stress, intercurrent illness, acute myocardial ischemia are excluded).
- Patients with paroxysmal symptoms, diagnostic yield is increased significantly by initiating collection during or shortly after paroxysm.

2. Plasma catecholamines are used as adjuncts to urinary studies. They must be obtained under strict conditions: basal state, supine position, and special collection tools. They represent secretion over a short period of time and are most useful if obtained during a paroxysm or in conjunction with provocative or suppression tests.

- Plasma catecholamines: adjuncts.
- Most useful if obtained during paroxysm or in conjunction with provocative or suppression tests.

3. Provocative testing with glucagon or histamine is potentially hazardous and has no place in routine evaluation. Very occasionally, it may be useful for normotensive patients with a history of paroxysmal symptoms suggestive of pheochromocytoma. In these patients, the provocative test needs to be done under strictly monitored circumstances and only after α-blockade has been instituted to prevent adverse cardiovascular effects. Plasma catecholamine levels >2,000 pg/mL within 3-5 min after administering 1 mg of glucagon IV point to the presence of pheochromocytoma. The clonidine suppression test is of limited usefulness. A 50% decrease in plasma catecholamines within 3 hours after administering 0.3 mg of clonidine points away from pheochromocytoma.

- Provocative testing with glucagon or histamine is potentially hazardous; has no place in routine evaluation.
- Clonidine suppression test has limited usefulness.

Localize the Pheochromocytoma

CT or MR imaging of the abdomen (if findings are negative, image the pelvis and thorax) is the mainstay of radiologic localization procedures. They have a >90% sensitivity and specificity. CT has better spatial resolution. MR is better characterization of mass, with pheochromocytomas showing high-signal intensity on T2-weighted images. Labelled MiBG is taken up by the chromaffin tissue and can be used as an adjunct to CT or MR imaging. Its advantages are that it can be used for whole-body scanning and is better at delineating extra-adrenal tumors and metastases. It may even be helpful in delineating the preclinical adrenal medullary hyperplasia. The disadvantages include a higher false-negative rate and the requirement of several days for completion.

- Localize the pheochromocytoma.
- CT or MR imaging of abdomen (if negative findings, image pelvis and thorax): mainstays of radiologic localization.
- CT: better spatial resolution.
- MR: better characterization of mass.
- Labelled MiBG is taken up by chromaffin tissue; used as adjunct to CT or MR imaging.

Treatment

Surgical excision of the tumor is curative. Medical treatment is used in preoperative preparation to diminish perioperative morbidity and mortality and on a chronic basis in surgical failures. α-Adrenergic blockade is the cornerstone of medical therapy and should be instituted as soon as the diagnosis is made. Phenoxybenzamine is the drug of choice to control the hypertension and to restore plasma volume. Start with a dose of 10 mg twice daily and increase every few days until the desired effect is obtained. Its major side effect is postural hypotension. Alternate drugs include prazosin, terazosin, labetalol, nifedipine, or ACE inhibitors. β-Blockade may be necessary to control tachyarrhythmias. They should only be used after adequate α-blockade. Propranolol 10 mg 3-4 times daily is usually adequate. For hypertensive emergencies, phentolamine, an α-blocker, is the drug of choice and can be given in 5-10-mg doses every 5-15 min as needed. Alternatively, nitroprusside or labetalol can be used. Long-term follow-up is important to assess for persistence, recurrence, or development of other manifestations of MEN IIA or IIB. If hypertension persists postoperatively, consider missed or metastatic pheochromocytoma, surgically induced renal ischemia, or underlying essential hypertension. For the inoperable pheochromocytoma, add metatyrosine, a competitive inhibitor of tyrosine hydroxylase, to the treatment.

- Surgical excision of the tumor is curative.
- Medical treatment: use preoperatively to diminish perioperative morbidity and mortality and on chronic basis in surgical failures.
- α-Adrenergic blockade: the cornerstone of medical therapy. Should be instituted as soon as diagnosis is made.
- β-Blockade: may be necessary to control tachyarrhythmias; use only after adequate α-blockade.
- For hypertensive emergencies: phentolamine (α-blocker) is the drug of choice.
- Long-term follow-up: important to assess for persis-

tence, recurrence, development of other manifestations of MEN IIA or IIB.

- If hypertension persists postoperatively, consider missed or metastatic pheochromocytoma, surgically induced renal ischemia, or underlying essential hypertension.

Incidentally Discovered Adrenal Mass

Small (1-6 cm) adrenal masses are found in up to 9% of unselected autopsies and in 0.7% of all abdominal CT scans. Most of these are nonfunctioning adenomas; a few are functioning adenomas or carcinomas of the adrenal cortex or medulla. Metastatic disease is frequent. The diagnostic approach should include:

1. Screening for pheochromocytoma. Measure 24-hour urinary metanephrines, vanillylmandelic acid, and fractionated catecholamines.
2. Screening for Cushing's syndrome. Use 1-mg overnight dexamethasone suppression test or a 24-hour urinary free cortisol.
3. Screening for primary aldosteronism. Use serum level of potassium in patients not taking diuretics and receiving >200 mEq of sodium per day.
4. For androgen-producing tumors, check serum dehydroepiandrosterone sulfate (DHEAS).
5. In addition, chest radiography to screen for carcinoma, tuberculosis, and fungal infection.
6. Assess size and nature of the mass on abdominal CT or MR.

- Screen for pheochromocytoma.
- Screen for Cushing's syndrome.
- Screen for primary aldosteronism.
- Check for androgen-producing tumors.
- Chest radiography.
- Assess size and nature of mass on abdominal CT or MR.

Management: surgical excision is indicated for functioning adrenal masses, large solid or solid-cystic masses (>6 cm in size), and cystic masses that have bloody contents on CT-guided needle aspiration. Otherwise, observation is indicated. The imaging study should be repeated in 3, 6, 12, and 24 months; an increase in size indicates need for surgical treatment.

- Surgical excision indicated for: functioning adrenal masses, large solid or solid-cystic masses (>6-cm size), cystic masses with blood contents on CT-guided needle aspiration.
- Otherwise, observation is indicated.

MALE GONADAL DISORDERS

Physiology

The male gonadal axis is shown in Fig. 11-13. The testis has two physiologic compartments: 1) the Leydig cells are endocrine cells whose main function is to secrete testosterone, and 2) the seminiferous tubules contain Sertoli cells and gametes and produce sperm. The full cycle of spermatogenesis takes 70-90 days. Sertoli cells also secrete inhibin.

- Two physiologic compartments of testis: Leydig cells and seminiferous tubules (Sertoli cells, gametes).
- Full cycle of spermatogenesis: 70-90 days.

Testosterone has two functions: 1) an endocrine function that includes development, growth, and maintenance of internal and external genitalia, secondary sex characteristics, libido and potency, pubertal growth spurt, and muscular development; and 2) a paracrine function, in which testosterone enters the adjoining seminiferous tubules and stimulates the early stages of spermatogenesis. Testosterone is a steroid that circulates in two forms: bound to a specific sex hormone-binding globulin (SHBG) and albumin (98%) and in a free form (2%). Testosterone acts intracellularly by binding to cytoplasmic- and nuclear-specific receptors. It also may function as a prohormone. Testosterone may undergo target-tissue transformation to dihydrotestosterone (DHT) by 5α-reductase (this occurs in such tissues as genitalia, prostate gland, and hair follicles) or to estradiol (E_2) by aromatase (as in the hypothalamus).

- Two functions of testosterone: endocrine and paracrine.
- Testosterone: a steroid circulating in bound (98%) and free (2%) forms.
- Also functions as a prohormone.
- Undergoes transformation to DHT by 5α-reductase in target tissue.
- Transformation to E_2 by aromatase.

A specific anterior pituitary cell, the gonadotrope, secretes the two pituitary hormones LH and FSH. These are glycoproteins consisting of α and β subunits. The α subunits are identical in the two hormones (and in TSH and hCG). The β subunit is hormone-specific and is responsible for its biologic effect. The system is regulated by one hypothalamic hormone, GnRH. GnRH is a decapeptide secreted in bursts every 70-90 min; it stimulates the production of LH and FSH by gonadotropes. The hypothalamic-pituitary-gonadal system is regulated by negative feedback as shown in Fig. 11-13. Inhibin has recently been isolated and characterized; it is a protein consisting of α and β polypeptide subunits and is synthesized by the Sertoli cells. Inhibin blocks GnRH-stimulated release of FSH. Activin, a newly described testicular peptide consisting of a dimer of the β-chains of inhibin, stimulates FSH secretion in vitro. The role of inhibin and activin in human physiology and disease states is not clear.

- Gonadotrope: specific anterior pituitary cell secreting LH and FSH.
- System is regulated by one hypothalamic hormone: GnRH.
- Inhibin is synthesized by Sertoli cells. Blocks GnRH-stimulated release of FSH.

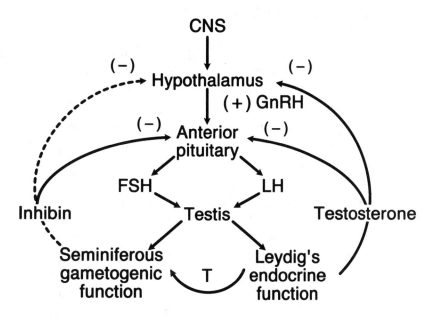

Fig. 11-13. Hypothalamic-pituitary-gonadal axis in males. CNS, central nervous system; FSH, follicle-stimulating hormone; GnRH, gonadotropin-releasing hormone; LH, luteinizing hormone; T, testosterone.

Sexual Development in Males

Testosterone is critical for the development of the male phenotype. Sex development in the male fetus proceeds in three phases: development of chromosomal sex, gonadal sex, and phenotypic sex. The chromosomal sex is 46,XY. In the presence of certain Y chromosome genes, the bipotential gonad develops into a testis. The fetus has bipotential internal and external genitalia; the internal genitalia are the wolffian and müllerian ducts. The fetal testes produce two hormones: testosterone and müllerian inhibitory factor (MIF). Testosterone is necessary for the development of the wolffian ducts into the male internal genitalia; MIF inhibits the development of the müllerian ducts. Testosterone is transformed by 5α-reductase in the bipotential external genitalia to DHT, which leads to the development of the male external genitalia.

- Three phases: development of chromosomal sex, gonadal sex, phenotypic sex.
- Chromosomal sex: 46,XY.
- In presence of certain Y chromosome genes, bipotential gonad develops into testis.
- Fetal testis produces two hormones: testosterone and MIF.
- Testosterone: necessary for development of wolffian duct.
- Testosterone transformed by 5α-reductase in bipotential genitalia to DHT. DHT leads to development of male external genitalia.

Laboratory Tests in Assessment of Male Gonadal Function

Semen analysis: normal volume, 2-5 mL; sperm count varies considerably but usually is >20 million/mL; motility, >60% at 2 hours; morphology, >60% normal forms. A normal semen analysis, with rare exceptions, rules out hypogonadism.

- Normal semen analysis, with rare exceptions, rules out hypogonadism.

Serum testosterone: measures bound (98%) and free (2%) testosterone. Its determinants are normal Leydig cell function and levels of SHBG. Low values indicate male hypogonadism. Serum level of testosterone may be low in eugonadal men with decreased SHBG, as in hypothyroidism, obesity, and acromegaly.

- Serum testosterone: determinants are normal Leydig cell function and levels of SHBG.

Serum free testosterone: measures the free biologically active fraction. It is not affected by conditions that modify SHBG levels.

Serum E_2: Low-normal or minimally increased levels may occur in primary testicular failure. Low levels in hypogonadotropism. Increased levels in hypogonadotropism due to estrogen-producing tumor.

Serum LH and FSH: LH and FSH are increased in patients with primary testicular failure and are "normal" or low in hypogonadotropism. Because of assay sensitivity limitations, values may be low in some eugonadal males. Always evaluate serum level of LH in relation to serum levels of testosterone and serum levels of FSH in relation to semen analysis. LH, and less so FSH, is secreted in a pulsatile pattern. Thus, for optimal evaluation, obtain 3 samples at 30- to 60-minute intervals and assay hormones in pooled sample.

- LH and FSH: increased in primary testicular failure.
- Normal or low in hypogonadotropism.
- Always evaluate serum level of LH in relation to serum level of testosterone.
- Evaluate serum levels of FSH in relation to semen analysis.

GnRH stimulation test: GnRH test does not help to distinguish between hypothalamic and pituitary causes of hypogonadotropism. Responses may be normal in pituitary disorders and absent in hypothalamic disorders. The test may sometimes be helpful in assessing pituitary reserve.

- GnRH test: does not help distinguish between hypothalamic and pituitary causes of hypogonadotropism.

hCG stimulation test: a provocative test to assess Leydig cell reserve; 4,000 IU are given intramuscularly daily for 4 days. Serum level of testosterone is measured before and on the 4th day of the test. It is useful in the differential diagnosis of cryptorchidism (normal response) from anorchia (no response).

Buccal smear: useful in the etiologic diagnosis of primary testicular failure. Presence of Barr bodies in >15% of mucosal cells in a male confirms the presence of an extra X chromosome (Klinefelter's syndrome and its variants), but the test results may be negative in Klinefelter's mosaics.

- Buccal smear: useful in etiologic diagnosis of primary testicular failure.

Karyotype: identifies sex chromosomal abnormalities, including mosaicism. However, it may not reveal mosaicism if this is present only in tissues other than those examined.

- Karyotype: identifies sex chromosomal abnormalities including mosaicism.

Testicular biopsy: useful in the diagnosis of severe oligospermia or azoospermia in males with normal testicular size and normal levels of testosterone and FSH. Such findings may be present in patients with spermatogenic arrest or ductal obstruction. Testicular biopsy and vasograms are needed for such differentiation.

Male Hypogonadism

Clinical Presentation

In adult males, hypogonadism can present as decreased libido, impaired potency, decreased ejaculate volume, infertility. Also, decreased energy and stamina; decreased sexual hair growth; and classic hypogonadal facies, with pallor and fine wrinkling around the mouth and eyes. There is also altered fat distribution, testicular atrophy, decrease in prostate size, osteoporosis, and gynecomastia. If hypogonadism develops acutely, hot flashes may occur.

In adolescents, hypogonadism presents as failure of sexual and physical maturation and sexual infantilism. There is absence of pubertal growth spurt, eunuchoid habitus, i.e., ratio of upper (crown to pubis)-to-lower (pubis to floor) segment is <1 and the ratio of span-to-height is >1, high-pitched voice, poor muscle development, and female pattern of fat distribution, also, small soft testes <2 cm in length and <2 mL in volume or gynecomastia. Note that small firm testes should suggest the presence of Klinefelter's syndrome and an associated anosmia/hyposmia points to Kallmann's syndrome.

The causes of male hypogonadism are outlined in Table 11-18.

Table 11-18.--Causes of Male Hypogonadism

Primary--testicular diseases (hypergonadotropic
 hypogonadism)
 Genetic and developmental
  Klinefelter's syndrome
  Male Turner's syndrome
  Noonan's syndrome
  46,XX male
  47,XYY male
  Functional prepubertal castrate
  Myotonia dystrophica
  Sertoli-cell-only syndrome
 Acquired
  Postpubertal testicular failure
  Cirrhosis
  Castration--trauma, surgery
  Irradiation
  Chemotherapy
 Male pseudohermaphroditism
  Complete
  Incomplete
   Androgen receptor defect
   5α-reductase deficiency
   Enzyme defect in testicular biosynthesis
   Lack of müllerian inhibitory factor
Secondary--hypothalamic-pituitary diseases
 (hypogonadotropic hypogonadism)
 Functional
  Systemic disease
  Malnutrition
  Anorexia nervosa
  Drugs
  Hyperprolactinemia
  Estrogen-producing tumors
  Thyroid disorders
  Adrenal disorders
 Organic
  Developmental
   Gonadotropin deficiency
    Isolated (Kallmann's syndrome, fertile eunuch
     syndrome)
    In association with deficiency of other pituitary
     hormones

Traumatic
Inflammatory
 Sarcoidosis
 Histiocytosis
 Granulomatous disease--tuberculosis
Degenerative--hemochromatosis
Vascular--carotid aneurysm
Neoplastic
 Pituitary tumors
 Craniopharyngioma
 Glioma
 Other primary and metastatic malignancies

Hypergonadotropic Hypogonadism

This may be congenital or acquired, and it may affect spermatogenic function, Leydig cell function, or both.

- Hypergonadotropic hypogonadism: may be congenital or acquired.
- May affect spermatogenic function and/or Leydig cell function.

Klinefelter's Syndrome

The basic defect in this common sex-chromosome anomaly (1:400-500) is the presence of one or more extra X chromosomes. The classic karyotype is 47,XXY. Variants include XXYY, poly X plus Y, and mosaicism. Pathologically, it is characterized by the development at puberty of seminiferous tubule hyalinization and clumping and varying levels of Leydig cell dysfunction. Clinically, it is characterized by small firm testes, gynecomastia, varying degree of testosterone deficiency and eunuchoidism, azoospermia, increased gonadotropin levels, and a positive buccal smear. Confirmation is by karyotyping of blood lymphocytes or testicular tissue. Patients with Klinefelter's syndrome have a slightly increased incidence of diabetes mellitus, chronic obstructive pulmonary disease, autoimmune disorders, varicose veins, malignancy of the breast, lymphoma, and germ cell neoplasm. The clinical picture may differ in variants and mosaics. If more than one X chromosome is present, the incidence of mental retardation and somatic abnormalities is increased. In mosaics, the clinical manifestations are less severe; if an XY line is present, fertility may be present. Infertility in classic Klinefelter's syndrome is irreversible. Testosterone therapy is given for androgen deficiency, and reduction mammoplasty is performed if the gynecomastia is a source of personal distress.

- Klinefelter's syndrome: basic defect is one or more extra X chromosomes.
- Classic karyotype is 47,XXY.
- Characterized pathologically by: seminiferous tubule hyalinization and clumping and varying levels of Leydig cell dysfunction.
- Characterized clinically by: small firm testes, gynecomastia, varying degree of testosterone deficiency and eunuchoidism, azoospermia, increased gonadotropin levels, and positive buccal smear.
- Confirmation: karyotyping of blood lymphocytes or testicular tissue.
- Clinical picture may differ in variants and mosaics.
- In classic Klinefelter's syndrome, infertility is irreversible.
- Testosterone therapy given for androgen deficiency.

Noonan's syndrome (Bonnevie-Ulrich): autosomal recessive; presence of Turner's stigmata in a patient with normal male karyotype; and primary testicular failure.

Acquired testicular disorders: first and foremost, impair spermatogenic function. Leydig cell failure occurs only in severe cases. Such disorders may include mumps orchitis in postpubertal males, chronic liver disease, and chronic renal failure. Testicular damage may result from irradiation: >6 Gy damage the seminiferous tubule and >8 Gy lead to Leydig cell damage. Cytotoxic agents, especially alkylating agents, damage spermatogenic function (consider sperm banking before therapy if fertility is an issue).

- Acquired testicular disorders: first and foremost, impair spermatogenic function.
- Only if severe, lead to Leydig cell dysfunction.

Sertoli-cell-only syndrome: azoospermia, testicular size somewhat reduced, normal or increased serum level of FSH, normal serum level of testosterone, no chromosome abnormality, no gynecomastia. Diagnosis is made by testicular biopsy. No treatment is available.

Myotonic dystrophy: 90% of men have testicular failure that is usually hypergonadotropic but may be hypogonadotropic in nature. Therapy consists only of testosterone therapy for Leydig cell failure.

Cryptorchidism: may be unilateral or bilateral; undescended testis may be intra-abdominal, inguinal, prescrotal, or ectopic. Associated indirect inguinal hernia (50%-90% of patients). Infertility is often present, even in unilateral cases; Leydig cell function is usually normal. Increased incidence of testicular cancer which is not reduced by surgical transposition. Correction should be performed by age 12 months; options include orchiopexy, endocrine therapy with GnRH, hCG, or both, or orchiectomy.

Aging in normal men: modest decrease in total and free testosterone; decreased spermatogenesis; modest increase in LH and FSH; increased incidence of sexual dysfunction; decreased muscle and bone mass. In summary, modest primary gonadal failure with reduction in spermatogenic and Leydig cell functions; fertility may not be affected.

Hypogonadotropic Hypogonadism

A hypothalamic-pituitary disorder may lead to decreased gonadotropin secretion and thus to decreased spermatogenesis and testosterone production. Rarely, it may be associated with isolated LH or FSH deficiency. It may be functional or organic and may or may not be associated with other primary function abnormalities (see section on Hypopituitarism).

- Hypogonadotropic hypogonadism: hypothalamic-pituitary disorder may lead to decreased gonadotropin secretion and thus decreased spermatogenesis and testosterone production.
- May be functional or organic.
- May or may not be associated with other pituitary function abnormalities.

Kallmann's Syndrome

Kallmann's syndrome is characterized by isolated hypogonadotropism plus anosmia/hyposmia. It is a congenital disorder, often familial, that is related to maldevelopment of the olfactory lobes and the GnRH-producing cells. Clinically, the patient presents with delayed puberty. Sexual infantilism, eunuchoidism, and occasionally a micropenis are present. Anosmia/hyposmia is present in 80% of patients. Other midline defects such as cleft lip or palate, color blindness, cryptorchidism, and skeletal abnormalities may also be present. Laboratory evaluation reveals hypogonadotropic findings. Other pituitary functions are normal. There may be unresponsiveness to a first single dose of GnRH; however, repeated GnRH stimulation leads to normal LH and FSH response. Therapy includes androgen replacement for sexual development and maintenance of sexual functions and secondary sex characteristics. Also, GnRH or gonadotropin therapy is warranted for fertility (is less effective if cryptorchidism is present).

- Kallmann's syndrome: isolated hypogonadotropism plus anosmia/hyposmia.
- Congenital disorder, often familial, and related to maldevelopment of olfactory lobes and GnRH-producing cells.
- Clinically, patient presents with delayed puberty.
- Anosmia/hyposmia is present in 80% of patients.
- Laboratory evaluation: hypogonadotropic findings; other pituitary functions are normal.
- Therapy: androgen replacement and GnRH or gonadotropin for fertility.

Acquired hypogonadotropism: remember hyperprolactinemia, which suppresses GnRH and presents with hypogonadotropism. Search for its cause. Therapy is with the dopamine agonist bromocriptine with or without androgen replacement. Evaluation and management of hypogonadotropic hypogonadism are outlined above (Hypopituitarism).

- Acquired hypogonadotropism: remember hyperprolactinemia, which suppresses GnRH and presents with hypogonadotropism.

Diagnostic Approach

Adult Male Hypogonadism

Diagnosis depends on assessing the clinical features, a semen analysis if feasible, and serum level of testosterone. For practical purposes, a normal semen analysis excludes hypogonadism. A low serum level of testosterone, total and free, points to hypogonadism (see below). Serum levels of LH and FSH determine whether the hypogonadism is primary testicular (hypergonadotropic) or secondary to hypothalamic-pituitary disease (hypogonadotropic). The cause of hypergonadotropism is usually obvious from the clinical setting. A karyotype is required to confirm sex and chromosome abnormalities. If the hypogonadism is hypogonadotropic, assess other pituitary functions and check the clinical setting for clues to functional disease (see Hypopituitarism). Among the functional disorders, the endocrine disorders of hyperprolactinemic syndrome, estrogen-producing tumors, and primary thyroid and adrenal disorders need to be considered. If functional hypogonadotropism has been excluded, perform CT or MR imaging of the hypothalamic-pituitary region and check visual fields if necessary.

- Diagnosis depends on: assessing clinical features, semen analysis if feasible, serum level of testosterone.
- Normal semen analysis (for practical purposes) excludes hypogonadism.
- Serum levels of LH and FSH: determine whether hypogonadism is primary testicular (hypergonadotropic) or secondary to hypothalamic-pituitary disease (hypogonadotropic).
- Cause of hypergonadotropism is usually obvious from clinical setting.
- If hypogonadism is hypogonadotropic, assess other pituitary functions and check clinical setting for clues to functional disease.
- If functional hypogonadotropism is excluded, image (CT/MR) hypothalamic-pituitary region and check visual fields if necessary.

Adolescent Male

The clinical setting and assessment of testicular volume are critical for the evaluation. If testicular volume is >4 mL, puberty has begun; observation and reassurance are indicated. If the volume is <4 mL, check serum levels of testosterone, LH, and FSH to document the disorder and to evaluate the axis level of dysfunction.

- Clinical setting and assessment of testicular volume are critical for evaluation.
- If testicular volume is >4 mL, puberty has begun.
- If volume is <4 mL, check serum levels of testosterone, LH, and FSH.

If hypogonadism is hypergonadotropic, diagnosis depends on clinical setting and karyotype. If it is hypogonadotropic, evaluate the sense of smell. Presence of anosmia/hyposmia, other midline congenital defects, and positive family history point to Kallmann's syndrome. If smell sensation is normal, check other pituitary functions and perform CT or MR imaging of the pituitary area. All the following point to constitutional delay of puberty: absence of other pituitary function abnormalities, no abnormality seen on imaging study, a positive family history of delayed but eventually normal puberty. Full pubertal development appears on follow-up examination. Presence of other pituitary function abnormalities and abnormal CT or MR findings point to organic hypothalamic-pituitary disorder (see above, Hypopituitarism).

- If hypergonadotropic, diagnosis depends on clinical setting and karyotype.

- If hypogonadotropic, evaluate sense of smell.
- If smell sensation is normal, check other pituitary functions and image (CT/MR) pituitary area.

Treatment of Male Hypogonadism

Androgen Therapy

In adults, androgen therapy is aimed at restoring and maintaining androgenic functions. In the hypogonadal pubertal male, it is designed to initiate and induce full pubertal development. It is important to remember that systemic testosterone cannot produce the high intratesticular levels of testosterone required to stimulate spermatogenesis. The drugs of choice for androgen replacement are testosterone enanthate or cypionate, long-acting 17-hydroxyl esters of testosterone. They are effective and safe. The usual dose is 200 mg intramuscularly every 10-20 days. Aggressive testosterone therapy in pubertal patients may lead to premature closure of the epiphyses and compromise adult height. The dose is 50-100 mg/2 weeks given intramuscularly and is generally increased to full replacement. Oral preparations available in the U.S. are all 17α-alkylated derivatives of testosterone. They are less effective, more costly, and can be associated with potentially serious side effects of hepatotoxicity, induction of peliosis hepatis, and hepatic tumors. Methyltestosterone is given in a dose of 25-50 mg daily by mouth or 10-25 mg daily buccally. Fluoxymesterone is given orally in a dose of 5-10 mg daily. Absolute contraindications for testosterone therapy are androgen-dependent tumors of the prostate and male breast. Relative contraindications include mental retardation, psychopathy, and elderly men with prostatism. Side effects include acne, mild weight gain, edema, increased erythropoiesis, and induction or worsening of obstructive sleep apnea.

- In adults, aims of androgen therapy: restore and maintain androgenic function.
- In hypogonadal pubertal males: to initiate and induce full pubertal development.
- Drugs of choice for androgen replacement: testosterone enanthate or cypionate.
- Aggressive testosterone therapy in pubertal patients may lead to premature closure of epiphyses and compromise adult height.
- Oral preparations: all 17α-alkylated derivatives of testosterone. Can have potentially serious side effects.
- Absolute contraindications for testosterone therapy are

androgen-dependent tumors of the prostate and male breast.

Gonadotropin or GnRH Therapy

The aim of gonadotropin or GnRH therapy is to induce spermatogenesis and establish fertility in hypogonadotropic patients. Therapy is expensive and requires multiple injections for gonadotropin therapy and pump administration for GnRH. For gonadotropin therapy, treatment is initiated with hCG alone in the dose of 2,000 IU subcutaneously or intramuscularly 3 times/week for 6-12 months. The aim is to increase intratesticular testosterone to induce maturation of the Sertoli cells and spermatogenesis. This is followed by the addition of human menopausal gonadotropin (hMG) in the dose of 75 IU intramuscularly or subcutaneously 3 times/week; spermatogenesis is completed and sperm may appear in the semen in 6-24 months. Although sperm counts are usually low in response to this therapy, fertility is restored in a substantial number of patients. After spermatogenesis is initiated, it may be maintained by hCG alone. In postpubertal patients with acquired hypogonadotropism, hCG alone may be sufficient to restore spermatogenesis. Pulsatile GnRH has been used successfully in patients with GnRH deficiency, such as Kallmann's syndrome. It requires a portable infusion pump with doses of GnRH given subcutaneously every 2 hours (to maintain gonadotrope responsiveness).

- Aim of therapy: to induce spermatogenesis and establish fertility in hypogonadotropic patients.
- Therapy is expensive.
- Requires multiple injections for gonadotropin therapy and pump administration for GnRH.
- For gonadotropin therapy: initiate treatment with hCG alone for 6-12 months.
- This is followed by addition of hMG.
- In postpubertal patients with acquired hypogonadotropism, hCG alone may be sufficient to restore spermatogenesis.
- Pulsatile GnRH: has been successful in patients with GnRH deficiency such as Kallmann's syndrome.
- Requires a portable infusion pump.

Anabolic Steroids and Athletes

Androgens have been and continue to be used to increase strength and performance in athletes. Because the potential risks outweigh the benefits, such androgen use should be strongly discouraged. Among the undesirable sequelae are hepatotoxicity, decreased spermatogenesis, and induction of hepatic tumors. The long-term effects of use of anabolic steroids are unknown.

- Such androgen use should be strongly discouraged.
- Undesirable sequelae: hepatotoxicity, decreased spermatogenesis, induction of hepatic tumors.

Male Infertility

Male infertility may result from 1) abnormal sperm count and quality; although this most commonly is "idiopathic" and related to impaired spermatogenesis, occasionally, it may be related to a well-defined disorder affecting the hypothalamic-pituitary-gonadal axis. 2) Ductal obstruction, which may be caused by congenital defects, vasectomy, postinfection obstruction, or cystic fibrosis. 3) Disorders of the accessory sex organs, ejaculation, or coital techniques. The major challenge in the etiologic diagnosis of azoospermia is to differentiate spermatogenic defects from ductal obstruction. An increased level of FSH points to a spermatogenic defect. However, FSH levels may be normal in both conditions. Diagnosis then depends on testicular biopsy and vasographic study.

- Male infertility may result from: abnormal sperm count and quality (is usually "idiopathic"); ductal obstruction; disorders of accessory sex organs, ejaculation, coital technique.
- Major challenge in etiologic diagnosis of azoospermia: differentiating spermatogenic defects from ductal obstruction. Determination of serum FSH level and, in some cases, testicular biopsy are needed to make the differentiation.

Varicocele is a common disorder affecting 10% of the general population. Its incidence in infertile men is 30%. It is usually left-sided (90% of men) and may be associated with infertility, decreased sperm count and motility, and abnormal morphology. Serum levels of testosterone, LH, and FSH are normal. Surgical repair improves fertility. Note that if the varicocele is right-sided, venous obstruction by malignancy and situs inversus should be ruled out.

- Varicocele is common; affects 10% of general population.
- Is usually left-sided (90%).
- May be associated with infertility.

- Serum levels of testosterone, LH, and FSH are normal.
- Surgical repair improves fertility.

Impotence

The causes of potency impairment are outlined in Table 11-19.

Table 11-19.--Causes of Impotence

Psychogenic, <50%
Vasculogenic--arterial, venous
Neurogenic--disorders of brain, spinal cord, or peripheral or autonomic nervous system
Endocrine
Diabetes mellitus
Neurogenic, vasculogenic, psychogenic, or mixed
Other endocrine disorders
Gonadal disorders
Hyperprolactinemia
Thyroid disorders
Adrenal disorders
Systemic disease
Renal failure
Liver disorder
Chronic bronchopulmonary disorders
Neoplastic disorders
Penile disorders--trauma, Peyronie's disease
Pharmacologic
Alcohol
Amphetamines, antidepressant agents, tranquilizers
Some antihypertensive drugs
Antiandrogens--cimetidine, spironolactone
Estrogens
Drugs associated with hyperprolactinemia

Diagnostic Approach

1) Careful history, physical examination, and selected appropriate laboratory studies can exclude or confirm many causes. 2) Endocrine evaluation includes measuring serum levels of testosterone, E_2, LH and FSH, prolactin, T_4 and TSH, and cortisol. 3) Screening test for vasculogenic impotence: intracavernous injection of a vasoactive drug such as papaverine, phentolamine, or prostaglandin E_1. Failure to achieve a normal response documents a vasculogenic disorder but does not distinguish between arterial and venous abnormalities. Additional vascular studies include duplex ultrasonography of the corpus cavernosum and penile arteriography (for arterial insufficiency) and cavernosometry and

cavernosography (for venous incompetence). 4) Evaluation for neurogenic impotence: presence of neurogenic bladder suggests diagnosis. Evaluate bulbocavernous reflex latency by EMG, and study somatosensory evoked response of the dorsal nerve to assess peripheral and sacral spinal function.

- Careful history, physical examination, selected appropriate laboratory studies.
- Endocrine evaluation: measure serum levels of testosterone, E_2, LH and FSH, prolactin, T_4 and TSH, cortisol.
- Screening test for vasculogenic impotence.
- Evaluation for neurogenic impotence.

Management

Treat the cause. Remove the offending drug or alcohol. Institute bromocriptine therapy for hyperprolactinemic disorders and testosterone therapy for hypogonadism. Recommend psychiatric counseling. Other available modalities include: 1) intracavernous pharmacotherapy; the risks include priapism (1%), corporal fibrosis (25%) with repeated injections, and hepatic dysfunction in those receiving papaverine; 2) external vacuum device or penile prosthesis; and 3) penile vascular surgery.

Gynecomastia

The causes of gynecomastia are outlined in Table 11-20.

Diagnostic Approach

If bilateral, rule out pseudogynecomastia (fatty enlargement). If unilateral, rule out tumors, especially carcinoma. Gynecomastia is identified by its firmness, fine nodularity, a central location posterior to the areola from which it spreads radially, and a well-defined outer border. Signs that should arouse suspicion of malignancy include eccentric location relative to the areola, unusual firmness, fixation, ulceration, bloody discharge from the nipple, and the presence of axillary lymphadenopathy. Mammography and excisional biopsy may be necessary for definitive diagnosis. A careful medical history, physical examination, and appropriate laboratory studies should rule out physiologic, pharmacologic, alcohol-related, and refeeding types of gynecomastia. Endocrine tests should include ones for testosterone, E_2, LH and FSH, βhCG, T_4 and TSH, DHEAS, prolactin, and, if needed, karyotyping.

- If bilateral gynecomastia, rule out pseudogynecomastia.
- If unilateral, rule out tumors.
- Signs that arouse suspicion of malignancy: eccentric location relative to areola, unusual firmness, fixation, ulceration, bloody discharge from nipple, axillary lymphadenopathy.
- Careful medical history, examination, appropriate laboratory studies to rule out: physiologic, pharmacologic, alcohol-related, refeeding types of gynecomastia.
- Endocrine tests: testosterone, E_2, LH and FSH, βhCG, T_4 and TSH, DHEAS, prolactin. Karyotype if needed.

Table 11-20.--Causes of Gynecomastia

Physiologic
Newborn
Adolescence
Aging
Pathologic
Decreased testosterone production
Primary testicular failure
Hypothalamic-pituitary testicular failure
Decreased testosterone action
Congenital
Acquired
Spironolactone, cimetidine
Increased estradiol production
hCG-producing tumors
Estrogen-producing tumors
Increased conversion of androgen to estrogen
Liver disease/alcohol
Thyrotoxicosis
Marked obesity
Hepatoma
Exogenous
Estrogenic drugs, alcohol
Refeeding gynecomastia
Hyperprolactinemic states
Uncertain causes
Methyltestosterone
Cytotoxic drugs
Amphetamine
Marihuana
Idiopathic

Management

Therapy may include reassurance, correction of underlying disorders, and tamoxifen (usually not helpful) or cosmetic surgery.

Female Gonadal Disorders

Physiology

The female gonadal axis is shown in Fig. 11-14. Function of the female gonadal system is characterized by cyclicity. Its dominant aspects are the ovarian cycle and endometrial menstrual cycle. The ovarian cycle is responsible for ovulation and the secretion of sex steroids and is under the control of the hypothalamic-anterior pituitary-gonadotropin axis.

- Cyclicity characterizes the function of the female gonadal axis during reproductive life.
- Ovarian cycle: responsible for ovulation and secretion of sex steroids.
- Under control of hypothalamic-anterior pituitary-gonadotropin axis.

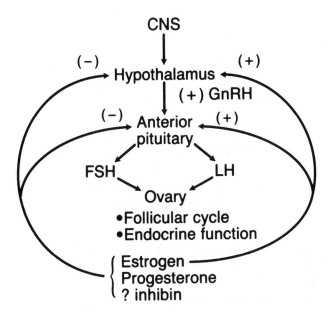

Fig. 11-14. Hypothalamic-pituitary-gonadal axis in females. Abbreviations same as in Figure 11-13.

The ovarian cycle consists of three phases: 1) follicular phase, primary follicle to mature graafian follicle; 2) ovulation; and 3) luteal phase dominated by the corpus luteum. If pregnancy does not occur, the corpus luteum regresses and another ovarian cycle is started. The hormone of the follicular phase is estradiol (E_2); luteal phase hormones are E_2 and progesterone. These hormones are responsible for the endometrial menstrual cycle. In the follicular phase, E_2 leads to proliferative endometrium. In the luteal phase, E_2 and progesterone lead to a secretory endometrium. With regression of the corpus luteum, steroid levels decrease, the endometrium is sloughed, and menstrual flow ensues.

- Three phases of ovarian cycle: follicular phase, ovulation, luteal phase.
- E_2: hormone of follicular phase.
- E_2 and progesterone: hormones of luteal phase.

The hypothalamic-pituitary unit controls the ovarian cycle. The hypothalamic decapeptide GnRH is secreted in bursts every 70-90 min. The anterior pituitary gonadotroph secretes the glycoproteins LH and FSH. Secretion of GnRH, LH, and FSH is cyclic. In the follicular phase, both gonadotropins are needed for follicular maturation and hormone secretion; LH leads to the synthesis of androgens by the thecal cells, and FSH promotes the growth of the granulosa cells and the aromatization of androgens to estrogens by these cells. A mid cycle LH peak causes ovulation. LH is needed for corpus luteum function. The female gonadal axis functions under negative and positive feedback. In general, steady or decreasing estrogen levels exert negative effects, increasing estrogen levels have positive effects, and the presence of both estrogen and progesterone has a negative effect. Documentation of ovulation is by 1) biphasic temperature curve (progesterone is thermogenic), 2) serial changes in cervical mucous and vaginal cell smear, 3) the presence of secretory endometrium on endometrial sampling, and 4) by the increase in the serum level of progesterone in the luteal phase.

- GnRH (hypothalamic decapeptide) is secreted in bursts every 70-90 min.
- GnRH, LH, FSH: secretion is cyclic.
- In follicular phase, both gonadotropins needed for follicular maturation and hormone secretion.
- Mid cycle LH peak causes ovulation.
- LH: needed for luteal function.
- Axis functions under negative and positive feedback.
- Document ovulation: biphasic temperature curve; presence of secretory endometrium on endometrial sampling; increase in serum levels of progesterone in luteal phase.

E_2 is secreted by the ovarian follicle and corpus luteum. It is responsible for: the initiation of female pubertal changes, development and maintenance of the genitalia and secondary sex characteristics, pubertal growth spurt and epiphyseal fusion, proliferative endometrium and receptive cervical mucus, breast duct development, negative and positive hypothalamic-pituitary feedback effect, and anabolic functions. Progesterone is secreted by the corpus luteum and is responsible for the secretory endometrium, hostile cervical mucus, breast and alveolar growth, hypothalamic-pituitary-gonadotropic axis feedback, and thermogenic effect. Androgens in females are responsible for libido, sexual hair growth, and anabolic functions.

Female sexual development has three phases: 1) chromosomal sex (46,XX in normal females); 2) gonadal sex, i.e., an ovary (absence of the Y chromosome and the presence of XX chromosomal constitution is necessary for full gonadal development); and 3) phenotypic sex. The ovary does not produce testosterone or MIF; therefore, the wolffian duct regresses and the müllerian duct develops into the female internal genitalia (fallopian tubes, uterus, and upper 2/3 of the vagina). In the absence of testosterone, no DHT is formed in the bipotential external genitalia and these structures develop into the female external genitalia.

- Three phases of female sexual development: chromosomal sex (46,XX), gonadal sex (ovary), phenotypic sex.
- Ovary does not produce testosterone or MIF.
- Without testosterone, no DHT is formed in bipotential external genitalia.

Amenorrhea

Etiology

The causes of amenorrhea are outlined in Table 11-21. Clinically, amenorrhea is best categorized as primary amenorrhea, which refers to absence of menarche in a phenotypic female who is at least 17 years old, and secondary amenorrhea, which refers to cessation of menstruation for at least 6 months in a woman with previously established menstrual function. Amenorrhea can result from impaired function of any component of the hypothalamic-pituitary-gonadal axis or from an anatomical abnormality of the genital tract. Outflow tract abnormalities are uncommon causes of primary or secondary amenorrhea. Developmental anomalies include imper-

Table 11-21.--Causes of Amenorrhea

Physiologic
    Premenarchal
    Pregnancy
    Postpartum state
    Postmenopausal
Pathologic
    Outflow tract disorders--genital tract aplasia, atresia, acquired destructive processes (e.g., Asherman's syndrome)
    Gonadal disorders
        Gonadal dysgenesis and its variants
        Other developmental disorders
        Autoimmune oophoritis and other destructive processes
        Polycystic ovaries
        Ovarian tumors
    Hypothalamic-pituitary disorders
        Functional
            Stress, diet, exercise
            Postpill
            Drugs
            Systemic disease
            Other endocrine disease
                Thyroid
                Adrenal
                Hyperprolactinemia
                Diabetes mellitus
        Delayed puberty
    Organic
        Isolated hypogonadotropism (e.g., Kallmann's syndrome)
        Hypopituitarism
            Various organic diseases--pituitary tumors, Sheehan's syndrome, hypophysitis

forate hymen, isolated absence of uterus, and vaginal aplasia or atresia. Acquired disorders include postabortive or postpartum endometritis, overzealous dilatation and curettage with destruction of the endometrial basal layer, and formation of adhesions and obliteration of the endometrial cavity (Asherman's syndrome and endometrial atrophy related to prolonged use of progestational agents or after treatment of endometriosis). Ovarian disorders, including developmental and acquired disorders, account for most of the causes of primary amenorrhea.

- Amenorrhea categorized clinically as primary and secondary amenorrhea.

- Can result from impaired function of any component of hypothalamic-pituitary-gonadal axis or from anatomical abnormality of genital tract.
- Outflow tract abnormalities: uncommon causes of primary or secondary amenorrhea.
- Ovarian disorders, developmental and acquired, account for most causes of primary amenorrhea.

Turner's 45/XO gonadal dysgenesis is the commonest cause of primary amenorrhea. It is estimated to affect 1 in 3,000 newborn females and is characterized by fibrous gonadal streaks, female phenotype, short stature, skeletal and developmental anomalies, and, in adolescent patients, primary ovarian failure and sexual infantilism. The physical abnormalities associated with Turner's syndrome include a webbed neck, low-set ears, multiple pigmented nevi, micrognathia, epicanthal folds, shield-like chest with microthelia, short metacarpals and metatarsals, an increased carrying angle at the elbows, renal developmental abnormalities, and cardiovascular anomalies (including coarctation of the aorta and aortic stenosis). In Turner's mosaics, patients have more than one sex chromosomal line, with commonest combination being 45/XO, 46/XX. The degree of ovarian dysgenesis varies depending on the ratio of XO to XX germ cells. Patients may present with primary or secondary amenorrhea. In cases of Turner's mosaics, the patients are not invariably short and may have few or many of the physical stigmata of Turner's syndrome, depending on which tissues get the XO chromosomal line.

- Turner's 45/XO gonadal dysgenesis: commonest cause of primary amenorrhea.
- Characterized by: fibrous gonadal streaks, female phenotype, short stature, skeletal and developmental anomalies, and, in adolescent patients, primary ovarian failure and sexual infantilism.
- Physical abnormalities associated with Turner's syndrome: renal developmental abnormalities and cardiovascular anomalies.
- Turner's mosaics: patients have more than one sex chromosomal line. Degree of ovarian dysgenesis varies depending on ratio of XO to XX germ cells.
- Turner's mosaics: patients may present with primary or secondary amenorrhea.

46/XX gonadal dysgenesis is characterized by a normal female karyotype, gonadal fibrous streaks, phenotypic female, and, in adolescent females, primary ovari-

an failure with failure of sexual maturation and primary amenorrhea. The patient has eunuchoidal features and does not have the physical stigmata of Turner's syndrome.

46/XY gonadal dysgenesis is characterized by fibrous streaks with a variable amount of testicular tissue, a female phenotype, and, in adolescent females, failure of normal sexual maturation and primary amenorrhea. Often, there is postpubertal virilization as a result of androgen secretion by the dysgenetic gonad. Such gonads are at an increased risk of neoplastic transformation; hence, gonadectomy is advisable as soon as the diagnosis is made.

True hermaphroditism is defined by the presence of both ovarian and testicular tissues in either the same or opposite gonads. The karyotype can be 46/XX or 46/XY, although some patients have mosaicism. The external genitalia are often ambiguous but can be distinctly female or male. The uterus is present in virtually all patients. At puberty, significant breast development occurs in most and menstruation in more than half of the patients. Some patients present with primary amenorrhea.

Testicular feminization is a hereditary disorder transmitted as an X-linked recessive trait that affects genetic males. It is characterized by peripheral tissue unresponsiveness to androgen (testosterone and dihydrotestosterone) due to androgen receptor abnormality. The vagina is often shallow, ending in a blind pouch. The testes may be inguinal and simulate an "inguinal hernia" or may be intra-abdominal. These male pseudohermaphrodites are raised as females. In adolescence, with the gonadotropin pubertal surge and increased estrogen production by the testes, normal breast and female secondary sexual maturation occurs except for the absence of sexual hair (which is androgen-dependent) and for primary amenorrhea. Gonadectomy is required after completion of pubertal development to forestall the development of neoplastic changes.

- Testicular feminization: affects genetic males.
- Characterized by peripheral tissue unresponsiveness to androgen (testosterone, dihydrotestosterone) due to androgen receptor abnormality.
- In adolescence, normal breast and female secondary sexual maturation occurs except for absence of sexual hair and for primary amenorrhea.
- Gonadectomy required after completion of pubertal development.

Ovarian disorders are common causes of secondary amenorrhea. The commonest disorder is polycystic ovary syndrome (see Hirsutism). Ovarian destructive processes are an uncommon cause of secondary amenorrhea and premature menopause. These processes include autoimmune oophoritis as part of polyendocrine autoimmune disease, various forms of mosaic gonadal dysgenesis that lead to premature exhaustion of the complement of ovarian follicles, abdominal irradiation, chemotherapy with such agents as cyclophosphamide and vincristine, and ovarian tumors that cause secondary amenorrhea by hormonal abnormalities (hypersecretion of estrogen, androgen, or hCG) or, if bilateral, by destruction of the ovarian tissue.

- Ovarian disorders: common causes of secondary amenorrhea.
- Commonest disorder: polycystic ovary syndrome.
- Ovarian destructive processes: uncommon cause of secondary amenorrhea and premature menopause.

Hypothalamic-pituitary disease can cause gonadotropin deficiency and amenorrhea by destruction of pituitary gonadotrophs or hypothalamic GnRH cell population by organic diseases of various origins or by functional suppression of these cells, commonly by a hyperprolactinemic state, nutritional disorder, and anorexia nervosa (see above, Hypopituitarism). Hypothalamic disorders are the least frequent causes of primary amenorrhea. Isolated deficiency of GnRH occurs in females but much less than in males. In some patients, it is associated with anosmia or hyposmia caused by hypoplasia or aplasia of the olfactory lobe (Kallmann's syndrome). This syndrome is familial and may be associated with midline craniofacial defects and other skeletal abnormalities. Constitutional delay in puberty can occur in females but less frequently than in males. It may be genetic, and a parent or a sibling may have experienced a similar delay. The patients have evidence of delayed growth throughout childhood and delayed bone age, but they ultimately progress through the normal stages of puberty. Organic hypothalamic-pituitary disease due to various causes is an uncommon cause of primary amenorrhea. In young adults, craniopharyngioma is the commonest space-occupying lesion; prolactinomas occur in this age group but are rare.

- Hypothalamic-pituitary disease can cause gonadotropin deficiency and amenorrhea by destruction of pituitary gonadotropin or hypothalamic GnRH cell population.
- Or, by functional suppression of these cells (by hyper-

prolactinemic state, nutritional disorder, anorexia nervosa).
- Hypothalamic disorders: the least frequent causes of primary amenorrhea.
- In young adults, craniopharyngioma is the commonest space-occupying lesion.

Hypothalamic-pituitary disorders are the commonest pathologic causes of secondary amenorrhea and may be either functional or organic. Functional hypogonadotropism results from hypothalamic amenorrhea caused by a defect in the cyclic center, inhibition of the mid cycle surge of GnRH and LH, and the failure of ovulation. This disorder is seen in anorexia nervosa and nutritional deficiency and in association with the following: physical exercise (e.g., running), various forms of emotional stress (e.g., young women in college, teenagers at camp, during bereavement), use of oral contraceptives, use of progestational agents, systemic disease, thyroid disorders, uncontrolled diabetes mellitus, hyperandrogenic state caused by adrenal or ovarian disorders, and estrogen-producing tumors. Postpill amenorrhea is common, accounting for about 30% of cases of secondary amenorrhea. It occurs in about 2% of women taking birth control pills who may or may not have had prepill menstrual irregularity. Of patients with postpill amenorrhea, 30% have hyperprolactinemia; some of these may have underlying pituitary adenoma. Generally, spontaneous recovery occurs in a few months unless a pituitary adenoma is present. Psychotropic drugs, especially the phenothiazine family, can cause hypogonadotropism by a direct effect at the hypothalamic level or secondary to hyperprolactinemia from the antidopaminergic effect of these drugs.

- Hypothalamic-pituitary disorders: commonest pathologic cause of secondary amenorrhea.
- May be functional or organic.
- Postpill amenorrhea is common, accounting for about 30% of cases of secondary amenorrhea.
- Of patients with postpill amenorrhea, 30% have hyperprolactinemia.
- Psychotropic drugs, especially phenothiazine family, can cause hypogonadotropism by direct effect at hypothalamic level or secondary to hyperprolactinemia.

Anorexia nervosa, a syndrome seen almost exclusively in young females, is manifested predominantly by weight loss, amenorrhea, and behavioral disorder. The age of onset is usually <25 years. Weight loss can be extreme and accompanied by a distorted and implacable attitude toward eating and weight. The patients deny their illness and fail to recognize their nutritional needs. Some may manifest unusual hoarding and handling of food. Bulimia (excessive food intake) and vomiting are seen in 50% of the patients. Amenorrhea occurs in all young female patients with anorexia nervosa, and in 25% of them, it precedes the weight loss. Other features include bradycardia, hypotension, constipation, impaired temperature regulation (inability to shiver and maintain body temperature in face of hypothermia or hyperthermia), lanugo hair growth, hypercarotenemia, and, in severe cases, dependent edema. Endocrine findings include hypogonadotropism, normal or increased serum levels of GH and low IGF-I, normal serum levels of T_4 and TSH but decreased levels of T_3 and increased reversed T_3 levels, serum cortisol levels that are generally increased and show normal suppressibility with dexamethasone, decreased 24-hour urinary 17-ketogenic and 17-ketosteroids, and normal serum level of prolactin.

- Anorexia nervosa: seen almost exclusively in young females.
- Predominant manifestations: weight loss, amenorrhea, and behavioral disorder.
- Amenorrhea occurs in all the young female patients, and in 25%, it precedes weight loss.
- Endocrine findings: hypogonadotropism, normal/increased GH serum level, low IGF-I, normal T_4 and TSH levels, decreased T_3 and increased reversed T_3 levels, cortisol levels in serum increased (normal suppressibility with dexamethasone), normal prolactin level in serum.

Primary hypothyroidism can lead to amenorrhea via three mechanisms: anovulation (in mild cases may lead to breakthrough bleeding and menorrhagia; in severe cases, to amenorrhea); hyperprolactinemia (can occur in 20%-30% of patients with primary hypothyroidism, can cause functional suppression of the hypothalamic-pituitary-gonadotropin axis); and associated autoimmune primary ovarian failure and consequent amenorrhea. Adrenal disorders can lead to amenorrhea through a hyperandrogenic state (congenital adrenal hyperplasia, Cushing's syndrome, adrenal tumors), through chronic adrenocortical insufficiency (by its effects on general health and nutrition), or by its association with autoimmune primary ovarian failure.

- Primary hypothyroidism can lead to amenorrhea.
- Three mechanisms: anovulation, hyperprolactinemia, associated autoimmune primary ovarian failure.

Hypogonadotropism can be the only manifestation of hypothalamic-pituitary organic disease or it can occur in association with other pituitary function abnormalities (see above, Hypopituitarism). Hyperprolactinemia is a common cause of secondary amenorrhea, accounting for 25%-40% of all cases. Postpartum pituitary necrosis (Sheehan's syndrome), previously a common cause, has declined in incidence with improvement in obstetric care.

- Hypogonadotropism can occur: as only manifestation of hypothalamic-pituitary disease or in association with other pituitary function abnormalities.
- Hyperprolactinemia: common cause of secondary amenorrhea (25%-40% of all cases).

Diagnostic Approach to Amenorrhea

Serum E_2: low values occur in hypogonadism of any cause. Because normal values may be found in anovulatory states, they may not be indicative of a normal gonadal axis.

- Low values: in hypogonadism of any cause.

Serum LH and FSH: these gonadotropins are secreted in a cyclic, pulsatile fashion; normal values vary depending on the phase of the ovulatory cycle. LH and FSH should always be evaluated in relation to menstrual function or serum E_2 levels. In hypogonadal females, high values indicate primary ovarian failure, but "normal" or low values indicate hypogonadism of hypothalamic-pituitary origin. A high LH/FSH ratio (>2) is common in polycystic ovarian syndrome.

- LH and FSH: always evaluate in relation to menstrual function or serum E_2 levels.
- Hypogonadal females: high values indicate primary ovarian failure; normal/low values indicate hypogonadism of hypothalamic-pituitary origin.

Serum prolactin: should always be assessed in the evaluation of amenorrhea. Hyperprolactinemia is a common cause of hypogonadotropism and points to a hypothalamic-pituitary disorder. Remember that the commonest cause of amenorrhea and hyperprolactinemia is pregnancy.

- Serum prolactin level: always assess it in evaluating amenorrhea.
- Commonest cause of amenorrhea and hyperprolactinemia: pregnancy.

The GnRH test: usually is not helpful in distinguishing between hypothalamic and pituitary causes of hypogonadotropism. The gonadotropin responses may be exaggerated, normal, or reduced in disorders of either the hypothalamus or pituitary.

- GnRH test: usually not helpful in distinguishing between hypothalamic and pituitary causes of hypogonadotropism.

Secondary Amenorrhea

1) Rule out physiologic amenorrhea: clinical setting and pregnancy test. 2) Rule out genital tract outflow disorders: evaluate clinical setting; in outflow disorders, progesterone test and estrogen/progesterone test results are negative. 3) Rule out hyperandrogenic state (see below, Hirsutism). 4) Measure serum levels of E_2, LH, and FSH to distinguish ovarian from hypothalamic-pituitary disorders. Low serum levels of E_2 and increased levels of FSH and LH point to primary ovarian failure; a karyotype is necessary in patients <35 years old. Low serum levels of E_2 and inappropriately low levels of LH and FSH point to hypothalamic-pituitary disorder. Rule out a functional disorder; if present, correct it; if periods resume, the diagnosis is functional disorder. If a functional disorder is not present or if its correction does not lead to the resumption of menstrual function, proceed with tests to rule out organic hypothalamic-pituitary disease. These include serum prolactin, other pituitary hormones, CT or MR imaging of the sella, and visual fields, if necessary. If an identifiable organic disease is found, treat it appropriately, but if no such organic disease is found, consider the amenorrhea to be of indeterminate cause and pursue long-term follow-up; an identifiable cause may become apparent in months or years.

- Rule out: physiologic amenorrhea, genital tract outflow disorders, hyperandrogenic state.
- Measure serum levels of E_2, LH, FSH to distinguish ovarian from hypothalamic-pituitary disease.
- Low levels E_2 and increased levels FSH and LH: primary ovarian failure.
- Low levels E_2 and inappropriately low levels FSH and LH: hypothalamic-pituitary disorder.

- Rule out functional disorder.
- If no functional disorder: perform tests to rule out hypothalamic-pituitary disease.
- If no organic disease: consider amenorrhea to be of indeterminate cause and pursue long-term follow-up.

Primary Amenorrhea

Evaluate the secondary sex characteristics: 1) If the sex characteristics are those of an adult female and pregnancy test results are negative, consider outflow obstruction (imperforate hymen), genital tract anomalies (such as absent uterus), or testicular feminization. Diagnosis depends on the clinical picture, pelvic examination, and use of pelvic ultrasonography. 2) If hyperandrogenic manifestations are present, proceed with work-up (as for hirsutism). 3) If sexually infantile, check serum levels of E_2, LH, and FSH and proceed as for secondary amenorrhea.

- Evaluate secondary sex characteristics.
- If adult female sex characteristics and negative results with pregnancy test: consider outflow obstruction, genital tract anomalies, testicular feminization.
- If sexually infantile: check serum levels E_2, LH, FSH and proceed as for secondary amenorrhea.

Management of Hypogonadal Females

It is important to identify and treat the cause. Reversing the cause of functional amenorrhea--e.g., restoring lost weight, reducing excessive physical exercise, surgical treatment for pituitary tumors, bromocriptine therapy for hyperprolactinemic disorders--usually restores normal menstrual function. If successful treatment of the cause is not possible, estrogen replacement is indicated.

- It is important to identify and treat the cause.
- If successful treatment of cause is not possible, estrogen replacement is indicated.

The goals of estrogen therapy include controlling vasomotor instability, preventing genitourinary atrophy, preserving secondary sex characteristics, preventing osteoporosis, reducing the risk of coronary artery disease (probable), and restoring a sense of well-being. Absolute contraindications to estrogen therapy include known or suspected estrogen-dependent neoplasm (breast or uterus), cholestatic hepatic dysfunction, active thromboembolic disorder, history of thromboembolic disorder associated with previous estrogen use, neuro-ophthalmologic vascular disease, and undiagnosed vaginal bleeding. Complications of estrogen replacement include: 1) increased risk of endometrial cancer which is dose- and duration-dependent (4x-8x); such cancer is usually stage I with no excess mortality; this risk is prevented by progestin supplementation; 2) possible risk of breast cancer; the weight of present evidence indicates no such increased risk; pretreatment breast examination and mammography (and annually thereafter) are essential; and 3) increased risk of surgical gallbladder disease.

- Complications of estrogen treatment: increased risk of endometrial cancer (prevented by progestin supplementation), possible risk of breast cancer, increased risk of surgical gallbladder disease.

Estrogen therapy can be administered orally, parenterally, topically, or transdermally. In women with a uterus and who need supplemental progestin, the therapy can be given sequentially or in combination. In sequential therapy, estrogen may be given as conjugated equine estrogen (or equivalent) in a dose of 0.625 mg daily in patients >45 years (or 0.9-1.25 mg in those <45 years) on days 1-25 of each month and supplemented with a progestin, such as medroxyprogesterone acetate in a dose of 5-10 mg/day, days 14-25 of each month. Such sequential therapy results in predictable cyclic withdrawal bleeding in 50%-60% of patients. For unpredictable bleeding, endometrial biopsy is indicated.

- Sequential therapy results in predictable cyclic withdrawal in 50%-60% of patients.
- For unpredictable bleeding: endometrial biopsy.

Combination therapy mimics oral contraceptive combinations. Its goal is to induce endometrial atrophy and amenorrhea in those who find cyclic withdrawal bleeding inconvenient or unacceptable. Conjugated equine estrogen is given in the same doses daily and medroxyprogesterone acetate in a dose of 2.5 mg daily. Most patients become amenorrheic in 4-6 months and can expect irregular spotting during that time.

- Combination therapy mimics oral contraceptive combinations.
- Goal: induce endometrial atrophy and amenorrhea in those who find cyclic withdrawal bleeding inconvenient or unacceptable.

Estrogen replacement therapy must be individualized and be given only after a thorough discussion with the patient about the pros and cons of the therapy. Start therapy as soon as possible after the diagnosis of estrogen deficiency and continue it indefinitely or until the cause has been reversed. No estrogen preparation is superior to the other, and the cardioprotective effect of transdermal estradiol is unproved. Supplemental progestin is indicated only for women who have a uterus; medroxyprogesterone acetate is preferred rather than 19-nortestosterone derivatives, because it is less likely to lower HDL-C levels. Before estrogen therapy is initiated, it is advisable to give medroxyprogesterone acetate, 10 mg daily for 10-14 days. If no withdrawal bleeding occurs, an atrophic endometrium is present (after ruling out pregnancy in appropriate setting) and estrogen therapy can be initiated. However, if withdrawal bleeding occurs, the endometrium is estrogen-primed and consideration should be given to performing endometrial biopsy to rule out endometrial hyperplasia before initiating estrogen replacement therapy.

- Estrogen replacement therapy: must be individualized.
- Give it only after thoroughly discussing the pros and cons.

Ovulation Induction

Hypogonadal women who desire fertility can receive treatment with clomiphene citrate, gonadotropin, or GnRH. The drug of choice for hyperprolactinemic infertility is the dopamine-agonist bromocriptine (see above, Hyperprolactinemic Syndrome and Prolactinomas).

Clomiphene citrate acts like an antiestrogen at the hypothalamic level and stimulates endogenous gonadotropin secretion. Its main use is in patients with chronic anovulation related to functional hypothalamic disorder and in patients with polycystic ovarian disease. It is given in a dose of 50 mg/day for 5 days; the dose can be increased by increments of 50 mg/day in successive cycles to a maximum of 250 mg/day for 5 days. An ovulatory surge occurs 5-12 days after completion of clomiphene and can be documented by basal body temperature or serum progesterone level. If needed, hCG can be given 7 days after last dose of clomiphene. Ovulation occurs in about 80% of patients, and 40%-50% achieve pregnancy. Multiple pregnancy rate (twins in most cases) occurs in <10% of patients. Side effects occur in <5% of patients and include vasomotor flushes, nausea or vomiting, abdominal discomfort, and visual symptoms. Symptomatic ovarian enlargement is rare.

- Clomiphene citrate: acts like antiestrogen at hypothalamic level.
- Stimulates endogenous gonadotropin secretion.
- Main use: patients with chronic anovulation related to functional hypothalamic disorder and patients with polycystic ovarian disease.

Gonadotropin therapy is indicated for patients with organic pituitary disease and for patients from whom a trial of clomiphene was unsuccessful. Gonadotropin therapy should be initiated and followed by an experienced reproductive endocrinologist: hMG, consisting of FSH and LH, or human FSH is given to achieve follicular development; hCG is then given to simulate the LH surge. This therapy is expensive and may have significant complications, including a 30% incidence of multiple pregnancies and ovarian hyperstimulation syndrome. The latter is the major side effect and consists of ovarian enlargement with multiple follicular cysts and edema, ascites, hypovolemia, and hemoconcentration. Gonadotropin therapy is monitored by measuring E_2 levels and pelvic ultrasonography. When hyperstimulation syndrome is present, conservative treatment is indicated; avoid pelvic examination because of danger of ovarian rupture. The condition resolves slowly over 7 days.

- Gonadotropin therapy: indicated for patients with organic pituitary disease and patients for whom a trial of clomiphene was unsuccessful.
- Therapy should be initiated and followed by an experienced reproductive endocrinologist.

GnRH therapy may be used for patients with a hypothalamic syndrome and intact pituitary gland. It is most effective in hypothalamic anovulation. Administer 5-20 μg (intravenously, subcutaneously, or by pump) every 90 min or so. Hyperstimulation is extremely unlikely. Its major disadvantage is the need for an elaborate setup.

- GnRH therapy: for patients with hypothalamic syndrome and intact pituitary gland.

Oral Contraceptives

Oral contraceptives are widely used and are of two types: 1) a combination of estrogen and progestin and 2) a progestin-only pill. The estrogen component is either mestranol or ethinyl estradiol, and the progestin component is one of six derivatives of 19-nortestosterone. Oral contraceptives inhibit GnRH secretion and the mid cycle LH surge. They also render the cervical mucus scanty, thick, and viscid and decrease fallopian tube motility, among other effects. Endometrial atrophy ensues (decreased vaginal menstrual flow) and vaginal epithelial maturation is decreased (increased incidence of candidial vaginitis). The failure rate is 0.1% in the first year.

- Two types of oral contraceptives: combination of estrogen and progestin and progestin-only.
- Oral contraceptives inhibit GnRH secretion and mid cycle LH surge.
- Failure rate in first year: 0.1%.

The metabolic effects of oral contraceptives include insulin resistance and impaired glucose tolerance, increased very-low-density lipoprotein and triglycerides, increased hepatic production of α_2-globulins (including angiotensinogen), and increase in blood coagulation factors and carrier proteins (e.g., TBG or transcortin). The complications of oral contraceptives are related principally to the estrogen component and include: increased risk (4x-10x) of thromboembolism, increased risk of coronary artery disease and strokes (advanced maternal age and smoking are major risk factors), increased frequency and severity of migraine headaches, hypertension (which is usually reversible), increased risk of development of hepatic adenoma (which may rupture and can be fatal), and postpill amenorrhea. The beneficial effects of oral contraceptives, in addition to contraception, include a decreased risk of benign breast disease, endometrial and ovarian cancer, and pelvic inflammatory disease. The relation of oral contraceptives to cervical cancer, pituitary tumors, and melanoma is unclear.

- Metabolic effects of oral contraceptives: insulin resistance and impaired glucose tolerance, increased very-low-density lipoprotein and triglycerides, increased hepatic production of α_2-globulins, increase in blood coagulation factors and carrier proteins.
- Complications: related principally to estrogen component.
- Complications include: increased risk of thromboembolism, coronary artery disease and strokes, increased frequency and severity of migraine headaches, hypertension, increased risk of hepatic adenoma, postpill amenorrhea.

The absolute contraindications to the use of oral contraceptives include thrombophlebitis and thromboembolic disorders, cardiovascular disease, impaired liver function, known or suspected estrogen-dependent tumors of the breast or uterus, pregnancy, and familial hypertriglyceridemia (for fear of precipitating pancreatitis). Oral contraceptives should be used very cautiously in women who smoke, are obese, or have varicose veins. If elective surgery is planned for a patient taking oral contraceptives, use of the medication is stopped 2 weeks preoperatively and resumed 2 weeks postoperatively.

Hyperandrogenic Syndrome: Hirsutism/Virilization

Sources of Circulating Androgens in Females

The sources of circulating androgens in females are shown in Fig. 11-15. Total serum testosterone includes free (1%-2%) and bound (98%-99%) components. Testosterone is bound to SHBG and albumin. In hyperandrogenic females, a high level of testosterone and a high level of DHEAS point to an adrenal origin, whereas a high level of testosterone and normal or slightly increased level of DHEAS point to ovarian origin of the hyperandrogenic state.

- Total serum testosterone: free (1%-2%), bound (98%-99%).
- In hyperandrogenic females: high level of testosterone and high level DHEAS point to adrenal
- origin.
  High level testosterone and normal/slightly increased level DHEAS point to ovarian origin.

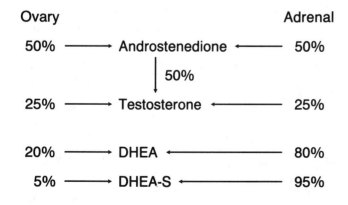

Fig. 11-15. Sources of circulating androgens in females. DHEA, dehydroepiandrosterone; DHEAS, dehydroepiandrosterone sulfate.

In hair follicles, testosterone is converted to dihydrotestosterone through the activity of 5α-reductase. Dihydrotestosterone is the active androgen in hair follicles. It is metabolized within the pilosebaceous unit to 3α-androstenediol glucuronide.

- In hair follicles, testosterone is converted to dihydrotestosterone via 5α-reductase.
- Dihydrotestosterone: active androgen in hair follicles.

Clinical Presentations

In order of increasing severity, the hyperandrogenic state may present with acne, hirsutism, menstrual and ovulatory disorders, defeminization, masculinization, and clitorimegaly.

- Clinical presentation in order of increasing severity: acne, hirsutism, menstrual and ovulatory disorders, defeminization, masculinization, clitorimegaly.

The causes of hyperandrogenicity are outlined in Table 11-22.

Table 11-22.--Causes of Hyperandrogenism

Exogenous--drugs
    Androgens
    Anabolic steroids
    Androgen-related progestin
    Metyrapone
Endogenous
    Neoplastic--autonomous production of androgens
        Ovarian tumors
        Adrenal tumors--benign, malignant
    Non-neoplastic--trophic hormone-dependent production
      of androgens
        Ovarian--LH-dependent
            Idiopathic hirsutism
            Polycystic ovaries
            Others/rare
        Adrenals--ACTH-dependent
            Late-onset congenital adrenal hyperplasia
                21-hydroxylase deficiency
                11-hydroxylase deficiency
                3β-ol-dehydrogenase deficiency
            Cushing's syndrome
            Hyperprolactinemic disorders

Diagnostic Approach

The most important clinical diagnostic clues relate to evaluation of the time of onset, tempo of progression, and severity of the hyperandrogenic state. In addition, search for pelvic or abdominal masses, features of Cushing's syndrome, and galactorrhea. A benign disorder is suggested by disease onset at puberty and a mild slowly progressive course. The rapid onset of disease at any age and a severe, rapidly progressive course point to a malignant disorder.

- Most important diagnostic clues relate to evaluating time of onset, tempo of progression, and severity of hyperandrogenic state.
- Benign disorder suggested by: onset at puberty, mild slowly progressive course.
- Malignant disorder suggested by: rapid onset at any age, severe rapidly progressive course.

The serum levels of testosterone and DHEAS are essential for diagnostic laboratory evaluation. Also, a screen for Cushing's syndrome (overnight 1-mg dexamethasone suppression test or 24-hour urinary free cortisol) and serum prolactin are also required. In selected patients and as guided by the clinical history and findings, determining the serum level of 17-hydroxyprogesterone with or without cosyntropin test for confirmation of congenital adrenal hyperplasia and determining the serum LH:FSH ratio for support of diagnosis of polycystic ovarian syndrome might be needed. Also in selected patients suspected of having neoplasm, pelvic ultrasonography and abdominal CT are necessary.

- Serum levels of testosterone and DHEAS: essential for diagnostic laboratory evaluation.
- Screen for Cushing's syndrome.
- Serum level of prolactin is required.

If plasma DHEAS is >7 ng/dL, the differential diagnosis is between adrenal tumor and late-onset congenital adrenal hyperplasia. Proceed with CT scan of the abdomen; if the findings are negative, proceed with serum 17-hydroxyprogesterone and cosyntropin test. Also, test for dexamethasone suppressibility of DHEAS.

- If plasma level of DHEAS is >7 ng/dL, differential diagnosis is between adrenal tumor and late-onset congenital adrenal hyperplasia.

Plasma levels of DHEAS that are <7 ng/dL exclude adrenal tumor and congenital adrenal hyperplasia. Proceed with measuring the serum level of testosterone; levels >200 ng/dL should raise the suspicion of ovarian tumor; pelvic ultrasonography and CT are required and, if necessary, laparoscopy and exploration. A serum level of testosterone <200 ng/dL points to polycystic ovarian syndrome.

- If plasma level of DHEAS is <7 ng/dL, measure serum level of testosterone.
- If serum level of testosterone is >200 ng/dL, suspect ovarian tumor.
- Serum level of testosterone <200 ng/dL, polycystic ovarian syndrome.

Idiopathic hirsutism. There is a modest increase in androgen production (mostly ovarian), with increased peripheral androgen production and increased sensitivity of the hair follicle. The hyperadrenogenicity is mild and LH-dependent. Also, the onset is at puberty and the disease has very slow progression; menstrual cycles are ovulatory; pelvic examination is normal. The serum levels of testosterone and DHEAS and the LH:FSH ratio are normal. Pelvic ultrasonographic findings are normal.

- Idiopathic hirsutism: modest increase in androgen production (mostly ovarian).
- Other features: LH-dependent, onset at puberty, very slow progression, menstrual cycles are ovulatory, normal serum level testosterone and DHEAS, and normal LH:FSH.

Polycystic ovarian syndrome is the commonest cause of hyperandrogenicity, but its pathogenesis is poorly understood. The ovaries are enlarged (70% of patients) and have multiple cysts and stromal thickening. Hyperandrogenicity is mild to moderate and is LH-dependent. Disease onset is at puberty and shows slow progression; hirsutism (70% of patients), menstrual abnormality (88%), infertility and anovulation (75%), and obesity (50%) are usually present. The serum level of testosterone is normal or modestly increased (70% of patients) and is nearly always <200 ng/mL. DHEAS levels are normal or mildly increased in 25% of patients, and the LH:FSH ratio is >2 in 75%. Changes seen on pelvic ultrasonography are characteristic (70%); hyperprolactinemia may be present in 25%-30% of patients. Serum levels of E_2 are normal; estrone levels are increased, and the risk of endometrial hyperplasia is increased.

- Polycystic ovarian syndrome: commonest cause of hyperandrogenicity.
- Hyperandrogenicity: mild to moderate, LH-dependent.
- Features: onset at puberty, slow progression, hirsutism (70%), menstrual abnormality (88%), infertility and anovulation (75%), and obesity (50%).
- Serum level of testosterone: normal or modestly increased (70%).
- Serum level DHEAS: normal or mildly increased.
- LH:FSH ratio is >2 in 75% of patients.
- Hyperprolactinemia in 25%-30% of patients.

Late-onset congenital adrenal hyperplasia may be of the "classic" type with severe enzyme deficiency and neonatal and postnatal presentation. It may also be "nonclassic" or "cryptic," in which the enzyme deficiency is mild and the presentation is pubertal or "late onset." Steroidogenic block may be of the 21-hydroxylase type (commonest), 11β-hydroxylase, or 3β-ol-dehydrogenase block. As a result of the steroidogenic block, cortisol secretion is decreased, ACTH is increased, and cortisol precursor build-up occurs with shunting toward androgen pathways. The presentation is usually at puberty. Serum levels of testosterone are increased except in 3β-ol-dehydrogenase. Serum levels of DHEAS are increased and 17-hydroxyprogesterone is increased in 21- and 11β-hydroxylase deficiency; 17-hydroxypregnenolone is increased in 3β-ol-dehydrogenase deficiency. All androgen abnormalities are ACTH-dependent and, hence, dexamethasone suppressible. 21-Hydroxylase deficiency, the commonest congenital adrenal hyperplasia, shows increased basal levels of 17-hydroxyprogesterone to >300 ng/dL; if normal, cosyntropin test is indicated; 30 min after the administration of ACTH, a value >1,200 ng/dL is diagnostic. Late-onset congenital adrenal hyperplasia is familial and may occur in 5%-20% of patients with features of polycystic ovaries.

- Nonclassic or cryptic type: enzyme deficiency is mild; presentation at puberty or late onset.
- Steroidogenic block: may be 21-hydroxylase (commonest type), 11-hydroxylase, or 3β-ol-dehydrogenase block.

- All androgen abnormalities are ACTH-dependent, hence dexamethasone suppressible.
- 21-Hydroxylase deficiency (commonest congenital adrenal hyperplasia): increased basal levels of 17-hydroxyprogesterone to >300 ng/dL. If normal, cosyntropin test is indicated; 30 min after giving ACTH, a value >1,200 ng/dL is diagnostic.

Endocrine Therapy

Endocrine therapy is temporizing and may need 6-12 months to show clinical effect. The goal is to decrease androgen production or to inhibit the androgen effect of hair follicles. Oral contraceptives are indicated for managing idiopathic hirsutism and polycystic ovaries. This therapy suppresses LH; increases SHBG; and inhibits DHT binding to its receptor. It is important to avoid the progestin norgestrel because of its androgenic effect. The primary role of glucocorticoid therapy is in the management of late-onset congenital adrenal hyperplasia, but it may be used also in polycystic ovaries if DHEAS levels are increased. Dexamethasone, 0.25-0.75 mg, or prednisone, 5-7.5 mg, is given at bedtime. The well-known risks of exogenous Cushing's syndrome and hypothalamic-pituitary-adrenal axis suppression may occur. In congenital adrenal hyperplasia, the efficacy of glucocorticoid therapy can be monitored by measuring the level of 17-hydroxyprogesterone. Spironolactone, the well-known aldosterone antagonist, is also an androgen receptor blocker and inhibitor of androgen action. It also decreases androgen production by its effect on steroidogenesis. The usual dose is 50-200 mg daily; spironolactone should be used only in conjunction with effective contraception. Cyproterone acetate is an antiandrogen that decreases dihydrotestosterone production and action. It also decreases LH release. It is given with topical or oral estrogen and is not available in the U.S.

- Endocrine therapy is temporizing.
- May need 6-12 months to show effect.
- Goal: decrease androgen production or inhibit androgen effect of hair follicles.
- Oral contraceptives: for managing idiopathic hirsutism and polycystic ovaries.
- Glucocorticoid therapy: primary role in managing late-onset congenital adrenal hyperplasia.
- Spironolactone: blocks androgen receptor and inhibits androgen action.

QUESTIONS
(See "Answers" section)

Multiple Choice

1. Secretion of growth hormone (GH) is stimulated by:
   a. Oral glucose
   b. L-Dopa
   c. Dexamethasone
   d. Metyrapone
   e. Somatostatin

2. Suprasellar extension of a pituitary tumor is likely to result in:
   a. Bitemporal hemianopsia
   b. Diplopia
   c. Facial pain
   d. Prolactin deficiency due to damage to pituitary stalk
   e. Nasopharyngeal mass

3. In familial multiple endocrine neoplasia (MEN) type I, pituitary tumors may be associated with:
   a. Pheochromocytoma
   b. Pseudohypoparathyroidism
   c. Tumors of the parathyroids and endocrine pancreas
   d. Medullary carcinoma of the thyroid
   e. Hyporeninemic hypoaldosteronism

4. Laboratory confirmation of the diagnosis of active acromegaly is best accomplished by:
   a. Failure of growth hormone levels to suppress to <2 ng/mL during a glucose tolerance test
   b. High somatostatin levels
   c. High serum level of phosphorus
   d. Presence of associated hyperprolactinemia responsive to bromocriptine therapy
   e. Growth hormone responds to an insulin tolerance test

5. Thyrotoxicosis due to a thyroid-stimulating hormone (TSH)-producing pituitary tumor may be associated with:
   a. Low ^{131}I uptake
   b. Atrophic thyroid
   c. Normal or high serum levels of TSH in the face of hyperthyroxinemia
   d. Exophthalmos
   e. High levels of thyroid-stimulating immunoglobulins

6. Subacute (granulomatous) thyroiditis is characterized by:
   a. Painless enlargement of the thyroid
   b. Hyperthyroidism with a high ^{131}I uptake
   c. Exophthalmos and pretibial myxedema
   d. High erythrocyte sedimentation rate and low ^{131}I uptake
   e. Permanent hypothyroidism

7. Which of the following facts is not true about hypoparathyroidism:
   a. May be caused by magnesium intoxication
   b. May be associated with hypocalcemia, hyperphosphatemia, and normal serum level of creatinine
   c. May be associated with other autoimmune endocrine disorders
   d. Chronic hypocalcemia may be associated with basal ganglia calcification and parkinsonian-like features
   e. Calcium and vitamin D are the mainstays of therapy

8. Which of the following is true about medullary carcinoma of the thyroid:
   a. Serum calcitonin levels are low and do not respond to pentagastrin stimulation
   b. Hypocalcemic tetany is a common abnormality because calcitonin inhibits bone resorption
   c. It may occur in association with primary hyperparathyroidism, pheochromocytoma, or mucosal neuromas
   d. It can cause Cushing's syndrome because of ectopic production of cortisol
   e. It may be familial, and serum thyroglobulin is the screening test of choice

9. Thyrotoxicosis caused by painless silent thyroiditis is characterized by:
   a. High ^{131}I uptake
   b. High antimicrosomal antithyroid antibodies
   c. Special predilection to occur in the postpartum period and to recur with subsequent pregnancies
   d. High levels of thyroid-stimulating immunoglobulins
   e. Eventual permanent hypothyroidism in most of the patients

10. Which of the following is not compatible with a diagnosis of euthyroid sick syndrome:

a. Increased levels of serum reverse T_3

b. Increased serum level of thyroxine (T_4)

c. Suppressed serum thyroid-stimulating hormone (TSH)

d. Increased serum level of triiodothyronine (T_3)

e. Reversibility of thyroid function abnormalities with recovery from the acute nonthyroidal illness

11. Gestational diabetes

a. Is the occurrence of pregnancy in a patient with insulin-dependent diabetes mellitus

b. Is the discovery of diabetes during pregnancy in a woman without a history of diabetes

c. Is always followed by established diabetes

d. May be treated with a sulfonylurea if hyperglycemia is mild

e. Can be detected by checking fasting plasma glucose at each trimester

12. Which is the preferred treatment for a patient with insulin-dependent diabetes mellitus who received insulin pump therapy and who has blood glucose values of 100 mg/dL at bedtime and 200 mg/dL fasting?

a. Reduce basal insulin infusion rate

b. Reduce presupper insulin bolus

c. Measure glucose at 3 a.m. (120 mg/dL) and increase basal insulin infusion rate

d. Double size of bedtime snack and increase presupper insulin dose

e. Add sulfonylurea at bedtime

13. A 45-year-old woman pharmacist experienced recurrent neuroglycopenic symptoms more than 5 hours after the last ingestion of food. At the time of Whipple's triad, plasma concentrations of insulin and C peptide were distinctly elevated. Which additional test would lead to a diagnosis?

a. Plasma proinsulin

b. Insulin antibodies

c. Plasma sulfonylurea

d. Ultrasonography of the pancreas

e. Mixed meal study

14. What is a reasonable next step in management of an obese 43-year-old male laborer with increased thirst and urination and a random plasma glucose of 315 mg/dL?

a. Oral glucose tolerance test using a 75-mg glucose load

b. Obtain two fasting plasma glucose values

c. Treat with a hypocaloric diet and recheck fasting plasma glucose within 3-7 days

d. Treat with insulin

e. Treat with sulfonylurea

15. Aldosterone secretion by the zona glomerulosa of the adrenal cortex is stimulated by:

a. Decreased blood volume

b. Hypokalemia

c. Metyrapone

d. Angiotensin-converting enzyme inhibitor

e. Dexamethasone

16. Which of the following facts is true about patients with Klinefelter's syndrome?

a. 46,XY karyotype

b. Testes normal in size and consistency

c. Small firm testes and azoospermia

d. Low serum levels of luteinizing hormone (LH) and follicle-stimulating hormone (FSH)

e. Fertility can be restored by pulsatile gonadotropin-releasing hormone (GnRH) therapy

17. Classic Turner's syndrome (45/XO) is characterized by:

a. Anosmia and hypogonadotropic hypogonadism

b. Precocious isosexual puberty

c. Shortness of stature which responds to therapy with estrogen

d. Fibrous gonadal streaks and hypergonadotropic hypogonadism

e. Short vagina and absence of female internal genitalia

18. Which of the following statements is true about Addison's disease (primary adrenocortical failure)?

a. Adrenal cortex increases cortisol secretion in response to 3-day stimulation by synthetic ACTH administration

b. Autoimmune disorder is the commonest cause, and one should look for associated other autoimmune endocrinopathies

c. Biochemical abnormalities of cortisol deficiency include hyperglycemia and hypocalcemia

d. Females with this disorder have hirsutism, acne, and high serum level of DHEAS

e. Aldosterone secretion is low because of low

angiotensin II level

19. Kallmann's syndrome is characterized by:
    a. Hypogonadism due to lack of gonadotropin-releasing hormone (GnRH)
    b. Panhypopituitarism
    c. Testes show hyalinization of the seminiferous tubules and irreversible azoospermia
    d. A hypothalamic mass is usually evident on MR scanning
    e. Karyotype is 46,XX

True/False
20. The prevalence of diabetes mellitus
    a. Is about 5% of the U.S. population
    b. Is higher in Hispanics, Native Americans, and African Americans
    c. Is equally divided between non-insulin-dependent and insulin-dependent diabetes mellitus
    d. Is close to 100% concordant in twins with insulin-dependent diabetes mellitus
    e. Is related to HLA type in insulin-dependent diabetes mellitus

21. The symptoms of central diabetes insipidus are worsened by subsequent development of ACTH deficiency and hypocortisolinism.

22. Primary hypothyroidism can be associated with hyperprolactinemia and a sellar mass. Such findings should prompt neurosurgical consultation and transsphenoidal surgery.

23. Factitial thyrotoxicosis due to surreptitious ingestion of triiodothyronine (T_3) is associated with absence of goiter, low free thyroxine index (FTI), and low ^{131}I uptake.

24. Familial hypocalciuric hypercalcemia is parathyroid hormone-dependent and is complicated in most patients by renal stones and parathyroid bone disease.

25. Sulfonylureas
    a. Should not be used during pregnancy
    b. Are effective in nonpregnant patients with insulin-dependent diabetes mellitus
    c. May be effective in combination with insulin in some patients with non-insulin-dependent diabetes mellitus
    d. Have minimal risk of hypoglycemia
    e. Should not be used in a patient with creatinine >2 mg/dL or abnormal liver function
    f. Should be given in divided dosage in the higher dose range

26. Symptoms of hypoglycemia:
    a. Are absent in artifactual hypoglycemia
    b. Occur in response to rapid decrease in glycemia
    c. Are nonspecific
    d. Are preceded by counterregulatory hormone release
    e. Are sufficient alone to diagnose the presence of hypoglycemia
    f. Differ between insulin-mediated and non-insulin-mediated hypoglycemia

27. In hypogonadotrophic hypogonadism, the testes can respond to gonadotropin therapy by increasing testosterone production and restoration of spermatogenesis.

28. In Cushing's syndrome caused by adrenal adenoma, the hypercortisol state is usually associated with normal or increased serum level of ACTH and suppressibility with high-dose (8 mg) dexamethasone test.

CHAPTER 12
ETHICS IN MEDICINE

Udaya B. S. Prakash, M.D.
William F. Dunn, M.D.

DEFINITION

Medical ethics is a set of principles that attempts to guide physicians in their relationships with patients and others. These principles are based on moral values shared by both the lay society (may vary from culture to culture) and the medical profession. Several oaths reflect physicians' beliefs and principles, including the Declaration of Geneva (1983), World Medical Association International Code of Medical Ethics (1983), American Medical Association Principles of Medical Ethics (1973), and the American College of Physicians Ethics Manual (1989). The Hippocratic oath is of major historical significance. Its principles form the framework for many of our current ethical standards, including beneficence, nonmaleficence, confidentiality, and active euthanasia. From its model come oaths sworn by many graduating physicians today.

ETHICAL DILEMMAS

Ethical issues in medicine are as dynamic as the scientific and technical progresses in medicine. In fact, the relentless advances in medical science are greatly responsible for the dynamism in medical ethics. These factors are partly accountable for ethical dilemmas. Furthermore, changes in societal mores and laws also have an impact on the ethical issues in medicine. An ethical dilemma can be defined as a predicament in which there is no clear course to resolve the problem of conflicting moral principles because of credible evidence both for and against a certain action. Increasing emphasis is being placed on medical ethics in the certifying and licensing examinations for physicians.

- Ethical dilemma: predicament in which there is no clear course to resolve the problem of conflicting moral principles because of credible evidence both for and against a certain action.
- Ethical issues in medicine are dynamic and will continue to change.

PRINCIPLES OF MEDICAL ETHICS

- The four major tenets are 1) autonomy, 2) beneficence, 3) nonmaleficence, and 4) justice.

1. Autonomy

This tenet involves respecting the patient's right to self-determination and the pursuit of one's own life plan. Autonomy implies "decisional capability" (the term "competence" is avoided here because of its competing legal definition). Decisional capability is the ability to deliberate about the available information and to draw inferences. Clinical evidence of confusion, disorientation, and psychosis resulting from organic diseases, metabolic disturbances, and iatrogenic interference can adversely affect decision-making ability. In clinical practice, the lack of decisional capability should be proved, and not presumed. Decisionally capable patients have the right to refuse medical therapy, even at the risk of death. If a previously decisionally capable patient had indicated, clearly and convincingly, whether life-sustaining therapy should be administered or withheld in the event of permanent unconsciousness, that wish should be respected (see "Living Will," page 302), unless it was subsequently clearly rescinded.

- Autonomy: respecting patient's right to self-determination and pursuit of one's own life plan.
- Implies "decisional capability," i.e., the right to refuse medical therapy, even at the risk of death.
- Lack of decisional capability should be proved, and not presumed.

Substituted Judgment

This is the ability of family members or other duly appointed person(s) to make therapeutic decisions on behalf of the patient, on the basis of what they believe the patient, if decisionally capable, would have chosen.

Surrogate Decision Maker

The surrogate represents the patient's interests and previously expressed wishes in the context of the medical issues. The surrogate is optimally designated by the patient before critical illness. One type of surrogate is the durable power of attorney, in which a legally binding proxy directive authorizes a designated individual to speak on behalf of the patient. The second type of surrogate is the patient's family, physician, or the court. The third type is a moral surrogate (usually a family member) who best knows the patient and has the patient's best interest at heart. Difficulties may arise when the moral surrogate is not the legal surrogate. Dialogue between the physician and surrogate is important.

- Optimally, surrogate is designated by patient before critical illness.

Living Will

This is a type of "advance directive" or "health care declaration." This document commonly includes a declaration of "durable power of attorney for health care matters (proxy)." The living will reflects the patient's autonomy. It can aid greatly in medical decision making, but it becomes ineffective if vaguely written or applied to patients with uncertain prognoses. Legal reliability may vary from state to state, and all clinicians should be aware of state-specific statutes regarding advance directives. Any decisionally capable person 18 years or older can have a living will.

- Living will: a type of "advance directive" or "health care declaration."
- The living will reflects patient's autonomy.
- Legal reliability may vary from state to state.

Disclosure

To make the principle of autonomy function, the physician must provide adequate and truthful information for decisionally capable patients to make medical decisions. In clinical reasoning, the physician must consider ethical issues as well as the patient's values and preferences. For example, even though folklore remedies are without scientific basis for treating advanced malignancies, and are considered unethical as primary therapy by the physician, the patient may not agree. If the patient wants unconventional treatment, the physician cannot simply dismiss the issue without well-reasoned and convincing discussion with the patient. A more serious issue is the availability of more than one acceptable form of therapy for a disease. In a patient with a cancer amenable to surgical resection, chemotherapy or radiation may provide a similar long-term outlook, albeit with different complications and side effects. However, the physician may be biased toward one of the three treatments. In this situation, it is the duty of the physician to set aside personal bias and provide detailed information on each treatment and its potential complications and to allow the well-informed patient to express personal preferences. If the physician assumes sole responsibility in the decision making (even though the patient is capable of analyzing the alternatives and coming to a reasoned conclusion), the important aspects to the patient may be overlooked or underestimated, including the impact of various treatments on the patient's quality of personal life, occupation, and social and economic aspects. The final plan should reflect an agreement between a well-informed patient and a well-informed, sympathetic, and unbiased physician.

- Physician must provide adequate and truthful information for decisionally capable patients to make medical decisions.
- Physician must consider ethical issues as well as the patient's values and preferences.

Informed Consent

This is voluntary acceptance of physician recommendations by decisionally competent patients or surrogates who have been furnished with ample truthful information regarding risks, benefits, and alternatives and who clearly indicate their comprehension of the information. Informed consent is essential when performing new, innovative, nonstandard surgical procedures and research procedures. Informed consent from surrogates is necessary to perform autopsy (except in specific instances such as coroners' cases) or to practice intubation, placement of intravascular lines, or other procedures on the newly dead. The amount of information needed by the patient to give informed consent is not that which the physician feels is adequate (Professional Practice Standard), but that which the average prudent person would need to make a decision (Reasonable Person Standard). In rare exceptions the physician can treat a patient without truly informed consent (e.g., an emotionally unstable patient who requires urgent treatment but informing the patient of the details may produce further problems). Many "informed consent" forms in clinical use do not meet the Reasonable Person Standard and are therefore of no value morally or legally.

- Amount of information needed by patient is that which the average prudent person would need to make a decision (Reasonable Person Standard).
- Many "informed consent" forms do not meet Reasonable Person Standard and are therefore of no value morally or legally.

Confidentiality

Patient confidentiality provides the patient the right to keep medical information solely within the realm of the physician-patient relationship. The physician is obliged to maintain the medical information in strict confidence. Exceptions to this include instances when data, if not released to appropriate agencies, have the potential to cause greater societal harm. Typical examples may include positive results of human immunodeficiency virus (HIV) test, or a sputum culture positive for *Mycobacterium tuberculosis*. Patients who voluntarily request HIV test should be informed by the physician that the result, if positive, will be automatically reported to the appropriate health agency. Confidentiality may also be broached when patients ask about hereditary diseases in their parents or siblings.

- Physician is obliged to maintain medical information in strict confidence.
- Exceptions include instances when data, if not released to appropriate agencies, may cause greater societal harm (e.g., positive HIV test, positive sputum culture for *Mycobacterium tuberculosis*).

Group-Specific Beliefs

Certain religious practices preclude or compromise accepted medical practices. The principle of autonomy allows that adult patients who refuse life-saving measures

(e.g., blood transfusion) should be allowed to maintain their religious practices. However, in cases involving children, the courts have overruled the religious objections.

- Adult patients who refuse life-saving measures (e.g., blood transfusion) should be allowed to maintain their religious practices.

2. Beneficence

This is acting to benefit patients by preserving life, restoring health, relieving suffering, and restoring or maintaining function. The physician (acting in good faith) is obligated to help patients attain their own interests and goals as determined by the patient, **not** the physician.

- Beneficence: preservation of life, restoration of health, relief of suffering, and restoration or maintenance of function.

Implied Consent

The principle of implied consent is invoked when true informed consent is not possible because the patient (or surrogate) is unable to express a decision regarding treatment, specifically, in emergency situations in which physicians are compelled to provide medically necessary therapy, without which harm would result. This clarifies that there is a duty to assist a person in urgent need of care. This principle has been legally accepted and it provides the physician a legal defense against battery (though not negligence).

- Implied consent is invoked when true informed consent is not possible.

Incurable Disease and Death

Probably the most distressing aspect of medical practice is the encounter with a patient who has incurable disease and in whom premature death is inevitable. The physician and patient (or surrogate) must formulate appropriate goals of therapy, choose what measures should be taken to maintain life, and decide how aggressive these measures ought to be. It is important to remind oneself that the patient is under enormous mental anguish and physical stress and that the ability to make solid decisions may be clouded. Furthermore, the decision(s) made by the patient may be guided by his or her understanding (whether adequate or not) of the medical condition and prognosis; religious beliefs; financial status; and other personal wishes. The patient may seek counsel from family, friends, and clergy as well as the attending physician.

- In incurable disease, recognize that patient is under enormous mental anguish and physical stress.
- Ability of patient to make solid decisions may be clouded.

The following guidelines are suggested in dealing with incurable disease and death. The patient and family (if patient so desires) must be provided ample opportunity to talk with the physician and ask questions. An unhurried openness and "willing-to-listen" attitude on the part of the physician are critical for a positive outcome. Patients often find it easier to share their feelings about death with their physician, who is likely to be more objective and less emotional, than with family and friends. Nevertheless, the physician should not remain or "appear" completely detached from the patient's feelings and emotions. Even an attempt on the part of the physician to enter the "inner" feelings of the patient will have a soothing, if not therapeutic, effect.

- The patient and family must be provided every opportunity to talk with the physician and ask questions.
- An unhurried openness and "willing-to-listen" attitude on the part of the physician are critical for a positive outcome.

The physician should assume the responsibility to furnish or arrange for physical, emotional, and spiritual support. Adequate control of pain, maintenance of human dignity, and close contact with the family are crucial. The emotional and spiritual support available through local clergy (as appropriate, given the patient's personal beliefs) should not be underestimated. At no other time in life is the reality of human mortality so real as in the terminal phases of disease. It is always preferable to allay the anxiety of the dying patient through adequate emotional and spiritual support rather than by sedation. The physician should constantly remind herself or himself that despite all the medical technology that surrounds the patient, the patient must not be dehumanized.

- Adequate pain control, maintenance of human dignity, and close contact with family are crucial.
- Despite all the technology that surrounds the patient, human-to-human contact should be most important aspect of treatment.
- It is always preferable to allay anxiety by adequate emotional and spiritual support rather than by sedation.

Control of Pain

The principle of beneficence calls for relief of suffering. Adequate analgesia, particularly in patients with incurable disease, is the responsibility of the physician. If death ensues in a terminally ill patient because of respiratory depression from analgesia, the physician has not acted immorally. Patients allowed to die after removal from ventilators are commonly treated in this fashion. Nevertheless, it is necessary to stress that the primary objective of analgesia is relief of pain and not the hastening of death, even in terminally ill patients.

- Beneficence calls for relief of suffering.
- Adequate analgesia, particularly in patients with incurable disease, is responsibility of the physician.
- Physician has not performed immorally if death in a terminally ill patient is result of respiratory depression from analgesic therapy; euthanasia is not the goal.

Conflict of Interest

The principle of beneficence requires that the physician not engage in activities that are not in the patient's best interest. This is considered to be a significant problem in the United States. Some studies have suggested that physicians' prescribing practices are influenced by financial and other significant rewards from drug companies. If the physician does not ardently avoid areas of potential conflict of interest (because of the principle of beneficence), the result may be maleficence.

3. Nonmaleficence

This principle is based on "do no harm, prevent harm, and remove harm." Under this principle come unprofessional behavior; verbal, physical, and sexual abuse of patients; and uninformed and undisclosed experimentation on patients with drugs and procedures with the potential to cause harmful side effects. Breach of physician-patient confidentiality which results in harm to the patient is another example of maleficence.

- Nonmaleficence: "do no harm, prevent harm, and remove harm."

4. Justice

Every patient deserves and must be provided optimal care as warranted by the underlying medical condition. Allocation of medical resources fairly and according to medical need is the basis for this principle. The decision to provide optimal medical care should be based on the medical need of each patient and the perceived medical benefit to the patient. The patient's social status, ability to pay, or perceived social worth should not dictate the quality or quantity of medical care. The physician's clear-cut responsibility is to the patient's well-being (beneficence). Physicians should not make decisions about individual care of their patients based on larger societal needs. The bedside is not the place to make general policy decisions.

- Justice: allocation of medical resources fairly and according to medical need.
- Physician should not make decisions about individual care of patients based on larger societal needs.

"DO NOT RESUSCITATE" (DNR)

DNR orders affect administration of cardiopulmonary resuscitation (CPR) only; other therapeutic options should not be influenced by the DNR order. Every person whose medical history is unclear or unavailable should receive CPR in the event of cardiopulmonary arrest. CPR is not recommended when it merely prolongs life in a patient with terminal illness. Of paramount importance are the patient's knowledge of the extent of disease and prognosis, the physician's estimate of the potential efficacy of CPR, and the wishes of the patient (or surrogate) regarding CPR as a therapeutic tool. However, if, in the physician's judgment, CPR would be futile, multiple physician groups, including the American Medical Association's Council on Ethical and Judicial Affairs, have recommended that CPR not be offered; however, the extent of legal support for this recommendation is as yet unclear. The DNR order should be reviewed frequently because clinical circumstances may dictate other measures (e.g., a patient with terminal cardiomyopathy who had initially turned down heart transplantation and wanted to be considered a "DNR candidate" may change her or his mind and now opt for the transplantation). Physicians should discuss the appropriateness of CPR or DNR with patients at high risk for cardiopulmonary arrest and with the terminally ill. The discussion should optimally take place in the outpatient setting, during the initial period of hospitalization, and periodically during hospitalization, if appropriate. DNR orders (and rationale) should be entered in the patient's medical records.

- DNR orders affect CPR only.
- Other therapeutic options should not be influenced by the DNR order.

- Every patient should be considered a candidate for CPR unless clear indications exist otherwise.
- CPR is not recommended when it merely prolongs life in a patient with terminal illness.
- DNR order should be reviewed frequently.
- DNR orders (and rationale) should be entered in patient's medical records.

PATIENT SELF-DETERMINATION ACT OF 1990

This federal act requires hospitals, nursing homes, and hospices to advise patients at admission of their right to accept or refuse medical care and to execute an advance directive. Managed care organizations and home health care agencies must provide the same information to each of their members at the time of enrollment. These organizations are required to 1) document whether patients have advance directives, 2) implement advance directive policies, and 3) educate their staffs and communities about advance directives.

- Hospitals, nursing homes, and hospices should advise patients, on admission, of their right to accept or refuse medical care and to execute an advance directive.

WITHHOLDING AND WITHDRAWING LIFE SUPPORT

This decision may be compatible with beneficence, nonmaleficence, and autonomy. The right of a decisionally capable person to refuse lifesaving hydration and nutrition was upheld by the U.S. Supreme Court (Table 12-1), but a surrogate decision maker's right to refuse treatment for decisionally incapable persons can be restricted by states. Brain death is not a necessary requirement for withdrawing or withholding life support. The value of each medical therapy (risk:benefit ratio) should be assessed for each patient. The American Medical Association has issued certain guidelines, and one of them states that a life-sustaining medical intervention can be limited without the consent of patient or surrogate when the intervention is judged to be futile. The extent to which these guidelines will be upheld by legal authorities is as yet unclear, as evidenced by a recent state court ruling in Minnesota (Table 12-1). When appropriate, the withholding or withdrawal of life support is best accomplished with input from more than one experienced clinician.

- Withholding or withdrawing life support does not conflict with the principles of beneficence, nonmaleficence, and autonomy.
- Brain death is not a necessary requirement for withdrawing or withholding life support.

PERSISTENT VEGETATIVE STATE

This is a chronic state of unconsciousness (loss of self-awareness) lasting for more than a few weeks, characterized by the presence of wake/sleep cycles, but without behavioral or cerebral metabolic evidence of possessing cognitive function or of being able to respond in a learned manner to external events or stimuli. The body retains functions necessary to sustain vegetative survival, if provided nutritional and other supportive measures--note that the U.S. Supreme Court has ruled that there is no distinction between artificial feeding and hydration versus mechanical ventilation (Table 12-1).

- Persistent vegetative state: unconsciousness (loss of self-awareness) lasting for more than a few weeks.
- U.S. Supreme Court ruling states that there is no distinction between artificial feeding and hydration versus mechanical ventilation.

DEFINITION OF DEATH

Death is irreversible cessation of circulatory and respiratory function **or** irreversible cessation of all functions of the entire brain, including the brain stem. Clinical criteria (at times substantiated by electroencephalographic [EEG] testing or assessment of cerebral perfusion) permit the reliable diagnosis of "cerebral death."

Table 12-1.--Pertinent Legal Rulings

Case, yr	Legal issue	Court	Decision
Quinlan, 1976	PVS--discontinuation of mechanical ventilation, previously articulated directive	New Jersey Supreme Court	Discontinuation (based on right to privacy)
Brophy, 1986	PVS--discontinuation of gastrostomy feedings, previously articulated directive	Massachusetts Supreme Court	Discontinue feedings (based on autonomy)
Bouvia, 1986	Severely impaired, refusal of nasogastric tube feedings by a decisionally capable patient	California Court of Appeals	Removal of nasogastric tube (based on autonomy)
Corbett, 1986	PVS--discontinuation of nasogastric tube feedings, no predefined directive(s)	Florida Court of Appeals	Discontinue feedings (based on right to privacy)
Cruzan, 1990	PVS--state of Missouri required "clear and convincing" evidence of individual's wishes before allowing withdrawal of life support	U.S. Supreme Court	States have right to restrict exercise of right to refuse treatment by surrogates; decisionally capable patients may refuse life-sustaining therapy, including hydration, nutrition, and mechanical ventilation
Wanglie, 1991	PVS--family wished continued support despite objections to continued life-sustaining therapy by the physicians and institution	Minnesota Supreme Court	Continuation (based on autonomy, substituted judgment)

PVS, persistent vegetative state.

The family should be informed of the brain death but should not be asked to decide whether further medical therapy should be continued. One exception is when the patient had earlier directed the family to make certain decisions, such as organ donation, in case of brain death.

Once it is ascertained that the patient is "brain dead" and that no further therapy can be offered, the primary physician, preferably after consultation with another physician involved in the care of the patient, may withdraw supportive measures.

The imminent possibility for harvesting organs for transplantation should in no way affect any of the above-outlined decisions. When organ donation is possible after the determination of brain death, the family should be approached, preferably before cessation of cardiac function, regarding organ donation.

- Death: irreversible cessation of circulatory and respiratory function **or** irreversible cessation of all functions of entire brain, including brain stem.
- EEG not necessary to establish death.

AUTHORS' NOTE

Laws concerning ethical issues in medicine continue to evolve, reflecting changing attitudes of society. It is certain that legal decisions will continue to influence the practice of medicine. Many states have no directly applicable statutes or court cases relating to difficult ethical issues in medical practice. Although this review is meant as a guide, for further information regarding state-specific mandates the individual practitioner is referred to the appropriate state medical society.

QUESTIONS
(See "Answers" section)

Multiple Choice

1. While you are making medical rounds, a nurse urgently calls you to see an 80-year-old severely emaciated and sick patient in whom cardiopulmonary arrest has occurred. The nurse has left the room and you have no medical information about the patient (you have not been caring for this patient). Which of the following is the most appropriate measure?
   a. Leave the room and tell the nurse to bring in the medical record
   b. Immediately begin cardiopulmonary resuscitation
   c. First, find out whether there is a "do not resuscitate" order written
   d. Call the patient's physician to obtain more information
   e. First, obtain electrocardiogram and arterial blood gas values

2. Your patient, a 30-year-old woman with leukemia refractory to multiple drugs, has been judged incurable by several specialists. No further therapy is available, and death within a few weeks is inevitable. The patient asks you whether she is dying. Which of the following is the correct response?
   a. Say an emphatic "yes"
   b. Tell the patient that "everything is going to be all right"
   c. Step out of the room and inform the husband, whom you have not met yet, of the inevitability of death
   d. Request the priest or chaplain to discuss this issue with the patient
   e. Have the nurse who has been caring for the patient inform the patient

3. A 13-year-old is brought to the emergency room following a motorcycle accident. Severe, continuous blood loss is noted (hemoglobin value is 4.6 g/dL). The parents refuse a blood transfusion because of their religious belief. They want to take the patient home. Which of the following options would you choose?
   a. Dismiss the patient against medical advice
   b. Avoid blood transfusion and manage with intravenous fluids

c. Contact the hospital's legal department for advice
d. Start immediate transfusion using whole blood
e. Request the hospital chaplain to reason with the parents

4. A 56-year-old man presents with unstable angina and requires urgent coronary angiography. He has a history of severe paranoid schizophrenia and expresses his apprehension about intravenous contrast dye (there is no history of prior administration of intravenous dye) and demands detailed information regarding the procedure. Before the procedure, you should do which of the following?
a. Do not tell the patient anything about angiography
b. Provide detailed information on angiography
c. Reassure patient without describing details of angiography
d. Start medical therapy and cancel angiography
e. Request the angiographer to discuss the details with the patient

5. You have been performing annual physical examinations on a 54-year-old man for the past 6 years. Despite your instructions, he continues to smoke and is noncompliant with the treatment program for his hypertension and diabetes mellitus. Which of the following options would you choose when you see him next?
a. Continue to examine him annually
b. Admonish him to evoke a sense of guilt and embarrassment
c. Refuse to see him again
d. Tell him to find another physician
e. Stop all treatment because he is noncompliant

True/False

6. A 55-year-old married male executive comes for annual physical examination. As part of the blood tests, he requests human immunodeficiency virus (HIV) serology and requests you to keep the result confidential. The HIV serology result is positive. Which of the following procedures are appropriate?
a. Inform the patient of the result
b. Inform the patient's insurance company
c. Inform the patient's children
d. Notify the local health agency
e. Inform the patient's wife
f. Inform the patient's employer

7. A 60-year-old man is admitted because of acute diverticulitis complicated by peritonitis, and he requires emergency surgery. He is a very poor surgical risk because of underlying coronary disease, chronic obstructive pulmonary disease, hypertension, and diabetes mellitus complicated by renal failure. He is confused and unable to answer your questions. He has no relatives, friends, or living will. Which of the following statements are true for this patient?
a. A risky surgery cannot be undertaken without informed consent
b. You can assume the role of moral surrogate
c. You cannot proceed with surgery without finding the legal guardian
d. Postpone surgery until your legal department decides the correct action
e. In many situations, informed consent has no value
f. Surgery in this high-risk patient implies maleficence

CHAPTER 13

GASTROENTEROLOGY I

Thomas R. Viggiano, M.D.

GASTROINTESTINAL AND PANCREATIC DISORDERS

ESOPHAGUS

Esophageal Function

The upper esophageal sphincter (or cricopharyngeus muscle) and the muscle of the proximal one-third of the esophagus are striated muscle under voluntary control. There is a transition from skeletal to smooth muscle in the mid-esophagus. In the distal one-third of the organ, the muscle is smooth muscle that is under voluntary control. The lower esophageal sphincter is a zone of circular muscle located in the distal 2-3 cm of the esophagus. To transport food from the mouth through the negative pressured chest into the positive pressured abdomen, the esophagus must transport food against a pressure gradient. To prevent reflux of gastric contents, the lower esophagus has a sphincter for unidirectional flow.

- The esophagus must transport food against a pressure gradient.

Normal Motility

After a person swallows, the upper esophageal sphincter relaxes within 0.5 sec. A primary peristaltic wave then passes through the body of the esophagus at a rate of 1-5 cm/sec, generating an intraluminal pressure of 40-100 mm Hg. Within 2 sec after the swallow, the lower esophageal sphincter relaxes and stays relaxed until the wave of peristalsis passes through it. Then, the lower esophageal sphincter contracts again to maintain its resting tone. Two major symptom complexes result if the esophagus is unable to perform its two major functions: dysphagia (transport dysfunction) and reflux (lower esophageal sphincter dysfunction).

- Dysphagia--transport dysfunction.
- Reflux--lower esophageal sphincter dysfunction.

Dysphagia

Dysphagia is the defective transport of food and is usually described as "sticking." Odynophagia is pain on swallowing. The two causes of dysphagia must be distinguished: mechanical (obstructed lumen) and functional (motility disorder). Answers to three questions frequently suggest the diagnosis: 1) what type of food produces the dysphagia, 2) what is the course of the dysphagia, and 3) is there heartburn (Fig. 13-1)?

Mechanical Cause

Mechanical obstruction occurs if the lumen is <12 mm. With mechanical obstruction, the course is progressive; dysphagia for solids is greater than for liquids, and there is weight loss.

- Mechanical obstruction: progressive course, weight loss, solids greater than liquids.

1. Stricture--Peptic stricture results from prolonged reflux and is usually a short (<2-3 cm long) narrowing in the distal esophagus.

- Peptic stricture results from prolonged reflux, usually in the distal esophagus.

Barrett's esophagus is a stricture in the mid-esophagus that may occur with an ulcer. This stricture is also due to reflux and, thus, is acquired and not congenital. Normal squamous mucosa is replaced by columnar

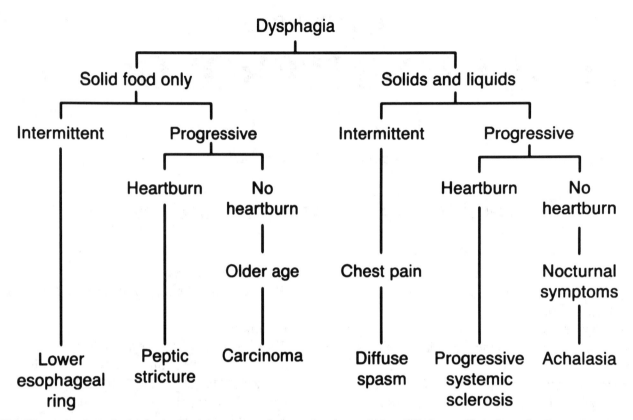

Fig. 13-1. Diagnostic scheme for dysphagia. Obtaining anwers to three questions (see text) often yields the most likely diagnosis. (From MKSAP VI: Part 1:44, 1982. American College of Physicians. By permission.)

epithelium, which has 30x increased risk to develop malignancy.

- Barrett's esophagus: stricture in mid-esophagus.
- It is a complication of chronic reflux.
- It has a 30x increased risk for malignancy

Lye stricture--Alkali is more injurious to the esophagus than acid (in postgastrectomy patients, alkaline reflux can produce severe esophagitis). Do not induce vomiting after lye ingestion. Stricture tends to occur at the three physiologic narrowings where the initial passage of the corrosive may have been delayed. Bougienage after 3-4 weeks may prevent occurrence of stricture. There is increased incidence of cancer.

- Postgastrectomy alkaline reflux can produce severe esophagitis.
- Do not induce vomiting after lye ingestion.
- Lye stricture is associated with increased incidence of cancer.

2. Tumor--Benign. Leiomyoma is the commonest benign tumor. It is usually asymptomatic. Recognize the appearance of this tumor on barium swallow fluo-

roscopy. Perform endoscopy even if classic changes are seen on barium swallow.

Malignant. Recognize the appearance of malignant tumors on barium swallow fluoroscopy. Also, know the conditions that predispose to esophageal (squamous) cancer--achalasia, lye stricture, Plummer-Vinson syndrome, tylosis, smoking, alcohol. The male:female ratio for esophageal malignancy is 4:1. Of the malignant tumors, 50% are squamous and 50% are adenocarcinoma. Progressive dysphagia with weight loss is usually seen. Diagnosis is established by endoscopy with biopsy and cytology. Prognosis--5-Year survival is only 7%-15%, 28% have lung metastases, and 25% have liver metastases. Treatment: squamous carcinoma is more radiosensitive than adenocarcinoma. Surgery is difficult for proximal lesions. Surgery and preoperative irradiation are used for distal 1/3 lesions. Palliation: laser endoscopy, bougienage, tube placement. Chemotherapy: no agents are known to be beneficial. Squamous carcinoma can produce ectopic PTH, thus hypercalcemia does not mean the tumor is unresectable. Barrett's esophagus gives rise to adenocarcinoma.

- Know the radiographic appearance of leiomyoma and

esophageal cancer.

- Conditions that predispose to cancer: achalasia, lye stricture, Plummer-Vinson syndrome, tylosis, smoking, alcohol.
- Esophageal cancers are usually unresectable; palliative treatment.
- 5-Year survival is only 7%-15%.

3. Ring--A mucosal ring is a mucosal membrane that marks the junction of the esophageal and stomach mucosa. Muscular rings are rare. It presents as intermittent dysphagia for solids or as a sudden obstruction from food bolus (steak house syndrome). Know the radiographic appearance. Treatment is dilatation.

- Ring: intermittent dysphagia and food bolus impaction.
- Know its radiographic appearance.
- Treatment is dilatation.

4. Web--A web is a membrane of squamous mucosa that occurs anywhere in the esophagus. It presents as intermittent dysphagia. Plummer-Vinson syndrome: cervical esophageal web, iron deficiency anemia, 15% chance of oropharyngeal or esophageal cancer.

- Web presents as intermittent dysphagia.
- Plummer-Vinson syndrome: cervical esophageal web, iron deficiency anemia, 15% chance of oropharyngeal or esophageal cancer.
- Intermittent dysphagia is caused by rings, webs, or motility disorders.

Functional Cause

With functional obstruction (motility disorders), there is dysphagia for solids and liquids, intermittent course, and weight loss may or may not occur. The three important motor abnormalities of the esophagus are achalasia, diffuse esophageal spasm, and scleroderma.

1. Achalasia--Denervated esophagus (degeneration of Auerbach's ganglion cells). Chest radiography shows air fluid level. Barium swallow fluoroscopy shows dilated esophagus with beak-like tapering. Motility pattern: incomplete relaxation of the lower esophageal sphincter (most important); hypertensive lower esophageal sphincter (usually does not have reflux); and aperistalsis in body (a later finding). Always endoscopically examine patients with achalasia. Cancer of the esophagogastric junction may present with radi-

ographic appearance and motility pattern of achalasia. A clue would be an older patient with dysphagia and heartburn. Treatment is with pneumatic dilatation and not bougienage. Pneumatic dilatation is as effective as Heller myotomy.

In Brazil, the parasite *Trypanosoma cruzi* (Chagas' disease) produces a neurotoxin that destroys the myenteric plexus. Esophageal dilatation identical to achalasia, megacolon, and megaloureter are seen in Chagas' disease.

- Functional obstruction: intermittent dysphagia for solids and liquids.
- Achalasia: chest radiograph shows air fluid level.
- Dilated esophagus with beak-like tapering on barium swallow fluoroscopy.
- Most important motility pattern in achalasia: incomplete relaxation of lower esophageal sphincter.
- Always endoscopically examine patients with achalasia.
- Treat achalasia with pneumatic dilatation and not with bougienage.
- Chagas' disease has esophageal dysfunction identical to that of achalasia.

2. Diffuse esophageal spasm--It usually presents as chest pain but may cause intermittent dysphagia. It is aggravated by stress and hot or cold liquids. Barium swallow fluoroscopy shows corkscrew esophagus, which is normal in the elderly (presbyesophagus). Motility: simultaneous contractions of high amplitude in the body of the esophagus. If the patient is asymptomatic during test, motility may be normal. The lower esophageal sphincter is hypertensive or has defective relaxation in 1/3 of patients. Medical treatment (nitrates, anticholinergics, nifedipine) has unpredictable results. Surgical treatment is long myotomy.

- Diffuse esophageal spasm usually presents as chest pain.
- It is aggravated by stress and hot or cold liquids.
- Barium swallow fluoroscopy shows corkscrew esophagus.
- Medical treatment has unpredictable results.

3. Scleroderma--Associated with Raynaud's phenomenon or physical findings (skin changes). Barium swallow fluoroscopy shows a common esophagogastric tube. Motility: aperistalsis in the body of the esoph-

agus and lower esophageal sphincter incompetence (severe reflux). Scleroderma and mixed connective tissue disease are associated with dysphagia in 75% of the cases. Systemic lupus erythematosus and dermatomyositis are associated with dysphagia in only 5% of cases.

- With scleroderma, aperistalsis in body of the esophagus.
- Lower esophageal sphincter incompetence (severe reflux) in scleroderma.

Oropharyngeal Dysphagia

Oropharyngeal dysphagia is the result of faulty transfer of the food bolus from the oropharynx to the esophagus caused by disorders of either neural regulation or skeletal muscle (Table 13-1). It presents as high esophageal dysphagia associated with coughing, choking, or nasal regurgitation. Structural causes include cervical osteophytes, goiter, lymphadenopathy, and Zenker's diverticulum. After recognizing that oropharyngeal dysphagia is present, other associated symptoms may lead to diagnosis of the underlying illness (e.g., a young person with oropharyngeal dysphagia, central scotoma, and neurologic symptoms has multiple sclerosis).

- Oropharyngeal dysphagia is the result of faulty transfer of a food bolus from the oropharynx to the esophagus due to neuromuscular disorders.
- It is a high esophageal dysphagia associated with coughing, choking, or nasal regurgitation.

Table 13-1.--Causes of Oropharyngeal Dysphagia

Muscular disorders	Neurologic disorders	Structural causes
Amyloidosis	Amyotrophic lateral sclerosis	Cervical osteophytes
Dermatomyositis	Cerebral vascular accident	Cricopharyngeal dysfunction
Hyperthyroidism	Diphtheria	Goiter
Hypothyroidism	Huntington's disease	Lymphadenopathy
Myasthenia gravis	Multiple sclerosis	
Myotonia dystrophica	Parkinson's disease	
Oculopharyngeal myopathy	Polio	
Stiff-man syndrome	Tabes dorsalis	
	Tetanus	

Gastroesophageal Reflux Disease

It is generally accepted that reflux of gastric contents occurs when the lower esophageal sphincter pressure is <10 mm Hg. Internists should know which agents alter lower esophageal sphincter pressure.

Reflux

The lower esophageal sphincter is the major barrier to reflux. This sphincter is a 2- to 4-cm-long specialized segment of circular smooth muscle in the terminal esophagus. The pressure of this sphincter varies markedly during the day, but the normal resting pressure is 15-30 mm Hg. Swallowing causes the pressure to drop promptly (within 1-2 sec after the onset of swallowing) and for the sphincter to remain relaxed until the peristaltic wave passes over it. The sphincter then contracts to maintain the increased resting pressure that prevents reflux. Pressure of the lower esophageal sphincter decreases significantly for 2 hr after a meal. Some gastroesophageal reflux occurs in everyone during the day but does not cause symptoms or esophagitis. Patients with clinically symptomatic reflux or inflammation show transient lower esophageal sphincter relaxations of unknown cause and have more frequent and longer lasting episodes of reflux. Various causes of change in lower esophageal sphincter pressure are listed in Table 13-2.

- Reflux of gastric contents occurs when lower esophageal sphincter pressure is <10 mm Hg.
- Lower esophageal sphincter pressure decreases for 2 hr after a meal.
- Patients with clinically symptomatic reflux show transient lower esophageal sphincter relaxations.
- Know which agents decrease lower esophageal sphincter pressure.

Table 13-2.--Changes in Lower Esophageal Sphincter Pressure

Increase	Decrease
Endogenous cause	Endogenous cause
Gastrin (pharmacologic doses)	Secretin
Glucagon	Motilin
	Cholecystokinin
	Progesterone
Exogenous cause	Exogenous cause
Protein meal	Diet
Antacids	Alcohol
Cholinergic drugs	Caffeine
Metoclopramide	Carminatives (spearmint, peppermint)
	Chocolate
	Fatty meal
	Smoking (nicotine)
	Theophylline
	Drugs
	Anticholinergic drugs
	Calcium channel blockers
	Nitrates
	α-Adrenergic antagonists
	β-Adrenergic agonists
	Morphine
	Diazepam
	Benzodiazepine

The degree of tissue damage is the real concern in gastroesophageal reflux disease. Multiple factors that determine whether reflux esophagitis occurs include 1) lower esophageal sphincter pressure, 2) volume of gastric contents, 3) rate of gastric emptying (if delayed reflux), 4) potency of refluxate (acid, pepsin, bile), 5) efficiency of esophageal clearance (motility, salivary, bicarbonate), and 6) resistance of esophageal tissue to injury and ability to repair.

The evaluation of esophagitis is designed to answer four important questions (Table 13-3): Does the patient have esophagitis and, if so, to what extent? Does the patient have reflux and, if so, how severe? Are the patient's symptoms due to reflux? What is the mechanism of reflux?

Internists should know how to use tests that evaluate reflux in a cost-effective way. In most patients, the medical history is sufficiently typical to warrant a trial of therapy without conducting expensive tests. Additional testing should be performed in patients with an atypical history, refractory symptoms, or possible complications of esophagitis.

- In most patients, the medical history is sufficiently typical to warrant a trial of therapy without tests.
- Testing should be performed in patients with an atypical history, refractory symptoms, or possible complications of esophagitis.

Table 13-3.--Evaluation of Esophagitis

Question	Tests for reflux (more sensitive one is listed first)
Is reflux present?	pH probe; isotope scan
Is esophagitis present?	Biopsy; endoscopy
Are symptoms due to reflux?	Acid perfusion (Bernstein test)
Mechanism of reflux?	Motility

Esophageal Tests

1. Barium swallow fluoroscopy--Reflux is found in 60% of patients with esophagitis but also in 25% of controls. It is a qualitative test and does not distinguish

between "normal" and abnormal reflux. Upper gastrointestinal radiography is used primarily as a screening test to exclude other diagnoses (e.g., ulcer) and to identify complications of reflux (e.g., strictures, ulcers, Barrett's esophagus). Patients with reflux and dysphagia should have barium esophagography first.

- Reflux is found in 60% of patients with esophagitis but also in 25% of controls.
- Patients with reflux and dysphagia should have barium esophagography first.

2. Esophagoscopy--This is the most definitive test if gross inflammation is present. However, 40% of patients may have symptomatic reflux with no gross inflammation. This is the preferred first test in long-standing cases of reflux to rule out Barrett's esophagus. It is also the first test for patients with reflux without dysphagia.

- Esophagoscopy is the test preferred first in long-standing cases of reflux to rule out Barrett's esophagus.
- It is first test for patients with reflux without dysphagia.

3. Esophageal biopsy--In patients with reflux but without gross esophagitis, the basal cell layer and papillae are elongated. Esophagoscopy and biopsy are about 100% sensitive for detecting reflux. With Barrett's esophagus, it is important for the biopsy sample to include the mucosa to detect dysplasia (premalignant changes).

- Biopsy may detect esophagitis when gross inflammation is not present.
- With Barrett's esophagus, it is important for biopsy sample to include the mucosa.

4. 24-Hour pH monitoring--Monitoring the pH in the distal esophagus of patients during a 24-hr period after their normal routine allows a more physiologic evaluation of reflux during daily activities. Reflux is determined by a pH that is <4; findings are positive when the pH is <4 more than 5% of the time. This test is valuable in patients with atypical symptoms, reflux symptoms, a nondiagnostic evaluation, or pulmonary symptoms.

- 24-Hour pH monitoring allows a more physiologic

evaluation of reflux during daily activities.
- Positive test: esophageal pH is <4 more than 5% of the time.
- This test is valuable in patients with atypical symptoms.

5. Acid perfusion (Bernstein test)--Saline perfusion for 10 min should not cause symptoms; next, switch to 0.1N HCl to see if the pain is reproduced. If heartburn and chest pain occur after acid instillation, treat for reflux.

- If heartburn and chest pain occur after acid instillation, treat for reflux.

6. Esophageal manometry--Manometry is reserved for patients with suspected esophageal motility disorders or with refractory reflux preoperatively.

- Esophageal manometry is reserved for suspected esophageal motility disorders.

Atypical Presentation and Complications of Gastroesophageal Reflux Disease

Atypical presentations include noncardiac chest pain, pulmonary (asthma and aspiration pneumonia), and hoarseness and cough.

Complications include ulceration, bleeding, stricture, aspiration, Barrett's esophagus, and carcinoma.

Treatment of Reflux

Treatment of gastroesophageal reflux disease is divided into three phases:

Phase 1 therapy--Lifestyle modifications: elevate head of bed 6 inches; modify diet so there is less fat and more protein; three meals a day; no eating for several hours before reclining; weight loss if overweight; and avoidance of specific foods (fatty foods, chocolate, alcohol, citrus juices, tomato products, coffee, carminatives). The patient should stop smoking and avoid alcohol. Avoid drugs that decrease lower esophageal sphincter pressure: anticholinergics, sedatives, tranquilizers, theophylline, progesterone or progesterone-containing birth control pills, nitrates, β-adrenergic agonists, and calcium channel blockers. Therapy is with antacids or alginic acid, 30 min after meals and at bedtime.

Phase 2 therapy--Therapy includes drugs that decrease gastric acid output: H_2 blockers, all are equally effective. A dose twice daily (bid) is preferable for treating gastroesophageal/reflux disease, e.g., cimetidine, 400 mg bid; ranitidine, 150 mg bid; famotidine, 20 mg bid; nizatidine, 150 mg bid. Omeprazole: reserve for cases refractory to H_2 receptor blockers. Drugs that increase lower esophageal sphincter pressure and esophageal clearance--cisapride, metoclopramide, bethanechol--have a limited role in treating reflux and often cause side effects.

Phase 3 therapy--This therapy includes antireflux surgery, which is reserved for patients who are refractory to medical therapy or who develop complications. Nissen fundoplication is the preferred operation; fundoplication increases lower esophageal sphincter pressure.

- Phase 1 therapy: modify lifestyle, avoid drugs that decrease lower esophageal sphincter pressure, and use antacids as the first line of treatment.
- Phase 2 therapy: H_2 blockers in twice daily doses are effective in most patients; use omeprazole in patients refractory to H_2 blockers.
- Do not use anticholinergics to treat reflux.
- Antireflux surgery is reserved for patients who are refractory to medical therapy or who develop complications.

Noncardiac Chest Pain

Chest pain is a frightening symptom, and patients are often referred to internists and gastroenterologists when cardiac evaluation does not have positive findings. Internists must understand the limitations of the diagnostic studies used to evaluate noncardiac chest pain. First, significant cardiac disease must be ruled out. Esophageal pain may be secondary to a motor disorder or a sensitive mucosa. Gastroesophageal reflux disease is the commonest cause of noncardiac chest pain, but the esophagus is only one of several possible causes. Esophageal spasm can closely mimic angina. Esophagogastroduodenoscopy rules out mucosal disease, i.e., inflammation, neoplasms, and chemical injury. Examine esophageal motility to look for motor disorders, e.g., esophageal spasm, "nutcracker esophagus." Therapy for noncardiac chest pain includes avoidance of precipitants. Antacids may be beneficial in patients with inflammation. Sublingual nitroglycerin or calcium channel blockers are sometimes helpful in motor disorders, but their efficacy is unproven. If appropriate, reassure patient that cardiac disease is not present.

- For noncardiac chest pain, rule out significant cardiac

disease.
- Gastroesophageal reflux disease is the commonest cause of noncardiac chest pain.
- Esophageal spasm can closely mimic angina.
- Esophagogastroduodenoscopy rules out mucosal disease.
- Sublingual nitroglycerin or calcium channel blockers sometimes are helpful.

Infections of the Esophagus

Patients with immunodeficiency disorders (AIDS), diabetes mellitus, malignancies (especially lymphoma and leukemia), and esophageal motility disorders are susceptible to opportunistic infections of the esophagus. These infections present as odynophagia. The most important infections to recognize are *Candida*, herpes, and cytomegalovirus. *Candida* infection: barium radiography shows small nodule in the upper 1/3 of the esophagus, and endoscopy shows cottage cheese-like plaques. Diagnosis is made by seeing pseudohyphae on KOH preparations. Treatment is with nystatin or clotrimazole for colonization and ketoconazole or fluconazole for esophagitis. Rarely, amphotericin B is used. Herpes infection: barium radiography and endoscopy show small discrete ulcers without plaques. Diagnosis is based on finding intranuclear inclusions (Cowdry's type A bodies). Cytomegalovirus infection: radiography and endoscopy show severe inflammation with large ulcers. Intranuclear inclusions may be seen but viral cultures are unreliable. Treatment is with ganciclovir.

Other Esophageal Problems

Medication-Induced Esophagitis

Medication-induced esophagitis presents as odynophagia or dysphagia and is more likely to occur if there is abnormal motility, stricture, or compression (left atrial enlargement). It is more common in the elderly and is recognized as inflammation in the mid-esophagus with sparing of the distal esophagus. Medications commonly associated with esophagitis include tetracycline, doxycycline, quinidine, potassium, ferrous sulfate, and ascorbic acid.

- Mid-esophageal inflammation is associated with abnormal motility, stricture, or compression and is more common in the elderly.
- Medicines responsible for esophagitis: tetracycline, doxycycline, quinidine, ferrous sulfate, ascorbic acid.

Mallory-Weiss Syndrome

Mallory-Weiss syndrome is mucosal laceration at the esophagogastric junction. It accounts for about 10% of upper gastrointestinal tract bleeding: 75% of patients have a history of retching or vomiting before bleeding, 72% have diaphragmatic hernias, and 90% stop bleeding. Vasopressin, endoscopic injection, or electrocautery may control bleeding. Surgical treatment for persistent bleeding.

- Mallory-Weiss syndrome: mucosal laceration at esophagogastric junction.
- Accounts for about 10% of upper gastrointestinal tract bleeding.
- 75% of patients have a history of retching and vomiting before bleeding.

Esophageal Perforation

Esophageal perforation commonly occurs after dilatation in an area of stricture. Spontaneous perforation of the esophagus (Boerhaave's syndrome) follows violent retching, often after an alcoholic binge. It also occurs after heavy lifting, defecation, seizures, and forceful labor (childbirth). The commonest site of perforation is the left posterior part of the distal esophagus. If pleural fluid is present, it may have an increased concentration of amylase. Zenker's diverticulum, cervical osteophytes (difficult intubations), and endoscopy (intubation) are causes of perforation of the cervical esophagus.

- Esophageal perforation commonly occurs after dilatation.
- Boerhaave's syndrome follows violent retching, often after an alcoholic binge.

STOMACH

Helicobacter pylori

The discovery of the relationship of *Helicobacter pylori* with ulcer disease has revoluntionized our thinking in this area. In 1982, a gram-negative, microaerophilic curved bacillus was successfully cultured from gastric biopsy specimens of patients with gastritis. Originally named *"Campylobacter pylori,"* this "new" organism was subsequently found to have significant differences from most true *Campylobacter* species and was subsequently named *"Helicobacter pylori."*

H. pylori has an age-related prevalence, occurring in

10% of the general population younger than age 30 and in 60% older than age 60. *H. pylori* is also more prevalent in blacks and Hispanics, poor socioeconomic groups, and institutionalized persons. Most likely, these bacteria are transmitted from person to person, although a common source infection cannot be dismissed. Evidence of person-to-person transmission includes clustering with families, higher than expected prevalence in institutionalized persons, transmission by endoscopy and biopsy, and a higher prevalence of infection among gastroenterologists.

H. pylori is found in almost all patients with gastritis without another cause, in 90%-95% of patients with duodenal ulcer, and in about 80% of patients with gastric ulcer. These bacteria are not found in gastritis of known cause, and their eradication or suppression is accompanied by resolution of the gastritis. It is generally accepted that *H. pylori* is responsible worldwide for chronic type B (antral) gastritis.

- *H. pylori* is present in 90% of patients with duodenal ulcer.
- *H. pylori* is present in 80% of patients with gastric ulcer.
- *H. pylori* is present in almost all patients with chronic type B gastritis without another cause.

Also, eradication of *H. pylori* hastens the healing of active duodenal ulcer and decreases the recurrence rate of duodenal ulcers and gastric ulcers. Recently, several studies have shown that infection with *H. pylori* is associated with an increased risk of gastric adenocarcinoma. Though there is mounting evidence that these bacteria are a significant pathogenic factor in gastritis, duodenal ulcer, gastric ulcer, and gastric cancer, there still is no proof that they cause any of these conditions.

- Eradication of *H. pylori* hastens healing rate and decreases the recurrence rate of duodenal ulcer.
- Eradication of *H. pylori* decreases the recurrence rate of gastric ulcer.
- *H. pylori* is associated with an increased risk of gastric adenocarcinoma.

Currently, the treatment of *H. pylori* is controversial. There are several recent reports of a significant response rate (70%-80%) after treatment with one antibiotic and an antisecretory agent. However, there is concern about the potential emergence of resistant organisms. Most investigators agree that treatment should include triple therapy with two antibiotics and a bismuth subsalicylate preparation. Many still recommend that treatment only be given to patients with culture-proved infections who are enrolled in controlled studies. Others recommend that *H. pylori* be eradicated in 1) patients with *H. pylori* infection who have had two or more episodes of symptomatic duodenal or gastric ulcer, 2) patients who are resistant to ordinary antisecretory treatment, 3) patients who have recurrent ulcer while receiving antisecretory treatment.

Treatment is not advocated for ulcers associated with nonsteroidal anti-inflammatory drugs, first episodes of ulcers, ulcers associated with the Zollinger-Ellison syndrome or massive hypersecretion, or treatment of nonulcer dyspepsia. Further studies are needed to determine whether treatment of chronic gastritis decreases the incidence of gastric cancer.

Peptic Ulcer Disease

Peptic ulcer disease is a heterogeneous group of disorders characterized by increased acid production or diminished mucosal resistance. The differences between duodenal ulcer and gastric ulcer should be recognized.

Gastric Ulcer

In the U.S., duodenal ulcer is 4x more common than gastric ulcer, which is rare before age 40 and has a peak incidence at age 55-65.

Pathophysiologic abnormalities--No convincing evidence for motility defects, and the evidence for duodenogastric reflux is conflicting. Other factors: prostaglandins, cytoprotection; mucosal blood flow, role of gastric mucosal ischemia; mucus and bicarbonate, possibly decreased amounts; acid and pepsin, most patients with gastric ulcer have acid secretory rates within the normal range. The exact role of *Helicobacter pylori* is unclear.

- Most patients with gastric ulcers have normal acid secretory rates.

Anatomical predisposition--Gastric ulcers usually occur on the lesser curve near the angulus, at the junction of oxyntic and antral mucosa.

- Gastric ulcers usually occur on the lesser curve near the angulus.

Environmental factors--Aspirin, nonsteroidal anti-

inflammatory drugs, and bile reflux damage the gastric mucosal barrier. Nonsteroidal anti-inflammatory drugs also inhibit prostaglandin synthesis. Smoking--Pathogenesis is unclear. Infectious agents--*Helicobacter pylori* and cytomegalovirus. Alcohol causes gastritis, but there is no definite evidence that stress, alcohol, or caffeine causes chronic gastric ulceration.

- Nonsteroidal anti-inflammatory drugs, aspirin, bile reflux, and smoking predispose to gastric ulceration.
- No definite evidence that stress, alcohol, corticosteroids, or caffeine causes gastric ulceration.

Natural history--65%-70% of ulcers heal in 12 weeks with placebo, and rate of recurrence in patients receiving placebo for up to 12 months is 55%-89%. Most ulcers recur in the same area. More than 2-3 recurrences are uncommon. Complications include bleeding, perforation, and obstruction. Clinical manifestations include pain frequently relieved by meals.

Diagnosis--Radiology can detect 90% of gastric ulcers. Criteria suggesting a benign gastric ulcer are Hampton line (a radiolucent line partially or completely traversing the orifice of the ulcer), folds radiating to the edge of an ulcer crater, an ulcer collar (a translucent band intervening between the ulcer crater and the lumen of the stomach). Criteria suggesting malignancy are negative filling defect in the ulcer crater or at its upper or lower margins and abnormal folds near the base.

- Barium radiography detects 90% of gastric ulcers.
- Negative filling defects in the ulcer crater or at its upper or lower margins suggest malignancy.
- Abnormal folds near base of the ulcer also suggest malignancy.

Endoscopy is indicated if there is a radiologically diagnosed gastric ulcer (3%-7% of malignant ulcers appear benign), a large ulcer (>2.5 cm), or an appearance not typically benign. It is also indicated after 8 weeks of therapy.

Medical therapy--Healing occurs in 60%-90% of cases treated for 6-8 weeks. Generally, healing rates are similar with H_2 blockers, antacids, sucralfate, and omeprazole. Healing is not increased with combined therapy (e.g., H_2 blockers plus antacids). Medical restrictions include eliminating or decreasing aspirin, nonsteroidal anti-inflammatory drugs, and smoking. Treatment of *H. pylori* is controversial.

● No increased healing with combination therapy.

Follow-up--If pain is not relieved within 2 weeks, add another medication. Repeat radiography or endoscopy in all patients to document healing. Refer for surgical treatment if ulcer is not healed in 12 weeks (allow 16 weeks if ulcer is large). For recurrent ulcers, the therapy used initially is usually adequate for treating recurrences. Surgical indications are patients with ulcer refractory to therapy, recurrent ulcer on maintenance therapy, complications, and malignancy. Prevention of recurrence: in most patients, recurrence can be treated with separate courses. Chronic maintenance is indicated for patients who would be at high risk if a recurrent ulcer became complicated by perforation or bleeding (e.g., patients with heart disease) and for those with previous complication of a gastric ulcer.

● Repeat radiography or endoscopy in all patients to document healing.
● Surgical treatment is indicated for patients with ulcer refractory to therapy, recurrent ulcer on maintenance therapy, complications, and malignancy.
● Maintenance treatment for patients with previous complication or at high risk for complication with recurrent ulcer.

Duodenal Ulcer

Epidemiology--Lifetime prevalence is about 10% for U.S. males and 4% for females. Risk factors--No convincing data that diet is a factor. Although alcohol is associated with mucosal lesions, it does not cause duodenal ulcer. Aspirin and nonsteroidal anti-inflammatory drugs induce acute injury and cause ulcers, perforation, and bleeding. The effect of corticosteroids is controversial, but the risk seems to be minimal. Cigarette smoking increases risk for duodenal ulcer and impairs ulcer healing. Caffeine causes dyspepsia but not ulcers. *H. pylori* increases risk for duodenal ulcer. There is a higher incidence of these ulcers if there is also chronic lung disease, cirrhosis, or chronic renal failure.

● Prevalence (U.S.): males, 10%; females, 4%.
● Aspirin, nonsteroidal anti-inflammatory drugs, smoking, and *H. pylori* increase risk for duodenal ulcer.
● No evidence that diet, alcohol, steroids, caffeine, or stress increase risk for duodenal ulcer.
● Chronic lung disease, cirrhosis, and chronic renal failure increase the risk for duodenal ulcer.

Pathogenesis and pathophysiology are dependent on acid and peptic activity. The ulcers are rare if acid secretion is <10 mEq/hr, but they can occur in cases of hypersecretion. Mucosal resistance is also a factor. The pathophysiologic abnormalities are complex and likely do not involve a single process. Proposed abnormalities include increased parietal cell and chief cell mass, increased basal secretory drive, increased postprandial secretory drive, rapid gastric emptying, and impaired mucosal defense.

● Duodenal ulcer is rare if acid secretion is <10 mEq/hr.

Diagnosis--80%-90% of ulcer craters can be detected on an optimal radiograph of the upper gastrointestinal tract. With routine radiographic techniques, 50% of duodenal ulcers may be missed. Endoscopy detects 85%-95% of gastroduodenal lesions with a specificity generally >90%. In patients with simple dyspepsia, a trial of antacids of H_2 blockers for 1-2 weeks is indicated in the appropriate clinical setting. Follow-up endoscopy to document healing in asymptomatic patients is not necessary for duodenal ulcer.

● 80%-90% of ulcer craters can be detected on an optimal radiograph of the upper gastrointestinal tract.
● Specificity is generally >90% with endoscopy.
● Follow-up endoscopy to document healing is not necessary for duodenal ulcer if patient is asymptomatic.

Natural history--Duodendal ulcer is a recurring, chronic disease, and 50%-80% of patients have recurrence within 6-12 months of initial healing. There is seasonal variation: the ulcers are more common in fall and spring.

● 50%-80% of patients have recurrence within 6-12 months.

Medical treatment--Eliminate factors impairing healing, including smoking, aspirin, and nonsteroidal anti-inflammatory drugs. H_2 receptor antagonists are all equally effective. Side effects: antiandrogen, gynecomastia, and impotence are usually seen only with high doses of cimetidine. Drug interactions: cimetidine inhibits cytochrome P450 system and affects the therapeutic effects of theophylline, lidocaine, phenytoin, and warfarin. Omeprazole inhibits H^+/K^+ ATPase pump responsible for acid secretion and irreversibly inactivates the enzyme. In normal subjects, it can produce anacidity. It is the drug of choice in Zollinger-Ellison syndrome and medically refractory reflux esophagitis. Anticholinergics have a limited role in duodenal ulcer. Do not use them in cases of gastroesophageal reflux disease or gastric ulcer. They decrease basal acid secretion by 40%-50% but are limited by their side effects (dry mouth, blurred vision).

The mechanism of antacids may not entirely be secondary to acid neutralization. Other factors may be the binding of bile acids, inactivation of pepsin, or enhanced mucosal resistance to injury. Side effects: Mg^{++}-diarrhea, aluminum hydroxide hypophosphatemia, and constipation. Prostaglandins (e.g., misoprostol) are produced by the gastroduodenal mucosa and have a role in mucosal resistance to injury. Prostaglandins of the E and I groups inhibit acid secretion. They are effective in preventing nonsteroidal anti-inflammatory drug-induced ulcers. Side effects: crampy abdominal pain and diarrhea. Sucralfate is a sulfated disaccharide complex with aluminum hydroxide. It does not alter gastric acid or pepsin secretion and is not effective in preventing nonsteroidal anti-inflammatory drug-induced ulcers.

- Cimetidine inhibits cytochrome P450; may develop toxicity from theophylline, lidocaine, phenytoin, and warfarin.
- Omeprazole is the drug of choice in Zollinger-Ellison syndrome and refractory gastroesophageal reflux disease.
- Do not use anticholinergics in gastroesophageal reflux disease or gastric ulcer.
- Misoprostol, but not sucralfate, prevents nonsteroidal anti-inflammatory drug-induced ulcers.

Refractory Ulcers

Twenty percent of peptic ulcers fail to heal in 4 weeks, but half of these heal with an additional 4 weeks of therapy. They are refractory if healing is not evident after 8-12 weeks, which is the case in 5% of ulcers. Symptoms may persist after healing, so documentation of the ulcer is necessary. Management--Treat for 8 weeks (or longer), check serum level of gastrin and salicylate (look for low level of uric acid). Prescribe larger doses of H_2 blockers at night or use omeprazole. Treat *H. pylori*.

- Refractory ulcer: failure to heal after 8-12 weeks of therapy.
- 5% of ulcers are refractory.
- Consider treatment for *H. pylori*.
- Exclude Zollinger-Ellison syndrome.

Recurrent Ulcers

Recurrence does not depend on the length of the initial treatment or on the dose/potency of the agent. Maintenance therapy does reduce recurrences--cimetidine 400 mg qhs, 60%-85% without recurrence; placebo, 17%-39% without recurrence. Between 15% and 20% of patients require more antisecretory efficacy than that achieved with cimetidine (400 mg at night) to prevent recurrence. Treatment for *H. pylori* decreases recurrence of duodenal and gastric ulcers.

Complications of Peptic Ulcer Disease and Indications for Surgery

Intractability is the most common reason for surgery. Confirmation of the presence of ulcer is necessary. Approximately 15% of patients with peptic ulcer disease have severe symptoms requiring surgical treatment.

- Intractability is the common reason for surgery.
- 15% of patients have severe symptoms requiring surgical treatment.

Hemorrhage occurs in 15%-20% of ulcer patients and is most common in patients in the 6th decade. Eighty percent of patients relate a history of symptomatic ulcer disease before the onset of bleeding. Hemorrhage is more common with gastric ulcer than with duodenal ulcer, possibly because of an older patient population and use of nonsteroidal anti-inflammatory drugs. More than 50% of those treated medically hemorrhage again in 10-15 years.

- 15%-20% of ulcer patients hemorrhage.
- Hemorrhage is most common in elderly persons taking nonsteroidal anti-inflammatory drugs.
- >50% of those treated medically hemorrhage again in 10-15 years.

Perforation is a less common complication than hemorrhage and more common than obstruction. Pyloroduodenal perforation is more common than gastric perforation. The preferred procedure for treating perforation is closure of the perforation and proximal selective gastric vagotomy.

- Pyloroduodenal perforation is more common than gastric perforation.

Penetration is the erosion of the ulcer through the wall

without leakage of the digestive contents into the peritoneal cavity. The common one is a posterior penetrating ulcer into the pancreas, mimicking pancreatitis. Penetrating ulcers require aggressive treatment and may be refractory.

Gastric outlet obstruction is a complication in 2% of all ulcer patients. In 90% of them, it is caused by duodenal ulcer and in 4%-5%, by gastric ulcer. Only 25%-35% respond to medical management and >90% of responders subsequently require surgical treatment.

- Gastric outlet obstruction is caused by duodenal ulcer in 90% of patients and by gastric ulcer in 4%-5%.

Peptic Ulcer Surgery

The objectives of an operation for peptic ulcer disease are 1) effectiveness (low recurrent rate), 2) safety (low mortality rate), and 3) preservation of the digestive apparatus (low morbidity, few complications). Operations alter the pathophysiology of peptic ulcer disease by: 1. Reducing stimuli for HCl secretion--Vagotomy eliminates the direct cholinergic stimulus. Antrectomy eliminates gastrin-mediated HCl secretion. 2. Reducing parietal cell mass--Antrectomy eliminates gastrin's trophic effect on parietal cells. Subtotal gastrectomy reduces the parietal cell mass by the amount resected. Total gastrectomy is not indicated for peptic disease. It is indicated for cancer and gastric bleeding (previously for Zollinger-Ellison syndrome) (Table 13-4).

- Vagotomy eliminates the direct cholinergic stimulus.
- Antrectomy eliminates gastrin-mediated HCl secretion and eliminates gastrin's trophic effect on parietal cells.
- Parietal gastrectomy reduces parietal cell mass.
- Total gastrectomy is not indicated for peptic disease but is indicated for cancer and gastric bleeding.

Table 13-4.--Results of Ulcer Operation

Procedure	Mortality, %	% complications	% ulcer recurrence	2nd operation
Gastroenterostomy	...	...	34	70% gastrectomy
Gastrectomy (BI, BII)	3	20% dumping, diarrhea	5	Vagotomy, remove retained antrum
Truncal vagotomy/ pyloroplasty	1	15% dumping, bilious vomiting	15	Re-vagotomize, antrectomy
Truncal vagotomy/ antrectomy[*]	<1	25% dumping, diarrhea	1	Re-vagotomize
Selective (gastric) vagotomy/pyloroplasty	<1	20% dumping 6% diarrhea	5	Re-vagotomize, antrectomy
Parietal cell vagotomy	<1	5% dumping	5-20 (rising with follow-up)	Re-vagotomize, antrectomy

[*]Preferred for obstruction and acute hemorrhage.

Postgastrectomy Syndromes

Early: 1) Duodenal stump leakage--Sudden, severe abdominal pain 3-6 days postoperatively and associated fever, leukocytosis, and abdominal rigidity. The patient is at higher risk if the duodenum is severely inflamed. 2) Bleeding--If within 24 hours: failure to ligate vessel or coagulopathy. If 4-7 days: anastomotic slough. 3) Gastric retention--Motility disorders may persist for 2 weeks postoperatively. Use gastroscopy to rule out obstruction; treatment is with nasogastric suction.

Late: Recurrent ulcer (anastomotic ulcer) occurs on intestinal side, usually within 2 cm of anastomoses. Differential diagnoses include inadequate vagotomy, inad-

equate operation, retained antrum, hyperplasia of G cells, and Zollinger-Ellison syndrome.

Work-up includes: 1) obtaining operative and pathology reports--Was stomach resected to the duodenum? Were vagal trunks identified? 2) Performing gastric acid studies--If basal acid output is <2 mEq/hr (Hollander test is not useful). 3) Determine gastrin level--Normal is <300 pg/mL; if >1,000 pg/mL, it indicates Zollinger-Ellison syndrome; if 300-1,000 mg/mL the gastrin stimulation test needs to be performed.

Dumping syndrome--Early: diaphoresis, tachycardia, hypotension, giddiness, abdominal cramps, and diarrhea occur within 15-30 min after eating. Vasomotor symptoms are due to release of vasoactive substances (bradykinin, serotonin) into portal blood and decreased circulating blood volume. Treatment--Frequent small meals low in carbohydrates. Dumping syndrome--Late: faintness, sweating, and coldness occur 1-3 hours after a meal. It resembles insulin reaction because the symptoms are due to a reactive hypoglycemia. Treatment--Frequent small meals low in carbohydrates. Somatostatin has relieved symptoms.

- Dumping syndrome--Early: diaphoresis, tachycardia, hypotension, giddiness, abdominal cramps, and diarrhea.
- Dumping syndrome--Late: faintness, sweating, and coldness due to hypoglycemia.
- Treatment: frequent small meals low in carbohydrates. Trial of somatostatin.

Diarrhea--Postgastrectomy diarrhea may result from many mechanisms. Malabsorption is caused by bacterial overgrowth or unmasking of a latent sprue or lactase deficiency. Postvagotomy diarrhea results from rapid gastric empleting, poor mixing of digestive enzymes, and decreased motility. It may be treated by frequent small meals low in carbohydrate and bulk (cholestyramine may help if rapid transit of bile acids is present). A special cause of diarrhea is gastrocolic fistula.

- Postgastrectomy diarrhea may result from malabsorption and postvagotomy diarrhea.

Gastrocolic fistula or gastrojejunocolic fistula-- Abdominal pain that may be relieved by diarrhea, usually malabsorption. Differential diagnosis is recurrent ulcer, cancer, or Crohn's disease. Colon radiography is the best test (upper gastrointestinal tract radiography detects only 50% of the fistulas).

- Colon radiography is the best test because upper gastrointestinal tract radiography detects only 50% of the fistulas.

Afferent loop syndromes: 1) Early--Postprandial bilious vomiting occurs 15-30 min after eating and is associated with nausea and abdominal discomfort. It occurs after Billroth II and results from partial obstruction of the afferent loop. Bile and pancreatic juice accumulate in the afferent loop, which eventually contracts and empties into the stomach. 2) Late (blind loop syndrome)--

Bacterial overgrowth occurs in the afferent loop and causes malabsorption as bile salts are deconjugated and megaloblastic anemia as bacteria use vitamin B_{12}. Treatment is to convert Billroth II to Billroth I or Roux-en-Y.

- Afferent loop syndrome (early) occurs after Billroth II and results from partial obstruction of the afferent loop.
- Blind loop syndrome is due to bacterial overgrowth in afferent loop.

Alkaline reflux gastritis--Abdominal pain, anemia, bilious vomiting. It is caused by the reflux of bile into the stomach. Gastroscopy shows inflammation on the gastric side of anastomoses. It is more frequent with larger resections (i.e., more frequently with Billroth II than with Billroth I than with pyloroplasty). Medical treatment-- Aluminum hydroxide gel (Amphojel) and cholestyramine are often unsuccessful. Surgical treatment is conversion to Roux-en-Y (good result in 90%-95%).

- Alkaline reflux gastritis: abdominal pain, anemia, bilious vomiting; caused by reflux of bile.

Anemia--Iron deficiency is the commonest cause of anemia and results from blood loss, bypass of duodenum where iron is absorbed, and decreased acid, which prevents conversion of the ferric form of iron to the ferrous form, which is better absorbed. Treatment--Ferrous sulfate and vitamin C (also, treat inflammation to prevent blood loss). Vitamin B_{12} deficiency is caused by loss of intrinsic factor with gastric resection, gastritis, or bacterial overgrowth. Folate deficiency is due to poor intake.

- Iron deficiency is the commonest cause of anemia.
- Vitamin B_{12} deficiency: caused by loss of intrinsic factor with gastric resection.
- Folate deficiency: due to poor intake.

Weight loss most commonly is caused by a small gastric reservoir, but always rule out malabsorption and its causes (bacterial overgrowth, sprue, fistula).

Gastric stump cancer occurs 15-20 years postoperatively.

Osteomalacia--Decreased calcium and vitamin D absorption after duodenal bypass.

Susceptibility to infections (especially TB) is due to decreased acid.

Zollinger-Ellison Syndrome

Etiology and Pathogenesis

Zollinger-Ellison syndrome is acid hypersecretion secondary to a gastrinoma usually located in the pancreatic head. The duodenal wall is the commonest extrapancreatic site (13%). The gastrinoma is solitary in 50% of cases. Two-thirds of them are malignant but usually indolent. Approximately 25% of patients with gastrinoma have multiple endocrine neoplasia syndrome type I. These patients usually have multiple gastrinomas. Increased gastric parietal cell mass is 2x-3x that of patients with duodenal ulcer.

- Zollinger-Ellison syndrome: acid hypersecretion secondary to gastrinoma.
- The gastrinoma is usually located in the pancreatic head.
- Two-thirds of them are malignant but usually indolent.
- Approximately 25% of the patients have multiple endocrine neoplasia syndrome type I.

Clinical Features

From 90% to 95% of patients with Zollinger-Ellison syndrome develop ulceration, 75% in the duodenal bulb. Diarrhea may precede ulcer symptoms. Diarrhea (present in 1/3 of the patients) is caused by large amounts of HCl secreted into the gastrointestinal tract, increased intestinal secretion, and reduced jejunal absorption. Steatorrhea may occur because of inactivation of pancreatic lipase and precipitation of bile salts. Vitamin B_{12} deficiency occurs secondary to acidic interference with intrinsic factor activity.

- Zollinger-Ellison syndrome: 90%-95% of patients develop ulceration, 75% in the duodenal bulb.
- Diarrhea may precede ulcer symptoms (present in 1/3 of patients).
- Steatorrhea may occur.

Gastrinoma should be considered (check serum level of gastrin) when any of the following are found: multiple ulcers in the upper gastrointestinal tract; ulcers distal to the first portion of the duodenum, intractable ulcers, recurrence postoperatively, unexplained secretory diarrhea, family history of peptic ulcer disease, history of parathyroid or pituitary tumors, gastric acid hypersecretion or hypergastrinemia, ulcer and hypercalcemia, or ulcer and diarrhea.

Diagnosis

Gastric acid secretion--Basal acid output is >15 mEq/hr, and the ratio of basal acid output to maximal acid output is >60%. The increase in acid output is proportionally less than in normal subjects in response to exogenous stimulation (only 1/3 of patients). Barium studies show prominent gastric rugal folds. The serum level of gastrin is the most sensitive and specific diagnostic test, but hypergastrinemia is seen in other disorders. Acid hypersecretion should be determined before conducting a provocative test. Secretin test--Normal values in patients with duodenal ulcer. Secretin decreases or has no effect on serum gastrin. In patients with Zollinger-Ellison syndrome, a dramatic increase in serum gastrin is seen. Levels increase promptly by at least 200 pg/mL. Findings are positive in 95% of those with gastrinoma. Standard meal--In Zollinger-Ellison syndrome, serum levels of gastrin do not increase or increase only slightly, but in gastrin cell hyperplasia, the increase is striking.

- Basal acid output is >15 mEq/hr.
- Barium studies show prominent gastric rugal folds.
- Serum level of gastrin: most sensitive and specific test, but hypergastrinemia is seen in other disorders.
- Secretin test: normal values in patients with duodenal ulcer; in Zollinger-Ellison syndrome, gastrin increases in 95% of cases.

Tumor localization intraoperatively is difficult, and the tumor is not found in 40%-45% of patients. Selective arteriography detects 1/3 of the tumors. Computed tomographic (CT) scanning also detects 1/3 of them. Together, arteriography and CT scanning detect 44% of gastrinomas. Transhepatic portal venous sampling gives results comparable to those of CT.

- Localization intraoperatively is difficult.
- Selective arteriography detects 1/3 of the tumors.
- CT scanning detects 1/3 of the tumors.

Treatment

Medical treatment--H_2-receptor antagonists induce ulcer healing in 80%-85% of cases, often requiring high doses (5-9 g/day). With long-term treatment, as many as 50% of patients have failure with H_2 blockers. Omeprazole heals 90%-100% of ulcers in 4 weeks. Somatostatin decreases serum levels of gastrin and gastric acid secretion.

- H_2-receptor antagonists produce healing in 80%-85% of cases.
- Omeprazole heals 90%-100% of ulcers in 4 weeks.
- Somatostatin decreases serum levels of gastrin and gastric acid secretion.

Surgical treatment--Approximately 20%-25% of gastrinomas can be completely removed surgically. Surgical exploration, with intent to resect, should be done except in patients with extensive metastatic disease, surgical contraindications, or with multiple endocrine neoplasia type I syndrome. If the gastrinoma cannot be localized or resected, options include total gastrectomy and proximal gastric vagotomy (reduces gastric acid secretion and H_2-blocker requirements).

- 20%-25% of gastrinomas can be completely removed surgically.
- Surgical exploration should be done except in patients with extensive metastatic disease, surgical contraindications, or with multiple endocrine neoplasia type I syndrome.

Prognosis

If resection is curative, life expectancy will be normal. If there are sporadic unresectable gastrinomas, the average life expectancy is 2 years.

Stress Ulcers

Underlying conditions for stress ulcers are trauma, sepsis, and serious illness. Most of the hemorrhages occur 3-7 days after the traumatic event. If no prophylactic treatment is given, 10%-20% of patients in Intensive Care Units have hemorrhaging. Burns, especially those involving >35% of the body, cause Curling's ulcer. Central nervous system trauma produces Cushing's ulcer, which is seen in 50%-75% of head injury patients. Cushing's ulcer tends to be deep and to perforate more often than others.

- Underlying conditions for stress ulcers: trauma, sepsis, serious illness.
- Hemorrhaging occurs 3-7 days after the traumatic event.
- If no prophylactic treatment is given, 10%-20% of patients in Intensive Care Units develop hemorrhaging.
- Burns involving >35% of body have greater tendency to produce Curling's ulcer.
- Stress ulcers are seen in 50%-75% of head injury patients.

Prophylaxis against bleeding is to keep pH >4.0. Antacids clearly decrease the incidence of bleeding over that of placebo. H_2-receptor antagonists are equally as effective as antacids and sometimes easier to use. Sucralfate is as effective as antacids and H_2 blockers according to some studies. Also, sucralfate may decrease nosocomial pneumonia in ventilator-dependent patients because gastric pH is not lowered (decreased bacterial overgrowth). Prostaglandins may have a role in prophylaxis. Enteral feedings can maintain intragastric pH >3.5. If antacids cannot be used, use H_2 blockers or sucralfate; combination treatment may be helpful.

- Prophylaxis: keep pH >4.0.
- Antacids, H_2-receptor antagonists, and sucralfate decrease incidence of bleeding.
- Sucralfate may decrease nosocomial pneumonia in ventilator-dependent patients.

Medical therapy for bleeding, acute gastric mucosal ulcers: correct the underlying predisposing condition. In general, upper gastrointestinal tract bleeding stops about 85% of the time. Some advocate use of iced saline lavage or intragastric levarterenol. Angiographic therapeutic techniques include intra-arterial vasopressin and transcatheter embolization. Endoscopic techniques are electrocautery (bicap heater probe) and laser photocoagulation. Surgical therapy for bleeding acute gastric mucosal ulcers must be considered when blood requirement is >4-6 units per 24-48 hr. Mortality rate for all forms of surgical therapy is 30%-40%.

Nonerosive Nonspecific Chronic Gastritis

Chronic gastritis is divided into two types: type A and type B. Type-A, or autoimmune, gastritis involves the body and fundus of the stomach. A subset of patients develops atrophic gastritis (inflammation of the gland zone with variable gland loss). Pernicious anemia with hypochlorhydria or achlorhydria and megaloblastic anemia may result. Antiparietal cell antibodies are found in 90% of patients. Intrinsic factor antibodies are seen less commonly. Other autoimmune diseases such as Addison's disease and Hashimoto's thyroiditis are often present. Gastrin concentrations in the serum are increased. Gastric carcinoid tumors rarely develop. Gastric polyps occur, and intestinal metaplasia may be precursor to gastric adenocarcinoma.

- Type-A gastritis is associated with pernicious anemia

and other autoimmune disorders.

- Serum levels of gastrin are increased.
- Type-A gastritis is associated with gastric carcinoids, polyps, and adenocarcinoma.

Type-B gastritis involves the antrum and is associated with *H. pylori* infection. Serum levels of gastrin are normal. Gastric ulcers and duodenal ulcers occur commonly, and there is increased incidence of gastric adenocarcinoma.

- Type-B gastritis is associated with *H. pylori* infection.
- Serum levels of gastrin are normal.
- Type-B gastritis is associated with gastric and duodenal ulcers and adenocarcinoma.

Gastric Cancer

In the 1940s, gastric cancer was the commonest malignant disease in the U.S. Since then, the decrease in incidence has been dramatic. Japan has the highest mortality rate from gastric cancer. Migration studies show a decrease in incidence in migrants from high-risk areas to low-risk areas and a suggestion of increased risk in persons moving from low-risk to high-risk areas. Environmental factors include diet--increased association with starch, pickled vegetables, salted fish/meat, smoked foods, increased salt consumption, and nitrate and nitrite consumption. Genetic factors include blood group A, which has a 2x-3x greater incidence among relatives. The population at risk are persons older than 50 years. The male:female ratio is as high as 2:1. Also, it is more common in lower socioeconomic groups.

- Dramatic decrease in the incidence of gastric cancer in the U.S. since the 1940s.
- Decreased incidence in migrants from high-risk areas.
- Increased association with starch, pickled vegetables, salted fish/meat, smoked foods, increased salt consumption, and nitrate and nitrite consumption.
- A 2x-3x greater incidence among relatives.

Possible Precancerous Lesions/Situations

1) Chronic atrophic gastritis and intestinal metaplasia are frequently found in patients with gastric cancer (one study showed gastric cancer in 10% of those with atrophic gastritis followed up for 20 years compared with 0.6% in those with normal mucosa or superficial gastritis). However, both conditions are found frequently in older persons without gastric carcinoma. A subtype of intestinal metaplasia, with marked cell differentiation and production of sulfomucin (type IIb), may be the only type associated with gastric cancer. 2) Chronic benign gastric ulcer rarely progresses to cancer. 3) Pernicious anemia--previous autopsy studies showed incidence of 10%. Recent endoscopic screening study of 123 patients with pernicious anemia showed prevalence of gastric neoplastic lesions of 8.1%. 4) Postgastrectomy carries increased risk, although surveillance endoscopy is not necessary.

- Chronic atrophic gastritis is frequently found in patients with gastric cancer.
- A subtype of intestinal metaplasia, with production of sulfomucin (type IIb), is associated with gastric cancer.
- Chronic benign gastric ulcer rarely progresses to cancer.
- Pernicious anemia incidence of 10%.
- Postgastrectomy: increased risk.

Clinical Aspects

Gastric cancer is often asymptomatic, but abdominal discomfort and weight loss are the common presenting complaints. Physical examination is often unrevealing, but up to 30% of patients have an epigastric mass. Perform endoscopy, with multiple (7-8) biopsies and CT scanning of abdomen (to identify extragastric extension).

- Abdominal discomfort and weight loss are common presenting complaints.
- 30% of patients have an epigastric mass.
- Perform endoscopy, with multiple (7-8) biopsies.

Treatment and Prognosis

For local disease--Resection, often requires total gastrectomy for tumor-free margins. Omentum and spleen (splenic hilus nodes) are often removed in curative resection. For disseminated disease--Surgical treatment is only necessary for palliation. Response to chemotherapy is generally poor. The only consistent factor is extent of disease. Five-year survival is 90% if the tumor is confined to the mucosa and submucosa, 50% if the tumor is through the serosa, and 10% if the tumor involves lymph nodes.

- Gastric cancer often requires total gastrectomy.
- Surgical treatment is only necessary for palliation.

Gastric Polyps

Gastric polyps are rare; 0.5% incidence in an autopsy series. The two types of polyps are hyperplastic and adenomatous. Hyperplastic polyps are more common and premalignant. No therapy is needed. Adenomatous polyps are premalignant, especially if >2 cm in size. They most often occur in achlorhydric stomachs, i.e., pernicious anemia, and are usually localized in the antrum. If pedunculated, the polyp can be endoscopically removed.

- Hyperplastic polyps are more common and not premalignant.
- Adenomatous polyps are premalignant, especially if >2 cm in size.

Gastroduodenal Dysmotility Syndromes

Symptoms that suggest abnormal gastric motility (i.e., gastroparesis) include nausea, vomiting, bloating, early satiety, dyspepsia, heartburn, anorexia, weight loss, and food avoidance. The specific cause of abnormal gastric motor function is unknown but is believed to be related to autonomic neuropathy. Diabetes mellitus is probably the commonest medical cause of symptomatic gastric motor dysfunction. Conditions causing gastroparesis are listed in Table 13-5.

- Nausea, vomiting, bloating, early satiety, dyspepsia, heartburn, anorexia, weight loss, and food avoidance suggest abnormal gastric motility.
- It is believed to be related to autonomic neuropathy.
- Diabetes mellitus: commonest medical cause of symptomatic gastric motor dysfunction.

Table 13-5.--Conditions Causing Gastroparesis

Acute conditions	Chronic conditions
Anticholinergic drugs	Amyloidosis
Hyperglycemia	Diabetes mellitus
Hypokalemia	Gastric dysrhythmias
Morphine	Pseudo-obstruction
Pancreatitis	Scleroderma
Surgery	Vagotomy
Trauma	

Treatment: Currently several prokinetic drugs are available in the U.S. These drugs normalize and/or augment motility, with an accompanying enhancement of aboral movement of luminal contents. Metoclopramide is a dopamine antagonist and a cholinergic agonist that increases the rate and amplitude of antral contractions. It crosses the blood-brain barrier and frequently causes such side effects as drowsiness, athetosis, and prolactin release. Domperidone is a selective dopamine antagonist that works only on peripheral receptors in the gut. It has no cholinergic effects and fewer side effects. Cisapride facilitates the release of acetylcholine from the myenteric plexus (local cholinergic agonist). It does not antagonize dopamine and has few side effects. Bethanechol is a systemic cholinergic agonist with side effects. It may be useful in low dosage in combination with other agents. Erythromycin stimulates both cholinergic and motilin receptors.

- Domperidone is a selective dopamine antagonist.
- Cisapride is a selective cholinergic agonist.
- Erythromycin stimulates both cholinergic and motilin receptors.

Percutaneous endoscopic gastrostomy--easy to place, allows long-term access for enteral feeding. Complications include aspiration, plugging of the tube, tube migration, and leakage around the tube.

SMALL INTESTINE

Diarrhea

Patients use the term "diarrhea" to refer to any increase in the frequency, fluidity, or volume of the stool or any change in its consistency. Normally, stools are generally solid and brown, but these features may vary with diet. Frequency of stools varies among persons from 1-3 stools daily to 2-3 stools weekly. Blood, pus (leukocytes), and oil are not present in normal stools (Table 13-6).

Table 13-6.--Normal Stool Composition

		Electrolytes, mEq/L	
Weight	<200 g	Na^+	40
Percent water	65-80	K^+	90
Fat	<7 g	Cl^-	15
Nitrogen	<2.5 g	HCO_3^-	30

Physicians define diarrhea as an increase in stool weight or volume. Because a stool is 65%-80% water, stool weight is proportional to stool water. Dietary fiber content influences water content of stool and, thus, stool weight can vary according to the diet of a culture. In the U.S., normal daily stool weight is <200 g/day and normal stool volume is <200 mL/day (compared with <400 g/day and 400 mL/day, respectively, in rural Africa).

It is important to understand normal daily intestinal fluid balance. Each day, 9-10 L of isotonic fluid is presented to the proximal small intestine (2 L, diet and 8 L, endogenous secretions). The small bowel absorbs most of the fluid (7-9 L), and the colon absorbs all the 1-2 L presented to it each day except <200 mL and forms a soft solid stool. There is considerable reserve because the maximal absorptive capacity of the small bowel is 12 L/day, and 4-6 L/day for the colon.

Mechanisms of Diarrhea

Osmotic diarrhea occurs when water-soluble molecules are poorly absorbed, remain in the intestinal lumen, and retain water in the intestine. Osmotic diarrhea follows ingestion of an osmotically active substance and stops with fasting. Stool volume is <1 L/day, and the stool has an anion gap--stool osmolality is greater than the sum of electrolyte concentrations. Often, stool pH is <7.0. Clinical examples of osmotic diarrhea include lactase deficiency, sorbitol foods, saline cathartics, and antacids.

- In osmotic diarrhea, stool volume is <1 L/day.
- Diarrhea stops with fasting.
- Stool has an anion gap.
- Causes osmotic diarrhea: lactase deficiency, sorbitol foods, and antacids.

In secretory diarrhea, fluid and electrolyte transport are abnormal, i.e., the intestine secretes rather than absorbs fluid. Stool volume is >1 L/day and its composition is similar to that of extracellular fluid so there is no anion gap. The diarrhea persists despite fasting and often presents with hypokalemia. Clinical examples of secretory diarrhea include bacterial toxins, hormonal tumors, surreptitious laxative ingestion, bile acid diarrhea, and fatty acid diarrhea.

- In secretory diarrhea, stool volume is >1 L/day.
- There is no anion gap.
- Diarrhea persists despite fasting.
- Causes of secretory diarrhea: bacterial toxins, hormonal tumors, surreptitious laxative ingestion, bile acid diarrhea, and fatty acid diarrhea.

In exudative diarrhea, membrane permeability is abnormal, and there is exudation of serum proteins, blood, or mucus into the bowel from sites of inflammation, ulceration, or infiltration. The diarrhea is small volume and may be associated with bloody stools. Examples include invasive bacterial pathogens (*Shigella, Salmonella*, etc.) and inflammatory bowel disease.

- Exudative diarrhea: abnormal membrane permeability.
- Diarrhea is small volume.
- Invasive bacterial pathogens (*Shigella, Salmonella*, etc.) and inflammatory bowel disease.

Motility disorders: both rapid transit (inadequate time for chyme to contact absorbing surface) and delayed transit (bacterial overgrowth) can cause diarrhea. Rapid transit occurs after gastrectomy and intestinal resection and in hyperthyroidism and carcinoid syndrome. Delayed transit occurs with structural defects (strictures, blind loops, small-bowel diverticuli) or underlying illnesses that cause visceral neuropathy (diabetes) or myopathy (scleroderma), i.e., pseudo-obstruction.

- Rapid transit: causes diarrhea because of malabsorption.
- Delayed transit: causes diarrhea because of bacterial overgrowth.

Mixed mechanisms: Many disease processes may have more than one mechanism for causing diarrhea, e.g., generalized malabsorption has osmotic and secretory components (fatty acids cause secretion in the colon).

Clinical Approach

It is useful to differentiate small-bowel ("right-sided") diarrhea from colonic ("left-sided") diarrhea (Table 13-7). Right-sided diarrhea is large in volume, with a modest increase in the number of stools. Symptoms attributed to inflammation of the rectosigmoid are absent and proctoscopic examination findings are normal. Left-sided diarrhea presents as frequent small volume stools with obvious evidence of inflammation, and proctosigmoidoscopic examination usually confirms inflammation. Left-sided diarrhea usually suggests an exudative mechanism, whereas the mechanism for right-sided diarrhea is nonspecific.

Acute Diarrhea

Acute diarrhea is abrupt in onset and usually resolves in several days (3-10 days). It is self-limited, and the cause usually is not found (? viral). No evaluation is necessary unless there are bloody stools and fever or infection is suspected (e.g., travel history, common source outbreak). If these conditions exist, do not treat with antimotility agents. Begin the work-up with stool studies for ova and parasites and proctosigmoidoscopy. Recognize the common situations that predispose to specific infections (see infectious diarrhea below).

- For acute diarrhea, no evaluation is necessary unless there are bloody stools and fever or infection is suspected.
- Do not administer antimotility agents if there are bloody stools and fever or if infection is suspected.

Table 13-7.--Right-Sided and Left-Sided Diarrhea: Contrasts in Clinical Presentation

Right-sided or small-bowel diarrhea	Left-sided diarrhea
Reservoir capacity intact	Reservoir capacity decreased
Large stool volume	Small amounts of stool
Modest increase in number	Frequency
No urgency	Urgency
No tenesmus	Tenesmus
No mucus	Mucus
No blood	Blood

Chronic Diarrhea

Chronic diarrhea is an initial episode lasting longer than 4 weeks or diarrhea that recurs after the initial episode. The commonest cause of chronic diarrhea is irritable bowel syndrome, but always rule out lactase deficiency. Be able to differentiate organic diarrhea from functional diarrhea (Table 13-8).

- Commonest cause of chronic diarrhea is irritable bowel syndrome.
- Always rule out lactase deficiency in suspected irritable bowel syndrome.
- Differentiate organic diarrhea from functional diarrhea.

Chronic Watery Diarrhea

The evaluation of chronic watery diarrhea usually requires distinguishing secretory diarrhea from osmotic diarrhea (Table 13-9). This can be done by collecting stools and measuring volume, osmolality, and electrolyte content and observing the patient's response to fasting.

- Evaluation of chronic watery diarrhea requires distinguishing secretory diarrhea from osmotic diarrhea.

Anatomy of Nutrient Absorption

The sites of nutrient, vitamin, and mineral absorption are the following: 1) the duodenum absorbs iron, magnesium, folate, water-soluble vitamins, and monosaccharides; 2) the jejunum absorbs fatty acids, amino acids, monosaccharides, and water-soluble vitamins; and 3) the ileum absorbs monosaccharides, fatty acids, amino acids, fat-soluble vitamins (A, D, E, K), vitamin B_{12}, and conjugated bile salts.

The distal small bowel can adapt to absorb nutrients. The proximal small bowel cannot adapt to absorb vitamin B_{12} or bile salts. Fat absorption is the most complex process. Dietary fat consists mostly of triglycerides that must be digested by pancreatic lipase to fatty acids and glycerol, which are solubilized by micelles for absorption. The fatty acids and monoglycerides are reesterified by intestinal epithelial cells into chylomicrons that are absorbed into the circulation by lymphatic vessels (Table 13-10).

- The distal small bowel can adapt to absorb nutrients.
- The proximal small bowel cannot adapt to absorb vitamin B_{12} or bile salts.

Suspect malabsorption if the medical history suggests steatorrhea, or if there is diarrhea with weight loss (especially if intake is adequate), chronic diarrhea of indeterminate nature, or nutritional deficiency (know the symptoms and signs of malabsorption) (Table 13-11).

- Diarrhea with iron deficiency anemia (evaluation for blood loss is negative) = proximal small bowel, e.g., sprue.
- Diarrhea with metabolic bone disease = decreased calcium and protein, thus, proximal small bowel.
- Hypoproteinemia with normal fat absorption suggests "protein-losing enteropathy." If eosinophilia is present, eosinophilic gastroenteritis; if lymphopenia is present, intestinal lymphangiectasia.
- Oil droplets (neutral fat) or muscle fibers (undigested protein) present in stool = pancreatic insufficiency (maldigestion).
- Serum levels of calcium, magnesium, and iron are usu-

Table 13-8.--Features Differentiating Organic Diarrhea From Functional Diarrhea

	Organic diarrhea	Functional diarrhea
Weight loss	Often present	Not present
Duration of illness	Variable (weeks to years)	Usually long (>6 months)
Quantity of stool	Variable but usually large (>200 g/24 hr)	Usually small (<200 g/24 hr)
Presence of blood in stool	May be present	Never present (unless from hemorrhoids)
Timing when diarrhea occurs	No special pattern	Usually in the morning but rarely wakes patient
Fever, arthritis, skin lesions	May be present	Not present
Emotional stress	No relation to symptoms	Usually precedes or coincides with symptoms
Cramping abdominal pain	Often	May be present

From Matseshe JW, Phillips SF: Chronic diarrhea: a practical approach. Med. Clin. North Am. 62:141-154, Jan 1978. By permission of WB Saunders Company.

Table 13-9.--Typical Findings in Osmotic and Secretory Diarrheas

	Osmotic diarrhea	Secretory diarrhea
Daily stool volume, L	<1	>1
Effect of 48-hr fasting	Diarrhea stops	Diarrhea continues
Fecal fluid analysis		
Osmolality, mOsm	400	290
Na + K x 2*, mEq/L	120	280
Solute gap†	>100	<50

*Multiplied by 2 to account for anions.

†Calculated by subtracting ([Na] + [K]) x 2 from osmolality.

From Krejs GJ, Hendler RS, Fordtran JS: Diagnostic and pathophysiologic studies in patients with chronic diarrhea. *In* Secretory Diarrhea. Edited by M Field, JS Fordtran, SG Schultz. Bethesda, MD, American Physiological Society, 1980, pp 141-151. By permission of publisher.

Table 13-10.--Mechanisms of Fat Malabsorption

Alteration	Mechanism	Disease state
Defective digestion	Inadequate lipase	Pancreatic insufficiency
Impaired micelle formation	Duodenal bile salt concentration	Common duct obstruction or cholestasis
Impaired absorption	Small-bowel disease	Sprue and Whipple's disease
Impaired chylomicron formation	Impaired β-globulin synthesis	Abetalipoproteinemia
Impaired lymphatic circulation	Lymphatic obstruction	Intestinal lymphangiectasia and lymphoma

Table 13-11.--Causes of Symptoms in Malabsorption

Extra-gastrointestinal symptom	Result of
Muscle wasting, edema	Decreased protein absorption
Paresthesias, tetany	Decreased vitamin D and calcium absorption
Bone pain	Decreased calcium absorption
Muscle cramps	Weakness, excess potassium loss
Easy bruisability, petechiae	Decreased vitamin K absorption
Hyperkeratosis, night blindness	Decreased vitamin A absorption
Pallor	Decreased vitamin B_{12}, folate, or iron absorption
Glossitis, stomatitis, cheilosis	Decreased vitamin B_{12} or iron absorption
Acrodermatitis	Zinc deficiency

ally normal in pancreatic insufficiency. Serum levels of albumin may also be normal.

- Howell-Jolly bodies (if there is no history of splenectomy) or dermatitis herpetiformis suggests celiac sprue (small-bowel biopsy is not diagnostic for sprue, but the response to gluten-free diet is).
- Fever, arthralgias, neurologic symptoms = Whipple's disease.

Helpful hints in the medical history, physical examination, or laboratory results may suggest the possibility of diarrhea or malabsorption (Table 13-12). Other hints in the history might include 1) age--youth suggests lactase deficiency inflammatory bowel disease or sprue, 2) travel--parasites, toxigenic agents (exposure to contaminated food or water), 3) drugs--laxatives, antacids, antibiotics, colchicine, lactulose, 4) family history--celiac sprue, inflammatory bowel disease, polyposis coli, lactase deficiency.

Medical history: previous surgery (short-bowel syndrome, dumping syndrome, blind loop syndrome, postvagotomy diarrhea, and ileal resection), radiation, systemic disease.

Table 13-12.--Associated Symptoms of Systemic Illnesses Causing Diarrhea

Symptom or sign	Diagnosis to be considered
Arthritis	Ulcerative colitis, Crohn's disease, Whipple's disease, *Yersinia* infection
Marked weight loss	Malabsorption, inflammatory bowel disease, cancer, thyrotoxicosis
Eosinophilia	Eosinophilic gastroenteritis, parasitic disease
Lymphadenopathy	Lymphoma, Whipple's disease
Neuropathy	Diabetic diarrhea, amyloidosis
Postural hypotension	Diabetic diarrhea, Addison's disease, idiopathic orthostatic hypotension
Flushing	Malignant carcinoid syndrome
Proteinuria	Amyloidosis
Peptic ulcers	Zollinger-Ellison syndrome
Hyperpigmentation	Whipple's disease, celiac disease, Addison's disease, pancreatic cholera, eosinophilic gastroenteritis

From Fine KD, Krejs GJ, Fordtran JS: Diarrhea. *In* Gastrointestinal Disease: Pathophysiology Diagnosis Management. Fourth edition. Edited by MH Sleisenger, JS Fordtran. Philadelphia, WB Saunders Company, 1989, pp 290-316. By permission of publisher.

Diseases Causing Diarrhea

Osmotic Diarrhea

Lactase deficiency: lactose is normally split by lactase into glucose and galactose, which are absorbed in the small bowel. In lactase deficiency, lactose is not absorbed in the small intestine but enters the colon, where it is fermented in the lumen by bacteria to lactic acid. The result is diarrhea of low pH and increased intestinal motility. The commonest disaccharidase deficiency is lactase deficiency. "Acquired" lactase deficiency (genetic?) is common in Orientals, blacks, Eskimos, and people from the Middle East. Diarrhea, abdominal cramps, and flatulence occur after ingestion of dairy products. There is improvement with diet. The pH of the stool is <6.0. Lactose tolerance test--Blood sugar increases <20 mg/100 mL after lactose ingestion. Abnormal H_2 breath test. Jejunal biopsy results are normal (disaccharidase levels are decreased). Lactose intolerance can occur in any clinical setting where the intestinal mucosa is damaged.

- Lactase deficiency: lactose is not absorbed in the small intestine.
- Diarrhea of low pH and increased intestinal motility.
- The commonest disaccharidase deficiency is lactase deficiency.
- Diarrhea, abdominal cramps, flatulence occur after ingestion of dairy products.
- Abnormal H_2 breath test.
- Patients on a weight reduction diet who drink diet soda or chew sugarless gum may develop osmotic diarrhea from sorbitol.

Secretory Diarrhea

Watery diarrhea, hypokalemia, achlorhydria--The WHDA or Verner-Morrison syndrome, also called "pancreatic cholera": it is a massive diarrhea (5 L/day) with dehydration and hypokalemia. The patient may have other multiple endocrine adenomatosis tumor (hypercalcemia, hyperglycemia). This diarrhea is associated with a non-beta islet cell tumor of the pancreas. Vasoactive intestinal peptide is the commonest mediator, followed by prostaglandin, secretin, and calcitonin. Clinical recognition is by pancreatic scan/angiography and measurement of hormone levels. Treatment is with somatostatin or operation.

- Pancreatic cholera: massive diarrhea, dehydration, hypokalemia.
- Patients may have other multiple endocrine adenomatosis tumor.
- It is associated with a non-beta islet cell tumor of the pancreas.

Carcinoid syndrome: results from tumors of enterochromaffin cells of neural crest origin; 90% of the tumors are in the terminal ileum. There is episodic facial flushing (lasting up to 10 min), watery diarrhea, wheezing, right-sided valvular disease (endocardial fibrosis), and hepatomegaly. If the gut is normal, look for bronchial tumors or gonadal tumors. Dietary tryptophan is converted into serotonin (causes diarrhea, abdominal cramps [intestinal hypermotility], nausea, and vomiting), histamine (responsible for the flushing), and other chemicals (bradykinin, ACTH). Carcinoid syndrome means that hepatic metastases are present. The diagnosis of carcinoid syndrome is made by finding elevated urinary levels of 5-hydroxyindoleacetic acid (5-HIAA) and by liver biopsy. This syndrome is not associated with hypertension. Treatment is with octreotide.

Laxative abuse: of the population over age 60, 15%-30% take laxatives regularly. This is laxative abuse. With surreptitious laxative ingestion, patients complain of diarrhea but do not admit taking laxatives. In referral centers, this is the commonest cause of watery diarrhea. Proctoscopy reveals melanosis coli. Barium enema shows "cathartic colon"--dilated, hypomotile, absent haustra. Laxatives causing melanosis coli include anthracene derivatives (senna, cascara, aloe). Diagnosis--Stool phenophthalein. Address underlying emotional problems.

- Proctoscopy reveals melanosis coli.
- Barium enema shows "cathartic colon," i.e., dilated, hypomotile, absent haustra.
- Address underlying emotional problems.

Bile Acid Malabsorption

Bile acid malabsorption is caused by ileal resection or disease. The diarrhea due to bile acid malabsorption may produce two different clinical syndromes, each requiring a different treatment. 1) Limited resection (<100 cm).

Malabsorbed bile acids enter the colon and stimulate secretion. Liver synthesis can compensate, so bile acid concentration in the upper small bowel is greater than the critical micelle concentration. No steatorrhea. Fecal fat is <20 g/24 hr. Treat with cholestyramine, which binds bile acids. 2) Extensive resection (>100 cm)--Bile acids are severely malabsorbed and enterohepatic circulation is interrupted. This limits synthesis, and the liver cannot compensate. Bile acid concentration is decreased in the upper small bowel, micelles cannot be formed, and fat malabsorption results. The malabsorbed fatty acids themselves stimulate secretion in the colon. Treat with low-fat diet (<50 g/day), medium chain triglycerides. Cholestyramine would further decrease bile acid concentration and increase steatorrhea.

- Limited resection: treat with cholestyramine.
- Extensive resection: treat with low-fat diet, medium chain triglycerides.

Bacterial Overgrowth

The proximal small intestine is usually sterile. The major defense mechanisms in the proximal small bowel are gastric acid, normal peristalsis (the most important defense), and intestinal IgA. When defenses are altered, bacterial overgrowth results. The mechanism of steatorrhea is deconjugation of bile acids by bacteria that normally are not present in the proximal intestine. Deconjugation of the bile acids changes the ionization coefficient, and the deconjugated bile acids can be passively absorbed in the proximal small bowel. Normally, conjugated bile acids are actively absorbed distally in the ileum. As a result, the critical micellar concentration is not reached, and mild steatorrhea results from the intraluminal deficiency of bile acids.

- Normal peristalsis is the most important defense in the proximal small bowel.
- Deconjugated bile salts can be absorbed passively.
- Mild steatorrhea results from the intraluminal deficiency of bile acids.

Clinical features of bacterial overgrowth are steatorrhea (10-20 g/day), vitamin B_{12} malabsorption (macrocytic anemia), positive jejunal cultures (>10^5 organisms), abnormal bile acid breath test. Breath test--bile acid breath test)--^{14}C-labeled bile acids release $^{14}CO_2$ when deconjugated by bacteria in the gut. This test has low sensitivity (20%-30% false-negative).

Associated conditions--Postoperative (blind loops, enteroenterostomy, gastrojejunocolic fistula), structural (diverticula, strictures, fistulas), motility disorders (scleroderma, pseudo-obstruction), achlorhydria (atrophic gastritis, gastric resections; achlorhydria corrects with antibiotics) and impaired immunity. Two types of the latter are hypogammaglobulinemic sprue (no plasma cells in lamina propria, and flat villi on small-bowel biopsy) and nodular lymphoid hyperplasia associated with IgA deficiency--know radiographic appearance--predisposes to *Giardia lamblia* infection.

- Diarrhea, vitamin B_{12} deficiency, and above conditions suggest bacterial overgrowth.

Infectious Diarrheas

The toxigenic and invasive causes of bacterial diarrhea and the associated features are outlined in Tables 13-13 and 13-14.

Staphylococcus aureus: The diarrhea is of rapid onset; it lasts for 24 hours. There is no fever, vomiting, or cramps. The toxin is ingested in egg products, cream, and mayonnaise. Treatment is supportive.

Clostridium perfringens ("Church picnic"): The toxin is ingested in precooked foods, usually beef and turkey. Heat-stable spores produce toxins. Although the bacteria are killed and the toxin is destroyed, the spores survive. When food is rewarmed, the spores germinate, producing toxin. The diarrhea is worse than the vomiting and is later in onset. It lasts 24 hours. Treatment is supportive.

E. coli ("Traveler's diarrhea"): The toxin is ingested in water and salads. It is a plasmid-mediated enterotoxin. Treatment is supportive. Prophylaxis is with doxycycline and bismuth subsalicylate (Pepto-Bismol). *E. coli* may be important in nursery epidemic diarrhea.

Vibrio cholerae: The toxin is ingested in water. It is the only toxigenic bacterial diarrhea in which antibiotics clearly shorten the duration of the disease. Treatment is with tetracycline.

Bacillus cereus: The source of the toxin is fried rice in oriental restaurants. One type has rapid onset and resembles *S. aureus* infection; the other type has a slower onset and resembles *C. perfringens* infection. The diagnosis is made by isolating the organism from contaminated food and by the medical history. Treatment is supportive.

Other toxigenic bacteria: *C. botulinum* produces a neurotoxin that is ingested in improperly home-processed vegetables, fruits, and meats. It interferes with the release of acetylcholine from peripheral nerve endings. *C. difficile*--See antibiotic/pseudomembranous colitis.

- Toxigenic bacterial diarrhea: watery; no fecal leukocytes.
- *S. aureus*: rapid onset.
- *C. perfringens*: "church picnic diarrhea," precooked foods, later in onset.
- *E. coli*: "traveler's diarrhea."
- *B. cereus*: fried rice in oriental restaurants.

Bacterial Diarrhea (Invasive)

Shigella: It is often acquired outside the U.S. Bloody diarrhea is characteristic, and fever and bacteremia occur. Diagnosis is based on positive stool and blood cultures. Treatment is with ampicillin. Resistant strains are emerging for which chloramphenicol is an alternative. (Plasmids are responsible for antibiotic deactivation resistance.)

Salmonella (non-*typhi*): In U.S., *Salmonella typhimurium* is the most common agent. The toxin is ingested with poultry. Fever is present. The absence of bloody diarrhea is the main characteristic that distinguishes it from *Shigella* infection. Diagnosis is based on positive stool culture. Treatment is supportive. Do not use antibiotics, which prolong the carrier state and do not affect the course of the disease. Use antibiotics only if blood cultures are positive.

Vibrio parahaemolyticus: The toxin is ingested with undercooked shellfish. This infection is increasing in frequency in the U.S. (it is common in Japan). Fever and bloody diarrhea are the chief characteristics. Diagnosis is based on positive stool culture. Antibiotics are of questionable value in treating this infection, but erythromycin may be most effective.

E. coli: Invasive *E. coli* is rare. It presents as fever and bloody diarrhea with profound toxicity.

S. aureus (enterocolitis): Diagnosis is based on positive stool culture or Gram's stain, which shows predominance of gram-positive cocci and a paucity of other organisms.

- Invasive bacterial diarrhea: fever, bloody stools, and fecal leukocytes.
- *Shigella*: bloody diarrhea.
- *S. typhimurium*: no bloody diarrhea; treat with antibiotics only if blood cultures are positive.
- *V. parahaemolyticus*: undercooked shellfish, bloody diarrhea.

Table 13-13.--Causes of Bacterial Diarrhea: Toxigenic

Organism	Onset, hr	Mediated by cyclic Amp	Fever	Intestinal secretion
Staphylococcus aureus	1-6	+	-	+
Clostridium perfringens	8-12	-	±	+
Escherichia coli	12	+	+	+
Vibrio cholerae	12	+	Due to dehydration	++++
Bacillus cereus	1-6	+	-	+
	12-24	+	-	++++

Table 13-14.--Causes of Bacterial Diarrhea: Invasive

Organism	Fever	Bloody diarrhea	Bacteremia	Antibiotic effective
Shigella	+	+	+	+
Salmonella	+	-	-	-
Vibrio parahaemolyticus	+	+	-	+(?)
Escherichia coli	+	-	-	-
Staphylococcus aureus (enterocolitis)	+	+	±	+
Yersinia enterocolitica	+	+	+	?
Campylobacter	+	+	±	+
Vibrio vulnificus	+	+	+	+

"Newer" Enteric Bacterial Pathogens

Yersinia enterocolitica: The spectrum of disease includes acute enteritis and chronic enteritis. Acute enteritis is similar to shigellosis and usually lasts 1-3 weeks. It is characterized by fever, diarrhea, leukocytosis, and fecal leukocytes. Chronic enteritis is found especially in children. There is diarrhea, failure to thrive, hypoalbuminemia, and hypokalemia. Other features are acute abdominal pain (mesenteric adenitis), right lower quadrant pain, tenderness, nausea, and vomiting. It mimics appendicitis or Crohn's disease. This gram-negative rod is hardy and can survive in cold temperatures. It grows on special medium (cold enriched). It is an invasive pathogen. Fecal-oral transmission in water and milk (isolate the patient).

Extraintestinal manifestations are nonsuppurative arthritis and ankylosing spondylitis (in HLA-B27). Skin manifestations are erythema nodosum and multiforme. Thyroid manifestations are Graves' disease and Hashimoto's disease. Multiple liver abscesses and granulomata are present.

Treatment is with aminoglycosides, trimethoprim-sulfamethoxazole (Bactrim): The bacteria are variably sensitive to tetracycline and chloramphenicol. Beta lactamases are frequently produced. Penicillin resistance is common.

- *Y. enterocolitica* infection: acute abdominal pain (differential diagnosis includes appendicitis and Crohn's disease).
- Fecal-oral transmission in water and milk.
- Manifestations include nonsuppurative arthritis and ankylosing spondylitis (in HLA-B27).

Campylobacter jejuni: These are comma-shaped, motile, microaerophilic gram-negative bacilli. Transmission is linked to infected water, unpasteurized milk, poultry, sick dogs, and infected children. Incubation period is 2-4 days before invasion of the small bowel. Infection results in presence of blood and leukocytes in the stool. It may mimic granulomatous or idiopathic ulcerative colitis. It may also mimic small-bowel secretory diarrhea, with explosive, frequent watery diarrhea due to many species that produce a cholera-type toxin. The diarrhea usually lasts 3-5 days but may relapse. Antibiotic treatment is with erythromycin when severe, but treatment often is not needed. Postdiarrheal illnesses are hemolytic uremic syndrome and postinfectious arthritis.

- *C. jejuni:* infected water, unpasteurized milk, poultry, sick dogs, infected children.

- May mimic granulomatous or idiopathic ulcerative colitis.
- Diarrhea: usually lasts 3-5 days but may relapse.

Enterohemorrhagic *E. coli*: There is a grossly bloody stool and abdominal pain but no fever. Hemolytic uremic syndrome--large quantities of Shiga-like toxin that is difficult to detect. A useful marker is the inability to ferment sorbitol. Food: hamburger.

- Grossly bloody stool and abdominal pain but no fever.
- May cause hemolytic uremic syndrome.
- Hamburger.

Vibrio vulnificus (noncholera): The organisms are extremely invasive and produce necrotizing vasculitis, gangrene, and shock. They are routinely isolated from seawater, zooplankton, and shellfish along the Gulf of Mexico and both coasts of the U.S., especially in the summer. Two clinical syndromes are 1) wound infection, cellulitis, fasciitis, or myositis after exposure to seawater or cleaning shellfish, and 2) septicemia after ingesting raw shellfish (oysters). Patients at high risk for septicemia include those with liver disease, congestive heart failure, diabetes, renal failure, immunosuppressive states, or hemochromatosis. Treatment is with tetracycline.

- *V. vulnificus* is extremely invasive, producing necrotizing vasculitis, gangrene, and shock.
- Wound infection, cellulitis, fasciitis, or myositis occurs after exposure to seawater or cleaning shellfish.
- Septicemia occurs after ingesting raw shellfish (oysters).

Aeromonas hydrophilia: Previously, the pathogenicity of the bacteria was questioned. Although the infection is often mistaken for that of *E. coli*, *A. hydrophilia* is now recognized as an increasingly frequent cause of diarrhea after swimming in fresh or salt water. The organism produces several toxins. Treatment is with trimethoprim-sulfamethoxazole and tetracycline.

Malabsorption Due to Diseases of the Small Intestine

Celiac Sprue

Celiac sprue is a gluten-sensitive enteropathy. It presents in children as growth retardation, and in adults as an iron deficiency that is unresponsive to iron given orally. Osteomalacia can be present without steatorrhea if the proximal small bowel is involved. Splenic atrophy and abnormal blood smear with Howell-Jolly bodies may be clues to the diagnosis in 10%-15% of cases. Skin manifestation is dermatitis herpetiformis. Small-bowel biopsy is *not* diagnostic, but response to gluten-free diet is diagnostic. If the patient is unresponsive to the diet, review diet for inadvertent gluten ingestion. If unresponsive after 10-15 years of successful dietary management, rule out lymphoma (especially if there is also abdominal pain).

- Celiac sprue: iron deficiency that is unresponsive to iron given orally; osteomalacia with or without steattorrhea.
- Splenic atrophy and abnormal blood smear with Howell-Jolly bodies may be clues to the diagnosis in 10%-15% of cases.
- Lymphoma is a late complication.

Tropical Sprue

In tropical sprue, the diarrhea occurs 2-3 months after travel to the tropics. After 6 months, megaloblastic anemia develops because of folate deficiency and possible coexisting vitamin B_{12} deficiency. The infectious agents are *Klebsiella* and *E. coli*. Small-bowel biopsy shows blunted villi similar to celiac sprue. Treatment is with tetracycline (250 mg four times daily) and folate with or without vitamin B_{12}.

- Tropical sprue: diarrhea and megaloblastic anemia after travel to the tropics.
- Cause: coliforms bacteria (*Klebsiella* more than *E. coli*).
- Treatment: tetracycline (250 mg 4 times daily) and folate with or without vitamin B_{12}.

Whipple's Disease

Whipple's disease is a systemic infectious disease involving the CNS, heart, kidneys, and small bowel. It is caused by gram-positive bacilli. Small-bowel biopsy shows PAS-positive granules in the macrophages. Suspect Whipple's disease in patients with recurrent arthritis, pigmentation, adenopathy, or CNS symptoms (dementia, myoclonus, ophthalmoplegia, visual disturbances, coma, seizures). Treatment is with tetracycline or with minocycline if CNS symptoms develop.

- Suspect Whipple's disease in patients with recurrent arthritis, pigmentation, adenopathy, and CNS symptoms.

- Small-bowel biopsy shows PAS-positive granules in the macrophages.
- Treatment: tetracycline or minocycline if CNS symptoms develop.

Eosinophilic Gastroenteritis

Patients with eosinophilic gastroenteritis have a history of allergies (asthma, etc.) and food intolerances and episodic symptoms of nausea, vomiting, abdominal pain, and diarrhea. Laboratory findings include eosinophilia, iron deficiency anemia, and steatorrhea or protein-losing enteropathy. Small-bowel radiographs show coarse folds and filling defects, and biopsy shows infiltration of the eosinophils in the mucosa and, occasionally, absence of villi. Rule out parasitic infection. Treatment with steroids produces a rapid response.

- Mucosal eosinophilic gastroenteritis: allergies, food intolerances, and eosinophilia, and episodic intestinal symptoms.
- Rule out parasitic infection.
- Steroids produce a rapid response.

Systemic Mastocytosis

Systemic mastocytosis is a proliferation of mast cells in the skin (urticaria pigmentosa), bones, lymph nodes, and parenchymal organs. Histamine is released, and 50% of patients have gastrointestinal symptoms, i.e., diarrhea and peptic ulcer. "Bath pruritus" (itching after hot bath) is a clue to the diagnosis.

- Systemic mastocytosis causes urticaria pigmentosa.
- 50% of patients have gastrointestinal symptoms.
- "Bath pruritus" is a clue to the diagnosis.

Intestinal Lymphangiectasia

Intestinal lymphangiectasia is a disorder due to lymphatic obstruction. Hypoplastic lymphatics cause lymph to leak into the intestine. The clinical features are edema (often unilateral leg edema), chylous peritoneal or pleural effusions, and steatorrhea or protein-losing enteropathy. Laboratory findings include lymphocytopenia (average, 600/mm^3) due to enteric loss. All serum proteins are decreased, including immunoglobulins. Small bowel radiographs show edematous folds, and small bowel biopsy shows dilated lacteals and lymphatics in the lamina propria which may contain lipid-laden macrophages. The same biopsy findings are seen in obstruction of mesenteric nodes (lymphoma, Whipple's disease, Crohn's disease),

obstruction of venous inflow to the heart (constrictive pericarditis, severe right-sided heart failure). Diagnosis is based on abnormal small-bowel biopsy findings and documented enteric protein loss. Treatment is with low fat diet and medium chain triglycerides (enters portal blood rather than lymphatics). Occasionally, surgical excision of the involved segment is useful if the lesion is localized.

- Intestinal lymphangiectasia: unilateral lymphedema of the leg and chylous peritoneal or pleural effusions.
- Lymphocytopenia universal.
- Decreased serum proteins.
- Small-bowel biopsy shows dilated lacteals and lymphatics.
- Treatment: low fat diet and medium chain triglycerides.

Amyloidosis

Systemic amyloidosis is characterized by a diffuse deposition of an amorphous eosinophilic extracellular protein polysaccharide complex in tissue. The major sites of amyloid deposition are blood vessel walls and the mucous membranes and muscle layers of the intestine. Any portion of the gut can be involved. Amyloid damages tissues by infiltration (muscle and nerve infiltration causes motility disorders, malabsorption) and ischemia (obliteration of vessels causes ulceration and bleeding). Intestinal dysmotility can produce diarrhea, constipation, pseudo-obstruction, megacolon, and fecal incontinence. Clinical findings in amyloidosis include macroglossia, hepatomegaly, cardiomegaly, proteinuria, and peripheral neuropathy. Pinch (post-traumatic) purpura or periorbital proctoscopic purpura occurs. Diagnosis--Small-bowel radiography shows symmetric, sharply demarcated thickening of the valvulae conniventes. Fat aspirate confirms diagnosis in 90%-95% of cases and rectal biopsy in 70%-85%.

Miscellaneous Small-Bowel Disorders

Meckel's diverticulum, the persistence of the vitelline duct, is the most frequent developmental abnormality of the gut. It is usually found within 100 cm from the ileocecal valve on the antimesenteric border of the ileum. It contains all layers of the intestinal wall and so is a true diverticulum. The mucosa is usually ileal but may be gastric (pancreatic, intestinal). Complications include obstruction due to intussusception and volvulus around the band fixing the diverticulum to the bowel wall. Benign (leiomyomas) and malignant (carcinoids, leiomyosarcoma) tumors have been found in diverticula. Diverticulitis is uncommon. Incarceration in an indirect inguinal hernia (Littre's hernia) and perforation that causes peritonitis may occur. Hemorrhage is the common complication and results from ulceration of the ileal mucosa adjacent to the gastric mucosa. This accounts for 50% of lower gastrointestinal tract bleeding in children and young adults. Radiography usually is not helpful in making the diagnosis. A nuclear scan (parietal cells concentrate technetium) may show the diverticulum, but false-positive and false-negative results can occur.

- Meckel's diverticulum is the most frequent developmental abnormality of the gut.
- It accounts for 50% of the lower gastrointestinal tract bleeding in children and young adults.

Aortoenteric fistula: A history of gastrointestinal tract bleeding in a patient who has had a previous aortic graft demands immediate evaluation to rule out an enteroenteric fistula. If the patient presents with massive bleeding, do not attempt endoscopy or arteriography. Emergency surgery is indicated.

- If patient presents with massive bleeding, do not attempt endoscopy or arteriography. Emergency surgery is indicated.

Chronic Intestinal Pseudo-Obstruction

Pseudo-obstruction is a syndrome characterized by the clinical findings of mechanical bowel obstruction but without occlusion of the lumen. The two types are primary and secondary. The primary type, also called idiopathic pseudo-obstruction, is a visceral myopathy or neuropathy. The secondary type is due to underlying systemic disease or precipitating causes.

Idiopathic (primary) pseudo-obstruction is associated with recurrent attacks of nausea, vomiting, cramping abdominal pain, distension, and constipation, which are of variable intensity and duration. If it is a familial cause, the patient will have a positive family history and the condition will be present at a young age. Esophageal motility is abnormal (achalasia) in most patients. Occasionally, urinary tract motility is abnormal, and diarrhea or steatorrhea results from bacterial overgrowth. Upper gastrointestinal tract and small-bowel radiographs show dilatation of the bowel and slow transit (not mechanical obstruction).

- Idiopathic pseudo-obstruction is due to a familial cause or to sporadic visceral myopathy or neuropathy.
- Recurrent attacks have variable frequency and duration.
- Abnormal esophageal motility occurs in most patients.
- Steatorrhea is caused by bacterial overgrowth.

Secondary pseudo-obstruction is due to underlying systemic disease or precipitating causes. These causes include the following (significant causes to remember are in italics):

1. Diseases involving the intestinal smooth muscle--*amyloidosis*, scleroderma, systemic lupus erythematosus, myotonic dystrophy, and muscular dystrophy.
2. Neurologic diseases--*Parkinson's disease*, Hirschsprung's disease, Chagas' disease, and familial autonomic dysfunction.
3. Endocrine disorders--*myxedema* and hypoparathyroidism.
4. Drugs--*antiparkinsonian medications* (*L-dopa*), phenothiazines, tricyclic antidepressants, ganglionic blockers, clonidine, and narcotics.

Approach to the Patient With Chronic Intestinal Pseudo-Obstruction

First, a mechanical cause for obstruction must be ruled out. Second, look for an underlying precipitating cause such as metabolic abnormalities, medications, or an underlying associated disease. If a familial idiopathic cause is suspected, assess esophageal motility. Suspect scleroderma if intestinal radiography shows large-mouth diverticula of the small and large intestines. Suspect amyloidosis if the skin shows palpable purpura and proteinuria and neuropathy are present.

- Secondary pseudo-obstruction is due to an underlying systemic disease or precipitating cause.
- Scleroderma presents as large-mouth diverticula of the intestine.
- Amyloidosis presents with palpable purpura, proteinuria, and neuropathy.

Inflammatory Bowel Disease

"Idiopathic inflammatory bowel disease" refers to two disorders of unknown cause: chronic ulcerative colitis and Crohn's disease. Other possible causes of inflammation, especially infection, should be excluded before making the diagnosis of idiopathic inflammatory bowel disease.

Ulcerative colitis is a mucosal inflammation involving only the colon. Crohn's disease is a transmural inflammation that can involve the intestine anywhere from the esophagus through the anus. The rectum is involved in about 95% of patients with ulcerative colitis and in only 50% of those with Crohn's disease. Ulcerative colitis is a continuous inflammatory process extending from the anal verge to more proximal colon (depending on the extent of the inflammation). Crohn's disease is a segmental inflammation in which inflamed areas alternate with virtually normal areas. Ulcerative colitis usually presents as frequent bloody bowel movements with minimal abdominal pain, whereas Crohn's disease presents with fewer bowel movements, less bleeding, and, more commonly, abdominal pain. Crohn's disease is associated with intestinal fistula and fistula to other organs as well as perianal disease. Ulcerative colitis does not form fistulas; perianal disease is uncommon. Strictures of the intestine are common with Crohn's disease but rare in ulcerative colitis (when they are present, they suggest cancer).

- Ulcerative colitis involves only the colon.
- Crohn's disease can involve the intestine anywhere from the esophagus through the anus.
- Ulcerative colitis is a continuous process.
- Crohn's disease is a segmental inflammation.
- Ulcerative colitis has frequent bloody bowel movements.
- Crohn's disease has fewer bowel movements, less bleeding, and more abdominal pain.
- Crohn's disease is associated with intestinal fistula, strictures, and perianal disease.

Extraintestinal Manifestations of Inflammatory Bowel Disease

Arthritis occurs in 10%-20% of patients, usually monoarticular or pauciarticular involvement of large joints. Joint symptoms mirror bowel activity, i.e., joints flare when colitis flares and joints improve as colitis improves. Also, ankylosing spondylitis (relationship with HLA-B27) and sacroiliitis--which are usually progressive and do not improve when colitis improves--can develop.

- The joint symptoms mirror bowel activity.
- Anklyosing spondylitis and sacroiliitis can develop.

Skin lesions occur in 10% of patients. The three types of lesions are erythema nodosum, pyoderma gangrenosum, and aphthous ulcers of the mouth. All these skin conditions usually improve with treatment of colitis. Severe, refractory skin disease is an indication for surgery.

- The skin lesions are erythema nodosum, pyoderma gangrenosum, and aphthous ulcers of the mouth.

Eye lesions occur in 5% of patients. The lesion is usually episcleritis and/or uveitis. These usually improve with treatment of inflammatory bowel disease.

Liver disease also occurs in 5% of patients. Primary sclerosing cholangitis is more common in chronic ulcerative colitis than in Crohn's disease. If alkaline phosphatase level is increased in patient with inflammatory bowel disease, the work-up for primary sclerosing cholangitis includes ultrasonography, endoscopic retrograde cholangiopancreatography, and liver biopsy.

- If elevated alkaline phosphatase with inflammatory bowel disease, rule out primary sclerosing cholangitis.

Renal stones occur in 5%-15% of patients. In Crohn's disease with malabsorption, calcium oxalate stones occur. In chronic ulcerative colitis, uric acid stones are secondary to dehydration and loss of bicarbonate in the stool, leading to acidic urine.

Indications for Colonoscopy

Colonoscopy is indicated for evaluating the extent of the disease and for stricture (biopsy) and filling defect (biopsy). It is also indicated for differentiating Crohn's colitis from ulcerative colitis when the two are otherwise indistinguishable. Another indication is for monitoring by random mucosal biopsy the development of dysplasia or cancer.

- Know the indications for colonoscopy in inflammatory bowel disease.

Toxic Megacolon

In patients with active inflammation, avoid the causes of toxic megacolon, including aerophagia, opiates, anticholinergics, hypokalemia, and barium enema.

- In patients with active inflammation, avoid the causes of toxic megacolon.

Treatment of Ulcerative Colitis

Medical: Sulfasalazine (azulfidine) was the mainstay of treatment. 5-Aminosalicylic acid (ASA) (the active agent) is bound to sulfapyridine (vehicle). Colonic bacteria break the bond, releasing 5-ASA. 5-ASA is not absorbed but stays in contact with the mucosa and exerts its anti-inflammatory action. The efficacy of 5-ASA may be related to its ability to inhibit the lipoxygenase pathway of arachidonic acid metabolism or to its ability to function as an oxygen free radical scavenger (further studies are needed). It is effective in acute disease and in maintaining remission. Side effects (male infertility, malaise, nausea, pancreatitis, rashes, headaches, hemolysis, impaired folate absorption, hepatitis, aplastic anemia, and exacerbation of colitis) occur in 30% of patients who take sulfasalazine and are related to the sulfapyridine moiety. 5-ASAs are a group of new drugs that deliver 5-ASA to the intestine in various ways. They eliminate sulfa toxicity but are more expensive than sulfasalazine. Two of these drugs are mesalamine and olsalazine. Mesalamine can be given topically (Rowasa suppositories, Rowasa enema) or orally (Asacol, 5-ASA coated with acrylic polymer which releases 5-ASA in the terminal ileum, and Pentasa, ethyl cellulose coating releases 50% of the 5-ASA in the small bowel). Olsalazine consists of two 5-ASA molecules conjugated with each other. Bacteria break the bond, releasing 5-ASA into the colon.

Aminosalicylates are used for mild to moderately active ulcerative colitis and in Crohn's disease. Topical forms are useful in proctitis or left-sided colitis; systemic forms are used for pancolitis. Although 80%-90% of patients do not tolerate sulfasalazine, they do tolerate oral 5-ASA preparations. Side effects include hair loss, pancreatitis (often in patients who developed pancreatitis while taking sulfasalazine), reversible worsening of underlying renal disease, and exacerbation of colitis.

- Sulfasalazine is effective in acute disease and in maintaining remission.
- Sulfasalazine: side effects occur in 30% of patients.
- Aminosalicylates are equally effective but more expensive; they are useful in 80%-90% of patients intolerant to sulfasalazine.

Corticosteroids--topical preparations should be used twice daily for patients with active mild to moderate disease that is limited to the distal colon. Corticosteroids should be added to the regimen of patients with more proximal disease if systemic steroids and sulfasalazine do not control the attacks. Up to 50% of the dose can be absorbed (depending on the preparation used and its vehicle). Oral preparations are indicated in active pancolonic disease of moderate severity in doses of 40-60 mg once daily or 20-40 mg daily in cases of mild disease that are unresponsive to topical steroids and sulfasalazine. Prednisolone, the active metabolite, is the preferred form of drug in patients with cirrhosis (these patients may not be able to convert inactive prednisone to prednisolone). For patients with a prompt response to oral steroids, the dose may be gradually tapered at a rate not to exceed a 5-mg reduction in the total dose every 3-7 days. Intravenous preparations should be used in large doses (prednisolone, 100 mg in divided doses) for up to 10-14 days in severely ill patients. At that time, if there is improvement, it should be possible to convert the medication to oral steroids (60-100 mg per day). If there is no improvement, surgical intervention (colectomy) is required. Steroids are not believed to prevent relapse and therefore should not be used after the patient has complete remission and is symptom-free.

- Prescribe topical preparations twice daily for patients with active mild to moderate disease that is limited to the distal colon.
- Corticosteroids should be added to the regimen of patients with more proximal disease if systemic steroids and sulfasalazine have not controlled the attacks.
- Oral preparations are useful in active pancolonic disease of moderate severity.
- Intravenous preparations are used for severely ill patients.

Total parenteral nutrition does not alter the clinical course of an ongoing attack. Indications for its use include: 1) severe dehydration and cachexia with marked fluid and nutrient deficits, 2) excessive diarrhea that has failed to respond to standard therapy for chronic ulcerative colitis, and 3) debilitated patients undergoing colectomy. Opiates (or their synthetic derivatives) and anticholinergics are contraindicated in chronic ulcerative colitis because they are ineffective and can contribute to the development of toxic megacolon.

- Total parenteral nutrition does not alter the clinical course of the ongoing attack.
- Use of opiates and anticholinergics is contraindicated in chronic ulcerative colitis.

Surgical: Surgical treatment is curative in chronic ulcerative colitis. Indications for colectomy are severe intractable disease, acute life-threatening complications (perforation, hemorrhage, toxic megacolon unresponsive to treatment), symptomatic colonic stricture, and suspected or documented colon cancer. Other indications include intractable moderate-to-severe colitis, refractory uveitis or pyoderma gangrenosum, growth retardation in pediatric patients, cancer prophylaxis, or inability to taper a regimen to low doses of steroids (i.e., <15 mg/day) over a period of 2-3 months. Procedures include a proctocolectomy with an ileoanal anastomosis, Koch pouch, or conventional Brooke ileostomy.

- Surgical treatment is curative in chronic ulcerative colitis.

Treatment of Crohn's Disease

Medical: For sulfasalazine, see Treatment of Ulcerative Colitis above. This drug is more effective for colonic disease than for small-bowel disease, although 5-ASA products designed to be released and activated in the small bowel may prove to be effective in the colon. Sulfasalazine does not have an additive effect or a steroid-sparing effect when used with corticosteroids, nor does it maintain remission in Crohn's disease as it does in ulcerative colitis. Nothing is effective in the prophylaxis of Crohn's disease.

- Sulfasalazine is more effective for colonic disease than for small-bowel disease.
- It does not have an additive effect or sparing effect when used with corticosteroids.
- It does not maintain remission in Crohn's disease.

Corticosteroids, see Treatment of Ulcerative Colitis above. The agents that most quickly control an acute exacerbation of Crohn's disease are corticosteroids. They are the most useful drugs for treating small-bowel Crohn's disease.

Azathioprine, in the National Crohn's Disease Cooperative Study, was not significantly different from placebo with regard to therapeutic response. However, this study has been criticized because azathioprine was given for a short period of time and its potential beneficial effect may have been missed--4-6 months are needed to realize any benefit from immunosuppressive drugs like azathioprine or 6-mercaptopurine. Azathioprine is associated with a higher rate of lymphoma than 6-mercaptopurine.

- Azathioprine is not significantly different from placebo with regard to therapeutic response.
- It is associated with a higher rate of lymphoma than 6-mercaptopurine.

6-Mercaptopurine, the active metabolite of azathioprine, has a steroid-sparing effect. Its use should be reserved for patients with active disease who are taking steroids when there is no need to reduce the steroid dose (or to maintain a given dose in the face of worsening disease activity).

- 6-Mercaptopurine is the active metabolite of azathioprine.
- It has a steroid-sparing effect.

Metronidazole (at a dose of 20 mg/kg) is quite effective for treating perineal disease. Six weeks may be needed for the therapeutic effect to become manifest; unfortunately, recurrences often occur when the drug dose is tapered or discontinued, leading to chronic therapy. It is as effective as sulfasalazine for disease of the colon. If a patient is unresponsive to sulfasalazine, it is worthwhile switching to metronidazole, but not vice versa. It is less effective for small-bowel disease. Side effects include glossitis, metallic taste, vaginal and urethral burning sensation, neutropenia, dark urine, urticaria, disulfiram (Antabuse) effect, and paresthesias.

- Metronidazole is quite effective for perineal disease.
- Recurrences are frequent when the drug dose is tapered or discontinued.
- It is as effective as sulfasalazine for disease of the colon.

Nutrition--bowel rest per se does not have any role in achieving remission in Crohn's disease. However, providing adequate nutritional support does help facilitate remission--any form of nutritional support is acceptable as long as it is adequate in amount. Adequate nutrition can be essential in maintaining growth in children with severe Crohn's disease.

Surgical: If Crohn's disease is present during exploration for presumed appendicitis, the acute ileitis should be left alone (many of these patients do not develop chronic Crohn's disease). An appendectomy can be performed if the cecum and appendix are free of disease. Of the Crohn's patients receiving surgical treatment, 70%-90% require reoperation within 15 years (many within the first

5 years after the initial operation). The anastomotic site is the most likely site for recurrence of disease. Indications for surgical treatment include intractable symptoms, acute life-threatening complications, obstruction, unhealed fistulas that cause complications, abscess formation, and malignancy.

- 70%-90% of Crohn's patients operated on require reoperation within 15 years.
- The anastomotic site is the most likely site for disease recurrence.

GASTROINTESTINAL MANIFESTATIONS OF AIDS

Gastrointestinal symptoms occur in 30%-50% of North American and European patients with AIDS and in nearly 90% of the patients in developing countries. The most frequent gastrointestinal tract symptom is diarrhea, which is often chronic and associated with weight loss. Dysphagia, odynophagia, abdominal pain, and jaundice are less frequent. Gastrointestinal tract bleeding is rare. The goal of evaluation is to identify treatable causes of infection or symptoms.

- The majority of AIDs patients with diarrhea have one or more identifiable pathogens.
- Some have no identifiable cause despite extensive evaluation. This may represent idiopathic AIDS enteropathy or, as yet, unidentified pathogens.

The gastrointestinal tract in AIDS is predisposed to a spectrum of viral, bacterial, fungal, and protozoan pathogens.

Viral

Cytomegalovirus

Cytomegalovirus is one of the most common and potentially serious opportunistic pathogens. It most commonly affects the colon and esophagus, although the entire gut, liver, biliary tract, and pancreas are susceptible. There is a patchy or diffuse colitis that may progress to ischemic necrosis and perforation. Symptoms: watery diarrhea and fever; less commonly, hematochezia and abdominal pain. Diagnosis: biopsy specimens show cytomegalic inclusion cells with surrounding inflammation (owl's eye). Treatment: ganciclovir, 5 mg per kg twice daily for 14-21 days. If resistant, use foscarnet.

Herpes Simplex Virus

The three gastrointestinal tract manifestations of herpes simplex virus infection in patients with AIDS are perianal lesions (chronic cutaneous ulcers), proctitis, and esophagitis. The organs affected are the colon and esophagus. Symptoms: perianal lesions are painful; proctitis causes tenesmus, constipation, and inguinal lymphadenopathy; and esophagitis causes odynophagia, with or without dysphagia. Diagnosis: cytologic identification of intranuclear (Cowdry's type A) inclusions in multinucleated cells. Diagnosis is confirmed by viral cultures. Treatment: acyclovir given orally or intravenously.

Adenovirus

Adenovirus recently has been reported to cause diarrhea. The organ affected is the colon. Symptoms: watery, nonbloody diarrhea. Diagnosis: culture and biopsy. Treatment: none.

Bacteria

Mycobacterium avium-intracellulare

Infection of the gut occurs in patients with disseminated disease. The small intestine is affected more commonly than the colon. Symptoms: fever, weight loss, diarrhea, abdominal pain, and malabsorption. Diagnosis: acid-fast organisms in the stool and tissue confirmed by culture from stool and biopsy specimens. Treatment: multiple drug therapy with ethambutol, rifampin, ciprofloxacin, and clarithromycin.

Salmonella (typhimurium and enteritidis)

Treatment is with amoxicillin, trimethoprim-sulfamethoxazole, or ciprofloxacin.

Shigella flexneri

Treatment is with trimethoprim-sulfamethoxazole, ampicillin, or ciprofloxacin.

Campylobacter jejuni

Treatment is with erythromycin or ciprofloxacin.

Salmonella, Shigella flexneri, and Campylobacter jejuni have a substanitally higher incidence of intestinal infection, bacteremia, and prolonged or recurrent infections in AIDS patients because of antibiotic resistance or compromised immune function or both.

Fungi

Candida albicans

In AIDS patients, *Candida* causes locally invasive mucosal disease in the mouth and esophagus. Disseminated candidiasis is rare because neutrophil function remains relatively intact. The presence of oral candidiasis in persons at risk for AIDS should alert the physician to possible HIV infection. If oral candidiasis is present, endoscopy is required to confirm esophageal involvement. Symptoms: odynophagia suggests esophageal involvement. Diagnosis: histologic examination shows hyphae, pseudohyphae, or yeast forms. Treatment: nystatin, ketoconazole, fluconazole, or amphotericin.

Histoplasma capsulatum

Histoplasma capsulatum is an important opportunistic infection in AIDS patients who reside in endemic areas. Colonic involvement is more common than small bowel involvement. Symptoms: diarrhea, weight loss, fever, and abdominal pain. The diagnosis is established by culture. Colonoscopy may show inflammation and ulcerations and histologic examination with Giemsa staining shows intracellular yeast-like *Histoplasma capsulatum* within lamina propria macrophages. Treatment: amphotericin or itraconazole.

Protozoa

Cryptosporidium

Cryptosporidium is among the commonest enteric pathogens, occurring in 10%-20% of patients with AIDS and diarrhea in the U.S. and in 50% of those in developing countries. The organs affected are the small and large intestines and the biliary tree. Symptoms: voluminous watery diarrhea, severe abdominal cramps, weight loss, anorexia, malaise, and low-grade fever. Biliary tract obstruction has been reported. Diagnosis: microscopic identification of organisms in stool specimens with modified acid-fast staining or specific *Cryptosporidium* stains. Organisms may also be identified in biopsy specimens or in duodenal fluid aspirates. Treatment: none is known.

Isospora belli

Isospora belli is the more common cause of diarrhea in developing countries. It resembles *Cryptosporidium* oocysts. The small intestine is affected primarily, but the organisms can be identified throughout the gut and in other organs. Symptoms: watery diarrhea, cramping abdominal pain, weight loss, anorexia, malaise, and fever. Diagnosis: oval oocysts in stool seen with modified Kinyoun acid-fast stain. Biopsy specimen from small intestine may show organisms in the lumen or within cytoplasmic vacuoles in enterocytes. *Isospora belli* oocysts contain two sporoblasts and differ from *Cryptosporidium* oocysts, which are small, round, and contain four sporozoites. Treatment: trimethoprim-sulfamethoxazole.

Microsporidia (enterocytozoon bieneuisi)

Microsporidia are emerging as an important pathogen; the organisms have been identified in up to 33% of AIDS patients with diarrhea. The organ affected is the small intestine. Symptoms: watery diarrhea with gradual weight loss but no fever and no anorexia. Diagnosis: based on electron microscopic identification of round-to-oval meront (proliferative) and sporont (spore-forming) stages of Microsporidia in the villous but not crypt epithelial cells of the duodenum and jejunum. There are reports of positive stool specimens with Giemsa staining. Treatment: none known.

Entamoeba histolytica

Treatment is with metronidazole.

Giardia lamblia

Treatment is with metronidazole.

Blastocystis hominis

Because there is no evidence that *Blastocystis hominis* is pathogenic, it does not need to be treated.

The rates of symptomatic infection with *Entamoeba histolytica*, *Giardia lamblia*, and *Blastocystis hominis* are not significantly higher than in non-HIV patients. *Entamoeba histolytica* is a nonpathogenic commensal in most patients with AIDS. Giardiasis may require prolonged treatment, as in other immunocompetent persons.

DIAGNOSTIC EVALUATION OF PATIENTS WITH AIDS WHO HAVE DIARRHEA

Initial studies include 1) examination for stool leukocytes; 2) stool cultures for *Salmonella* species, *Shigella flexneri*, and *Campylobacter jejuni* (at least three specimens); 3) stool examination for ova and parasites (using saline, iodine, trichrome, and acid-fast preparations), and 4) stool assay for *Clostridium difficile* toxin. Additional studies include 1) gastroscopy to inspect tissue, aspirate luminal material, and obtain biopsy specimens; 2) examining duodenal aspirate for parasites and culture; 3) duodenal biopsy specimens cultured for cytomegalovirus and mycobacteria; 4) colonoscopy to inspect tissue and obtain biopsy specimens; 5) biopsy specimens cultured for cytomegalovirus, adenovirus, mycobacteria, and herpes simplex virus; 6) biopsy specimens stained with hematoxylin-eosin for protozoa and viral inclusion cells, with methenamine silver or Giemsa stain for fungi, and with Fite for mycobacteria.

If the initial studies and the additional studies listed above do not yield a diagnosis, then there is controversy about further evaluation. Most experts advocate empiric treatment with loperamide (Imodium). Others recommend that biopsy specimens from the duodenum be examined with electron microscopy for Microsporidia or from the colon for adenovirus. I favor empiric treatment with loperamide, because there is no treatment for either Microsporidia or adenovirus.

COLON

Pseudomembranous Enterocolitis

This is a necrotizing inflammatory disease of the intestines characterized by the formation of a membrane-like collection of exudate overlying a degenerating mucosa. Associated conditions are colon obstruction, uremia, ischemia, intestinal surgery, and all antibiotics (except vancomycin).

Antibiotic Colitis

The symptoms of antibiotic colitis are fever, abdominal pain, and diarrhea (mucus and blood), which occurs usually 1-6 weeks after antibiotic therapy. Sigmoidoscopy shows pseudomembranes and friability. Biopsy reveals inflammation and microulceration with exudation. The condition usually remits, but it recurs in 15% of cases. Complications include perforation and megacolon. Pathogenesis--The antibiotic alters colonic flora so there is overgrowth of *Clostridium difficile*. The toxin produced by *C. difficile* is cytotoxic, causing necrosis of the epithelium and exudation (pseudomembranes). Diagnosis--Toxin assay is positive in 98% of cases, and cultures are positive in about 75%. Radiography reveals pseudomembranes. Proctoscopic findings may be normal or show classic pseudomembranes. Treatment--Discontinue use of antibiotics and provide general supportive care (fluids, etc.). Avoid use of antimotility agents. If no response, metronidazole, 250 mg three times daily,

is 80% effective and inexpensive. Vancomycin, 125 mg four times daily, is also 80% effective but very expensive. If the patient is very ill, cholestyramine binds toxin. For first recurrence, same antibiotic can be used or the drug can be switched. For multiple recurrences, add cholestyramine and prolong the course of treatment with antibiotics.

- Antibiotic colitis: symptoms include fever, abdominal pain, diarrhea 1-6 weeks after antibiotic therapy.
- Toxin assay is positive in 98% of patients.
- Culture is positive in 75%.
- Metronidazole is the initial treatment.
- 15% have recurrence.

Radiation Colitis

Radiation injury usually affects both the colon and the small bowel. Endothelial cells of small submucosal arterioles are very radiosensitive and respond to large doses of radiation by swelling, proliferating, and undergoing fibrinoid degeneration. The result is an obliterative endarteritis. Disease spectrum--1) Acute disease occurs during or immediately after radiation; the mucosa fails to regenerate, and there is friability, hyperemia, and edema. 2) Subacute disease occurs 2 to 12 months after radiation. Obliterative endarteritis produces progressive inflammation and ulceration. 3) Chronic disease consists of fistulas, abscesses, strictures, and bleeding from intestinal mucosal vessels. Predisposing factors include 1) other diseases that produce microvascular insufficiency, e.g., hypertension, diabetes mellitus, atherosclerosis, and heart failure, because they accelerate the development of vascular occlusion; 2) total radiation dose of 40-50 Gy; 3) previous chemotherapy; 4) adhesions; 5) previous surgery and pelvic inflammatory disease; and 6) age, the elderly are more susceptible. Radiography of acute disease shows fine serrations of bowel, and of chronic disease, stricture of the rectum. Endoscopy shows atrophic mucosa with telangiectatic vessels. Treatment--Endoscopic coagulation is effective.

- Radiation colitis involves both the colon and the small bowel.
- The endothelial cells of the small submucosal arterioles are very radiosensitive.
- The result is obliterative endarteritis.
- Predisposing factors: hypertension, diabetes mellitus, atherosclerosis, chemotherapy, and >40 Gy of radiation.
- The rectum is most commonly involved.

Ischemia

Review of Vascular Anatomy

The celiac trunk supplies the stomach and duodenum. The superior mesenteric artery supplies the jejunum, ileum, and right colon. The inferior mesenteric artery supplies the left colon and rectum.

Acute Ischemia

The symptoms of acute ischemia are sudden severe abdominal pain, vomiting, and diarrhea (with or without blood). Early in the course of ischemia, physical examination findings are normal, but later findings indicate peritonitis. Risk factors include severe atherosclerosis, congestive heart failure, atrial fibrillation (source of emboli), hypotension, and oral contraceptives.

There are several syndromes. 1) Acute mesenteric ischemia is due to obstruction of the superior mesenteric artery in 80% of cases. Most (95%) emboli lodge in this artery because of laminar flow, vessel caliber, and the angle it takes off from the aorta. The clue to search for emboli is atrial fibrillation. This syndrome results in a loss of small bowel and produces short-bowel syndrome. Radiography shows ileus, small-bowel obstruction, and, later, gas in the portal vein. The treatment is embolectomy, which has a 90% mortality rate. 2) Ischemic colitis is due to poor perfusion. It commonly involves areas of the colon between adjacent arteries, i.e., "watershed areas," such as the splenic flexure and rectosigmoid. This syndrome presents with abdominal pain and rectal bleeding. Radiography: thumbprinting of watershed areas is characteristic on radiography. The treatment is supportive, and if the condition deteriorates, surgical resection. 3) Nonocclusive ischemia is due to poor tissue perfusion caused by inadequate cardiac output. It can involve both the small and the large bowel. Its distribution does not conform to an area supplied by a major vessel. It occurs in patients with cardiac failure or anoxia or who are in shock. It is questioned whether digitalis causes mesenteric vasoconstriction.

- Acute superior mesenteric artery syndrome is usually due to emboli.
- Ischemic colitis: diagnosis is based on radiographic finding of thumbprinting of watershed areas.

Chronic Ischemic Colitis

Chronic ischemic colitis is uncommon. Symptoms include postprandial pain and fear of eating (weight loss).

At least two of three major splanchnic vessels must be occluded. It is associated with hypertension, diabetes mellitus, and atherosclerosis. Abdominal bruit is a clue to the diagnosis. Angiography is diagnostic in about 50% of cases and shows a stenotic area in two of three major vessels. Treatment is with surgical revascularization.

Occlusion of the superior mesenteric vein accounts for approximately 10% of the cases of bowel ischemia. Risk factors include hypercoagulable states such as polycythemia vera, liver disease, pancreatic cancer, intra-abdominal abscess, and portal hypertension. It presents as abdominal pain that gradually becomes severe. Diagnosis is based on angiographic findings. Treatment is surgical.

- Chronic ischemic colitis is associated with hypertension, diabetes mellitus, atherosclerosis.
- Mesenteric venous thrombosis occurs with hypercoagulable states.

Amebic Colitis

The colon is the usual site of the disease initially. Symptoms vary from none to explosive bloody diarrhea with fever, tenesmus, and abdominal cramps. Proctoscopy shows discrete ulcers with undermined edges and normal adjacent mucosa. If an exudate is present, swab and make wet mount preparations for trophozoites. Indirect hemagglutination is useful for invasive disease. Radiography shows concentric narrowing of the cecum in 90% of cases. Treat with metronidazole (Flagyl). *Entamoeba histolytica* is the only pathogenic ameba.

- The colon is the initial site of disease.
- Proctoscopy shows discrete ulcers with undermined edges.
- Radiography shows concentric narrowing of the cecum in 90% of cases.
- *Entamoeba histolytica* is the only pathogenic ameba.

Tuberculosis

Tuberculosis presents as diarrhea, a change in bowel habits, and rectal bleeding. The ileocecal area is the most commonly involved site. Radiography shows a contracted cecum and ascending colon and ulceration. Proctoscopy reveals deep and superficial ulcers. The rectum may be spared. A hypertrophic ulcerating mass may be seen. Biopsy samples stained with Ziehl-Neelsen stain are positive for acid-fast bacilli. All cases are associated with pulmonary or miliary tuberculosis.

- Tuberculosis is associated with diarrhea, change in bowel habits, rectal bleeding.
- The ileocecal area is commonly involved.
- Deep and superficial ulcers are characteristic findings.
- All cases are associated with pulmonary or miliary tuberculosis.

Streptococcus bovis endocarditis is associated with colon disease (diverticulosis or cancer). The colon should be evaluated.

Irritable Bowel Syndrome

Colon motility (and small bowel motility) is the only abnormality. Gas production is not increased. Always rule out lactase deficiency. It is a diagnosis of exclusion (requires negative evaluation).

Nontoxic Megacolon (Pseudo-Obstruction)

Acute pseudo-obstruction of the colon occurs postoperatively (nonabdominal operations) and with spinal cord injury, sepsis, uremia, electrolyte imbalance, and drugs (narcotics, anticholinergics, and psychotropic agents). When the cecum is >13-14 cm in diameter, the risk of perforation increases. Obstruction should be ruled out with Hypaque enema. Treatment includes placement of a nasogastric tube, discontinue drug therapy, correction of metabolic abnormalities, and, if needed, colonoscopic decompression or cecostomy.

Chronic pseudo-obstruction of the colon is seen in disorders that cause generalized intestinal pseudo-obstruction.

Congenital Megacolon

Congenital megacolon (Hirschsprung's disease) occurs in 1 of 5,000 births. There is increased incidence with Down's syndrome. Congenital megacolon usually becomes manifest in infancy; however, it can present in adulthood. There is a variable length of aganglionic segment from the rectum to the proximal colon (usually confined to rectum or rectosigmoid). The diagnosis is usually made at birth because of meconium ileus or obstipation. If the diagnosis is made in an adult, the patient has a history of chronic constipation. Colon radiographs show a characteristically narrowed distal segment and a dilated proximal colon. Rectal biopsy shows aganglionosis. Anorectal manometry shows loss of the anorectal reflex. Treatment: sphincter-saving operations.

- Congenital megacolon: increased incidence with Down's syndrome.

- In adult, chronic constipation.
- Colon radiographs show characteristically narrowed distal segment and dilated proximal colon.
- Rectal biopsy shows aganglionosis.
- Motility: absent and rectal inhibitory reflex.

Lower Gastrointestinal Tract Bleeding

The evaluation of rectal bleeding should begin with the digital examination, anoscopy, and proctosigmoidoscopy. If a definitive diagnosis cannot be made, next perform a barium enema or arteriography, depending on the nature of the bleeding. The inability to cleanse the colon appropriately during active bleeding makes the barium enema difficult to perform and interpret. Some advocate use of nuclear scanning if the activity of the bleeding is uncertain. With active bleeding, angiography is the diagnostic procedure of choice. It is also indicated for patients with recurrent episodes of rectal bleeding who have had normal results on previous standard tests, i.e., barium enema or colonoscopy. Colonoscopy is not useful if lower gastrointestinal tract bleeding is torrential, but it may be of some benefit if there is a slower rate of bleeding. Colonoscopy is valuable for evaluating patients with unexplained rectal bleeding and persistently positive findings on tests for occult blood in the stool.

- Initial evaluation of rectal bleeding: digital examination, anoscopy, and proctosigmoidoscopy.
- If activity of bleeding is uncertain, try bleeding scan.
- Colonoscopy is not useful if there is torrential lower gastrointestinal tract bleeding.
- Angiography is the procedure of choice for active bleeding.

The important causes of lower gastrointestinal tract bleeding are:

- Angiodysplasia--it usually involves the right colon and small bowel and may respond to endoscopic treatment.
- Diverticular disease--there is usually bleeding without other symptoms.
- Inflammatory bowel disease (colitis)--5% of patients present with this.
- Ischemic colitis--painful and bloody diarrhea.
- Cancer--it rarely causes significant bleeding.
- Meckel's diverticulum--it is the commonest cause of lower gastrointestinal tract bleeding in young patients. It is usually painless.
- Hemorrhoids--they are usually present as rectal outlet bleeding.

Evaluation of lower gastrointestinal tract bleeding: stabilize the patient, perform proctoscopy to rule out rectal outlet bleeding, and obtain nasogastric tube aspirate or use esophagogastroduodenoscopy to rule out upper gastrointestinal tract bleeding. Radionuclide-tagged red blood cell scan may help determine if bleeding is occurring, but it may not precisely localize the bleeding site. If there is active bleeding, perform angiography. If bleeding stops or occurs at a slow rate, perform colonoscopy. If the patient is young, perform Meckel's scan.

Treatment: If angiography localizes the bleeding site, vasopressin, infusion, or embolization may be useful. If the bleeding is found by colonoscopy, epinephrine injection, electrocoagulation, or laser coagulation may be useful. If bleeding is massive or if significant bleeding continues, surgical management is needed.

Diverticular Disease of the Colon

Definitions

Diverticula are acquired herniations of the mucosa and submucosa through the muscular layers of the colonic wall. *Diverticulosis* is the mere presence of uninflamed diverticula of the colon. *Diverticulitis* is the inflammation of one or more diverticula. The diagnosis and management of the complications of diverticular disease are outlined in Table 13-15.

Diverticulitis

Microperforation or macroperforation of the diverticulum with subsequent peridiverticular inflammation is necessary to produce diverticulitis. The severity of the clinical symptoms depends on the extent of the inflam-

Table 13-15.--Diagnosis and Management of Complications of Diverticular Disease

Complication	Symptoms	Findings	Treatment
Diverticulitis	Pain, fever, and constipation or diarrhea (or both)	Palpable tender colon, leukocytosis	Liquid diet, with or without antibiotics or elective surgery
Pericolic abscess	Pain, fever (with or without tenderness), or pus in stools	Tender mass, guarding leukocytosis, soft tissue mass on abdominal films or ultrasonography	Nothing by mouth, intravenous fluids, antibiotics, early surgical treatment with colostomy
Fistula	Depends on site: dysuria, pneumaturia, fecal discharge on skin or vagina	Depends on site: fistulogram, methylene blue	Antibiotics, clear liquids, colostomy, and, later, resection
Perforation	Sudden severe pain, fever	Septic patient, leukocytosis, free air	Antibiotics, nothing by mouth, intravenous fluids, immediate surgical treatment
Liver abscess	Right upper quadrant pain, fever, weight loss	Tender liver, tender bowel or mass, leukocytosis, alkaline phosphatase, lumbosacral scan (filling defect)	Antibiotics, surgical drainage, operation for bowel disease
Bleeding	Bright red or maroon blood, or clots	Blood on rectal exam, sigmoidoscopy, colonoscopy, angiography	Conservative: blood transfusion if needed, with or without operation

mation. Free perforation is infrequent (diverticula are invested by longitudinal muscle and mesentery). Local perforations may dissect along the colon wall and form intramural fistulas. The clinical presentation is left lower quadrant pain, fever, abdominal distension, constipation, and occasionally a palpable tender mass. Treatment includes resting the bowel or using a low fiber diet and antibiotics and obtaining an early surgical consultation.

Indications for surgical treatment during the acute phase include the development of generalized peritonitis, an enlarging inflammatory mass, fistula formation, colonic obstruction, inability to rule out a carcinoma in an area of stricture, or recurrent episodes of diverticulitis.

- Diverticulitis: the clinical symptoms depend on the extent of inflammation.

- Free perforation is infrequent.
- Clinical presentation: left lower quadrant pain, fever, abdominal distension, constipation, and occasionally a palpable tender mass.
- Treatment: rest bowel; give antibiotics and obtain a surgical consultation.

Angiodysplasia

Angiodysplasia is a common and increasingly recognized cause of lower gastrointestinal tract bleeding in elderly patients. Acquired vascular ectasias are believed to be associated with aging. Angiodysplasia is associated with cardiac disease, especially aortic stenosis. It usually involves the cecum and the ascending colon. There are no associated skin or visceral lesions. The ectasias appear to be due to the chronic, partial, intermittent, and low-grade obstruction of submucosal veins where they penetrate the colon. Obstruction is from muscle contraction and distension of the cecum. Colon radiography is of no diagnostic value. Angiography localizes the extent of involvement. Colonoscopy may show lesions. Apply cautery.

- Acquired vascular ectasias are associated with aging.
- Angiodysplasia is associated with cardiac disease, especially aortic stenosis.
- It usually involves the cecum and ascending colon.
- Colonoscopy may show lesions. Apply cautery.

Colon Polyps

Types of epithelial polyps include: 1) hyperplastic polyps--metaplastic, completely differentiated glandular elements; they are benign . 2) Hamartomatous polyps--mixture of normal tissues; they are benign. 3) Inflammatory polyps--epithelial inflammatory reaction; they are benign. 4) Adenomatous polyps--failure of differentiation of glandular elements. They are the only neoplastic (premalignant) polyp. The three types of adenomatous polyps are tubular adenoma, mixed (tubulovillous) adenoma, and villous adenoma (syndrome of hypokalemia, profuse mucus). The risk of cancer in any adenomatous polyp depends on two features: size >1 cm and presence of villous elements. If a polyp is found on flexible sigmoidoscopy and biopsy shows hyperplastic polyp, no further work-up is needed. If biopsy shows adenomatous polyp, perform colonoscopy to look for additional polyps and to perform polypectomy.

- Adenomatous polyps are the only neoplastic (premalignant) polyp; there are three types.

- The risk of cancer in any adenomatous polyp depends on: size >1 cm and presence of villous elements.
- If biopsy shows adenomatous polyp, perform colonoscopy.

Hereditary Polyposis Syndromes

Only those polyposis syndromes associated with adenomatous polyps have risk of cancer.

Familial polyposis: adenomatous polyps of the colon. More than 95% of the patients develop colorectal carcinoma. There are no extra-abdominal manifestations except for bilateral congenital hyperplasia of the retinal pigment epithelium. Diagnosis is based on family history and documentation of adenomatous polyps. Screening of all family members is indicated, and colectomy is indicated before malignancy develops.

- More than 95% of patients with familial polyposis develop colorectal carcinoma.
- There are no extra-abdominal manifestations.
- Colectomy is indicated before malignancy develops.

Gardner's syndrome: adenomatous polyps involving the colon, although the terminal ileum and proximal small bowel are rarely involved. More than 95% of the patients develop colorectal cancer. Extraintestinal manifestations include congenital hypertrophy of the retinal pigment epithelium; osteomas of the mandible, skull, and long bones; supernumerary teeth; soft tissue tumors; thyroid and adrenal tumors; and epidermoid and sebaceous cysts. Screening of family members is indicated, and colectomy should be performed before malignancy develops.

- More than 95% of patients with Gardner's syndrome develop colorectal cancer.
- There are extraintestinal manifestations.
- Screening of family members is indicated.

Turcot-Despres syndrome: adenomatous polyps of the colon associated with malignant gliomas and other brain tumors. Autosomal recessive inheritance.

Polyposis Syndromes Not Associated With Risk of Cancer

Peutz-Jeghers syndrome: hamartomas of the small intestine and less commonly of the stomach and colon. Pigmented lesions of the mouth, hands, and feet are associated with ovarian sex cord tumors and tumors of the proximal small bowel.

- Peutz-Jeghers syndrome: hamartomas of the small intestine.
- Pigmented lesions of the mouth, hands, and feet.

Juvenile polyposis: hyperplastic polyps involving the colon and, less commonly, the small intestine and stomach. It presents as gastrointestinal tract bleeding or intussusception with obstruction.

- Only adenomatous polyps are premalignant.
- Perform colectomy for diffuse polyposis only if they are adenomatous.
- Screen family of patients with heritable polyposis syndromes only if the polyps are adenomatous.
- All the above syndromes are autosomal dominant except Turcot-Despres syndrome.

Colorectal Cancer

Epidemiology

Epidemiology is important in etiologic theories. Colorectal carcinoma is the second most common cancer in the U.S. There are 100,000 new cases and 60,000 deaths annually. Six percent of Americans eventually develop colon cancer. The mortality rate has not decreased since the 1930s. The incidence varies widely among different populations; it is highest in "westernized" countries. Compared with past rates, rates for cancer of right colon and sigmoid are increased but decreased for the rectum: cecum/ascending colon, 25%; sigmoid, 25%; rectum, 20%; transverse colon, 12%; rectosigmoid, 10%; and descending colon, 6%.

- Colorectal cancer is the second most common cancer in the U.S.
- There are increased rates for cancer of the right colon and sigmoid colon.

Etiology

The role of the environment as a cause of colorectal cancer is supported by regional differences and migrant studies of incidence. Diet--High fat diet increases the risk and may enhance cholesterol/bile acid content of bile which is converted by colonic bacteria to compounds that may promote tumors. High fiber diet is protective. Increased stool bulk may dilute carcinogens/promoters and decrease exposure by decreasing transit time. Fiber components may bind carcinogens or decrease bacterial enzymes that form toxic compounds. Charbroiled

meat/fish and fried foods contain possible mutagens. Antioxidants (vitamins A and C), selenium, vitamin E, yellow-green vegetables, and calcium may protect against cancer.

- High fat diet increases the risk of colorectal cancer.
- High fiber diet has a protective effect.
- Charbroiled meat/fish and fried foods contain possible mutagens.

Genetic Factors

Certain oncogenes amplify or alter gene products in colon cancer cells. Aneuploidy is characteristic of more aggressive tumors. The carbohydrate structure of colonic mucus is altered in colon cancer. Cell-cell interaction possibly has a role in cancer development. Also, genetic predisposition has a role in many colon cancer patients. Familial adenomatous polyposis syndromes are autosomal dominant. There is autosomal dominant inheritance of cancer family syndromes (cancer of other sites as well as of the colon) and hereditary site-specific colon cancer. Colorectal cancer appears in the 40-50 age group (20 years earlier than in the general population). Discrete polyps may precede cancer but not diffuse polyposis. Genetic susceptibility in the general population also has a role, e.g., a 3x increased risk of colorectal cancer in first-degree relatives of patients with sporadic colorectal cancer.

- Aneuploidy is characteristic of more aggressive tumors.
- Genetic predisposition to cancer exits in many colon cancer patients.
- Familial adenomatous polyposis is autosomal dominant.
- There is a 3x increased risk of colorectal cancer in first-degree relatives of patients with sporadic colorectal cancer.

Risk Factors for Colorectal Cancer

The risk factors for colorectal cancer include the following: 1) age greater than 40--the risk increases sharply at age 40, doubles each decade until age 60, and peaks at age 80. 2) Personal history of adenoma or colon cancer--the risk increases with the number of adenomas; 2%-6% patients with colon cancer have synchronous colon cancer and 1.1%-4.7% have metachronous cancers. 3) Family history of colon cancer. 4) Inflammatory bowel disease--dysplasia precedes cancer. Cancer rate begins to increase after 7 years of chronic ulcerative colitis and increases

10% per decade of disease. After 25 years the risk is 30%. The risk is greatest for universal colitis. The risk is delayed a decade in left-sided colitis and is negligible in ulcerative proctitis. Cancer risk is *not* related to severity of the first attack, disease activity, or age at onset. Cancer arising in chronic ulcerative colitis has a prognosis similar to that of other colon cancers. The rate of colon cancer is also increased 4x-20x in Crohn's colitis or ileocolitis. 5) Personal history of female genital or breast cancer carries a 2x increased risk of colon cancer.

- Risk factor: age greater than 40.
- Risk increases with the number of adenomas.
- 2%-6% of patients with colon cancer have synchronous colon cancer and 1.1%-4.7% have metachronous cancers.
- Cancer rate begins to increase after 7 years of chronic ulcerative colitis.
- After 25 years, the risk is 30%.
- The risk is greatest for universal colitis.
- Crohn's colitis: the rate of colon cancer is increased (4x-20x).

Pathology and Prognostic Indicators

Cancer arises in the epithelium and invades transmurally to penetrate the bowel wall and then enters the regional lymphatics to reach distant nodes. Hematogenous spread is via the portal vein to the liver.

Surgical-pathogen stage of primary tumor--The depth of invasion and the extent of regional lymph node involvement are important in determining prognosis.

Modified Dukes' classification (Astler-Coller, 1954): A--mucosa, submucosa (80% 5-year survival); B1--into, not through, the muscularis propria without nodal involvement (65%); B2--through the bowel wall without regional nodal involvement (43%); C1-B1 with regional nodes involved (53%); C2-B2 with regional nodes involved (15%); and D--distant metastases (5%-10%).

The extent of regional node involvement and prognosis: 1-4 nodes, 35% recur; and >4 nodes, 61% recur.

Other pathologic features and prognosis include: 1) ulcerating/infiltrating tumor is worse than exophytic/polypoid tumor; 2) poorly differentiated is worse than highly differentiated histology; 3) venous/lymphatic invasion has a poor prognosis, as does aneuploidy.

Clinical features and prognosis: a high preoperative level of carcinoembryonic antigen is associated with high recurrence rate and a shorter time before recurrence occurs. Poor prognosis if present with obstruction/perforation.

Prognosis is worse in younger than in older patients.

- The depth of invasion and the extent of regional lymph node involvement are important in determining prognosis.
- High preoperative level of carcinoembryonic antigen is associated with high recurrence and a shorter time before recurrence.
- Poor prognosis if present with obstruction/perforation.
- The prognosis is worse in younger than in older patients.

Diagnosis

The clinical presentation is that of a slow growth pattern. Disease may be present for 5 years before symptoms appear. The symptoms depend on the location of the disease. A proximal colon tumor may present with symptoms of anemia, abdominal discomfort, or a mass. The left colon is narrower, and patients may present with obstructive symptoms, change in bowel habits, and rectal bleeding.

If cancer is suspected, perform air-contrast barium enema and flexible sigmoidoscopy or colonoscopy. If cancer is detected with air-contrast barium enema or flexible sigmoidoscopy, colonoscopy is needed to rule out synchronous lesions.

Metastatic survey includes physical examination, evaluation of liver-associated enzymes, and chest radiography. Image the liver if levels of liver-associated enzymes are abnormal. Preoperative level of carcinoembryonic antigen aids in prognosis and follow-up.

- Proximal colon disease: presenting symptoms may be anemia, abdominal discomfort, or mass.
- Left colon disease: obstructive symptoms, change in bowel habits, and rectal bleeding.
- Preoperative level of carcinoembryonic antigen aids in prognosis and follow-up.

Treatment

For most cases, surgical resection is the treatment of choice. This includes wide resection of the involved segment (5-cm margins) with removal of lymphatic drainage. In rectal carcinoma, low anterior resection is performed if an adequate distal margin of at least 2 cm can be achieved; this rectal sphincter-saving operation does not make the prognosis worse in comparison with abdominal perineal resection. The primary tumor is usually resected even if there are distant metastases so as to prevent obstruction/bleeding.

- For most cases, surgical resection is the treatment of choice.

Postoperative Management--No Apparent Metastases

Repeat colonoscopy in 6-12 months and then every 3 years if the findings are negative. Annually test for occult blood in stool.

Adjuvant chemotherapy: 5-fluorouracil and levamisole decrease recurrence by 41% and mortality by 33% in colonic stage C; they may be beneficial for stage B2. Radiotherapy plus 5-fluorouracil decreases the recurrence rate in rectal cancer stages B2 and C, but it is not clear if there is any survival advantage.

- Repeat colonoscopy in 6-12 months and then every 3 years if the findings are negative.
- Annual testing for occult blood in stool.
- 5-Fluorouracil and levamisole decrease recurrence by 41% and mortality by 33% in colonic stage C.

Prevention of Colorectal Carcinoma

Primary prevention--The steps to be taken in primary prevention are not known, although epidemiologic data indicate that a high fiber, low fat diet is reasonable. Secondary prevention--Identify and eradicate premalignant lesions and detect cancer while it is still curable. Screening includes occult blood screening and sigmoidoscopy. With occult blood screening, earlier stage lesions are detected, but this has not decreased mortality. The Hemoccult test has a 20%-30% positive predictive value for adenomas and 5%-10% for carcinomas. With sigmoidoscopy, earlier stage lesions are detected, and the removal of adenomas results in lower than expected incidence of rectosigmoid cancers, but none show decreased mortality. Flexible sigmoidoscopy detects 2x-3x more neoplasms than rigid proctoscopy.

Recommendations for screening--1) For average risk (i.e., anyone not in high-risk group): annual rectal examination after age 40; annual occult blood test after age 50; sigmoidoscopy after age 50 (every 3-5 years after negative findings on two examinations 1 year apart). 2) For prior adenoma or carcinoma: annual occult blood testing; colonoscopy every year until normal x 2, then every 3 years. 3) For familial adenomatous polyposis: annual sigmoidoscopy beginning at puberty until polyposis is diagnosed, then colectomy. 4) For hereditary nonpolyposis cancer syndromes: colonoscopy at age 20; then annual Hemoccult test and colonoscopy every 3 years.

5) For first-degree relative with colorectal cancer: annual occult blood test and periodic sigmoidoscopy beginning at age 40. 6) For a woman with breast/genital cancer: annual occult blood test and periodic sigmoidoscopy. 7) For ulcerative colitis: annual colonoscopy and multiple biopsies starting after 7 years of universal chronic ulcerative colitis or after 15 years of left-sided chronic ulcerative colitis; dysplasia indicates the need for more frequent endoscopic follow-up and may lead to colectomy.

- Earlier stage lesions can be detected but early detection has not been shown to decrease mortality.
- Flexible sigmoidoscopy detects 2x-3x more neoplasms than rigid proctoscopy.

PANCREAS

Embryology

The pancreas develops in the 4th week of gestation as a ventral and dorsal outpouching or bud from the duodenum. Each bud has its own duct. As the duodenum rotates, the buds appose and join and the ducts anastomose. Pancreas divisum results from failure of the ducts of the dorsal and ventral pancreas to fuse. This may predispose to acute pancreatitis. In annular pancreas, part of the ventral pancreas encircles the duodenum (usually the second part, proximal to the ampulla) and causes obstruction.

- Pancreas divisum: failure of dorsal and ventral pancreas to fuse. May predispose to acute pancreatitis. Be able to recognize this condition on radiographs.
- Annular pancreas: part of ventral pancreas encircles the duodenum (usually the second part, proximal to the ampulla) and causes obstruction. Be able to recognize this on radiographs.

Classification of Pancreatitis

Acute--reversible inflammation. 1) Interstitial pancreatitis accounts for 80% of cases. Perfusion of the pancreas is intact. It is less severe, with <1% mortality. 2) Necrotizing pancreatitis accounts for 20% of cases. It is more severe, with 10% mortality if sterile and 30% if infected.

Chronic--irreversible (i.e., structural disease, with endocrine or exocrine insufficiency). It is documented by pancreatic calcifications, ductal abnormalities (by endoscopic retrograde cannulization of pancreas [ERCP]), scarring seen on biopsy, endocrine insufficiency (diabetes), and exocrine insufficiency (malabsorption).

- Acute interstitial pancreatitis: perfusion is intact, mortality is <1%.
- Acute necrotizing pancreatitis: perfusion is compromised, mortality is 10% if sterile and 30% if infected.
- Chronic pancreatitis is documented by pancreatic calcifications, ductal abnormalities, endocrine insufficiency (diabetes), and exocrine insufficiency (malabsorption).

Acute Pancreatitis

In acute pancreatitis, activation of pancreatic enzymes causes autodigestion of the gland. Clinical features are abdominal pain, nausea and vomiting ("too sick to eat"), ileus, peritoneal signs, hypotension, and abdominal mass (pseudocyst).

Etiologic Factors

Alcohol is the commonest cause and gallstones the second common cause. The third common cause is idiopathic (approximately 10%). The following drugs cause pancreatitis: azathioprine, 6-mercaptopurine, L-asparaginase, hydrochlorothiazide diuretics, sulfonamides, sulfasalazine, tetracycline, furosemide, estrogens, valproic acid, pentamidine (both parenteral and aerosolized), and the antiretroviral drug dideoxyinosine (ddI). Know these drugs.

The evidence that the following drugs may also cause pancreatitis is less convincing and not definite: corticosteroids, nonsteroidal anti-inflammatory drugs, methyldopa, procainamide, chlorthalidone, ethacrynic acid, phenformin, nitrofurantoin, enalapril, erythromycin, metronidazole, nonsulfa-linked aminosalicylate derivates (such as 5-aminosalicylic acid and interleukin-2).

Other causes: hypertriglyceridemia may cause pancreatitis if the triglycerides are >1,000. Look for types I, IV, and V hyperlipoproteinemia and for associated oral contraceptive use. Hypertriglyceridemia may mask hyperamylasemia. Hypercalcemia may also cause pancreatitis; look for underlying multiple myeloma, hyperparathyroidism, or metastatic carcinoma. In immunocompetent patients, mumps and coxsackievirus cause acute pancreatitis. In AIDS patients, acute pancreatitis has been reported with cytomegalovirus infection. Ductus divisum, or incomplete fusion of the dorsal and ventral pancreatic ducts, may predispose to acute pancreatitis in some people, although this is a controversial matter.

- In nonalcoholic patients with acute pancreatitis, renew all medications, check lipid levels and calcium levels, and rule out gallstones.
- Know which medications definitely cause acute pancreatitis.

Clinical Presentation

Pain may be mild to severe; it is usually sudden in onset and persistent. The pain typically is located in the upper abdomen, with radiation to the back. Relief may be obtained by bending forward or sitting up. Exacerbation of the pain is common with ingestion of food or alcohol. The absence of pain is a poor prognostic feature, because these patients usually present with shock.

Fever, if present, is low grade, rarely exceeding 101°C in the absence of complications.

Volume depletion--Most patients are hypovolemic, because fluid accumulates in abdomen.

Jaundice--Patients with pancreatitis may have a mild elevation in total bilirubin, but they are not usually clinically jaundiced. When jaundice is present it usually represents obstruction of the common bile duct by stones, compression by pseudocyst, or inflamed pancreatic tissue.

Dyspnea--A wide range of pulmonary manifestations may be seen. In over half of all cases of acute pancreatitis, some degree of hypoxemia is present. This is usually from pulmonary shunting. Patients often have atelectasis and may develop pleural effusions.

- Fever >101°C suggests infection.

Diagnosis of Acute Pancreatitis

Serum amylase--An increase in serum level of amylase is the most useful test for acute pancreatitis. The level of amylase increases 2-3 hours after an attack and remains elevated for 3-4 days. The magnitude of the elevation does not correlate with the clinical severity of the attack. Serum amylase levels may be normal in some (<10%) patients because of alcohol or hypertriglyceridemia. Persistent elevation suggests a complication, e.g., pseudocyst, abscess, ascites. Serum amylase is cleared by the kidney. Urine amylase level remains elevated after serum amylase level returns to normal. Isoenzyme identification may aid in distinguishing between salivary (nonpancreatic) and pancreatic sources. Serum lipase may help distinguish between pancreatic hyperamylasemia and an ectopic source (lung, ovarian, or esophageal carcinoma). Lipase levels are also elevated longer than amylase levels after acute pancreatitis.

Nonpancreatic hyperamylasemia--Parotitis; renal failure; macroamylasemia; intestinal obstruction, infarction, perforation; ruptured ectopic pregnancy; diabetic ketoacidosis; drugs (such as morphine); burns; pregnancy; and neoplasms (lung, ovary, esophagus).

- If presentation for pancreatitis is classic but amylase value is normal, repeat amylase test, check urine amylase and serum lipase levels, and scan the abdomen.
- Persistent hyperamylasemia suggests a complication.
- If amylase is mildly elevated and there is a history of vomiting but no signs of obstruction, perform esophagogastroduodenoscopy to rule out a penetrating ulcer.

Physical findings: 1) Vital signs--tachycardia and orthostasis. 2) Skin--fat necrosis and xanthelasmas. Grey Turner's sign (flank discoloration) or Cullen's sign (periumbilical discoloration) suggests retroperitoneal hemorrhage. 3) Abdomen--often it is less impressive than the amount of pain the patient is having.

- Be able to recognize metastatic fat necrosis.
- Grey Turner's sign and Cullen's sign suggest retroperitoneal hemorrhage.

Laboratory findings: 1) Chest radiography--An isolated left pleural effusion strongly suggests pancreatitis. Infiltrates may represent aspiration pneumonia or adult respiratory distress syndrome. 2) Abdominal flat plate--Look for sentinel loop (dilated loop of bowel over pancreatic area) and colon cutoff sign (abrupt cutoff of gas in the transverse colon). Pancreatic calcifications indicate chronic pancreatitis. 3) Ultrasonography is the procedure of choice in acute pancreatitis, although in the presence of ileus, air in the bowel may obscure visualization of the pancreas. Ultrasonographic examination gives information about the pancreas and is the best method for delineating stones. However, it is not a good method for use in obese patients. 4) CT scan is the next step when visualization of the pancreas is poor with ultrasonography. It gives the same information as ultrasonography, is slightly less sensitive in picking up stones and texture abnormalities, involves radiation, and is more expensive. CT scan is indicated in critically ill patients to rule out necrotizing pancreatitis and is the better imaging choice in obese patients. 5) ERCP has no role in the diagnosis of acute pancreatitis and should be avoided, because it may cause infection. Occasionally, when acute pancre-

atitis is caused by common bile duct obstruction, endoscopic papillotomy may be performed to relieve the obstruction.

- An isolated left pleural effusion on chest radiography is strongly suggestive of acute pancreatitis.
- On abdominal flat plate, be able to recognize the sentinel loop sign, colon cutoff sign, and pancreatic calcifications.
- Ultrasonographic examination is the procedure of choice in patients with mild acute pancreatitis, in thin patients, and to rule out gallstones.
- CT scan is indicated in seriously ill patients to rule out necrotizing pancreatitis and in obese patients.
- ERCP has no role in the diagnosis of acute pancreatitis.

Treatment

Supportive care is the backbone of treatment, with monitoring for and treatment of complications when they occur. Fluids--Restore and maintain intravascular volume; this usually can be accomplished with crystalloids and peripheral intravenous catheters. Monitor blood pressure, pulse, urine output, daily intake and output, and weight. Eliminate medications that may cause pancreatitis. Use of a nasogastric tube does not shorten the course or severity of pancreatitis. But it should be used in case of ileus or severe nausea and vomiting. Analgesics--Meperidine (Demerol), 75-125 mg given i.m. every 3-4 hours, is preferred, especially over morphine, because it causes less sphincter of Oddi spasm. The efficacy of antisecretory drugs such as H_2 blockers, anticholinergics, somatostatin, or glucagon has not been documented. Total parenteral nutrition is unnecessary in most cases of pancreatitis. Peritoneal dialysis does not change the overall mortality, although it may decrease early mortality in severe pancreatitis.

- Supportive care is the backbone of treatment.
- Eliminate medications that may cause pancreatitis.
- Nasogastric tube does not shorten the course or severity of pancreatitis.
- Meperidine (Demerol) is preferred because it causes less sphincter of Oddi spasm.

Complications

A local complication is phlegmon, a mass of inflamed pancreatic tissue. It may resolve. Pseudocysts, a fluid collection within a nonepithelial-lined cavity, should be expected if there is persistent pain and persistent hyper-amylasemia. In 50%-80% of cases, this resolves within 6 weeks without intervention. Pancreatic abscess usually develops 2-4 weeks after the acute episode and presents as fever (>101°C), persistent abdominal pain, and persistent hyperamylasemia. If a pancreatic abscess is not drained surgically, the mortality rate is virtually 100%. Give antibiotics effective for gram-negative and anaerobic organisms. Jaundice is due to common bile duct obstruction. Pancreatic ascites results from disruption of the pancreatic duct or a leaking pseudocyst.

- A local complication of pancreatitis should be suspected if fever, persistent pain, or persistent hyper-amylasemia occurs.

A systemic complication is respiratory distress syndrome, a well-recognized complication of acute pancreatitis. Circulating lecithinase probably splits fatty acids off lecithin, producing a faulty surfactant. Pleural effusions occur in approximately 20% of patients with acute pancreatitis. If aspirated, a high amylase content is found. Fat necrosis may be due to elevated levels of serum lipase.

- Adult respiratory distress syndrome is a complication of acute pancreatitis.
- Pleural effusions occur in approximately 20% of patients with acute pancreatitis and have a high amylase content.

Assessment of Severity

Most patients with acute pancreatitis recover without any sequelae. The overall mortality rate of acute pancreatitis is 5%-10%, and death is most often secondary to hypovolemia and shock, respiratory failure, pancreatic abscess, or systemic sepsis. Ranson's criteria are reliable for predicting mortality in acute pancreatitis (Table 13-16). Mortality--less than 3 signs, 1%; 3-4 signs, 15%; 5-6 signs, 40%; and 7 or more signs, 100%.

- Most patients with acute pancreatitis recover without any sequelae.

Chronic Pancreatitis

Chronic use of alcohol (at least 10 years of heavy consumption) is the commonest cause of chronic pancreatitis. Gallstones and hyperlipidemia usually do not cause chronic pancreatitis.

Hereditary pancreatitis is autosomal dominant with variable penetrance. Onset is before age 20, although 20% of patients may present later than this. It is marked by recurring abdominal pain, positive family history, and pancreatic calcifications. It may increase the risk for pancreatic cancer.

Trauma with pancreatic ductal disruption causes chronic pancreatitis. Protein calorie malnutrition is the commonest cause of chronic pancreatitis in Third World countries.

- Chronic pancreatitis is commonly caused by alcohol but seldom by gallstones or hyperlipidemia.
- Hereditary pancreatitis is seen in young people with a positive family history and pancreatic calcifications.
- Protein calorie malnutrition is the commonest cause of chronic pancreatitis in Third World countries.

Table 13-16.--Ranson's Criteria

Admission	48 hours
Age >55 yr	pO_2 <60 mm Hg
Leukocyte count >15,000	Hematocrit decrease >10%
Glucose >200	Blood urea nitrogen increase >5 mg/dL
Aspartate aminotransferase >250	
Lactate dehydrogenase >350	Calcium <8 mg/dL
	Estimated fluid sequestration >6 L

From Ranson JHC: Acute pancreatitis: surgical management. *In* The Exocrine Pancreas: Biology, Pathobiology, and Diseases. Edited by VLW Go, JD Gardner, FP Brooks, E Lebenthal, EP DiMagno, GA Scheele. New York, Raven Press, 1986, pp 503-511. By permission of publisher.

Triad of Chronic Pancreatitis

The triad consists of pancreatic calcifications, steatorrhea, and diabetes mellitus. Pancreatic calcifications--Diffuse calcification is due to hereditary, alcohol, or malnutrition. Local calcification is due to trauma, islet cell tumor, or hypercalcemia. By the time steatorrhea occurs, 90% of the gland has been destroyed and lipase output has decreased by 90%.

- Chronic pancreatitis presents as abdominal pain, pancreatic calcification, steatorrhea, diabetes mellitus.

Laboratory Diagnosis

Amylase and lipase levels may be normal. Stool fat is >10 g per 24 hours on a 48-72-hour stool collection while the patient is on a 100-g fat diet.

Pancreatic function tests: CCK/secretin stimulation--secretin given intravenously and submaximal CCK, with aspiration of duodenal contents and marker.

Bentiromide test--Para-aminobenzoic acid (PABA) conjugated with N-benzoyl tyrosine (Bentiromide) is given orally. If chymotrypsin activity is adequate, the molecule is cleaved and PABA is absorbed and excreted in the urine. This test requires a normal small intestine (normal D-xylose test) and is useful only in severe steatorrhea.

CT scan shows calcifications, irregular pancreatic contour, dilated duct system, or pseudocysts.

ERCP reveals protein plugs, segmental duct dilatation, and alternating stenosis and dilatation with obliteration of branches of the main duct.

- Amylase and lipase levels may be normal, but evidence for structural disease or endocrine or exocrine insufficiency is present.
- 90% of the gland must be damaged for steatorrhea to occur.

Pain

The mechanism of the pain is not clearly defined; it may be due to ductular obstruction. One-third to one-half of patients have a reduction in pain after 5 years. The possibility of coexistent disease such as peptic ulcer should be considered. Abstinence from alcohol may relieve pain. Analgesics, aspirin or acetaminophen, are used occasionally with the addition of codeine (narcotic addiction is a frequent complicating factor). Celiac plexus blocks relieve pain for 3-6 months, but long-term efficacy is disappointing. A trial of pancreatic enzyme replacement for 1-2 months should be tried. Women with idiopathic chronic pancreatitis are most likely to respond. Surgery should be considered only after conservative measures have failed. Patients with a dilated pancreatic duct may respond favorably to a longitudinal pancreatojejunostomy (Puestow procedure).

- Abstinence from alcohol may relieve pain.
- Narcotic addiction is a frequent complicating factor.
- A 1-2-month trial of pancreatic enzyme replacement is worthwhile. Women are most likely to respond.
- Surgical treatment: only after conservative measures have failed.

Malabsorption

Patients have malabsorption not only of fat but also of

essential fatty acids and fat soluble vitamins. The goal of enzyme replacement is to maintain body weight. Diarrhea will not resolve. Enteric-coated or microsphere enzymes are designed to be released at an alkaline pH, thus avoiding degradation by stomach acid. Their advantage is that they contain larger amounts of lipase. The disadvantages are that they are expensive and bioavailability is not always predictable.

Pancreatic Cancer

Pancreatic carcinoma is more common in men than in women. It usually presents between the ages of 60 and 80 years. The 5-year survival rate is <2%. Risk factors include diabetes, chronic pancreatitis, carcinogens, benzidine, cigarette smoking, and high fat diet. Pancreatic carcinoma usually presents late in the course of the disease. Patients may have a vague prodrome of malaise, anorexia, and weight loss. Symptoms may be overlooked until the development of pain or jaundice.

- Courvoisier's sign: painless jaundice with a palpable gallbladder suggests pancreatic cancer.
- Trousseau's sign: recurrent migratory thrombophlebitis is associated with pancreatic cancer.
- Recent-onset diabetes and nonbacterial (thrombotic) "marantic" endocarditis.

Routine laboratory blood analysis has limited usefulness. Patients may have increased levels of liver enzymes, amylase, and lipase or anemia, although this is variable. Tumor markers are also nonspecific. Ultrasonography is 80% sensitive in localizing pancreatic masses, as is abdominal CT. Either imaging method may be used in conjunction with fine-needle aspiration or biopsy to make a tissue diagnosis. ERCP is used if the ultrasonographic or CT results are inconclusive. It has a sensitivity >90%. ERCP also allows aspiration of pancreatic secretions for cytologic analysis. The "double duct" sign is a classic presentation, with obstruction of both the pancreatic and the bile ducts.

- Ultrasonography and CT are 80% sensitive in localizing pancreatic masses.
- ERCP has a sensitivity >90%.

Surgical treatment is the only hope for cure; unfortunately most lesions are nonresectable. The criteria for resectability are tumor <2 cm, absence of lymph node invasion, and absence of metastasis. Survival is the same for total pancreatectomy and the Whipple procedure: 3-year survival, 33%; 5-year survival, 1%; and operative mortality, 5%.

Radiation therapy may have a role as a radiosensitizer in unresectable cancer. However, survival is unchanged. Chemotherapy has also been disappointing and studies have not consistently shown improved survival.

Cystic Fibrosis

Because patients with cystic fibrosis are living longer, internists should know the common intestinal complications of this disease. Exocrine pancreatic insufficiency (malabsorption) is the common (85%-90%) and most important complication. Endocrine pancreatic insufficiency (diabetes) occurs in 20%-30% of the patients. Rectal prolapse occurs in 20%, and a distal small-bowel obstruction from thick secretions occurs in 15%-20%. Focal biliary cirrhosis develops in 20%.

- Pancreatic insufficiency occurs in 85%-90%.

Pancreatic Endocrine Tumors

Zollinger-Ellison syndrome is a non-beta-cell islet tumor of the pancreas that produces gastrin, causing gastric acid hypersecretion. This results in peptic ulcer disease (see section on Stomach).

Insulinoma is the commonest islet cell tumor--a beta-cell islet tumor that produces insulin, which causes hypo-

glycemia. The diagnosis is based on finding increased fasting plasma levels of insulin and hypoglycemia. CT scanning or arteriography may be useful in localizing the tumor.

Glucagonoma is an alpha-cell islet tumor that produces glucagon. It presents with diabetes, weight loss, and a classic skin rash, migratory necrolytic erythema. The diagnosis is based on finding increased glucagon levels and failure of blood sugar to increase after injection of glucagon.

Pancreatic cholera is a pancreatic tumor that produces VIP, which causes watery diarrhea (see Secretory Diarrhea).

Somatostatinoma is a delta-cell islet tumor that produces somatostatin, which inhibits insulin, gastrin, and pancreatic enzyme secretion. The result is diabetes mellitus and diarrhea. The diagnosis is based on finding increased plasma levels of somatostatin. Octreotide (Sandostatin) is useful in treating these tumors because it prevents the release of hormone and antagonizes target organ effects.

- Zollinger-Ellison syndrome: non-beta-cell islet tumor of the pancreas.
- Insulinoma: commonest islet cell tumor.
- Pancreatic cholera: pancreatic tumor that produces VIP, which causes secretory diarrhea.
- Octreotide prevents hormone release and antagonizes hormone effects.

QUESTIONS
(See "Answers" section)

Multiple Choice

1. All the following conditions predispose to the development of esophageal cancer except for:
   a. Lye stricture
   b. Smoking
   c. Alcohol
   d. Diffuse esophageal spasm
   e. Achalasia

2. The symptom complex of oropharyngeal dysphagia is suggested to the clinician by the presence of all the following except for:
   a. High esophageal (cervical) dysphagia
   b. Aspiration
   c. Epigastric pain
   d. Nasal regurgitation with swallowing
   e. Choking with swallowing

3. All the following decrease lower esophageal sphincter pressure except:

a. Alcohol
b. Caffeine
c. Anticholinergic agents
d. Calcium channel blockers
e. Protein

4. All the following medications have been implicated in medication-induced esophagitis except for:
   a. Ferrous sulfate
   b. Quinidine
   c. Potassium
   d. Anticholinergic agents
   e. Tetracycline

5. All the following conditions have been associated with an increased frequency of peptic ulcer disease except:
   a. Nonsteroidal anti-inflammatory drugs
   b. Cigarette smoking
   c. Corticosteroids
   d. Cirrhosis
   e. Chronic pulmonary disease

6. All the following clinical entities have an osmotic mechanism for diarrhea except:
   a. Surreptitious laxative ingestion
   b. Saline cathartics
   c. Antacids
   d. Sorbitol foods
   e. Lactase deficiency

7. All the following are seen in malabsorption secondary to pancreatic insufficiency except:
   a. Edema
   b. Bone pain
   c. Alopecia
   d. Easy bruisability
   e. Night blindness

8. Extraintestinal manifestations of inflammatory bowel disease include all of the following except:
   a. Celiac sprue
   b. Arthritis
   c. Primary sclerosing cholangitis
   d. Renal stones
   e. Episcleritis or uveitis

9. All the following are indications for colonoscopy in the evaluation of inflammatory bowel disease except:

a. To evaluate extent of disease
b. To perform biopsy of a stricture
c. To evaluate iron deficiency anemia
d. To differentiate Crohn's colitis from ulcerative colitis
e. To monitor for development of dysplasia or cancer.

10. All the following conditions have been associated with the development of pseudomembranous colitis except:
    a. Uremia
    b. Ischemia
    c. Intestinal surgery
    d. Antibiotics
    e. Foreign travel

11. All the following polyps have an increased risk of cancer except for:
    a. A solitary 2-cm tubular adenoma
    b. A solitary 2-cm villous adenoma
    c. Gardner's syndrome
    d. Familial polyposis
    e. Juvenile polyposis

12. All the following have been associated with precipitation of toxic megacolon except:
    a. Proctoscopy
    b. Barium enema
    c. Anticholinergic agents
    d. Opiates
    e. Hypokalemia

13. All the following confirm the diagnosis of chronic pancreatitis except:
    a. Pancreatic calcifications
    b. Chronic abdominal pain
    c. Abnormal pancreatogram
    d. Diabetes mellitus
    e. Malabsorption

14. All the following drugs have been associated firmly with acute pancreatitis except:
    a. Corticosteroids
    b. 6-Mercaptopurine
    c. Azathioprine
    d. Furosemide
    e. L-Asparaginase

15. All the following are nonpulmonary features of cys-

tic fibrosis except:
a. Focal biliary cirrhosis
b. Rectal prolapse
c. Meconium ileus
d. Celiac sprue
e. Pancreatic insufficiency

True/False

16. With regard to *Helicobacter pylori*, indicate whether the following are true or false:
    a. Not commonly found in asymptomatic people
    b. The commonest cause of histologic gastritis
    c. A common and important factor in peptic ulcer disease
    d. Important for the development of adenocarcinoma of the stomach
    e. If eradicated, does not improve healing rate of ulcers
    f. If eradicated, prevents recurrence of ulcers.

17. Concerning infectious diarrhea; indicate whether the following are true or false:
    a. *Bacillus cereus* is associated with fried rice in oriental restaurants
    b. *Salmonella* is associated with poultry
    c. *Vibrio parahaemolyticus* is associated with ingestion of shellfish
    d. Antibiotics shorten the duration of traveler's diarrhea
    e. Antibiotics shorten the duration of cholera
    f. Antibiotics shorten the duration of *Salmonella* infection

18. With regard to colorectal cancer, indicate whether or not the following are risk factors:
    a. Age
    b. Hyperplastic polyps
    c. Ulcerative colitis
    d. Diverticulosis
    e. Female genital cancer
    f. Breast cancer

19. With regard to treating inflammatory bowel disease, indicate whether the following are true or false:
    a. Corticosteroids are useful for maintenance therapy in Crohn's disease and ulcerative colitis
    b. Left-sided ulcerative colitis may be treated with topical aminosalicylates or steroids
    c. Severe attacks of ulcerative colitis usually require high doses of corticosteroids
    d. Immunosuppressive agents may be effective for chronically active steroid-dependent disease
    e. Bowel rest is more effective than elemental diet
    f. Antibiotic therapy appears to be more effective in ulcerative colitis than in Crohn's disease

20. With regard to malabsorption, indicate whether the following are true or false:
    a. The presence of oil droplets in the stool suggests pancreatic insufficiency
    b. The presence of undigested meat fibers in the stool suggests intestinal disease
    c. Vitamin B_{12} deficiency may be seen in intestinal disease and pancreatic disease
    d. Iron deficiency anemia commonly occurs with pancreatic insufficiency
    e. Blunted villi on small-bowel biopsy are diagnostic for celiac sprue
    f. Small-bowel biopsy that shows PAS-positive organisms in macrophages is seen in Whipple's disease

NOTES

CHAPTER 14
GASTROENTEROLOGY II

John J. Poterucha, M.D.

HEPATOBILIARY DISORDERS

VIRAL HEPATITIS

Hepatitis A

Hepatitis A virus (HAV) is a small RNA virus that accounts for 20%-25% of acute hepatitis in developed countries. The disease generally is transmitted by the fecal-oral route and has an incubation period of 15-50 days. Spread is more common in overcrowded areas with poor hygiene and poor sanitation. Ingestion of raw shellfish can cause epidemics. Hepatitis caused by HAV is generally mild, especially in children who often have a subclinical or nonicteric illness. Infected adults are more ill and usually develop jaundice. Rarely, HAV may cause fulminant hepatitis. The prognosis is excellent. Chronic liver disease does not develop from HAV. A serum IgM anti-HAV is present during acute illness, generally persists for 2-6 months, and is followed by IgG anti-HAV, which offers immunity from further infection. Because the virus is usually cleared from the feces before onset of jaundice, isolation of patients generally does not halt the spread of infection. Immune serum globulin should be given for household contacts of infected patients. When a common source of food-borne infection is identified, serum globulin should be given to those exposed. A hepatitis A vaccine has been developed but is not available in the U.S.A.

- HAV is transmitted by fecal-oral route.
- Incubation period is 15-50 days.
- Ingestion of raw shellfish can cause epidemics.
- Prognosis is excellent.
- Chronic liver disease does not develop.
- IgM anti-HAV is present during acute illness.
- Give immune serum globulin for household contacts.

Hepatitis B

Hepatitis B virus (HBV) is a DNA virus with a surface and core. The core consists of a core antigen and "e" antigen. The disease is transmitted parenterally or by sexual contact. In high carriage areas, e.g., certain areas of Asia, infants may acquire infection from the mother during childbirth. High-risk groups in U.S.A. include intravenous drug users, persons with multiple sexual contacts, and health-care workers. Clinical course of HBV infection varies. Most infections in adults are subclinical, and even when symptomatic, disease resolves within 6 months. During acute hepatitis, symptoms (when present) are generally more severe than those of HAV. Jaundice rarely lasts >4 weeks. Some patients may have preicteric symptoms of "serum sickness," including arthralgias and urticaria. These symptoms may be related to immune complexes, which can also lead to polyarteritis and glomerulonephritis.

- HBV is transmitted parenterally or by sexual contact.
- Infants may acquire infection from mothers.
- High-risk groups: intravenous drug users, persons with multiple sexual contacts, health-care workers.
- Most infections in adults are subclinical.
- Jaundice rarely lasts >4 weeks.

HBV is not directly cytopathic and hepatocellular necrosis is due to host immune response to viral-infected cells. This inflammatory response accounts for HBV symptoms. Thus, patients with symptomatic HBV are more likely to "clear" the virus than those with subclinical infection. For example, patients with fulminant hepatitis B who recover rarely develop chronic hepatitis B. Viral markers in blood during self-limited infection with

HBV are shown in Figure 14-1.

- Host immune response: causes hepatocellular necrosis and accounts for HBV symptoms.
- Patients who recover from fulminant hepatitis B rarely develop chronic hepatitis B.

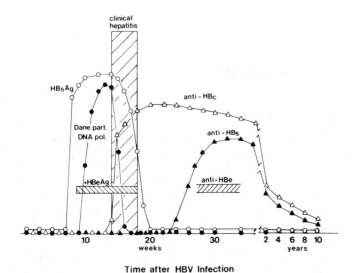

Fig. 14-1. Viral markers in blood during self-limited hepatitis B virus infection. (From Robinson WS: Biology of human hepatitis viruses. *In* Hepatology: A Textbook of Liver Disease. Vol 2. Second edition. Edited by D Zakim, TD Boyer. Philadelphia, WB Saunders Company, 1990, pp 890-945. By permission of publisher.)

Note that IgM anti-HBc is nearly always present during acute hepatitis B, and 5%-6% of patients with acute HBV lack hepatitis B surface antigen (HBsAg). This is especially true in fulminant hepatitis B. HBV-DNA and hepatitis B e antigen (HBeAg) correlate with ongoing viral replication and indicate infectivity. Patients with hepatitis B mutants may have high HBV-DNA levels but lack HBeAg. Such patients are generally found in the Mediterranean and Far East and may have a severe course. Commonly encountered serologic patterns of HBV are shown in Table 14-1.

Ten percent of patients acquiring HBV as adults and 90% of those infected as neonates do not clear HBsAg from the serum within 6 months and, thus, become chronic carriers. Chronicity is more common in patients with a defect of the immune system. Most chronic carriers of HBsAg have a good prognosis. Histologically, their livers are essentially normal. Chronic liver disease due to HBV may lead to cirrhosis and liver failure. Patients with chronic HBV liver disease may also have relapse, with development of fatigue and abnormal liver findings.

Conversion from an HBeAg-negative state to HBeAg-positivity can occur. Patients with chronic HBV liver disease, particularly if cirrhosis is present, are at high risk for development of hepatocellular carcinoma and should be screened with liver ultrasonography and alpha-fetoprotein determinations every 6 months.

- IgM anti-HBc is nearly always present during acute hepatitis B.
- HBV-DNA and HBeAg correlate with ongoing viral replication and indicate infectivity.
- 10% of patients acquiring HBV as adults and 90% of those infected as neonates do not clear HBsAg.
- Most chronic carriers of HBsAg: good prognosis and essentially normal livers histologically.
- Chronic liver disease due to HBV may lead to cirrhosis.
- Patients with HBV chronic liver disease are at high risk for development of hepatocellular carcinoma.

Patients with chronic hepatitis B are candidates for therapy with interferon-α. About 30%-40% will have a response manifested by loss of HBeAg and HBV-DNA. A few patients will also clear HBsAg. The patients more likely to respond to interferon include those with relatively recent diagnosis of chronic hepatitis B, high serum levels of aminotransferases, active hepatitis without evidence of cirrhosis on biopsy, and low serum levels of HBV-DNA. Those patients with HBV who respond to interferon often have transient elevation of aminotransferases after about 8 weeks of treatment. A brief period of pretreatment with corticosteroids may improve response in those with only mildly elevated levels of aminotransferases. Corticosteroids otherwise have no role in treating HBV liver disease.

Hepatitis D

The delta agent is a small RNA particle that requires the presence of HBsAg to cause infection. Hepatitis D virus (HDV) infection can occur simultaneously with acute HBV (coinfection) or may infect a chronic HBsAg carrier (superinfection). HDV is strongly associated with intravenous drug abuse. Infection with HDV should only be considered in patients with HBsAg and is diagnosed by anti-HDV seroconversion. Acute delta hepatitis is self-limited but may cause fulminant hepatitis. Like HBV, HDV recurs in the transplanted liver.

- Delta agent requires presence of HBsAg to cause infection.
- HDV is strongly associated with i.v. drug abuse.

Table 14-1.--Common Serologic Patterns of Hepatitis B Virus

HBsAg	Anti-HBs	Anti-HBc	HBeAg	Anti-HBe	Interpretation
+	-	IgM	+	-	Acute HBV infection, high infectivity
+	-	IgG	+	-	Chronic HBV infection, high infectivity
+	-	IgG	-	+	Late-acute or chronic HBV infection, low infectivity
+	+	+	±	±	HBsAg of one subtype and heterotypic anti-HBs (common)
					Process of seroconversion from HBsAg to anti-HBs (rare)
-	-	IgM	±	±	Acute HBV infection
					Anti-HBc window
-	-	IgG	-	±	Low-level HBsAg carrier
					Remote past infection
-	+	IgG	-	±	Recovery from HBV infection
-	+	-	-	-	Immunization with HBsAg (after vaccination)
					Remote past infection (?)
					False-positive

From Dienstag JL, Wands JR, Isselbacher KJ: Acute hepatitis. *In* Harrison's Principles of Internal Medicine. Twelfth edition. Edited by JD Wilson, E Braunwald, KJ Isselbacher, RG Petersdorf, JB Martin, AS Fauci, RK Root. New York, McGraw-Hill, 1991, pp 1322-1337. By permission of publisher.

- Consider this infection only in patients with HBsAg.
- Diagnosed by anti-HDV seroconversion.
- Like HBV, HDV recurs in transplanted liver.

Hepatitis C

In early 1970s, most patients with post-transfusion hepatitis (PTH) were found to have no serologic markers for either HAV or HBV infection. Thus, PTH was referred to as non-A, non-B hepatitis. In 1989, a single-stranded RNA virus was identified that accounts for most cases of PTH. This is the hepatitis C virus (HCV). In addition to a history of blood transfusions, other risk factors for acquiring HCV infection include parenteral drug abuse and needlestick exposure. However, 40%-50% of HCV patients have no identifiable risk factors and 50%-60% of previously classified "cryptogenic" cirrhosis is due to HCV. The most common presentation of HCV infection is a chronic, asymptomatic elevation of aminotransferases. A characteristic feature of chronic HCV is fluctuation in liver enzymes. The correlation between symptoms and degree of hepatic inflammation is poor. First-generation ELISA tests only became positive a mean of 24 weeks after infection. Also, false-positives occurred in patients with high levels of gamma globulin, as in autoimmune hepatitis. Second-generation ELISAs have increased sensitivity and specificity. The recombinant immunoblot assay (RIBA) is a supplemental test for patients who are anti-HCV positive by ELISA. HCV-RNA can be measured by polymerase chain reaction.

- HCV, a single-stranded RNA virus, causes most cases of PTH.
- Risk factors: blood transfusions, parenteral drug abuse, needlestick exposure.
- 40%-50% of HCV patients have no identifiable risk factors.
- Common presentation: chronic, asymptomatic elevation of aminotransferases.
- Characteristic feature: fluctuation in liver enzymes.

Chronic infection develops in at least 50% of patients with HCV infection, and in 20%, it progresses to cirrhosis. Patients with HCV-induced cirrhosis are at increased risk for development of hepatocellular carcinoma. Chronic HCV infection may be associated with cryoglobulinemia. Interferon-α at a dose of 3 million units given subcutaneously three times weekly for 6 months normalizes alanine aminotransferase levels in 40%-50% of patients, but 50% of them have relapse within 6 months after discontinuation of therapy. Patients with cirrhosis are less likely to respond to interferon.

- Chronic infection develops in 50% of infected patients.
- Cirrhosis develops in 20%.
- HCV patients with cirrhosis are at increased risk for hepatocellular carcinoma.
- Chronic HCV infection may be associated with cryoglobulinemia.
- Interferon-α normalizes aminotransferase levels in 40%-50% of patients.
- Patients with cirrhosis are less likely to respond to interferon.

Hepatitis E

Hepatitis E virus (HEV) is an enterically transmitted RNA virus. It can cause acute hepatitis in patients from India, Pakistan, Mexico, Southeast Asia, and travelers returning from these regions. Clinically, hepatitis E resembles hepatitis A. A notable exception is the high risk of fulminant hepatitis E in women who acquire infection during third trimester of pregnancy. Chronic hepatitis E does not occur. Hepatitis A, B, and E are compared in Table 14-2.

- HEV is an enterically transmitted RNA virus.
- It resembles hepatitis A.

- High risk of fulminant hepatitis E in women who acquire infection during third trimester of pregnancy.

Miscellaneous

Epstein-Barr virus, cytomegalovirus, and herpes viruses can all cause acute viral hepatitis, which is most serious in immunocompromised patients.

AUTOIMMUNE HEPATITIS

"Autoimmune hepatitis" (AH) was previously called "autoimmune *chronic* active hepatitis" because it required 3-6 months of abnormal liver enzymes. However, AH can present as acute hepatitis. Classically, AH affects young persons (10-20 years), mainly women. The onset is usually insidious, and initial liver biopsy may show cirrhosis in some patients.

By definition, patients with AH should have no history of drug-related hepatitis, HBV, HCV, or Wilson's disease. Immunoserologic markers, including antinuclear antibody (ANA), smooth muscle antibody, soluble liver antigen antibodies, and antibodies to liver/ kidney microsomal (LKM) antigens, are often seen and may help separate patients into certain groups. There is an association with certain HLA-types. Associated conditions include Hashimoto's thyroiditis, Coombs' positive hemolytic anemia, diabetes, and glomerulonephritis. Marked increases in serum gamma globulin levels are common, and

Table 14-2.--Comparison of Hepatitis A, B, and E

Feature	Hepatitis A	Hepatitis B[*]	Hepatitis E
Incubation	15-45 days (mean, 30)	30-180 days (mean, 60-90)	14-60 (mean, 40)
Onset	Acute	Often insidious	Acute
Age preference	Children, young adults	Any age	Young adults
Transmission			
Fecal-oral	+++	-	+++
Sexual	±	++	±
Percutaneous	Unusual	+++	-
Severity	Mild	Often severe	Mild
Prognosis	Generally good	Worse with age, debility	Good
Chronicity	None	Occasional (5%-10%)	None
Prophylaxis	Ig	Hepatitis B immune globulin, HBV vaccine	?
Carrier	None	0.1%-30%[†]	None

[*]Concomitant delta hepatitis is similar to hepatitis B, but more severe outcomes are favored.
[†]Varies considerably throughout the world.
From Dienstag JL, Wands JR, Isselbacher KJ: Acute hepatitis. *In* Harrison's Principles of Internal Medicine. Twelfth edition. Edited by JD Wilson, E Braunwald, KJ Isselbacher, RG Petersdorf, JB Martin, AS Fauci, RK Root. New York, McGraw-Hill, 1991, pp 1322-1337. By permission of publisher.

aminotransferases are generally 4-10 times normal. Corticosteroids (30-40 mg/day) produce improvement in 60%-80% of patients. Changes in results of liver tests and gamma globulin are often dramatic. Azathioprine can be added to allow use of lower doses of prednisone. The prednisone dose should be reduced to control symptoms and maintain serum level of aminotransferases below five times normal. Even after excellent response to corticosteroids, relapse often occurs and control of AH often requires maintenance therapy. Although corticosteroids do not seem to prevent progression to cirrhosis, they improve survival in patients with severe disease.

- Classically, AH affects young persons (10-20 years old), mainly women.
- Onset is usually insidious.
- Should be no history of drug-related hepatitis, HBV, HCV, or Wilson's disease.
- Immunoserologic markers are often seen.
- Marked increases in serum gamma globulin levels are common.
- 60%-80% of patients improve with corticosteroids.
- Changes in results of liver tests and gamma globulin are often dramatic.
- Control of AH often requires maintenance therapy.

ALCOHOLIC LIVER DISEASE

Alcoholic Hepatitis

Alcoholic hepatitis is a histologic diagnosis characterized by fatty change, degeneration, and necrosis of hepatocytes (with or without Mallory bodies) and inflammatory infiltrate of neutrophils. Almost all patients have increased intralobular connective tissue, and they may have cirrhosis. Clinically, patients may be asymptomatic or jaundiced and critically ill. Common symptoms include anorexia, nausea, vomiting, abdominal pain, and weight loss. The most common sign is hepatomegaly, which may be accompanied by ascites, jaundice, fever, splenomegaly, and encephalopathy. AST is elevated in 80%-90% of cases but is almost always <400 U/L. Aminotransferases of >400 U/L are not a feature of alcoholic liver disease and a search for other causes (i.e., ingestion of acetaminophen) should be pursued. The AST:ALT ratio is frequently >2. Leukocytosis is seen, particularly in severely ill patients.

- Alcoholic hepatitis is a histologic diagnosis.

- It is characterized by: fatty change, degeneration, and necrosis of hepatocytes (± Mallory bodies) and inflammatory infiltrate of neutrophils.
- Common symptoms: anorexia, nausea, vomiting, abdominal pain, weight loss.
- Commonest sign: hepatomegaly, which may be accompanied by ascites, jaundice, fever, splenomegaly, encephalopathy.
- Elevated AST (almost always <400 U/L) in 80%-90% of cases.
- AST:ALT is frequently >2.
- Leukocytosis in severely ill patients.

Bad prognostic markers include encephalopathy, spider angiomata, ascites, renal failure, prolonged prothrombin time, and bilirubin >20 mg/dL. Many patients have progression to cirrhosis, particularly if alcohol intake is not curtailed. Corticosteroids may be beneficial as acute treatment of alcoholic hepatitis, particularly in patients with severe disease characterized by encephalopathy and markedly prolonged prothrombin time.

- Bad prognostic markers: encephalopathy, spider angiomata, ascites, renal failure, prolonged prothrombin time, bilirubin >20 mg/dL.
- Corticosteroids may be beneficial in severe disease.

Alcoholic Cirrhosis

Cirrhosis is defined histologically by fibrosis with nodular parenchymal regeneration. Typically, the cirrhosis of alcoholics is micronodular. Only 60% of patients with alcoholic cirrhosis have signs or symptoms of liver disease. Most patients with cirrhosis have no history of alcoholic hepatitis. Women are more predisposed to cirrhosis from alcoholism; this may be related to gastric mucosal levels of alcohol dehydrogenase. Liver enzymes may be relatively normal in cirrhosis without alcoholic hepatitis. Concomitant HCV infection is common in patients with alcoholic liver disease. Prognosis of alcoholic cirrhosis depends on whether patients continue to drink and whether there are symptoms (jaundice, ascites, gastrointestinal bleeding) of chronic liver disease. The 5-year survival for patients without ascites, jaundice, or hematemesis and who abstain is 89%. For those with symptoms and who continue to drink, the 5-year survival is 34%. Although propylthiouracil can produce improved survival in patients with stable alcoholic liver disease, most hepatologists do not advocate its use. Liver transplantation is an option for patients with end-stage alcoholic liver disease as long as they have abstained from alcohol for ≥1 year.

- Cirrhosis of alcoholics is micronodular.
- Only 60% of patients with alcoholic cirrhosis have signs or symptoms of liver disease.
- Women are more predisposed to cirrhosis from alcoholism.
- Liver enzymes may be relatively normal.
- 5-Year survival for patients without ascites, jaundice, or hematemesis and who abstain is 89%.
- 5-Year survival for those with symptoms and continue to drink is 34%.
- Liver transplantation is an option.

Fatty Liver

Fatty liver is the morphologic change seen most commonly in alcoholic liver disease and it may be seen in patients who do not abuse alcohol but have diabetes or obesity.

- Fatty liver is commonly seen in alcoholic liver disease.
- Fatty liver is also seen in patients who do not drink but have diabetes or obesity.

CHRONIC CHOLESTATIC LIVER DISEASES

Primary Biliary Cirrhosis

Primary biliary cirrhosis is a chronic, progressive, cholestatic liver disease primarily affecting middle-aged women. Its cause is unknown but appears to involve an immunologic disturbance resulting in small bile duct destruction. Many patients are identified because of asymptomatic increase of alkaline phosphatase. Common early symptoms are pruritus and fatigue. Patients also may have symptoms due to Hashimoto's thyroiditis or sicca complex. Biochemical features include increased alkaline phosphatase and IgM levels. Later, bilirubin increases, serum albumin decreases, and prothrombin time is prolonged. Steatorrhea may occur because of progressive cholestasis. Fat-soluble vitamin deficiencies and metabolic bone disease are common.

- Primary biliary cirrhosis primarily affects middle-aged women.
- Common early symptoms: pruritus and fatigue.
- Alkaline phosphatase and IgM levels increase.
- Fat-soluble vitamin deficiencies and metabolic bone disease are common.

Circulating antimitochondrial antibodies (AMA) occur in 90%-95% of patients. They are directed against autoantigens, called M2, on inner mitochondrial membranes. The classic histologic lesion is granulomatous infiltration of septal bile ducts. Treatment of primary biliary cirrhosis is generally symptomatic. Cholestyramine may be helpful for itching. Fat-soluble vitamin deficiencies should be addressed. Cyclosporin A, colchicine, and methotrexate are suggested as treatment options to arrest disease progression, but data about them are not conclusive. Results of liver tests improve after treatment with ursodeoxycholic acid (histologic improvement is also seen in some cases).

- AMA occur in 90%-95% of patients.
- Classic histologic lesion: granulomatous infiltration of septal bile ducts.
- Treatment is generally symptomatic.
- Results of liver tests improve after use of ursodeoxycholic acid.

Primary Sclerosing Cholangitis

Primary sclerosing cholangitis (PSC) is a chronic cholestatic liver disease characterized by obliterative inflammatory fibrosis of extra- and intrahepatic bile ducts. An immune mechanism has been implicated. Patients may have an asymptomatic increase in alkaline phosphatase or progressive fatigue, pruritus, and jaundice. Bacterial cholangitis is uncommon unless biliary tract surgery or instrumentation has been performed previously. Cholangiography establishes the diagnosis of PSC, showing short strictures of bile ducts with intervening segments of normal or slightly dilated ducts, producing a beaded appearance. This cholangiographic appearance can be mimicked by that of AIDS cholangiopathy (due to cytomegalovirus or cryptosporidium) and ischemic cholangiopathy after intra-arterial infusion of fluorodeoxyuridine.

- PSC: obliterative inflammatory fibrosis of extra- and intrahepatic bile ducts.
- Immune mechanism is implicated.
- Asymptomatic increase in alkaline phosphatase.
- Bacterial cholangitis is uncommon.
- Cholangiography establishes diagnosis.
- AIDS cholangiopathy mimics cholangiographic appearance of PSC.

The most commonly associated disease accompanying PSC is chronic ulcerative colitis. Ulcerative colitis occurs in 70% of patients with PSC and may antedate, accompany, or even follow the diagnosis of PSC. Proctocolectomy done for ulcerative colitis has no effect on the development of PSC. Patients with PSC are at higher risk for bile duct cancer; its development may be indicated by rapid clinical deterioration, with jaundice, weight loss, and abdominal pain. Treatment for PSC is generally supportive. Surgical reconstruction or percutaneous or endoscopic balloon dilatation of bile duct strictures may offer palliation, especially in patients with recurrent cholangitis. Ursodeoxycholic acid is being investigated as a treatment. Many patients have progressive liver disease and require liver transplantation.

- Ulcerative colitis occurs in 70% of patients with PSC.
- Proctocolectomy has no effect on development of PSC.
- PSC patients are at higher risk for bile duct cancer.
- Treatment for PSC is generally supportive.
- Many patients require liver transplantation.

HEREDITARY LIVER DISEASES

Genetic Hemochromatosis

Hemochromatosis is a genetically transmitted disorder of iron metabolism characterized by iron overload. The basic defect may be inappropriately high absorption of iron from the gastrointestinal tract. Because the gene for hemochromatosis is linked closely to HLA loci, HLA typing within a family may help identify susceptible members of a kindred. Genetic hemochromatosis is transmitted in an autosomal recessive manner. In the general population, heterozygote frequency is 10%. Only homozygotes manifest progressive iron accumulation.

- Genetic hemochromatosis is a disorder of iron metabolism.
- It is characterized by iron overload.
- High absorption of iron by gastrointestinal tract.
- Autosomal recessive transmission.
- Only homozygotes have progressive iron accumulation.

Patients usually present with end-stage disease. Peak incidence is between the ages of 40 and 60. Iron overload is manifested more often in men, because women are somewhat protected by menstrual losses of iron. Clinical features include arthropathy, hepatomegaly, skin pigmentation, diabetes, cardiac dysfunction, and hypo-

gonadism. Routine liver biochemistry studies generally show little disturbance. Serum level of iron is elevated and transferrin saturation is >90%. Serum levels of ferritin are high, and levels >1,000 suggest hemochromatosis. Increased iron and ferritin levels also occur in other liver diseases, particularly alcoholic liver disease. Liver biopsy with quantitation of hepatic iron concentration is the standard method for diagnosing hemochromatosis. Generally, hepatic iron levels in hemochromatosis are >10,000 $\mu g/g$ dry weight.

- Patients usually present with end-stage disease.
- Iron overload is more common in men.
- Clinical features: arthropathy, hepatomegaly, skin pigmentation, diabetes, cardiac dysfunction, hypogonadism.
- Serum levels of ferritin are high.
- Standard for making diagnosis: liver biopsy with quantitation of hepatic iron concentration.

Hemochromatosis is treated by depleting excessive iron stores by repeated phlebotomies. Standard recommendation is to remove 500 mL per week to point of mild anemia. Maintenance program of 4-8 phlebotomies per year is required. When initiated in precirrhotic stage, removal of iron can render liver normal and may improve cardiac function and diabetes. Treatment does not reverse arthropathy, hypogonadism, or eliminate increased risk (30%) of hepatocellular carcinoma. All first-degree relatives of patients should be screened for evidence of iron overload.

- Hemochromatosis is treated with repeated phlebotomies.
- Iron removal can render liver normal.
- Treatment does not reverse arthropathy, hypogonadism, or eliminate increased risk (30%) of hepatocellular carcinoma.
- First-degree relatives should be screened.

Wilson's Disease

Wilson's disease is an autosomal recessive disorder characterized by increased amounts of copper in tissues. The basic defect involves an inability to prepare copper for biliary excretion. The liver is chiefly involved in children, but neuropsychiatric manifestations are prominent in older patients. The Kayser-Fleischer ring is a brownish pigmented ring at the periphery of the cornea. It is not invariably present and is more frequent in patients with neurologic manifestations. Hepatic forms of Wilson's disease include fulminant hepatitis (often accompanied by hemolysis and renal failure), chronic active hepatitis, and insidiously developed cirrhosis. Development of hepatoma is rare. Neurologic signs include tremor, rigidity, altered speech, and changes in personality. Fanconi's syndrome and premature arthritis may occur.

- Wilson's disease: autosomal recessive disorder characterized by increased copper in tissues.
- Basic defect: inability to prepare copper for biliary excretion.
- Kayser-Fleischer ring: brownish pigmented ring at periphery of cornea.
- This ring is more frequent in patients with neurologic manifestations.
- Hepatoma is rare.
- Neurologic signs: tremor, rigidity, altered speech, changes in personality.

Evidence of hemolysis (total bilirubin elevated out of proportion to direct bilirubin), low or normal level of alkaline phosphatase, and low serum level of uric acid (due to Fanconi's syndrome) suggest Wilson's disease. Diagnosis is established on basis of low serum level of copper, low level of ceruloplasmin, and increased urinary copper. Ceruloplasmin levels can be misleading--they can be increased by estrogen or biliary obstruction and decreased by liver failure of any cause. High concentrations of copper in liver are found in Wilson's disease; similarly high values can also occur in cholestatic syndromes. Penicillamine chelates and increases urinary excretion of copper. It is the treatment of choice. Initiate treatment at 1.2 g/day. Failure of treatment should not be diagnosed until after 2 years of treatment have been given. All siblings of patients should be screened for copper. Trientine is an alternative to penicillamine. Zinc inhibits gastrointestinal absorption of copper and can be used as adjunctive therapy. Liver transplantation corrects the metabolic defect of Wilson's disease.

- Diagnosis: low level of serum copper, low level ceruloplasmin, increased urinary copper.
- Ceruloplasmin levels can be misleading.
- High concentrations of liver copper: in Wilson's disease and cholestatic syndromes.
- Penicillamine: treatment of choice; it increases urinary excretion of copper.
- Alternative treatment: trientine

- Liver transplantation corrects metabolic defect.

Alpha₁-Antitrypsin Deficiency

Alpha₁-antitrypsin (AIAT) is synthesized in the liver. The gene is on chromosome 14. M is the common normal allele, and Z and S are frequent abnormal alleles. Intrahepatic accumulation of AIAT in ZZ phenotype causes liver disease; however, disease occurs in only 10%-20% of ZZ patients. During first 6 months of life, patients often have history of cholestatic jaundice that resolves. In later childhood or early adulthood, cirrhosis may develop. Prevalence of cirrhosis in patients with MZ phenotype is increased, but the risk is small. Hepatoma can complicate AIAT deficiency, especially in males. Diagnosis of AIAT deficiency is made by determining AIAT phenotype. Serum levels of AIAT may be variable and unreliable. Liver transplantation corrects the metabolic defect and changes recipient's phenotype to that of the donor.

- Intrahepatic accumulation of AIAT causes liver disease.
- During first 6 months of life, cholestatic jaundice that resolves.
- Hepatoma can complicate AIAT deficiency, especially in males.
- Diagnosis is made by determining AIAT phenotype.
- Liver transplantation corrects metabolic defect.

FULMINANT HEPATIC FAILURE

Fulminant hepatic failure is defined as hepatic failure with encephalopathy developing <8 weeks after onset of jaundice in patients with no history of liver disease. Its common causes are listed in Table 14-3. Poor prognostic markers include a drug-induced cause (other than acetaminophen), older age, grade 3 or 4 encephalopathy, acidosis, and prothrombin time >50 seconds. Treatment is supportive, and steroids offer no benefit. Patients should be transferred to a medical center where liver transplantation is available.

- Fulminant hepatic failure: hepatic failure with encephalopathy developing <8 weeks after onset of jaundice and no history of liver disease.
- Poor prognostic markers: drug-induced (not acetaminophen), older age, grade 3 or 4 encephalopathy, prothrombin time >50 seconds.
- Steroids offer no benefit.

DRUG-INDUCED LIVER DISEASE

Drugs cause toxic effects in the liver in many ways, often mimicking naturally occurring liver disease. Most drug-induced liver disorders are idiosyncratic and not dose-related; 2% of cases of jaundice in hospitalized patients and 25% of cases of fulminant hepatitis are drug-induced. Consequently, all drugs that have been used by a patient with liver disease must be identified. Histologic classification of drug-induced liver disease and examples are given in Table 14-4.

Table 14-3.--Common Causes of Fulminant Hepatic Failure

Infective
  Hepatitis virus A, B, C(?), D, E
  Herpes simplex
Drug reactions and toxins
  Halothane
  Isoniazid-rifampicin
  Antidepressants
  Nonsteroidal anti-inflammatory drugs
  Valproic acid
  Acetaminophen overdose
  Mushroom poisoning
  Herbal remedies
Ischemic
  Ischemic hepatitis
  Surgical "shock"
  Acute Budd-Chiari syndrome
Metabolic
  Wilson's disease
  Fatty liver of pregnancy
  Reye's syndrome
Miscellaneous (rare)
  Massive malignant infiltration
  Severe bacterial infection

From Sherlock S, Dooley J: Diseases of the Liver and Biliary System. Ninth edition. Oxford, Blackwell Scientific Publications, 1993, p 102. By permission of publisher.

Acetaminophen toxicity may occur at relatively low doses in alcoholics, because alcohol induces hepatic microsomal P-450 enzymes, which metabolize acetaminophen to its toxic metabolite. Disulfiram can also cause fulminant hepatitis. Amoxicillin-clavulinic acid causes severe cholestatic hepatitis, and valproic acid, tetracycline, and AZT can cause severe steatosis. Amiodarone may cause hepatotoxicity, whose histologic features can mimic those of alcoholic liver disease. Methotrexate in a total dose >2 g can cause hepatic fibrosis; some physicians advocate annual liver biopsies in patients receiving long-term methotrexate for psoriasis or rheumatoid arthritis. Intravenous cocaine can cause massive necrosis and death. Adenomas can occur with long-term use of oral contraceptives. Lovastatin commonly causes mild increases in aminotransferase.

- Most drug-induced liver disorders are idiosyncratic, not dose-related.
- 2% of cases of jaundice (hospitalized patients) and 25% of cases of fulminant hepatitis are drug-induced.
- Identify all drugs that have been used by a patient with liver disease.
- In alcoholics, acetaminophen toxicity may occur at relatively low doses.
- Amoxicillin-clavulinic acid causes severe cholestatic hepatitis.
- Amiodarone may cause hepatotoxicity.
- Total dose of methotrexate >2 g can cause hepatic fibrosis.
- Cocaine i.v. can cause massive necrosis.
- Long-term use of oral contraceptives can cause adenomas.

LIVER TUMORS

Hepatocellular Carcinoma

The risk of hepatocellular carcinoma is increased in cirrhosis of nearly any cause but particularly if due to HBC, HCV, hemochromatosis, and alcoholic liver disease. Alpha-fetoprotein is increased in only 50% of patients with hepatocellular carcinoma. Common metastatic sites are lymph nodes, lungs, bone, and brain. Paraneoplastic syndromes include gynecomastia, hypercalcemia, hypoglycemia, polycythemia, and clubbing. Surgical resection is the treatment of choice, presuming hepatic reserve is sufficient to permit resection. Liver transplantation is complicated by high rate of recurrence. Percutaneous alcohol ablation may be useful for small tumors (this is experimental).

- Risk is increased in cirrhosis of nearly any cause.
- Alpha-fetoprotein is increased in 50% of patients with hepatocellular carcinoma.
- Common metastatic sites: lymph nodes, lungs, bone, brain.
- Paraneoplastic syndromes: gynecomastia, hypercal-

Table 14-4.--Histologic Patterns and Corresponding Examples of Drug-Induced Liver Disease

Pattern	Example
Zonal necrosis	Acetaminophen, carbon tetrachloride
Nonspecific hepatitis	Aspirin, oxacillin
Viral hepatitis-like lesion	Isoniazid, methyldopa
Granulomatous hepatitis	Quinidine, allopurinol
Chronic hepatitis	Methyldopa, nitrofurantoin
Fibrosis	Methotrexate
Cholestasis	
Inflammatory	Chlorpromazine, erythromycin estolate
Bland	Estrogens, anabolic steriods
Fatty liver	
Large globules	Ethanol, corticosteroids
Small droplets	Tetracycline, valproic acid
Vascular lesions	
Hepatic vein thrombosis	Oral contraceptives
Veno-occlusive disease	Certain antitumor agents
Noncirrhotic portal hypertension	Vinyl chloride monomer
Peliosis hepatis	Anabolic steroids
Tumors	
Adenoma	Oral contraceptives, androgens
Focal nodular hyperplasia	Oral contraceptives
Carcinoma	Oral contraceptives, androgens
Angiosarcoma	Vinyl chloride monomer

From Bass NM, Ockner RK: Drug-induced liver disease. *In* Hepatology: A Textbook of Liver Disease. Vol 2. Second edition. Edited by D Zakim, TD Boyer. Philadelphia, WB Saunders Company, 1990, pp 754-791. By permission of publisher.

cemia, hypoglycemia, polycythemia, clubbing.
- Treatment of choice: surgical resection.
- Liver transplantation is complicated by high recurrence rate.

Cholangiocarcinoma

The incidence of cholangiocarcinoma is increased in patients with PSC, *Clonorchis* infection, and history of choledochal cysts (Caroli's disease). Cholangiocarcinoma can be difficult to diagnose, especially in patients with PSC.

Adenoma

Adenomas are associated with use of oral contraceptives. They can present with acute right upper quadrant pain and hemodynamic compromise because of bleeding.

Cavernous Hemangioma

Cavernous hemangioma is commonest benign tumor of the liver. CT scan with contrast agent can often be diagnostic.

Metastases

Metastases are more common than primary tumors of the liver. Frequent primary sites are colon, stomach, breast, lung, and pancreas. Surgical resection of isolated colon cancer metastases has limited effect on long-term survival.

COMPLICATIONS OF END-STAGE LIVER DISEASE

Ascites

The pathogenesis of ascites is disputed but probably involves a combination of decreased effective circulatory blood volume (underfill theory) and inappropriate renal sodium retention with expansion of plasma volume (overfill theory). The initial event may be vasodilatation. Patients with ascites generally have a low urinary sodium. Treatment of ascites involves sodium restriction, diuretics, and (occasionally) fluid restriction. Bed rest is often helpful initially. Generally, spironolactone (100-200 mg/day) is used initially, although a low dose of furosemide (20-40 mg) is often added. The goal is to increase urinary sodium and allow loss of 1 L of ascitic fluid (1 kg weight) per day. Paracentesis is indicated for diagnostic purposes and should be done therapeutically in patients with tense ascites or with respiratory compromise from abdominal distention. Large-volume paracentesis (up to 10 L) combined with 6 g albumin per liter of ascitic fluid removed is safe and well tolerated, particularly in patients who also have peripheral edema.

- Pathogenesis of ascites probably involves combination of decreased effective circulatory blood volume and inappropriate renal sodium retention with expansion of plasma volume.
- Patients generally have low urinary sodium.
- Treatment: sodium restriction, diuretics.
- Large-volume paracentesis is safe and well tolerated.

Pleural effusion occurs in 6% of patients with cirrhosis and is right-sided in 67%. Edema usually follows ascites and is related to hypoalbuminemia and possibly increased pressure on the inferior vena cava by intra-abdominal fluid. The sudden onset of ascites in young patients should raise the possibility of hepatic venous outflow obstruction (Budd-Chiari syndrome).

Tests most useful for determining the cause of ascites are measurements of total protein and the serum-ascitic fluid albumin gradient [albumin (serum) minus albumin (ascites)]. Albumin gradient >1.1 g/dL almost always indicates portal hypertension. Ascites secondary to portal hypertension induced by congestive heart failure can be distinguished from cirrhotic ascites because congestive heart failure usually has ascitic fluid protein >2.5. Exudative ascites from cancer or tuberculosis generally has ascitic fluid protein >2.5 and albumin gradient of <1.1 (Table 14-5).

Refractory ascites is uncommon. Most physicians advocate therapeutic paracentesis as needed. Peritoneovenous shunts are complicated by disseminated intravascular coagulation and shunt malfunction and, in comparison with diuretics and paracentesis, do not improve survival.

- Pleural effusion occurs in 6% of patients with cirrhosis and is right-sided in 67%.
- Sudden onset of ascites in young patients raises possibility of hepatic venous outflow obstruction (Budd-Chiari syndrome).
- Albumin gradient >1.1 g/dL almost always indicates portal hypertension.
- Peritoneovenous shunts do not improve survival.

Table 14-5.--Use of Single Measurements to Determine Cause of Ascites

	Serum-ascites albumin gradient, g/dL	Ascites protein, g/dL
Cirrhosis	>1.1	<2.5
Congestive heart failure	>1.1	>2.5
Malignancy	<1.1	>2.5

Spontaneous Bacterial Peritonitis

Spontaneous bacterial peritonitis (SBP) occurs in 10%-20% of cirrhotic patients with ascites. SBP is defined as a bacterial infection of ascitic fluid without any intra-abdominal source of infection. Fever, abdominal pain, and abdominal tenderness are classic symptoms; however, many patients have few or no symptoms. SBP should be suspected in any patient with cirrhotic ascites. For all patients, diagnostic paracentesis is advisable as initial step. Coagulopathy and thrombocytopenia should not prohibit performing diagnostic paracentesis. Cell count, Gram's stain, and culture of ascitic fluid should be performed on all patients. Bedside inoculation of blood culture bottles with ascites increases diagnostic yield. SBP is more common in patients with large-volume ascites and those with a low ascitic fluid protein (<1.5 g). Also, blood of all SBP patients should be cultured, because almost 50% will be positive. Variants of SBP are listed in Table 14-6.

Generally, all variants should be treated with 5-10 days of third-generation cephalosporin. Response to antibiotics should be assessed by repeat paracentesis 48 hours after initiation of therapy. The polymorphonuclear count should fall by 50% and cultures should be sterile. The hospital mortality rate of SBP is 50%-70%, and even if a patient survives hospitalization, the 1-year mortality rate is 60%-80%. A polymicrobial infection of ascitic fluid should prompt a search for an intra-abdominal focus of infection; SBP nearly always involves only one organism.

- SBP occurs in 10%-20% of cirrhotic patients with ascites.
- Classic symptoms: fever, abdominal pain, abdominal tenderness.
- Many patients have few or no symptoms.
- Bedside inoculation of blood culture bottles with ascites increases diagnostic yield.
- SBP is more common in cases of large-volume ascites and in those with low ascitic fluid protein (<1.5 g).
- All varients of SBP should be treated with 5-10 days of third-generation cephalosporin.
- SBP nearly always involves only one organism.

Hepatorenal Syndrome

Hepatorenal syndrome consists of renal failure with normal tubular function in patients with cirrhosis. Differential diagnosis is given in Table 14-7. Hepatorenal syndrome is difficult to distinguish from prerenal azotemia; thus, a brief trial of colloid expansion may be needed. Hepatorenal syndrome is often precipitated by vigorous diuretic therapy. Treatment is supportive. After liver transplantation is performed, kidney function returns to normal.

- Hepatorenal syndrome: renal failure with normal tubular function in cirrhotic patient.
- It is difficult to distinguish from prerenal azotemia.
- It is often precipitated by vigorous diuretic therapy.
- After liver transplantation, kidney function returns to normal.

Portal Systemic Encephalopathy

Portal systemic encephalopathy is a reversible decrease in the level of consciousness in patients with severe liver disease. Disturbed consciousness, personality change, intellectual deterioration, and slowed speech are common manifestations. Electroencephalogram is often abnormal and patients often have asterixis (flapping tremor). The grading system commonly used for portal systemic encephalopathy is given in Table 14-8.

The sudden development of portal systemic encephalopathy in patients with stable cirrhosis should prompt a search for bleeding, infection, or electrolyte disturbances; however, simple precipitating events may include increased dietary protein or constipation. Serum or arterial levels of ammonia are usually increased.

Table 14-6.--Variants of Spontaneous Bacterial Peritonitis

	Ascitic fluid poly-morphonuclear cells, mL	Ascitic fluid cultures
Spontaneous bacterial peritonitis	>250	Positive
Culture-negative neutrocytic ascites	>250	Negative
Bacterascites	<250	Positive

Table 14-7.--Differential Diagnosis for Hepatorenal Syndrome

	Prerenal azotemia	Hepatorenal syndrome	Acute renal failure
Urinary sodium concentration, mEq/L	<10	<10	>30
Urine to plasma creatinine ratio	>30:1	>30:1	<20:1
Urinary osmolality	At least 100 mOsm > plasma osmolality	At least 100 mOsm > plasma osmolality	Equal to plasma osmolality
Urinary sediment	Normal	Unremarkable	Casts, debris

From Epstein M: Functional renal abnormalities in cirrhosis: pathophysiology and management. In Hepatology: A Textbook of Liver Disease. Vol 2. Second edition. Edited by D Zakim, TD Boyer. Philadelphia, WB Saunders Company, 1990, pp 493-512. By permission of publisher.

Table 14-8.--Grading System for Portal Systemic Encephalopathy

Grade of encephalopathy	Level of consciousness	Neurologic abnormalities	EEG abnormalities
0	Normal	None	None
1	Trivial lack of awareness	Slight tremor Uncoordination	Symmetric slowing (5-6 cps)
	Personality change Day-night reversal	Asterixis	Triphasic waves
2	Lethargic	Asterixis	Symmetric slowing
	Inappropriate behavior	Abnormal reflexes	Triphasic waves
3	Asleep but arousable	Asterixis	Symmetric slowing
	Confused when awake	Abnormal reflexes	Triphasic waves
4	Unarousable	Babinski response Decerebrate posture Pupillary responses preserved	Very slow (2-3 cps) delta activity

cps, cycles per second; EEG, electroencephalogram.
From Schafer DF, Jones EA: Hepatic encephalopathy. *In* Hepatology: A Textbook of Liver Disease. Vol 1. Second edition. Edited by D Zakim, TD Boyer. Philadelphia, WB Saunders Company, 1990, pp 447-460. By permission of publisher.

Ammonia levels are often used to follow the course of treatment. Treatment consists of dietary protein restriction and lactulose. Lactulose has a laxative effect to decrease the nitrogenous compounds presented to the liver. It also acidifies gut contents, thereby "trapping" ammonia as NH^{4+}, but it is unclear whether this is important. Oral neomycin offers no benefit over lactulose.

- Portal systemic encephalopathy: reversible decrease in level of consciousness in patients with severe liver disease.
- EEG is often abnormal.
- Patients often have asterixis, or flapping tremor.
- Sudden development of portal systemic encephalopathy: look for bleeding, infection, or electrolyte disturbances.
- Ammonia levels are often used to follow course of treatment.
- Treatment: dietary protein restriction, lactulose.

Variceal Hemorrhage

Esophageal varices are collateral vessels that develop because of portal hypertension. Varices can occur in other parts of the gut. Isolated gastric varices without esophageal varices can occur with sinistral (left-sided) portal hypertension due to splenic vein thrombosis. Most cirrhotic patients with varices do not hemorrhage, but a first hemorrhage has a 30%-50% mortality. Bleeding is generally massive. Early endoscopy is indicated for diagnosis

and treatment. Endoscopic therapy consists of sclerotherapy or band ligation. Vasopressin in combination with nitroglycerin decreases portal venous pressure and may help stop the hemorrhage.

- Esophageal varices are collateral vessels that develop because of portal hypertension.
- Most cirrhotic patients with varices do not hemorrhage.
- First hemorrhage: 30%-50% mortality.
- Bleeding is generally massive.
- Early endoscopy is indicated for diagnosis and treatment.

Recurrent bleeding occurs in 80%-100% of cases. Propranolol given orally can help prevent rebleeding, although most physicians advocate sclerotherapy or banding until varices are obliterated. Patients with refractory bleeding are candidates for shunting. Surgical shunts have a high rate of mortality and morbidity and are complicated by portal systemic encephalopathy. Transjugular intrahepatic portal systemic shunt (TIPS) is a new technique performed by vascular radiologists. It involves creating a tract (with expandable stents) between a branch of the hepatic vein and a branch of the portal vein via access from the jugular vein. TIPS is effective in controlling bleeding and has the advantage of avoiding an operation. Incidence of portal systemic encephalopathy after TIPS is 10%-40%, but it usually can be controlled with medical therapy.

- Rebleeding occurs in 80%-100% of cases.
- Patients with refractory bleeding are candidates for shunting.
- Incidence of portal systemic encephalopathy after TIPS is 10%-40%.

CHOLESTASIS AND BILIARY TRACT DISEASE

Cholestasis is broadly defined as a failure of normal bile flow. Alkaline phosphatase levels are usually elevated. Bilirubin can be increased in cholestasis. Although bilirubin can be increased in hepatocellular disorders (e.g., hepatitis), it may be normal in cholestatic diseases. When alkaline phosphatase is elevated without hyperbilirubinemia, the liver origin of the alkaline phosphatase can be confirmed by either alkaline phosphatase isoenzymes or gamma glutamyl transferase elevations. Intrahepatic cholestasis is often due to medications or focal hepatic lesions. Extrahepatic cholestasis can be due to tumors, stones, or benign strictures. Acute biliary obstruction, usually due to a common bile duct stone, may be accompanied by marked transient elevations in aminotransferases. Hyperbilirubinemia without other markers of cholestasis may be due to hemolysis, resorption of hematomas, or massive transfusions. The commonest cause of isolated indirect hyperbilirubinemia is Gilbert syndrome, which is easily confirmed by showing a decline in bilirubin after patient has eaten. Usually, the medical history and ultrasonography (to detect dilated biliary system) identify whether cholestasis is intrahepatic or obstructive. Ultrasonography is more likely to show dilated bile ducts in patients with obstruction if bilirubin is ≥ 10 mg/dL and/or jaundice has been present for ≥ 10 days.

- Cholestasis is failure of normal bile flow.
- Alkaline phosphatase levels are usually elevated.
- Acute biliary obstruction may be accompanied by marked transient elevations in aminotransferases.
- Gilbert syndrome: commonest cause of isolated indirect hyperbilirubinemia.
- Medical history and ultrasonography usually identify whether cholestasis is intrahepatic or obstructive.

Gallstones and Cholecystitis

Gallstones can be cholesterol or pigment. Cholesterol gallstones occur when bile is supersaturated with cholesterol relative to bile salts. Excessive cholesterol secretion (females, obesity, exogenous estrogens) or defi-

cient bile acid secretion (terminal ileal disease or resection, bile acid sequestrant therapy) can lead to cholesterol gallstones. Pigment stones can occur with hemolysis or cirrhosis, but there usually is no identifying cause. Ultrasonography is 90%-97% sensitive for detecting gallstones. Cholecystitis may be suggested by gallbladder contraction, marked distention, surrounding fluid, or wall thickening. Ultrasonography also offers the opportunity to detect dilated bile ducts. Radionuclide biliary scanning is helpful in diagnosing cystic duct obstruction with cholecystitis if performed during an episode of pain. Positive test results are marked by nonvisualization of the gallbladder despite biliary excretion of radioisotope.

- Cholesterol gallstones occur when bile is supersaturated with cholesterol.
- Pigment stones can occur with hemolysis or cirrhosis.
- Ultrasonography is 90%-97% sensitive for detecting gallstones.
- Radionuclide biliary scanning helps diagnose cystic duct obstruction with cholecystitis.

Asymptomatic gallstones require no therapy, even in high-risk patients. Patients with episodes of biliary colic or acute cholecystitis should have cholecystectomy. Laparoscopic cholecystectomy is the procedure of choice. High surgical risk patients can undergo percutaneous cholecystostomy as a temporary measure. Nonsurgical therapies for stones include percutaneous extraction, oral dissolution with ursodeoxycholic acid or chenodeoxycholic acid, or direct contact dissolution via gallbladder catheter with methyl-tert butyl ether (MTBE). Ursodeoxycholic acid should only be used for small CT-radiolucent cholesterol stones. It needs to be given for 6-24 months.

- Asymptomatic gallstones require no therapy.
- Procedure of choice: laparoscopic cholecystectomy.
- Use ursodeoxycholic acid for only small CT-radiolucent cholesterol stones.

Bile Duct Stones

Most bile duct stones originate in the gallbladder, although a few patients have primary duct stones. CT and ultrasonography are relatively insensitive for common bile duct stones and diagnosis usually requires cholangiography accomplished via endoscopic retrograde cholangiopancreatography (ERCP). Patients can have minimal or no symptoms due to common bile duct stone or they can have life-threatening cholangitis with abdominal pain, fever, and jaundice. Patients with common bile duct stones should have them removed. This can be done in 90% of cases via ERCP. Urgency of the procedure depends on clinical presentation. Patients with minimal symptoms can have elective ERCP, but those with cholangitis and fever unresponsive to antibiotics should have urgent endoscopic treatment.

- Most bile duct stones originate in the gallbladder.
- Diagnosis of common bile duct stones usually requires cholangiography.
- Common bile duct stones should be removed.
- Urgent endoscopic treatment is needed if cholangitis and fever are unresponsive to antibiotics.

Laparoscopic removal of common bile duct stones is not established. Patients who are to have laparoscopic cholecystectomy should have preoperative ERCP if there is a good possibility of common duct stones (i. e., patients with a history of cholangitis, jaundice, or gallstone pancreatitis or those with elevated values on liver tests). If patient has common bile duct stones and gallbladder stones, the options are open cholecystectomy and common bile duct exploration, laparoscopic cholecystectomy and ERCP with sphincterotomy and stone extraction, or ERCP alone while leaving the gallbladder in situ. For high surgical risk patients, the last-named option is reasonable. Patients with gallbladder stones who have papillotomy and clearance of their duct stones have only 10% chance of having further problems with their gallbladder stones.

- Patients with gallbladder stones who have papillotomy and clearance of their duct stones have only 10% chance of further problems with their gallbladder stones.

Benign Biliary Tract Strictures

Most benign biliary strictures are iatrogenic. They were especially common in the early days of laparoscopic cholecystectomy. Such strictures are best treated surgically.

Malignant Biliary Obstruction

Malignant biliary obstruction is usually due to carcinoma of the head of the pancreas, bile duct cancer, or metastatic cancer to hilar nodes. If the disease is unresectable, palliative endoscopic or percutaneous stenting is as effective as surgical bypass. One exception is impending duodenal obstruction at which time operation offers the opportunity for bypass of both biliary and duodenal obstruction. A major complication of stenting is occlusion of the stents, which occurs in 1-6 months.

- Usual causes of malignant biliary obstruction: carcinoma of the head of the pancreas, bile duct cancer, metastatic cancer to hilar nodes.
- Palliative endoscopic or percutaneous stenting is as effective as surgical bypass.
- Major complication of stenting: occlusion of the stents.

Gallbladder Carcinoma

Gallbladder carcinoma has a strong association with calcified (porcelain) gallbladder. For this reason, cholecystectomy is best for calcified gallbladder.

Sphincter of Oddi Dysfunction

Sphincter of Oddi dysfunction is a poorly defined entity characterized by right upper quadrant pain without any structural cause. Patients with typical biliary-type pain, elevated values on liver tests during the pain, a dilated common bile duct, and delayed drainage of contrast after cholangiography often improve after sphincterotomy. Patients without all these criteria generally have a poor or variable response to sphincterotomy.

QUESTIONS
(See "Answers" section)

Multiple Choice

1. An 82-year-old man has a 2-day history of upper abdominal pain, dark urine, and light stools. Three weeks previously he had an acute myocardial infarction. Findings on the initial physical examination were notable for a temperature of 38.2°C and jaundice. The white blood cell count was 16,000/mL, with 14% bands. Bilirubin was 8.0/5.0 mg/dL; aspartate aminotransferase, 93 U/L, and alkaline phosphatase, 111 U/L. Ultrasonography demonstrated multiple small gallstones and no dilated bile ducts. He was given antibiotics intravenously, but the next morning his temperature was 39.4°C, and the white blood cell count was 22,000/mL; bilirubin, 9.4 mg/dL; aspartate aminotransferase, 443 U/L; and alkaline phosphatase, 150 U/L. Which of the following is the next appropriate step:
   a. Surgical consultation for laparoscopic cholecystectomy
   b. Surgical consultation for open cholecystectomy
   c. Hepatitis serologies
   d. Endoscopic retrograde cholangiography
   e. Continued observation

2. A 46-year-old asymptomatic Asian man has a long history of a positive hepatitis B surface antigen (HBsAg) and wants to know whether he should be treated with alpha-interferon. His alanine aminotransferase (ALT) is 134 U/L; bilirubin, 1.2/0.3 mg/dL; and platelets, 90,000 x 10^9/L. The alpha-fetoprotein is 280 ng/mL (normal, 0-20 ng/mL). Which of the following is the next appropriate step:
   a. Computed tomography or ultrasonography of the liver
   b. Alpha-interferon 5 MU three times weekly
   c. Repeat the alpha-fetoprotein measurement in 6 months
   d. Begin corticosteroid therapy followed by alpha-interferon
   e. Perform a percutaneous liver biopsy

3. All the following statements are true about hepatitis C virus (HCV) except:
   a. HCV accounts for 90% of post-transfusion hepatitis
   b. Chronic hepatitis is common after HCV infection
   c. Nearly all patients have a history of parenteral exposure
   d. Fluctuating aminotransferase levels are characteristic of HCV infection
   e. There is an increased risk of hepatocellular carcinoma in HCV-induced cirrhosis

4. Complications of chronic cholestatic liver disease include all the following except:
   a. Metabolic bone disease
   b. Hypercholesterolemia
   c. Steatorrhea
   d. Cardiomyopathy
   e. Fat-soluble vitamin deficiencies

5. A 50-year-old alcoholic man presents with jaundice and lethargy. Physical examination findings are notable for temperature of 37.9°C, confusion, jaundice, asterixis, spider angiomata, ascites, and splenomegaly. Hemoglobin is 10.3 g/dL; leukocytes, 2,600/μL; platelets, 68,000/μL; bilirubin, 12.4 mg/dL; AST, 1,004 U/L; and ALT, 938 U/L. Which of the following is inappropriate:
   a. Methylprednisolone, 32 mg/day
   b. Diagnostic paracentesis
   c. Tests for HBsAg, IgM anti-HBc, IgM anti-HAV
   d. Lactulose
   e. Blood and urine drug screen, including a search for acetaminophen

True/False

6. With regard to primary sclerosing cholangitis and inflammatory bowel disease, indicate whether the following are true or false:
   a. Less than 50% of patients with primary sclerosing cholangitis have inflammatory bowel disease
   b. Less than 50% of patients with inflammatory bowel disease have primary sclerosing cholangitis
   c. Successful treatment of inflammatory bowel disease usually prevents progression of primary sclerosing cholangitis
   d. The incidence of primary sclerosing cholangitis is similar in patients with ulcerative colitis and Crohn's disease
   e. Patients with primary sclerosing cholangitis have an increased risk of bile duct cancer
   f. The steatorrhea seen in patients with primary sclerosing cholangitis and chronic ulcerative colitis is due to the colitis.

7. With regard to ascites, indicate whether the following are true or false:

   a. A serum-ascites albumin gradient >1.1 is characteristic of ascites of portal hypertension

   b. Patients with high protein ascites are more likely to develop spontaneous bacterial peritonitis than those with low protein ascites

   c. A patient with cirrhotic ascites and an ascitic fluid leukocyte count of 2,000/mm^3 should receive treatment for spontaneous bacterial peritonitis even if the results of Gram staining and culturing are negative

   d. An ascites protein concentration >2.5 g/dL usually distinguishes malignant ascites from ascites due to congestive heart failure

   e. A single episode of bacterial peritonitis due to *E. coli* in a patient with cirrhotic ascites should prompt endoscopic studies of the upper and lower gastrointestinal tract to search for an origin of the infection

   f. Negative findings on cytologic examination of ascitic fluid effectively exclude ascites related to hepatocellular carcinoma

NOTES

CHAPTER 15

GENERAL INTERNAL MEDICINE

Scott C. Litin, M.D.

INTERPRETATION OF DIAGNOSTIC TESTS

Diagnostic test assessment takes into account two sets of characteristics: those pertaining to the test itself (sensitivity and specificity) and the pretest likelihood that the disease is present in the person being tested (prevalence of disease in a population). When a diagnostic test is applied to a population at risk for the abnormal condition, patients in the studied population can be assigned to one of four groups (Table 15-1):

True-positive = disease present, abnormal test result.

False-positive = disease absent, abnormal test result.

False-negative = disease present, normal test result.

True-negative = disease absent, normal test result.

Table 15-1.--2-By-2 Table

Diagnostic test result		Target disorder		
		Present	Absent	
	Positive	True + a	False + b	a+b
	Negative	c False -	d True -	c+d
		a+c	b+d	a+b+c+d

Prevalence = (a+c)/(a+b+c+d)
Test characteristics
    Sensitivity = a/(a+c)
    Specificity = d/(b+d)
Frequency-dependent properties
    PPV = a/(a+b)
    NPV = d/(c+d)

When data are displayed in a 2-by-2 table, the following test characteristics can be defined (Table 15-1):

1. Sensitivity

    Positive in disease (PID).

    True positivity rate--proportion of patients with the target disorder who have positive test result.

    2-By-2 table with definition = a/(a+c).

    Screening tests attempt to maximize sensitivity to avoid missing a person with the disease.

    Characteristic of test--not affected by population characteristics.

2. Specificity

    Negative in health (NIH).

    True negativity rate--proportion of patients having no disease who have negative findings on screening test.

    2-By-2 table definition = d/(b+d).

    Confirmatory tests used in follow-up of screening try to maximize specificity to avoid incorrectly labeling healthy person as having disease.

    Characteristic of test--not affected by population characteristics.

3. Positive predictive value

    When a patient's illness is evaluated by interpreting a diagnostic test, the 2-by-2 table is read horizontally, not vertically. Therefore, in judging the value of a diagnostic test, it is not essential to know its sensitivity and specificity but whether a patient with positive test results has the disease, i.e., how well the test results predict a disease when compared with the standard for that particular disease. Thus, the horizontal properties of the diagnostic test are of primary interest. Among all patients with a positive diagnostic test result, (a+b), in what proportion, a/(a+b), has the diagnosis been correctly predicted or ruled in? This proportion is the positive predictive value (PPV).

- PPV is the proportion of patients who test positive who have the disease.
- This provides information most useful in clinical practice.
- PPV is affected by prevalence of disease in population.
- 2-By-2 table definition = a/(a+b).

4. Negative predictive value

It is also important to know the percentage of patients with a negative test result, (c+d), who actually do not have the disease. This proportion, d/(c+d), is the negative predictive value (NPV).

- NPV is the proportion of patients who test negative and have no disease; it is prevalence-dependent.
- 2-By-2 table definition = d/(c+d).

5. Prevalence

PPV and NPV of diagnostic test depend on proportion of persons with the disease among the entire group of persons to whom test is applied. This proportion, (a + c)/(a+b+c+d), is the prevalence.

How to Construct a 2-by-2 Table

Sensitivity, specificity, and predictive values of normal and abnormal test results can be calculated with even a limited amount of information. For example, suppose a new diagnostic test gives abnormal results in 90% of patients who have the disease and normal results in 95% of patients who are disease-free and, furthermore, the prevalence of the disease in the population to which the test is applied is 10%. This provides the following information:

$$sensitivity = 90\%$$
$$specificity = 95\%$$
$$prevalence = 10\%$$

This test is now ready to be applied to a group of patients by filling in a 2-by-2 table (Table 15-2). The calculation is easier if the test is applied to a large number of patients, e.g., 1,000, and a+b+c+d = 1,000.

Because the prevalence of the disease is 10%, 100 patients have the disease (0.1 x 1,000 = 100, or a+c = 100). Of the patients, 90%, or 900, are disease-free (0.9 x 1,000 = 900, or b+d = 900).

Because the sensitivity of the test is 90%, of the 100 patients with disease, 90% have an abnormal test result (a = 0.9 x 100 = 90) and 10% have a normal result

(c = 0.1 x 100 = 10).

Specificity of 95% means that of the 900 patients who are disease-free, 95% have a normal test result (d = 0.95 x 900 = 855) and 5% have an abnormal test result (b = 0.05 x 900 = 45).

The 2-by-2 table (Table 15-2) shows that 135 patients (a+b) have an abnormal test result; however, only 90 of these 135 patients actually have the disease. Therefore, the PPV of an abnormal test is a/(a+b) = 90/135 = 66.7%, i.e., only two-thirds of all patients with abnormal findings will actually have the disease. Similarly, one can determine that 865 patients (c+d) have a normal test result: 855 of these 965 patients are disease-free. Therefore, the NPV of the test is d/(c+d) = 855/865 = 98.8%.

Table 15-2.--2-By-2 Table for Test With 90% Sensitivity, 95% Specificity, and 10% Prevalence

		Disease present	Disease absent	
Diagnostic test result	Positive	90 a	45 b	135 a+b
	Negative	c 10	d 855	c+d 865
		a+c	b+d	a+b+c+d
Total		100	900	1,000

Prevalence = (a+c)/(a+b+c+d) = 100/1,000 = 10%
Test characteristics
   Sensitivity = a/(a+c) = 90/100 = 90%
   Specificity = d/(b+d) = 855/900 = 95%
Frequency-dependent properties
   PPV = a/(a+b) = 90/135 = 66.7%
   NPV = d/(c+d) = 855/865 = 98.8%

Clinicians should be able to perform these simple calculations. The PPV and NPV of test results, not the sensitivity and specificity, are important in internal medicine.

For example, if the prevalence of the disease in the clinician's population is 4% instead of 10%, PPV and NPV can be recalculated. PPV of abnormal test results falls to 42.9%, quite different from the 66.7% above, although the sensitivity and specificity of the test (90% and 95%, respectively) have not changed (Table 15-3).

- The most important factor in interpreting an abnormal

test result in a patient is the prevalence of the disease in the population being tested.

- High-risk populations (high prevalence of disease) tend to improve the PPV of an abnormal test result.
- Low-risk populations (screening tests) make the NPV of a normal test result look impressive.

Table 15-3.--2-By-2 Table for Test With 90% Sensitivity, 95% Specificity, and 4% Prevalence

		Disease present	Disease absent	
Test result	Positive	36 a	48 b	84 a+b
	Negative	c 4	d 912	c+d 916
		a+c	b+d	a+b+c+d
	Total	40	960	1,000

Prevalence = (a+c)/(a+b+c+d) = 40/1,000 = 4%

Test characteristics

  Sensitivity = a/(a+c) = 36/40 = 90%

  Specificity = d/(b+d) = 912/960 = 95%

Frequency-dependent properties

  PPV = a/(a+b) = 36/84 = 42.9%

  NPV = d/(c+d) = 912/916 = 99.5%

PREOPERATIVE MEDICAL EVALUATION

The Art of Medical Consultation

This section is concerned with advice given by an internist to a surgeon in assessing preoperative risk in managing perioperative problems (J. Gen. Intern. Med. 2:257-269, 1987). Guidelines for the internist to optimize compliance with the advice are listed below:

1. Limit the number of recommendations to five or fewer.
2. Focus on crucial recommendations and avoid diluting management plan with trivial suggestions.
3. Be specific, especially regarding drug dosages. Recommend not only which drug to use but specify dose and frequency of administration.
4. Advice about therapy (i.e., initiating or discontinuing drug therapy) is heeded more often than diagnostic suggestions (i.e., ordering tests).
5. Labor-intensive advice that requires the surgeon to do something (look at a blood smear, perform a

procedure, etc.) is poorly heeded. If such tasks must be performed, the medical consultant should do them personally.
6. Oral communication with the surgeon usually enhances compliance.
7. Follow-up visits and notes further improve compliance.

Successfully communicating one's assessment and plan is an art. A three-step approach--diagnosis/treatment/prognosis--is often helpful.

1. Diagnosis--the internist creates a problem list that is a table of contents for anyone involved in the care of patient. It is particularly useful to anesthesiologists and surgeons.
2. Treatment--the internist offers recommendations that will diminish the surgical risks associated with patient's problem. The emphasis is on therapeutics aimed only at diminishing surgical risk.
3. Prognosis--the internist states the surgical and anesthetic risk for each problem (often available in published literature). When this information is lacking, the internist has to substitute personal judgment.
4. The internist should comment on the cumulative risk for a patient with multiple medical problems, such as cardiac, pulmonary, and liver disease. The risk in such patients may become prohibitive.

- Diagnosis--a problem list.
- Treatment--recommendations only for decreasing surgical risk.
- Prognosis--surgical and anesthetic risk for each problem.
- Internist should comment on cumulative risk for patient with multiple medical problems.

Risks of Anesthesia and the Operation

The risk of dying in the perioperative period (i.e., intraoperatively or within 48 hours postoperatively) is about 0.3% of all operations. Deaths occur during three periods--anesthetic induction (10%), intraoperatively (35%), and in the first 48 hours postoperatively (55%). The American Society of Anesthesiologists (ASA) has published a classification scheme to aid clinicians (Table 15-4). This classification is subjective, and many physicians favor a systematic assessment as opposed to a global impression. However, ASA class IV and V patients have roughly 100 times the mortality of class I patients for a surgical procedure. Also, an emergency procedure roughly doubles the risk in any ASA classification of patients.

- Risk of dying in perioperative period is 0.3% of all operations.

- Three periods in which deaths (%) occur: anesthetic induction (10%), intraoperatively (35%), and within 48 hours postoperatively (55%).

Table 15-4.--American Society of Anesthesiologists Classification of Anesthetic Mortality Within 48 Hours Postoperatively

Class	Physical status	48-Hour mortality
I	Normal healthy person < 80 years old	0.07%
II	Mild systemic disease	0.24%
III	Severe but not incapacitating systemic disease	1.4%
IV	Incapacitating systemic disease that is a constant threat to life	7.5%
V	Moribund patient not expected to survive 24 hours, regardless of surgery	8.1%
E	Suffix added to any class indicating emergency procedure, e.g., IE, IIE, IIIE	Doubles risk

From MKSAP IX: Part C, Book 4, 1991. American College of Physicians. By permission.

Many physicians have mistakenly thought that spinal anesthesia is safer than general anesthesia in high-risk patients. From a cardiopulmonary standpoint, this is not true. Spinal anesthesia may be associated with wide fluctuations in blood pressure, anxiety, and less control of the airway and ventilation. Thus, it is inappropriate for the internist to write, "patient too ill for general anesthesia; okay if done under spinal." The final decision about the type of anesthesia is the responsibility of the anesthesiologist.

- From cardiopulmonary point of view, spinal anesthesia is not safer than general anesthesia.
- Spinal anesthesia may be associated with wide fluctuations in blood pressure.
- The final decision about the type of anesthesia is the responsibility of the anesthesiologist.

The type of operation performed is also an important determinant of morbidity and mortality. Procedures associated with low risk include eye surgery, oral surgery, dilatation and curettage, hysterectomy, and herniorrhaphy. Certain other procedures are associated with a higher risk, including craniotomy and cardiovascular operations. Other operations would be considered intermediate risk.

- Low-risk procedures are eye surgery, oral surgery, dilatation and curettage, hysterectomy, and herniorrhaphy.
- Higher risk procedures are craniotomy and cardiovascular operations.

- Other procedures are of intermediate risk.

However, the importance of associated disease in determining surgical risk may outweigh the nature of the procedure or the type of anesthesia used in predicting outcome. The following sections discuss risk assessment and management strategies grouped by organ system.

Pulmonary Risks and Management

Pulmonary complications (hypoventilation, atelectasis, and pneumonia) occur in about one-third of patients postoperatively and account for 50% of overall perioperative mortality. Patients at definite risk for pulmonary complications include smokers, patients with chronic obstructive pulmonary disease, obesity, thoracic surgery, and upper abdominal surgery. Patients with probable increased risk include those >70 years whose duration of anesthesia is >2 hours or who currently have respiratory infection.

- Pulmonary complications account for 50% of overall perioperative mortality.

Preoperative pulmonary function testing should be part of the evaluation of high-risk patients. The interpretation of these tests regarding risk assessment is controversial. However, most authors agree that the simple spirometric measurement of forced expiratory volume in 1 second (FEV_1) is probably as good a predictor as any of surgical risk. If the FEV_1 is >2 L, the patient can safely undergo the surgical procedure. If the FEV_1 is between 1 and 2 L, the risk of postoperative pulmonary complications is increased. A FEV_1 <1 L is indicative of high risk of postoperative pulmonary complication.

- FEV_1 is a good predictor of surgical risk.
- FEV_1 >2 L, patient can safely undergo procedure.
- FEV_1 <1 L, high risk of postoperative pulmonary complication.

Several measures have been advocated to decrease the pulmonary risks. Preoperative measures to decrease pulmonary risk include instruction in respiratory maneuvers, cessation of cigarette smoking, use of bronchodilators, antibiotic treatment of chronic bronchitis, and chest physiotherapy. Postoperative measures include chest physiotherapy and inspiratory maneuvers, minimization of postoperative narcotic analgesia, and early mobilization of elderly patients.

Cardiac Risks and Management

A risk-factor index, the Goldman index, was devised through a prospective analysis of patients >40 years old undergoing noncardiac general surgery in an attempt to allow clinicians to estimate cardiac risk after clinical assessment (N Engl J Med 297:845-850, 1977). This scale has been validated prospectively and has formed the framework of preoperative cardiac evaluation (Tables 15-5 and 15-6).

Myocardial infarction (MI) is the most feared perioperative complication. Of perioperative MIs, 50% are fatal and 60% are silent. The risk of perioperative MI peaks on the third postoperative day. Patients with recent MIs are at the greatest risk for perioperative MIs. The risk of perioperative MI without cardiac disease = 0.2%. The risk of perioperative MI in patients with recent MI (<3 months) = 27%; if the MI occurred 3-6 months ago, 11%; and if the MI was >6 months ago, 5%. With hemodynamic catheters and aggressive intensive care management, the perioperative MI rate of patients with recent MI could be markedly decreased (MI < 3 months = 5.7%; MI 4 to 6 months = 2.3%). However, the standard recommendation is to delay nonemergent surgery for at least 6 months after MI.

- Of perioperative MIs, 50% are fatal and 60% are silent.
- The risk of perioperative MI peaks on 3rd postoperative day.
- Patients with recent MI are at greatest risk for perioperative MI, but this rate can be decreased with hemodynamic catheters and aggressive intensive care management.
- Standard recommendation--delay nonemergent surgery for at least 6 months after MI.

Cardiac Evaluation for Patients Undergoing Vascular Surgery

Vascular operations place the greatest stress on the heart (cross-clamping abdominal aorta, peripheral arterial bypass grafts, etc.). The prevalence of coronary artery disease (CAD) is much higher in vascular surgical patients (~60%) than in the general surgical population (10%-15%). Thus, the Goldman criteria (Tables 15-5 and 15-6) fail to predict complications accurately in vascular surgical patients. For this group, new predictive rules are needed because of the difference in the prevalence of disease. Adequate exercise levels indicate a low rate of cardiac complications in patients who can exercise on a treadmill to >5 METs or on a bicycle ergometer to > 400 kg/m per minute. For those unable to exercise, lack of redistribution on dipyridamole or adenosine thallium scans is predictive of a low rate of complications.

- Vascular operations place the greatest stress on the heart.
- Prevalence of CAD is higher in vascular surgical patients (60%) than in general surgical population (10%-15%).
- Goldman criteria do not accurately predict the complications in vascular surgical patients.
- Adequate exercise levels in these patients indicate a low rate of complication.
- Inability to exercise but lack of redistribution on dipyridamole or adenosine thallium scans indicates a low rate of complications.

To help select patients in need of further study before vascular surgery, five clinical factors have been described: 1) age >70 years, 2) Q-wave on EKG, 3) history of angina pectoris, 4) history of ventricular ectopy requiring treatment, and 5) diabetes mellitus. When these clinical variables were applied to a group of patients, the following complications were noted:

1. No clinical variables--only 3.1% had postoperative ischemic events.
2. Three or more clinical variables--50% had postoperative ischemic events.
3. One or two clinical variables--a further risk subdivision could be made on basis of result of dipyridamole thallium scan.

Table 15-5.--The Goldman Cardiac Risk-Index for Noncardiac Surgery

Clinical variable	Point assessment
History	
Age >70 years	5
Recent myocardial infarction (≤6 mo)	10
Physical examination	
Ventricular gallop or jugular venous pressure ≥12 cm H_2O	11
Significant valvular aortic stenosis	3
Electrocardiogram	
Rhythm other than sinus or atrial ectopy on preoperative tracing	7
More than 5/min ectopic ventricular beats on any tracing preoperatively	7
Poor general medical condition (any of the following)	
PO_2 <60 mm Hg or PCO_2 >50 mm Hg	
Serum potassium <3.0 meq/L or bicarbonate <20 meq/L	
Blood urea nitrogen >50 mg/dL or creatinine >3.0 mg/dL	3
Chronic liver disease	
Noncardiac debilitation	
Surgical procedure	
Intraperitoneal, intrathoracic, aortic	3
Emergency	4
Maximum score	53

From MKSAP IX: Part C, Book 4, 1991. American College of Physicians. By permission.

Table 15-6.--Cardiac Complications Stratified by the Goldman Risk Index

Risk-index class	Point score	No or minimal complication, %	Severe complications, %	Cardiac death, %
I	0-5	99	0.6	0.2
II	6-12	96	3	1
III	13-25	86	11	3
IV	≥26	49	12	39

From MKSAP IX: Part C, Book 4, 1991. American College of Physicians. By permission.

a. If scan showed no redistribution--only 3.2% had perioperative ischemic events.

b. If scan showed redistribution--30% had perioperative ischemic events.

On the basis of these factors and the extensive literature on the topic, the following are concluded:

- Vascular disease is a marker for CAD.
- CAD is a major cause of perioperative and long-term mortality in vascular surgical patients.
- Perioperative cardiac complication rates are low if:
  There are no clinical indicators of CAD.
  The patient can achieve an adequate exercise capacity.
  No redistribution is present on dipyridamole thallium scan.

  Absence of ischemia on preoperative ambulatory ECG monitoring.
- In selected patients, perioperative and long-term mortality is decreased by treatment intervention directed at CAD.

Monitoring for Perioperative Myocardial Ischemia

In high-risk patients undergoing noncardiac surgery, early postoperative myocardial ischemia is an important correlate of adverse cardiac outcomes. Patient subgroups who are at high risk for postoperative ischemia and who might benefit most from intensive Holter monitoring in the postoperative period can be identified preoperatively: left ventricular hypertrophy, CAD, diabetes, hypertension, and digoxin use. By identifying high-risk patients and monitoring them postoperatively with real-time monitors with alarms triggered by ST-segment depression, ischemia could be identified instantaneously so rapid intervention could potentially prevent clinical ischemia events. However, this hypothesis is as yet unstudied and unproven, and these interventions, if performed in all at-risk patients, would drive up costs tremendously!

- Early postoperative myocardial ischemia is an important correlate of adverse cardiac outcome in high-risk noncardiac surgical patients.

Valvular Heart Disease

Patients with valvular heart disease present specific risks in noncardiac surgery. Significant aortic stenosis is associated with a "fixed" cardiac output that cannot increase in response to surgical stress. Though such patients have a minimal risk with local anesthesia, spinal anesthesia is at increased risk because of the frequent induction of vasodilatation that can cause cardiovascular collapse. Although general anesthesia can be performed with acceptable risks in selected patients with severe aortic stenosis, conventional wisdom is to repair the valve preoperatively (when possible) in patients with critical aortic stenosis.

- Significant aortic stenosis is associated with a "fixed" cardiac output that cannot increase with surgical stress.
- Although selected patients with severe aortic stenosis can undergo general anesthesia, the valve should be repaired preoperatively when possible in those with critical aortic stenosis.

When mitral regurgitation is present, the status of left ventricular function is of primary importance. Patients with mitral regurgitation tolerate vasodilatation well.

- Patients with mitral regurgitation tolerate vasodilatation.
- Patients with valvular heart disease should receive endocarditis prophylaxis in accordance with the standard recommendations of the American Heart Association.

Anticoagulation Issues in Patients With Mechanical Prosthetic Heart Valves Undergoing Noncardiac Surgery

Check with the surgeon first to see whether the intensity of anticoagulation needs to be altered. Procedures such as teeth extractions, cataract surgery, and other minor operations can be performed safely with therapeutic levels of anticoagulation. Often, other factors must be considered

when determining a risk/benefit assessment regarding continuous anticoagulation in patients with mechanical prosthetic heart valves. It is well-known that prosthetic valves in the mitral position are more thrombogenic than aortic prostheses, regardless of the type of valve. Generally, older ball-cage valves (Starr-Edwards) are more thrombogenic than standard disk valves (St. Jude); the least thrombogenic are the bioprosthetic valves. After a risk/benefit assessment is made, one can elect to do the following:

1. Discontinue warfarin therapy for several days before the procedure to allow the prothrombin time (PT) to normalize (outpatient setting) and reinstitute therapy shortly postoperatively.
2. Reduce the warfarin dose (outpatient setting) to maintain the patient in a lower or subtherapeutic range during the procedure.
3. Discontinue warfarin therapy and institute heparin therapy (inpatient setting). Heparin use can be discontinued 4 hours preoperatively and reinstituted, along with oral anticoagulation therapy, when considered safe after the procedure.

For most situations, option #1 or #2 can be safely undertaken at great cost savings because of fewer hospitalization days and not significantly increasing patient risk. Preoperative heparin therapy is recommended only for those cases in which the risk of surgical bleeding with anticoagulation therapy and the risk of thromboembolism without anticoagulation therapy is high (i.e., major surgery in the setting of a thrombogenic mitral valve prosthesis).

- Teeth extractions, cataract surgery, and other minor operations can be performed safely with therapeutic levels of anticoagulation.
- Prosthetic valves in mitral position are more thrombogenic than aortic prostheses.
- Older ball-cage valves are more thrombogenic than standard disk valves.
- Bioprosthetic valves are least thrombogenic.
- Anticoagulation in the setting of mechanical prosthetic heart valves significantly lowers the incidence of thromboemboli but never lowers this incidence to zero.

Congestive Heart Failure

Patients with congestive heart failure (CHF) have an incidence of perioperative pulmonary edema ranging from 3% (New York Heart Association class I) to 25% (class IV). Patients with a prior history of CHF but no preoperative evidence of this disorder have a 6% incidence of perioperative pulmonary edema. Although preoperative CHF is the greatest risk factor for development of pulmonary edema, 50% of those who develop this complication have no history of CHF. Most patients who develop CHF perioperatively do so in the first hour after termination of anesthesia. CHF should be aggressively treated preoperatively, and the therapy for chronic compensated CHF should be maintained in the perioperative period.

- Incidence of perioperative pulmonary edema is from 3% to 25% in patients with CHF.
- Greatest preoperative risk for developing pulmonary edema is CHF.
- If CHF develops perioperatively, it usually does so in 1st hour after anesthesia is terminated.
- Treat CHF aggressively preoperatively, and in perioperative period, maintain therapy for chronic compensated CHF.

Hypertension

When hypertension is stable and diastolic blood pressure is ≤110 mm Hg, no benefit is derived from postponing elective surgery to achieve better control. If diastolic blood pressure is >110 mm Hg, it should be stabilized for several days preoperatively to diminish risk.

- If diastolic blood pressure is >110 mm Hg, it should be stabilized for several days preoperatively.

Hematologic Risk and Management

Patients with poorly controlled polycythemia vera have a high surgical morbidity and mortality secondary to an excess of thromboembolic events and decrease in oxygen transport secondary to high blood viscosity. In polycythemia vera, phlebotomy should be performed to decrease the hematocrit to <45% before elective surgery. Platelet counts <50,000/mm^3 or >1,000,000/mm^3 should be evaluated with bleeding times and corrected preoperatively. A platelet count of 50,000/mm^3 usually provides adequate hemostasis for most surgical procedures. If the count is <20,000/mm^3, spontaneous bleeding is common. A bleeding time, activated partial thromboplastin time (APTT), and PT should be determined preoperatively only if the medical history and physical examination results indicate increased bleeding risk, such as previous bleeding with major or minor surgery, easy bruising, or a family history of bleeding disorder.

- Patients with poorly controlled polycythemia vera have high surgical morbidity and mortality because of throm-

boembolic events and high blood viscosity.
- In polycythemia vera, perform phlebotomy to decrease hematocrit to <45% before elective surgery.
- Platelet count of 50,000/mm^3 usually provides adequate hemostasis for most operations.
- Preoperatively determine bleeding time, activated partial thromboplastin time, and prothrombin time only if medical history and physical examination indicate increased bleeding risk.

Liver Risks and Management

Patients with chronic liver disease, particularly those with progressive hepatic failure, possess a high operative risk. Preoperatively, the internist should concentrate on correcting electrolyte abnormalities and abnormal clotting variables, reducing ascites, treating encephalopathy, and improving the patient's nutritional status.

Endocrinologic Risks and Management

Thyrotoxic patients are at high risk for surgical complications, such as arrhythmias, high output CHF, and death. Thyroid storm occurs in 20%-30% of patients. Thus, elective surgery should be postponed and treatment (antithyroid drugs or radioiodine) should be given for at least 3 months until the patient is euthyroid. If surgery is emergent, a thyrotoxic patient should be pretreated with propranolol, propylthiouracil, potassium iodide, and hydrocortisone. The hypothyroid patient can undergo surgical procedures at very low risk. Severely myxedematous patients should receive thyroxine replacement therapy, careful monitoring, and supportive therapy, including free water restriction and diuretics.

- Thyrotoxic patients are at high risk for surgical complications.
- This condition should be treated for 3 months or until patient is euthyroid before any elective operation is performed.
- In case of emergency operation, pretreat with propranolol, propylthiouracil, potassium iodide, and hydrocortisone.

Patients with diabetes mellitus have a greater risk of surgical complications due to underlying cardiovascular and cerebrovascular disease. It is preferable to have the patient in moderate diabetic control preoperatively to diminish the risk of infection. Remember that the patient may not be able to recognize signs and symptoms of hypoglycemia in the perioperative period. Thus, oral hypoglycemic agents are withheld, the insulin dose is cut in half on the operative day, and the serum glucose level should be maintained in the 150-250 mg/dL range in the perioperative period.

- In cases of diabetes mellitus, there is greater risk of surgical complications because of underlying cardiovascular and cerebrovascular disease.
- Withhold oral hypoglycemic agents, cut insulin dose in half on day of operation, and maintain serum glucose level at 150-200 mg/dL in perioperative period.

To be on the safe side, a steroid prep should be given to any patient who has received suppressive doses of corticosteroids for 2 weeks or more during the past year.

Nutrition

Perioperatively, malnourished patients have increased complications related to wound infection, pneumonia, respiratory insufficiency, and adversely affected cellular and humoral immune function. In nutritional assessment, clinical judgment of malnutrition is as accurate as objective measurements. Thus, detailed laboratory measurements of albumin and other substances are usually not necessary. There is some rationale in giving preoperative nutritional supplementation to malnourished patients.

Thromboembolism Prophylaxis

Although all surgical patients are at some risk for venous thromboembolic disease, certain patients form a high-risk subset, including elderly patients, patients undergoing prolonged anesthesia or surgery, patients with previous venous thromboembolic disease, prolonged immobilization or paralysis, malignancy, obesity, varicosities, or estrogen use. Very reasonable guidelines for thromboembolism prophylaxis in surgical patients to decrease the overall risk of deep venous thrombosis or pulmonary embolism are given in Table 15-7.

Table 15-7.--Perioperative Prophylaxis for Thromboembolism

Surgery	Risk, %	Therapy
General	15-35	Heparin[*] Pneumatic compression
Orthopedic Hip fracture or arthroplasty	40-55	Warfarin[†] or ALD-heparin[‡] Dextran 70 Pneumatic compression
Gynecologic Benign Malignant	5-15 15-35	Heparin Pneumatic compression Dextran 70 Same
Urologic Open prostatectomy	20-50	Heparin Pneumatic compression

[*]Heparin--5,000 units given subcutaneously 2 hours preoperatively and every 8-12 hours thereafter until patient is ambulatory.
[†]Warfarin--10 mg the night before surgery, 5 mg the night of surgery, and subsequent daily dosing to achieve a prothrombin ratio of 1.2-1.3 until the patient is ambulatory, or similar therapy beginning 10-14 days preoperatively and continued until full ambulation.
[‡]ALD-heparin (adjusted low-dose heparin)--escalation from 3,500-5,000 units, given every 8 hours beginning 2 days before surgery, to achieve an activated partial thromboplastin time ratio of 1.2-1.3 until full ambulation.
From MKSAP IX: Part C, Book 4, 1991. American College of Physicians. By permission.

Antimicrobial Therapy

Antibiotics are given perioperatively to prevent infection of normally sterile tissues by direct contamination during the surgical procedure. The risk of wound infection depends largely on type of operation. "Clean" operations are ones in which the gastrointestinal, genitourinary, and respiratory tracts are not entered and there is no surrounding inflammation. Previously, this type of procedure did not require prophylactic antibiotics because the risk of infection was only about 5%, as opposed to a much higher risk in other procedures requiring prophylactic antibiotics to prevent wound infection (clean-contaminated, contaminated, and dirty operations). However, antibiotic prophylaxis may be indicated for some commonly performed, simple, clean procedures such as inguinal hernia repair and breast surgery. Also, a short course of prophylactic therapy (one dose of antibiotic preoperatively and no more than one dose postoperatively) is as effective as longer regimens and less likely to be associated with toxicity or development of resistant organisms.

Preoperative Laboratory Tests

Few laboratory tests should be ordered solely because an operation is planned. In the absence of symptoms, signs, or risk factors for a disease, results of routinely ordered tests are usually normal, and when abnormal, they are usually ignored. Authors looking at specific preoperative tests have suggested that chest radiography, ECG, PT, APTT, and bleeding time are not justified as "routine" preoperative tests. In the cost-effective climate of modern medical practice, tests should be performed for specific clinical indications and not because a patient is being seen in the outpatient clinic, hospital, or operating room.

- Chest radiography, ECG, PT, APTT, and bleeding time are not "routine" preoperative tests.
- Tests should be performed for specific clinical indications.

Geriatric Surgical Patients

The number of surgical procedures performed on elderly patients has steadily increased. Elderly patients comprise 15% of the population but account for one-third of all surgical procedures, half of all emergency surgical procedures, and three-quarters of overall surgical mortality. Age is an independent risk factor for perioperative cardiovascular morbidity. The Goldman index scale (Tables 15-5 and 15-6) also underestimates the cardiac risk in geriatric patients, who, like vascular surgical patients, have a much higher prevalence of CAD. Also, as with patients undergoing vascular surgery, geriatric patients scheduled for a high-risk procedure should have a thoughtful cardiac evaluation. In certain instances, this might include exercise assessment to provide guidance. Most elderly patients have at least one associated chronic medical illness. This fact and the pathophysiologic effects of aging on the cardiovascular and pulmonary systems probably explain why geriatric patients have a higher perioperative mortality rate than younger patients. Intervention aimed at meticulously looking for and treating postoperative complications (anemia, infection, pneumonia) leads to improved outcomes (less postoperative delirium, fewer hospital days, etc.) in geriatric patients.

- Elderly patients account for one-third of all surgical procedures.
- Age is independent risk factor for perioperative cardiovascular morbidity.
- Geriatric patients have much higher prevalence of CAD.
- Geriatric patients have a higher perioperative mortality rate.

Perioperative Medication Management

The internist tailors perioperative drug therapy to individual circumstances with particular attention to three factors:

1. Have the indications and doses for the specific drug been clearly defined?
2. What are the likely anesthetic and surgical interactions and complications?
3. Is a clinically important withdrawal syndrome likely, and how can it be managed safely?

Most drugs used in managing chronic medical conditions can and should be continued through the perioperative period. Often, patients can receive medications with sips of water on the morning of surgery and resume oral medications or parenteral substitution later in the day. Should particular questions occur about the continuation of a specific drug, communicate with the anesthesiologist.

- Most drugs for chronic medical conditions should continue to be used through the perioperative period.

CURRENT CONCEPTS IN ANTICOAGULATION THERAPY

International Normalized Ratio

What Is Its Significance?

The international normalized ratio (INR) was developed to standardize reporting of the PT assay test results. This was necessary because of the variability in the responsiveness of the different thromboplastins used as reagents throughout the world. The international sensitivity index (ISI) is the value representative of the responsiveness of a given thromboplastin to the reduction of vitamin K-dependent coagulation factors. The variations in ISI between different thromboplastins are due to differences in their manufacture and source and in method of preparation. A more responsive thromboplastin produces less rapid stimulation of coagulation factors, producing a greater prolongation of the PT for a given reduction in clotting factors. A less responsive thromboplastin activates residual clotting factors more rapidly and results in a less prolonged PT, despite a comparable decrease in clotting factors. Therefore, with use of a more responsive thromboplastin, a lower dose of warfarin is required to maintain the PT at a desired ratio than the dose required with a less responsive thromboplastin--i.e., an acceptable PT ratio using a very responsive thromboplastin might give a false sense of security in a patient who is actually at risk for clotting. If a less responsive thromboplastin were used, that same ratio might give a false sense of security in a patient who is actually at risk for major bleeding. The INR is simply an exponential mathematical transformation of PT (usually reported in seconds) into a ratio value.

- INR standardizes reporting of PT assay test results.

How Can the INR be Calculated?

The INR is calculated from the patient's PT ratio, which is a simple calculation, and the ISI, which is more complicated. The ISI is calculated by the manufacturer of the thromboplastin or by the laboratory performing the test. The formula is

$$INR = \left(\frac{Patient\ PT}{Control\ PT}\right)^{ISI}$$

How Does the INR Help in Clinical Practice?

The ISI of most thromboplastins used in the U.S. varies from 1.8 to 2.8. Because there is no "typical" North American thromboplastin, the earlier habit of using PT ratios has inadvertently left many patients at risk due to over or under anticoagulation. The use of the INR offers several advantages listed below:

- Smooth regulation of anticoagulant therapy.
- Benefit to patients who travel, because there is consistency among laboratories using different types of thromboplastin.
- Standardization of anticoagulant therapy in clinical trials and scientific publications.

What Are Recommended INR Therapeutic Ranges for Oral Anticoagulant Therapy?

These ranges are summarized in Table 15-8. In short, an INR of 2.0-3.0 is used for all indications except for mechanical prosthetic heart valves, which require a slightly higher INR of 2.5-3.5.

Table 15-8.--Recommended INR Therapeutic Ranges for Oral Anticoagulant Therapy

Indication	INR
Prophylaxis of venous thrombosis (high-risk surgical procedure)	2.0-3.0
Treatment of venous thrombosis	2.0-3.0
Treatment of pulmonary embolism	2.0-3.0
Prevention of systemic embolism	2.0-3.0
Tissue heart valves	2.0-3.0
Acute myocardial infarction (to prevent systemic embolism)	2.0-3.0
Valvular heart disease	2.0-3.0
Atrial fibrillation	2.0-3.0
Recurrent systemic embolism	2.0-3.0
Mechanical prosthetic heart valves (high risk)	2.5-3.5

Antithrombotic Therapy for Venous Thromboembolic Disease

Guidelines for anticoagulation in patients with venous thromboembolic disease are summarized in Table 15-9.

Anticoagulation in Prosthetic Heart Valves

What Are the Recommendations for Anticoagulation in Patients With Mechanical Prosthetic Heart Valves?

It is strongly recommended that all patients with mechanical prosthetic heart valves receive warfarin. Levels of warfarin that prolong INR to 2.5-3.5 are recommended. Levels of warfarin producing an INR <1.8 have a high risk of thromboembolic events, and levels that increase INR to >4.5 have a high risk of excessive bleeding. Dipyridamole (375-400 mg/day) in addition to warfarin may have an additive effect without any increase in bleeding. Aspirin (100 mg/day) in addition to warfarin may have additive effect without increasing the risk of major bleeding, although minor bleeding may be increased.

- All patients with mechanical prosthetic heart valves should receive warfarin.
- Use warfarin levels that prolong INR to 2.5-3.5.
- Warfarin levels that 1) produce INR <1.8 have high risk of thromboembolic events or 2) increase INR >4.5 have high risk of excessive bleeding.
- Dipyridamole plus warfarin may have additive bene-

fit without increased bleeding.
- A low dose of aspirin plus warfarin may have addi-

tive benefit without causing major bleeding (may increase minor bleeding).

Table 15-9.--Guidelines for Anticoagulation in Patients With Venous Thromboembolic Disease

Deep venous thrombosis or pulmonary embolus	Guidelines for anticoagulation
Suspected	Give heparin 5,000 U i.v. and perform imaging study
Confirmed	Rebolus with heparin 5,000-10,000 U i.v. and start maintenance infusion at 1,300 U/hour (heparin 20,000 U in 500 mL 5% dextrose in H_2O, infused at 33 mL/hour)
	Check activated partial thromboplastin time at 6 hours to keep its value between 1.5 and 2.5 times control
	Check platelet count daily
	Start warfarin therapy on day 1 at 10 mg daily for first 2 days, then administer warfarin daily at estimated daily maintenance dose
	Stop heparin therapy after 5 to 7 days of joint therapy when INR is 2.0-3.0 off heparin
	Anticoagulate with warfarin for 3 months at an INR of 2.0-3.0

What Is Recommended if a Patient With a Prosthetic Heart Valve Has a Systemic Embolism Despite Adequate Therapy With Warfarin (INR 2.5-3.5)?

Such patients might benefit from the addition of aspirin (100-160 mg/day) to the warfarin. Dipyridamole (400 mg/day) in addition to warfarin is an alternative option. Finally, some patients may respond to slight increase in warfarin dose, thus increasing INR to 3.0-4.5.

- No regimen ever lowers the risk of systemic embolization to zero!

What Are the Recommendations for Anticoagulation in Patients With Bioprosthetic Heart Valves?

It is recommended that all patients with bioprosthetic valves in the mitral position receive warfarin therapy (INR, 2.0-3.0) for the first 3 months. Anticoagulant therapy of patients with bioprosthetic valves in the aortic position who are in sinus rhythm is optional during the first 3 months. Certain patients with bioprosthetic valves have underlying conditions (i.e., atrial fibrillation, left atrial thrombus) that require long-term warfarin therapy to prevent systemic emboli. Among patients with bioprosthetic heart valves who are in sinus rhythm, long-term therapy with aspirin (325 mg daily) may offer protection against thromboembolism and appears reasonable for patients without contraindication.

- Patients with bioprosthetic valves in mitral position

receive warfarin therapy (INR, 2.0-3.0) for 1st 3 months.
- Patients with bioprosthetic valves who have atrial fibrillation or left atrial thrombus require long-term warfarin therapy to prevent systemic emboli.
- Long-term therapy with aspirin may protect patients with bioprosthetic heart valves who are in sinus rhythm against thromboembolism.

Hemorrhagic Complications of Anticoagulation

When the Anticoagulant Effect of Warfarin Needs to Be Reversed, What Is the Best Way to Do This?

The anticoagulant effect of warfarin can be reversed by stopping treatment, administering vitamin K, or replacing vitamin K-dependent coagulation factors with fresh frozen plasma. When warfarin therapy is discontinued, no significant effect is seen on INR for 2 or more days, because of the half-life of warfarin (36 to 42 hours) and the delay before newly synthesized functional coagulation factors replace dysfunctional coagulation factors.

Administering vitamin K lowers the INR more rapidly, depending on the dosage of vitamin K and severity of the anticoagulant effect. When high doses of vitamin K (10-15 mg i.v.) are used, reversal is rapid and seen by about 6 hours. The downside is that patients often remain resistant to warfarin for up to a week, making continued warfarin treatment difficult. This problem can be overcome by using much lower dosages of vitamin K given intravenously (0.5-1.0 mg).

- Anticoagulant effect of warfarin can be reversed by stopping treatment, giving vitamin K, or replacing vitamin K-dependent coagulation factors with fresh frozen plasma.
- Replacement of vitamin K-dependent coagulation factors with fresh frozen plasma produces an immediate effect and is the treatment of choice in cases of life-threatening bleeding or serious warfarin overdosages.

Are There Certain Patient Characteristics That Increase the Risk of Hemorrhagic Complications of Anticoagulant Treatment?

A strong relationship between intensity of anticoagulant therapy and risk of bleeding has been reported in patients receiving treatment for deep venous thrombosis and prosthetic heart valves. The concurrent use of drugs that interfere with hemostasis and produce gastric erosions (aspirin, NSAID) increases risk of serious upper gastrointestinal tract bleeding. However, low doses of aspirin (100 mg/day) may have only minimal gastric side effects and can increase the efficacy of warfarin without significantly increasing risk of major bleeding. Other drugs such as trimethoprim-sulfamethoxazole and disulfiram inhibit the clearance of warfarin, thus potentiating its effect. Still other agents such as broad-spectrum antibiotics have the potential of augmenting anticoagulant effect of warfarin by eliminating bacterial flora, thereby producing vitamin K deficiency. Several comorbid disease states associated with increased bleeding during warfarin therapy are treated hypertension, renal insufficiency, and cerebrovascular disease.

- Relationship between intensity of anticoagulant therapy and risk of bleeding is strong.
- Concurrent use of drugs that interfere with hemostasis and produce gastric erosions increases risk of serious upper gastrointestinal tract bleeding.
- Trimethoprim-sulfamethoxazole and disulfiram inhibit clearance of warfarin, potentiating its effect.
- Broad-spectrum antibiotics eliminate bacterial flora, thus augmenting warfarin's anticoagulant effect.

Cerebrovascular Disorders

What Are the Recommendations for Patients With Symptomatic Carotid Stenosis?

Carotid endarterectomy performed by experienced surgeons is superior to medical therapy for preventing stroke after an anterior circulation transient ischemic attack (TIA) or minor stroke in appropriately selected patients. In several trials, patients with >70% carotid stenosis without major operative risk factors had a significant reduction in their risk of stroke over the subsequent 2 years compared with that of medical controls.

What Is the Recommended Mode of Therapy for TIAs and Minor Strokes?

Aspirin is effective in doses from 75 mg to 1,300 mg/day in preventing recurrent symptoms or stroke. For patients who are not candidates for carotid endarterectomy (posterior circulation symptoms, major medical problems, unfavorable anatomy), aspirin treatment is strongly recommended. Ticlopidine is slightly more effective than aspirin but is significantly more expensive and more toxic. At this time, ticlopidine is recommended only for patients who are aspirin-sensitive or for those having recurrent ischemic events during aspirin therapy.

What Is Appropriate Therapy During a Progressing Ischemic Stroke?

No therapy is known to have a positive effect during these situations. Many physicians believe it might be reasonable to anticoagulate with heparin for 3-5 days in this setting, especially if the ischemic stroke involves the vertebrobasilar circulation. Others simply recommend aspirin.

What Therapy Is Suggested After a Completed Thrombotic Stroke?

Use of anticoagulants in patients with completed thrombotic strokes is either of no value or actually harmful. Some studies support aspirin therapy after minor thrombotic stroke. One study reported ticlopidine, 500 mg/day, was superior to placebo in patients with moderate to severe strokes. However, because of cost and toxicity of ticlopidine, aspirin is recommended initially. Ticlopidine should be considered only for aspirin-intolerant patients or patients with ischemic symptoms during aspirin therapy.

What Is Recommended Therapy After Acute Cardioembolic Stroke?

In nonhypertensive patients with small to moderate-sized embolic strokes, a computed tomographic scan should be done 48 hours or more after the onset of stroke to document the absence of spontaneous hemorrhagic transformation. If no hemorrhage is seen, institute heparin therapy followed by warfarin, at a dose that prolongs the

PT to an INR of 2.0-3.0. If the patient had a large embolic stroke but is deemed a potential anticoagulation candidate, anticoagulant therapy should be postponed 7-14 days because of the predisposition in these patients to hemorrhagic transformation.

TREATMENT OF HYPERLIPIDEMIA

Case

A 55-year-old man with stable class II angina is referred for consideration of drug treatment for hyperlipidemia. He is otherwise healthy. He quit smoking cigarettes 2 years previously and has no other known risk factors for CAD. He has closely followed the advice of a dietician for the past 3 months, but his cholesterol levels have shown no significant decrease. His most recent values are: total cholesterol, 240 mg/dL; HDL-C, 35 mg/dL; and triglycerides, 75 mg/dL.

Discussion

The evidence is that lowering cholesterol also lowers risk of CAD. Recent evidence shows that lowering cholesterol level lowers the risk of CAD and is associated with decreased progression of coronary artery lesions as well as increased regression of these lesions.

The National Cholesterol Education Program Report defined high-risk status as definite CAD or two of the following risk factors:

- Male sex.
- Positive family history of CAD at age <55 years.
- Smoker.
- Hypertension.
- HDL <35 mg/dL.
- Diabetes mellitus.
- Severe obesity, >30% overweight.
- History of definite occlusive cerebrovascular or peripheral vascular disease.

LDL-cholesterol is used to monitor patients with hypercholesterolemia and is calculated from the following formula:

$$LDL\text{-}C = (total\ cholesterol) - (HDL\ cholesterol) - (triglycerides/5).$$

In this case, LDL-C = (240) - (35) - (75/5). Therefore, this patient's LDL-C = 190 mg/dL.

Secondary causes of hyperlipidemia should be ruled out in all patients. Secondary causes of hyperlipidemia may be caused by diseases (hypothyroidism, diabetes, uremia, obstructive liver disease), drugs (corticosteroids, progestins, thiazides, beta-blockers), or diet (alcohol abuse, increased saturated fats).

- Rule out secondary causes of hyperlipidemia in all patients.

After secondary causes are ruled out, the first line of treatment is intensive diet therapy. This should be intitiated in patients without CAD or risk factors if LDL-C ≥160 mg/dL, and for patients with CAD or at least two risk factors if LDL-C ≥130 mg/dL.

If trial of diet therapy fails to lower serum cholesterol levels adequately, drug therapy should be considered. Based on coronary regression studies, many experts suggest patients with known CAD be treated for LDL-C levels ≥130 mg/dL. Other high-risk patients without CAD are considered if LDL-C is ≥160 mg/dL and low-risk patients are considered if LDL-C is ≥190 mg/dL.

- If diet therapy fails to lower cholesterol to goal level, consider drug therapy.

If hypolipidemic drugs are used, choice of drug depends on mechanism of action, side effect profile, efficacy, and cost. In general, the following drugs alone or sometimes in combination are recommended.

1. For patients with elevated LDL-C--bile acid sequestrants, nicotinic acid, and HMG CoA reductase inhibitors.
2. For patients with elevated LDL-C and elevated triglycerides--nicotinic acid, gemfibrozil, and HMG CoA reductase inhibitors.
3. For patients with isolated hypertriglyceridemia if treatment is indicated--nicotinic acid and gemfibrozil.

Drug therapy for hyperlipidemia must be individualized. In general, positive effect is gained and few side effects experienced by starting therapy with low doses of medication and increasing slowly if necessary. No studies yet support use of drug therapy in the elderly.

QUESTIONS

(See "Answers" section)

Multiple Choice

1. A blood test available to help identify patients with prostate cancer has a sensitivity of 75% and a specificity of 80%. The estimated prevalence of prostate cancer in your referral male population is 10%. If a patient has positive results on the blood test, what is the chance that he has prostate cancer?
   a. 12%
   b. 29%
   c. 75%
   d. 91%
   e. 97%

2. By using the same numbers as in question 1, if a patient has negative results on the blood test, what is the chance that he is free of prostate cancer?
   a. 12%
   b. 29%
   c. 75%
   d. 91%
   e. 97%

3. A 70-year-old man with controlled atrial fibrillation, stable angina, and diabetes is to undergo prostate surgery next week. His medications include digoxin, atenolol, isosorbide, aspirin, and insulin. Which of the following would be appropriate preoperative management:
   a. Continue treatment with atenolol, and avoid withdrawing its use
   b. Discontinue treatment with digoxin preoperatively
   c. Recommend spinal anesthesia to decrease the surgical risk in this patient
   d. Discontinue treatment with aspirin 1 day preoperatively to decrease risk of bleeding
   e. Continue treatment with insulin at usual preoperative dose

4. A 60-year-old man who smoked presents for a health screening evaluation. His total cholesterol is 260 mg/dL; HDL cholesterol, 20 mg/dL, and triglycerides, 300 mg/dL. Which of the following pertaining to his hyperlipidemia is not correct:
   a. His LDL cholesterol is 180 mg/dL
   b. He should be examined for secondary causes of hyperlipidemia
   c. His low HDL cholesterol is a risk factor for coronary artery disease
   d. He should be instructed in an intensive diet program
   e. Should diet fail to change his lipid profile, the most appropriate drug to initiate treatment would be a bile acid sequestrant

5. Which of the following is not associated with increased bleeding risk in patients receiving warfarin:
   a. Concurrent use of trimethoprim-sulfamethoxazole
   b. Concurrent use of acetaminophen
   c. Concurrent use of disulfiram
   d. Renal insufficiency
   e. Concurrent use of nonsteroidal anti-inflammatory drugs

True/False

6. With regard to preoperative medical evaluation, indicate whether the following are true or false:
   a. The risk of dying in the perioperative period is about 0.3% when all operations performed in the U.S. are considered
   b. An emergency operation roughly doubles surgical risk
   c. Upper abdominal surgery does not increase the risk for pulmonary complications
   d. Chest radiography should routinely be performed in all patients receiving general anesthesia
   e. Diastolic blood pressure >95 mm Hg is associated with an increased surgical risk
   f. Mild hypothyroidism is associated with a high risk of surgical complications

7. With regard to the International Normalized Ratio (INR), indicate whether the following are true or false:
   a. The INR was developed to standardize reporting of prothrombin time assay results
   b. The INR allows for consistency between laboratories that use different types of thromboplastin
   c. The INR allows for standardization of anticoagulation therapy in clinical trials and in reporting results
   d. The therapeutic INR for heparin anticoagulation is between 1.5 and 2.5
   e. The therapeutic INR for warfarin anticoagulation in mechanical heart valves is between 2.0 and 3.0
   f. The INR is an exponential mathematical transformation of the prothrombin time (seconds) into a ratio value

NOTES

CHAPTER 16
GENETICS

Virginia V. Michels, M.D.

Genetic factors play a role in the development of many types of human disease. Genetic determinants may be single gene defects, mitochondrial mutations, chromosome abnormalities, or multifactorial.

CHROMOSOME ABNORMALITIES

Approximately a sixth of all birth defects and cases of congenitally determined mental retardation are due to chromosome abnormalities. Chromosome abnormalities occur in about 1 in 180 live births. One-third of these abnormalities involve an abnormal number (aneuploidy) of non-sex chromosomes (autosomes). Factors known to result in a higher-than-average risk for having a child with autosomal aneuploidy are maternal age ≥35 years and having previously had an affected child. Prenatal diagnosis by karyotyping of fetal cells obtained by amniocentesis or chorionic villus sampling can be offered to pregnant women who are at increased risk.

- Chromosome abnormalities occur in 1 in 180 live births.
- Risk factors for autosomal aneuploidy: maternal age ≥35 years, having had an affected child.

Down Syndrome

The most common autosomal aneuploidy syndrome in term infants is Down syndrome (incidence, 1 in 880). The most serious consequence of Down syndrome is mild-to-moderate mental retardation (average IQ, about 50). Forty percent of patients with Down syndrome have a congenital heart defect, most frequently ventricular septal defect or atrioventricular canal defect, although other congenital heart defects may occur. Males with Down syndrome are usually sterile, but affected females are fertile and have a very high risk of having an affected child. Most persons with Down syndrome have trisomy 21 as a result of a new mutation nondisjunctional event; in these cases, the risk to the parents of having another affected child is 1%-2% or higher, depending on maternal age. In 3% of persons with Down syndrome, a translocation chromosome abnormality is present, in which the extra chromosome 21 is attached to another chromosome, most commonly 14 (Fig. 16-1). These translocation chromosomes may be inherited in an *unbalanced* form from a parent carrying a *balanced* form of the translocation; these parents have a 5%-15% risk of having another affected child. For identification of these high-risk families, chromosome analysis should be done on all patients with Down syndrome. Even if the parents have completed their childbearing, the karyotype of the affected individual should be determined so that other relatives (e.g., adult siblings) can be counseled. The same principles are presumed to be true for other autosomal aneuploidy syndromes.

- Most common autosomal aneuploidy syndrome in term infants is Down syndrome.
- Most serious consequence of Down syndrome is mild-to-moderate mental retardation.
- Most frequent heart defect in Down syndrome is ventricular septal defect or atrioventricular canal defect.
- Males with Down syndrome are often sterile, but females are fertile.
- Most persons with Down syndrome have trisomy 21.

Sex Chromosome Aneuploidy Syndromes

Approximately 35% of chromosome abnormalities in

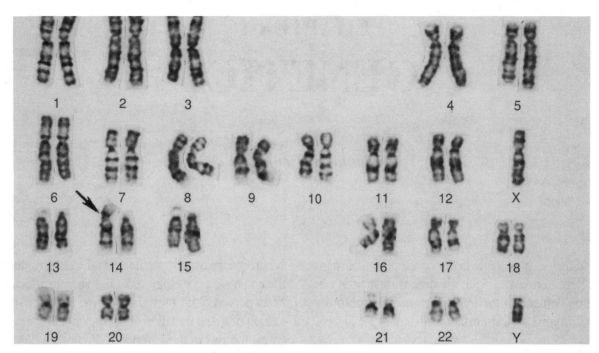

Fig. 16-1. Karyotype 46,XY,-14,+t(14;21)(p11;q11) from patient with Down syndrome. Extra chromosome 21 material is translocated to a chromosome 14. Result is robertsonian translocation. (Karyotype courtesy of G. Dewald, Ph.D.)

live-born infants involve sex chromosome aneuploidy. These infants may have an additional X or Y chromosome or be lacking one. Patients with 47,XXX or 47,XYY karyotypes usually have no major birth defects or mental retardation, although the mean IQ may be 90 rather than 100. These patients usually are detected incidentally. Similarly, patients with a 47,XXY karyotype (Klinefelter syndrome) have a mean IQ of about 90 but also have small testes, infertility, and a tall eunuchoid body habitus. Patients with a 45,X karyotype (Turner syndrome) or its variants--one structurally abnormal X, such as 46,X,r(X) (Fig. 16-2)--or mosaicism for an X or Y chromosome--such as 45,X/46,XX--usually are mentally normal but have a risk of approximately 30% for a congenital heart defect. Bicuspid aortic valve with or without coarctation of the aorta is particularly common. Short stature, webbed neck, increased number of pigmented nevi, failure to develop secondary sexual characteristics, short 4th or 5th metacarpals or metatarsals, renal malformations, and increased risk for thyroid disease are also variably present. Ordinarily, parents of patients with sex chromosome aneuploidy are not at increased risk for having another affected child, and these parents do not routinely need chromosome analyses.

- 46,XXY karyotype (Klinefelter syndrome): small testes, infertility, tall eunuchoid body habitus.
- 45,X karyotype (Turner syndrome): usually mental-

ly normal, 30% risk of congenital heart defect, and commonly bicuspid aortic valve.
- Other possible features of 45,X karyotype: short stature, webbed neck, increased number of pigmented nevi, no secondary sex characteristics, short 4th or 5th metatarsals or metacarpals.

Other Chromosome Abnormalities

Thirty-four percent of chromosome abnormalities involve structural changes such as deletions, duplications, inversions, or translocations. The translocations may be balanced (no net loss or gain of genetic material) or unbalanced. People with balanced translocations are usually phenotypically normal and healthy but may be at increased risk for miscarriages or their children may have birth defects. Patients with net loss or gain of genetic material by any of the mechanisms listed above have phenotypic abnormalities that usually include mental retardation and frequently other major or minor birth defects. Parents of all patients with a structural chromosome abnormality should have chromosome analyses to determine whether they are carriers of a balanced translocation.

- Parents of all patients with a structural chromosome abnormality should have chromosome analyses.

Fragile X-Linked Mental Retardation

The fragile X-linked mental retardation syndrome

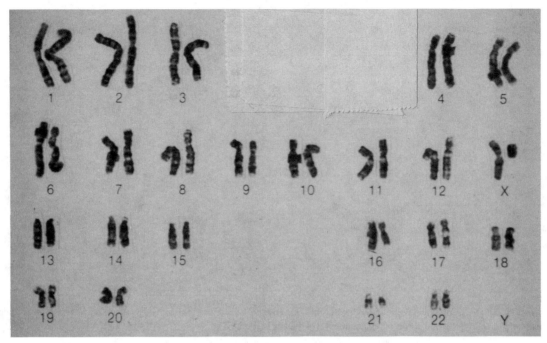

Fig. 16-2. Karyotype 46,X,r(X) from patient with Turner syndrome. (Karyotype courtesy of G. Dewald, Ph.D.)

occurs in about 1 in 1,000 males. This unusual chromosome abnormality is characterized by a visible fragile site on the long arm of an X chromosome at band 27 when the lymphocytes are cultured in media deficient in folic acid (Fig. 16-3). The fragile site is never observed in all cells, and the frequency may be as low as 4%. Affected males may be physically normal or have a long, thin face with prominent jaw, large simplified ears, and enlarged testes. The degree of mental retardation ranges from mild to profound. An occasional male is clinically normal and is referred to as a "transmitting" male. Carrier females may be phenotypically normal or mildly retarded and dysmorphic; occasionally they are moderately or severely retarded. Some carrier females do not express the fragile site cytogenetically. Initially puzzling aspects of this syndrome included the observations that transmitting males had daughters who, although obligate carriers, rarely showed signs of the disease. However, these daughters could have typically affected sons. This now can be explained by the discovery of a DNA trinucleotide repeat (CGG) that is more likely to expand and thereby become more abnormal during transmission through a female. Direct DNA analysis of the size of the trinucleotide repeat is a more accurate method than standard cytogenetic analysis for detection of carrier females.

- Fragile X: fragile site on long arm of X chromosome at band q27.

- Males with fragile X: may be physically normal or have long, thin face, prominent jaw, large ears, enlarged testes, mild to profound mental retardation.
- Carrier females: phenotypically normal or mildly retarded and dysmorphic.
- To detect carrier females: direct DNA analysis of trinucleotide repeat is most accurate.

PATTERNS OF INHERITANCE

Autosomal Dominant

In autosomal dominant inheritance, the responsible gene is located on one of the autosomes and the gene overrides its homologue in terms of clinical effect. Therefore, one copy of the gene is sufficient for the trait to be expressed or for the disease to be present, and heterozygotes have the disease. There is a 50% chance that any child born to an affected person will inherit the abnormal gene.

- Autosomal dominant inheritance: responsible gene is located on autosome and overrides its homologue.
- 50% chance that child of affected person will inherit abnormal gene.

The severity of the disease caused by the abnormal gene may be uniform for some conditions, such as achon-

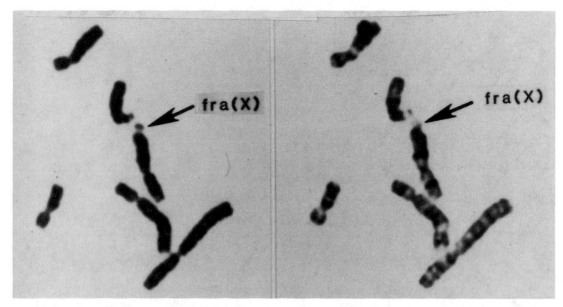

Fig. 16-3. Chromosome analysis from patient with fragile X syndrome. Fragile site is visible on long arm of X chromosome at band q27 when lymphocytes are cultured in media deficient in folic acid. (Photograph courtesy of G. Dewald, Ph.D.)

droplasia, but the severity may be variable for other conditions, such as neurofibromatosis and Marfan syndrome. This difference of severity is referred to as "variable expression." In contrast, the term "incomplete penetrance" means that some persons who have inherited the gene show no signs of it. Obviously, the clinical decision regarding whether a person has signs of the gene defect depends on the thoroughness of the examination and the sensitivity of the investigative techniques. For example, many families with hypertrophic cardiomyopathy were thought to include members with incomplete penetrance until asymptomatic patients were examined with echocardiography. Although transmission of a disease through members of either sex through multiple generations of a family strongly suggests autosomal dominant inheritance, it is important to remember that autosomal dominant diseases can occur without a positive family history. This can occur because of incomplete penetrance, incorrect assignment of paternity, new mutation, or somatic mosaicism. New mutation events represent changes in the genetic material of the individual egg or sperm that gives rise to the fetus. Although the risk for siblings of a person whose disease arose by new mutation is not increased over that of the general population, the risk for the offspring still is 50%. Somatic mosaicism refers to the possibility that one of the parents has the gene defect in only some cells, including the reproductive cells (germinal mosaicism), such that the person has no or few signs of the disease but potentially can transmit the disease to one or more children.

- In autosomal dominant inheritance, disease severity may be uniform or variable.
- Incomplete penetrance: no signs of abnormal gene in a person who has inherited it.
- Somatic mosaicism: person has gene defect in only some cells.

Some of the diseases with autosomal inheritance are listed in Table 16-1 and summarized on the following pages.

Ehlers-Danlos Syndromes

Type I

There may be up to 15 forms of Ehlers-Danlos syndrome. Type I, or gravis type, was the first described and serves as a prototype for discussion of this group of genetically heterogeneous disorders. The syndrome is inherited as an autosomal dominant condition, and the basic defect in type I disease has not been defined. The disorder is characterized by velvety textured, hyperextensible, fragile skin that splits easily and heals poorly, resulting in wide, thin scars. Many tissues are friable, which is an important consideration when surgical procedures are considered. Even fetal membranes are affected and frequently rupture before term, resulting in premature birth. "Molluscoid pseudotumors" are areas of sagging, wrinkled, redundant skin that may develop over the knee and elbow joints. Small fat- or mucin-containing spherules may be present in the subcutaneous tissue and may be calcified. The joints are hyperextensible and prone to

Table 16-1.--Diseases With Autosomal Dominant Inheritance

Achondroplasia

Amyloidosis (many types)

Ehlers-Danlos syndrome, types I, II, III, VI, VIII, some type IV and VII

Huntington chorea

Hypertrophic cardiomyopathy

LEOPARD syndrome

Low-density lipoprotein (LDL) receptor deficiency (hypercholesterolemia)

Marfan syndrome

Multiple endocrine neoplasia, types I, IIa, and IIb

Myotonic dystrophy

Neurofibromatosis, types 1 and 2

Noonan syndrome[*]

Osler-Weber-Rendu disease (hereditary hemorrhagic telangiectasia)

Osteogenesis imperfecta, types I and IV, most type II

Polycystic kidney disease (some forms are autosomal recessive)

Porphyria (several types)

Pseudoxanthoma elasticum (some forms are autosomal recessive)

Spherocytosis

Tuberous sclerosis

Von Hippel-Lindau disease

Von Willebrand disease

[*]Most cases are sporadic, but there is good evidence that they have new-mutation autosomal dominant disease.

dislocations. Pes planus, scoliosis, degenerative arthritis, visceral diverticulosis, and spontaneous pneumothorax may occur.

- Ehlers-Danlos type I is autosomal dominant condition.
- Features: velvety textured, hyperextensible, fragile skin.
- Joints are hyperextensible and prone to dislocation.
- Associated conditions: pes planus, scoliosis, degenerative arthritis, visceral diverticulosis, spontaneous pneumothorax.

Involvement of small blood vessels results in easy bruisability. Mitral valve prolapse may occur in 50% of patients. Dilatation of the aortic root or pulmonary artery and prolapse of the tricuspid valve may occur. Vascular rupture is relatively rare.

- Ehlers-Danlos type I: mitral prolapse occurs in 50%.

- Vascular rupture is uncommon.

Type II

Ehlers-Danlos syndrome type II, or mitis type, is similar to type I but milder; it also is inherited as an autosomal dominant disorder. A significant number of patients have mitral valve prolapse. It is uncertain whether this disorder results from a mutation at the same locus as for type I.

- Ehlers-Danlos type II is milder than type I.

Type III

The joint hypermobility of Ehlers-Danlos syndrome type III, or benign familial hypermobility syndrome, is similar to that in type I and may result in joint dislocations. However, skin hyperextensibility and scarring are minimal or absent. There is a wide range of expression both within and between families. Families with the mildest manifestations merge with the general population in terms of normal variation in joint mobility. It is an autosomal dominant disorder.

- In Ehlers-Danlos type III, joint hypermobility is similar to that in type I.
- Skin hyperextensibility and scarring are minimal or absent.

Type IV

Ehlers-Danlos syndrome type IV, or vascular type, is genetically heterogeneous with both autosomal dominant and autosomal recessive forms. It is usually due to deficiency of type III collagen synthesis or secretion in skin, aorta, uterus, and intestine. This is the most severe form of Ehlers-Danlos syndrome and is characterized by rupture of large arteries, the colon, or the gravid uterus. Angiography and other invasive procedures may precipitate vascular or organ rupture and should be done only after careful consideration of the risk:benefit ratio. Mitral valve prolapse frequently is present. In some patients the skin is extremely thin, allowing visualization of the underlying venous network (Fig. 16-4). Despite this, there is a tendency to form keloid scars and contractures. In contrast to other forms of Ehlers-Danlos syndrome, the skin and connective tissues may not be hyperextensible. Occasional complications include spontaneous pneumothorax and severe periodontal disease. This defect is expressed in cultured skin fibroblasts, so prenatal diagnosis theoretically is possible. Although it has been suggested that type III collagen also is deficient in some patients with congenital cerebral aneurysms or acquired abdominal aortic aneurysms who do not have classic Ehlers-Danlos syndrome, demonstrable defects occur in only a very small proportion of patients.

- Ehlers-Danlos type IV has both autosomal dominant and autosomal recessive forms.
- It is due to deficiency of type III collagen synthesis.
- Angiography and other invasive procedures may precipitate vascular or organ rupture.
- Mitral valve prolapse is frequently present.
- Occasional complications: spontaneous pneumothorax and severe periodontal disease.

Type V

Ehlers-Danlos syndrome type V is an X-linked recessive disease that may be associated with lysyl oxidase deficiency, although this has not been a universal finding. Skin hyperextensibility is severe, but joint hypermobility is mild to moderate. Mitral and tricuspid valve prolapse or insufficiency may be present.

- Ehlers-Danlos type V is X-linked recessive disease.

Type VI

Ehlers-Danlos syndrome type VI is called the ocular type because blindness from retinal detachment or ocular rupture is a serious complication. In some cases the disease is due to an autosomal recessively inherited deficiency of procollagen lysyl hydroxylase. Severe scoliosis, recurrent joint dislocations, aortic rupture, and gastrointestinal hemorrhage also can occur. Prenatal diagnosis is possible only in families with a documented biochemical defect.

- Ehlers-Danlos type VI is called ocular type.
- Blindness from retinal detachment is a complication.
- Some cases are autosomal recessive.
- Scoliosis, joint dislocations, aortic rupture, gastrointestinal hemorrhage can occur.

Type VII

Ehlers-Danlos syndrome type VII, or arthrochalasis multiplex congenita, is characterized by extreme joint laxity and dislocations. Some patients have defective conversion of procollagen to collagen, which is an autosomal recessive defect. However, others have structural abnormalities of half their α-2 chains of type I collagen

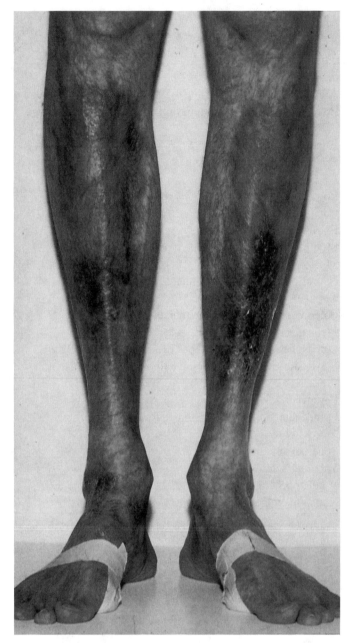

Fig. 16-4. Thin, prematurely aged-appearing skin in young man with Ehlers-Danlos syndrome type IV.

which interfere with the enzymatic conversion of procollagen to collagen; this is an autosomal dominant condition.

- Ehlers-Danlos type VII can be autosomal recessive or autosomal dominant.

Type VIII

Ehlers-Danlos syndrome type VIII is similar to types I and II but includes particularly severe periodontal disease. It is an autosomal dominant disorder, and the basic defect is unknown.

- Ehlers-Danlos type VIII is autosomal dominant.

There is marked genetic heterogeneity in all the Ehlers-Danlos syndromes that have been chemically defined. An equal degree of heterogeneity probably will be found in the more common types I, II, and III.

Hypertrophic Cardiomyopathy

Isolated hypertrophic cardiomyopathy frequently is inherited as an autosomal dominant disorder. In two series of 30 patients and 14 patients, 93% had an affected parent or child or both when studied by echocardiography. A lower proportion of familial cases had been reported previously, but echocardiography had not been used to study relatives. Regardless of the exact proportion of familial cases, it is clear that a significant number are inherited and that investigation of first-degree relatives is necessary. Even if parents are normal by echocardiography, the possibility of new mutation cannot be excluded, and children born to an affected parent must be considered to be at risk and should be evaluated. The possibility of an autosomal dominant disorder can never be excluded on the basis of a negative family history.

- Isolated hypertrophic cardiomyopathy is autosomal dominant.
- Investigation of first-degree relatives is necessary.
- Children of affected parents are at risk.

As with any autosomal dominant disorder, the risk of passing the abnormal gene to each offspring is 50%. Although there is a high degree of penetrance, families with incomplete penetrance have been reported. The course of the disease may be variable, even within a family; therefore, the age at onset cannot be predicted precisely. It is not rare to study a child who presents with symptoms and to discover, after family investigations, that an asymptomatic parent is affected.

- In hypertrophic cardiomyopathy, risk of passing gene to each offspring is 50%.
- Course of disease is variable.
- Age at onset cannot be predicted.

Hypertrophic cardiomyopathy with or without outflow obstruction has been observed within single families. This is compelling evidence that they are different manifestations of the same disease.

Approximately 50% of families with hypertrophic car-diomyopathy have a defect in the β cardiac myosin heavy-chain gene on chromosome 14q. However, other families have not shown linkage to this locus, a finding demonstrating genetic heterogeneity.

- About 50% of families with hypertrophic cardiomyopathy have defect in β cardiac myosin heavy-chain gene.

Marfan Syndrome

The Marfan syndrome is relatively common; its incidence is 1 in 20,000. It is an autosomal dominant disorder with extremely variable expression, and approximately 20% of cases arise by new mutation. There are no well-documented instances of nonpenetrance.

- Marfan syndrome is relatively common--1 per 20,000.
- It is autosomal dominant disorder.
- About 20% of cases arise by new mutation.

The disease involves the musculoskeletal, cardiovascular, and ocular systems. Skeletal abnormalities include tall stature, a low upper:lower segment ratio because limbs are relatively long compared with the trunk, scoliosis or kyphosis, and pectus deformities. These features result from overgrowth of the tubular bones. Increased joint laxity and hyperextensibility are common, but occasionally patients have limited extension of fingers and elbows. The face may be long and the palate highly arched. This "marfanoid habitus" may be present in patients with other disorders such as other connective tissue dysplasias, mucosal neuroma syndrome (multiple endocrine neoplasia type IIb or III), Stickler syndrome, and homocystinuria. The characteristic body habitus is never sufficient evidence for making the diagnosis of Marfan syndrome in the absence of other characteristic features or a well-documented family history of Marfan syndrome.

- Marfan syndrome involves musculoskeletal, cardiovascular, and ocular systems.
- Skeletal abnormalities: tall stature, low upper:lower segment ratio, scoliosis or kyphosis, pectus deformities.
- Increased joint laxity and hyperextensibility are common.

The ocular abnormalities associated with Marfan syndrome include subluxation of the lenses, myopia, and retinal detachment. As the most specific ocular feature, dislocation of the lenses is very helpful in making the diagnosis of Marfan syndrome, although ectopia lentis also can occur in other disorders such as homocystinuria and Weill-Marchesani syndrome. Dislocations occur in 50%-80% of patients; the lens frequently is displaced upward, but this is not always the case. Gross dislocations may be evident without the aid of special equipment, but lesser degrees of dislocation may be evident only by slit-lamp examination. Therefore, all patients suspected of having Marfan syndrome must have a complete ophthalmologic evaluation, including slit-lamp examination. Patients with Marfan syndrome should have frequent ophthalmologic examinations to permit early detection of complications such as retinal detachment or glaucoma.

- Ocular abnormalities of Marfan syndrome: subluxation of lenses, myopia, retinal detachment.
- Dislocation of lenses is helpful for diagnosis; ectopia lentis can occur in homocystinuria and Weill-Marchesani syndrome.
- Dislocations occur in 50% -80% of cases.
- All patients must have ophthalmologic evaluation.

The life expectancy of patients with Marfan syndrome is shortened because of cardiovascular disease. The most common manifestation is mitral valve prolapse with or without mitral regurgitation. Dilatation of the ascending aorta is the next most common cardiovascular disorder; it may lead to aortic regurgitation, aortic rupture, or dissecting aneurysm. Although <70% of patients have evidence of cardiovascular disease on physical examination, >80% have abnormalities detected by echocardiography.

- Life expectancy in Marfan syndrome is shortened by cardiovascular disease.
- Most common cardiovascular manifestations are mitral valve prolapse and dilatation of ascending aorta.
- More than 80% of patients have abnormalities found on echocardiography.

Mitral valve prolapse in patients with Marfan syndrome initially may involve only the posterior leaflet; it may be late systolic or pansystolic and often is progressive. Prophylactic antibiotic therapy for bacterial endocarditis is warranted. The prevalence of mitral valve prolapse is similar in males and females. In one retrospective series of 166 patients who had had echocardiography before age 22 years, 8 patients died as a result of mitral valve regurgitation and the complication developed in an additional 15 patients. Mitral insufficiency may be present in infants with Marfan syndrome. Acute onset of severe mitral regurgitation due to rupture of chordae tendineae may occur even in childhood. Mitral valve prolapse in a patient with a "marfanoid" body habitus is not a sufficient basis for the diagnosis of Marfan syndrome in the absence of a positive family history of Marfan syndrome or other characteristic findings. Patients with some forms of Ehlers-Danlos syndrome and nonspecific connective tissue dysplasias can have a similar body habitus, joint laxity, and mitral valve prolapse.

- Mitral valve prolapse in Marfan syndrome is progressive.
- Prophylactic antibiotic for bacterial endocarditis is warranted.

In two series, aortic abnormalities were found in 60%-90% of patients with Marfan syndrome. In children and adults, the diameter of the aortic root usually is abnormal in proportion to body surface area. Aortic dilatation is progressive, with symmetric involvement in the region of the sinus of Valsalva and sinotubular ridge. The maximal aortic root diameter is several centimeters superior to the level of aortic leaflet insertion. A greater degree of aortic root dilatation is positively correlated with aortic regurgitation and dissection. Progression of aortic root dilatation may be due to the strain of left ventricular ejection, and β-adrenergic blockers may protect against progressive dilatation. In a controlled study, patients with aortic root dilatation who were given propranolol to decrease left ventricular inotropy by 30% had a significantly lesser degree of dilatation and less morbidity. However, in a study of hemodynamic indices measured by cardiac catheterization, acute administration of β-adrenergic blockers did not reduce hemodynamic loading on an already dilated aortic root, and this may even be deleterious.

- Aortic abnormalities occur in 60%-90% of cases of Marfan syndrome.
- Aortic dilatation is progressive.

Although surgical risks are increased in patients with Marfan syndrome because of tissue friability, surgical treatment frequently is successful for mitral and aortic regurgitation and for aortic dissection. In one series of 41 patients who had a total of 79 operations for aneurysms or valvular insufficiencies, the early mortality rate was

3%; 62% survived at least 15 years. This study spanned 16 years, and 7 of the 11 late deaths may have been prevented by surgical techniques that now are available.

- Surgical risks are increased in Marfan syndrome.
- Surgical treatment is often successful for mitral and aortic regurgitation and aortic dissection.

Patients with Marfan syndrome are prone to traumatic aortic rupture, so contact sports and strenuous exercise should be avoided. The risk of cardiovascular complications during pregnancy poses a special problem for women with Marfan syndrome. Acute aortic dissection may occur before, during, or after labor. A retrospective review of one series of patients suggested that the risk of maternal death was "low in patients with minimal preexisting vascular disease" but the risk may be "significant" in those with moderate degrees of aortic root dilatation. Therefore, aortic root diameter must be considered when counseling women who are considering childbearing. Some physicians advise women with aortic root dilatation not to become pregnant. Those who decide to become pregnant should receive care appropriate for high-risk obstetric patients.

- Patients with Marfan syndrome should avoid contact sports and strenuous exercise (risk of aortic rupture).
- In pregnant women with Marfan syndrome, aortic dissection may occur before, during, or after labor.
- Some physicians advise women with aortic root dilatation not to become pregnant.

Additional features sometimes associated with Marfan syndrome include decreased amounts of subcutaneous tissue, skin striae, inguinal hernias, pneumothorax, and degenerative joint disease.

In addition to physical examination, the diagnostic evaluation of patients suspected of having Marfan syndrome should include chest radiography, ophthalmologic examination (including slit-lamp evaluation of the lenses), and echocardiography. A thorough family history should be obtained. For patients with a well-documented family history of Marfan syndrome, characteristic involvement of the skeletal, cardiovascular, or ocular organ systems may be sufficient for the diagnosis to be made. However, in patients without a positive family history, the patient must have the characteristic body habitus and either aortic root dilatation or ectopia lentis. In those with ectopia lentis, homocystinuria must be exclud-

ed. In patients with the characteristic body habitus and mitral valve prolapse but without aortic root dilatation, the diagnosis cannot be made definitely. If skin hyperextensibility, poor skin and wound healing, or atrophic skin scarring is present, the patient probably has a form of Ehlers-Danlos syndrome. If no other abnormality is present, it may be impossible to exclude the diagnosis of Marfan syndrome, and subsequent evaluations are warranted.

- Diagnostic evaluation for Marfan syndrome includes chest radiography, ophthalmologic evaluation, echocardiography.

First-degree relatives should be evaluated even if they have no obvious stigmata of Marfan syndrome. Families have been observed in which a child presented with obvious phenotypic features of Marfan syndrome and a parent was found to be affected only after echocardiography revealed aortic dilatation or slit-lamp examination revealed ectopia lentis.

The basic cause of Marfan syndrome is a defect in fibrillin; the gene encoding fibrillin is on chromosome 15q15-21. This discovery potentially makes presymptomatic and prenatal diagnosis possible in families known to have the disease, and in the near future it also may allow for diagnostic testing in patients with equivocal signs of the disease.

- Cause of Marfan syndrome is defect in fibrillin.

Myotonic Dystrophy

Myotonic dystrophy, the most common form of muscular dystrophy in adults, has an incidence of approximately 1 per 8,000-20,000. The inheritance pattern is autosomal dominant with extremely variable expression. Although average age at onset is in the second to third decade of life, the disease may be evident at birth or first be noticed in the seventh decade. The disease is characterized by myotonia, muscle atrophy and weakness, ptosis of the eyelids, and expressionless facies resulting from particularly severe involvement of facial and temporal muscles. Rate of progression of the disease is variable, but disability is usually severe within 15-20 years after onset. Associated abnormalities may include premature frontal baldness, testicular atrophy or menstrual irregularities, gastrointestinal symptoms related to smooth muscle involvement, and cardiac disease. Distinctive refractile posterior subcapsular cataracts often are evident by slit-lamp examination. Although glucose intolerance is common, overt diabetes mellitus occurs in only about 6% of patients.

- Myotonic dystrophy is most common form of muscular dystrophy in adults.
- Incidence is 1 in 8,000-20,000.
- Autosomal dominant inheritance with extremely variable expression.
- Age at onset is usually second to third decade of life.
- Characteristics: myotonia, muscle atrophy and weakness, ptosis of eyelids, expressionless facies.
- Disability is severe within 15-20 years after onset.
- Associated abnormalities: premature frontal baldness, testicular atrophy or menstrual irregularities, gastrointestinal symptoms, cardiac disease.
- Diabetes mellitus occurs in 6% of patients.

The diagnosis is based on clinical findings and a typical electromyographic pattern characterized by prolonged rhythmic discharges. The gene for myotonic dystrophy is located on chromosome 19 at band q13, and genetic counseling is warranted for the patient and family. First-degree relatives should be investigated. The risk for children born to an affected parent is 50%. The molecular basis of most cases of myotonic dystrophy is expansion of a CTG trinucleotide repeat sequence in a gene encoding a protein kinase. Thus, direct DNA-based diagnosis of the disease is possible in some cases. Affected females also need to be aware of the additional risk of having an affected infant with severe, sometimes fatal, hypotonia and mental deficiency. This infantile form of the disease does not occur when the father is the affected parent.

- Diagnosis of myotonic dystrophy is based on clinical and electromyographic findings or DNA analysis.
- Genetic counseling is warranted for patients and family members with myotonic dystrophy.
- First-degree relatives should be investigated.

Cardiac disease is present in approximately two-thirds of patients with myotonic dystrophy, and sudden death may occur. There is prolongation of the P-R or QRS interval, and there are changes in the T wave and ST segment. Intra-atrial and His-Purkinje conduction may be prolonged, and heart block may require implantation of a pacemaker. There seems to be degeneration of the conducting tissue before other cardiac muscle is involved.

If general anesthesia is required, caution must be taken. Many affected patients have alveolar hypoventilation resulting in a serious risk of postanesthetic respiratory depression, which can occur several hours after the patient seems to be alert and stable.

- Cardiac disease occurs in 2 of 3 patients with myotonic dystrophy, and sudden death may occur.
- Many patients have alveolar hypoventilation.

Neurofibromatosis

Type 1

Neurofibromatosis type 1 is an autosomal dominant disorder with an incidence of approximately 1 in 3,000-4,000. Approximately 50% of patients have the disease because of a new mutation. The disorder has markedly variable expression but very high penetrance. The diagnosis is based on two or more of the following clinical criteria: six or more café-au-lait macules of ≥1.5 cm in diameter (in a child, five or more that are 0.5 cm), axillary or inguinal freckling, two or more Lisch nodules of the iris, two or more neurofibromas or one plexiform neurofibroma, a definitely positive family history, or one of these and one of the uncommon characteristic manifestations such as orbital or sphenoid wing dysplasia, optic or other central nervous system glioma, renal artery dysplasia with or without abdominal aorta coarctation, or tibial pseudofracture. Additional, less specific signs of the disease may include pheochromocytoma and scoliosis. Fewer than 10% of patients develop malignancy, often neurofibrosarcoma. The gene has been identified and seems to be a GTPase-activating protein involved in the *ras* signaling process. The gene is very large, and multiple different mutations have been identified; there is no evidence for non-allelic heterogeneity. Because of the multitude of different mutations, there is no clinically useful DNA-based test for direct diagnosis. However, linkage analysis can be used for presymptomatic or prenatal diagnosis in informative families (see Linkage Analysis, page 411).

- Neurofibromatosis type 1 is autosomal dominant.
- Incidence is 1 in 3,000-4,000.
- Disorder has markedly variable expression but very high penetrance.
- Fewer than 10% of patients develop malignancy (often neurofibrosarcoma).
- Multiple different mutations have been identified.

Type 2

Neurofibromatosis type 2 is an autosomal dominant disorder that is genetically distinct from neurofibromatosis type 1. The gene has been localized to the long arm of chromosome 22 and was recently identified. DNA-based diagnosis is possible on a research basis but not yet widely available. The disorder is characterized by acoustic neuromas, usually bilateral, with or without other central nervous system gliomas, subcapsular posterior cataracts, and café-au-lait macules.

- Neurofibromatosis type 2 is autosomal dominant.
- Characteristics: acoustic neuromas, sometimes nervous system gliomas, subcapsular cataracts, café-au-lait macules.

Osteogenesis Imperfecta

Historically, osteogenesis imperfecta has been divided into four types. Type I is the most common form of osteogenesis imperfecta tarda, and type IV tends to be more severe. Osteogenesis imperfecta congenita includes types II and III. Type II is lethal in the perinatal period, whereas type III may be compatible with prolonged survival with extreme crippling and short stature. The disease is characterized by multiple bone fractures, and some patients have opalescent teeth, blue sclerae, and child- or adult-onset hearing loss. Some patients have increased bruisability. The clinical expression is extremely variable between and within families. Multiple defects in the genes encoding the α-1 and α-2 chains of type I collagen have been reported, and thus the disease is extremely heterogeneous at the DNA level.

Types I and IV, most type II, and some type III osteogenesis imperfecta cases are autosomal dominant. Mitral valve prolapse is increased in frequency but infrequently progresses to significant regurgitation. The mean aortic root diameter is slightly but significantly increased, and aortic regurgitation occurs in 1%-2% of patients.

Tuberous Sclerosis

Tuberous sclerosis is an autosomal dominant disorder with variable expression and high penetrance. Approximately 50% of cases arise by new mutation. It is characterized by cortical or retinal tubers, seizures, mental retardation in <50%, depigmented "ash leaf" macules, facial angiofibromas, dental pits, subungual or periungual fibromas, shagreen patches, and renal cysts or angiomyolipomas. Cardiac rhabdomyomas are more frequent in the fetus and infant and often resolve with age.

Pulmonary fibrosis resulting in a "honeycomb" appearance by radiography is more frequent in young women and tends to progress rapidly. Central nervous system astrocytomas may occur. The gene defect remains unidentified, but there is good evidence for non-allelic heterogeneity, with one locus on chromosome 9 and another on chromosome 16.

- Tuberous sclerosis is autosomal dominant and has high penetrance.
- About 50% of cases arise by new mutation.
- Characteristics: cortical or retinal tubers, seizures, mental retardation in <50%, "ash leaf" macules, angiofibromas, subungual or periungual fibromas, shagreen patches, renal cysts or angiomyolipomas.

Von Hippel-Lindau Disease

Von Hippel-Lindau disease is characterized by retinal, spinal cord, and cerebellar hemangioblastomas, cysts of the kidneys, pancreas, and epididymis, and renal cysts and cancers. Other manifestations include hemangioblastomas of the medulla oblongata, cysts and hemangiomas of other visceral organs, pancreatic cancer, and pheochromocytomas.

- Characteristics of von Hippel-Lindau disease: retinal, spinal cord, and cerebellar hemangioblastomas; cysts of kidneys, pancreas, and epididymis.

Retinal hemangioblastomas often are the earliest manifestation of von Hippel-Lindau disease. The mean age at diagnosis is 21-28 years, but they can occur as early as 4 years. Initially, the lesion appears as a small red dot that may enlarge at a variable rate to appear as a gray disk or globular, red tumor. The lesions leak, and localized retinal detachment is frequent. Large lesions may be obscured by exudate or gliosis, or they may calcify. Multiple or bilateral lesions occur in 20%-58% of patients, and 16%-36% of those with retinal lesions have diminished vision.

- Retinal hemangioblastomas may be earliest manifestation of von Hippel-Lindau disease.

Hemangioblastomas of the central nervous system in von Hippel-Lindau disease are benign, and associated morbidity is due to space-occupying effects. They occur most frequently in the cerebellum and spinal cord but also can be in the medulla oblongata and rarely in the cerebrum. The average age at onset of symptoms is 30 years.

- Hemangioblastomas of central nervous system in von Hippel-Lindau disease are benign tumors with morbid effects.

Renal cysts, hemangiomas, and benign adenomas are usually asymptomatic. Rarely, cysts are so extensive as to mimic polycystic kidney disease and cause renal failure. The cysts vary in size from a few millimeters to >2 cm; they are bilateral in 60% and frequently multiple. Renal clear cell cancers are bilateral or multiple in 40%-87% of cases, causing death in 33% of patients at a mean age of 44.5 years.

- Renal cysts, hemangiomas, and benign adenomas are usually asymptomatic in von Hippel-Lindau disease.
- Renal cancer is a major cause of death.

Most pancreatic cysts are asymptomatic. They rarely lead to diabetes mellitus or steatorrhea. Pancreatic disease, including cystadenocarcinoma or islet cell tumors, tends to cluster in certain families.

Adrenal cysts, adenomas, and cortical hyperplasia are asymptomatic. Pheochromocytomas are bilateral in 17%-34% of patients, and the average age at diagnosis is 25-34 years. Pheochromocytomas tend to cluster within certain families, but linkage studies have shown that families with and without pheochromocytomas have defects of the same gene.

- Pheochromocytomas of von Hippel-Lindau disease cluster within certain families.

Many male patients with von Hippel-Lindau disease have benign, asymptomatic epididymal lesions, although occasionally fertility is impaired. An epididymal cyst in a relative at risk is not sufficient by itself to diagnose von Hippel-Lindau disease.

Inheritance is autosomal dominant, and the risk for any child born to an affected person is 50%. Expression is variable, but penetrance is complete in thoroughly evaluated families. Males and females are affected equally.

- Von Hippel-Lindau disease is autosomal dominant.

Patients with a hemangioblastoma should have a review of the family history, computed tomography or magnetic resonance imaging of the head and upper spine, oph-

thalmologic examination, and computed tomography or ultrasonography of the abdomen. Patients with bilateral epididymal cysts or polycystic pancreas should also be screened, and it should be considered in patients with pheochromocytomas, polycystic kidneys, or renal cancer. Patients with von Hippel-Lindau disease need annual physical and ophthalmologic examinations, peripheral blood cell count, urinalysis, computed tomography or magnetic resonance imaging of the head, and computed tomography or ultrasonography of the abdomen. Evaluation of urinary catecholamines is reasonable, particularly if the patient is hypertensive or has a family history of pheochromocytoma. Patients should have genetic counseling, and first-degree relatives should have physical and ophthalmologic examinations beginning at age 4 years, imaging of the head and spine at 11 years, and imaging of the abdomen at 18 years. It is unknown at what age one can safely discontinue screening for at-risk members. Presymptomatic and prenatal diagnosis by use of linked DNA markers is available. The gene that causes von Hippel-Lindau disease was recently identified and is localized to chromosome 3p25-26.

Autosomal Recessive

Autosomal recessive disease also occurs because of abnormal genes that are located on the autosomes. However, one copy of the abnormal gene is not sufficient to cause disease, and heterozygotes (carriers) are not clinically different from the general population. When two persons who are heterozygotes for a given gene defect mate, the children are at 25% risk of inheriting the abnormal gene from both parents and, thus, of having the disease.

- Autosomal recessive inheritance: abnormal genes are located on autosomes, but one copy of gene is not sufficient to cause disease.
- Heterozygotes (carriers) are not clinically different from general population.

Because the heterozygous state may be transmitted silently through many generations before the chance mating of two heterozygotes occurs, it is not surprising that there rarely is a family history of the disease in previous generations. The occurrence of multiple affected siblings within a family suggests autosomal recessive inheritance; however, because of the small average family size in this country, many autosomal recessive diseases seem to occur as isolated cases.

The risk for the children of a person who has an autosomal recessive disease depends on the frequency of the abnormal gene in the population. Except for common diseases such as cystic fibrosis or sickle cell anemia, the risk is usually small, provided that this person does not marry a relative or a person who has a family history of the same disease.

Many diseases that are caused by an identified metabolic defect, such as homocystinuria, are autosomal recessive diseases due to an enzyme deficiency. When the enzymatic defect is established, carrier testing and prenatal diagnosis sometimes are possible.

Some of the diseases with autosomal recessive inheritance are listed in Table 16-2 and summarized on the following pages.

Table 16-2.--Diseases With Autosomal Recessive Inheritance

Alkaptonuria
α_1-Antitrypsin deficiency
Cystic fibrosis
Familial Mediterranean fever
Friedreich ataxia
Gaucher disease
Glycogen storage disease, types I, II, III, IV, V, VII
Hemochromatosis
Homocystinuria
Oculocutaneous albinism
Phenylketonuria
Pseudoxanthoma elasticum (some forms are autosomal dominant)
Refsum disease
Sickle-cell disease
Tay-Sachs disease
α- and β-Thalassemia
Wilson disease

Friedreich Ataxia

This is an autosomal recessive disorder. The first sign of the disease is ataxic gait. The mean age at onset is approximately 12 years. Dysarthria, hypotonic muscle weakness, loss of vibration and position senses, and loss of deep tendon reflexes develop subsequently. In some patients, diabetes mellitus, nystagmus, optic atrophy, dementia, respiratory dysfunction due to kyphoscoliosis, and decreased sensory nerve conduction velocities also develop.

- Friedreich ataxia is autosomal recessive.
- First sign of disease is ataxic gait.
- Mean age at onset is 12 years.
- Dysarthria, hypotonic muscle weakness, loss of vibration and position senses, and loss of deep tendon reflexes develop subsequently.

In one series, 60 of 82 patients with Friedreich ataxia had clinical evidence of cardiac dysfunction 4 months to 4 years before death, and 56% died of heart failure. The mean age at death was 36.6 years. Cardiac arrhythmias, particularly atrial fibrillation, were common and occurred in 50% of fatal cases. At autopsy, most cases had marked thickening of the left ventricle with extensive interstitial fibrosis and focal degeneration of muscle fibers. Muscle fibers were hypertrophied and many had large nuclei. The cardiomyopathy may be of the hypertrophic type with subaortic stenosis.

- Cardiac arrhythmias occur in 50% of fatal cases of Friedreich ataxia.

The risk for a sibling being affected is 25%. The basic biochemical defect remains unknown. However, the gene has been localized to chromosome 9q12-21.1 by genetic linkage studies of affected families. This evaluation potentially allows for prenatal or presymptomatic diagnosis of cases in which one affected child already has been diagnosed.

- Risk of Friedreich ataxia in sibling of affected person is 25%.

Gaucher Disease

Gaucher disease is an autosomal recessive disorder due to deficiency of the enzyme glucocerebrosidase, which results in lipid storage in the spleen, liver, bone marrow, and other organs. Type 1 (non-neuronopathic) disease is most frequent in Ashkenazi Jews (carrier frequency, 1 in 10). The disease may be asymptomatic at any age or present in childhood or adulthood with splenomegaly, hepatosplenomegaly, thrombocytopenia, anemia, degenerative bone disease, or pulmonary disease. Type 2 (infantile, neuronopathic) has no ethnic predisposition, and type 3 (juvenile form) has intermediate clinical signs. The first sign of neurologic involvement in types 2 and 3 is supranuclear ophthalmoplegia.

- Gaucher disease is autosomal recessive.

- Disease is due to deficiency of the enzyme glucocerebrosidase.
- Type 1 is most frequent in Ashkenazi Jews.
- Type 2 has no ethnic predisposition.
- First sign of neurologic involvement in types 2 and 3 is supranuclear ophthalmoplegia.

Enzyme replacement is effective treatment for non-neuronopathic forms of the disease, but it is not yet known whether it is effective for patients with neurologic involvement.

- Enzyme replacement therapy is effective for non-neuronopathic Gaucher disease.

Glycogen Storage Diseases

Glycogen storage disease type I is due to deficiency of the enzyme glucose-6-phosphatase. It is characterized by hypoglycemia, hypercholesterolemia, hyperuricemia, lactic acidosis, short stature, hepatomegaly, and delayed onset of puberty. Adults with this disease may develop malignant hepatomas, premature coronary disease, pancreatitis, gout, and renal disease.

- Glycogen storage disease type I is due to deficiency of the enzyme glucose-6-phosphatase.
- Characteristics: hypoglycemia, hypercholesterolemia, hyperuricemia, lactic acidosis, short stature, hepatomegaly, delayed puberty.

Glycogen storage disease type II (Pompe disease) is an autosomal recessive disorder due to deficiency of the lysosomal enzyme α-1,4-glucosidase (acid maltase). The infantile form is characterized by hypotonia, macroglossia, and progressive cardiomyopathy resulting in death within the first year of life. The electrocardiogram is characterized by high-voltage QRS complexes in all leads and a short P-R interval. Cardiac catheterization frequently reveals biventricular hypertrophy with left outflow tract obstruction. The myocardium is different histologically from the myocardium in isolated hypertrophic cardiomyopathy. There is evidence of glycogen storage with vacuolation of heart muscle. Histologic examination of tissues such as liver and kidney may reveal engorged lysosomes, but in muscle the lysosomes may have ruptured and cytoplasmic glycogen is seen. The diagnosis can be confirmed by determination of α-1,4-glucosidase activity in skeletal muscle or leukocytes. Prenatal diagnosis through enzyme analysis of amniotic fluid cells is possible.

- Glycogen storage disease type II is autosomal recessive.
- Disease is due to deficiency of the enzyme α-1,4-glucosidase.
- Characteristics of infantile form: hypotonia, macroglossia, progressive cardiomyopathy.

Juvenile and adult forms of glycogen storage disease type II also exist. The presenting characteristic is skeletal muscle weakness, and cardiac involvement usually is absent or minimal. At least one patient had a cardiac arrhythmia that required implantation of a ventricular pacemaker, but her echocardiogram showed no cardiomegaly.

- Characteristics of juvenile and adult forms of glycogen storage disease: skeletal muscle weakness, minimal or absent cardiac involvement.

Glycogen storage disease type III is due to an autosomal recessively inherited deficiency of amylo-1,6-glucosidase (debrancher) activity. The enzyme is deficient in liver, and in some patients also in skeletal muscle, cultured skin fibroblasts, and leukocytes. Clinically, the disorder is characterized by hepatomegaly and growth retardation that resolves at puberty. There may be hypoglycemia and hyperlipidemia. Skeletal muscle weakness may develop in adult life. Cardiomyopathy, when present, may be life-threatening and mimic hypertrophic cardiomyopathy. Histologic evaluation of cardiac tissue reveals increased intracellular glycogen with no disarray of myofibers or myofibrils. Deficiency of the enzyme has been documented in cardiac muscle from one patient.

- Glycogen storage disease type III is autosomal recessive.
- Disease is due to deficiency of amylo-1,6-glucosidase activity.
- Characteristics: hepatomegaly, growth retardation that resolves at puberty.

Hemochromatosis

Clinical features of the disease may be gray-brown skin pigmentation, cardiomyopathy, hepatomegaly with fibrosis or cirrhosis, diabetes mellitus, hypogonadism, and bone demineralization. The disease is due to tissue damage by iron overload, although the extent of iron overload in an organ does not always correspond to the severity of tissue damage. Biochemical abnormalities include increased serum iron and ferritin levels, increased transferrin saturation, and increased urinary iron excretion, especially in response to deferoxamine administration. The hemochromatosis gene is linked to the HLA complex on chromosome 6, and this linkage association was instrumental in proving the autosomal recessive inheritance pattern.

- Features of hemochromatosis: gray-brown skin pigmentation, cardiomyopathy, hepatomegaly, diabetes mellitus, hypogonadism, bone demineralization.
- Disease is due to tissue damage by iron overload.
- Disease is autosomal recessive.

The risk for siblings of an affected patient is 25%, and therefore all should be screened for biochemical evidence of the disease. Patients with iron overload should have phlebotomy until the excess iron is removed, regardless of whether clinical signs of the disease are present. The risk for offspring of affected individuals is relatively low (approximately 1 in 36) but is not negligible because of the relatively high gene frequency in the general population. Therefore, offspring should be screened to determine whether they are at risk for the disease. Some advocate population screening.

- Siblings of patients with hemochromatosis have risk of 25% for the disease.
- Offspring of patients with hemochromatosis need to be screened.

Heart disease occurs in 15%-20% of patients with clinically evident hemochromatosis, and the earliest signs may be electrocardiographic changes characterized by decreased QRS amplitude and T-wave flattening or inversion. Later, congestive heart failure and arrhythmias may occur. The heart condition sometimes resolves after phlebotomy.

- Heart disease occurs in 15%-20% of patients with hemochromatosis.

Homocystinuria

The classic form of homocystinuria is due to autosomal recessively inherited deficiency of cystathionine β-synthase. The gene is expressed in skin fibroblasts and amniocytes, so prenatal diagnosis by determination of enzyme activity in amniocytes is feasible.

- Homocystinuria is autosomal recessive disease.
- Disease is due to deficiency of cystathionine β-synthase.

The incidence of the disease is approximately 1 per 200,000. Clinically, it is characterized by tall stature with a low upper segment:lower segment ratio, pectus deformities, scoliosis, genu valgum, pes planus, and a highly arched palate. Lens dislocation is progressive, and the direction of displacement is usually, but not always, downward. Myopia, retinal detachment, secondary glaucoma, fair hair and skin, cutaneous flushing, and hernias may be present. Approximately 50% of patients are mentally retarded, but this is variable even within a sibship. The electroencephalogram may be abnormal, and some patients have seizures, focal neurologic signs, and hemiatrophy of the brain. Acute episodes of "nervousness" or schizophrenic behavior may occur. Osteoporosis with a tendency to fractures and "codfish"-shaped, collapsed vertebrae may be evident radiographically. None of the features are present consistently in all patients, and some affected individuals appear normal.

- Incidence of homocystinuria is about 1 per 200,000.
- Clinical features: tall stature, pectus deformities, scoliosis, genu valgum, pes planus, highly arched palate.
- Lens dislocation is progressive.
- About 50% of patients are mentally retarded.
- "Nervousness" or schizophrenic behavior may occur.
- Osteoporosis and "codfish"-shaped, collapsed vertebrae may be seen on radiographs.

Cardiovascular abnormalities include arterial or venous thrombosis, angina pectoris, coronary occlusions at a young age, renal artery narrowing resulting in hypertension and renal atrophy, cerebrovascular accidents, thrombophlebitis, and pulmonary emboli. Dilatation of the pulmonary artery and left atrial endocardial fibroelastosis have been reported. Thrombi are particularly likely to occur after operation, venipuncture, or catheterization.

- Cardiovascular abnormalities of homocystinuria: arterial or venous thrombosis, angina pectoris, coronary occlusions at young age.
- Thrombi are likely after operation, venipuncture, catheterization.

Histologic examination of the arteries reveals marked fibrous thickening of the intima. Aortic intimal fibrosis may be severe enough to mimic coarctation. Medial changes consist of thrombosis and dilatation with widely spaced, frayed muscle fibers. The elastic fibers of the large arteries may be fragmented, and dilatation of the ascending aorta has been observed. No consistent platelet defect has been noted.

The disease sometimes may be diagnosed by positive results of urinary nitroprusside test and confirmed by the more sensitive method of elevated urinary homocystine excretion by amino acid chromatography. Levels of plasma homocystine and its precursor, methionine, are increased. The goal of treatment is to lower the plasma homocystine level, which seems to result in slower progression and fewer symptoms of the disease; 50% of patients respond to pyridoxine therapy (25-1,000 mg/day). Supplemental folate also should be given because patients who are potentially capable of responding to pyridoxine may not do so in the presence of folate deficiency. A low-protein, low-methionine diet can be useful, but adults find it difficult to comply with this. For infants, a low-methionine formula is available. Betaine and penicillamine also have been reported to be of benefit in decreasing plasma homocystine levels.

- In homocystinuria, levels of plasma homocystine and its precursor, methionine, are increased.
- Goal of treatment: lower plasma homocystine level.

A rare form of homocystinuria is due to deficiency of *N*-methyltetrahydrofolate-homocysteine methyltransferase. Affected patients have additional neurologic symptoms, and the plasma methionine levels may be normal. Patients with homocystinuria due to abnormal cobalamin metabolism also have normal plasma methionine levels and may have methylmalonic acidemia and megaloblastic anemia.

Pseudoxanthoma Elasticum

There are two hereditary forms of pseudoxanthoma elasticum: autosomal dominant and autosomal recessive. Both forms are characterized by yellowish skin papules, especially on the neck and flexural areas, angioid streaks and choroiditis of the retina, and vascular complications, including angina pectoris, claudication, calcification of peripheral arteries, and renal vascular hypertension. In one series of patients, 19% had angina pectoris, 14% had calcification of peripheral arteries, and 18% had intermittent claudication. The age at onset of complications is variable, and they may occur in early adolescence. Endocardial thickening may result in deformity of the valves, and the conduction system also may be involved, resulting in arrhythmias. Histologically, the arteries show fragmented elastic fibers with granular deposits in place of amorphous elastin. The basic defect is not known but seems to be either an intrinsic abnormality of elastin or secondary destruction of elastin.

- Two hereditary forms of pseudoxanthoma elasticum: autosomal dominant and autosomal recessive.
- Characteristics: yellowish skin papules, angioid streaks and choroiditis of retina, vascular complications.

Refsum Disease

Refsum disease is an autosomal recessive neurodegenerative disease characterized by cerebellar ataxia, hypertrophic polyneuropathy, and retinitis pigmentosa. Deafness, ichthyosis, and cardiac conduction defects are frequently present. Onset of the disorder may be in infancy or middle age, and the course is progressive. Cerebrospinal fluid protein concentration is increased, and phytanic acid accumulates in serum and organs. Hypertrophic interstitial neuritis and degenerative changes of nuclei and fiber tracts are observed histologically in the brain stem. The electrocardiogram is characterized by a prolonged P-Q interval and ST-segment and T-wave changes. Impaired atrioventricular conduction, bundle-branch block, and sudden death from cardiac arrhythmia may occur. Myocardial fibrosis has been reported.

- Refsum disease is autosomal recessive.
- Characteristics: cerebellar ataxia, hypertrophic polyneuropathy, retinitis pigmentosa.
- Frequently present: deafness, ichthyosis, cardiac conduction defects.

Phytanic acid is a fatty acid present in dairy products and fat from grazing animals. Patients with Refsum disease are deficient in the catabolic enzyme phytanic acid α-hydroxylase, which results in accumulation of ingested phytanic acid in fatty deposits in the involved organ systems. The enzyme deficiency is expressed in cultured skin fibroblasts, and prenatal diagnosis is possible.

- Patients with Refsum disease are deficient in phytanic acid α-hydroxylase.

Dietary restriction of phytanic acid results in clinical improvement and stabilization of the disease. Electrocardiographic changes sometimes resolve after treatment. Plasmapheresis removes phytanic acid from the body and may allow liberalization of the diet; it can be extremely valuable in the management of acutely ill patients.

Tay-Sachs Disease

Tay-Sachs disease is an autosomal recessive disease due to deficiency of hexosaminidase A. The classic infantile form of the disease is rapidly fatal and is due to storage of ganglioside GM_2 in neural tissue. It is particularly common in people of Ashkenazi Jewish ancestry; the carrier frequency is 1 in 30. Therefore, screening for carriers by determination of enzyme activity in serum (or leukocytes, particularly in pregnant women, in whom the serum level is unreliable) is recommended in this population. Prenatal diagnosis is available when both the mother and father are carriers.

- Tay-Sachs disease is autosomal recessive.
- Disease due to deficiency of hexosaminidase A.

Rare juvenile and adult forms of the disease exist and may present with ataxia, upper motor neuron disease, or other neurologic disorders. These late-onset variants have less of an ethnic predisposition.

X-Linked Recessive

X-linked recessive diseases are caused by abnormal genes located on the X chromosome. Female heterozygotes, who have one abnormal gene on one X chromosome and one normal gene on the other X chromosome, usually are clinically normal. Exceptions may occur because of the phenomenon of lyonization, in which one X chromosome is inactivated at random early in fetal life; if the normal gene is inactivated in a critical number of cells, the woman may have symptoms or clinical signs of the disease. However, the disease usually is less severe than in males. The likelihood of clinical signs of the disease developing in a female varies by disease. For example, it is rare for female carriers of hemophilia VIII to have severe bleeding problems, but it is relatively common for carriers of ornithine carbamoyltransferase (ornithine transcarbamoylase) deficiency to have intermittent symptoms.

- X-linked recessive diseases are caused by abnormal genes on X chromosome.
- Development of clinical signs of disease in female varies by disease.

Males who inherit the abnormal gene have no corresponding genetic loci on the Y chromosome and therefore are referred to as "hemizygotes." Any male child born to a heterozygous female is at 50% risk for having the disease; female children are at 50% risk for inheriting the gene and being carriers. All the daughters of affected males are carriers, and all the sons are unaffected (i.e., male-to-male transmission cannot occur).

- Males with abnormal gene are called "hemizygotes."
- Male child of heterozygous female has 50% risk of disease.
- Female child is at 50% risk of inheriting the gene.

X-linked recessive diseases also may arise by new mutation affecting either the mother or the afflicted son. Genetic counseling is difficult in these situations because if the mother represents the new mutation the risk for her future male children is 50%. However, if the child represents the new mutation, there is no significant risk for siblings of that child. New advances in DNA-based diagnosis have resulted in opportunities for carrier detection for some diseases which circumvent problems created by lyonization.

Some of the conditions with X-linked recessive inheritance are listed in Table 16-3 and summarized on the following pages.

Table 16-3.--X-Linked Recessive Conditions

Adrenoleukodystrophy ("X-linked" form)
Chronic granulomatous disease (many cases; autosomal recessive forms are less common)
Color blindness
Duchenne and Becker muscular dystrophy
Fabry disease
Glucose-6-phosphate dehydrogenase deficiency
Hemophilia A and B
Ocular albinism
Rickets, hypophosphatemic
Testicular feminization

Duchenne and Becker Muscular Dystrophy

Duchenne muscular dystrophy is one of the most common types of muscular dystrophy; its incidence is approximately 1 in 3,500 newborn males. It is an X-linked recessive disease, and approximately a third of the cases arise by new mutation. Progressive skeletal weakness beginning at 2 to 5 years of age, with death in the late teens or 20s, is characteristic. The diagnosis is made on the basis of clinical findings and markedly increased creatine kinase levels. The muscle biopsy findings are relatively non-specific. Becker muscular dystrophy has later onset.

- Incidence of Duchenne muscular dystrophy is 1 in 3,500 newborn males.
- Duchenne muscular dystrophy is X-linked recessive.
- Skeletal weakness at 2 to 5 years of age is characteristic.

The genetic defect that results in both Duchenne and Becker muscular dystrophies involves the dystrophin gene located on chromosome X at band p2l. Approximately two-thirds of patients have a submicroscopic partial gene deletion, and the rest have undetected deletions, duplications, or other abnormalities. The dystrophin gene is very large, consisting of at least 60 exons and 1,800 kilobases. The entire gene has been cloned. The protein product of this gene, dystrophin, is a rod-shaped cytoskeletal protein that is predominantly localized to the surface membrane of striated muscle cells. Identification of the molecular defect has resulted in improved ability to determine carrier status in female relatives by DNA analysis. This is a significant improvement over carrier testing by measurement of creatine kinase levels, because levels are increased in only 70% of obligate carriers. DNA analysis also can be used for prenatal diagnosis. All mothers, sisters, and children of patients with Duchenne or Becker muscular dystrophy should have genetic counseling.

- Mothers, sisters, and children of patients with Duchenne or Becker muscular dystrophy need genetic counseling.

The heart disease in patients with Duchenne muscular dystrophy is characterized by significant changes in systolic time intervals suggestive of compromised left ventricular function. There are histologic changes characterized by multifocal dystrophic areas with fibrosis and loss of myofilaments. These changes are most marked in the posterobasal segment and contiguous lateral and inferior walls of the left ventricle.

- Heart disease in Duchenne muscular dystrophy involves changes in systolic time intervals.

Fabry Disease

Fabry disease is a lysosomal storage disease due to deficiency of α-galactosidase A. The inheritance pattern is X-linked recessive, although females may have less severe signs of the disease than males. Glycosphingolipids accumulate in the endothelium, perithelium, and smooth muscle of blood vessels. There is less accumulation in ganglion cells, myocardial cells, reticuloendothelial cells, and connective tissue cells.

- Fabry disease is due to deficiency of α-galactosidase A.
- Disease is X-linked recessive.
- Females may have less severe signs than males.

The first signs of the disease may be telangiectatic angiokeratomas of the skin and mucous membranes. Acroparesthesias and episodes of severe burning pain in the palms and soles with proximal radiation also may occur in childhood and adolescence. Whorl-shaped corneal opacities and cataracts develop. In adulthood, cardiovascular and renal diseases are the major causes of morbidity and mortality. Cardiac problems, including ischemia, infarction, congestive heart failure, mitral insufficiency, and aortic stenosis, may result from progressive glycosphingolipid infiltration. Systemic hypertension due to infiltration of renal parenchymal vessels may aggravate the cardiac disease. Electrocardiography may show signs of left ventricular hypertrophy, ST-segment changes, and T-wave inversion. Occasionally, patients have arrhythmias and a short P-R interval.

- First signs of Fabry disease may be telangiectatic angiokeratomas of skin and mucous membranes.
- Acroparesthesias may occur in childhood and adolescence.
- Whorl-shaped corneal opacities and cataracts develop.
- In adults, cardiovascular and renal diseases develop.

The interventricular septum and posterior left ventricular wall may be thickened. Cardiomegaly, especially involving the left atrium and ventricle, is observed. The right atrium and ventricle may be dilated. Myocardial cells show extensive glycosphingolipid deposited around the nucleus and between myofibrils. Endothelial cells and smooth muscle cells are hypertrophied. The mitral valve frequently is thickened and has normal or thick papillary muscles; the tricuspid valve may be involved, but the aortic and pulmonary valves usually are normal. Lipid-filled cells are seen within the fibrous tissue of involved valves.

Neurologic signs result from small-vessel involvement in the brain. The most frequent cause of death is renal failure.

Dilantin and carbamazepine are useful for treating the pain. Renal transplantation can prolong life. The gene has been cloned, and prenatal diagnosis is possible.

MITOCHONDRIAL MUTATIONS

Mitochondria each contain several circular copies of their own genetic material, mitochondrial DNA. This mitochondrial DNA is approximately 16,000 base pairs in length and encodes for transfer-RNAs and several proteins involved in the mitochondrial respiratory chain. Many mitochondrial enzymes, including some others of the respiratory chain complex, are encoded by nuclear DNA and transported into the mitochondria. Mitochondrial DNA mutations cause Leber's optic atrophy and the multisystem syndromes of multiple episodes of lactic acidosis and stroke (MELAS) and myoclonic epilepsy with ragged red fibers (MERRF). Many cases of Kearns-Sayre syndrome (cardiomyopathy and ophthalmoplegia) are due to mitochondrial mutations. Mitochondrial disorders can arise as new mutations or be maternally inherited; only the egg contributes mitochondria to the zygote, the sperm does not. Mitochondrial mutations may be homoplasmic (present in all mitochondrial DNA) or heteroplasmic (present in only some of the mitochondrial DNA). Accumulation of acquired mutations may contribute to the aging process, and mitochondrial mutations may play a role in the pathogenesis of ischemic heart disease.

- Mitochondrial DNA mutations cause Leber's optic atrophy and multisystem syndromes.
- Many cases of Kearns-Sayre syndrome are due to mitochondrial mutations.
- Only the egg contributes mitochondria to the zygote; sperm does not.

MULTIFACTORIAL CAUSATION

Multifactorial means that the disease or trait is determined by the interaction of environmental influences and a polygenic (many gene) predisposition. Human conditions that may have multifactorial causation include many common birth defects--such as congenital heart defects, cleft lip and palate, and neural tube defects--and many common diseases--such as diabetes mellitus, asthma, hypertension, and coronary artery atherosclerosis.

- Multifactorial causation: disease or trait is due to environmental influences and polygenic predisposition.
- Birth defects that may have multifactorial causation: congenital heart defects, cleft lip and palate, neural tube defects.
- Diseases that may have multifactorial causation: diabetes mellitus, asthma, hypertension, coronary artery atherosclerosis.

The multifactorial model predicts that there will be a tendency for familial aggregation of the condition but without a strict mendelian pattern of inheritance. Familial aggregation also can be due to common environmental factors, so familial aggregation by itself is not sufficient to prove multifactorial causation.

Because familial aggregation exists for multifactorial disorders, it is implicit that the occurrence risk will be increased for members of an affected family over that of the general population. As expected, the risk is highest for first-degree relatives (parents, siblings, children) who have half of their genes in common. The risk is less for second-degree relatives (grandparents, aunts, uncles, grandchildren, nephews, nieces) who share one-quarter of their genes. The risk decreases exponentially thereafter; third-degree relatives (great-grandparents, cousins, great-grandchildren) share only one-eighth of their genes. Empiric (observed) risk figures for some well-studied multifactorial disorders fit well with the predicted risks.

The genetic liability in multifactorial causation is due to the cumulative effect of many genes, each having a small effect, rather than to the effect of one major gene. These genes create a liability that presumably is continuously distributed within the population. If the genetic liability is strong enough, under an unfortunate set of environmental circumstances the disorder will occur.

- Genetic liability in multifactorial causation is due to cumulative effect of many genes.

For many multifactorial conditions, there is a difference in predilection between males and females which could result directly from genetic differences or from different internal (e.g., hormonal) or external environmental factors. Furthermore, if a member of the less commonly affected sex has the condition, his or her genetic liability was probably greater and therefore the risk for his or her relatives is greater. Similarly, if a person has a more severe form of the disease, the risk for relatives is higher. For disorders in which disease frequency increases with age, earlier onset sometimes implies a greater risk for relatives. Finally, the greater the number of affected individuals within the family, the higher the risk for other relatives. There also are racial differences in the frequency of many disorders of multifactorial causation.

When the inheritance pattern of any disease is being determined, the possibility of genetic heterogeneity always must be considered. For example, there are both autosomal dominant and multifactorial causes of atrial septal defect which may be indistinguishable clinically. Failure to recognize that different genetic diseases can cause the same or similar clinical entities can result in confusion when determining risks.

Table 16-4 lists some conditions of multifactorial causation.

Table 16-4.--Conditions of Multifactorial Causation

Atherosclerosis
Atopic disease or allergy
Cancer
Cardiac defects (congenital)
Cleft lip or palate
Diabetes mellitus
Hypertension
Neural tube defects
Schizophrenia

PRESYMPTOMATIC AND PRENATAL DIAGNOSIS OF GENETIC DISEASE BY DNA ANALYSIS

Presymptomatic and prenatal diagnosis of genetic diseases utilizing peripheral blood specimens or specimens obtained by amniocentesis or chorionic villus sampling has become a routine part of clinical practice because of the identification of the basic genetic defect underlying numerous mendelian conditions and the capability for direct DNA diagnosis. In addition, even when the causative genetic defect has not yet been identified, knowledge of its chromosome localization may allow for diagnosis by linkage analysis. Because individual genes are too small to be seen microscopically, standard chromosome analysis generally is not helpful even when the gene has been localized to a specific chromosome region.

The DNA-based laboratory procedures used for diagnosis, the limitations of the tests, and the importance of an accurate clinical diagnosis and family history are described below. A discussion of the prenatal diagnosis of Duchenne muscular dystrophy (DMD) provides an excellent example of these issues. Although the following examples describe prenatal diagnosis, the same principles apply to presymptomatic diagnosis.

Importance of an Accurate Clinical Diagnosis and Family History

The importance of a correct diagnosis in the index patient when diagnosis by DNA analysis is being contemplated cannot be overemphasized. This criterion is in contrast to many instances of genetic diagnosis by chromosome analysis in which the cytogeneticist usually can be relied on to note most abnormalities (fragile X and subtle deletions are examples of exceptions) regardless of the exact indication for the study. This approach is possible because the procedure of chromosome analysis involves examination of all 46 chromosomes in a given cell to look for gross structural changes. In contrast, it is impossible to systematically examine each of a person's 100,000 genes to detect all abnormalities.

- It is impossible to systematically examine each of a person's 100,000 genes.

The laboratory's process of detection of even one abnormal gene must be directed by the precise clinical diagnosis. The DNA-based assays are specific for the disease being studied, and abnormalities elsewhere in the genome will not be detected. Thus, if the incorrect assay is chosen because of an incorrect clinical diagnosis, the disease-causing mutation will not be detected. For example, if a pregnant woman's brother and uncle are believed to have DMD but the correct diagnosis is X-linked Emery-Dreifuss muscular dystrophy, the wrong DNA analysis will be performed and may result in an erroneous prediction as to whether the fetus is affected. It is the responsibility of the physician to obtain medical records or to arrange for one of the affected relatives to be examined to confirm the reported diagnosis, and the physician may want the assistance of a medical geneticist or other specialist in this process.

In addition to confirmation of the diagnosis, an accurate family pedigree is necessary. It is important to know whether the index patient represents a sporadic case or whether other family members also are affected. This information must be considered in the determination of whether DNA diagnosis is possible and in the interpretation of the results of DNA analysis. In sporadic cases, diagnosis by linkage analysis (see below), which is based on tracking the mutation through the family, may be impossible.

● Accurate family pedigree is necessary for diagnosis.

In these sporadic cases, diagnosis often can be established only for diseases for which direct DNA diagnosis is possible. In contrast, in families with multiple affected members, direct DNA diagnosis is the first diagnostic choice when possible, followed by linkage analysis if the mutation cannot be directly identified. For other diseases, linkage studies are the only option. For example, in DMD, approximately 60% of patients have a deletion identifiable by techniques in routine use for clinical testing. If a deletion is detected in a sporadic patient with DMD, it usually is possible to determine whether the mother is a carrier and, if so, direct DNA diagnosis can be applied for her male fetuses. If a deletion cannot be detected in a sporadic patient with DMD, then specific prenatal diagnosis is not possible for the mother's future children, although exclusion of a disease may still be possible by use of linked markers. The mother of a sporadic patient with DMD has a prior risk for being a carrier of approximately 2 in 3, and the options include fetal sex determination followed by termination of all male fetuses, although at least 2 of 3 would be expected to be unaffected, or termination of fetuses that inherited the same markers as the index patient, in which at least 1 of 3 would be unaffected.

● In families with multiple affected members, direct DNA diagnosis is first diagnostic choice.

Alternatively, if there are multiple affected family members with DMD, the issue of new mutation is not a concern. If a deletion is detected in these multiplex families, this is the simplest approach for testing male fetuses of women at risk within the family. However, if a deletion is not detected, then blood specimens can be collected from multiple family members for linkage analysis (Fig. 16-5).

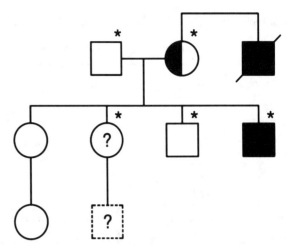

Fig. 16-5. Sample pedigree of family with males with Duchenne muscular dystrophy (shaded symbols). Carrier females are shown with half-shaded symbols. Members for whom blood was requested for DNA linkage analysis are marked with an asterisk. Squares, males; circles, females; line through square indicates that person is deceased; dashed-line square indicates male fetus. Note that blood for DNA from pregnant woman's father and unaffected brother is helpful for DNA linkage studies. Most laboratories offering these tests assist the referring physician in determining which family members need testing.

Linkage Analysis

Linkage analysis for prenatal diagnosis is based on the biologic fact that individual units of genetic material (genes) are situated in linear order on one of the 24 types of chromosomes (22 autosomes plus the X and Y chromosomes). The word "alleles" refers to the different forms of genetic material at the same gene locus, for example, the A and B alleles at the ABO blood group locus. Genes located on different chromosomes segregate independently, so there is a 50% chance that an individual egg or sperm will contain the same or different alleles encoded within these two chromosomal loci (Fig. 16-6).

● "Alleles" are different forms of genetic material at same gene locus.

Genes located on the same chromosome are *syntenic*. During the pairing of homologous chromosomes during meiosis, crossovers can occur between genes even if they are located on the same chromosome. The average number of crossovers per chromosome per meiosis is two. Genes located far apart on the same chromosome are more likely to be separated by crossovers than are genes located close together. If the genes are so far apart that they are separated by crossovers at least 50% of the time, then these genes are not linked even though they are syntenic, and they exhibit random segregation (Fig. 16-7).

● Genes located on same chromosome are *syntenic*.

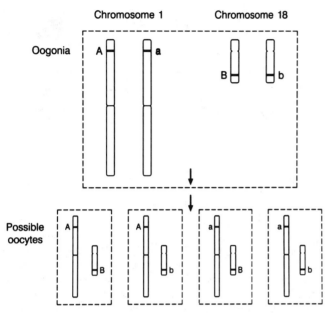

Fig. 16-6. Random segregation of gene locus on chromosome 1 in relation to gene locus on chromosome 18. There is a 50% chance that allele A will segregate with allele B or allele b. These loci are not syntenic and do not demonstrate linkage.

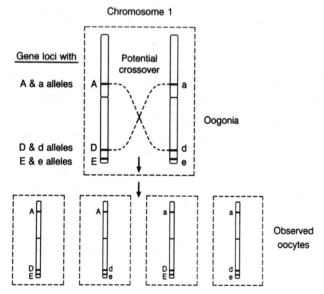

Fig. 16-7. Three gene loci on chromosome 1. Locus with alleles A and a is located at sufficient distance from loci with alleles Dd and Ee that random segregation occurs. However, loci with alleles Dd and Ee always show D and E together or d and e together (not drawn to scale). Loci for Dd and Ee do not show random segregation and thus are linked.

Of course, linkage is not an all-or-none phenomenon. There is the potential for crossover to occur between any two gene loci, and this could happen in 20% of meioses, 2% of meioses, or 0.2% of meioses, for example, depending on the "distance" between them. Although physical distance is correlated with the likelihood of crossover, other factors such as location of the genes adjacent to the chromosome centromere and sex of the individual also influence the likelihood of crossover. Therefore, a measure of the functional likelihood of crossover, a centimorgan (cM), is used to describe the observed recombination rate. Thus, if crossovers occur in 10% of meioses, the loci are said to be 10 cM apart. On average, 1 cM corresponds to approximately 1,000 kilobases of DNA. The degree of linkage of specific genes must be generated from clinical observations in numerous families.

For tests used in clinical practice, it is important to know the frequency of crossovers occurring between the disease gene and the marker gene, because this is one factor that limits the accuracy of the test. If the disease gene and the marker gene are 2 cM apart, it is important for the patient to know that the accuracy will be less than 98%. The use of flanking markers, i.e., markers on both sides of the gene, if available, can help circumvent the problem of undetected crossovers. Although known genes sometimes are used for markers, more commonly DNA segments of unknown function are used for markers. These "anonymous" DNA segments, like genes themselves, can be highly variable in their nucleotide sequence. These normal variations are located extensively throughout the genome and can be recognized by one of many different kinds of bacterial enzymes that cut DNA at specified sites. DNA polymorphisms located within the gene of interest are less likely to show recombination with the mutation site than those located adjacent to the gene (Fig. 16-8).

● The accuracy of linkage-based diagnosis is variable from one disease to another, depending on how tightly the disease gene and marker DNA are linked.

The size of the DNA fragments generated by these cutting enyzmes varies among individuals because of normal variations in our DNA sequences. These different-sized fragments are referred to as restriction fragment length polymorphisms. These can be separated by size by electrophoresing them on a gel. Once separated by size, the DNA fragments can be transferred to a nylon membrane as part of the procedure known as Southern blot analysis.

Southern Blot Procedure

After a patient's DNA has been extracted from peripheral blood lymphocytes, subjected to enyzme cutting, and

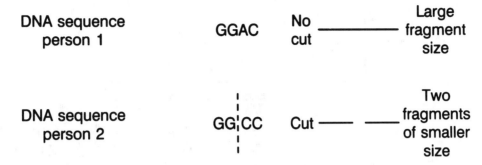

Fig. 16-8. Bacterial restriction enzyme *HAE* III. There are hundreds of types of bacterial enzymes that recognize and cleave specific DNA sequences. Appropriate enzyme that provides most information for DNA markers near disease gene of interest will be selected by the laboratory performing the test. Resulting fragments of differing sizes in different persons are restriction fragment length polymorphisms.

electrophoresed to separate different sizes of DNA fragments, a radioactive probe for the disease gene or for the marker DNA segments is applied and hybridizes to the complementary DNA sequences of interest. The fragments then can be visualized on x-ray film. An example of linkage analysis by Southern blotting in a family with DMD is shown in Figure 16-9.

In addition to linkage analysis, Southern blotting can be used in some cases for direct detection of deletion or duplication types of mutations, or for single-base mutations if the enzyme restriction site is directly altered by the mutation. An example of direct detection of a deletion in a patient with DMD is shown in Figure 16-10.

Polymerase Chain Reaction

Another method of DNA diagnosis that has had great impact on clinical practice is the polymerase chain reaction (PCR). The PCR involves replication of a specific, relatively small segment of DNA in an exponential fashion, so that up to a billion copies are produced. One uses known DNA sequences from within the area of interest, and these known DNA sequences allow creation of synthetic oligonucleotides that serve as primers to hybridize with the patient's DNA sequence to initiate the amplification process (Fig. 16-11).

The multiple copies of the DNA segment that are produced by the PCR then can be identified by various techniques, including direct visualization after gel electrophoresis. This allows detection of mutations in the patient's DNA. For example, the PCR can be used for detection of mutations in specific regions of the dystrophin gene for the diagnosis of DMD and other diseases.

Diseases Amenable to DNA Diagnosis

The number of diseases diagnosable by DNA analysis is increasing as additional disease genes are localized or identified and cloned. Humans are believed to have approximately 100,000 genes; currently, approximately 2,000 genes have been mapped. Diseases for which DNA diagnosis is available are listed in Tables 16-5 through 16-7, but these lists will change rapidly.

Table 16-5.--Autosomal Dominant Diseases Diagnosable by DNA Analysis

Amyloidosis, some forms
Familial adenomatous polyposis coli
Familial hypercholesterolemia (low-density lipoprotein receptor defects)
Huntington disease
Multiple endocrine neoplasia, types I, II, and IIb or III
Myotonic dystrophy
Neurofibromatosis, type 1
Osteogenesis imperfecta, some forms
Polycystic kidney disease
Retinoblastoma
Von Willebrand disease

Furthermore, when diagnosis is based on linkage, some families may not have the necessary number of family members available to allow for informative DNA analysis. Other families may have a sufficient number of family members who are willing to participate but the DNA markers in common usage to study their specific gene defect may not be informative in a particular family. An example of this problem is shown in Figure 16-12.

Thus, the physician who encounters a clinical situation for the first time which may be amenable to DNA-based diagnosis should discuss the testing procedure and

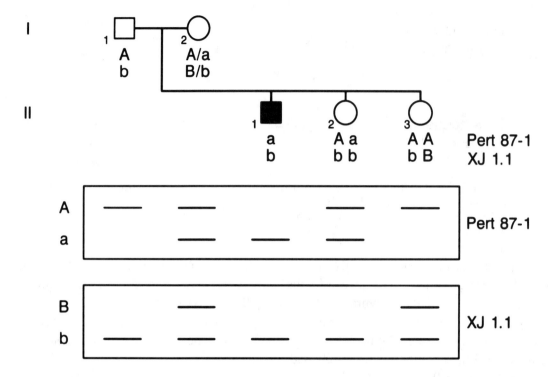

Fig. 16-9. Representation of a family segregating for Duchenne muscular dystrophy and data for two probes that detect restriction fragment-length polymorphism, Pert 87-1 and XJ 1.1. Bottom half of figure represents Southern blot analysis of these two probes with arbitrary designation of alleles A/a for Pert 87-1 and B/b for XJ 1.1. Square, normal male; circle, female; shaded symbol, affected individual. Sister II.3 of affected male II.1 inherited Ab haplotype from her father and AB haplotype from her mother. Because her brother has ab haplotype, it can be predicted that she is not a carrier and her fetus is not at increased risk. Although sister II.2 did inherit the ab haplotype, it cannot be determined with certainty that she is a carrier because it is not known whether the mutation arose in brother or whether mother is a carrier. Sister II.2 could elect prenatal diagnosis, with the realization that males who inherit the ab haplotype might be affected or unaffected, whereas those who inherit the Ab haplotype would most likely be unaffected.

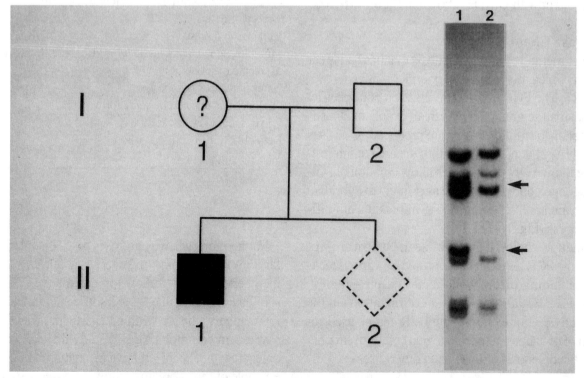

Fig. 16-10. Mother (I.1) of this patient (II.1) with sporadic Duchenne muscular dystrophy wanted to know whether she was a carrier or whether a new mutation had occurred in her son, because of her concern for the risk for future children. Southern blot analysis detected a deletion in her son (II.1) (lane 2 as compared to control in lane 1). By densitometry, the mother seemed to have less than the expected amount of DNA (not shown) corresponding to her son's deletion. Thus, she was diagnosed as being a carrier for the dystrophy and can be offered specific prenatal diagnosis. If no deletion had been detectable (by various methods), then her carrier status could not have been determined.

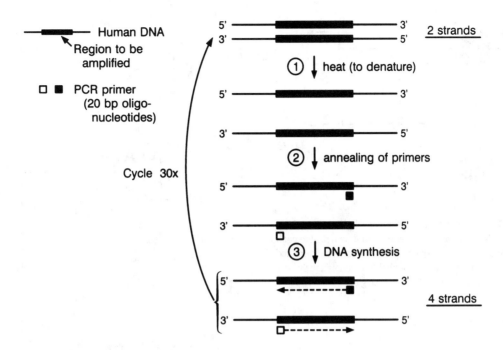

Fig. 16-11. PCR is used to make multiple copies of short segment of DNA of interest. DNA from patient is denatured to single-stranded DNA in the presence of oligonucleotide primers. DNA sequences of these primers are made to specification to anneal with DNA sequences on both sides of DNA segment of interest. DNA between these primers is then synthesized, and entire process can be repeated automatically.

Table 16-6.--Autosomal Recessive Diseases Diagnosable by DNA Analysis	Table 16-7.--X-Linked Diseases Diagnosable by DNA Analysis
α_1-Antitrypsin deficiency	Alport syndrome (X-linked form)
Carbamoyl-phosphate synthetase I deficiency	Duchenne or Becker muscular dystrophy
Congenital adrenal hyperplasia (21-hydroxylase deficiency)	Fragile X-linked mental retardation
Cystic fibrosis	Friedreich ataxia
Gaucher disease	Hemophilia A and B
Glycogen storage disease, type VI (Hers disease)	Lesch-Nyhan syndrome
Phenylketonuria	Ornithine transcarbamoylase deficiency
Sickle cell disease	Wiskott-Aldrich syndrome
Tay-Sachs disease	X-linked ichthyosis
α- and β-Thalassemia	X-linked lymphoproliferative disease

its limitations with the laboratory personnel or a geneticist familiar with the details of the specific disease testing before a detailed discussion of the prenatal diagnosis with the patient. Ideally, these discussions should take place before a woman becomes pregnant. For example, if a woman provides a family history of a brother with DMD and she is deciding whether to have a child, it would be prudent to confirm the diagnosis and get a detailed family history to determine whether prenatal diagnosis seems feasible rather than simply stating that prenatal diagnosis is possible. This woman would be in a difficult situation if she became pregnant while assuming that prenatal diag-

nosis was possible only to find out later that prenatal diagnosis was not possible because her brother was a sporadic case or is deceased and she has no detectable deletion. Parenthetically, deletions can be much more difficult to detect in a woman heterozygous for an X-linked disease than in a hemizygous affected male.

● DNA-based diagnoses cannot be used for all families, even when DNA tests for a specific disease are available.

An example of an X-linked disease has been used throughout this discussion, but the same general princi-

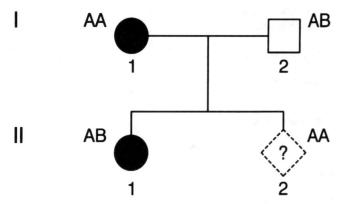

Fig. 16-12. Mother (I.1) and first child (II.1) are affected by autosomal dominant disease. Marker alleles linked to this disease are shown next to each person's symbol. Because mother's genotype is AA, it cannot be determined whether the fetus inherited the chromosome with the A marker and the disease gene or the other A marker without the disease gene. This family is said to be noninformative.

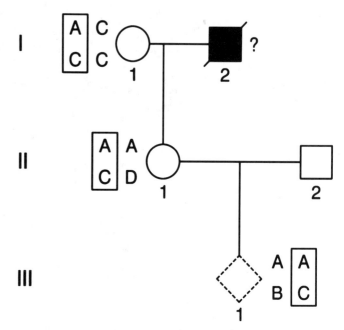

Fig. 16-13. Pregnant woman's father (I.2) died of Huntington disease. It cannot be determined whether mother (II.1) has inherited the gene for Huntington disease, but her fetus has inherited alleles of maternal grandmother (I.2), so it can be predicted that fetus will be unaffected. Woman's status remains uncertain.

ples apply to autosomal dominant and recessive diseases. Prenatal diagnoses of cystic fibrosis, sickle cell disease, and the thalassemias are particularly important because of their high frequency. Virtually all cases of sickle cell disease and most cases of thalassemia can be diagnosed by direct DNA analysis with the PCR without the need for linkage analysis. Direct DNA analysis with the PCR of the phenylalanine 508 mutation, which accounts for approximately 70% of cystic fibrosis mutations, is possible; however, the remaining 30% of mutations are so diverse that more extensive gene testing or linkage analysis is necessary.

Occasionally, linkage analysis can be applied even if the affected family member is deceased or represents a sporadic case. If multiple alleles are analyzed that flank the site of the gene defect, it may be possible to deduce the marker genotype of the deceased person by studying other family members. This type of analysis has been accomplished for DMD, Huntington disease, and familial adenomatous polyposis, as shown in Figure 16-13.

Another potential pitfall in prenatal diagnosis by DNA analysis is genetic heterogeneity. For example, most patients with autosomal dominant polycystic kidney disease have a gene defect linked to markers on chromo-

some 19. However, up to 10% of families have a phenotypically similar disease due to a different, nonallelic genetic mutation that does not show linkage to these markers. Thus, in the minority of families linkage cannot be performed for presymptomatic or prenatal diagnosis; if the family is not recognized to be one of the "unlinked" families, an erroneous diagnosis may be made. There are numerous other examples of this type of genetic heterogeneity, including retinitis pigmentosa, spinocerebellar ataxias, and Charcot-Marie-Tooth disease.

It is anticipated that the rapid advances made in molecular genetics in the past several years will accelerate as the genetic bases of additional diseases are identified and newer techniques for molecular diagnosis become available.

- Genetic heterogeneity can confound DNA linkage studies.

GLOSSARY

Autosome: Chromosome other than sex chromosome.

Chromosome: Long strands of double-stranded DNA that encode genes and that are associated with a protein framework. Normal human has 46 chromosomes per cell.

Deletion: Structural abnormality in which part of a chromosome is missing.

Duplication: Structural abnormality in which an extra copy of part of a chromosome is present.

Gene: A portion of DNA molecule that codes for a specific RNA or protein product.

Hemizygote: A person who has a gene form on one chromosome but no homologous chromosome with a corresponding gene site. The term usually refers to males because they have only one X chromosome.

Heterozygote: A person who has different gene forms at a given site on two homologous chromosomes.

Homozygote: A person who has the same gene forms at a given site on two homologous chromosomes.

Inversion: Structural abnormality characterized by reversal of a segment within the chromosome.

Karyotype: The chromosome complement of an individual person.

Linkage (genetic linkage): Physical proximity of two gene loci on the same chromosome such that segregation is nonrandom.

Phenotype: The observable biochemical or physical characteristics of an individual as determined by genetic material and environment.

Proband: The index patient.

Recurrence: Occurrence of another case of a specific condition in the same family.

Translocation: Structural abnormality characterized by transfer of a piece of one chromosome to another chromosome.

QUESTIONS
(See "Answers" section)

Multiple Choice

1. The risk for a 28-year-old woman to have a child with Down syndrome after having had one child with a 47, XY,+21 karyotype is approximately:
   a. 1 in 800
   b. 2 in 100
   c. 15 in 100
   d. 1 in 4
   e. 1 in 2

2. All of the following are diagnostic criteria for Marfan syndrome except:
   a. Long-limbed body habitus
   b. Aortic root dilatation
   c. Predisposition for venous thrombosis
   d. Ocular lens dislocation
   e. Scoliosis

3. All of the following describe the genetic aspects of myotonic dystrophy except:
   a. Autosomal dominant inheritance
   b. Variable expression
   c. Anticipation
   d. Autosomal recessive inheritance
   e. Trinucleotide repeat expansion

4. For women who carry the gene for an X-linked reces-

sive disease, which one of the following statements is correct?

a. 50% of children will have the disease
b. 50% of daughters will have the disease
c. 50% of sons will have the disease
d. 100% of sons will have the disease
e. 100% of children will have the disease

5. Specific DNA prenatal diagnosis of Duchenne muscular dystrophy for a male fetus can be established in all of the following cases except:
a. Affected brother is deceased; mother has no detectable mutation
b. Affected brother and mother have detectable mutation
c. Affected brother has detectable mutation; mother does not
d. Affected uncle and mother have detectable mutation
e. Affected brother is deceased; mother has detectable mutation

True/False

6. Mutations in mitochondrial DNA:
a. Are paternally inherited
b. Are maternally inherited
c. Are always homoplasmic
d. Always arise as new mutations
e. Always cause disease

7. The following are characteristic of neurofibromatosis type I in some patients:
a. Optic gliomas
b. Café-au-lait macules
c. Pheochromocytoma
d. Renal cancers
e. Pancreatic cancers

CHAPTER 17
GERIATRICS

Darryl S. Chutka, M.D.

DEMOGRAPHICS

The age at which a person becomes elderly is not fixed. People age at different rates and at times, and the chronologic age does not match the physiologic age. The process of aging begins when one is born, and from that time on, a combination of changes takes place--both anatomically and physiologically--that results in the changes of aging. In addition to these changes, various disease states occur and result in further changes in the person. Fortunately, most organs have the reserve capability to handle the changes due to normal aging and many disease states.

The demographics of aging suggest that with time those older than 65 years will represent a larger proportion of our population. Currently, the elderly represent about 12% of our population. If current trends continue, this number is expected to double during the next 40 years. Two important terms to understand are "life expectancy" and "life span." Life expectancy has increased as our culture progresses through time. Currently, life expectancy is about 84 years for women and 80 years for men. This increase is primarily because of improved nutrition, sanitation, and immunizations. Much of the increase in life expectancy is due to the reduction in premature mortality in children and young adults and not to a decrease in the mortality of the elderly. Although life expectancy has shown an increase with time, life span has remained fixed at approximately 100-110 years. More people are living closer to the end of their life span and fewer are dying prematurely. This is known as "rectangularization of the survival curve." The elderly can be divided into three groups: the "young-old" (65-75 years), "middle-old" (75-85 years), and "old-old" (>85 years). The "old-old" is the fastest growing segment of the population.

The sex ratio (M:F) decreases with advancing age. Of the group of people >65 years, there are approximately 75 men for every 100 women. Among those >85 years, there are only 50 men for every 100 women. Over two-thirds of the elderly live in a family setting with their spouse or children. Only 5% of those >65 years reside in a nursing home; although with advancing age, this percentage increases (20% of those >85 years).

- People >65 years represent about 12% of our population.
- Life expectancy has increased primarily because of improved nutrition, sanitation, and immunizations.
- Life expectancy has increased with time; life span has not.
- The "old-old" (>85 years) is the fastest growing segment of the population.
- Only 5% of those >65 years live in a nursing home.

HEALTH CARE FINANCING

The cost of health care for the elderly is substantial. It is estimated that the elderly account for 36% of U.S. health care costs. Those >65 years have 4x the number of physician visits and 4x-5x the length of hospital stays as those <65 years. Most of the health care cost for the elderly is for hospital care (40%). The costs for physician visits (20%) and long-term care (20%) are also substantial. Financing long-term care can be particularly difficult for the elderly. Many assume Medicare will provide coverage when in fact it covers little (2%). Half of all long-term care financing is provided by individual patients or their families. Medical assistance through Medicaid for those in financial need covers 40% of the cost. Long-term care insurance provides only 5% of the cost.

- The elderly account for 36% of U.S. health care costs.
- The elderly have 4x the number of physician visits and 4x-5x the length of hospital stays.
- Most of the financing for long-term care is by private pay. Medicare provides coverage for only 2%.

ASSISTIVE DEVICES

Assistive devices are very important for many of the elderly in allowing them to maintain their independence and mobility. These devices often allow many to live independently and often delay or prevent their being institutionalized. Before recommending an assistive device, one needs to take several factors into account. Patients must accept the fact that they have an impairment and that the assistive device will help. The device must also be affordable, properly fitted, and easy to use.

Walkers and canes are very useful for elderly patients with sensory impairments, weakness or pain of the lower extremities, or problems maintaining balance. Canes can support up to 25% of body weight and are most useful for those with unilateral leg weakness or pain. The cane should be fitted so that the elbow is flexed at a 20°-30° angle. Walkers can support up to 50% of body weight, depending on the type used. Parkinsonian patients often have a tendency to fall backward and do well with walkers that have wheels on the front. Persons with significant upper extremity weakness often benefit most from four-wheeled walkers.

- Assistive devices are important in maintaining independence and mobility.
- Walkers and canes benefit those with unilateral disabilities of the lower extremities or sensory impairments.
- Canes can support up to 25% and walkers 50% of body weight.

VISION CHANGES

A combination of anatomical and physiologic changes related to aging and various disease states that are common in the elderly frequently cause decreased vision. It is estimated that a substantial number of nursing home residents have significant vision loss and that at least 25% are legally blind. The commonest eye problem in the elderly population is presbyopia, causing difficulty with close focus. It is caused by decreased lens flexibility due to continued addition of cells to the lens throughout life. Cataracts also become more common with advancing age; actually they begin forming fairly early in life, but the progression varies from person to person. Chronic open-angle glaucoma produces a slowly progressive loss of peripheral vision that often is not noticed by the patient until a significant amount of vision is lost. Open-angle glaucoma rarely has symptoms until peripheral vision is lost. If this disease is watched for, it can be diagnosed and effectively treated before significant vision loss occurs. Acute angle-closure glaucoma is much less common than chronic open-angle glaucoma; however, patients present to physicians much sooner because of the associated symptoms. In acute angle-closure glaucoma, obstruction to aqueous humor outflow results in a rapid increase in intraocular pressure, producing symptoms of eye pain, blurred vision with halos around lights, and nausea. The pupil dilates and is unresponsive to light. Urgent treatment is needed to prevent vision loss.

The decision to treat a patient with glaucoma is not based solely on the amount of ocular tension. Treatment is started when there is evidence of vision loss or physical evidence of ocular damage, such as cupping of the optic disks. The options for treatment of glaucoma are several. Pilocarpine causes pupillary constriction and opens the trabecular meshwork, resulting in an increase in aqueous humor flow. β-Blockers such as timolol decrease the production of aqueous humor. Epinephrine decreases the production of aqueous humor and increases its flow. Carbonic anhydrase inhibitors act by decreasing the production of aqueous humor. Trabeculoplasty by laser is often performed when the glaucoma cannot be adequately controlled medically. It results in increased aqueous humor outflow.

HEARING CHANGES

Hearing loss, either conductive or sensorineural, is common with increasing age because of a combination of physiologic and environmental effects (e.g., exposure to loud noise). Causes of conductive hearing loss include cerumen impaction, perforation of the tympanic membrane, cholesteatoma, Paget's disease, and otosclerosis. Causes of sensorineural hearing loss include problems with the inner ear or dysfunction of the neurologic components of audition (auditory nerve, brain stem, auditory pathways in the brain). The incidence of hearing loss, especially of high frequencies (presbycusis), increases significantly among persons >65 years. Noise-induced hearing loss produces a similar high-frequency hearing loss. Presbycusis is more complex than simple high-frequency tone loss. The ability to discriminate speech is worse than predicted for the amount of pure tone lost. Patients with presbycusis have the most difficulty in appreciating consonant sounds.

- Hearing loss may be either conductive or sensorineural.
- Presbycusis results in both loss of high frequency tones and loss of sound discrimination.

RHEUMATOLOGIC PROBLEMS

Rheumatologic problems are among the commonest complaints of the elderly. These diseases tend to be chronic and often accumulate with time. Whereas most of these diseases are not life-threatening, they commonly cause an alteration in lifestyle and lead to significant disability. Osteoarthritis is extremely common among the elderly and is present in >80%. It produced joint symptoms that vary with time and the degree of activity. Osteoarthritis usually can be differentiated from rheumatoid arthritis by the medical history and findings on physical examination. Osteoarthritis does not tend to produce systemic symptoms, which are common in rheumatoid arthritis. Joint inflammation, although seen in osteoarthritis, is more pronounced in rheumatoid arthritis. Osteoarthritis and rheumatoid arthritis both are chronic diseases. Patients have variability in their disease activity; however, acute worsening of a specific joint should make a physician suspicious of a superimposed crystalline arthritis (gout or pseudogout) or septic arthritis, both of which are seen occasionally in those with underlying chronic joint disease.

- Osteoarthritis is the commonest rheumatologic disease among the elderly.
- Acute joint symptoms in patients with osteoarthritis or rheumatoid arthritis may represent crystalline or septic arthritis.

Osteoarthritis

Osteoarthritis has a typical radiographic appearance that includes asymmetrical narrowing of the joint space, the presence of osteophytes, subchondral sclerosis, and cystic changes in the bone. Systemic symptoms do not occur. Joint pain is common with joint use and weight-bearing activity. Rest usually provides relief from this pain. Osteoarthritis most commonly involves the hands, especially the distal and proximal interphalangeal joints, knees, and hips. It tends to spare the metacarpophalangeal joints of the hand, wrists, elbows, and ankles.

- Radiographs of osteoarthritis show asymmetrical narrowing of the joint space.

Rheumatoid Arthritis

Rheumatoid arthritis is often found in elderly patients, most commonly as a chronic disease that was acquired earlier in life. It can also develop later in life and usually falls into one of two groups. It may present as typical rheumatoid arthritis with symmetrical distal joint inflammation, positive rheumatoid factor, and a propensity to progress with time. The second form is rather common in the elderly and presents with proximal joint pain and stiffness, very similar to polymyalgia rheumatica; rheumatoid factor is often negative. In contrast to osteoarthritis, rheumatoid arthritis patients have systemic symptoms. Radiographs of joints involved with rheumatoid arthritis characteristically show symmetrical narrowing of the joint space. Elderly patients receive the same therapeutic agents as younger patients: nonsteroidal anti-inflammatory drugs, chloroquine, methotrexate, gold, and low doses of steroids.

- Approximately 10% of the cases of rheumatoid arthritis develop in persons >65 years.
- Radiographs of rheumatoid arthritis show symmetrical narrowing of the joint space.

Crystalline Arthropathy

Crystalline arthropathy is common in the elderly population. Whereas gout tends to be more common in men and involves more distal joints, especially the great toe, pseudogout is more common in women and tends to involve more proximal joints, especially the knee.

Gout is a monoarticular arthritis caused by intra-articular deposition of uric acid crystals. It is associated with the hyperuricemia produced by thiazide diuretics. Gouty attacks may be precipitated by stressful events such as surgery, various severe illnesses, or trauma. Urate crystals are long and needle-like in shape. They are negatively birefringent with polarizing microscopy. Treatment for an acute attack of gout is nonsteroidal anti-inflammatory drugs. Colchicine given orally or intravenously may be used in patients who should not receive nonsteroidal anti-inflammatory drugs. Long-term therapy for gout may include low doses of daily colchicine, allopurinol, or probenecid. Long-term treatment usually is not initiated until after several acute episodes of gout have occurred. Treatment of asymptomatic hyperuricemia is rarely necessary. Treatment is often started when initiating chemotherapy for various hematologic malignancies.

- Gout is a monoarticular arthritis; it is more common in men.
- Gout is associated with use of thiazides.
- The urate crystals are negatively birefringent with polarizing microscopy.

Pseudogout (calcium pyrophosphate deposition disease) is also a monoarticular arthritis that most frequently involves the knee and wrist. As with gout, an acute attack can occur with surgery, trauma, or illness. Radiographs of joints with pseudogout often show linear articular calcification. The calcium pyrophosphate crystals are rectangular in shape and exhibit positive birefringence with polarizing microscopy. Treatment of an acute attack is with nonsteroidal anti-inflammatory drugs or steroids given intra-articularly in the affected joints.

- Pseudogout is a monoarticular arthritis and commonly involves the knee.
- The calcium pyrophosphate crystals are positively birefringent with polarizing microscopy.

Polymyalgia Rheumatica and Temporal Arteritis

Polymyalgia rheumatica and temporal arteritis are diseases that occur more commonly in women than in men and that are seen in persons >50 years old. Patients with polymyalgia rheumatica describe stiffness, aching, and weakness of proximal muscles, especially in the morning. They may also complain of nonspecific malaise, fatigue, and anorexia with weight loss. Low-grade fever may also occur. Although the patients commonly describe weakness, muscle strength is normal when tested. The diagnosis is usually suspected on the basis of the classic history obtained from the patient; no specific laboratory test is diagnostic for the disease. Patients usually have an increased erythrocyte sedimentation rate and, occasionally, mild anemia. The levels of muscle enzymes (creatinine kinase, aspartate aminotransferase) are not increased. The response to treatment is very characteristic and often can be used to support the diagnosis. Treatment with low doses of steroids (prednisone, 15-20 mg/day) results in dramatic improvement in the symptoms, often within 24 hours. After treatment has been initiated, the steroid dose can be gradually tapered, using the patient's clinical response and erythrocyte sedimentation rate as indicators of disease activity.

- Polymyalgia rheumatica is more common in women.
- Although patients complain of weakness, muscle strength is normal.
- Laboratory findings include an increased erythrocyte sedimentation rate and mild anemia.
- Patients respond dramatically to treatment with steroids.

Temporal arteritis develops in about 15% of patients with polymyalgia rheumatica. Systemic symptoms include low-grade fever and fatigue; anorexia with weight loss is common. More than 50% of the patients have unilateral or bilateral headache. Many patients also have scalp and bitemporal tenderness and jaw claudication secondary to facial artery involvement with disease. Vision loss, including unilateral or bilateral visual blurring, visual field loss, diplopia, and blindness, may occur. It is the most worrisome symptom. As with polymyalgia rheumatica, temporal arteritis is usually suspected on the basis of the patient's description of the symptoms. Few findings are documented on physical examination. Some patients have tender, swollen, and/or pulseless temporal arteries. Rarely, bruits may be heard over medium-sized arteries involved with disease. Although there is no diagnostic laboratory test specific for temporal arteritis, almost all patients have significantly increased erythrocyte sedimentation rate, often >100 mm/hour. Mild anemia may also be present. After temporal arteritis is suspected, the diagnosis should be confirmed with temporal artery biopsy; however, treatment should not be withheld pending results of the biopsy. A generous piece (4-5 cm) of the temporal artery should be obtained, initially on the side of the patient's symptoms. If the findings are negative, a similar biopsy should be performed on the contralateral side. The inflammatory changes in the artery may be spotty or confined to a small portion of the artery, occasionally causing difficulty in confirming the diagnosis pathologically. Treatment consists of high doses of steroids (prednisone, 60 mg/day) and may be started before the biopsy sample is obtained, assuming it is to be done in the next 24-48 hours. Prednisone should be tapered by assessing the patient's clinical response to treatment and the erythrocyte sedimentation rate.

- Temporal arteritis develops in about 15% of patients with polymyalgia rheumatica.

- Patients with polymyalgia rheumatica should not have temporal artery biopsies unless they have symptoms of temporal arteritis.
- Temporal arteritis commonly presents with a unilateral or bilateral headache.
- Vision loss is the most worrisome symptom.
- The erythrocyte sedimentation rate is usually increased.

THYROID DISEASE

Most elderly patients with hyperthyroidism present with typical findings; however, a significant minority have somewhat atypical symptoms. Some elderly develop anorexia with weight loss, altered stool frequency (either diarrhea or constipation), or cardiovascular abnormalities, including hypertension, increased angina, myocardial ischemia, congestive heart failure, and atrial fibrillation. Other symptoms that may develop include apathy, depression, tremor, and myopathy. Ophthalmopathy, lid lag, and increased perspiration are relatively uncommon in the elderly. The development of a goiter with hyperthyroidism is noted in only about 60% of the elderly. The commonest cause of hyperthyroidism in the elderly is Graves' disease. Radioiodine therapy is the safest and most economical treatment for hyperthyroidism in elderly patients.

- Hyperthyroidism associated with goiter is uncommon in the elderly.
- Graves' disease is the commonest form of hyperthyroidism in the elderly.

The diagnosis of hypothyroidism in elderly patients is often made by finding low levels of total (serum) thyroxine (T_4) or an increased sTSH on laboratory testing of asymptomatic patients. The common symptoms of hypothyroidism are vague (constipation, cold intolerance, dry skin) and often attributed to the many "symptoms of aging." Almost all the patients have hypothyroidism due to primary thyroid failure rather than to pituitary or hypothalamic insufficiency. The commonest cause of hypothyroidism in the elderly is Hashimoto's thyroiditis. Treatment should begin with a low dose of thyroid supplement (25-50 µg/day), increasing the dose by 25 µg every 3-4 weeks. Patients with coronary artery disease should receive an even lower starting dose and more gradual dose increments. It takes approximately 6-8 weeks for a given dose of thyroid supplement to equilibrate. The sTSH should be checked after about 8 weeks to assess whether the supplement dose is correct. Thyroid hormone requirements decrease with advancing age, most require 75-100 µg/day; however, some elderly require as little as 50 µg/day. Subclinical hypothyroidism can be found in approximately 15% of the elderly. These patients are clinically euthyroid and have a low-normal total (serum) T_4 level and a slightly elevated sTSH level. Whether to treat these patients is a matter of controversy. Most physicians do not treat unless symptoms of hypothyroidism develop or the sTSH level continues to increase.

- Hypothyroidism is often difficult to detect in the elderly.
- Most cases of hypothyroidism are due to primary thyroid failure rather than to pituitary or hypothalamic disease.
- Hashimoto's thyroiditis is the commonest cause of hypothyroidism.
- Very low starting doses and very gradual dose increments should be used in hypothyroid patients with coronary artery disease.

Euthyroid sick syndrome is common in elderly hospitalized patients. They are clinically euthyroid, but with low serum levels of T_3 and T_4, and a low-normal level of sTSH. Laboratory values tend to return to normal after the patient has recovered from the illness. The syndrome may be caused by a decreased amount of thyroid-binding protein and a substance that inhibits T_4 binding.

DEMENTIA

Approximately 10%-20% of the population >65 years old have some degree of dementia. The number increases with advancing age and has been reported to be as high as 50% in those >90 years. Up to 30% of elderly patients referred for memory impairment have a treatable condition, most often depression. The commonest form of irreversible dementia is Alzheimer's disease (50%-70%), followed by multi-infarct dementia (15%-25%). Reversible dementias include depression (pseudodementia), drug toxicity, hypothyroidism, vitamin B_{12} deficiency, normal-pressure hydrocephalus, subdural hematoma, and neurosyphilis. Dementia involves considerably more than loss of memory. Other cognitive functions that are affected include judgment, abstract thinking, attention, ability to learn new material, and, eventually, recognition and production of speech. Personality changes frequently accompany dementia, and patients may have paranoia and delusional thoughts and show agitation and aggressiveness.

- 10%-20% of persons >65 years old have some form of dementia (50% of those >90 years).
- 30% of the elderly referred for memory impairment have a treatable condition, often depression.
- The commonest cause of irreversible dementia is Alzheimer's disease.

The diagnosis of Alzheimer's disease cannot be confirmed until postmortem examination; no laboratory test, including computed tomographic (CT) scan of the head, is specific for the disease. The evaluation of a demented patient involves establishing the existence of cognitive impairment and performing baseline tests to follow future deterioration. Evaluation is also important to rule out reversible dementias. None of the medications commonly used in the management of demented patients dramatically improves cognitive function. Medications such as sedative-hypnotics or major tranquilizers frequently help resolve some of the abnormal behaviors (agitation, delusions, hallucinations, etc.), but they often worsen memory and orientation. Major tranquilizers may also cause movement disorders (tardive dyskinesia), thus contributing to falls.

- No laboratory test is specific for diagnosis of Alzheimer's disease.
- Evaluation is important for ruling out reversible dementias.
- Medications commonly used in the management of dementia do not improve memory or orientation.

The evaluation of a patient with dementia includes taking a medical history and performing a physical (including neurologic) examination and general laboratory tests: thyroid function test, syphilis serology, and determination of vitamin B_{12} level. Also, CT scanning of the head is done to rule out mass lesions in the central nervous system (not to check for cerebral atrophy). There is no association between the presence of cerebral atrophy and dementia. Psychometric evaluation is also useful, especially when following progress of the patient. Electroencephalography (EEG) and lumbar puncture are performed only in unusual circumstances and are rarely necessary.

The neuropathologic findings in Alzheimer's disease include neuronal plaques (dystrophic neurons) and neu-rofibrillary tangles (neurons containing abnormal microtubule protein). However, these neuropathologic findings are not specific to Alzheimer's disease but are also seen in lesser amounts in patients who do not have dementia.

Other dementias are: 1) dementia associated with Parkinson's disease--up to 40% of parkinsonian patients develop dementia; 2) Pick's disease, which has an earlier onset than Alzheimer's disease and is associated with atrophy of the frontal and temporal lobes; 3) Creutzfeldt-Jakob disease, a rapidly progressive dementia with associated myoclonic jerks; 4) Huntington's disease, which is autosomal dominant and has early onset of symptoms (usually in 30s-40s); the patients eventually have choreiform movements; and 5) AIDS dementia, which affects up to 50% of people with AIDS.

Delirium is an acute confusional disorder that is frequently mistaken for dementia. It is associated with a decreased level of consciousness, hallucinations, and delusions. Its several causes include 1) many common medical illnesses (urinary tract infection, sepsis, pneumonia, etc.) in patients with limited organ reserve function or organ failure; 2) drugs, including sedative-hypnotics, anticholinergic agents, nonsteroidal anti-inflammatory drugs, β-blockers, and antipsychotic agents; 3) metabolic disturbances, such as hyper- or hypoglycemia and hypercalcemia; 4) hypoxia; and 5) hypotension. Patients with delirium frequently have a preexisting mild (often unrecognized) dementia.

PULMONARY CHANGES

Pulmonary function declines with advancing age, likely because of a combination of the normal anatomical and physiologic changes of aging, injury from various environmental exposures (tobacco, air pollution), and disease states that affect the lung. Changes in the shape of the lungs contribute to the changes in pulmonary physiology. The apical-to-base length of the lungs decreases but the anterior-to-posterior length increases with age. The bronchioles and alveolar ducts increase in diameter, decreasing alveolar surface area. The aged lungs also have reduced compliance because of decreased lung elasticity. These anatomical and physiological changes result in a decrease in efficiency of air exchange, reduced air flow rates, and alterations in lung volumes. The changes that occur include decreases in mucociliary clearance, vital capacity, 1-second forced expiratory volume, maximal breathing capacity, and diffusing capacity. The lung residual volume and alveolar-arterial oxygen gradient increase with age.

- Pulmonary function declines with age because of a combination of changes due to aging, environmental exposure, and disease.
- Changes in lung shape contribute to changes in pulmonary physiology.

RESPIRATORY DISEASE

Pneumonia is one of the top 10 causes of death among the elderly and is the cause of death in 15% of nursing home residents. The bacterial organisms that cause pneumonia change with advancing age. Elderly patients have increased numbers of gram-negative bacteria as part of their normal oral flora. They also have an increased likelihood of aspirating their oral secretions, which probably contribute to the increased incidence of pneumonias caused by gram-negative and anaerobic bacteria. The likely cause of a pneumonia depends on the setting in which the patient acquired the infection. Overall, *Streptococcus pneumoniae* is the commonest etiologic organism, but *Haemophilus influenzae*, other gram-negative bacteria, and anaerobes are more common among those in nursing homes and hospitals. Treatment for the pneumonia must reflect the most likely etiologic agent.

Appropriate treatment for pneumonia acquired in an outpatient setting or nursing home would be a second-generation cephalosporin. Many of these infections are due to *S. pneumoniae*. After this diagnosis is established, either by blood culture or sputum culture, the treatment can be switched to penicillin given intravenously, although a small percentage of organisms are now penicillin-resistant. For pneumonia acquired in a hospital, additional coverage is needed for gram-negative and atypical bacteria. Acceptable treatment includes a third-generation cephalosporin with erythromycin given intravenously. Because of the high mortality of pneumonia, many believe that elderly nursing home patients should be hospitalized to initiate treatment. If the patient's condition is not very toxic and appears stable, pneumonia can be treated in the nursing home if the patient is watched closely.

- Pneumonia is among the top 10 causes of death among the elderly.
- Elderly patients have a greater number of gram-negative bacteria as part of their normal oral flora.
- Aspiration is more likely to occur in elderly persons.

- Treatment must reflect the likely causal organisms.

Tuberculosis, after declining in frequency for many years, is increasing in frequency. It is more common with advancing age. Most cases of tuberculosis are due to reactivation of a previous infection rather than being newly acquired disease. It is thought that about 4% of patients with a positive PPD (tuberculin test) eventually develop active tuberculosis. Tuberculosis is suspected on the basis of clinical findings, which at times may be subtle and include fatigue, anorexia with weight loss, and cough. Chest radiography may also help in suspecting the disease. Confirmation of the disease requires evaluation of sputum or gastric washings for the presence of acid-fast organisms. Cultures may take up to 6 weeks to become positive. Patients should start receiving treatment with three antituberculin drugs, including isoniazid (INH), ethambutol, and rifampin, until the results of sensitivity testing are known. If the tuberculosis organism is not a resistant strain, the patient may receive treatment with two drugs, usually INH and rifampin. Drug-induced hepatotoxicity is common with advancing age and must be watched for carefully.

On admission to a nursing home, the patient should be administered a 2-stage PPD. If the initial PPD is negative, a second PPD should be applied 2 weeks later. Up to 15% of additional positive reactors are identified with this method. In those with a positive PPD, chest radiography should be performed. If the findings are negative and the patient is asymptomatic, no treatment should be initiated unless it can be shown that the patient has converted to a positive PPD within the last 2 years. If the chest radiographic findings are abnormal, sputum and gastric washings should be obtained and cultured. Patients should receive treatment if their PPD is positive and they have had exposure to another patient with active tuberculosis. Treatment options include the following: 1) isoniazid (300 mg/day) and rifampin (600 mg/day) for 9 months; and 2) isoniazid (300 mg/day), rifampin (600 mg/day), and pyrazinamide (30 mg/kg daily) for 2 months, then isoniazid and rifampin for another 4 months.

Chemoprophylaxis for persons >35 years consists of isoniazid for 6-12 months. It is indicated if the PPD is >10 mm and if 1) there has been conversion to a positive PPD within the last 2 years, 2) the patient is an intravenous drug user, or 3) the patient has a coexisting medical problem (silicosis, previous gastrectomy, weight loss >10% of ideal body weight, chronic obstructive pulmonary disease, chronic renal failure, or diabetes mellitus) or is immunocompromised (including patients taking steroids).

- Tuberculosis is increasing in frequency.
- Most tuberculosis in the elderly is due to reactivation of disease rather than to new infection.
- Patients admitted to a nursing home should have a 2-stage PPD test.

IMMUNIZATIONS

Pneumococcal pneumonia vaccine is effective against 23 of the commonest strains of *S. pneumoniae*, which account for 80% of the strains that commonly cause pneumonia. Because of decreasing effectiveness, revaccination is now being advised after 6 years. The influenza vaccine is changed on a yearly basis, depending on the prevalent strain. It should be given annually to high-risk persons, those >65 years old, and those in frequent close contact with the elderly. It takes about 2-3 weeks to develop immunity to influenza after receiving the vaccine. Any of the elderly who are unvaccinated during an influenza epidemic should be given amantadine or rimantadine. Tetanus immunization consists of an initial series of three injections, then a booster every 10 years.

OSTEOPOROSIS

Osteoporosis and its complications are extremely common problems among the elderly. Hip fractures and vertebral compression fractures are common causes of morbidity and mortality. Peak bone density is achieved at about age 30, with men having a higher bone density than women at all ages. After age 30, bone density gradually declines throughout the rest of the lifetime. Loss of estrogen, either because of an operation (oophorectomy) or menopause, causes a more rapid decline in bone density. The diagnosis of osteoporosis is usually made clinically. The following help establish the diagnosis: 1) presence of multiple risk factors (advanced age, female, Caucasian, low calcium intake through much of one's lifetime, thin build, steroid use, tobacco use, alcohol use, Northern European ancestry, prolonged inactivity, and positive family history for osteoporosis); 2) ruling out secondary causes (glucocorticoid excess, hypogonadism, hyperthyroidism, hyperparathyroidism, osteomalacia, myeloma); 3) physical examination findings (loss of height, increased thoracic kyphosis); and 4) radiographic findings of osteope-

nia or vertebral compression fractures. Bone density can be measured by several techniques (single- or dual-photon absorptiometry, quantitative CT scan). Bone density can be used to assess the risk of fractures, to check progression of disease, and to assess response to treatment. No simple laboratory tests are available that can confirm the diagnosis of osteoporosis.

The treatment of osteoporosis is disappointing and, currently, is best aimed at prevention. Premenopausal women require 1,000 mg/day of elemental calcium; postmenopausal women, 1,500 mg/day. Currently, the most effective treatment is adequate calcium intake, weight-bearing exercise, adequate vitamin D (600-800 IU/day), and estrogen replacement therapy, especially when initiated shortly after menopause. Progestin should be used with estrogen to reduce the risk of endometrial cancer, unless the patient has had a hysterectomy. Although calcitonin increases bone density, it may not reduce the risk of bone fractures. Its significant cost also limits its use.

- Osteoporosis is common with advancing age as bone density declines.
- Hip and vertebral compression fractures are common causes of morbidity and mortality.
- No simple laboratory tests are available to confirm the diagnosis of osteoporosis.

OSTEOMALACIA

Osteomalacia is caused by a deficiency of vitamin D. It may be due to inadequate intake of vitamin D, lack of exposure to the sun, or malabsorption. Osteomalacia results in defective bone mineralization. Radiographically, it appears osteopenic and can look like osteoporosis. Laboratory findings include decreased levels of calcium, phosphorus, $1,25(OH)_2D_3$, and increased levels of alkaline phosphatase.

URINARY INCONTINENCE

Urinary incontinence is quite common among the elderly, involving at least 15% of those living independently and about 50% of those in institutions. It causes multiple medical, social, and economic complications and is a common reason for nursing home placement. Incontinence may lead to urinary tract infection, skin breakdown, social isolation, and depression. Understanding urinary incontinence requires a knowledge of the anatomy of the urinary tract and of the physiology of micturition. Failure to appreciate this information results in inaccurate diagnosis and ineffective treatment.

Anatomy

Sympathetic nerves innervate the internal sphincter and the detrusor muscle of the bladder. Stimulation of these nerves produces increased internal sphincter tone and relaxation of the detrusor muscle. Stimulation of the parasympathetic nerves that innervate the detrusor muscle causes it to contract. Somatic (pudendal) nerves innervate the external sphincter. Their stimulation produces increased tone in the external sphincter.

The detrusor muscle consists of three muscular layers. Its functions include urine storage (relaxed detrusor) and urine emptying (contracted detrusor). The internal sphincter is a smooth muscle under involuntary control. The external sphincter is striated muscle under voluntary control. It contracts in response to transient increases in intra-abdominal pressure (cough, sneeze, etc.). The external sphincter rapidly fatigues and has little importance in maintaining continence.

The brain causes stimulation of the sympathetic nerves when urine storage is desired and stimulation of the parasympathetic nerves when bladder emptying is desired. The spinal cord transmits sensory (ascending) signals to the brain and motor (descending) signals to the bladder.

Effects of Age

The changes in the urinary system that occur with aging do not cause urinary incontinence; incontinence is not a normal change due to aging. However, the changes that occur with aging can contribute to the problem of incontinence. These changes include smaller bladder capacity, early contractions of the detrusor muscle, decreased ability to suppress detrusor muscle contractions and postpone urination, and increased nocturnal urine production.

Medications Affecting Urination and Continence

Medications that can affect urination and continence include 1) potent diuretics, which cause brisk filling of the bladder; 2) anticholinergic agents that can impair detrusor muscle contraction; 3) sedative-hypnotics that may cause confusion; 4) narcotics that impair detrusor muscle contraction; 5) α-adrenergic agonists that increase internal sphincter tone; 6) α-adrenergic antagonists that decrease internal sphincter tone; and 7) calcium channel blockers that decrease detrusor muscle tone.

Established Incontinence

Patients are more likely to have incontinence treated effectively if it is of recent onset. Although established incontinence is more difficult to treat, it can be managed with significant benefit to the patient. Overactivity of the detrusor muscle is a common cause of established incontinence, accounting for 40%-70% of cases. It causes early detrusor contractions at low bladder volumes. Symptoms include urinary frequency and urgency, with losses of small-to-moderate urine volumes. Nocturia often occurs. Detrusor overactivity is seen with central nervous system disease (mass lesions, Parkinson's disease, stroke) or bladder irritation (infection, benign prostatic hyperplasia, fecal impaction, atrophic urethritis).

- Detrusor overactivity is common in the elderly, accounting for 40%-70% of cases of urinary incontinence.
- Detrusor overactivity may be seen with central nervous system disease or disorders that cause bladder irritation.

Overflow incontinence is uncommon. It is seen with outflow obstruction (benign prostatic hyperplasia, tumor) or detrusor underactivity/hypotonic bladder (autonomic neuropathy). Symptoms are low urine flow and frequent urinary dribbling.

- Overflow obstruction is uncommon.
- It is seen with urinary outflow obstruction or a hypotonic detrusor.

Outlet incompetence (stress incontinence) is common in women and rare in men (unless sphincter damage has occurred). It is caused by pelvic floor laxity and lack of bladder support, resulting in small losses of urine with transient increases in intra-abdominal pressure (cough, sneeze, etc.).

- Outlet incompetence is common in women and rare in men.

Functional incontinence is the inability of normally continent patients to reach toilet facilities in time. Often, it is due to medications and some limitation of mobility (restraints, hemiparesis).

Evaluation of Incontinence

Evaluation of incontinence includes taking a medical history and performing a physical examination and several simple laboratory tests. The history should include determining: the amount of urine lost, precipitating factors, whether symptoms of obstruction exist, and mobility status. Also, document symptoms of neurologic disease, associated disease states, menstrual status and parity, and medications used.

Physical examination of the abdomen should evaluate bladder distension and possible abdominal masses. In examining the pelvis, check for uterine, bladder, or rectal prolapse; atrophic vaginitis; and pelvic masses. The rectal examination should document any masses, fecal impaction, sphincter tone, and prostate enlargement or nodules. A neurologic examination should be performed to search for disease of the central nervous system or of the spinal, autonomic, or peripheral nerves.

Laboratory tests that should be conducted include 1) urinalysis and urine culture to check for infection, pyuria, and hematuria; 2) blood urea nitrogen and creatinine determination to assess renal function; 3) calcium and glucose measurements to assess polyuric states; 4) occasionally, intravenous pyelography and/or renal ultrasonography may be performed to check for hydronephrosis, which may occur with chronic bladder outlet obstruction; and 5) postvoid residual bladder volume to estimate the degree of bladder emptying. Urodynamics usually are not necessary to establish the diagnosis of incontinence. Often, the urodynamic test results do not fit the clinical picture. Many elderly with no incontinence have abnormal urodynamics, and many with incontinence have normal urodynamics. These studies are often indicated when patients have medically confusing histories or more than one type of incontinence. Cystometry measures bladder volume and pressure and can be used to detect uninhibited detrusor muscle contractions, lack of bladder contractions, and bladder sensation. Voiding cystourethrography measures the urethrovesical angle and residual urine volume. Uroflow measures urinary flow rate, and electromyography evaluates the external sphincter and detects detrusor-sphincter dyssynergia.

Treatment of Incontinence

The treatment of detrusor overactivity is aimed at suppressing the early detrusor contractions. Behavioral training is often successful. Also, medications that inhibit parasympathetic stimulation of the bladder muscle are effective. The anticholinergic drugs that are used are oxybutynin, flavoxate, and imipramine. Calcium channel blockers, used as smooth muscle relaxants, may also be tried.

The treatment of overflow incontinence is aimed at providing complete bladder drainage from a bladder that either is not adequately contracting or has significant outflow obstruction. When treating a hypotonic bladder, medications work by increasing the tone of the detrusor muscle (cholinergic agonists). Treatment of obstruction includes operation (transurethral resection of the prostate) and use of α-adrenergic antagonists (prazosin, terazosin, or doxazocin), which decrease the tone of the internal sphincter. An external urinary catheter is of little benefit, because it does not drain the bladder. An indwelling catheter or intermittent catheterization is occasionally necessary.

The treatment of outlet incompetence is aimed at restoring the normal posterior urethrovesical angle of 90°-100° either surgically or medically, by increasing the tone of the internal sphincter medically (α-adrenergic agonists). Hormonal therapy helps restore the mucosa of the urethra, increasing its resistance. The drugs that are used include α-adrenergic agonists (pseudoephedrine, phenylpropanolamine, and imipramine). Topical estrogens are the hormonal agents used. Other treatments include operation and pelvic floor (Kegel) exercises.

Urologic Consultation

In most elderly patients, the diagnosis of urinary incontinence can be established without urodynamic studies or evaluation by a urologist. The following conditions indicate the need for urologic evaluation: high postvoid residual urine volume, outflow obstruction, significant uterine or bladder prolapse, abnormal findings on prostate examination, recurrent urinary tract infections, hematuria, unknown diagnosis, or failure to improve with treatment.

Use of Urinary Catheters

External (condom) catheters have a slight risk of infection and problems with long-term use. They have minimal benefit in overflow incontinence. Intermittent catheterization has a small risk of infection with each insertion. It is useful with temporary incontinence. Use postvoid residual volumes as a guide in determining the frequency of catheterization. Intermittent catheterization has limited use in chronic incontinence of nursing home patients due to expense and in those with limited manual dexterity who will self-catheterize. Indwelling catheters eventually cause significant bacteriuria. The chronic use of suppressive antibiotics is not recommended because it results in infections caused by resistant organisms. Antibiotic treatment should be reserved for symptomatic infections only.

USE OF MEDICATIONS IN THE ELDERLY

More than 30% of all prescriptions are written for persons >65 years old. Medications are a common cause of iatrogenic disease in the elderly, and they tend to cause more frequent and more severe adverse effects than they do in younger patients. Thus, it is important to know about dosing elderly patients and about selecting drugs that are better tolerated by the elderly. Changes occur in the pharmacokinetics and pharmacodynamics in the elderly and affect how medications are handled.

- More than 30% of all prescriptions are written for persons >65 years old.
- Changes occur in the pharmacokinetics and pharmacodynamics in the elderly.

Pharmacokinetic changes with aging include changes in drug absorption, distribution, metabolism, and excretion. Drug absorption is decreased in the elderly because of villous atrophy in the small bowel (resulting in a reduced surface area for the absorption of medications), reduced blood supply to small bowel, and decreased gastric acidity (some medications require an acid medium for adequate absorption). Although these mechanisms have little clinical importance, they may slightly decrease the rate of medication absorption. Drug distribution does play a major role in altered pharmacokinetics. With advancing age, adipose stores increase, which results in an increased volume of distribution for fat-soluble drugs. Water stores decrease, resulting in a smaller volume of distribution for water-soluble drugs. Plasma proteins decrease in many elderly persons, resulting in less protein-bound (inactive) drug and more nonprotein-bound (active) drug. Drug metabolism is reduced because of a decrease in the liver metabolism of drugs, which is due to decreases in liver size and weight, blood supply, number of functioning hepatocytes, and microsomal enzyme activity. Drug clearance also decreases with age. Renal function tends to decline with age, although the variability among persons is great. This is due to a reduction in glomerular filtration rate and renal plasma flow (up to 30%). The serum level of creatinine is not a good measure of renal function in the elderly, because creatinine is a product of muscle breakdown. The elderly have decreased lean body mass with advancing age; therefore, less creatinine is produced. Thus, it is possible to have a normal serum level of creatinine in an elderly patient who has as much as a 30% reduction in renal function. An estimation of the creatinine clearance (CrCl) can be calculated by the following formula:

$$CrCl \ (mL/min) = \frac{(140 - age) \times weight \ (kg)}{72 \times serum \ creatinine \ (mg/dL)}$$

Pharmacodynamic changes also occur with aging and have an effect on the action of medications. These changes involve age-related alterations in receptor responsiveness, i.e., receptors for various drugs may be more or less responsive to different medications. Receptors are more responsive in relation to benzodiazepines and opiates and less responsive with regard to adrenergic agonists and antagonists. More or less of the drug is needed to achieve the same effect as in younger patients.

Adverse drug effects are common in the elderly, frequently causing serious complications. Elderly patients often have limited organ reserve function and are unable to respond as younger persons can to the adverse effect.

SLEEP DISORDERS IN THE ELDERLY

Changes occur in sleep with aging. Some of these changes are due to the normal physiology of aging, others to associated disease states, and some to specific sleep disorders that are more common among the elderly.

Sleep Physiology

Sleep stages 1 and 2 represent the light stages of sleep. The percentage of sleep spent in these stages increases with age. As a result, the elderly are aroused more easily by noise, light, or various disease symptoms (e.g., pain) and have an increased number of nighttime awakenings. Sleep stages 3 and 4 are considered the deep stages of sleep. Deep-stage sleep decreases with age; thus, the elderly have a less restful sleep. Rapid eye movement (REM) sleep also decreases with age, with fewer and shorter REM periods. Sleep latency (the time required to fall asleep) increases with age, making it increasingly difficult for elderly persons to fall asleep.

Sleep Disorders

Some sleep disorders increase in frequency with age. Nocturnal myoclonus is the unilateral or bilateral twitching of the legs that occur after a person falls asleep. Although the patient is usually not aware of these twitchings, the bed partner is. Nocturnal myoclonus results in multiple nocturnal awakenings, often interrupting and shortening deep-stage sleep.

Restless leg syndrome, another sleep disorder, is the

uncomfortable sensation in the legs that occurs before a person falls asleep. This sensation is relieved by moving the legs or by walking. It results in increased sleep latency. Restless leg syndrome is often associated with nocturnal myoclonus.

Sleep apnea has three forms: obstructive, central, and mixed. The obstructive form is relatively common in the elderly. Sleep apnea causes multiple (can be hundreds of episodes) nighttime awakenings. It is more common in males (30:1) and obese persons. In addition to interfering with sleep, it may produce pulmonary and systemic hypertension. Currently, the most effective treatment is nasal continuous positive airway pressure. Sleep apnea is made worse with the use of sedative-hypnotic medications.

Medications for Insomnia

Medications for insomnia are useful for short-term use only. They are not beneficial for chronic insomnia and may increase apneic spells in those with sleep apnea. If a sedative-hypnotic medication is to be used in an elderly patient, short-acting or intermediate-acting drugs are advised (Table 17-1). Drugs with longer half-lives tend to be more lipid-soluble, and they often have active metabolites. They may accumulate when used on a nightly basis and produce daytime somnolence. Drugs with shorter half-lives tend to be less lipid-soluble and to have minimally active or inactive metabolites. Any of the sedative-hypnotic medications may worsen confusion and/or memory, especially in patients with some underlying cognitive impairment.

Table 17-1.--Sedative-Hypnotic Drugs for Elderly Patients

Long-acting	Intermediate-acting	Short-acting
Diazepam	Temazepam	Oxazepam
Flurazepam	Lorazepam	Triazolam
Clonazepam	Estazolam	
Chlordiazepoxide		

QUESTIONS
(See "Answers" section)

Multiple Choice

1. An elderly demented man is brought to the clinic for evaluation of urinary incontinence. Because of his dementia, the medical history elicited from the patient is unreliable. The nursing home staff reports that the patient is chronically wet. On examination, the prostate is 2x-3x symmetrically enlarged. The next step in the evaluation of this patient's incontinence should be:
   a. Postvoid urinary residual volume
   b. Cystometric studies
   c. Fluoroscopy of the urethra while the patient is voiding
   d. Electromyography of the internal urinary sphincter
   e. Empiric trial of oxybutynin

2. Which of the following statements is *not* true about the demographics of the elderly?
   a. Life span has not significantly increased in the last 50 years
   b. About 5% of persons older than 65 reside in a nursing home
   c. Medicare covers the costs of about 1/2 of all the elderly in a nursing home
   d. Persons older than 85 are the fastest growing segment of the population
   e. Life expectancy has significantly increased in the last 100 years

3. Which of the following statements about glaucoma is *not* true?
   a. Symptoms develop insidiously with open-angle glaucoma
   b. Presenting symptoms of open-angle glaucoma are often loss of peripheral vision

c. Eye pain is more characteristic of closed-angle glaucoma

d. Anticholinergic medications may precipitate an attack of closed-angle glaucoma

e. Pilocarpine, by dilating the pupil and increasing aqueous drainage, is an effective treatment for glaucoma

4. Which of the following is true of temporal arteritis in the elderly?

a. A normal erythrocyte sedimentation rate does not rule out temporal arteritis

b. A small biopsy is adequate because pathologic changes found in the artery are diffuse

c. Treatment with high doses of steroids should be withheld until after temporal artery biopsy is performed.

d. Because temporal arteritis can coexist with polymyalgia rheumatica, temporal artery biopsy should be performed in patients with polymyalgia rheumatica

e. Temporal arteritis is more common in men than in women

5. Which of the following is true about patients with Alzheimer's disease?

a. They have neurofibrillary tangles that are not found in other types of dementia

b. Head CT scan should be performed to look for cerebral atrophy

c. There is a characteristic loss of dopamine, a central nervous system neurotransmitter

d. Patients may improve with antidepressant treatment

e. No evidence of genetic transmission has been found

True/False

6. Benzodiazepines, antihistamines, and alcohol usually decrease sleep latency.

7. Cystometry is most useful for establishing the diagnosis in urinary stress incontinence.

NOTES

CHAPTER 18

HEMATOLOGY

Thomas M. Habermann, M.D.

ANEMIAS

Evaluation of Anemias

A pragmatic approach to anemias is critical.

The complete blood cell count (CBC) is the most commonly ordered blood test. The measured values of the CBC include the total counts for red blood cells (RBCs), platelets, and white blood cells (WBCs) and the volumes of RBCs, platelets, WBCs, and hemoglobin. The calculated values include the hematocrit, mean corpuscular volume, mean corpuscular hemoglobin, mean corpuscular hemoglobin concentration, and red cell distribution width. These values help to differentiate thalassemia from iron deficiency anemia (Tables 18-1 and 18-2).

In a nonreferral practice, iron deficiency anemia is the cause of up to 90% of all hypochromic-microcytic anemias (color plate 18-1). Of the remaining 10%, the thalassemic syndromes are more common than the other rare forms of the hypochromic-microcytic anemias. The anemia of chronic disease, however, is variable, depending on whether the setting is inpatient or outpatient and whether a community-based or a referral center. The

Table 18-1.--Differentiation of Microcytic Anemias on Basis of Blood Values

| | Type of anemia | |
	Thalassemia	Iron-deficiency
RBC count	$>5.0 \times 10^{12}/L$	$<5.0 \times 10^{12}/L$
Red cell distribution width	<16	>16
MCV-RBC-(5 x Hb-3.4)	Negative	Positive

Hb, hemoglobin; MCV, mean corpuscular volume; RBC, red blood cell.

Table 18-2. Comparison of Hypochromic-Microcytic Anemias

Disease state	MCV	Red blood cells	% transferrin saturation	Ferritin, µg/L	Marrow iron
Iron deficiency anemia	Decreased	Decreased	<15	Low	Absent
Anemia of chronic disease	Normal or decreased	Decreased	<15 or normal	Normal or increased	Normal or increased
Thalassemia minor	Decreased	Usually increased	Normal	Normal or increased	Normal

MCV, mean corpuscular volume.

Modified from Savage RA: Cost-effective laboratory diagnosis of microcytic anemias of complex origin. ASCP check sample H84-10(H-153). By permission of American Society of Clinical Pathologists.

CBC and other laboratory values provide further information for differentiating these entities (Table 18-2). These studies often provide the major clues to the type of anemia. One must always be concerned about blood loss. The evaluation of stool for blood loss is essential in the initial work-up and may also provide clues to a combined anemia. A laboratory approach to microcytic anemias is outlined in Figures 18-1 and 18-2.

Erythropoietin

Erythropoietin is a glycoprotein that acts through specific receptors on RBC precursors. It is produced primarily in the kidneys, although a small amount is produced in the liver. There are no preformed stores. The gene is located on chromosome 7. Recombinant human erythropoietin is identical to native erythropoietin, and antibodies have not been reported. There is an inverse relationship between the circulating concentration of erythropoietin and the hemoglobin or hematocrit value. Regulation is linked to an oxygen sensor, not peripheral catabolism. Serum erythropoietin levels are not influenced by age or sex. The higher hemoglobin value in men seems to be due to androgenic steroids. Erythropoietin levels are low, never absent, in chronic renal failure, polycythemia rubra vera, rheuma-

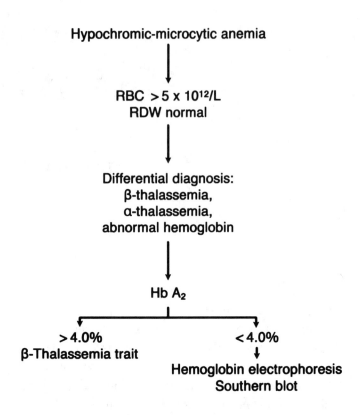

Fig. 18-1. Algorithm for approach to diagnosis of hypochromic-microcytic anemias with an increased total red blood cell (RBC) count. Hb, hemoglobin. (Modified from Savage RA: Cost-effective laboratory diagnosis of microcytic anemias of complex origin. ASCP check sample H84-10(H-153). By permission of American Society of Clinical Pathologists.)

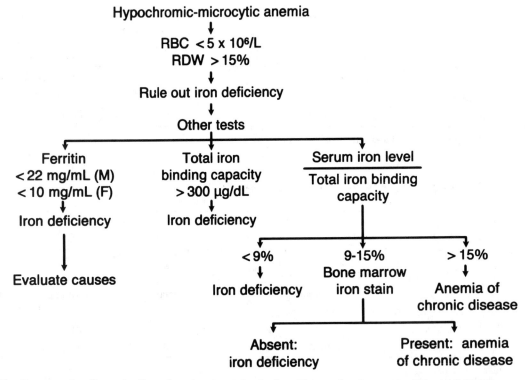

Fig. 18-2. Algorithm for approach to diagnosis of hypochromic-microcytic anemias with normal or decreased red blood cell (RBC) counts. RDW, red cell distribution width. (Modified from Savage RA: Cost-effective laboratory diagnosis of microcytic anemias of complex origin. ASCP check sample H84-10(H-153). By permission of American Society of Clinical Pathologists.)

toid arthritis, and human immunodeficiency virus (HIV) infection. Zidovudine can increase the serum erythropoietin value. High erythropoietin levels are present in marrow hypofunction (pure RBC aplasia), deficiency states (iron deficiency), tumor, autonomous production (hepatocellular carcinoma), and high altitude.

Anemias of cancer may respond to erythropoietin, particularly multiple myeloma, lymphoma, and solid tumors; it is also useful after bone marrow transplantation. Erythropoietin has been used with efficacious results in the autologous blood donor setting, especially in women and in persons who donate >4 units.

- Erythropoietin: a glycoprotein produced in kidney; it acts through specific receptors on RBC precursors.
- Gene is located on chromosome 7.
- Its level is low in renal failure, polycythemia rubra vera, rheumatoid arthritis, and HIV infection.
- Its level is high in pure RBC aplasia, iron deficiency, tumors, high altitude.

In evaluating patients with erythrocytosis, a normal or low erythropoietin value associated with an increased RBC mass does not prove autonomous erythropoiesis.

Hemolytic Anemia

First, it is essential to determine the presence of hemolytic anemia as manifested by laboratory evidence of an increased rate of erythropoiesis and laboratory evidence of increased RBC destruction. Second, specific causes should be sought. Hemolytic anemias may be Coombs-negative or Coombs-positive.

The initial evaluation includes a history and physical examination, CBC, morphology, and reticulocyte count. Conditions found during the work-up that can be mistaken for hemolysis include hemorrhage, recovery from deficiency states, metastatic carcinoma, and myoglobinuria. Studies of a family's hematologic history are important.

Inheritance Patterns

Membrane defects and unstable hemoglobin diseases are autosomal dominant. Most enzymopathies are autosomal recessive. The commonest enzymopathy, glucose-6-phosphate dehydrogenase deficiency, is sex-linked, as is phosphoglycerate kinase deficiency.

- Membrane defects and unstable hemoglobin diseases are autosomal dominant.

- Most enzymopathies are autosomal recessive.
- Glucose-6-phosphate dehydrogenase deficiency is sex-linked.

Laboratory Findings

The CBC abnormalities in autoimmune hemolytic anemia include anemia, thrombocytosis, or thrombocytopenia. The presence of autoimmune hemolytic anemia and autoimmune thrombocytopenia is called Evans's syndrome. The reticulocyte value is usually persistently elevated, reflecting an enhanced bone marrow response. The bilirubin value is usually 1 to 5 µg/dL and almost exclusively unconjugated or indirect. The direct bilirubin should be less than 15% of total if the bilirubin value is >4 µg/dL. The haptoglobin concentration is usually low with no compensatory increased rate of synthesis, and the lactate dehydrogenase level is elevated.

Peripheral Smear (Differential Diagnosis)

Spherocytes (color plate 18-2) are associated with hereditary spherocytosis, burns, *Clostridium* infections, autoimmune hemolytic anemia, and hypophosphatemia. Basophilic stippling occurs in lead poisoning, β-thalassemia, and arsenic poisoning. Hypochromia occurs in thalassemia and lead poisoning. Target cells are present in thalassemia, hemoglobin C and E, obstructive jaundice or hepatitis, lecithin-cholesterol-acyltransferase deficiency, and the splenectomy state (color plate 18-3). Agglutination is present in cold agglutinin disease (color plate 18-4). Stomatocytes are associated with acute alcoholism and are also found as an artifact. Acanthocytes (color plate 18-5) are present in chronic liver disease, abetalipoproteinemia, malabsorption, and anorexia nervosa. Heinz bodies are present in glucose-6-phosphate dehydrogenase deficiency.

Schistocytes: Microangiopathic Hemolytic Anemia

In microangiopathic hemolytic anemia, the RBCs are fragmented and deformed in the peripheral blood (color plate 18-6). The fragmentation is caused by fibrin deposits in small blood vessels leading to mechanical hemolysis. The results of the Coombs' test are negative. Patients with microangiopathic hemolytic anemia are often thrombocytopenic.

Microangiopathic hemolytic anemia is associated with thrombotic thrombocytopenic purpura, hemolytic uremic syndrome, malignant hypertension, pulmonary hypertension, acute glomerulonephritis, acute renal failure, renal allograft rejection, preeclampsia, eclampsia, disseminated intravascular coagulopathy, collagen vascular diseases, scleroderma, systemic lupus erythematosus, Wegener's syndrome, periarteritis nodosa, carcinomatosis, small gastric carcinomas, hemangiomas, and Kasabach-Merritt syndrome and as a toxic effect of mitomycin C.

Differential Diagnosis of Intravascular Hemolysis

The differential diagnosis includes transfusion reactions from ABO antibodies, microangiopathic hemolytic anemia, paroxysmal nocturnal hemoglobinuria, paroxysmal cold hemoglobinuria, autoimmune hemolytic anemia (uncommon), cold agglutinin syndrome, immune complex drug-induced hemolytic anemia, infections (including falciparum malaria and clostridial sepsis), and glucose-6-phosphate dehydrogenase deficiency.

- Most hemolysis is extravascular.

In intravascular hemolysis, hemoglobin is released into the plasma. It rapidly combines with haptoglobin, which transports it to the liver. When haptoglobin is depleted, hemoglobinemia results, and plasma turns pink-red in color at concentrations of 50-100 mg/dL.

Hemoglobinuria occurs when the plasma hemoglobin is >25 mg/100 mL. The urine may become pink, red, brown, or black. Other causes of red urine include beets, phenazopyridine (Pyridium), porphyrinuria, and myoglobinuria. Hemosiderinuria is the result of desquamation of renal tubular cells.

Coombs-Positive Hemolytic Anemia

Positive results with Coombs' test indicates the presence of C3 and/or IgG on RBCs. Twenty percent to 80% of warm antibody autoimmune hemolytic anemias are secondary. The Coombs' test gives positive results in 8%-15% of all hospitalized patients, and studies reveal no cause in 95% of these patients. Hemolytic transfusion reactions and drug-related causes are important causes of a positive Coombs' reaction.

- Coombs' test: detects presence of C3 and/or IgG on RBCs.
- The cause of positive findings on Coombs' test is unknown in 95% of hospitalized patients.
- Transfusion-related and drug-related causes are important causes of positive Coombs' reaction.

Drug-Induced Hemolytic Anemia (Mechanisms)

Autoantibody mechanism (methyldopa)--This is dose-related, and about 0.3%-0.8% of patients develop hemolysis. Hemolysis occurs in 18 weeks to 4 years. The direct Coombs' test becomes positive in 3-6 months and is IgG in high titer. There is no anamnestic response to rechallenge. Discontinuation of use of the drug usually leads to a rapid reversal in hemolysis. The mechanism of action is related to an altered cellular immune system, with a block in the activation of suppressor T cells. Other drugs with a similar mechanism known to cause autoimmune hemolytic anemia include procainamide, ibuprofen, and cimetidine.

Drug-adsorption (hapten) immunohemolytic anemia (penicillin)--This complication requires high doses of drug for >7 days. The onset is subacute at 7-10 days. A high titer of penicillin antibody is always present in the serum. A positive Coombs' test develops in 3% of patients and is related to dose in that at 2 million units per day 30% of patients are positive and at 10 million units per day, 100% of patients are positive. A penicillin allergy is not necessarily present. Drug-absorption hemolytic anemia may be fatal if not detected early. Other drugs, including cephalosporins, tetracycline, quinidine, and cisplatin, may cause autoimmune hemolytic anemia by the same mechanism.

Immune-complex mechanism (innocent bystander) (stibophen)--An antidrug antibody forms first and reacts with the drug to form an immune complex. The antidrug antibody complex is then absorbed on the RBCs. The cell-bound complex may activate complement, causing intravascular hemolysis. The Coombs' test is positive because of the presence of complement on the RBC surface. Clinically, a small quantity of drug is sufficient to cause autoimmune hemolytic anemia if there is previous exposure. Acute intravascular hemolysis with hemoglobinemia and hemoglobinuria is the usual clinical course. Drugs implicated in this type of autoimmune hemolytic anemia include quinidine, quinine, phenacetin, acetaminophen, aminosalicylate (PAS), isoniazid (INH), streptomycin, rifampin, methadone, probenecid, insulin, sulfonylureas, hydralazine, hydrochlorothiazide, sulfa drugs, triamterene, and melphalan. Immune hemolytic anemia and renal failure are seen in patients taking captopril, hydrochlorothiazide, rifampin, dipyrone, and mitomycin C.

- Autoantibody mechanism: methyldopa.
- Drug-adsorption mechanism: penicillin.

- Immune-complex mechanism: stibophen, quinine, quinidine.
- Some drugs produce autoimmune hemolytic anemia by more than one mechanism.

The treatment of warm autoimmune hemolytic anemia includes the following. The first general principle is to treat the underlying disease and discontinue the use of drugs that have been implicated in hemolysis. If the patient is clinically stable, do not transfuse blood. Avoid transfusion in patients with autoimmune hemolytic anemia. If the patient is symptomatic and studies show improvement in symptoms if the hemoglobin is >8 g/dL, transfuse with packed RBCs only if angina, cardiac decompression, or neurologic symptoms (e.g., lethargy, weakness, confusion, or obtundation) are present. If transfusion is required, then transfuse with the most compatible RBCs by crossmatch with type-specific ABO and Rh blood. The major risk of transfusion is the formation of autoantibodies to foreign RBC antigens by previous transfusions and pregnancies.

If steroids are given, the dose of prednisone should be 60-80 mg/day. Most patients respond in 7 days. If the patient has a relapse during tapering of the drug, return to the previous dose. About 50% of patients with idiopathic autoimmune hemolytic anemia require other therapy. Splenectomy is required in about 60% of cases. Immunosuppressive drugs such as cyclophosphamide (60 mg/m^2 per day) or azathioprine (80 mg/m^2 per day) are the next line of therapy.

Cold Agglutinin Syndrome (Primary Cold Agglutinin Disease)

Cold agglutinin syndrome is characterized by the presence of agglutination, hemolytic anemia, a positive Coombs' test response, chronic anemia, and a "monotonous" prognosis. Autoantibodies are maximally reactive at low temperatures. The degree of hemolysis depends on the thermal amplitude: the higher the titer, the more likely to bind complement. The clinical signs and symptoms are related to small vessel occlusion and include acrocyanosis of the ears, tip of the nose, toes, and fingers. Hepatosplenomegaly is uncommon. This should be differentiated from Raynaud's phenomenon (Table 18-3).

Table 18-3.--Comparison of Cold Agglutinin Syndrome and Raynaud's Phenomenon

	Raynaud's phenomenon	Cold agglutinin syndrome
Skin color	White to blue to red	Dusky blue, then normal or blanch
Area affected	One or two fingers	All digits equally
Complication		Gangrene may occur

The peripheral blood smear shows agglutination of RBCs that disappears if prepared at 37°C (color plate 18-4). Agglutinated RBCs clump together. In rouleaux, the cells stack up on one another (color plate 18-7). The anemia is mild to moderate, and the Coombs' test is positive. The cold agglutinin titer is >1:1,000. Therapy includes avoidance of the cold. Steroids are less effective in cold than in warm autoimmune hemolytic anemia. Splenectomy is generally ineffective. Some patients may respond to immunosuppressive drugs such as cyclophosphamide or chlorambucil. Plasma exchange is not very effective but should be considered if the patient is acutely ill, because IgM is intravascular.

- Cold agglutinin syndrome: agglutination and hemolytic anemia.
- Acrocyanosis of ears, tip of nose, toes, fingers; differentiate from Raynaud's phenomenon.
- Positive Coombs' test response and cold agglutinin titer >1:1,000.

Immunology of Cold Agglutinins

An IgM antibody exhibits a reversible thermal-dependent equilibrium reaction with RBCs and is favored at lower temperatures. A monoclonal kappa protein is seen in cold agglutinin syndrome, chronic lymphocytic leukemia, multiple myeloma, lymphoma, and Waldenström's macroglobulinemia. In secondary diseases, there is a polyclonal light chain reaction with a high thermal cold agglutinin of anti-I specificity (*Mycoplasma pneumoniae*) or a high thermal amplitude cold agglutinin of anti-i specificity (infectious mononucleosis, cytomegalovirus, and lymphoma) are identified.

Mycoplasma pneumoniae (anti-I)--In patients with

Mycoplasma pneumoniae, 50% have cold agglutinins >1:64, most have splenomegaly, and acrocyanosis is unusual. The course of this complication generally resolves in 2-3 weeks, but fatalities have been reported. Treatment includes keeping the patient warm and treating the infection with tetracycline or erythromycin.

Infectious mononucleosis (anti-i)--Of patients with infectious mononucleosis, 40%-50% have cold agglutinins and 3% have autoimmune hemolytic anemia. The onset occurs by 13 days in 67% of patients. The duration of hemolysis is <1 month in 75% of patients and 1-2 months in 25%. Hepatosplenomegaly is present in 71% of patients. Steroids are of distinct value in treating this disorder, as may be splenectomy.

Paroxysmal Cold Hemoglobinuria (Complement-Mediated Lysis)

Paroxysmal cold hemoglobinuria is the least common cause of autoimmune hemolytic anemia. Results of the Donath-Landsteiner test are positive. This condition can be idiopathic or secondary. The secondary causes include syphilis (congenital and late), mononucleosis, mycoplasma, chicken pox, mumps, and measles. Measles is the commonest secondary cause. Clinical manifestations include shaking chills, fever, malaise, abdominal pain, back pain, and leg pain. There is rapid and severe anemia. The prognosis is good. This condition resolves after the infection clears. Treatment includes protection from the cold, treatment of the underlying disease, and possibly a short course of steroids.

Coombs-Negative Hemolytic Anemias

The differential diagnosis includes the enzymopathies, glucose-6-phosphate dehydrogenase deficiency, pyruvate kinase deficiency, paroxysmal nocturnal hemoglobinuria, hereditary spherocytosis, and thrombotic thrombocytopenic purpura.

Glucose-6-Phosphate Dehydrogenase Deficiency

This is the commonest RBC enzyme deficiency. It is inherited on the X chromosome and is sex-linked. All enzymopathies are autosomal recessive except glucose-6-phosphate dehydrogenase and phosphoglycerate kinase, which are sex-linked. In males, it is present in 12% of blacks, 20%-32% of Greeks, and 0.4% of Italians. In females, one X chromosome is inactivated, and the gene is present on both, so the activity ranges from 0%-100% with a mosaic population. Patients with falciparum malaria have a selective advantage because of the production

of parasite-encoded glucose-6-phosphate dehydrogenase. The oxidation of hemoglobin leads to the formation of methemoglobin, and sulfhemoglobin may be a product, with precipitation, condensation, and attachment of the denatured portion to the inside of the membrane-forming Heinz bodies. The normal enzyme has a half-life of 62 days, but reticulocytes have a half-life of 124 days and aged cells have a half-life of 31 days. Therefore, in an acute hemolytic state, the glucose-6-phosphate level may be within normal limits. There is individual variability to oxidant stress. It is not possible to stimulate the enzyme with methylene blue or ascorbic acid to counteract the formation of methemoglobin; these may actually exacerbate the anemia.

- Glucose-6-phosphate dehydrogenase deficiency: commonest RBC enzyme deficiency; inherited on X chromosome.
- Falciparum malaria provides some protection.
- More common in Italian men than in black men than in Caucasian men
- Half-life: normal, 62 days; reticulocytes, 124 days; and aged cells, 31 days.

In the steady state, there is no anemia or RBC defect. There is an increased risk of hemolysis in patients with concurrent renal or hepatic disease, viral and bacterial infections, diabetic acidosis, and low levels of blood glucose. Even a mild infection can produce hemolytic anemia, and this is more common than drug provocation. The organisms commonly associated with this complication are *Salmonella*, *Escherichia coli*, pneumococcus, *Rickettsia*, and viral hepatitis. Favism is seen only in Caucasians and not in blacks.

- No anemia or RBC defect in the steady state.

Drugs commonly causing hemolytic anemia in glucose-6-phosphate dehydrogenase deficiency include antimalarial agents (primaquine, chloroquine), dapsone, sulfonamides (sulfanilamide, sulfamethoxazole, sulfapyridine, sulfasalazine), nitrofurantoin, diazoxide, and nitrites (which are derived from nitrates from nitroglycerin, fertilizer-contaminating home wells, and amyl nitrate).

- Important to look for cause, particularly drugs.

Abnormal laboratory findings include intravascular hemolysis, methemoglobinemia, and methemalbuminenia (highly specific for intravascular hemolysis). The presence of Heinz bodies on supravital staining is a good screening test, but the absence of these bodies does not rule out the diagnosis. Reticulocytosis rarely masks the deficiency in Caucasians but it may in blacks and heterozygous females. The glucose-6-phosphate dehydrogenase assay is the definitive test. Treatment includes treating the underlying infection and withdrawing use of the offending drug.

- Heinz bodies on blood smear (supravital stain).
- Treat underlying infections and withdraw offending drugs.

Other Enzymopathies

About 35 distinct enzymopathies have been identified, and most of them are accepted as an etiologic basis for RBC dysfunction. Two deficiency states comprise the largest number: glucose-6-phosphate dehydrogenase and pyruvate kinase. With the exception of glucose-6-phosphate dehydrogenase deficiency, potentially symptomatic enzymopathies are uncommon. Treatment is supportive and empirical. Other enzymopathies include unstable hemoglobins, glucose phosphate isomerase, pyrimidine 5'-nucleotidase, and triosephosphate isomerase deficiencies. In a study on a referral population, only 35% of patients who were referred for an enzyme deficiency work-up had an identifiable enzyme deficiency.

Paroxysmal Nocturnal Hemoglobinuria

Paroxysmal nocturnal hemoglobinuria is a chronic disease caused by an unidentifiable RBC defect. Patients with this condition have a median survival of 10 years. It is a clonal disorder in which blood cells are unusually sensitive to activated complement and are lysed. Lysis is complement-mediated. Hemolysis occurs at night because this is when people become more acidotic. The disorder is characterized by abnormal pluripotent stem cells, reticulocytopenia, leukopenia, or thrombocytopenia due to lysis by complement. Normal and abnormal cells occur simultaneously in most patients. A distinct class of membrane proteins is selectively deleted from the plasma membranes of maturing cells. Defects that affect cells in paroxysmal nocturnal hemoglobinuria are related to the omission of membrane lipid phosphotidylinositol membrane proteins. This involves deficiencies in the surface molecules that normally regulate activation of C3B and C5-9 in the complement cascade. There is a decrease in a membrane protein that regulates

the alternate complement pathway on normal blood cells, decay-accelerating factor. Also, the activity of red blood cell acetylcholinesterase is decreased.

Clinically, the disorder is characterized by a chronic hemolytic anemia with hemoglobinuria and hemoglobinemia (intravascular hemolysis). Venous thrombosis of the portal system, brain, and extremities is associated with 50% of the deaths in paroxysmal nocturnal hemoglobinuria. Episodes of severe pain in the abdomen and back in conjunction with painful or difficult swallowing may occur.

Complications include acute nonlymphocytic leukemia in 5%-10% of patients (paroxysmal nocturnal hemoglobinuria clone disappears), aplastic anemia (association of aplastic anemia, splenomegaly, and relative reticulocytosis suggests diagnosis), venous thrombosis (Budd-Chiari syndrome is the major cause of death). Budd-Chiari syndrome is manifested by abdominal pain, tender hepatomegaly, nausea, vomiting, fever, and increased levels of lactate dehydrogenase, serum glutamic-oxaloacetic transaminase, gamma-glutamyltransferase, and conjugated bilirubin. Hepatic venography is important in making the diagnosis. Treatment includes emergent heparinization, a long-term course of anticoagulation, and fibrinolytic therapy.

Diagnosis--The sucrose hemolysis test can give false-positive results but is a good inexpensive screening test. The Ham test acid hemolysis test is the best confirmatory test.

Treatment--Iron therapy: a burst of erythropoiesis can be seen if the patient is iron deficient; however, in most cases, iron may be given safely. Androgen therapy stimulates bone marrow and is of most benefit if the bone marrow is hypoplastic. Prednisone (alternate-day therapy, 15-40 mg) may inhibit activation of complement by the alternate pathway. Prednisone is of no benefit if the bone marrow is hypoplastic or there is mild hemolysis. Discontinue treatment with steroids if no effect occurs in 6 weeks. Transfusions: Initially, transfuse with packed RBCs. If complicated by hemolysis, washed or frozen RBCs should be given. A hemolytic crisis may be initiated by infections. Treatment may include steroids, transfusion, and hydration to prevent renal failure. For venous thrombosis, the treatment of choice is heparin, which may activate alternate pathway of complement. Painful episodes are managed with narcotics and rehydration. Bone marrow transplantation is indicated in severe aplastic anemia. Antithymocyte globulin is effective in the management of paroxysmal nocturnal hemoglobinuria.

- Paroxysmal nocturnal hemoglobinuria: a chronic disease caused by an unidentifiable RBC defect.
- Venous thrombosis is associated with 50% of deaths.
- Intravascular hemolysis with hemoglobinuria and hemoglobinemia.
- Leukemia occurs in 5%-10%; aplastic anemia.
- Diagnosis: Ham test and sucrose hemolysis test.

Hereditary Spherocytosis

Hereditary spherocytosis is an autosomal dominant disorder in which splenomegaly is invariably present. It is caused by an underlying defect in the RBC membrane cytoskeleton caused by a partial deficiency in one or more of the components called spectrin and band 4.1. Osmotic fragility of RBCs is increased. The clinical features include jaundice, splenomegaly, negative results with Coombs' test, spherocytes, and increased osmotic fragility. Gallstones are present in 43%-85% of patients. Treatment is splenectomy, which invariably causes cessation of hemolysis. It should be performed after the first decade of life.

- Hereditary spherocytosis: autosomal dominant as well as sporadic.
- Splenomegaly occurs in most patients; cholelithiasis in 43%-85%.
- Other features: negative results with Coombs' test; increased osmotic fragility.
- Treatment: splenectomy after first decade of life.

Thrombotic Thrombocytopenic Purpura

Thrombotic thrombocytopenic purpura is a syndrome rather than a disease. Classically, it is characterized by the pentad of anemia, thrombocytopenia, neurologic signs, fever, and renal abnormalities. The anemia is normochromic-normocytic with microangiopathic hemolytic features (color plate 18-6). The Coombs' test gives negative results. Prothrombin time, activated partial thromboplastin time, and fibrinogen are normal. The cause of this syndrome is unknown in more than 90% of patients. It is related to pregnancy and use of oral contraceptives.

Clinically, thrombocytopenia is associated with bleeding in 96% of cases, petechiae and purpura, retinal bleeding, hematuria, gingival bleeding, melena, menorrhagia, hematemesis, and hemoptysis. Neurologic signs consist of remittent and frequent changes, including headache, coma, mental changes, paresis, seizure/coma, aphasia, syncope, visual symptoms, dysarthria, vertigo, agitation,

confusion, and delirium. Renal abnormalities include a creatinine level of >1.5 in less than 20% of cases. Azotemia is an unfavorable prognostic sign. An abnormal urinary sediment with proteinuria, hematuria, pyuria, or casts was present in 82% in one series.

The pathologic findings are characterized by widespread intraluminal hyaline vascular occlusions with platelet aggregates and fibrin with no inflammatory changes in terminal arterioles or capillaries in virtually any organ. The preferred biopsy site is the bone marrow. Other sites to consider for biopsy are the gingiva, skin, petechial spot, muscle, and lymph nodes.

The treatment of choice is plasmapheresis with the replacement of fresh frozen plasma (plasma exchange). Other ancillary treatments include dipyridamole (400-600 mg/day), aspirin (with a dose from 300 mg twice a week to 600-1,200 mg/day), and prednisone (dose of 60 mg/kg per day). The overall response rate to therapy is 80%-90%.

- Thrombotic thrombocytopenic purpura: the pentad of anemia, fever, thrombocytopenia, neurologic signs, and renal abnormalities.
- Cause is unknown; exclude oral contraceptives and pregnancy as etiologic factors.
- Features: Coombs' test gives negative results, microangiopathy, normal prothrombin time, activated partial thromboplastin time, and fibrinogen.

Adult Hemolytic Uremic Syndrome

Adult hemolytic uremic syndrome is characterized by microangiopathic hemolytic anemia (anemia and thrombocytopenia) with a creatinine level >3 mg/dL. There is no fever or neurologic signs. The pathologic findings are similar to those in thrombotic thrombocytopenic purpura but are limited to only the kidneys. It is often preceded by an acute infective process. There is a much higher morbidity and mortality rate in adults, and adult hemolytic uremic syndrome is best managed as thrombotic thrombocytopenic purpura is in adults.

Sickle Cell Anemia

Sickle cell anemia is the commonest heritable hematologic disease affecting humans. The gene must be inherited from both parents. It occurs in black Africans and rarely in Caucasians. About 8% of blacks carry the sickle cell gene, with the disease occurring in 1/625 of them. There is a selective advantage from *Plasmodium falciparum* malaria, with preferential sickling of only the parasitized cells. Hemoglobin S is different from hemoglobin A in the substitution of valine for glutamic acid at the sixth position, resulting in abnormalities in polymerization (or gelation) with deoxygenation that leads to sickling. The end result of the polymerization is a permanently altered membrane protein. Two-thirds of the RBCs are removed by extravascular mechanisms.

Sickling is promoted by low oxygen tension, low pH, increased 2,3-diphosphoglycerate, high cellular concentration hemoglobins, loss of cell water, hemoglobin C, hemoglobin D, and HbO-ARAB. Sickling is retarded by hemoglobin A, hemoglobin F (at least 30%), hemoglobin J, and α-thalassemia.

Symptoms are not present unless the patient is older than 6 months. Vaso-occlusive disease develops between the ages of 12 months and 6 years. Acute crises are due to recurrent obstruction of the microcirculation by intravascular sickling. Laboratory testing is not helpful. Atypical symptoms should suggest pneumonia, pulmonary infarct, acute pyelonephritis, or cholecystitis.

Bone and joint crises: bone and joint symptoms include gnawing pain and swelling of the elbows and knees. Radiographs may show bone infarcts and periostitis, but these do not appear until symptoms subside. Infarcts and periostitis may be documented with bone scans. Abdominal crises: small infarcts of mesentery and abdominal viscera with symptoms of 4-5 days' duration. This is a nonsurgical problem if bowel sounds are present.

Central nervous system crises: children and young adults are more susceptible. Children have infarcts, and adults characteristically have hemorrhages. Do not perform angiographic procedures unless the patient has been prepared with RBCs. The therapy for these crises is immediate exchange transfusion. Chronic transfusion therapy is indicated in this complication to maintain hemoglobin S <30%, because the risk of recurrent episodes is >50%.

Pulmonary crises: acute chest syndrome accounts for 20% of deaths. Clinical aspects include fever, chest pain, tachypnea, increased WBC count, and pulmonary infarcts. Age makes a difference in cause. In children, infected segments enhance local sickling, so sickling is a secondary phenomenon. The causative organisms include pneumococcus, *Mycoplasma, Haemophilus, Salmonella,* and *Escherichia coli.* In adults, sickling tends to be a primary event, with no signs of infection.

Aplastic crises: usually follow a febrile illness, with disappearance of reticulocytes and normoblasts. They last 5-10 days. Hemolytic crises: may occur in patients with concomitant glucose-6-phosphate dehydrogenase deficiency, hereditary spherocytosis, and mycoplasmal pneumonia.

Infectious crises are the most frequent cause of death of patients younger than 5 years. The organisms include *Streptococcus pneumoniae* of the blood and spinal fluid (70% of patients). Normally, 80% of the cases of meningitis are caused by *Haemophilus influenzae* in this age group. At ages older than 5 years, gram-negative bacteria predominate, with osteomyelitis caused by *Staphylococcus,* pneumococcus, and *Salmonella.* The causes of infections/infectious crises include decreased IgM, defective alternate pathway, deficiency phagocytosis-promoting peptide tuftsin, and impaired splenic function. The challenge with *Streptococcus pneumoniae* is not followed by appropriate opsonin production.

Chronic manifestations--There is a progressive lag in growth and development after the first decade of life and a chronic destruction of bone and joints, with ischemia and infarction of the spongiosa. The vertebrae become fish-mouthed. Avascular necrosis is common in multiple joints. Ocular manifestations include stasis and occlusion of small vessels that is nonproliferative or proliferative. They may require laser photocoagulation. Cardiovascular manifestations include cardiomegaly, flow murmurs, and a pansystolic murmur with click that mimics mitral regurgitation. Restrictive lung disease may develop. Hepatobiliary manifestations include hepatomegaly with the pathologic features of distended sinusoids, periportal fibrosis, and hemosiderin pigment. Marked hyperbilirubinemia may be due to hepatitis, intrahepatic sickling, choledocholithiasis, or coexistent glucose-6-phosphate dehydrogenase deficiency. There is an increased incidence of pigmented gallstones in 30%-60% of adults, with symptoms in 10%-15%. Renal manifestations include papillary necrosis, hyposthenuria by age 6-12 months (disruption of countercurrent multiplier system, nocturia, enuresis), hematuria (ulcer in renal pelvis, urate stones), nephrotic syndrome secondary to fecal segmental glomerulonephropathy, tubular damage secondary to small infarcts, and priapism. Leg ulcers may occur.

In pregnancy, there is no increase in disease manifestations, but there is an increase in maternal mortality of 20% and fetal mortality of 20%. Early complications of pregnancy include thrombophlebitis, pyelonephritis, and hematuria. Late complications include major infarcts of the lung, kidney, and brain; toxemia; congestive heart failure; and postpartum endometritis. In the U.S., 31% of the patients die by age 14. To live beyond age 40 is unusual.

Laboratory findings include anemia (range 5.5-9.5 g/dL), sickled cells, cigar cells, ovalocytes, targets, basophilic stippling, polychromatophilia, reticulocytes (8%-12%), and hyposplenia with Howell-Jolly bodies. A persistent increase in the WBC count of 12,000-15,000 is characteristic. On hemoglobin electrophoresis, hemoglobin S moves more slowly than hemoglobin A.

Treatment--The primary treatment is prevention. Infection, fever, dehydration, acidosis, hypoxemia, cold, and high altitude should be avoided. Acetaminophen is indicated for fever because aspirin contributes to an acid load. A temperature >105°F means infection, and infection is uncommon if the temperature is <102°F. Prophylactic use of penicillin is beneficial. Vaccines, including pneumococcal, influenza A, and *Haemophilus*, are indicated, as is folate supplementation, especially in pregnancy. Iron chelation is recommended if the transfusion requirement is high. Splenectomy is recommended for those children who survive the initial splenic sequestration crisis. This is the only indication for splenectomy. Blood transfusion and exchange transfusion are the most effective means of treatment available. The hemoglobin S cells should be reduced to <30%. These modalities are especially indicated for the following: history of cerebral vascular accidents, progressive retinopathy, renal or cardiac decompensation preoperatively, and pregnancy (at 30-34 weeks, maintain hemoglobin >10 g/dL). Short-term transfusion therapy is indicated in acute chest syndrome. Other indications for transfusion are priapism, protracted hematuria, and chronic skin ulcers. In vaso-occlusive crises, the cornerstone of treatment includes fluids and correction of urinary sodium losses. Other important considerations are treatment of infections: penicillin in children and coverage for *Staphylococcus* in adults. Analgesics are essential. Blood transfusions do not modify the course. No useful drugs are available. Prenatal diagnosis may be made by analysis of amniotic fluid or chorionic villi biopsy, which is preferred to fetal blood sampling.

Sickle cell trait occurs in 8% of American blacks. There is no anemia, RBC abnormalities, increased risk of infections, or increased mortality; 35%-45% of hemoglobin is hemoglobin S. Associations with sickle cell trait include hematuria, splenic infarction at high altitude (over 10,000 feet), hyposthenuria, bacteriuria, pyelonephritis in pregnancy, and reduced mortality from *Plasmodium falciparum* infection.

In hemoglobin SC disease, the patients have only hemoglobin S and C, with an absence of hemoglobin A and normal or increased levels of hemoglobin F. The disorder is less severe than sickle cell disease with three exceptions: proliferative retinopathy, aseptic necrosis of femoral heads, and acute chest syndrome secondary to fat emboli in the final months of pregnancy. There is mild anemia; in 10% of patients, the hemoglobin is <10 g/dL. Sickle cells are rare on the peripheral blood smear, and 50% of the cells in the peripheral blood are target cells. The spleen remains functional.

Hemoglobin S/β-thalassemia is less severe than sickle cell disease. The spleen remains functional, but retinopathy is more common.

MALIGNANCIES

Chronic Lymphocytic Leukemia

Chronic lymphocytic leukemia is a lymphoproliferative disorder of mature lymphocytes (color plate 18-8). It is the commonest form of leukemia in patients 60 years and older; 90% of patients are older than 50. Chronic lymphocytic leukemia is more of an accumulative than a proliferative disorder of long-lived immunologically incompetent cells. It is rare in the Orient. The two staging classifications are outlined in Tables 18-4 and 18-5.

Predictors of survival include stage, response to initial treatment, WBC count >50,000, abnormal chromosomes, and lymphocyte doubling time (unfavorable if <12 months).

Complications include recurrent infection; 50% of patients have hypogammaglobulinemia. Fever in chronic lymphocytic leukemia is secondary to infection and not to chronic lymphocytic leukemia. The exception is Richter's syndrome. Immunologic complications include autoimmune hemolytic anemia (in 10% of patients); immune-mediated thrombocytopenia (in <5%), which is IgG-mediated and is treated with steroids; and pure RBC aplasia.

- Fever = infection (except for Richter's syndrome).
- Hypogammaglobulinemia in 50% of patients with recurrent infection.
- Autoimmune hemolytic anemia in 10%.
- Thrombocytopenia in <5%.
- Prophylactic gamma globulins are indicated for gamma globulin levels <0.3 g/dL with or without previous infection.

Chronic lymphocytic leukemia is associated with

Table 18-4.--Staging: Rai Classification

Stage	Characteristics	No. patients	Median survival time, mo	No. patients[*]	Median survival time, mo
0	Peripheral (>15,000) lymphocytosis, bone marrow lymphocytosis (>40%)	22	>150	79	129
I	Lymphocytosis, lymphadenopathy	29	101	154	74.4
II	Lymphocytosis, splenomegaly	39	71	203	58.2
III	Lymphocytosis, anemia with hemoglobin <11, excluding AIHA	21	19	127	28.1
IV	Lymphocytosis, thrombocytopenia	14	19	105	19.3

[*]Six combined series.

Data from Rai KR, Sawitsky A, Cronkite EP, Chanana AD, Levy RN, Pasternack BS: Clinical staging of chronic lymphocytic leukemia. Blood 46:219-234, 1975.

Table 18-5.--Classification of International Workshop on Chronic Lymphocytic Leukemia

Clinical stage	Features
A	No anemia or thrombocytopenia and fewer areas of lymphoid enlargement. (Spleen, liver, and lymph nodes in cervical, axillary, and inguinal regions.) A(0), A(I), or A(II).
B	No anemia or thrombocytopenia with three or more involved areas. B(I) or B(II).
C	Anemia (<10 g/dL) and/or thrombocytopenia regardless of the number of areas of lymphoid enlargement. C(III) or C(IV).

From International Workshop on CLL: Chronic lymphocytic leukaemia: proposals for a revised prognostic staging system. Br J Haematol 48:365-367, 1981. By permission of Blackwell Scientific Publications.

increased incidence of solid tumors of the lung and skin (basal cell, squamous cell). Other hematologic malignancies associated with chronic lymphocytic leukemia include Richter's syndrome, which is chronic lymphocytic leukemia that has transformed into large cell lymphoma and is characterized by fevers, massive asymmetrical adenopathy, splenomegaly, and a poor outcome. Also, patients may develop secondary drug-induced acute non-lymphocytic leukemia. Infectious complications include *Staphylococcus aureus*, pneumococci, *Pseudomonas, Klebsiella, Pneumocystis*, cytomegalovirus, *Candida*, herpes simplex, and herpes zoster.

Laboratory findings: lymphocytes are usually monotonous, small, and may be clefted; 97% express common B-cell antigens CD19 and CD20, surface immunoglobulins IgM or IgM and IgD, and coexpress T-cell-specific antigen CD5. Chromosomal abnormalities are found in 55% of patients. Of these, trisomy 12 is the common one. Structural abnormalities of chromosomes 13 and 14 are also seen. Patients with chromosome abnormalities are likely to have a worse prognosis. To date, there is no evidence of pure clonal remissions or cure. The median survival time is 5 years from the onset of treatment.

- Trisomy 12 is the commonest chromosomal abnormality.

Specific treatment--Survival is better if chronic lymphocytic leukemia responds to treatment. Chlorambucil and/or prednisone is the initial treatment of choice. The overall response is 60%-70%. Prednisone alone is indicated in immune-related anemia and thrombocytopenia. Fludarabine is the treatment of choice for chronic lymphocytic leukemia in relapse. Splenectomy is recommended for refractory immune complications, massive splenomegaly, and hypersplenism. Other options include systemic chemotherapy with cyclophosphamide, vincristine, doxorubicin (Adriamycin), and prednisone.

Treatment guidelines--Rai classification:

Stage 0--No treatment.

Stage I and stage II--Treat only if symptomatic from bulky lymphadenopathy or hepatosplenomegaly or WBC count is >50,000. If the disease is stable and there is no impairment of job status, no treatment is necessary. There is no documentation of an increase in survival with early treatment. In fact, one study has shown an increased risk of secondary malignancies with no increase in survival.

Stage III and stage IV--Short median life expectancy, invariably symptomatic. Treat all patients to alleviate symptoms and to improve life expectancy.

Treatment guidelines--International Workshop classification:

Stage A--Observe.

Stage B--Some patients will need treatment, as outlined in stages I and II indications above.

Stage C--Treat all patients.

- Treat patients with Rai stages III and IV disease and International Workshop stages B and C.
- Overall response rate to chlorambucil and/or prednisone is 60%-70%.
- Fludarabine is the treatment of choice for patients who have relapse.

Hairy-Cell Leukemia

Hairy-cell leukemia is characterized by an insidious onset of cytopenias without constitutional symptoms. At some time during the course of the disease, 90% of patients have splenomegaly. The hairy cell cytoplasmic projections are "hairy" with multiple, thin, or blunt projections (color plate 18-9). The cells contain tartrate-resistant acid phosphatase (positive TRAP stain). Most are B-cell in nature and clonal, as demonstrated by light- and heavy-chain immunoglobulin gene rearrangements. Hairy-cell leukemia accounts for <2% of all leukemias. The cause is not known.

- Hairy-cell leukemia: cytopenias.
- Splenomegaly is common.
- Hairy cells have cytoplasmic projections.

- B-cell in nature and clonal.
- Constitutes <2% of all leukemia.

Clinical characteristics--The symptoms are related to cytopenias, infections, and splenomegaly.

- Middle-aged patients.
- Splenomegaly in 90% of patients.
- Infections related to cytopenias.

Laboratory findings reveal anemia, thrombocytopenia, neutropenia, and pancytopenia. More than 75% of patients have anemia, thrombocytopenia, and neutropenia. The bone marrow yields a dry tap on bone marrow aspiration; biopsy specimens are hypercellular with diffuse infiltration. Hairy cells may or may not be seen in the peripheral blood.

- Cytopenias in 75% of patients.
- Bone marrow: dry tap.
- Hairy cells may not be seen in peripheral blood smear.

Complications--Infection is the major cause of death. Infection should be considered when a previously stable patient develops new symptoms. Fever is not a manifestation of the disease but indicates an underlying infection. Localized pyogenic infections are more common, e.g., bacterial pneumonia, urinary tract infections, and infections of the skin. The incidence of atypical mycobacterial infections is increased. There is a higher incidence of viral infections, fungal infections, parasitic diseases, toxoplasmosis, histoplasmosis, coccidiosis, and pneumocystis. Bleeding and vasculitis (skin, joint, erythema nodosum) are other complications.

- Infection is the major cause of death.
- Fever denotes infection.
- Atypical mycobacterial infections.

Treatment--Observation may be indicated for patients who are asymptomatic with very mild cytopenias. Indications for intervention include significant cytopenia, serious or recurrent infections associated with neutropenia, bleeding secondary to thrombocytopenia, splenic infarction, vasculitis, and increasing number of hairy cells. 2-Chlorodeoxyadenosine produces complete remission in 85%-88% of patients after a single 7-day continuous, intravenous infusion. Other treatments include alpha recombinant interferon, which produces a 13% complete remission after 18 months of subcutaneous treatments, and 2'deoxycorformycin, which produces complete remission in 75% of patients, with a relapse rate of 10%. Splenectomy only improves peripheral blood cell counts and has no effect on the bone marrow. The only indications for splenectomy are a very large spleen and patchy bone marrow involvement in a young patient, splenic infarct, and profound life-threatening bleeding secondary to thrombocytopenia.

- 2-Chlorodeoxyadenosine is the treatment of choice in hairy-cell leukemia.
- Other treatments include splenectomy, alpha recombinant interferon, and 2'deoxycorformycin.

Lymphadenopathy

The differential diagnosis of lymphadenopathy and fever with or without splenomegaly includes the following:

1. Infectious mononucleosis, Epstein-Barr virus, cytomegalovirus, and toxoplasmosis.
2. Syphilis, subacute bacterial endocarditis, sarcoidosis, *Salmonella*, tuberculosis, and acquired immune deficiency (AIDS).
3. Hodgkin's disease, non-Hodgkin's lymphoma, angioimmunoblastic lymphadenopathy, mixed essential cryoglobulinemia, systemic mastocytosis, chronic lymphocytic leukemia, myelofibrosis, Waldenström's macroglobulinemia, and multiple myeloma.
4. Systemic lupus erythematosus and rheumatoid arthritis.
5. Kawasaki disease, Whipple's disease, serum sickness, and Kaposi's sarcoma.

Hodgkin's Disease

The diagnosis of Hodgkin's disease is based on the presence of Reed-Sternberg cells, which typically have two or more nuclei with prominent nucleoli, giving the cells the appearance of owl's eyes (color plate 18-10). The cause is unknown, although 20%-50% of patients have the Epstein-Barr virus incorporated into the genome. The staging classification is outlined in Table 18-6, and the staging procedures in Table 18-7.

- Hodgkin's disease: the presence of Reed-Sternberg cells with characteristic pathologic features.
- 20%-50% of patients have the Epstein-Barr virus incorporated into genome.
- The histologic subtype is not an independent prognostic factor if appropriate treatment is given.

Table 18-6.--The Cotswolds Staging Classification of Hodgkin's Disease

Classification	Description
Stage I	Involvement of a single lymph node region or lymphoid structure
Stage II	Involvement of two or more lymph node regions on the same side of the diaphragm (the mediastinum is considered a single site, whereas hilar lymph nodes are considered bilaterally)
Stage III	Involvement of lymph node regions or structures on both sides of the diaphragm
Stage III-1	With or without involvement of splenic, hilar, celiac, or portal nodes
Stage III-2	With involvement of para-aortic, iliac, and mesenteric nodes
Stage IV	Involvement of one or more extranodal sites in addition to a site for which the designation "E" has been used
	Designations applicable to any disease stage
A	No symptoms
B	Fever (temperature >38°C), drenching night sweats, unexplained loss of >10% of body weight within the preceding 6 months
X	Bulky disease (a widening of the mediastinum by more than 1/3 or the presence of a nodal mass with a maximal dimension >10 cm)
E	Involvement of a single extranodal site that is contiguous or proximal to the known nodal site
CS	Clinical stage
PS	Pathologic stage (as determined by laparotomy)

From Lister TA, Crowther D: Staging for Hodgkin's disease. Semin Oncol 17:696-703, 1990. By permission of WB Saunders Company.

Table 18-7.--Staging Procedures for Hodgkin's
Disease

History and examination: identification of B symptoms

Imaging procedures: plain chest radiography, computed tomography of the thorax, computed tomographic scan of the abdomen and pelvis, and bipedal lymphangiography

Hematologic procedures: full blood cell count with differential, determination of erythrocyte sedimentation rate, and bilateral bone marrow aspiration and biopsy

Biochemical procedures: tests of liver function and measurement of serum albumin, lactate dehydrogenase, and calcium

Special procedures: laparotomy, ultrasonographic scanning, magnetic resonance imaging, gallium scanning, technetium bone scanning, and liver-spleen scanning

Staging laparotomies: performed only if radiation therapy is the desired treatment, so is not indicated in clinical stage IIIB to IVB patients; the detection of intra-abdominal disease would alter the choice of therapy. Patients should not have adverse features for relapse, such as a large mediastinal mass. The risk of abdominal involvement in females younger than 35 years with nodular sclerosing Hodgkin's disease and high cervical neck nodes is low

---

Modified from Lister TA, Crowther D: Staging for Hodgkin's disease. Semin Oncol 17:696-703, 1990. By permission of WB Saunders Company.

Radiation therapy--Patients with pathologic stages I and II disease are traditionally managed with radiation therapy, as outlined in Table 18-8.

Chemotherapy--Complete remission rates with chemotherapy are 70%-90%; the relapse rate is 33%. The cure rate is 50%-66%. Studies are evaluating different programs of MOPP, MOPP-ABVD, ABVD, and other alternatives. In recent trials, ABVD, MOPP-ABVD, and MOPP-ABV had higher complete remission rates than MOPP. (MOPP: nitrogen mustard, vincristine [Oncovin], prednisone, and procarbazine; ABV: doxorubicin [Adriamycin], bleomycin, and vinblastine [Velban]; D, DTIC.)

Complications of survival include pneumococcal sepsis in 7% of patients after splenectomy, anthracycline cardiomyopathy, preleukemia or dysmyelopoietic syndromes, acute nonlymphocytic leukemia in 3.3%-10%, diffuse aggressive lymphomas, infertility, hypothyroidism, thyroid carcinoma, avascular necrosis, and solid tumors (lung, stomach).

Autologous bone marrow transplantation--Indications include failure to achieve complete remission with chemotherapy, progressive disease during initial therapy, relapse in <1 year of treatment with chemotherapy, more than two relapses, B symptoms at relapse, and relapse after initial treatment of stage IV disease. Of all patients treated with autologous bone marrow transplant, 33% have a 3-year disease-free survival.

Regimens commonly used are CBV (cyclophosphamide, carmustine [BCNU], etoposide [VP16]) and cyclophosphamide/total body irradiation. Death rate from toxicity is 7%-15%.

- Complete remission in 70%-90%.
- Cure in 50%-90% with initial therapy.
- Complications of survival include acute nonlymphocytic leukemia, anthracycline cardiomyopathy, infertility, diffuse aggressive lymphomas, and solid tumors.

Non-Hodgkin's Lymphomas

Non-Hodgkin's lymphomas are clinically, morphologically, and immunologically a diverse group of lymphoproliferative disorders. A classification for non-Hodgkin's lymphoma is outlined in Table 18-9.

Staging--History and physical examination, CBC, erythrocyte sedimentation rate, LDH, liver function tests, measure serum albumin and calcium, chest radiograph, computed tomographic scan of the abdomen with or without chest, and bilateral bone marrow.

Table 18-8--Initial Treatment of Hodgkin's Disease

Stage	Type	Response
IA	Radiation therapy (mantle and para-aortic)	93% freedom from progression
IIA	Radiation, extended field (mantle and para-aortic)	82% freedom from progression
IIIA1	Radiation	
IIIA2, IIIB, IV	Chemotherapy	

Table 18-9.--Non-Hodgkin's Lymphomas

Classification	
Low grade	Malignant lymphoma: small lymphocytic
	Malignant lymphoma: follicular, predominantly small cleaved cell
	Malignant lymphoma: follicular, mixed small cleaved and large cell
Intermediate-grade	Malignant lymphoma: follicular, predominantly large cell
	Malignant lymphoma: diffuse, small cleaved cell
	Malignant lymphoma: diffuse, mixed small and large cell
	Malignant lymphoma: diffuse large cell
High grade	Malignant lymphoma: large cell immunoblastic
	Malignant lymphoma: lymphoblastic
	Malignant lymphoma: small noncleaved cell
Miscellaneous	Composite malignant lymphoma
	Mycosis fungoides
	Extramedullary plasmacytoma
	Unclassified
	Other

Modified from The Non-Hodgkin's Lymphoma Pathologic Classification Project: National Cancer Institute sponsored study of classification of non-Hodgkin's lymphoma: summary and description of a working formulation for clinical usage. Cancer 49:2112-2135, 1982. By permission of American Cancer Society.

Low-Grade Non-Hodgkin's Lymphoma

Most cases of low-grade non-Hodgkin's lymphomas are stage IIIA and IVA at presentation. These lymphomas have long survival times but are not curable. They are very responsive to initial treatment. The median age range of the patients is 50-60 years. The median survival rates exceed 8-10 years. Most patients with advanced low-grade non-Hodgkin's lymphoma cannot be cured by routine therapy. The initial management of the asymptomatic patient with no B symptoms or bulky disease is observation. Drugs used in the treatment of low-grade non-Hodgkin's lymphoma include chlorambucil and prednisone; cyclophosphamide, vincristine, and prednisone; and other experimental therapeutic interventions. If the patient is younger than 50 years, consider autologous bone marrow transplantation after initial induction therapy or at first relapse.

Intermediate-Grade Non-Hodgkin's Lymphoma

Intermediate-grade non-Hodgkin's lymphoma is a curable disease, but survival is short if patients do not respond to initial therapy. The complete remission rates are 53%-86%, and the cure rates are 30%-65%. The prognosis is worse if the patient is older than 60 years, has stage III or IV disease, has more than one extranodal site, is Eastern Cooperative Oncology Group (ECOG) performance status ≥ 2, or has an elevated serum level of LDH (International Non-Hodgkin's Lymphoma Prognostic Factors Project). Treat all patients who are candidates for therapy. CHOP (cyclophosphamide, doxorubicin [Adriamycin], vincristine, and prednisone) chemotherapy is currently the standard treatment. For patients in relapse, autologous bone marrow transplantation results in a 20%-40% prolonged disease-free survival with apparent cure.

- Intermediate-grade lymphoma is curable.
- CHOP chemotherapy is currently the standard of care in initial management.
- Worse prognosis: age >60, stage III/IV disease, >1 extranodal site, ECOG performance status ≥ 2, elevated serum level of LDH.

Monoclonal Gammopathies

The differential diagnosis of monoclonal gammopathies includes monoclonal gammopathies of undetermined significance and malignant monoclonal gammopathies. The malignant gammopathies include multiple myeloma (IgG, IgA, IgD, IgE, and free light chains): overt multiple myeloma, smoldering multiple myeloma, plasma cell leukemia, nonsecretory myeloma, and osteosclerotic myeloma. Also plasmacytoma (solitary plasmacytoma of bone, extramedullary plasmacytoma); malignant lymphoproliferative diseases (Waldenström's [primary] macroglobulinemia, malignant lymphoma); heavy chain diseases; and amyloidosis (primary, with myeloma).

Monoclonal Gammopathies of Undetermined Significance

In this condition, the M-protein level is <3 g/dL in the serum, and there are <10% plasma cells in the bone marrow. The serum level of creatinine is normal, and either a small amount of M protein or no M protein occurs in the urine. There is no anemia or osteolytic bone lesions. Twenty-three percent of the patients may have progression to a malignant monoclonal gammopathy.

Multiple Myeloma

In multiple myeloma, 10% or more plasma cells are found in the bone marrow (color plate 18-11). At least one of the following must be present: M protein in the serum >3 g/dL, M protein in the urine, osteolytic bone lesions. Anemia, hypercalcemia, or increased creatinine level are present in variable numbers of patients.

Clinical features include bone pain (66% of patients), renal insufficiency (50%), hypercalcemia (30%), weakness, fatigue, and spinal cord compression (5%). The incidence of pneumococcal pneumonia, gram-negative infections, and herpes zoster is increased. The CBC resembles that of normochromic-normocytic anemia. Radiographs show punched-out lytic lesions, osteoporosis, and fractures.

Treatment--Because multiple myeloma is not curable, treatment should be delayed until evidence of progression develops, the patient becomes symptomatic, or treatment is necessary to prevent imminent complications. Controversy exists as to whether melphalan and prednisone taken orally or a combination of intravenously and orally administered alkylating agents should be used (M2 protocol melphalan, cyclophosphamide, carmustine, vincristine, and prednisone). With melphalan and prednisone, a 50%-60% objective response is seen.

- Plasma cells: <10% in monoclonal gammopathies of undetermined significance; >10% in myeloma.
- M protein: <3 g/dL in monoclonal gammopathies of undetermined significance; ≥3 g/dL in myeloma.
- Myeloma: bone pain (66% of patients), renal dysfunction (50%), hypercalcemia (30%), spinal cord compression (5%).
- Myeloma: punched-out bone lesions, pneumococcal infection.

Amyloidosis

Patients with amyloidosis present with fatigue, weight loss, hepatomegaly, macroglossia, renal insufficiency, proteinuria, nephrotic syndrome, congestive heart failure, orthostatic hypotension, carpal tunnel syndrome, and peripheral neuropathy. Amyloidosis is classified as primary, secondary (chronic infections, autoimmune disease), familial, associated with aging, amyloidosis of endocrine glands with medullary carcinoma, and amy-

loidosis with multiple endocrine neoplasia type II. Treatment with melphalan and prednisone has an 18% response rate in primary amyloidosis. Pathologic characteristics--Primary amyloidosis consists of the variable region of immunoglobulin light chains; secondary amyloidosis consists of protein A.

Acute Leukemias

The cause of acute leukemia is unknown in most cases, but there are many associations, including idiopathic aplastic anemia, paroxysmal nocturnal hemoglobinuria, myeloproliferative disorders, preleukemic syndromes, radiation, benzene, cytotoxic chemotherapy, Down syndrome, Fanconi's syndrome, and ataxia-telangiectasia. The classic syndrome of patients who have been exposed to alkylating agents (melphalan, cyclophosphamide, chlorambucil) is pancytopenia in 10-36 months, with the chromosome abnormalities of monosomy 5 and 7. It is refractory to standard treatment regimens.

- Alkylating agents should be used in benign diseases, with consideration of the risk of development of acute myelogenous leukemia, non-Hodgkin's lymphoma, bladder cancer, and other solid tumors.
- Recently described secondary leukemias are those related to topoisomerase II inhibitor agents.
- High incidence of neoplasms in Down syndrome, Fanconi's syndrome, ataxia-telangiectasia.

Acute Nonlymphocytic Leukemia (Acute Myelogenous Leukemia)

The median age of patients with acute nonlymphocytic leukemia (color plate 18-12) is 65 years. Fifty percent of patients have symptoms for >3 months. Good prognostic signs include females <40 years old; chromosome abnormalities of t(8,21), t(15,17), inversion 16, or normal chromosomes; and obtaining complete remission with one cycle of induction chemotherapy. Poor prognostic signs include age >40; preleukemic phase; the chromosome abnormalities of monosomy 5, monosomy 7, t(9,22), trisomy 8, 11q-, and complex cytogenetic patterns; and poor general physical condition or underlying health problems.

For patients who present with extreme leukocytosis (WBC >100,000) with acute leukemia, the initial complication of most concern is cerebral hemorrhage. Emergency treatment includes hydration, alkalinization of urine, allopurinol (600 mg), hydroxyurea (6-8 g orally), cranial irradiation (4-6 Gy), and leukopheresis followed by the treatment of the specific type of leukemia.

- Acute nonlymphocytic leukemia: median age of patients is 65 years; 50% have symptoms >3 months.
- Good prognosis in patients <40 years old, chromosomal abnormalities t(8,21), t(15,17), inv16, or normal chromosomes, obtaining complete remission with one cycle of induction chemotherapy.

Therapy--Platelet transfusions are required throughout the course of the treatment. Early empiric broad-spectrum antibiotic coverage for fevers is essential.

Induction chemotherapy:

1. Cytarabine (cytosine arabinoside) with an anthracycline agent (daunorubicin or idarubicin)--The complete remission rate is 55%-85%, with the potential for cure in 20% of patients. Despite substantial recent advances, most patients with acute myelogenous leukemia eventually have relapse and most do so within 1 year. Of patients who have relapse after induction and consolidation therapy, 30%-50% achieve a second remission.

2. *Trans*-retinoic acid (Atra)--M3 acute myelogenous leukemia (promyelocytic acute nonlymphocytic leukemia) (color plate 18-13) with a t(5,17) translocation: *trans*-retinoic acid results in a 90% complete remission rate. These patients then need to be treated with cytarabine or a daunorubicin-type program. This is the first malignancy in which a chromosomal alteration has served as the target for induction chemotherapy.

Intensification therapy with a program such as high-dose cytosine arabinoside is superior to maintenance therapy.

The following generalizations may be made about allogeneic bone marrow transplantation in acute nonlymphocytic leukemia. Generally, after 2 years of complete remission, the risk of relapse is lower. Transplantation in cases of relapse is age-dependent: patients <30 years old have a better prognosis than those >30. Allogeneic bone marrow transplantation in early relapse or in second remission is almost as efficacious as transplantation in first complete remission. Recommendations--If the patient is <55 years old, consider bone marrow transplant in first remission of HLA match with poor prognostic factors. In those patients without poor risk factors and not on study, perform transplantation in early relapse or second remission. Results--Currently, the disease-free survival at 5 years for patients undergoing transplanta-

tion in first remission is 50%; in first relapse, 30%; and in second remission, 28%.

Acute Lymphoblastic Leukemia

Acute lymphoblastic leukemia (color plate 18-14) is commonest in children with complete remission rates >90% and with long-term disease-free survivals of 60%-70%. In adults, this leukemia is less common, with remission rates of up to 75%; however, most patients will relapse. Clinical presentation--One-third of patients present with bleeding, and 25% have symptoms for >3 months. Bone pain, lymphadenopathy, splenomegaly, and hepatomegaly are more common in acute lymphoblastic leukemia than in acute nonlymphocytic leukemia. Splenomegaly, lymphadenopathy, and hepatomegaly occur in 3/4 of the patients (compared with 1/2 of patients with acute myelogenous leukemia).

Prognostic factors--The best prognosis is in children 3-10 years old. After the age of 20, survival time continues to decrease with increasing age and shorter complete remission durations. Poor prognostic factors include age, WBC count >30 x 10^9/L, null cell phenotype, specific chromosome abnormalities, and achievement of remission after >4 weeks of intensive chemotherapy. Chromosomal abnormalities--80%-90% of adults have chromosome abnormalities. Normal chromosomes have the best prognosis. The poorest prognosis is associated with t(9,22); t(4,11); t(8,14); and t(1,19). Also, t(9,22) has <15% survival at 5 years and is present in 25% of adults but only 2%-3% of children. Chromosome abnormalities are independent of age, WBC count, immunotype.

Treatment:

1. Induction--The three agents commonly used include vincristine, prednisone, and anthracyclines along with one or more of the following: L-asparaginase, cytarabine, methotrexate, or cyclophosphamide. The complete remission rate is 75%.

2. Intensification/postinduction therapy is commonly used. Long-term relapse-free survival of 10%-42% in adults. The use of allogeneic bone marrow transplant in first complete remission results in a 40%-63% disease-free survival at 2-10 years. Trials are under way for evaluating autologous bone marrow transplant.

3. Relapse--Allogeneic or autologous bone marrow transplants are of benefit in patients who achieve a second complete remission. After a second complete remission and then allogeneic transplant, the

disease-free survival ranges from 26% to 54% at various time periods. At second complete remission and then autologous transplant, the disease-free survival ranges from 23% to 31% at various periods of time.

Myeloproliferative Disorders

The myeloproliferative disorders are polycythemia rubra vera, agnogenic myeloid metaplasia, essential thrombocythemia, and chronic granulocytic leukemia. Their characteristic features are given in Table 18-10. The myeloproliferative disorders are interrelated: polycythemia rubra vera converts to agnogenic myeloid metaplasia in 10% of cases. Essential thrombocythemia converts to agnogenic myeloid metaplasia in 5% of cases. Acute myelogenous leukemia is a complication of polycythemia rubra vera (10% of cases), essential thrombocythemia (15%), agnogenic myeloid metaplasia (20%), and chronic myelogenous leukemia (70%).

- The myeloproliferative disorders are polycythemia rubra vera, agnogenic myeloid metaplasia, essential thrombocythemia, and chronic granulocytic leukemia.
- Myeloproliferative disorders are interrelated.

Table 18-10.--Characteristic Features of Chronic Myeloproliferative Disorders

Characteristic	Polycythemia rubra vera	Agnogenic myeloid metaplasia	Primary thrombocythemia	Chronic granulocytic leukemia
Increased red cell mass	Yes	No	No	No
Myelofibrosis	Later	Yes	Rare	Later
Thrombocytosis	Variable	Variable	Yes	Variable
bcr-abl Oncogene	No	No	No	Yes

From Petitt RM, Silverstein MN: Current clinical management of primary thrombocythemia. Contemp Intern Med Jan 1991, pp 46-52 By permission of Aegean Communications.

Chronic Myelogenous Leukemia (Chronic Granulocytic Leukemia)

Chronic myelogenous leukemia constitutes 20%-30% of all leukemias and is characterized by an acquired defect of clonal origin at the pluripotential cell level. There is a pool of granulocyte precursors with the capacity for normal maturation (color plate 18-15). The Philadelphia chromosome, t(9,22), is the hallmark of this disease. The translocation results in the formation of a chimeric *bcr-abl* gene. The disease terminates in a maturation block or blast crisis. New chromosomal abnormalities appear and reappear. Different cell types can be seen, including myeloblasts (50%-60% of patients), megakaryoblasts (15%), B lymphoblasts, erythroblasts (10%), monoblasts, myelomonocytic blasts, and basophilic blasts.

Clinical features--Before the advent of allogeneic bone marrow transplantation, the median survival was 3.5 years after diagnosis. Prognostic factors are different in multiple series. In one study, a good prognosis (61-month median survival versus 34 months) was associated with a spleen size of 0-6 cm and 0%-10% circulating blasts. A poor prognosis was associated with an age >45 years and platelet count >70,000. The chronic phase is characterized by <10% blasts in blood and bone marrow and is of 2-3 years' duration. Symptoms include malaise, dyspnea, anorexia, fever, night sweats, weight loss, abdominal fullness, easy bruising, bleeding, gout, priapism, and hypermetabolism. Splenomegaly is present in 85% of patients.

Laboratory findings--Leukocytosis with <10% blasts in the chronic phase of disease and WBC count of 100,000 are common. Granulocytes in all stages of maturation are present on peripheral blood smear, with basophilia and eosinophilia. The number of platelets is increased, with large bizarre forms present on peripheral blood smears. The hemoglobin concentration ranges from 9 to 12 g/dL. The leukocyte alkaline phosphatase score is low or absent. The differential diagnosis of a low or absent leukocyte alkaline phosphatase score includes paroxysmal nocturnal hemoglobinuria, infectious mononucleosis, and aplastic anemia. The vitamin B_{12} level is increased because of increased transcobalamin I. Other findings include pseudohyperkalemia, pseudohypoglycemia, and false-positive increase in acid phosphatase in the serum. The bone marrow is hyperplastic, with myelofibrosis in 10%-40% of patients.

- Chronic myelogenous leukemia: acquired defect of clonal origin.
- Philadelphia chromosome, t(9,22), is the hallmark of the disease.
- WBC count is usually >100,000; granulocytes in all stages of maturation; platelets usually >400,000.
- Bone marrow shows hyperplasia; myelofibrosis in 10%-40% of patients.
- Leukocyte alkaline phosphatase score is low or absent in chronic myelogenous leukemia, paroxysmal nocturnal hemoglobinuria, infectious mononucleosis, aplastic anemia.
- Increased vitamin B_{12}; elevated acid phosphatase.

Treatment--Conventional chemotherapy has not appreciably prolonged survival. There is little evidence that any patient has been cured by conventional therapy, including hydroxyurea and multiagent regimens. The three agents used in the initial treatment of chronic myelogenous leukemia are hydroxyurea, busulfan, and alpha recombinant interferon. Although hydroxyurea is used more commonly, it is no more effective than busulfan. However, hydroxyurea is the treatment of choice for high blast counts and leukostasis lesions, and it is safe in thrombocytopenia. Moreover, it has fewer side effects than busulfan. Recovery after an overshoot is more rapid than with busulfan. Continued maintenance therapy is necessary. Megaloblastic RBCs appear in the peripheral blood. Hydroxyurea should be used in all patients who are considered candidates for bone marrow transplantation, because of the risk of interstitial pneumonitis and veno-occlusive disease with busulfan. Busulfan is effective in this disease. The dose of busulfan must be reduced by 50% at a WBC count of 20,000, and its use must be stopped when the WBC count reaches 10,000-12,000. Its side effects include thrombocytopenia, leukopenia, prolonged bone marrow myelosuppression, increased skin pigmentation, pulmonary toxicity, amenorrhea, germinal cell atrophy, fetal malformations, veno-occlusive disease of liver, and a wasting syndrome. Alpha recombinant interferon suppresses the Philadelphia chromosome. Hematologic responses are 40%-80%, with cytogenetic remissions in the range of 10%-40%. The median survival is >60 months. Ongoing trials are comparing interferon alpha with hydroxyurea.

The treatment of "blast crisis" includes allopurinol, fluids, hydroxyurea, cranial radiation, and leukocyte apheresis.

- Accelerated phase at 30-36 months; the chronic phase converts to an accelerated or blast phase (75%), which is characterized by blast counts >20%; increase in anemia, thrombocytopenia, basophilia, and leukocyte alkaline phosphatase score; splenomegaly; lymphadenopathy; bone pain; cerebral hemorrhage; fever; headache; and myelofibrosis. Cytogenetic abnormalities precede condition by 6 months.
- If treated with busulfan or hydroxyurea, 10%-15% of patients die in the first year and about 26% per year thereafter.
- Toxicity of busulfan: prolonged myelosuppression, pulmonary toxicity, veno-occlusive disease of liver.
- Alpha recombinant interferon suppresses the Philadelphia chromosome.
- Intensive treatment in patients with chronic granulocytic leukemia does not postpone or prevent blast crisis or appreciably improve survival.
- Currently, the only curative regimen is autogeneic bone transplantation.

Allogeneic bone marrow transplantation should be performed in the chronic phase, within the first 6-12 months in patients <55 years old who have an HLA-identical match or an identical twin. The only curative regimen to date is high-dose chemotherapy with total body irradiation followed by transplantation of allogeneic bone marrow from HLA-identical siblings. The actuarial probability of survival at 3 years is 63%.

Agnogenic Myeloid Metaplasia

Clinical features--Splenomegaly occurs in 100% of the patients and is the hallmark of agnogenic myeloid metaplasia. Other features are leukoerythroblastic peripheral blood smear (96% of patients), teardrop cells, and hypocellular marrow (85%). The basic event is the fibroblastic proliferation in bone marrow (color plate 18-16). Anemia may be caused by expanded plasma volume, ineffective erythropoiesis, blood loss, or hemolysis.

Pathologic features--The bone marrow reveals panhyperplasia with modest fibrosis to osteosclerosis. The spleen is pathologically characterized by extramedullary hematopoiesis in the sinusoids of red pulp. Hepatomegaly may occur in 70% of patients because of engorgement by blood, extramedullary hematopoiesis, or hemosiderosis.

- Agnogenic myeloid metaplasia: splenomegaly is its hallmark.
- Leukoerythroblastic peripheral blood smear in 96%.

- Teardrop cells.
- Basic event: fibroblastic proliferation of bone marrow.

Treatment--Observe the 20% of asymptomatic patients (80% will remain asymptomatic at 5 years). Medical therapy for anemia with symptoms includes the following:

1. Transfusion with packed RBCs if RBC mass is low (check RBC mass and plasma volume).
2. Androgens for ineffective erythropoiesis: testosterone enanthate (400-600 mg/week) or fluoxymesterone (10 mg three times daily). Response occurs in 40% of males and 32% of females. Poor response in long-existing disease and massive splenomegaly. Side effects are hirsutism and fluid retention.
3. Corticosteroids for hemolysis.
4. Check stool for occult blood loss due to esophageal varices and microinfarcts of gut.
5. Treat vitamin B$_{12}$ and folate deficiency if indicated.

Pressure symptoms occur in 23% of patients and may be managed with hydroxyurea or splenic irradiation.

1. 63% of patients respond to splenic irradiation but the response duration is short (3.5 months). Indications for splenic irradiation include splenic infarct, perisplenitis, and ascites from peritoneal implants.
2. Bleeding with or without thrombocytopenia may be managed with platelet transfusions.
3. Treat disseminated intravascular coagulopathy appropriately if present (may be present in up to 40% of patients).
4. Splenectomy is indicated in major hemolysis, pressure symptoms, life-threatening thrombocytopenia, portal hypertension, and life-threatening bleeding.

Prognosis--Overall survival is 60% at 5 years. Prognosis is good if patient is asymptomatic, hemoglobin concentration is >10, platelet count is >100,000, and liver is <5 cm below the costal margin.

Essential Thrombocythemia (Primary Thrombocythemia)

Essential thrombocythemia is a clonal hematologic disorder in which patients present with asymptomatic thrombocytosis, thromboembolic complications, or hemorrhagic problems.

Diagnosis--Platelet count is >600,000/mm^3; megakaryocytic hyperplasia in the bone marrow; splenomegaly; absence of the Philadelphia chromosome, which is a translocation between chromosome 9 and 22 (100% of patients); normal RBC mass (100%); and stainable iron in the bone marrow. Also, there is no other secondary cause of thrombocytosis, including acute or chronic inflammatory disease; acute or chronic bleeding; iron deficiency; chronic bone marrow stimulation (e.g., hemolysis); rebound after thrombocytopenia; disseminated malignancy; splenectomy, congenital asplenic, or functional hyposplenism; and intense exercise, parturition, trauma, epinephrine.

Treatment--Platelet apheresis should be used in the emergent management of acute bleeding or thrombosis. Patients <30 years old may be observed if there are no hemorrhagic or thrombotic problems, no significant trauma, and no emergency or elective surgery. Platelet apheresis is indicated in cases of elective surgery for patients of any age and in pregnant women during the course of delivery. Chronic treatments available for the management of essential thrombocythemia include hydroxyurea; anagrelide; antiaggregating agents for mild thrombotic symptoms, including aspirin and dipyridamole; radioactive phosphorus at a dose of 2.7 mCi/m^2; and alpha recombinant interferon.

Erythrocytosis

Polycythemia--The history, physical examination, CBC, arterial blood gases, leukocyte alkaline phosphatase score, and the marrow can determine the diagnosis in a high percentage of patients, as shown in Table 18-11. Every patient with unexplained erythrocytosis should have an intravenous pyelogram or CT scan of the abdomen.

The differential diagnosis of erythrocytosis with a normal oxygen saturation value includes the following: hypernephroma, renal adenoma, hydronephrosis, renal cyst, transplantation, Bartter's syndrome, cerebellar hemangioblastoma, adrenal cortical adenoma or hyperplasia, ovarian carcinoma, hepatoma, pheochromocytoma, uterine fibroids, and hemoglobinopathies.

- Polycythemia rubra vera: very low erythropoietin.
- Cerebral blood flow decreases at a hematocrit of >46.
- Smoking 1.5 packs of cigarettes per day can raise hematocrit to 60% (check carboxyhemoglobin).
- RBC mass returns to normal when smoking is stopped.

Table 18-11.--Differential Diagnosis of Erythrocytosis

	Polycythemia rubra vera	Stress erythrocytosis	Anoxic polycythemia	Tumor
History	Multiple symptoms	Nervous Hypertension Obesity	High-altitude COPD Fibrosis Congenital heart disease Sleep apnea Hemoglobinopathy	
Gout	Occasionally	Occasionally		
Other history	Postbathing pruritus[*]			
Examination	Plethora skin, mucous membrane	±Plethora	Cyanosis	No cyanosis, clubbing, or COPD
	Distention of retinal vein		Clubbing[*]	Mass in left upper quadrant
	Hepatomegaly (50%) Splenomegaly (75%);[*] not others			
Laboratory				
Oxygen saturation	Normal	Normal	<88% (±88%-92%)[*]	Normal
LAP score	+++ (almost invariably)[*]	Normal	Normal	Normal
Red blood cell mass	++	Normal	+ to ++	+ to ++
Plasma volume	Normal or slightly increased	Reduced	Normal	Normal
Excretory urogram	Normal	Normal	Normal	Tumor
Erythrocyte sedimentation rate	0-1[*]	Normal	Normal, low	
Bone marrow	Pancytosis	Erythrocytosis	Erythrocytosis	Erythrocytosis
Platelets	+ to ++ (50%)	Normal	Normal	± Normal

COPD, chronic obstructive pulmonary disease; LAP, leukocyte alkaline phosphatase.

[*]Most important differentiating factors.

Modified from Dameshek W: Comments on the diagnosis of polycythemia vera. Semin Hematol 3:214-215, 1966. By permission of WB Saunders Company.

Polycythemia Rubra Vera

Clinical features include weakness, postbathing pruritus, headache, dizziness, weight loss, joint symptoms, dyspnea, epigastric distress. Classification: category A, increased RBC mass, splenomegaly, normal arterial oxygen saturation; category B, platelet count >400,000, WBC >12,000 (no fever or infection), leukocyte alkaline phosphatase score >100, serum level of vitamin B$_{12}$ >900. The presence of all three criteria in category A establishes the diagnosis. If the patient has increased RBC mass (category A) with either of the other two category A criteria, then two of the four category B criteria are necessary to establish the diagnosis. Unfavorable prognostic signs are previous thrombotic disease, age >60 years, diabetes mellitus, vascular diseases, and hypertension.

Laboratory findings--The bone marrow is normal in up to 10% of patients; 90%-95% have absent iron stores in the bone marrow even if not phlebotomized. Cytogenetic abnormalities are present in 11%. The erythropoietin level is low. The Philadelphia chromosome in the bone marrow is negative. Morphologically, the bone marrow may resemble chronic myelogenous leukemia in 10%-40% of patients. The leukocyte alkaline phosphatase score is increased.

- The leukocyte alkaline phosphatase score may be increased in polycythemia rubra vera, leukemoid reactions, agnogenic myeloid metaplasia, idiopathic thrombocytopenic purpura, pregnancy, pyogenic infections, and stress erythrocytosis.

- Think of polycythemia rubra vera with microcytosis, absent iron stores, and splenomegaly.

Treatment in patients who are asymptomatic is phlebotomy to maintain hematocrit <42-45. Phlebotomize every 2-4 months, because there is 250 mg of iron in 1 pint of blood. If the normal daily absorption is 4 mg, then phlebotomizing every 2 months will maintain the hematocrit in an appropriate range. Start at 500 mL every other day for 3-6 phlebotomies and maintain hematocrit at 42-45 every 2-4 months. In the elderly, start at 250 mL phlebotomies. There is a risk of thrombosis in older patients with vascular lesions, with the rate and volume of phlebotomy, and in patients with a history of thrombosis. In patients with asymptomatic thrombocytosis, anagrelide reduces platelet count in 96% of those treated. Other agents available include hydroxyurea and alpha recombinant interferon.

In patients who are symptomatic or who are at risk for thrombosis, hydroxyurea, anagrelide, and ^{32}P are the treatments of choice. With ^{32}P, the number of platelets decreases in 2 weeks and the number of RBCs decreases in 1 month. This treatment is indicated for patients older than 60, because of the 2.3-fold risk of acute nonlymphocytic leukemia in younger patients treated with ^{32}P. Chlorambucil is not indicated because of a 5.3-fold risk of developing acute nonlymphocytic leukemia when compared with phlebotomy.

- Sequence of ordering tests in erythrocytosis.
  CBC: increased total RBC count and/or hematocrit on CBC. Arterial oxygen saturation: if oxygen saturation >92%, then check carboxyhemoglobin (smoker's polycythemia), RBC mass, plasma volume, erythropoietin level.

Oncogenes

Oncogenes are gene loci that have the potential to affect neoplastic transformation of cells. They were originally defined in viral systems. Most oncogenes identified to date have been detected in tumors induced by acute transforming viruses. Alkylating agents and radiation involve activation of many of the same cellular oncogenes that are homologous to the oncogenes carried by retroviruses. Many oncogenes have been shown to be associated with specific chromosomal breakpoints or translocations (Table 18-12). Therefore, a silent oncogene can come to be involved at an active chromosomal site, resulting in unregulated expression (cell division) or expression of an inappropriate cell type (cell differentiation). Also, there are proteins that convert an extracellular signal into an intracellular biochemical event, leading to a neoplastic event such as epidermal growth factor. Oncogenesis is likely a multistep process.

Oncogenes in virus-induced transformation-- Retroviruses: viral gene sequences encode a product thought to activate transcription of many different cellular genes. Examples include HTLV-I, causative agent in adult T-cell leukemia; HTLV-II, associated with one T-cell hairy-cell leukemia line; and Epstein-Barr virus infection, Burkitt's lymphoma, nasopharyngeal carcinoma, Hodgkin's disease. Oncogene activation may occur with rearrangements of an oncogene, mutation of an oncogene, or through altered expression of an oncogene.

- Oncogenes are gene loci with potential to affect neoplastic transformation of cells.
- Most known oncogenes have been detected in tumors induced by viruses.
- Many oncogenes are associated with chromosomal breakpoints or translocations.

Table 18-12.--Chromosome Rearrangement and Increase of Specific Oncogenes

Disease	Rearrangement	Oncogene
Burkitt's lymphoma	t(8,14)	c-*myc*
	t(8,22)	Translocation into transcriptionally active immunoglobulin heavy or light chain loci
Acute lymphocytic leukemia	t(8,14)	c-*myc*
Chronic granulocytic leukemia	t(9,22)	c-*abl*

COAGULATION

Prolonged Bleeding Time

The coagulation mechanism does not participate in the bleeding time. An abnormal bleeding time is a reflection of vascular defects, quantitative disorders of platelets (including thrombocytopenia and thrombocytosis), or functional disorders of platelets. Qualitative platelet defects result in an abnormal bleeding time but normal partial thromboplastin time, prothrombin time, thrombin time, and platelet count (except von Willebrand's disease and disseminated intravascular coagulopathy).

- Prolonged bleeding time differential diagnosis includes Glanzmann's thrombasthenia, von Willebrand's disease, Bernard-Soulier syndrome, disseminated intravascular coagulopathy, thrombocytopenia, storage pool disease, drugs (aspirin, etc.), and uremia.

von Willebrand's disease

von Willebrand's disease is the commonest inherited bleeding disorder; at least 20 subtypes have been described. The inheritance pattern is autosomal dominant with incomplete penetrance (parent of either sex). The bleeding is usually mild, but hemorrhage postoperatively can be severe. Mucocutaneous bleeding, epistaxis, easy bruising, and menorrhagia are characteristic, with occasional gastrointestinal tract bleeding, hematuria, and, rarely, hemarthroses.

To understand von Willebrand's disease, it is helpful to review platelet activity. The initial step of adhesion is followed by aggregation. Collagen and factor VIII-related antigen are involved in adhesion. Factor VIII-related antigen is found in plasma, platelets, and endothelial regions and is detected functionally by its ability to cause aggregation of washed platelets when ristocetin is administered. Aggregation requires ADP and thromboxane A_2. The activation of the clotting mechanism and generation of thrombin seem to result from the activation of the platelet membrane during adhesion and aggregation. Platelets make available platelet factor III and catalyze the activation of other coagulation factors. von Willebrand factor (vWF) is contained in endothelial cells, platelets, and plasma. The factor VIII complex is composed of the following: 1) VIII:C, the coagulant activity which is missing in hemophiliac plasma; this is decreased in hemophilia and von Willebrand's disease and circulates in the plasma with von Willebrand factor VIII (VIII vWF). 2) VIII C:Ag, antigenic determinants of VIII:C; this is

decreased in von Willebrand's disease and is normal in hemophilia. 3) VIII vWF antigen (vWF:Ag): Willebrand factor (vWF), this serves as a carrier for VIII:C and is the mediator of the initial platelet adhesion to the blood vessel wall. It is produced by megakaryocytes and vascular endothelial cells. The adhesive function is contained largely within large multimers. 4)VIII vWF activity: ristocetin cofactor, the activity necessary for ristocetin-induced platelet aggregation that is not present in von Willebrand's disease. 5) VIII R:Ag, antigenic determinant of VIII R:vWF and/or VIII R:RCo; factor VIII-related antigen is important in adherence, and it is likely that the activities of VIII R:vWF and VIII R:RCo are properties of this protein. All platelet-related activities of the VIII molecule are referred to as "vWF." vWF plays an essential role in the adhesion of platelets to the subendothelium. Factor VIII coagulant activity and vWF activity reside in two separate molecules that are noncovalently bound in the plasma. Therefore, von Willebrand's disease represents a defect in hemostasis involving the interaction of the platelet membrane glycoprotein, subendothelial tissues, and vWF. There is either decreased synthesis, decreased release, or abdominal production of vWF.

The many distinct variants can be divided into different subtypes. Type I is characterized by a quantitative abnormality in vWF. It is the commonest type and is autosomal dominant in inheritance pattern. The total amount of circulating vWF multimers are $\leq$50%. The distribution and function of vWF are normal. Type II is characterized by a qualitative abnormality in vWF. Type IIA and IIB are characterized by an absence of more functionally potent, large high molecular weight vWF multimers from plasma. There is a decrease in the total vWF and VIII:C levels. A number of variants exist. Type IIC is characterized by quite abnormal multimers. Heterozygous vWD disease is characterized clinically by mild to moderate bleeding. It is autosomal dominant in inheritance pattern. The laboratory diagnosis of von Willebrand's disease includes prolonged bleeding time, reduced VIII:C, VIII:vWF antigen (vWF:Ag), vWF activity (ristocetin-cofactor activity), normal platelet aggregation except in the presence of ristocetin, and a mildly prolonged partial thromboplastin time.

Treatment--Mild and moderate cases of von Willebrand's disease require treatment only at the time of an operation or bleeding. For menorrhagia, birth control pills are effective. For dental extractions, local hemostasis and local fibrinolytic agents are effective. In pregnancy, there is no need to transfuse in mild to moderate cases of the disease, because the levels of vWF increase with the duration of pregnancy. The mainstays of treatment are 1-desamino-8-D-arginine vasopressin (DDAVP), factor VIII concentrates rich in vWF, and cryoprecipitate. DDAVP causes the release of preformed vWF multimers from the subendothelium and is useful in type I von Willebrand's disease. Repeated injections of this agent may cause hyponatremia. Rapid tachyphylaxis may develop. A trial should be conducted before it is used as primary therapy. The levels increase for 4-8 hours. This usually is only effective in type I von Willebrand's disease. For patients with type IIB von Willebrand's disease or for those with type I disease who have become transiently unresponsive to DDAVP, viral-inactivated factor VIII preparations rich in vWF are recommended. Cryoprecipitate from carefully selected and repeatedly tested donors is more desirable than cryoprecipitate from random donors.

Glanzmann's Thrombasthenia

Glanzmann's thrombasthenia results from a defect in the first phase of platelet aggregation, secondary to marked reduction or absent platelet glycoproteins IIb and IIIa. It is autosomal recessive in inheritance pattern. Early hemorrhagic complications occur in the neonatal period, and epistaxis, purpura, petechiae, and ecchymoses persist throughout life. The laboratory findings include no clumping of platelets on the peripheral blood smear, normal platelet number and morphology, and no aggregation with ADP, epinephrine, thrombin, or collagen. There is aggregation with ristocetin/factor VIII R:vWF. Treatment consists of nasal packing, local measures, and cryoprecipitate, with or without platelets, when local measures are not successful.

Bernard-Soulier Syndrome

Bernard-Soulier syndrome is the result of the absence of glycoprotein Ib complexes on the surface of human platelets that mediate ristocetin-induced vWF-dependent platelet aggregation. Glycoprotein Ib is the platelet receptor for vWF. It is more common in Caucasians and blacks and is autosomal recessive in inheritance pattern. This disorder is characterized by moderate to severe bleeding with surgery and menstruation. Bleeding typically is from mucous membranes, gums, and the gastrointestinal tract. The bleeding time is markedly prolonged. Characteristically, there is thrombocytopenia with giant platelets. The aggregation pattern is the opposite of that of Glanzmann's thrombasthenia with normal platelet aggregation with ADP, collagen, epinephrine, and thrombin but no aggregation with ristocetin.

Storage Pool Disease

Normally, ATP, ADP, serotonin, and calcium are stored by platelets and released from them. In storage pool disease, there is a marked decrease in platelet ADP and a lesser decrease in ATP. Because of the profound decrease in ADP, the amount released from the platelets is insufficient to bring uninvolved platelets into larger aggregates.

Disseminated Intravascular Coagulopathy

Disseminated intravascular coagulopathy is characterized by a dynamic process caused by many diseases with microvascular clotting secondary to thrombin deposition. The laboratory findings are variable. No single laboratory test can confirm or exclude the diagnosis, which depends on the clinical setting and laboratory findings. The manifestations vary from patient to patient and from time to time in the same patient. These may be of little clinical significance or cause life-threatening bleeding or clotting. The mortality rates range from 50% to 85%.

The pathophysiology of disseminated intravascular coagulopathy is complex. Thrombin is formed in the vascular system and alters platelets. The platelets aggregate, agglutinate, and secrete many products, resulting in thrombocytopenia and platelets that do not function well. Thrombin cleaves fibrinopeptides A and B from fibrinogen to form fibrin monomers. These monomers may complex with fibrinogen (polymerization) to form insoluble fibrin, which is deposited in capillaries and small blood vessels, resulting in microangiopathy. Activated factor XIII cross-links fibrin to make it more resistant to fibrinolysis. Thrombin increases the activity of factors V and VIII. Therefore, thrombin accounts for the decreased fibrinogen, platelets, and factors II, V, VIII, and XIII. Secondary fibrinolysis may occur. Activated factor XII leads to kallikrein production, resulting in the conversion of plasminogen to plasmin, which is capable of digesting fibrinogen, factors V, VIII, XIII, and complement. Fibrinogen is converted to X, Y, D, and E. The clinical picture depends on a balance: if thrombin activity is greater than plasmin activity, there is thrombosis; or, if plasmin activity is greater than thrombin activity, there is hemorrhage.

The following occur in acute disseminated intravascular coagulopathy: bleeding from wounds and periveni-puncture sites, ecchymoses, petechiae, hematomas, hematuria, intracranial hemorrhage, intrapleural hemorrhage, intraperitoneal hemorrhage, hemoptysis, vaginal melena, and hematemesis. Thromboembolic complications, as manifested by necrotic skin lesions, pulmonary emboli, acute arterial occlusions, ischemia, stroke, and myocardial infarction, may occur in 8% of patients. Thrombosis is more common than bleeding in chronic disseminated intravascular coagulopathy.

Causes--Infections are the primary cause (gram-negative and gram-positive organisms, e.g., *Staphylococcus*, *Streptococcus*, pneumococcus, typhoid, *Rickettsia*, viral, fungal, histoplasmosis, *Aspergillus*). Malignancies are the second most common cause: leukemia (acute progranulocytic [M3]), carcinomas of the pancreas, prostate, breast, and lymphoma. Surgery/trauma is the third leading cause. Other causes are liver disease, pregnancy, acute renal failure associated with cardiogenic shock, gun shots, endothelial injury (giant hemangiomas, aortic aneurysms, angiography), hemolytic transfusion reactions, burns, crush injuries, acidosis, and alkalosis.

Tests--The best screening study results are thrombocytopenia in 90% of patients, increased prothrombin time in 90% of patients, and hypofibrinogenemia in 70% of patients. The best available confirmatory test is the fibrin D-dimer assay, which detects fibrinogen fragments that are formed by the lysis of cross-linked fibrin.

● Screening tests for disseminated intravascular coagulopathy: thrombocytopenia (90%), increased prothrombin time (90%), hypofibrinogenemia (70%)

Treatment--The first goal in treatment is to treat the underlying disease. Then, the approach depends on the clinical situation. If the patient has a low level of fibrinogen, low platelet count, and/or low levels of clotting factor and is not bleeding or undergoing a surgical procedure, no treatment is necessary. If the patient is bleeding or undergoing a surgical procedure, treat with cryoprecipitate, fresh frozen plasma, and platelets. If the patient continues to bleed and the above measures do not cause an increase in coagulation factors, it may be necessary to continue factor and platelet replacement therapy and start a continuous infusion of heparin. If there is evidence of fibrin deposition (such as dermal necrosis in purpura fulminans, acral ischemia, or venous thromboembolism), heparin therapy is indicated. Other instances in which heparin is indicated are retained dead fetus with hypofibrinogenemia before induction of labor, excessive bleeding associated with giant hemangioma, promyelocytic leukemia, and mucinous adenocarcinoma. Heparin is not indicated in >95% of patients.

Coagulation and Liver Disease

The most important factor is the condition of the blood vessels. There is no tendency to bleed unless and until blood vessels are damaged, such as by needle, surgical procedure, or gastric acid. The three main coagulation patterns are: 1) portal hypertension, which is characterized by thrombocytopenia and normal coagulation-factor synthesis; 2) cholestasis, which results in impaired absorption of fat-soluble vitamins and an increase in prothrombin time and activated partial thromboplastin time; and 3) acute and chronic hepatocellular disease, which is characterized by a normal fibrinogen level (until late in the course of the disease), thrombocytopenia, and an increase in prothrombin time and activated partial thromboplastin time because of multiple factor deficiencies. Table 18-13 contrasts liver disease with disseminated intravascular coagulopathy.

Table 18-13.--Differences in Laboratory Findings in Liver Disease and Disseminated Intravascular Coagulopathy

Tests	Liver disease	Disseminated intravascular coagulopathy
Thrombocytopenia	Mild, decreased in 50% of cases, <50,000 uncommon	90% of cases
Increased prothrombin time	Common	90% of cases
Decreased fibrinogen	Late in disease	70% of cases
Factor V	Decreased	Regularly decreased
Factor VIII	Normal	Regularly decreased
Factors VII, X	Decreased	Normal

Factor-Deficiency States

Factor XI Deficiency (Hemophilia C)

This disorder is autosomal dominant in inheritance pattern and more common among persons of Jewish descent. Bleeding occurs after injury or operation. Laboratory findings include prolonged partial thromboplastin time and activated partial thromboplastin time but a normal prothrombin time. The treatment of choice is fresh frozen plasma.

Factor IX Deficiency (Christmas Disease, Hemophilia B)

This X-linked disorder accounts for 15% of all cases of hemophilia. It is clinically indistinguishable from factor VIII deficiency. The laboratory abnormalities include an abnormal partial thromboplastin time. The treatment for mild cases is fresh frozen plasma. Patients undergoing a surgical procedure or who have major bleeding should receive purified factor IX complex. There may be an increased risk of thrombosis, because of the presence of activated factors VII and X. Three other available products are KONȳNE, Proplex, and Profilnine, which are factor IX-complex products developed from a monoclonal antibody purifying process. They are safe from contamination with the AIDS virus, and the risk of hepatitis is significantly reduced.

Factor VIII Deficiency (Hemophilia A)

This disease results from a defect in factor VIII:C, is X-linked recessive in inheritance pattern, and accounts for 85% of cases of hemophilia. If a hemophiliac male has children from a normal female, all daughters are obligatory carriers and all sons are normal. If a normal male marries a carrier, each daughter has a 50% chance of being a carrier and each son has a 50% chance of having hemophilia. At birth, there are no bleeding manifestations; however, 50% of males bleed at the time of circumcision. Bleeding occurs in 75% of severely affected infants by age 18 months. The severity of hemophilia runs true in families. Severe hemophiliacs have less than 1% factor VIII and clinically have hemarthroses, atrophied muscles, and subcutaneous hematomas in the tongue and neck, and hematomas in the genitourinary and gastrointestinal tracts. Mild hemophiliacs have factor VIII levels of 5%-25% and may bleed heavily, even fatally postoperatively or after dental extractions unless the factor is adequately replaced.

Laboratory studies reveal an abnormal partial thromboplastin time, abnormal factor VIII:C, normal prothrombin time, normal bleeding time, and normal thrombin time. Treatment consists of factor VIII concentrate, which has a half-life of 8-12 hours. Current factor VIII:C concentrates are regarded as safe from HIV transmission. However, three highly purified products, all produced by monoclonal antibodies, are available and no cases of AIDS or hepatitis have been reported with the use of these products. There have been no seroconversions to HIV with any of the products in the U.S., including products that have been heated in aqueous solution, solvent-detergent treated, and/or immunoaffinity purified. Recombinant factor VIII products are also available. Always check Bethesda unit assay before any general surgery in patients with hemophilia. From 5% to 20% of hemophiliacs develop inhibitors (IgG antibodies) that inactivate factor VIII:C (Bethesda units). If the inhibitor is <3 Bethesda units/mL, then treat with higher doses or replacement therapy. If the value is higher (>10 Bethesda units), one can attempt to use prothrombin complex concentrates (II, VII, IX, X) to "bypass." Table 18-14 contrasts hemophilia A with von Willebrand's disease.

- Management of hemophilia A: a desmopressin trial should be undertaken in cases of mild-to-moderate hemophilia A.
- For other patients, factor VIII products that are heat treated, solvent-detergent treated, or immunoaffinity purified.

Table 18-14.--Differences Between Hemophilia A and von Willebrand's Disease

	Hemophilia A	von Wille-brand's disease
Inheritance	Sex-linked	Autosomal
Bleeding time	Normal	Prolonged
Factor VIII C	Decreased	Decreased
Factor VIII rag	Normal	Decreased
Ristocetin cofactor	Normal	Decreased

Acquired factor VIII deficiency states may occur and are secondary to the following causes: idiopathic, postpartum, collagen vascular diseases (rheumatoid arthritis, systemic lupus erythematosus, temporal arteritis), drug hypersensitivity (penicillin, sulfonamides), malignancies (lymphoproliferative, solid tumors), and old age. Clinically, bleeding is intramuscular, retropharyngeal, retroperitoneal, and cerebral. Also, hematuria occurs. The treatment is very difficult and requires the combination of steroids, plasmapheresis, prothrombin-complex concentrate, activated prothrombin-complex concentrate, and porcine factor VIII.

Factor XII deficiency is an autosomal recessive disorder in which thromboembolic complications are more important than bleeding complications. The activated partial thromboplastin time is abnormal, and the prothrombin time is normal.

Factor VII deficiency is characterized clinically by epistaxis, gingival bleeding, bleeding after trauma, menorrhagia, and hemarthroses. The activated partial thromboplastin time is normal, and the prothrombin time is abnormal.

Factor X deficiency is characterized by bleeding that

is the same as that in factor VII deficiency. An acquired factor X deficiency state may occur in amyloidosis. The activated partial thromboplastin time and prothrombin time are abnormal.

Factor V deficiency may be acquired in myeloproliferative disorders. Bruising occurs with severe bleeding postoperatively and at onset of menstruation. Treatment consists of administering platelets and fresh frozen plasma.

In factor XIII deficiency, there is a history of umbilical cord bleeding, ecchymoses, and prolonged hemorrhage from cuts. It is autosomal recessive in inheritance. All routine clotting tests, including bleeding time, may give normal results. Treatment is with fresh frozen plasma. Table 18-15 summarizes the hemorrhagic disorders.

Table 18-15.--Summary of Test Results in Hemorrhagic Disorders and Anticoagulant Therapy

	Prothrombin time	Activated partial thromboplastin time	Thrombin time	Fibrinogen	Bleeding time
Classic hemophilia A	Normal	Abnormal	Normal	Normal	Normal
von Willebrand's disease	Normal	Normal or abnormal	Normal	Normal	Abnormal
Afibrinogenemia	Abnormal	Abnormal	Abnormal	Absent	Normal
Hypofibrinogenemia	Normal	Normal	Normal	Low	Normal
Dysfibrinogenemia	Normal or abnormal	Normal or abnormal	Abnormal	Normal	Normal
Factor XIII deficiency	Normal	Normal	Normal	Normal	Normal
Heparin	Slightly abnormal	Abnormal	Abnormal	Normal	Normal or abnormal
Warfarin (Coumadin)	Abnormal	Normal or abnormal	Normal	Normal	Normal

Treatment of Factor Deficiency States

Circulatory overload problems must be taken into consideration when transfusing into patients materials used to treat deficiency states. The composition of these materials is given in Table 18-16. To control major bleeding or to prepare patients for a surgical procedure, it is advised that the plasma level of factor VIII be increased to 60% in patients with factor VIII deficiency. The number of factor VIII units is calculated by multiplying the patient's weight in pounds by 12 (example, 160 pounds x 12 = 1,920 units of factor VIII).

Fresh frozen plasma is a good source of all factors. It is used in treating congenital deficiencies in factors II, V,

VII, IX, X, XI, and XIII and multiple coagulation deficiencies, including oral anticoagulant overdose, liver disease, massive transfusion, disseminated intravascular coagulopathy, plasmapheresis, and vitamin K deficiency. One should suspect multiple coagulation factor deficiencies in patients with prolonged prothrombin times and partial thromboplastin times >1.5 times normal if not due to known coagulation factor deficiency or circulating lupus-like anticoagulant. In dosing fresh frozen plasma, 1-2 units is usually not sufficient to replace coagulation factors as in liver disease, which requires 3-9 units. The maximal effect declines 2-4 hours after transfusion. Purified antihemophilic concentrates are derived from

Table 18-16.--Composition of Materials Used to Treat Factor Deficiency States

Type	Volume, mL	Factor VIII units per container	Amount of protein per 100 factor VIII units, mg
Fresh frozen plasma	180-250	160-225	3,300
Cryoprecipitate	10-30	75-120	900
Antihemophilic factor	10-25	250-500	500

Modified from Huestis DW, Bove JR, Busch S: Practical Blood Transfusion. Third edition. Boston, Little, Brown and Company, 1981, p 295. By permission of authors.

fresh frozen plasma of paid donors and are lyophilized or freeze-dried in form. Complications include hepatitis and factor VIII inhibitors. Cryoprecipitate is a good source of V, VIII, and fibrinogen. The activity per gram of protein is 12-60 times that of fresh frozen plasma. One bag will increase the factor VIII level 2.5% or one bag per 6 kg of body weight twice a day in factor VIII deficiency. Factor IX complex contains factors II, VII, IX, and X. Activated factor IX-complex products include KONyNE and anti-inhibitor coagulant complex, heat treated (Autoplex T). This is indicated in severe factor IX deficiency and in the management of factor VIII inhibitors. Complications include hepatitis, disseminated intravascular coagulopathy, and thrombosis.

Hypercoagulable States

The differential diagnosis of hypercoagulable states includes polycythemia rubra vera, paroxysmal nocturnal hemoglobinuria, chronic disseminated intravascular coagulopathy, cryoglobulinemia, the lupus anticoagulant, and the deficiency states of protein S, protein C, antithrombin III. Protein S deficiency is more common than deficiency of protein C or antithrombin III. Routine coagulation assays fail to detect these patients. A 50% reduction in either protein S or C increases thrombotic tendencies. Family studies are requisite. Assays are available for all three. Protein S is a vitamin K-dependent factor that is required for expression of activated protein C anticoagulant activity. There is an increased incidence of thrombosis, with venous complications greater than arterial. Activated protein C destroys activated factors V and VIII and, thus, is a potent plasma anticoagulant. Activated protein C requires a second vitamin K-dependent factor, or cofactor, protein S. Antithrombin III deficiency is an uncommon cause of venous thromboembolism. The management of protein S deficiency, protein C deficiency, and antithrombin III deficiency requires heparin and

oral anticoagulant agents. There is an increased incidence of warfarin (Coumadin) necrosis that is a rare complication in nonhospitalized patients and occurs 2-10 days after initiating treatment with warfarin.

The lupus anticoagulant is a coagulation inhibitor of the activated partial thromboplastin time that does not correct with mixing experiments with equal volumes of normal plasma. This coagulation inhibitor is secondary to nonspecific IgG and IgM antibodies. It is phospholipid-dependent. The antiphospholipid antibody has some lupus anticoagulant antibody activity directed against phospholipids. Cardiolipin may be absent. This can cause false-positive VDRL results. The screening test is the prolonged activated partial thromboplastin time. Clinically, venous thrombosis of the lower extremities is more common than arterial thrombosis. This is associated with pregnancy, atypical stroke syndrome in younger adults, chronic skin ulcers, and, in patients <45 years old, surviving myocardial infarction.

Warfarin

Warfarin limits the gamma-carboxylation of the vitamin K-dependent coagulation proteins II, VII, IX, X and anticoagulant proteins C and S, impairing their biologic function in blood coagulation. This drug is contraindicated in pregnancy and in patients with a hemorrhagic tendency such as thrombocytopenia or coagulation factor abnormalities, diastolic blood pressure >110 mm Hg, gastrointestinal lesions liable to bleed, severe liver disease, severe renal disease, malabsorption, subacute bacterial endocarditis, diverticulosis, or colitis. It is also contraindicated if the patient recently had a surgical procedure performed on the central nervous system or eye. The appropriate dose of warfarin is that which maintains the prothrombin time at an International Normalized Ratio (INR) of 2-3, which corresponds to a prothrombin time ratio of 1.3 to 1.5. The main complication is bleeding, which occurs in 2%-4% of patients. In patients with a prolonged prothrombin time with or without bleeding, use of the drug should be stopped for 24-72 hours. In patients who have taken a suicidal dose or have a suspected cerebral hemorrhage and who need no further anticoagulation, vitamin K given intravenously at a dose of 20-30 mg may be administered with fresh frozen plasma. Fresh frozen plasma may be administered to patients taking warfarin who require continued anticoagulation but who have life-threatening bleeding. Drugs that potentiate warfarin include those that prolong the prothrombin time, such as phenylbutazone, metronidazole, sulfinpyrazone, trimethoprim/sulfamethoxazole, and disulfiram. Drugs that inhibit platelet function, such as aspirin, may also potentiate the toxic effects of warfarin. Some drugs antagonize warfarin; e.g., cholestyramine reduces the absorption of warfarin. Other drugs, such as barbiturates, carbamazepine, and rifampin, increase the clearance of warfarin.

Heparin

Heparin inhibits thrombin by forming a heparin-antithrombin III complex. The heparin is then reused. In the initial treatment of deep venous thrombosis or pulmonary embolus, the goal is to prolong the activated partial thromboplastin time at a level of 1.5-2.5 times normal within the first 24 hours of treatment. If this is not accomplished, the risk of recurrent thromboembolism is 15-fold, and the risk persists for weeks. Heparin and warfarin may be given simultaneously and be overlapped for 5 days, after which treatment should be warfarin alone. Warfarin treatment should be maintained for 3 months if there are no risk factors. Heparin is indicated for the treatment of venous thrombosis and pulmonary emboli. It is also used to prevent venous thrombosis and pulmonary emboli (prophylactic doses of 5,000 U subcutaneously every 8-12 hours in cases of abdominal surgery or for medical patients with a history of thrombosis, prolonged bed rest, congestive heart failure, and cancer). A dose of 12,000 U is administered subcutaneously twice a day for the prevention of mural thrombosis after myocardial infarction. Heparin is indicated in the prevention of coronary artery rethrombosis after thrombolysis, and it is the treatment of choice in venous thrombosis and pulmonary emboli in pregnancy (15,000 U subcutaneously twice a day). Impedance plethysmography, ultrasonography, or venography may document this complication of pregnancy. Warfarin is contraindicated in pregnancy because of the risks of embryopathy, including nasal hypoplasia and central nervous system abnormalities. Heparin is indicated after treatment with thrombolytic therapy. The normal dose is a 5,000 U bolus followed by 30,000 to 35,000 U/24 hours by continuous infusion. Side effects include hemorrhage (which occurs in 6.8% of patients treated by continuous infusion), osteoporosis, and skin necrosis. A hypersensitivity reaction may convert antithrombin III from a slow inhibitor to a very rapid inhibitor.

Thrombolytic Therapy

The thrombolytic agents are streptokinase, urokinase, recombinant tissue plasminogen activator, and anisolyated streptokinase-plasminogen activator complex. Fibrin is the major target of thrombolytic therapy. Anticoagulation does *not* dissolve or prevent the growth of thrombi (even at recommended doses), eliminate the source of subsequent emboli in the deep veins during an acute attack, alleviate hemodynamic problems, prevent valvular damage, prevent persistent venous hypertension, or prevent persistent pulmonary hypertension. The primary role of anticoagulation is prophylaxis against further propagation of the clot.

Thrombolytic therapy lyses thrombi and emboli and restores the circulation to normal, normalizes hemodynamic disturbances, reduces morbidity, decreases systemic and mean pulmonary artery pressures at 72 hours, prevents venous vascular damage and subsequent venous hypertension in the lower extremities, and prevents permanent damage to the pulmonary vascular bed, reducing the likelihood of persistent pulmonary hypertension. Residual emboli usually persist with heparin therapy alone. Tissue plasminogen activator has a relative fibrin specificity; yet, significant fibrinolysis and bleeding may occur. There is an initial fibrinolysis of the plug followed by proteolysis of fibrinogen, V, and VIII. In general, venous thrombi are rich in fibrin and are potentially more suitable than platelet thrombi to fibrinolytic therapy. The age of the thrombus is also important in that it is essential to start these agents within 48 hours in cases of pulmonary emboli and in <7 days in cases of deep venous thrombosis. In cases of pulmonary emboli, this treatment improves hemodynamics and pulmonary perfusion; it may be indicated with more lobar pulmonary arteries or an equivalent amount of emboli in other vessels with or without shock or submassive emboli accompanied by shock or impending shock or persistent hypotension. In deep venous thrombosis, these agents may minimize valvular dysfunction and decrease the risk of recurrent and postphlebitic syndrome. If the timing is appropriate, these agents may be administered in thrombosis of the hepatic, renal, mesenteric, cerebrovenous, sinus, and central retinal veins. Of arterial disorders, acute myocardial infarction has been the most excessively studied. The SCAT 1 trial demonstrated that mortality was significantly lower in patients randomized to heparin after thrombolytic therapy in acute myocardial infarction. The GISSI 2 trial demonstrated a lower mortality rate after patients received streptokinase but not tissue plasminogen activator. The GUSTO trial revealed that a rapid infusion of tissue plasminogen activator with intravenously given heparin was most favorable.

Thrombolytic therapy is monitored with fibrinogen levels. The absolute contraindications to this therapy include active internal bleeding and a cerebral vascular accident within 2 weeks. Relatively major contraindications include the following if they have occurred within <10 days: major surgical procedure, obstetrical delivery, pregnancy, the first 10 days postpartum, organ biopsy, burns, skin grafts, previous puncture of noncompressible vessels, thoracentesis, paracentesis, gastrointestinal tract bleeding, ulcerative colitis, diverticulosis, serious trauma, systolic blood pressure >200 mm Hg, diastolic pressure >110 mm Hg, intracranial neoplasms, or thrombocytopenia. Relatively minor contraindications include a high likelihood of left-sided heart thrombus such as mitral stenosis with atrial fibrillation, subacute bacterial endocarditis, severe hepatic or renal disease, age >75 years, diabetic hemorrhagic retinopathy, active and progressive cavitating lung lesions, ulcerative cutaneous and mucous membrane lesions, recent intra-arterial diagnostic procedure except arterial blood gases. Bleeding may be superficial or internal; it occurs because of the indiscriminate lysis of fibrin. Thrombolytic agents are not substitutes for heparin and warfarin and, therefore, the morbidity is additive. Approaches to hemorrhage control include volume replacement, manual techniques, and RBC transfusions. If bleeding is massive, replace with cryoprecipitate, fresh frozen plasma, and discontinue use of heparin. With central nervous system bleeding, discontinue fibrinolytic therapy and administer cryoprecipitate and fresh frozen plasma. Avoid anticoagulant agents, aspirin, antiplatelet drugs, and dextran.

Aplastic Anemia

Aplastic anemia may develop as a consequence of a defect in the stem cell population, defective marrow environment, or immune suppression. This group of disorders with failure of hematopoiesis is characterized by peripheral pancytopenia, bone marrow hypocellularity, and absence of malignant or myeloproliferative diseases. No primary disease of hematopoietic tissue is evident.

Natural history--Before the use of allogeneic bone marrow transplantation and antithymocyte globulin, 80% of patients were not alive at 1-2 years, and 20% had partial recovery.

- Aplastic anemia: pancytopenia, hypocellular bone marrow, and absence of primary disease of hematopoietic tissue.
- 80% death rate at 2 years; full recovery uncommon without allogeneic bone marrow transplantation or antithymocyte globulin.

Clinical features include weakness, fatigue, easy bruising or bleeding, fever, and infections. Lymphadenopathy and splenomegaly are uncommon. In 40%-70% of patients, the cause of aplastic anemia is idiopathic. This is more frequent in adults. Drugs are the second most common cause of aplastic anemia. These include chloramphenicol, phenylbutazone, methylphenylethylhydantoin, trimethadione, sulfonamides, gold, and benzene. Paroxysmal nocturnal hemoglobinuria and infections are the third and fourth most common causes, respectively. Infectious hepatitis is the most common infection to cause aplastic anemia. Non-A, non-B, non-C hepatitis followed by hepatitis A are the most common types of hepatitis to cause aplastic anemia. Hepatitis B is the least common hepatitis that causes aplastic anemia. These patients have a poor prognosis. Other infectious agents causing aplastic anemia include Epstein-Barr viral infections, influenza, and mycobacterial infections. Ionizing irradiation may also be a cause.

If transfusion is needed, select nonrelated donors and use leukocyte-poor RBC transfusions and single-donor platelet transfusions. Transfusions should be given with considerable care and concern. Family members should not be donors, because they are more likely to sensitize the patient to minor histocompatibility antigens present in the donor but absent in the patient. The survival rate is better for those not receiving transfusion. Immunosuppressive treatments include antithymocyte globulin with or without cyclosporine. These are not curative. In a trial of moderate to severe aplastic anemia patients, 11 of the 21 treated with antithymocyte globulin alone had sustained improvement, whereas none of the 21 in the control population improved. The bone marrow transplantation success rate is 65% in young patients. This is the therapy of choice in all patients with a homozygous twin and should be considered immediately for all patients younger than 50 with severe aplastic anemia and an HLA match. Cyclosporine or corticosteroids, at a dose of 0.2-1.0 mg/kg daily, and androgens are other therapeutic modalities. Androgens are not effective in severe aplastic anemia. The toxic effects include virilization and hepatic toxicity. The 17-alpha derivative is responsible for hepatic adenomas and hepatocellular carcinoma.

- With severe aplastic anemia, avoid transfusions.
- If the patient is younger than 50 and has an HLA-matched donor or identical twin, perform bone marrow transplantation with cyclophosphamide and irradiation as preconditioning before transplantation if transfused. If older than 45-50 years and no HLA match, treat with antithymocyte globulin.

Neutropenia

The causes of neutropenia are multiple. Drug-induced neutropenia is associated with sulfonamides, semisynthetic penicillins (nafcillin, ampicillin), phenothiazines, nonsteroidal anti-inflammatory agents (indomethacin), and antithyroid medications (propylthiouracil, methimazole). Cyclic neutropenia is characterized by oscillations in the neutrophil counts every 19-23 days. It is a disorder of neutrophil production at a regulation phase. The typical clinical syndrome is manifested as furuncles, cellulitis, chronic gingivitis, and abscesses. Patients can predict the timing of successive episodes. Treatment involves timely antibiotics, avoidance of dental and surgical work at nadirs, oral hygiene, and dental care. Granulocyte colony-stimulating factor (filgrastim) may be effective in increasing the neutrophil count.

Neutropenia in the black population is common, and if patients are asymptomatic, this need not be evaluated further. Other causes of neutropenia include autoimmune neutropenia (which is secondary to an antibody), antigens, rheumatoid arthritis, and chronic active hepatitis.

Thrombocytopenia

Severe hemorrhage is unusual in thrombocytopenia; patients usually have only petechiae and menorrhagia. There is decreased platelet survival with increased platelet-associated IgG antibody, which is a panantibody that binds to autologous platelets, monologous platelets, and megakaryocytes. The spleen is the primary site of the antibody response. The differential diagnosis includes idiopathic thrombocytopenic purpura, drug-induced

thrombocytopenia, and secondary causes, including systemic lupus erythematosus (in which 14%-26% of patients develop thrombocytopenia), sarcoidosis, non-Hodgkin's lymphoma, chronic lymphocytic leukemia, viral infections, ovarian carcinoma, purpura of septicemia, Evans's syndrome, and post-transfusion purpura.

Post-transfusion purpura occurs 7-10 days after blood transfusion and is a complication of the transfusion of blood products from donors positive for the platelet antigen P1A[1] into P1A[1]-negative recipients previously sensitized to this antigen by pregnancy or transfusions. Treatment includes plasmapheresis and exchange transfusion; prednisone may be added to the regimen.

Idiopathic thrombocytopenic purpura is characterized by thrombocytopenia with a normal WBC count and hemoglobin (Table 18-17). The mean platelet volume is increased. Splenomegaly is present in only 10% of patients. If it is present, one should think of other causes. Bone marrow examination reveals a normal to increased number of megakaryocytes. Corticosteroids are the mainstay of treatment; 70% of patients initially respond, with about a 40% chance of long-term remission at an initial dose of prednisone of 1 mg/kg daily for up to 1 month. Steroids decrease antibody production in the reticuloendothelial system and decrease reticuloendothelial clearance. Patients who have relapse after a steroid-induced remission may respond to a repeat course of steroids. Splenectomy removes the predominant site of antibody production and platelet destruction and is followed by a 75% chance of long-term remission. Danazol decreases the number of phagocytic cell IgG Fc receptors. A slow infusion of vincristine or vinblastine may be given to patients who do not respond to the above measures. A high dose of gamma globulin blocks the Fc receptors of phagocytic cells and is used in emergency bleeding in acute idiopathic thrombocytopenic purpura, e.g., central nervous system bleeding. Other agents used in refractory cases include azathioprine (Imuran), cyclophosphamide, and colchicine.

In drug-induced thrombocytopenia, the pathophysiology is secondary to haptens bound to a carrier protein. Clinically, there is acute bleeding with a hemorrhage syndrome characterized by bleeding from mucous membranes, petechiae, and oozing after brushing the teeth. These problems subside after use of the drug is discontinued. Drug-induced thrombocytopenia subsides in 4-14 days except for gold, which may take much longer. (Viral-induced thrombocytopenia resolves in 2 weeks to 3 months.) Drugs implicated include heparin, quinidine,

Table 18-17.--Idiopathic Thrombocytopenic Purpura

Characteristics	Acute	Chronic
Presentation	Abrupt onset of petechiae, purpura, mucosal bleeding	Insidious petechiae, menorrhagia
Usual age	Children (2-6 years old)	Adults (20-40 years old)
Sex	Male = female	Female:male = 3:1
Antecedent infection	Common 85%	Uncommon
	Typically an upper respiratory tract infection	
Platelet count, x10^9/L	<20,000 x 10^9/L	30-80 x 10^9/L
Duration	2-6 weeks	Months to years
Spontaneous remission	80% within 6 months	Uncommon, fluctuates

From Lee GR, Bithell TC, Foerster J, Athens JW, Lukens JN: Wintrobe's Clinical Hematology. Vol 2. Ninth edition. Philadelphia, Lea & Febiger, 1993, p 1331. By permission of publisher.

quinine, gold salts, sulphonamides, procainamide, and rifampin. Heparin-induced thrombocytopenia has a variable incidence of 1%-30%. Heparin may enhance platelet aggregation; this mechanism has been implicated in thrombocytopenia and thrombosis. Venous thrombosis is more common than arterial thrombosis. The mechanism of action is immunologic, with heparin-specific IgG antibody and antibodies against a platelet-heparin complex. This complication is usually mild, and the patients are asymptomatic. It develops 3-15 days after therapy, with a median time of 10 days. It is not dose-related and can occur at very low doses. There are no reliable risk factors. Patients are at higher risk if there is a history of this problem. It is essential to pay attention to any substantial reduction in platelet counts while patients are taking heparin.

- Drug-induced thrombocytopenia subsides in 4-14 days except with gold.
- Viral-induced thrombocytopenia resolves in 2 weeks to 3 months.
- Heparin-induced thrombocytopenia is not dose-related.

Postsplenectomy State

Postsplenectomy complications include sepsis secondary to pneumococcus, meningococcus, *Haemophilus influenzae*, *Escherichia coli*, and *Staphylococcus aureus*. Hematologic features include such RBC abnormalities as Howell-Jolly bodies present on the peripheral blood smear. Leukocytes show a postsplenectomic surge and then return to normal numbers. Platelets also show a postsplenectomic surge; the value usually returns to normal in 1 month. If there is a history of splenectomy but no Howell-Jolly bodies on a peripheral blood smear, sus-

pect an accessory spleen and confirm it with a liver-spleen scan.

Spontaneous Splenic Ruptures

Spontaneous splenic ruptures have been reported to occur in infectious mononucleosis (color plate 18-17), cytomegalovirus infections, acute and chronic myelogenous leukemia, acute and chronic lymphocytic leukemia, myeloproliferative diseases, and non-Hodgkin's lymphoma.

Transfusion Reactions

The major transfusion reactions include acute hemolytic transfusion reactions, transfusions associated with anti-IgA antibodies, transfusion-associated adult respiratory distress syndrome, delayed hemolytic transfusion reactions, febrile transfusion reactions, urticarial transfusion reactions, and circulatory overload. Acute hemolytic transfusion reactions are the most life-threatening. The commonest cause is human error (51%), especially when blood is released on an emergency basis, and these are secondary to ABO mismatches. Other causes include antibodies not detected before transfusion, such as Kell, Duffy, and Kidd. ABO mismatches are less frequent when compared with Kell, Duffy, and Kidd and have virtually disappeared from transfusion reaction complications, but clerical error may play a role in these reactions. Intravascular hemolysis is caused by problems related to ABO, Kell, Duffy, and Kidd. Females are at greater risk than males, because sensitization through pregnancy leads to a higher frequency of preformed antibodies. Obstetrical complications with massive bleeding also predispose females. Age is a factor because older people receive more transfusions. Transfusion of large amounts of blood products given urgently also increases the risk. Clinically, there is pain at the intravenous site, apprehension, back pain, abdominal pain, fever, chills, chest pain, hypotension, nausea, flushing, and dyspnea. The Coombs' test gives positive results in all but anti-A. Complications include oliguria in 33.3% of cases, acute postischemic renal failure, and disseminated intravascular coagulopathy in 4%. In one series, the mortality rate was 17%. Treatment includes immediate termination of the transfusion, intravenous access, vigorous administration of fluids, and furosemide to increase renal cortical blood flow. It is difficult to differentiate between an acute hemolytic transfusion reaction and a febrile nonhemolytic transfusion reaction at the time fever occurs. Therefore, fevers occurring during transfusion should be worked up for hemolysis.

Transfusion reactions associated with anti-IgA antibodies and anaphylactic reactions are secondary to IgA deficiency, the development of a class-specific anti-IgA antibody, normal IgA levels with anti-IgA antibodies acquired through pregnancy or previous transfusions, and ataxia telangiectasia, in which 44% of patients have class-specific anti-IgA antibodies. The pathogenesis is secondary to anti-IgA antibodies of IgG type that are capable of binding complement. Clinically, patients develop apprehension, hives, hypotension, chest pain, abdominal pain, lumbar pain, flushing of the face and neck, dyspnea, and cyanosis. Wheezing, diarrhea, vomiting, unconsciousness, and chills may occur. Fevers are uncommon. The treatment includes stopping the transfusion and giving antihistamines and conventional anti-anaphylactic drugs. Transfusion policy for patients with this problem includes washed RBCs, frozen RBCs, and IgA-deficient plasma.

Transfusion-associated adult respiratory distress syndrome or transfusion-related acute lung injury is a complication of transfusion, with respiratory distress in 6 hours, hypotension, bilateral pulmonary infiltrates, normal pulmonary capillary wedge pressure, and fever. Recovery is rapid, occurring in 24-48 hours. Most blood donors implicated in this complication have had multiple pregnancies. Possible mechanisms include leukoagglutinating and lymphocytotoxic antibodies passively transfused from the donor to the recipient, resulting in polymorphonuclear-leukocyte-complement-triggered pulmonary edema. The treatment is supportive. Many patients require a ventilator with positive end-expiratory pressure, furosemide, and dopamine. This disorder may be misdiagnosed as circulatory overload.

Delayed hemolytic transfusion reactions occur because of the inability to detect clinically significant recipient antibodies before transfusion. This is less dramatic and less dangerous than acute hemolytic reactions and is more common in females. The recipient's plasma already contains antibody before transfusion because of previous transfusion, or previous pregnancy. It usually involves the Rh or Kidd systems, which become rapidly undetectable and increase quickly in titer on rapid stimulation. Results of the Coombs' test are positive. There is evidence of hemolysis. One-third of patients are asymptomatic, and the others present with anemia, chills, jaundice, and fever. Management consists of monitoring hemoglobin and renal output. Urticarial reactions are a complication of 1%-3% of all transfusions. Glottal edema and asthma are rarely associated. The cause is an antibody in the recipient against foreign-donor serum proteins. Treatment consists of stopping the transfusion, which is not absolutely necessary, and giving antihistamines (premedication with antihistamines if patient had previous reaction).

Febrile reactions are characterized by chills and fever an hour after the transfusion starts, with accompanying flushing, headache, tachycardia, and discomfort lasting 8-10 hours. This occurs in 1% of all transfusions. The causes include previous transfusions or pregnancy with acquired antibodies against donor leukocyte antigens, antiplatelet antibodies, and antiserum protein antibodies. Treatment consists of stopping the transfusion to evaluate the problem further, because one cannot initially distinguish a febrile reaction from a hemolytic transfusion reaction because both conditions may present with fever.

Circulatory overload may cause tightness in the chest, dry cough, and acute edema in patients with an already increased intravascular volume or decreased cardiac reserve. Management includes slowing the transfusion to 100 mL/hour, placing patient in sitting position, and giving diuretics.

Gaucher's Disease

Adults have type I Gaucher's disease, with no neurologic symptoms, splenomegaly, and no symptoms; 50% have anemia or thrombocytopenia. Bone lesions are present in 75%, with the femur being most common with an Erlenmeyer flask deformity. Avascular necrosis and pathologic fractures may occur. The pathogenesis is related to an accumulation of glucosylceramide due to deficient β-glucuronidase. The Gaucher cell is large and has an eccentric nucleus and fibrillar cytoplasm that is wrinkled like tissue paper (color plate 18-18). Treatment options include alglucerase (Ceredase) (an enzyme replacement therapy that is extraordinarily expensive), hemisplenectomy, and allogeneic bone marrow transplantation.

- Differential diagnosis of asymptomatic massive splenomegaly includes Gaucher's disease, agnogenic myeloid metaplasia, portal hypertension, splenic cyst, non-Hodgkin's lymphoma, and hairy-cell leukemia.

Porphyria

The porphyrias are autosomal dominant except congenital erythropoietic porphyria, which is autosomal recessive. Acute intermittent porphyria lacks skin lesions. It is important to check fecal porphyrins in protoporphyria, variegate porphyria, and coproporphyria. The porphyrias are compared in Table 18-18.

Cardiac Toxicity of Chemotherapeutic Agents

Doxorubicin (Adriamycin) has the greatest potential for cardiac toxicity. It is dose-limited at a dose of 450 mg/m^2 to 500 mg/m^2. The course is characterized by cardiomyopathy to congestive heart failure to death.

The pathologic features are characterized by a diffuse patchy myocardial cell degeneration that antedates any alteration in left ventricular function. Risk factors include age older than 70 years, coronary artery disease, hypertension, and the use of other cardiotoxic agents. Weekly and prolonged continuous infusion schedules may reduce the risk of toxicity. Acutely, there may be transient and reversible nonspecific ST-segment changes, decrease in ejection fraction, or arrhythmias. The dilated cardiomyopathy is dose-dependent: a 3.5% risk at a total dose of 400 mg/m^2 and 7% at a dose of 550 mg/m^2. The clinical features of the cardiomyopathy vary widely. Follow-up examination requires evaluating left ventricular ejection fraction by radionuclide ventriculography or echocardiography. The former is more sensitive.

- Doxorubicin has the greatest potential for cardiac toxicity.
- Incidence of cardiomyopathy is dose-dependent.
- Age >70 years, coronary artery disease, and previous radiation may potentiate toxicity.

Table 18-18.--Comparison of Porphyrias

Porphyria cutanea tarda	Acute intermittent porphyria	Porphyria variegata
	Features	
Most common	Increased urinary δ-aminolevulinic acid	South Africa, Holland
Iron overload	and porphobilinogen	Clinically: skin, sun-exposed,
Skin lesions on light-exposed	Triad of abdominal pain; neurologic	mechanical fragility; abdominal
areas	problems of polyneuropathy and	pain; neurologic problems (e.g.,
Hypertrichosis	paresis; psychiatric problem with	acute intermittent porphyria)
Increased uroporphyrins in urine	hallucinations, confusion, and psychosis	
	Associations	
Alcoholic liver disease	Drugs: sulfa, griseofulvin, phenytoin,	
Estrogens: females, males	progesterone, estrogen, barbiturates, alcohol,	
treated for prostatic carcinoma	lead, arsenic, ergot	
Hexachlorobenzene	Menstrual cycle	
	Infection	
	Decreased food intake	
	Treatment	
Phlebotomy, chloroquine	Hematin, large amounts of glucose,	Hematin, glucose
	chlorpromazine	

Superior Vena Cava Syndrome

Most cases (78%) of superior vena cava syndrome are caused by malignancy. Extrinsic compression of the thin superior vena cava, which has a low intravascular pressure, in a rigid compartment contributes to the pathophysiology of this syndrome. The causes include bronchogenic carcinoma (75% of cases, with small cell and squamous cell carcinoma most common), lymphoma (15%), testicular carcinoma (consider this if biopsy shows anaplastic or undifferentiated carcinoma; check β-subunit of human chorionic gonadotropin and alpha-fetoprotein), carcinoma, and adenocarcinoma of undetermined primary. The symptoms include suffusion of face and conjunctiva, dyspnea, facial swelling, other swelling, cough, dysphagia, syncope, orthopnea, stridor, and lethargy. Physical examination reveals thoracic vein distention, neck vein distention, facial edema, cyanosis, edema of upper extremities, paralyzed vocal cord, Horner's syndrome, and heart murmurs. The diagnosis is established by the history and physical examination. Superior vena cava venography is not useful. A tissue diagnosis is essential to establish a diagnosis precisely. Mediastinotomy is the safest way to obtain histologic diagnosis. If the syndrome is rapid in onset, then treatment must be rapid. In patients with lymphoma, testicular carcinoma, or small cell carcinoma of the lung, treat the underlying disease initially with chemotherapy. If life-threatening problems are present, such as tracheal obstruction or increased intracranial pressure, emergency radiation therapy may be necessary in any disorder presenting with superior vena cava syndrome. Steroids may be helpful. Initial treatment with radiation therapy is indicated in solid tumors, with a total dose of 30-50 Gy or a single dose of 7-12 Gy. Anticoagulation is indicated only if a blood clot has been implicated in the pathophysiology. Diuretics and surgical decompression are not indicated.

- For superior vena cava syndrome, establish a tissue diagnosis.
- Features: edema of the face and neck and venous engorgement of the upper torso.
- Medical emergency in certain situations; may require immediate radiation.

Hypercalcemia in Malignant Disease

Virtually any malignancy may lead to hypercalcemia. Specific causes include carcinomas of the breast and lung (squamous and large cell carcinoma are common and adenocarcinoma and small cell carcinoma are uncom-

mon causes), hypernephroma, other tumors (head and neck, cervix, prostate, neuroblastoma, hepatoma, and melanoma), lymphoma, Burkitt's lymphoma, multiple myeloma, Hodgkin's disease, and Waldenström's macroglobulinemia.

- Hypercalcemia in malignancy does not always denote advanced stage cancer.
- Lung malignancies of squamous cell and large cell lung cancer, myeloma are common causes.

Nonmalignant causes include primary hyperparathyroidism, thyroid disease (Graves' disease, myxedema), renal disease, acute renal failure, chronic renal failure, rhabdomyolysis, drugs (thiazides, lithium, calcium carbonate, tamoxifen, hypervitaminosis A and D), bed rest (fracture), trauma, watery diarrhea, miliary tuberculosis, hypophosphatasia, histiocytosis X, diuretic phase of acute tubular necrosis, granulomatous disorders (tuberculosis, sarcoid, cocci, berylliosis), adrenal insufficiency, acromegaly, pheochromocytoma, immobilization, hyperalimentation, familial, idiopathic mild alkali syndrome, and addisonian crisis.

The signs and symptoms include lassitude, somnolence, weakness, anorexia, nausea, vomiting, constipation, abdominal pain, peptic ulcer, pancreatitis, polyuria, polydipsia, poor intake, renal failure, hyporeflexia, Babinski's sign, myopathy, stupor, coma, occasional localizing signs, visual abnormalities, psychotic behavior, bradycardia, tachycardia, shortened QT interval, digitalis sensitivity, arrhythmias, hypertension, fractures, pain, skeletal deformities, loss of height, poor skin turgor, calcinosis, and band keratopathy. It is misdiagnosed as terminal disease, brain metastases, drug toxicity, renal failure, diabetes insipidus, acute abdomen, and intractable peptic ulcer disease. The diagnosis can be confirmed by measuring serum levels of parathyroid hormone (PTH). In cancer, these levels are low, and in primary hyperparathyroidism, the level is increased.

- Misdiagnoses include terminal disease, brain metastases, drug toxicity, renal failure, diabetes insipidus, acute abdomen, and intractable peptic ulcer disease.

The mechanisms of action of hypercalcemia are multiple. Osteolytic metastases may produce accelerated skeletal resorption. The tumor may secrete a polypeptide with PTH-like activity without osseous metastases. Local osteolytic factors can cause direct pressure. Prostaglandin PGE_2 is associated with the hypercalcemia of renal carcinoma, tumors of the parotid gland, lung cancer, adenocarcinoma of the pancreas, and metastatic carcinoma of unknown primary tumor. In these cases, there are no bone metastases, and the PTH levels are undetectable. Treatment includes indomethacin at a dose of 15-50 mg/day or aspirin at a dose of 1-4.8 g/day. Osteoclast activating factors are associated with multiple myeloma, lymphoma, and Burkitt's non-Hodgkin's lymphoma. There are non-PTH extracts from tumor in vitro that cause active bone resorption and regress with specific anti-tumor activity. Other factors include dehydration, mobilization, adrenal insufficiency secondary to tumor metastases, estrogens, androgens, progestins, and tamoxifen.

Most hypercalcemia is related to increased bone resorption. Intestinal absorption is low or low-normal in most cases. There usually is no increase in renal tubular reabsorption, but the kidney may be involved in hyperparathyroidism, breast cancer, metabolic alkalosis, and salt depletion. The course is short and rapidly progressive. There may be moderate to severe weight loss and no renal calculi; pancreatitis is rare. The serum level of calcium is >14 in 75% of patients. The serum level of alkaline phosphatase may be increased, normal, or decreased. Anemia and metabolic alkalosis may be present. The alkaline phosphatase level is elevated in 50% of patients but can be elevated in primary hyperparathyroidism. Hypophosphatemia can occur whether or not there is a PTH-secreting tumor. Hypoalbuminemia must be considered, and for every gram of albumin below 4, add 1 to the ionized calcium.

Treatment is multifaceted. The use of such precipitating factors as vitamins A and D, lithium, thiazides, absorbable antacids, and estrogens should be discontinued. The patient should be mobilized. Also, the patient should be hydrated with a minimum of 2.5-4 L of fluid in the first 24 hours. To each liter of normal saline, add 20-40 mEq of KCl and 10-20 mEq of magnesium. Experimentally, if the sodium is increased from 25 mEq to 250 mEq, calcium excretion is increased threefold and is not related to the glomerulofiltration rate. Treat the underlying disease. Glucocorticoids are especially efficacious in multiple myeloma, breast cancer, and non-Hodgkin's lymphomas. The typical dose is 80 mg of prednisone in divided doses daily. The mechanisms of action include antitumor effects, an antivitamin D effect, inhibition of prostaglandin synthesis or release, inhibition of osteoclast activating factor production, anti-PTH activity, and an inhibitory effect on osteoprogenitor cells. Furosemide should be administered after 2 L of fluid. The dosages are variable, ranging from 20 mg to 40 mg

up to every 4 hours. Furosemide blocks the tubular reabsorption of calcium, depletes sodium, depletes potassium, and depletes magnesium. The biphosphonates have an inhibitory effect on osteoclast function and viability. Etidronate at a dose of 7.5 mg/kg over 4 hours is given intravenously up to 7 days. This decreases calcium within 2 days. Pamidronate is given by intravenous infusion at a dose of 15-45 mg/day for up to 6 days. Alternatively, 90 mg may be given over 24 hours or it may be administered orally at a dose of 1,200 mg for up to 5 days. In general, the biphosphonates are more potent than calcitonin and less toxic than plicamycin. Plicamycin inhibits RNA synthesis in osteoclasts. There may be subjective improvement within 12 hours and improvement in the serum levels of calcium in 36 hours. The dose is 25 μg/kg over 4 hours and may be repeated once if necessary. Side effects include thrombocytopenia, hemorrhage, renal complications, increased liver enzymes, sudden arterial occlusion, and toxic epidermal necrolysis. Contraindications include thrombocytopenia and coagulopathy. Calcitonin may be administered subcutaneously or intramuscularly in the form of salmon calcitonin at a dose of 4 U/kg every 12 hours. The onset is rapid, but the response is moderate and unsustained. Gallium nitrate reduces the solubility of hydroxyapatite crystals to inhibit bone resorption. The dose is 200 mg/m^2 in 1 L of fluid intravenously over 5 days. This may be nephrotoxic. Use of phosphate should be restricted to extreme life-threatening hypercalcemia. Calcium phosphate complexes are deposited in vessels, lungs, and kidneys.

HEMOCHROMATOSIS
Hemochromatosis is the end result of a pathologic process that evolves over years.

- Endocrine dysfunction: 50% with diabetes at presentation and a minority have vascular sequelae; hypogonadism (decreased libido, impotence, and amenorrhea); hypopituitarism.
- Cardiac: congestive heart failure, arrhythmias.
- Skin: bronze, "slate gray."
- Arthropathy: chondrocalcinosis, bone cysts, irregularity.
- Hepatomegaly: cirrhosis.
- Lethargy, weight loss.
- The transferrin saturation is >62% early in life.

The gene responsible for hereditary hemochromatosis is coinherited with the HLA A3 antigen and the A3,

B7 and A3, B14 haplotypes. It is inherited as an autosomal recessive trait and involves 1/20,000 hospital admissions; 2-4/1,000 are affected in the general population. The male/female ratio is 10/1. Males present in the fourth to fifth decade. The transferrin saturation is >62% even early in life and before tissue iron loading occurs. The causes of hemochromatosis include hereditary hemochromatosis (idiopathic), secondary anemia and ineffective erythropoiesis (thalassemia major, thalassemia minor), hereditary spherocytosis, idiopathic refractory sideroblastic anemia and myelodysplasia, oral intake of iron (medicinal), liver disease (alcoholic cirrhosis, portal caval anastomosis), drugs (isoniazid, chloramphenicol), and copper deficiency.

The best screening test is a transferrin saturation >62%; it is reliable in identifying homozygotes. Urine iron is increased in the range of 5-20 mg/24 hours (normal, <2 mg/24 hours). Hepatic iron by dry weight is markedly increased at 200-1,800 µg/100 ng dry weight (normal, 30-140). The goal of treatment is to improve prognosis and the clinical course in patients with established liver damage. The mainstays of treatment are phlebotomy and chelation; 200 mg of iron are removed per phlebotomy unit. Patients initially have venesection twice weekly. Deferoxamine (10 mg/day by continuous infusion) is the chelation agent used most often. Features not altered by chelation include arthropathy, hypogonadism, development of hepatocellular carcinoma, and hepatic cirrhosis.

HEMATOLOGY OF ACQUIRED IMMUNE DEFICIENCY

In acquired immune deficiency (AIDS), there is an absolute reduction of T4 lymphocytes, with a relative reduction of the T4 to T8 ratio. Also, there is functional impairment of T4 lymphocytes. Whereas T8 lymphocytes may increase early in the disease in infections, they decrease in number late in the disease. Neutropenia may be due to autoimmune destruction with antigranulocyte antibodies in two-thirds of patients, decreased production, zidovudine (AZT), ganciclovir, trimethoprim-sulfamethoxazole, pentamidine, or antineoplastic chemotherapy. Neutrophil dysfunction is also manifested by decreased chemotaxis, granulation, and phagocytosis.

Anemia is a significant problem in HIV-infected patients, and the degree of anemia is a prognostic factor in the patients. HIV-associated RBC problems include decreased RBC production; 70% of AIDS patients have decreased erythropoietin levels. Approximately 25% of patients have positive results on the Coombs' test, but significant hemolysis is not common. Of patients treated with zidovudine, 30% develop significant anemia. Decreased RBC production is a principal cause. Erythropoietin has been used successfully. Anemia is also associated with infections from *Mycobacterium avium* complex, parvovirus, B19, *Mycobacterium tuberculosis*, and histoplasmosis. Anemia may be malignancy-related.

Thrombocytopenia occurs in 5%-15% of HIV-infected patients and is often detected early in the disease. Idiopathic thrombocytopenic purpura is usually accompanied by platelet-associated antibodies and responds to zidovudine (80% of patients), steroids (90%), splenic irradiation (60%), immunoglobulin given intravenously, and splenectomy (80%). Other HIV associations include thrombotic thrombocytopenic purpura, decreased platelet production, and peripheral platelet sequestration. Other non-HIV associations include therapy, infection, and malignancy. Coagulation disorders may complicate HIV disorders. The lupus-like anticoagulant is present in 20% of HIV patients, usually in association with opportunistic infections, and is rarely associated with thrombosis or bleeding. Other problems include increased vWF:Ag levels (with a poor prognosis if >200%), elevated level of tissue plasminogen activator (with a poor prognosis if >20 ng/mL), and an elevated fibrinogen level.

Non-Hodgkin's lymphoma is the second most common HIV-associated malignancy, occurring in 0.5%-1.0% of patients. Extranodal disease occurs in 66.6% of patients. There is also an increased risk of Hodgkin's disease among HIV patients.

PARVOVIRUS INFECTION

Parvovirus infection (B19), or fifth disease, is a highly contagious disease in children. Adults with this infection may develop a polyarthralgia syndrome or cytopenia. Abnormalities in the erythroid line include severe anemia, reticulocytopenia, and RBC hypoplasia in the marrow. Pancytopenia may occur. Immunoglobulin therapy administered intravenously may be of benefit.

REVIEW OF CHEMOTHERAPEUTIC AGENTS

Chemotherapeutic agents--alkylating agents, antibiotics, and hormones--and their effects are reviewed in Table 18-19.

Table 18-19.--Chemotherapy Agents

Drug	Toxic effects	Other
	Alkylating agents	
Carmustine	Delayed marrow suppression, nausea, vomiting, pulmonary, hepatic toxicity, secondary leukemia	Cumulative marrow suppression, crosses blood-brain barrier
Busulfan	Pulmonary fibrosis	Hepatic metabolism, renal excretion
Carboplatin	Marrow suppression, nausea and vomiting, less nephrotoxicity and neurotoxicity than cisplatin	Renal excretion
Chlorambucil	Pulmonary, secondary leukemia	Hepatic metabolism
Cisplatin	Nephrotoxicity, peripheral neuropathy, ototoxicity, magnesium depletion	Renal excretion
Cyclophosphamide	Leukopenia, cystitis, pulmonary fibrosis, syndrome of inappropriate ADH secretion, alopecia, nausea, vomiting	Hepatic metabolism to active compound, renal excretion lower dose with renal failure, late transitional cell carcinoma of bladder
Dacarbazine	Marrow suppression, flu-like syndrome, severe nausea and vomiting, fever	
Melphalan	Marrow suppression, secondary leukemia	Renal excretion, erratic oral absorption
Nitrogen mustard	Marrow suppression, nausea and vomiting, sterility, secondary leukemia	
Streptozocin	Diabetes, marrow suppression, severe nausea and vomiting, renal	Leads to pancreatic and endocrine insufficiency
	Antibiotics	
Bleomycin	Pulmonary fibrosis (threshold 400 μg/lifetime) but may recur at lower doses, fever and chills, myalgias, skin pigmentation, alopecia, adult respiratory distress syndrome with oxygen	Lower dose with renal insufficiency
Dactinomycin	Marrow suppression, radiation recall, nausea and vomiting, mucositis, alopecia	
Daunorubicin	Marrow suppression, radiation recall, cardio-myopathy, mucositis, nausea and vomiting, alopecia	Decrease dose by 50% if bilirubin >1.5 mg/dL or by 75% if bilirubin >3.0 mg/dL
Doxorubicin	Dose-related cardiomyopathy, marrow suppression, alopecia, nausea and vomiting, stomatitis, radiation recall	Hepatic metabolism, biliary excretion, decrease dose by 50% if bilirubin >1.5 mg/dL or by 75% if bilirubin >3.0 mg/dL
Mitomycin C	Delayed marrow suppression, nausea and vomiting, alopecia, hepatic toxicity, microangiopathic hemolytic anemia	Vesicant, alkylator, forms free radicals
Mitoxantrone	Marrow suppression, cardiac toxicity, nausea and vomiting, mucositis, alopecia, blue sclera and urine	

Table 18-19 (continued)

Drug	Toxic effects	Other
	Hormones	
Corticosteroids	Diabetes, hepatic toxicity, aseptic necrosis, adrenal insufficiency, myopathy, infection, osteoporosis, peptic ulcer disease, hypokalemia, psychosis, cataract	
Diethylstilbesterol (estrogen)	Feminization, hypertension, irregular menses, hepatic toxicity, thrombotic complications, fluid retention, morning sickness	
Flutamide	Gynecomastia, hepatic toxicity	
Fluoxymesterone	Masculinization, fluid retention, hepatic toxicity, irregular menses, erythrocytosis	
Leuprolide	Tumor flare, hot flashes, impotence, amenorrhea	LHRH agonist
Megestrol acetate	Thrombosis, menstrual irregularities, male impotence	

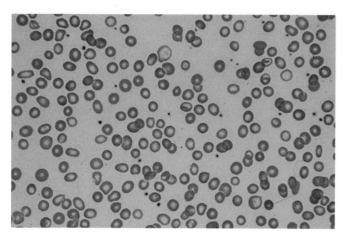

Color plate 18-1. Hypochromic-microcytic anemia. Small cells, <6 μm in diameter, with increased central pallor and assorted aberrations in size (anisocytosis) and in shape (poikilocytosis). (Courtesy of Curtis A. Hanson, M.D., Mayo Clinic.)

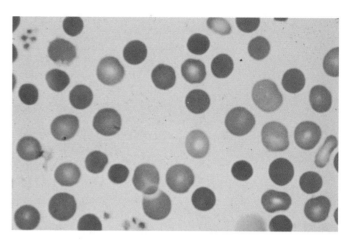

Color plate 18-2. Spherocytes. Smooth, small, and spheroidal darkly stained cells with minimal or no central pallor. (Courtesy of Curtis A. Hanson, M.D., Mayo Clinic.)

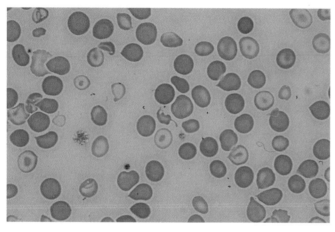

Color plate 18-3. Target cells. Red blood cells with a broad diameter and a dark center. (Courtesy of Curtis A. Hanson, M.D., Mayo Clinic.)

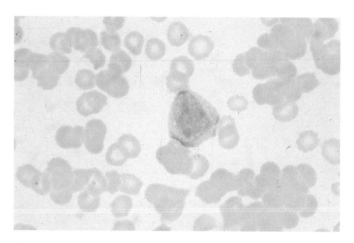

Color plate 18-4. Agglutination. Clumping of red blood cells.

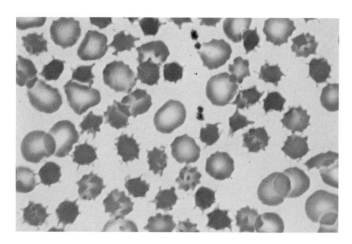

Color plate 18-5. Acanthocytes. Note the thin, thorny, or finger-like projections. (Courtesy of Curtis A. Hanson, M.D., Mayo Clinic.)

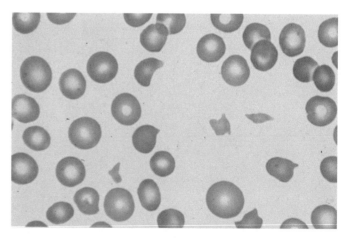

Color plate 18-6. Schistocytes. Fragmented red blood cells shaped like helmets, triangles, or kites. (Courtesy of Curtis A. Hanson, M.D., Mayo Clinic.)

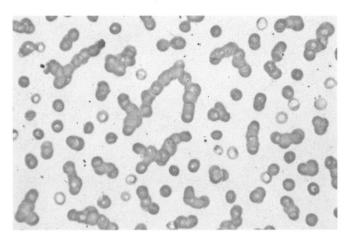

Color plate 18-7. Rouleaux. Stacking of red blood cells. (Courtesy of Curtis A. Hanson, M.D., Mayo Clinic.)

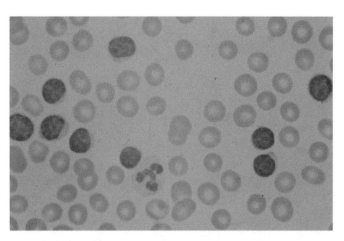

Color plate 18-8. Chronic lymphocytic leukemia. Large number of small and agranular mature lymphocytes whose nuclei are approximately the same size as red blood cells.

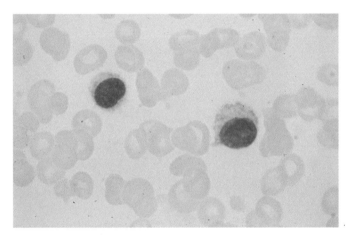

Color plate 18-9. Hairy-cell leukemia. Mature lymphocytes with eccentrically placed nuclei and pale cytoplasm that has characteristic projections.

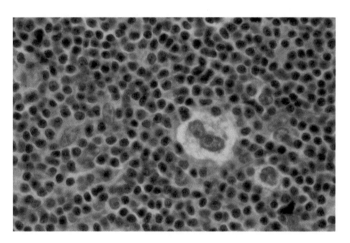

Color plate 18-10. Hodgkin's disease. A Reed-Sternberg cell, a binucleate large cell. (Courtesy of Curtis A. Hanson, M.D., Mayo Clinic.)

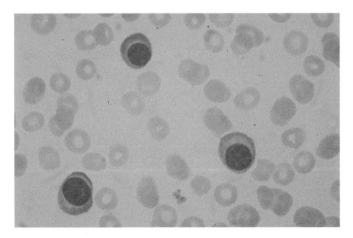

Color plate 18-11. Plasma cell. Note the eccentrically placed round nucleus; the copious, dark blue cytoplasm has a characteristic pale-staining area adjacent to the nucleus.

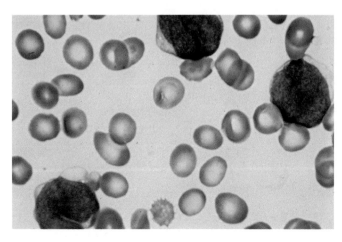

Color plate 18-12. Acute nonlymphocytic leukemia. Large pleomorphic cells with large nuclei and a barely visible nuclear membrane.

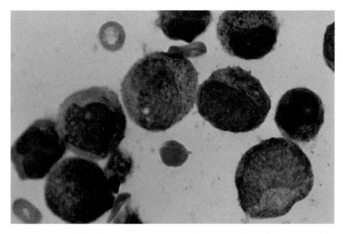

Color plate 18-13. Acute promyelocytic leukemia. Note the large nuclei; more than half of the leukemic cells have large atypical granulations. (Courtesy of Curtis A. Hanson, M.D., Mayo Clinic.)

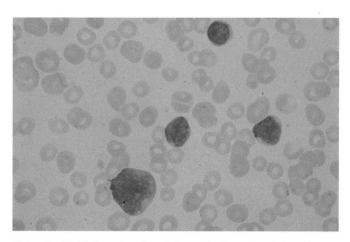

Color plate 18-14. Acute lymphocytic leukemia. Large, rounded, and indented nuclei with diverse shapes and scant, darker blue cytoplasm.

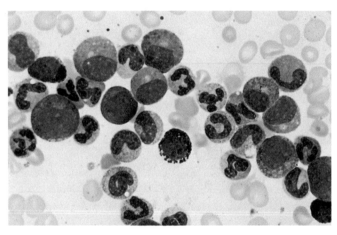

Color plate 18-15. Chronic myelogenous leukemia. Normal-appearing myeloid cells representing all stages of maturation, with a decreased number of erythropoietic cells and one basophil precursor in the center. (Courtesy of Curtis A. Hanson, M.D., Mayo Clinic.)

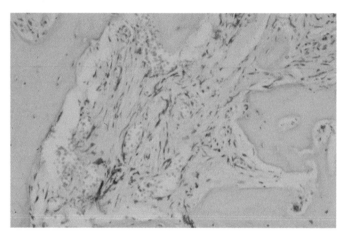

Color plate 18-16. Fibrosis. Bone marrow biopsy showing core diffusely replaced by fibrosis, with minimal normal hematopoietic elements present.

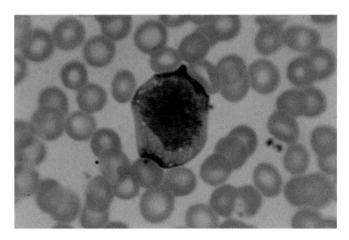

Color plate 18-17. Infectious mononucleosis. Large atypical lymphocyte has a large amount of pale cytoplasm, which may be vacuolated, and a large oblong nucleus.

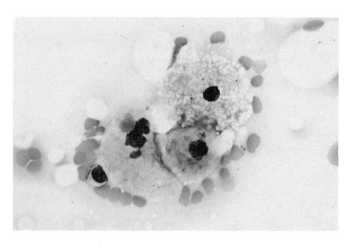

Color plate 18-18. Gaucher's cells. Large cell with characteristic pale, foamy, and fibrillar cytoplasm. (Courtesy of Curtis A. Hanson, M.D., Mayo Clinic.)

QUESTIONS
(See "Answers" section)

Multiple Choice

1. Low erythropoietin levels occur in all the following except:
   a. Chronic renal failure
   b. HIV infection
   c. Polycythemia rubra vera
   d. Iron deficiency
   e. Rheumatoid arthritis

2. Which of the following is calculated on the basis of the complete blood cell count?
   a. Red blood cell
   b. Mean corpuscular volume
   c. Red blood cell volume
   d. Platelet count
   e. Hemoglobin

3. In glucose-6-phosphate dehydrogenase deficiency:
   a. In a steady state, patients are typically anemic
   b. In an acute hemolytic state, the level of glucose-6-phosphate dehydrogenase may be normal
   c. Heinz bodies demonstrated with supravital staining are not present on a screening test
   d. Patients with cirrhosis and diabetes are not at increased risk for hemolysis
   e. Drugs more commonly provoke hemolysis than viral and bacterial infections

4. In hereditary spherocytosis:
   a. Results of the osmotic fragility test are normal
   b. Results of the Coombs' test are positive
   c. A deficiency of spectrin in the membrane cytoskeleton on SDS gel electrophoresis is characteristic
   d. The inheritance pattern is autosomal recessive
   e. There is no need to study family members

5. Thrombotic thrombocytopenic purpura is characterized by:
   a. A prolonged prothrombin time
   b. Thrombocytopenia
   c. Positive findings with fibrin-D dimer test
   d. A prolonged activated partial thromboplastin time
   e. An abnormal creatinine level in all patients

6. A 25-year-old woman had a low left supraclavicular node involved with Hodgkin's disease. Findings on computed tomographic scanning of the chest and abdomen, lymphangiography, and a formal staging laparotomy were all negative. The treatment of choice is:
   a. Observation, because there is no disease detectable after biopsy
   b. Radiation therapy in mantle and para-aortic fields
   c. Radiation therapy with mantle plus inverted Y fields
   d. MOPP (nitrogen mustard, vincristine [Oncovin], prednisone, procarbazine)
   e. MOPP-ABVD (MOPP-doxorubicin [Adriamycin], bleomycin, vinblastine, DTIC)

7. Which of the following is not associated with a low leukocyte alkaline phosphatase score?
   a. Chronic myelogenous leukemia
   b. Aplastic anemia
   c. Paroxysmal nocturnal hemoglobinuria
   d. Infectious mononucleosis
   e. Hairy-cell leukemia

8. A 50-year-old woman had a monoclonal protein in the serum with an M spike of 1.79 g/dL. The hemoglobin, calcium, and creatinine levels and metastatic bone survey were normal. The treatment of choice in this patient is:
   a. Observation
   b. CHOP (cyclophosphamide, vincristine, prednisone, and doxorubicin [Adriamycin])
   c. Melphalan and prednisone
   d. Interferon
   e. Melphalan, cyclophosphamide, carmustine, vincristine, and prednisone

9. Patients with recurrent infections and chronic lymphocytic leukemia should have which of the following laboratory evaluations?
   a. Absolute neutrophil count
   b. Bone marrow
   c. Serum protein electrophoresis
   d. Chromosome studies of bone marrow
   e. B and T peripheral blood cell typing studies

10. In the treatment of chronic lymphocytic leukemia:
    a. All patients should receive treatment because it is a malignancy
    b. All patients with lymphadenopathy and spleno-

megaly should receive treatment

c. Patients with a hemoglobin <11 g/dL or platelet count <100,000 should receive treatment

d. All patients with a white blood cell count >20,000 should receive treatment

e. All patients with 98% lymphocytes should receive treatment

11. Which of the following drugs potentiates warfarin?
   a. Barbiturates
   b. Cholestyramine
   c. Carbamazepine
   d. Rifampin
   e. Trimethoprim-sulfamethoxazole

12. Results of which of the following laboratory tests are abnormal in hemophilia A?
   a. Bleeding time
   b. Factor VIIIC
   c. Factor VIII ristocetin:antigen
   d. Factor IX level
   e. Fibrinogen level

13. Which of the following is not true about von Willebrand's disease?
   a. It is the most commonly inherited bleeding disorder
   b. The inheritance pattern is autosomal dominant with incomplete penetrance
   c. It is characterized by mucocutaneous bleeding, epistaxis, and menorrhagia
   d. Patients with mild disease do not bleed during a surgical procedure
   e. Type I von Willebrand's disease is characterized by a quantitative abnormality of von Willebrand factor.

14. Which of the following is indicated treatments in von Willebrand's disease except:
   a. Cryoprecipitate
   b. Birth control pills
   c. Desamino-D-arginine vasopressin
   d. Topical treatment in preparation for oral surgery
   e. Fresh frozen plasma

15. Which of the following laboratory tests is usually normal in von Willebrand's disease?
   a. Bleeding time
   b. Factor VIIIC

c. Partial thromboplastin time
d. Prothrombin time
e. VIII:von Willebrand antigen

16. Which of the following statements about the cause of aplastic anemia is true:
   a. The commonest cause in the U.S. is idiopathic
   b. Hepatitis B is the hepatitis that most commonly causes aplastic anemia
   c. Phenylbutazone, anticonvulsants, and sulfonamides are the most common causes of aplastic anemia
   d. Patients with paroxysmal nocturnal hemoglobinuria are not at increased risk for developing aplastic anemia
   e. X-linked lymphoproliferative syndrome patients are not at increased risk

17. The following is true about hemochromatosis:
   a. 2 to 4/100,000 persons in the general population are affected
   b. Arthropathy, hypogonadism, risk of hepatocellular carcinoma, and hepatic cirrhosis are reversed by chelation
   c. The transferrin saturation is >62% even early in life and before tissue iron loading occurs
   d. Diabetes is not common at presentation
   e. This entity is an autosomal dominant trait

18. Which of the following is not associated with thrombocytopenia:
   a. Heparin
   b. Septicemia
   c. Post-transfusion purpura
   d. Hemophilia A without HIV infection
   e. Bernard-Soulier syndrome

19. In patients presenting with thoracic vein distention, neck vein distention, and edema of the face:
   a. Superior vena cava venography is very useful
   b. Anticoagulation is indicated in all patients
   c. Mediastinotomy is one of the safest ways to obtain a histologic diagnosis
   d. Use of diuretics should be promptly implemented
   e. Surgical decompression should be attempted

20. Which of the following is false about the porphyrias?
   a. They are autosomal dominant in inheritance pattern except for congenital erythropoietic porphyria

b. Patients with acute intermittent porphyria do not have skin lesions

c. Porphyria cutanea tarda is associated with alcoholic liver disease and estrogens

d. Barbiturates, alcohol, and estrogens are not associated with exacerbations of acute intermittent porphyria

e. Acute intermittent porphyria may be exacerbated by estrogens

True/False

21. The following are consistent with a diagnosis of iron deficiency anemia:
    a. Macrocytic red blood cell indices
    b. Increase in ferritin
    c. Red blood cell count >5 x 10^{12}/L
    d. Red cell distribution width <16
    e. Hemoglobin A2 >4.0%
    f. Transferrin saturation >15%

22. Paroxysmal nocturnal hemoglobinuria is characterized by:
    a. Development of acute nonlymphocytic leukemia in 5%-10% of patients
    b. Aplastic bone marrow in 75% of patients
    c. Unusual venous thromboses
    d. Chronic hemolytic anemia with hemoglobinuria
    e. Episodes of severe pain in the back and abdomen
    f. Decrease in decay accelerating factor (DAF)

23. The major criteria for the diagnosis of polycythemia rubra vera are:
    a. Platelet count >400,000
    b. Splenomegaly
    c. Increased vitamin B_{12} level
    d. Normal oxygen saturation
    e. Elevated RBC mass
    f. Postbathing pruritus

24. The following are predictors of survival in intermediate histology non-Hodgkin's lymphoma:
    a. Age
    b. Sex
    c. Performance status
    d. LDH
    e. Stage
    f. Bone marrow involvement with nodal involvement

25. With regard to anticoagulants, which of the following are true or false?
    a. Heparin inhibits thrombin by forming a heparin-antithrombin III complex
    b. Warfarin limits the vitamin K-dependent coagulation proteins
    c. The vitamin K-dependent factors are II, VII, IX, X
    d. Warfarin affects protein C and S
    e. Warfarin forms a complex with antithrombin III
    f. Heparin is contraindicated in the management of deep venous thrombosis in pregnancy

26. A prolonged bleeding time may occur in:
    a. Glanzmann's thrombasthenia
    b. von Willebrand's disease
    c. Bernard-Soulier syndrome
    d. Uremia
    e. Hemophilia A
    f. Storage pool disease

27. In the treatment of aplastic anemia, which of the following are true or false?
    a. Related donors should be used for transfusion before transplantation
    b. Survival rates are not affected by transfusion before transplantation
    c. The treatment of choice in HLA-matched patients younger than 40 is antithymocyte globulin
    d. The treatment of choice in children with an HLA match is bone marrow transplant
    e. The response rate with antithymocyte globulin is about 50%
    f. Spontaneous remissions are common

28. With regard to transfusion reactions, which of the following are true or false?
    a. Ataxia telangiectasia patients may have class-specific anti-IgA antibodies that may cause transfusion reactions
    b. 50% of acute hemolytic transfusion reactions are caused by human error
    c. Females are at higher risk for acute hemolytic transfusion reactions
    d. Females have a higher risk of transfusion-associated adult respiratory distress syndrome
    e. Females have a higher risk of delayed hemolytic transfusion reactions
    f. Females have a higher risk of febrile transfusion reactions

NOTES

CHAPTER 19
HYPERTENSION

Gary L. Schwartz, M.D.

HYPERTENSION

Definition

Systolic blood pressures between 130 and 139 mm Hg and diastolic blood pressures between 85 and 89 mm Hg are considered high-normal. Hypertension is defined as average blood pressure ≥140/90 mm Hg. It is stratified further on the basis of pressure level (Table 19-1).

- Hypertension is average blood pressure ≥140/90 mm Hg.

Table 19-1.--Stages of Hypertension

Stage[*]	Degree	Blood pressure, mm Hg	
		Systolic	Diastolic
1	Mild	140-159	90-99
2	Moderate	160-179	100-109
3	Severe	180-209	110-119
4	Very severe	≥210	≥120

[*]Stage is defined by systolic *or* diastolic blood pressure.
Modified from Joint National Committee on Detection, Evaluation, and Treatment of High Blood Pressure: The Fifth Report of the Joint National Committee on Detection, Evaluation, and Treatment of High Blood Pressure (JNC V). Arch Intern Med 153:154-183, 1993.

Isolated systolic hypertension, mainly a problem of the elderly, is defined as systolic blood pressure ≥140 mm Hg with diastolic blood pressure ≤90 mm Hg. Secondary causes of isolated systolic hypertension include disorders associated with either increased cardiac output (anemia, thyrotoxicosis, arteriovenous fistula, Paget's disease of bone, beriberi) or increased cardiac stroke volume (aortic insufficiency, complete heart block).

- Isolated systolic hypertension affects mainly the elderly.
- Secondary cause: increased cardiac output (anemia, thyrotoxicosis, arteriovenous fistula, Paget's disease of bone, beriberi).
- Secondary cause: increased cardiac stroke volume (aortic insufficiency, complete heart block).

Epidemiology

Blood pressure increases with age. Systolic blood pressure increases throughout the seventh decade but diastolic blood pressure plateaus in the fifth decade. Hypertension is a major risk factor for cardiovascular morbidity and mortality (myocardial infarction, congestive heart failure, stroke, and renal disease). Risk is continuous and proportionate over both systolic and diastolic blood pressure levels. Systolic blood pressure is as good or better a predictor of risk than diastolic blood pressure. Hypertension is more common in men than in women and in blacks than in whites. For any given level, men have greater morbidity and mortality than women and blacks greater than whites. It is estimated that 50 million Americans have hypertension or are taking medication to lower blood pressure.

- Hypertension is a major risk factor for cardiovascular morbidity and mortality.
- Risk is continuous and proportionate over both systolic and diastolic blood pressure levels.
- Hypertension is more common in men than in women and in blacks than in whites.
- Men and blacks have greater morbidity and mortality.

In hypertensive patients, the most common causes of death are due to complications of coronary artery disease.

479

Factors that add to this risk are tobacco use, hyperlipidemia, diabetes, obesity, sedentary lifestyle, and family history of premature cardiovascular disease. Target organ damage (stroke, left ventricular hypertrophy, ischemic heart disease, congestive heart failure, renal disease) increases risk of cardiovascular events even if blood pressure is controlled. This is used to argue for early treatment of mild hypertension.

- The most common causes of death in hypertensive people are related to complications of coronary artery disease.
- Other risk factors for coronary artery disease: tobacco use, hyperlipidemia, diabetes, obesity, sedentary lifestyle, family history of premature cardiovascular disease.
- Target organ damage increases risk of cardiovascular events even if blood pressure is controlled.

Left ventricular hypertrophy is a powerful predictor of sudden death and myocardial infarction in hypertensive patients. Other factors associated with increased left ventricular muscle mass include increasing age, obesity, and increased physical activity. Echocardiography is more sensitive than electrocardiography in detecting left ventricular hypertrophy.

- Left ventricular hypertrophy is a powerful predictor of sudden death and myocardial infarction in hypertensive persons.
- Echocardiography is more sensitive than electrocardiography in detecting left ventricular hypertrophy.

Diagnosis

Because blood pressure varies, the diagnosis of hypertension requires several measurements made on different occasions. The patient should be at rest in the sitting position for at least 5 minutes before the measurement. Recent physical activity, use of tobacco or caffeine, or a full urinary bladder can transiently increase blood pressure. Some persons have elevated blood pressure when it is measured in a physician's office but have normal blood pressure at all other times. This is called office hypertension or white coat hypertension. Whether these people suffer the adverse consequences of hypertension is uncertain; therefore, they usually require no treatment initially, but need to be followed up and periodically assessed for target organ

damage. Older patients may have pseudohypertension, a falsely elevated systolic and diastolic blood pressure when measured by the cuff method; it is the result of a stiff vascular tree caused by atherosclerosis. Pseudohypertension may exist if the radial artery remains palpable after brachial artery occlusion by inflating the blood pressure cuff above systolic blood pressure level (Osler maneuver).

- Diagnosis of hypertension requires several measurements made on different occasions.
- Recent physical exercise, use of tobacco or caffeine, or a full urinary bladder can increase blood pressure.
- Office (white coat) hypertension: increased blood pressure only when measured in a physician's office.
- Older patients may have pseudohypertension, the result of a stiff vascular tree.

Evaluation

After the diagnosis of hypertension is established, 1) determine, if possible, duration and severity of hypertension and any previous therapies and reasons for discontinuation, 2) assess for target organ damage, 3) identify associated cardiovascular risk factors, and 4) consider the possibility of secondary hypertension. Secondary hypertension accounts for <5% of all cases of increased blood pressure.

- Secondary hypertension explains <5% of all cases of increased blood pressure.

Clues to secondary hypertension are features that are not consistent with essential hypertension. Essential hypertension usually occurs in the third or fourth decade. There is often a family history of hypertension. Usually, blood pressure is mildly increased initially and easily controlled with one or two medications. Target organ damage is rare and routine laboratory findings are normal. Blood pressure does not progress to higher levels over a short period of time. Factors inconsistent with essential hypertension are listed in Table 19-2.

- Recognition of secondary hypertension is important.

Drugs

Certain drugs can cause or aggravate hypertension or interfere with the action of antihypertensive medications. These drugs and their mechanism of action are listed in Table 19-3.

Table 19-2.--Factors Inconsistent With Essential Hypertension

Age at onset--before 20 or after 50 years
Blood pressure >180/110 mm Hg at time of diagnosis
Significant target organ damage at time of diagnosis
Hemorrhages and exudates on funduscopic examination
Renal insufficiency
Cardiomegaly
Features suggesting secondary hypertension
    Primary aldosteronism (unprovoked hypokalemia,
      Chvostek's sign, Trousseau's sign)
    Pheochromocytoma (labile blood pressure with sweating,
      tremor, tachycardia, pallor, neurofibromatosis, orofacial
      neuromas [MEN II])
    Renovascular disease (abdominal bruits)
    Cushing's disease (truncal obesity, pigmented stria)
    Coarctation of aorta (delayed/absent femoral pulses)
    Polycystic kidney disease (abdominal or flank masses,
      family history of renal disease)
    Poor response to appropriate three-drug therapy

- Certain drugs can cause or aggravate hypertension or interfere with the action of antihypertensive medications.
- Oral contraceptives induce sodium retention, increase renin substrate, and facilitate the action of catecholamines.
- Nonsteroidal anti-inflammatory drugs induce sodium retention by blocking formation of vasodilating, natriuretic prostaglandins.
- Tricyclic antidepressants block uptake of guanethidine and inhibit the action of centrally acting agents (methyldopa, clonidine).

Laboratory Studies

Routine laboratory tests should include: complete blood cell count, potassium, glucose, creatinine or BUN, uric acid, calcium, cholesterol (total and HDL), triglycerides, urinalysis, and electrocardiogram (ECG). Additional studies should not be performed unless abnormalities are identified on initial screening tests or the history or examination suggests a secondary form of hypertension.

Treatment

The goal of therapy is to eliminate the cardiovascular morbidity and mortality attributable to hypertension by reducing blood pressure to <140/90 mm Hg.

Nonpharmacologic Therapy

Nonpharmacologic therapy may be sufficient for patients with mild hypertension. It is adjunctive therapy for those with more severe hypertension. Restriction of daily sodium intake to 90 mEq (2 g sodium, 4 g salt) decreases blood pressure in some but not all hypertensive persons. Although salt sensitivity is more common among persons who are black, obese, elderly or who have low renin hypertension or higher blood pressure levels, the antihypertensive effect of many medications is enhanced by sodium restriction. Also, sodium restriction minimizes diuretic-induced potassium losses. The prevalence of hypertension is increased in the obese. A rise in blood pressure parallels weight gain and occasionally leads to hypertension. Weight loss may decrease blood pressure. Weight reduction to within 15% of ideal body weight is the goal, although losses of as little as 10 lb may produce a decrease in blood pressure. Restriction of daily alcohol intake to <2 oz is often associated with a decrease in blood pressure. Alcohol is a source of calories, and its use is often associated with poor compliance. Excessive alcohol intake may cause labile hypertension that is difficult to control in association with other symptoms (flushing, tachycardia) that suggest pheochromocytoma. Regular aerobic exercise may decrease blood pressure directly and by facilitating weight loss. Because coronary artery disease is the most common cause of mortality in hypertensive persons, all cardiovascular risks need to be addressed. The benefits of blood pressure reduction are diminished in smokers. Dyslipidemia (elevated LDL cholesterol, reduced HDL cholesterol, elevated triglycerides) and glucose intolerance coexist more often in hypertensive than in normotensive patients.

- Restriction of daily sodium intake to 90 mEq decreases blood pressure in some, not all, hypertensive persons.
- Weight reduction to within 15% of ideal body weight is the goal.
- Restriction of alcohol intake to <2 oz daily is often associated with a decrease in blood pressure.
- Regular aerobic exercise may decrease blood pressure directly.
- Address all cardiovascular risk factors.

Short-term trials have shown that biofeedback and relaxation training decrease blood pressure in a subset of hypertensives. Long-term effects of these modalities on blood pressure reduction have not been assessed. Short-term studies have shown that dietary supplementation

Table 19-3.--Drugs That Can Elevate Blood Pressure or Interfere With Antihypertensive Therapy

Drug	Mechanism
Oral contraceptives	Induce sodium retention
	Increased renin substrate
	Facilitate action of catecholamines
Alcohol (>2 oz daily)	Activation of sympathetic nervous system
	Increased cortisol secretion
	Elevated intracellular calcium levels
Sympathomimetics and amphetamine-like substances (cold formulas, allergy medications, diet pills)	Increase peripheral vascular resistance
	Interfere with action of guanethidine and guanadrel
Nonsteroidal anti-inflammatory drugs	Induce sodium retention by blocking formation of vasodilating, natriuretic prostaglandins, thus interfering with action of diuretics, β-blockers, and angiotensin converting enzyme inhibitors
Corticosteroids	Iatrogenic Cushing's disease
Tricyclic antidepressants	Block uptake of guanethidine
	Inhibit action of centrally acting drugs such as methyldopa and clonidine
Ephedrine	Competitive antagonist of guanethidine
Monoamine oxidase inhibitors (in combination with tyramine-- found in aged cheeses and some red wines)	Prevent degradation and metabolism of norepinephrine released by tyramine-containing foods
	Increase blood pressure when combined with reserpine/guanethidine
Cocaine	Vasoconstriction
	Interferes with action of adrenergic inhibitors
Marijuana	Increases systolic blood pressure

with potassium, calcium, and magnesium decreases blood pressure; however, potential dangers of long-term supplementation are unknown. Thus, the role of these cations in the treatment of hypertension is unclear.

A 6-month trial of nonpharmacologic therapy is appropriate for stage 1 hypertension. If nonpharmacologic therapy fails to reduce blood pressure to <140/90 mm Hg, drug treatment should be considered, especially in patients at increased risk because of additional cardiovascular risk factors or target organ changes. Also, significant changes in lifestyle (weight reduction, exercise, limitation of alcohol intake, sodium restriction) may allow tapering of an established drug program.

- A 6-month trial of nonpharmacologic therapy is appropriate for stage 1 hypertension.
- If this fails to reduce blood pressure to <140/90 mm Hg, consider drug treatment.

Pharmacologic Therapy

More than 50% of cases of stage 1 hypertension can be controlled with one drug. Important factors in selecting a drug for initial therapy are its 1) effectiveness as monotherapy, 2) side-effects, and 3) cost. Proper drug selection is important in maintaining long-term compliance.

Drugs appropriate for monotherapy are diuretics, β-blockers, calcium channel antagonists, ACE inhibitors, α-blockers, and α-β-blockers. Centrally acting α-agonists (clonidine, methyldopa, guanfacine, guanabenz) and traditional vasodilators (hydralazine, minoxidil) may be associated with pseudotolerance--i.e., reflex stimulation of the renin-angiotensin-aldosterone system and/or the sympathetic nervous system that causes fluid retention and loss of efficacy with prolonged use--and so ordinarily are not used as monotherapy. Centrally acting α-agonists are appropriate when used in combination with diuretics, whereas traditional vasodilators are best as a third drug in combination with diuretics and adrenergic inhibitors. Additional factors influencing drug selection include the recognition that certain drugs work better according to a patient's age and race (diuretics and calcium antagonists are more effective in blacks and the elderly, as are β-blockers and ACE inhibitors in whites and younger patients), the presence of concomitant diseases, and drug-drug interactions. If the first drug chosen fails to control blood pressure, discontinue its use and substitute a drug of a different class or add a second drug to the first. With combination therapy, make certain that the chosen drugs work in combination and that two drugs of the same class are not used simultaneously.

- Drugs for monotherapy: diuretics, β-blockers, calcium channel antagonists, ACE inhibitors, α-blockers, α-β-blockers.
- Centrally acting α-agonists ordinarily are not used as monotherapy but are appropriate in combination with diuretics.
- Traditional vasodilators are best as a third drug in combination with diuretics and adrenergic inhibitors.

Thiazide Diuretics

Thiazide diuretics have been the mainstay of treatment of mild-to-moderate hypertension. Concomitant diseases for which these drugs should be considered are edema states and congestive heart failure. Metabolic disturbances associated with their use are hypokalemia, hyperuricemia, hypercalcemia, hypomagnesemia, hyponatremia, glucose intolerance, and elevation of LDL cholesterol and triglycerides. Because of these potential adverse effects, relative contraindications to the use of thiazide diuretics include the coexistence of diet-controlled type II diabetes, gout, hyperlipidemia, cardiac arrhythmias, and ischemic heart disease. Drug interactions include potentiation of lithium toxicity (thiazides reduce renal clearance of lithium), lessening of the anti-coagulant effect of warfarin, enhancement of digitalis toxicity, and enhancement of the effects of skeletal muscle relaxants. Nonsteroidal anti-inflammatory drugs reduce the antihypertensive effect of thiazide diuretics. Use of these diuretics is associated with pancreatitis, vasculitis, mesenteric infarction, jaundice, and photosensitivity. Rarely, they cause blood dyscrasias. Thiazide diuretics are usually ineffective when serum creatinine is >2.0 mg/dL. An exception is indapamide, a thiazide-like diuretic that is effective in states of reduced renal function and that is less likely to elevate blood lipids. When serum creatinine is >2.0 mg/dL, the more potent loop diuretics or metolazone is more effective. Volume expansion is often etiologically important in hypertension associated with renal insufficiency.

- Metabolic disturbances associated with diuretics: hypokalemia, hyperuricemia, hypercalcemia, hypomagnesemia, hyponatremia, glucose intolerance, elevated LDL cholesterol and triglycerides.
- Drug interactions: potentiation of lithium toxicity, lessening of anticoagulant effect of warfarin, enhancement of digitalis toxicity, enhancement of effects of skeletal muscle relaxants.
- Use of diuretics associated with pancreatitis, vasculitis, mesenteric infarction, jaundice, photosensitivity.

Furosemide

The major indications for furosemide are hypertension associated with renal insufficiency and the need for a diuretic more potent than thiazides. Similar to thiazide diuretics, furosemide can cause hypokalemia, hyperuricemia, elevated fasting blood glucose and can reduce lithium clearance. Unlike thiazide diuretics, furosemide causes calciuresis. Potential adverse effects include reversible deafness and postural hypotension (especially in older patients). Furosemide reduces salicylate clearance and enhances the effects of skeletal muscle relaxants. It is synergistic when used with metolazone.

- Major indication for furosemide: hypertension associated with renal insufficiency.
- Furosemide can cause: hypokalemia, hyperuricemia, elevated fasting blood glucose, reduced lithium clearance, enhanced salicylate clearance, enhanced effect of skeletal muscle relaxants.
- Adverse effects: reversible deafness and postural hypotension.

Bumetanide

The actions of bumetanide are identical to those of furosemide, but bumetanide is a more potent diuretic (on a milligram per milligram basis).

Ethacrynic Acid

The actions and effects of ethacrynic acid are similar to those of furosemide. Although permanent hearing loss is a risk, ethacrynic acid is an alternative diuretic for patients with sulfa sensitivity.

Potassium-Sparing Diuretics

1. Spironolactone. Spironolactone is an aldosterone antagonist used specifically in patients with primary aldosteronism or with severe secondary aldosteronism. Its diuretic effect is antagonized by concomitant use of salicylates. Adverse effects include hyperkalemia, gynecomastia (but not breast cancer), and skin rash. Spironolactone is usually combined with thiazides to limit hypokalemia.

- Diuretic effect of spironolactone is antagonized by concomitant use of salicylates.
- Adverse effects: hyperkalemia, gynecomastia, skin rash.

2. Triamterene. Triamterene inhibits renal potassium wasting independent of aldosterone. Side effects include hyperkalemia and skin rash.

- Triamterene inhibits renal potassium wasting independent of aldosterone.

3. Amiloride. The actions of amiloride are similar to those of triamterene. Side effects are hyperkalemia, gastrointestinal distress, and skin rash.

Of the potassium-sparing diuretics, only spironolactone causes gynecomastia. In general, these drugs should be avoided in cases of renal failure and when ACE inhibitors are used.

- Avoid potassium-sparing diuretics in renal failure and when ACE inhibitors are used.

Adrenergic Inhibitors

When a diuretic alone fails to control blood pressure, an adrenergic inhibitor can be added. Adrenergic inhibitors are divided into centrally acting and peripherally acting drugs.

1. Peripherally acting inhibitors.
   a. Reserpine. Reserpine blocks transport of norepinephrine into storage granules in peripheral neurons, causing decreased sympathetic nervous system tone. Side effects include depression, nasal congestion, and stimulation of gastric acid secretion, which can precipitate or aggravate peptic ulcer disease. A history of depression or peptic ulcer disease should contraindicate its use.

- Major side effects of reserpine: depression, nasal congestion, stimulation of gastric acid secretion.

   b. Guanethidine. Guanethidine generally is used only as part of a combination drug program to treat resistant hypertension. It lowers blood pressure by causing degranulation of catecholamine storage granules in nerve endings. It does not enter the central nervous system. It has a long half-life. The maximum hypotensive effect of a given dose may not be manifested for 2-3 weeks. It should be given only once daily, and titration requires several weeks. Major side effects are postural hypotension, fluid retention, diarrhea, and retrograde ejaculation. Tricyclic antidepressants, antihistamines, and ephedrine interfere with its action. Guanadrel, a short-acting form of guanethidine, is easier to titrate to an effective dose because it has a shorter half-life.

- Major side effects of guanethidine: postural hypotension, fluid retention, diarrhea, retrograde ejaculation.
- Tricyclic antidepressants, antihistamines, ephedrine interfere with its action.

   c. Prazosin. Prazosin blocks the α_1-adrenergic receptor on vascular smooth muscle cells to blunt catecholamine-induced vasoconstriction. The first dose can precipitate hypotension and syncope; therefore, it should be given before bedtime. Longer acting peripheral α_1-blockers (doxazocin, terazosin) that allow single daily dosing are available. These drugs may lessen voiding symptoms associated with benign prostatic hypertrophy. Although use of α_1-blockers in the elderly is frequently associated with orthostatic hypotension, they do not have adverse metabolic side effects. Other side effects include gastrointestinal distress and, rarely, sedation and dry mouth.

- Because the first dose of prazosin can cause hypotension and syncope, it should be given before bedtime.
- Use in elderly is often associated with orthostatic hypotension but no adverse metabolic side effects.

    d. β-Blockers. Many β-blockers are available, differing in cardioselectivity (affinity for cardiac $β_1$ receptors greater than for noncardiac $β_2$ receptors), lipid solubility, and whether they have partial intrinsic (agonist) sympathomimetic activity (ISA). Non-ISA β-blockers lower blood pressure by reducing cardiac output, inhibiting sympathetically mediated renin release from the kidneys, and inhibiting central sympathetic outflow. β-Blockers with ISA activity do not reduce cardiac output and cause mild peripheral vasodilatation. As lipid solubility increases, more drug is metabolized by the liver, more of it enters the brain, and its duration of action is shorter. As lipid solubility decreases, the drug is mainly eliminated by renal excretion, less of it enters the brain, and its duration of action is longer. Very lipid soluble drugs are propranolol, metoprolol, and timolol. Intermediate lipid soluble drugs are pindolol and acebutolol. Least lipid soluble drugs are atenolol and nadolol.

- As lipid solubility increases, more drug is metabolized by the liver, more of it enters the brain, and its duration of action is shorter.
- As lipid solubility decreases, drug is eliminated mainly by renal excretion, less enters the brain, and its duration of action is longer.
- Very lipid soluble drugs: propranolol, metoprolol, timolol.
- Least lipid soluble drugs: atenolol and nadolol.

Cardioselective β-blockers include acebutolol, atenolol, and metoprolol. Cardioselectivity is relative; at high doses, all β-blockers are nonselective (block both cardiac $β_1$ and noncardiac $β_2$ receptors). β-Blockers with ISA activity are pindolol and acebutolol. Three β-blockers--propranolol, timolol, metoprolol--prevent sudden death and myocardial infarctions in patients with a history of myocardial infarction. β-Blockers should be considered for use in hypertensive patients with concomitant angina, supraventricular arrhythmia, glaucoma, migraine headaches, or hypertrophic cardiomyopathy. Contraindications to the use of β-blockers are asthma, congestive heart failure with reduced systolic function, disease of the conduction system of the heart, angina due to coronary vasospasm, Raynaud's phenomenon, severe occlusive peripheral vascular disease, pheochromocytoma (in absence of alpha blockade), and depression. Because β-blockers may mask the symptoms of hypoglycemia and delay recovery from it, caution is required when used in patients taking insulin. Side effects include cold extremities (non-ISA β-blockers), fatigue, insomnia, nasal congestion, and possibly depression.

- Cardioselectivity is relative; all β-blockers are nonselective at high doses.
- Propranolol, timolol, metoprolol prevent sudden death and myocardial infarction in patients with history of myocardial infarction.
- Contraindications: asthma, congestive heart failure with reduced systolic function, disease of conduction system of heart, angina due to coronary vasospasm, Raynaud's phenomenon, severe occlusive peripheral vascular disease, pheochromocytoma, depression.
- β-Blockers may mask hypoglycemia and delay recovery from it, so use them carefully in patients taking insulin.
- Side effects: cold extremities, fatigue, insomnia, nasal congestion, possibly depression.

    e. Labetalol. Labetalol is a combination of a nonselective β-blocker and a postsynaptic $α_1$-blocker. The ratio of α to β blocking action is between 1:3 and 1:7. It induces decreased cardiac output and peripheral vascular resistance. Labetalol can be used intravenously to treat hypertensive crisis. All the precautions applying to β-blockers apply to this drug. Orthostatic hypotension and scalp itching are its commonest side effects. It may interfere with metanephrine and catecholamine assays.

- Labetalol can be used intravenously.
- All precautions applying to β-blockers apply to labetalol.

- Common side effects: orthostatic hypotension and scalp itching.
- It may interfere with metanephrine and catecholamine assays.

    2. Centrally acting inhibitors.
        a. Methyldopa. Methyldopa inhibits central sympathetic outflow. Its side effects include sedation, dry mouth, hepatitis, fever, positive Coombs' test, hemolytic anemia, leukopenia, thrombocytopenia, and antinuclear antibody positivity. Doses should not exceed 3 g/day. Hemoglobin and liver enzymes should be checked periodically. Methyldopa potentiates lithium and haloperidol toxicity, increases prolactin levels with consequent breast stimulation, interferes with metanephrine assays, and can induce orthostatic hypotension (especially in the elderly).

- Methyldopa side effects: sedation, dry mouth, hepatitis, fever, positive Coombs' test, hemolytic anemia, leukopenia, thrombocytopenia, antinuclear antibody positivity.
- It potentiates lithium and haloperidol toxicity and increases prolactin levels.
- It can induce orthostatic hypotension, especially in the elderly.

        b. Clonidine. Clonidine also inhibits central sympathetic outflow and has the side effects of dry mouth and sedation, but it is not associated with liver toxicity or positive Coombs' test. Because sudden discontinuation of clonidine may induce rebound hypertension, accompanied by symptoms of tachycardia, flushing, and diaphoresis, it should be slowly tapered. (Rebound hypertension can occur with all centrally acting agents and with β-blockers.) Taper and discontinue use of clonidine preoperatively for anticipated surgical procedures in which the patient will not be able to take the medication. Alternatively, patients can be converted preoperatively to the transdermal form of clonidine. Treatment of rebound hypertension usually involves reinstituting clonidine therapy (or whatever agent was discontinued suddenly).

- Sudden discontinuation of clonidine may induce rebound hypertension.

- It should be tapered slowly.
- Taper and discontinue it preoperatively.

        c. Guanabenz. Guanabenz, a newer centrally acting α_2 agonist, is similar in action to clonidine and methyldopa. It may also have weak peripheral neuronal blocking properties. Its side effects are similar to those of clonidine and methyldopa, but, unlike methyldopa, it is not associated with liver toxicity or positive Coombs' test.

- Side effects of guanabenz are similar to those of clonidine and methyldopa.

        d. Guanfacine. Guanfacine, another new clonidine-like drug, can be given once daily and may have fewer central nervous system side effects.

Vasodilators

Vasodilators are usually used as step 3 agents in combination with a diuretic and an adrenergic inhibitor.

1. Hydralazine. Hydralazine decreases blood pressure by directly dilating arterioles. Doses should not exceed 200 mg daily. Its side effects include headache, palpitations, tachycardia, fluid retention, lupus-like syndrome, and peripheral neuropathy. Hydralazine should not be used in patients with a recent cerebral hemorrhage or a dissecting aortic aneurysm because of its tendency to increase cardiac output and cerebral blood flow.

- Hydralazine: direct dilatation of arterioles.
- Dose should not be >200 mg daily.
- Side effects: headache, palpitations, tachycardia, fluid retention, lupus-like syndrome, peripheral neuropathy.
- Do not give to patients with recent cerebral hemorrhage or dissecting aortic aneurysm.

2. Minoxidil. Minoxidil is a very potent, direct vasodilator used to treat severe hypertension with or without renal insufficiency. Its side effects include significant volume expansion with edema, hirsutism, and pericardial effusion. It may cause atrial fibrosis and pulmonary hypertension, but this has not been proven.

- Side effects: volume expansion with edema, hirsutism, pericardial effusion.

ACE Inhibitors

ACE inhibitors decrease blood pressure by inhibiting

the enzyme that converts angiotensin I to angiotensin II, a potent vasoconstrictor. These drugs are appropriate initial therapy for hypertension and work well in combination with other antihypertensive agents, particularly diuretics. Captopril is the only sulfhydryl-containing ACE inhibitor. Because it is eliminated by renal excretion, dose reduction is necessary in cases of renal insufficiency (this is true for most available ACE inhibitors). Side effects presumed to be due to the sulfhydryl group in captopril are skin rash, loss of taste, proteinuria with membranous glomerulonephropathy, and leukopenia. Leukopenia is more likely to occur in patients with collagen vascular disease and renal insufficiency. Side effects shared by all ACE inhibitors are orthostatic hypotension, hyperkalemia, cough, angioedema, and loss of renal function. In patients with bilateral renal artery stenosis, ACE inhibitors can precipitate acute renal failure because of disruption of autoregulation of glomerular filtration in the setting of severe renal ischemia.

- ACE inhibitors inhibit enzyme that converts angiotensin I to angiotensin II.
- ACE inhibitors are appropriate initial therapy for hypertension.
- Dose reduction is necessary in renal insufficiency.
- Side effects of captopril: skin rash, loss of taste, proteinuria with membranous glomerulonephropathy, leukopenia.
- Side effects of all ACE inhibitors: orthostatic hypotension, hyperkalemia, cough, angioedema, loss of renal function.

Calcium Channel Antagonists

Calcium channel antagonists are direct vasodilators. They are divided into dihydropyridines (nifedipine, nicardipine, isradipine, felodipine, and amlodipine) and nondihydropyridines (verapamil, diltiazem). These drugs can be used as initial therapy for hypertension in patients with concomitant ischemic heart disease and angina, variant angina due to coronary vasospasm, supraventricular arrhythmias (verapamil), Raynaud's phenomenon (nifedipine), and migraine headaches (verapamil). Verapamil (and to a lesser extent, diltiazem) has a negative effect on the proximal cardiac conduction system and is a negative inotrope. Verapamil should not be used in patients with conduction system disease (sick sinus syndrome, second degree or greater heart block) and should be avoided in patients with congestive heart failure (ejection fraction <40%). Verapamil in combination with β-blockers

can produce profound cardiodepression. Because it reduces the renal and nonrenal elimination of digoxin, verapamil increases the risk of digoxin toxicity. Quinidine and verapamil in combination can cause serious hypotension in patients with idiopathic hypertrophic subaortic stenosis.

- Calcium channel antagonists are direct vasodilators.
- Verapamil should not be used in sinus syndrome or second degree or greater heart block.
- Avoid using verapamil with congestive heart failure (ejection fraction <40%).
- Verapamil increases risk of digoxin toxicity.

Verapamil and other calcium channel antagonists can cause an increase in liver enzymes associated with hepatic necrosis. The commonest side effect of verapamil is constipation. Most of the side effects associated with nifedipine and other dihydropyridine calcium channel antagonists are related to their potent peripheral vasodilator properties. These side effects include headache, tachycardia, flushing, and edema. Cimetidine and other drugs decreasing blood flow to the liver may increase the biologic effects of calcium channel antagonists. All calcium channel antagonists are metabolized by the liver and dose adjustments may be necessary in the presence of liver disease. They can be safely used in renal insufficiency.

- Calcium channel antagonists can cause increase in liver enzymes associated with hepatic necrosis.
- Commonest side effect of verapamil: constipation.
- Other side effects: headache, tachycardia, flushing, edema.
- Calcium channel antagonists are metabolized by liver so dose adjustments are necessary in liver disease.

CAUSES OF SECONDARY HYPERTENSION

Renovascular Hypertension

Renovascular hypertension is the commonest form of potentially curable secondary hypertension. It occurs in 1%-2% of the hypertensive population. Stenosis of a renal artery increases renin production from the ischemic kidney. Renin acts on circulating renin substrate to produce angiotensin I, which is converted to angiotensin II, a potent vasoconstrictor, by ACE found in lung and other tissues. In addition to vasoconstriction, angiotensin II stimulates aldosterone production, which causes renal sodium retention and volume expansion. Angiotensin II also stimulates thirst and release of vasopressin.

- Renovascular disease: commonest form of potentially curable secondary hypertension.
- Renal artery stenosis increases renin production.
- Renin increases angiotensin II.
- Angiotensin II is a potent vasoconstrictor and stimulates aldosterone production, causing renal sodium retention and volume expansion.

Correcting renal ischemia eliminates the stimulus for excess renin release and often cures or lessens hypertension. In unilateral renal artery stenosis, prolonged hypertension eventually causes nephrosclerosis in the nonischemic kidney. If this occurs, relieving renal arterial stenosis may not cure hypertension. The longer the duration of hypertension before diagnosis, the less likely correction of renal ischemia will be beneficial for blood pressure control.

- Correcting renal ischemia eliminates excess renin release.
- Longer the duration of hypertension, less likely correction of renal ischemia will be beneficial.

Fibromuscular dysplasia is the commonest cause of renovascular hypertension in younger persons, especially women. Lesions usually affect the middle and distal portions of the main renal vessels, often extending into branches. Medial fibroplasia, the most common subtype in adults, has a classic string-of-beads appearance on angiography. Except for rare subtypes, fibromuscular dysplasia progresses slowly over time; however, dissection and thrombosis can occur.

- Fibromuscular dysplasia: commonest cause of renovascular hypertension in younger persons.
- It progresses slowly over time.

Atheromatous disease is the commonest cause of renovascular hypertension in older patients. Lesions usually are in the proximal third of the renal artery, often near the orifice. Although atheromatous renal artery disease may occur in 50%-75% of older persons with hypertension, it causes or aggravates hypertension less frequently. The disease is frequently bilateral and, in 50% of cases, progresses over time, even if blood pressure is controlled. Bilateral disease can progress and lead to end-stage renal disease.

- Atheromatous disease: commonest cause of renovascular hypertension in older persons.
- Disease is frequently bilateral and, in 50% of cases, progresses over time.

Clinical clues suggesting renovascular hypertension include: onset of hypertension before age 25 (consider fibromuscular dysplasia, especially in women); onset of hypertension after age 50 (consider atherosclerotic renal vascular disease); presentation of accelerated or malignant hypertension; sudden worsening of hypertension (renovascular hypertension superimposed on essential hypertension). The most important physical finding is an abdominal bruit, especially a high-pitched systolic/diastolic bruit in the upper abdomen or flank. However, 50% of patients with renovascular hypertension do not have this finding. Other physical clues include severe retinopathy of accelerated malignant hypertension or evidence of occlusive disease in other vascular beds. Laboratory abnormalities consistent with renovascular hypertension include hypokalemia (due to secondary aldosteronism) and, rarely, ischemia-induced polycythemia or nephrotic range proteinuria.

- For hypertension before age 25, consider fibromuscular dysplasia, especially in women.
- Most important physical finding: abdominal bruit.
- Laboratory abnormalities: hypokalemia, ischemia-induced polycythemia, nephrotic range proteinuria.
- For hypertension after age 50, consider atherosclerotic renovascular disease.

Decline of renal function with use of an ACE inhibitor or after sudden reduction of blood pressure may indicate bilateral renal artery disease or small vessel disease of the kidneys (nephrosclerosis). Atheroembolic renal disease may present with a sudden onset or worsening of hypertension and a subacute decline in renal function. Historical clues (e.g., occurrence after angiography or aortic surgery), physical findings (livedo reticularis, peripheral emboli), and laboratory abnormalities (increased erythrocyte sedimentation rate, anemia, hematuria, eosinophilia, eosinophiluria) help identify these patients.

- Sudden decline in renal function with use of ACE inhibitor may indicate bilateral renal artery disease.
- Sudden onset or worsening of hypertension and subacute decline in renal function may be due to atheroembolic renal disease.

In young patients with hypertension (even if not severe) of short duration who have suggestive clinical features, evaluation for renovascular hypertension is indicated, because identification and correction of renal artery stenosis can be performed with low risk of morbidity and mortality, and correction is associated with a high probability of cure. Evaluation for renovascular hypertension in older patients must be done on a selective basis. Selection should be restricted to those patients with suggestive clinical features whose blood pressure cannot be controlled medically or who have an unexplained, observed decline in renal function and who are considered reasonable risks for (and are willing to undergo) interventional therapy.

- In young patients with hypertension of short duration, evaluate for renovascular hypertension.
- Evaluation for renovascular hypertension in older patients must be done on selective basis.

Screening Tests

Intravenous Pyelography

Intravenous pyelography has been replaced by captopril renography as the initial screening test of choice. Characteristic abnormalities are: 1) unilateral reduction in renal mass, with pole-to-pole diameter of smaller kidney reduced by ≥1.5 cm; 2) delayed appearance of contrast agent in collecting system of ischemic kidney; 3) hyperconcentration of contrast agent in ischemic kidney on delayed films; 4) ureteral scalloping by collateral vessels; and 5) cortical thinning or irregularity. Sensitivity is 70%-75%; thus normal findings on intravenous pyelography do not exclude the diagnosis. It is a reasonable choice if renal obstruction, infarction, calculus disease, or parenchymal disease is of concern.

- Abnormalities on intravenous pyelography: unilateral reduction in renal mass (≥1.5-cm reduction in pole-to-pole diameter of smaller kidney), delayed appearance of contrast agent in collecting system of ischemic kidney (hyperconcentration of this agent in ischemic kidney), ureteral scalloping by collateral vessels, cortical thinning or irregularity.

Captopril Radionuclide Renal Scan

Many consider the captopril radionuclide renal scan the screening method of choice. Sensitivity of captopril renography is 90%; specificity is 90%-95%. Pretest treatment of patients with captopril increases the sensitivity

of the scan compared with that of standard renography. The rationale is that glomerular filtration in an ischemic kidney depends on the vasoconstricting effect of angiotensin II on the efferent arteriole of the nephron. Acute treatment with an ACE inhibitor causes efferent arteriolar dilatation, with loss of filtration pressure in the nephron. This causes a decline of glomerular filtration in the ischemic kidney, with less effects on renal blood flow. These changes are identified with the scanning technique. The renal scan is safe for patients with renal insufficiency or a history of contrast allergy. Its interpretive value is reduced by azotemia and bilateral or branch renal artery disease. Urinary outflow obstruction may mimic renal artery stenosis.

- Many consider captopril radionuclide scan the screening method of choice.
- Sensitivity of 90% and specificity of 90%-95%.
- It is safe for patients with renal insufficiency or history of contrast allergy.
- Urinary outflow obstruction may mimic renal artery stenosis.

Digital Venous Subtraction Angiography

Digital venous subtraction angiography uses contrast media but access to the circulation is through a peripheral vein. Thus, it can be performed safely as an outpatient procedure. It allows visualization of the proximal main renal arteries (usual location of atherosclerotic disease) in 90% of patients but is not good for assessing distal or branch renal arteries (usual location of fibromuscular dysplasia). This technique is expensive, and in 20%-30% of cases, renal arteries are not identified because of superimposition of abdominal vessels or patient motion. Sensitivity is 85%-90% and specificity is 85%-90%.

- Proximal main renal arteries are visible in 90% of patients.
- Not good for assessing distal or branch renal arteries.
- It is expensive.
- Renal arteries not identified in 20%-30% of cases.
- Sensitivity of 85%-90% (same for specificity).

Duplex Ultrasonography

Duplex ultrasonography is noninvasive and does not use contrast media. It should be considered for patients with renal insufficiency or history of contrast allergy. This method measures flow-velocity changes in renal vessels that occur with renal artery stenosis. However, in up to 50% of cases, one or both renal arteries cannot be visualized because of technical problems. Sensitivity is 80%-90% and specificity is 60%-80%.

- Consider duplex ultrasonography for patients with renal insufficiency or history of contrast allergy.
- In up to 50% of cases, one or both renal arteries cannot be visualized.
- Sensitivity of 80%-90% and specificity of 60%-80%.

Captopril Test

Acute blockade of angiotensin II formation by ACE inhibitors produces a reactive increase in plasma renin activity. The magnitude of this increase is greater in patients with renovascular hypertension than in those with essential hypertension. This is the basis for the captopril test. Use of antihypertensive agents that influence the renin-angiotensin-aldosterone axis must be discontinued several days before the test. Plasma renin activity is measured at baseline and at 60 minutes after administering captopril orally. Criteria for a positive test include: 1) post captopril plasma renin activity >12 ng/mL per hour, 2) absolute increase in plasma renin activity over baseline of ≥10 ng/mL per hour, and 3) ≥150% increase in plasma renin activity if baseline plasma renin activity is >3 ng/mL per hour or ≥400% if baseline renin activity is <3 ng/mL per hour. Results are compromised in presence of renal insufficiency. Sensitivity is 39%-100% and specificity is 72%-100%.

- Plasma renin activity is measured at baseline and at 60 minutes after administering captopril orally.
- With renal insufficiency, results are compromised.
- Sensitivity of 39%-100% and specificity of 72%-100%.

Renal Vein Renins

Lateralization of renal vein renins is the best predictor of a good interventional outcome in unilateral renal artery stenosis; however, because many factors can influence renin secretion and are difficult to control for, this is not a good screening test. It is invasive and expensive. Lateralization is present if the ratio of renin activity on the affected side compared with the normal side is 1.5:1.0 or greater. Sensitivity is 63%-77% and specificity is 60%-95%.

- Lateralization of renal vein renins: best predictor of good interventional outcome in unilateral renal artery stenosis.

- It is invasive and expensive.
- Lateralization is present if ratio of renin activity of affected side to normal side is 1.5:1.0 or greater.

Renal Arteriography

Renal arteriography is the standard method for identifying renal arterial lesions. Renal artery stenosis must be demonstrated in combination with clinical features and, in some cases, renal vein renins. If there are good clinical reasons to suspect disease, proceeding directly to arteriography is appropriate.

- Renal arteriography: the standard method for identifying renal arterial lesions.

Therapy for Renovascular Hypertension

Options for management of renovascular hypertension include medical and interventional therapies. Percutaneous balloon angioplasty and surgical procedures to relieve renal ischemia are the nonmedical treatments. Goals of interventional therapy are to cure or improve hypertension and to preserve renal function. Interventional therapy should be reserved for good surgical candidates. Medical therapy is reserved for patients not considered candidates for interventional therapy (because of extent or location of vascular lesions, medical/surgical risk, uncertainty about causative significance of lesion).

Percutaneous transluminal angioplasty is the treatment of choice for amenable lesions due to fibromuscular dysplasia. Its role in the management of atherosclerotic renovascular lesions is less well defined. Complications of angioplasty include groin hematoma, dye-induced azotemia, dissection of the renal artery, renal infarction, and, rarely, rupture of the renal artery with loss of the kidney and the need for immediate surgery. Cholesterol embolization is a risk in older patients with diffuse atherosclerosis.

- Angioplasty is treatment of choice for amenable lesions due to fibromuscular dysplasia.
- Its complications: groin hematoma, dye-induced azotemia, dissection of renal artery, renal infarction, and, rarely, rupture of renal artery.

Surgical treatment is best for cases of atheromatous renal artery disease. Kidneys ≤8 cm in pole-to-pole length should be removed, not revascularized, if intervention is indicated and removal will not jeopardize overall renal function.

● Surgical treatment is best for most cases of atheromatous renal artery disease.

Medical treatment of renovascular hypertension differs little from that of essential hypertension. Volume retention and vasoconstriction (due to activation of sympathetic nervous system and angiotensin II) both contribute to the hypertension. ACE inhibitors can precipitate acute renal failure if unrecognized bilateral renal artery stenosis is present. Medical treatment does not correct the underlying ischemia of the affected kidney, and decreasing systemic blood pressure without correcting renal vascular stenosis may aggravate further loss of renal function.

● Medical treatment of renovascular hypertension is similar to that of essential hypertension.
● If there is bilateral renal artery stenosis, ACE inhibitors can precipitate acute renal failure.
● Medical treatment does not correct underlying ischemia of affected kidney.

Renal Parenchymal Disease

Renal parenchymal disease is the commonest cause of secondary hypertension. At least three mechanisms are involved in the hypertension of renal disease: volume expansion, renin oversecretion, and decreased production of renal vasodilators (prostaglandins, kallikrein, kinin). Treatment should include sodium restriction and diuretics. Oversecretion of renin occurs in a small proportion of patients with chronic renal disease. In advanced renal insufficiency, avoid the use of lipid insoluble β-blockers, which rely on kidney for excretion. ACE inhibitors should be used with caution and in reduced dose because they can cause hyperkalemia and a further decline in renal function.

● Renal parenchymal disease: commonest cause of secondary hypertension.
● Treatment should include sodium restriction and diuretics.
● Renin oversecretion occurs in a small proportion of patients with chronic renal disease.
● Use ACE inhibitors cautiously and at reduced dose.

Primary Aldosteronism

Hypertension, hypokalemia, suppressed plasma renin activity, and increased aldosterone excretion form the syndrome of primary aldosteronism. Its main subtypes are unilateral aldosterone-producing adenoma and bilateral adrenal hyperplasia. Rarer subtypes are unilateral hyperplasia, glucocorticoid suppressible hyperplasia, and aldosterone-producing cortical carcinoma. Primary aldosteronism should be suspected in any hypertensive patient presenting with spontaneous hypokalemia or significant hypokalemia precipitated by usual dose diuretic therapy. One should consider other hypokalemic hypertensive syndromes: diuretics, renovascular hypertension, Cushing's disease, exogenous steroids, and ingestion of licorice containing glycyrrhizinic acid (renal cortisol catabolism inhibitor).

● Primary aldosteronism: hypertension, hypokalemia, suppressed plasma renin, increased aldosterone secretion.
● Main subtypes: unilateral aldosterone-producing adenoma and bilateral adrenal hyperplasia.
● Suspected in patients with spontaneous hypokalemia or significant hypokalemia precipitated by usual dose diuretic therapy.

Clinical Features

Clinical symptoms are uncommon. Significant hypokalemia may cause muscle weakness, cramps, headache, palpitations, polydipsia, polyuria, or nocturia. Hypertension is usually moderate but may be severe; it is often resistant to pharmacologic intervention. Retinal vascular changes of significant hypertension may be present. Trousseau's or Chvostek's signs may be present if marked alkalosis is associated with the hypokalemia. Peripheral edema is rare.

● Significant hypokalemia may cause muscle weakness, cramps, headache, palpitations, polydipsia, polyuria, or nocturia.
● Peripheral edema is rare.

Laboratory Features

Characteristic laboratory abnormalities include hypokalemia, mild metabolic alkalosis (serum bicarbonate >31 mEq/L), and relative hypernatremia (serum sodium concentration >142 mEq/L). Relative hypernatremia is related to decreased vasopressin release as the result of volume expansion, resetting of central osmostat for vasopressin release, altered thirst, and hypokalemia-induced suppression of vasopressin release or action. Mild increase in fasting blood glucose level is seen in about 25% of patients (hypokalemia suppresses insulin release). ECG may show changes of left ventricular hypertrophy and hypokalemia (prolongation of ST segment, U waves, and T-wave inversions).

- Laboratory abnormalities: hypokalemia, mild metabolic alkalosis, relative hypernatremia.
- In about 25% of patients, mild increase in blood glucose.
- ECG shows left ventricular hypertrophy and hypokalemia (prolongation of ST segment, U waves, T-wave inversions).

Diagnosis

Investigation of primary aldosteronism is divided into three series of studies: 1) screening for primary aldosteronism, 2) confirming the diagnosis, and 3) performing imaging studies and physiologic maneuvers to distinguish between the two main subtypes of primary aldosteronism. Screening studies should include measurement of serum sodium, potassium, upright plasma renin activity (PRA), and plasma aldosterone concentration (PAC). In a hypokalemic, hypertensive patient, a PAC to PRA ratio >20 suggests the diagnosis of primary aldosteronism. Diagnosis of primary aldosteronism rests on demonstrating hypokalemia, renin suppression, and increased aldosterone excretion in a sodium replete state (24-hour sodium excretion >200 mg) in hypertensive patients. Before initiating a diagnostic evaluation, the use of potentially interfering drugs must be discontinued and plasma volume status assessed. Spironolactone, estrogens, diuretics, prostaglandin synthetase inhibitors, sympathomimetics, and adrenergic inhibitors may influence the renin-angiotensin-aldosterone axis. Use of these medications must be discontinued for at least 6 weeks before investigation. If hypertension must be treated in the interim, guanadrel, α-blockers, or calcium channel antagonists may be used. After a high salt diet for 3 days (and with concomitant vigorous potassium supplementation), patients should submit a 24-hour urine collection for measurement of sodium, potassium, creatinine, and aldosterone. Creatinine can be used as an approximation of the adequacy of the collection. A 24-hour urine aldosterone >12 ng (when urine sodium is >200 mEq/24 hours) confirms the diagnosis of primary aldosteronism.

- In a hypokalemic, hypertensive patient, PAC to PRA ratio >20 suggests primary aldosteronism.
- Diagnosis of primary aldosteronism: hypokalemia, renin suppression, increased aldosterone secretion in a sodium replete state in hypertensive patient.
- Before diagnostic evaluation: discontinue interfering

drugs and assess plasma volume status.
- After a 3-day high salt diet, measure sodium, potassium, creatinine, and aldosterone in 24-hour urine collection.
- 24-Hour urine aldosterone >12 ng (if urine sodium is >200 mEq/24 hr) confirms diagnosis of primary aldosteronism.

Adenoma and bilateral hyperplasia must be distinguished. Removing an aldosterone-producing adenoma normalizes hypertension and hypokalemia in 70% of cases. Unilateral or bilateral adrenalectomy seldom corrects hypertension when bilateral adrenal hyperplasia is present. Adrenal CT scan is the initial study for distinguishing between subtypes. CT is effective in localizing adenomas >1 cm in diameter when the adrenal glands are imaged at 0.3-cm intervals. Generally, if a single adenoma >1 cm in diameter is clearly identified, surgical treatment is the choice. If no mass is identified, assume the diagnosis of bilateral hyperplasia and prescribe spironolactone or other potassium-retaining diuretics. Often, additional medications are needed for blood pressure control.

- Removing aldosterone-producing adenoma normalizes hypertension and hypokalemia in 70% of cases.
- Unilateral or bilateral adrenalectomy seldom corrects hypertension in cases of bilateral adrenal hyperplasia.
- Adrenal CT scan is initial study for distinguishing between subtypes.
- If single adenoma is >1 cm in diameter, treatment is surgical.
- If no mass is seen, prescribe spironolactone or other potassium-retaining diuretics.

If the results are equivocal, or the gland opposite that containing the presumed adenoma is abnormal, or if CT findings are normal in a young patient with severe hypertension and hypokalemia, sampling blood from the adrenal veins may distinguish between subtypes. In these settings, subspecialty consultation should be sought.

- If results are equivocal, sampling blood from adrenal veins may distinguish between subtypes.

Pheochromocytoma

Pheochromocytomas may arise wherever chromaffin cells are found. Of all pheochromocytomas, 80%-90% are in the adrenal glands, either unilaterally or bilaterally.

They also may occur anywhere along the sympathetic chain and occasionally in aberrant sites (frequently in the bladder or organ of Zuckerkandl). Pheochromocytomas are malignant in up to 15% of cases. Chromaffin cells synthesize catecholamines from tyrosine. Norepinephrine is the end product in all sites except in the adrenal medulla, where 75% of norepinephrine is metabolized further to epinephrine. Extra-adrenal tumors produce only norepinephrine, whereas adrenal pheochromocytomas may produce excess of one or both chemicals. Patients with tumors secreting predominantly epinephrine tend to have mainly systolic hypertension, tachycardia, sweating, flushing, and tremulousness and may present with hypotension. Patients with tumors secreting mainly norepinephrine tend to have both diastolic and systolic hypertension, less tachycardia, and fewer paroxysms of anxiety and palpitations.

- 80%-90% of pheochromocytomas are in adrenal glands.
- They may be anywhere along sympathetic chain.
- They are malignant in up to 15% of cases.
- Extra-adrenal tumors produce only norepinephrine.
- Adrenal pheochromocytomas produce excess of epinephrine or norepinephrine or both.

About 6% of pheochromocytomas are familial. There is a tendency for familial pheochromocytomas to be bilateral. The simple familial form is inherited as an autosomal dominant trait and is not associated with other glandular dysfunction. Multiple endocrine neoplasia type II syndrome consists of medullary carcinoma of the thyroid (elevated plasma calcitonin levels), pheochromocytoma, and hyperparathyroidism. Pheochromocytomas are associated with neurofibromatosis (cafe-au-lait spots) and von Hippel-Lindau syndrome (retinal angiomas, cerebellar hemangioblastomas).

- 6% of pheochromocytomas are familial.
- Familial tumors: tend to be bilateral.
- Multiple endocrine neoplasia type II: medullary carcinoma of thyroid, pheochromocytoma, and hyperparathyroidism.
- Pheochromocytoma associated with neurofibromatosis and von Hippel-Lindau syndrome (retinal angiomas, cerebellar hemangioblastomas).

Symptoms
Headache, sweating, or palpitations are common, and all may occur in paroxysms. Paroxysms of hypertension occur in <50% of patients; most patients have sustained hypertension. Exercise, bending, urination, defecation, induction of anesthesia, smoking, or infusion of intravenous contrast media can induce a paroxysm. Some patients have a history of weight loss and hypermetabolism. Others have both hypertension and orthostatic hypotension and some have retinopathy of accelerated hypertension.

- Common symptoms of pheochromocytoma: headache, sweating, palpitations.
- Exercise, bending, urination, defecation, induction of anesthesia, smoking, or infusion of contrast media can induce a paroxysm.
- Some patients have history of weight loss and hypermetabolism; others have both hypertension and orthostatic hypotension.

Screening
Patients who should be screened for pheochromocytoma are those with a history of paroxysmal hypertension, progressive or treatment-resistant hypertension, hypertension with diabetes, hypermetabolism and weight loss, marked hypertension in response to anesthesia induction, neurocutaneous lesions and hypertension, family history of pheochromocytoma, medullary carcinoma of the thyroid or hyperparathyroidism, and orthostatic hypotension. Patients with a history of paroxysmal symptoms and hypertension should also be screened for pheochromocytoma, as should children with hypertension. The best screening test is 24-hour urine metanephrine concentration. Because pheochromocytomas may secrete intermittently, multiple samples may be required. Urine should be collected immediately after a paroxysm. In addition to urine metanephrine concentration, urine VMA concentration and plasma and urine catecholamine concentrations should be measured in selected patients. Medications that can interfere with these assays include sympathomimetics, methyldopa, phenothiazines, tricyclic antidepressants, β-blockers, labetalol, and levodopa.

- Screening for pheochromocytoma: history of paroxysmal hypertension, progressive or treatment-resistant hypertension, hypertension with diabetes, hypermetabolism and weight loss, marked hypertension in response to anesthesia induction.
- Screen children with hypertension.
- Best screening test is 24-hour urine metanephrine con-

centration.

- Medications interfering with assays: sympathomimetics, methyldopa, phenothiazines, tricyclic antidepressants, β-blockers, labetalol, levodopa.

Diagnosis and Treatment

CT scanning should be the first test used to locate a tumor. Treatment is surgical. Preoperatively, administer α-blockers followed by β-blockers if needed for blood pressure and cardiac rhythm control. Patients with hypertensive crisis can be given α-blockers intravenously. β-Blockers can be used if tachycardia is excessive.

- Use CT first to locate tumor.
- Treatment is surgical.
- Preoperatively, administer α-blockers followed by β-blockers.

Coarctation of the Aorta

Coarctation of the aorta is commonly just beyond the take off of the left subclavian artery. It is detected most often in childhood but may escape detection until adulthood. The classic feature of coarctation is increased blood pressure in the upper extremities with low or unobtainable blood pressure in the lower extremities. The mechanism of hypertension involves volume expansion and inappropriate renin secretion. Symptoms of coarctation include headache, cold feet, and exercise-induced leg pain (claudication). Clinical signs include hypertension, murmurs in the front or back of the chest, visible pulsations in the neck or chest wall, and weak femoral pulses or delay when simultaneously palpating the radial and femoral pulse. Chest radiography can be diagnostic. Characteristic "3 sign" due to dilatation above and below the constriction plus notching of the ribs by enlarged collateral vessels may be identified. Diagnosis is proved by aortography, and treatment is surgical. Postoperative hypertension is usually transient and may be associated with mesenteric vasculitis and bowel infarction. Plasma renin activity levels are usually high. β-Blockers or ACE inhibitors are recommended treatments.

- Coarctation of the aorta is usually just beyond take off of left subclavian artery.
- Usually detected in childhood but may not be detected until adulthood.
- Classic feature: increased blood pressure in upper extremities and low/unobtainable blood pressure in lower extremities.

- Mechanism: volume expansion and inappropriate renin secretion.
- Symptoms: headache, cold feet, exercise-induced leg pain.
- Signs: hypertension, murmurs in front or back of chest, visible pulsations in neck or chest wall, weak femoral pulses.
- Chest radiography can be diagnostic.

Hypertension in Pregnancy

Normally, blood pressure decreases early in pregnancy and then gradually increases to pre-pregnant levels toward term. During pregnancy, renin substrate, renin activity, and aldosterone levels increase. Vessels during normal pregnancy are hyporesponsive to angiotensin, perhaps because of prostaglandins produced by the uteroplacental unit. Although aldosterone levels increase, renal sodium retention is not marked, probably because progesterone and prostaglandins are natriuretic. Progesterone is also a vasodilator. During normal pregnancy, plasma volume and cardiac output increase 50%-60% of baseline. Renal blood flow and glomerular filtration rate increase by 35%. Blood pressure decreases in normal pregnancy because of reduced peripheral vascular resistance. Other substances that increase during normal pregnancy are estrogen, deoxycorticosterone, and vasodilating prostaglandins produced by the uteroplacental unit.

- Blood pressure decreases early in pregnancy, gradually increasing to pre-pregnant levels toward term.
- Renin substrate, renin activity, and aldosterone increase.
- During pregnancy, vessels are hyporesponsive to angiotensin.
- Renal sodium retention is not marked, probably because progesterone and prostaglandins are natriuretic.
- In normal pregnancies, blood pressure decreases because of reduced peripheral vascular resistance.

Definition

Hypertension during pregnancy is when systolic blood pressure increases ≥30 mm Hg and diastolic blood pressure increases ≥15 mm Hg compared with values before 20 weeks' gestation. When previous blood pressure levels are unknown, a pressure of ≥140/90 mm Hg is abnormal. Four major hypertensive syndromes in pregnancy are 1) chronic hypertension--high blood pressure known to be present before pregnancy or diagnosed before 20th week of gestation, 2) preeclampsia-eclampsia (described below), 3) chronic hypertension with superimposed preeclampsia, and 4) transient hypertension (or gestational hypertension)--increase in blood pressure without significant edema or proteinuria, with return of blood pressure to normal within 10 days after delivery. This is a predictor for the future development of essential hypertension.

- Hypertension: systolic blood pressure increases ≥30 mm Hg and diastolic blood pressure increases ≥15 mm Hg compared with values before 20 weeks' gestation.
- Transient hypertension is a predictor for future development of essential hypertension.

Preeclampsia is characterized by the triad of hypertension, edema, and proteinuria developing after the 20th week of gestation. Eclampsia consists of these symptoms plus convulsions. Warning symptoms of eclampsia include headache, blurring of vision, epigastric pain, hyperreflexia, or cerebral symptoms. Risk of developing eclampsia is markedly increased in patients with severe proteinuria (>5 g), oliguria, or absolute blood pressures >160/110 mm Hg. Preeclampsia occurs more commonly in women who are relatively young or old to be pregnant, first pregnancy, twin pregnancy, obesity, diabetes, family history of eclampsia or preeclampsia in mother, renal disease, or pregnancy in the setting of chronic hypertension. Preeclampsia developing before the 20th week of gestation suggests the possibility of molar pregnancy, fetal hydrops, α-thalassemia, or renal disease.

- Preeclampsia: characteristic triad of hypertension, edema, and proteinuria after 20th week of gestation.
- Eclampsia: same symptoms as preeclampsia plus convulsions.
- Preeclampsia is more common in women relatively young or old for pregnancy, first or twin pregnancy, obesity, diabetes, family history of eclampsia or preeclampsia in mother, renal disease, pregnancy in setting of chronic hypertension.

The cause of preeclampsia is not well known. The best hypothesis involves underperfusion of the uteroplacental unit. Unlike normal pregnant women, those with preeclampsia are sensitive to the pressor effects of angiotensin. There is a marked rise in peripheral resistance. Renal blood flow and glomerular filtration rate are reduced. Vascular volume is reduced. There is often hemoconcentration. Placental prostaglandin levels fall. Uric acid is most often elevated and distinguishes patients with preeclampsia from those with chronic hypertension in pregnancy.

- Unlike normal pregnant women, those with preeclampsia are sensitive to pressor effects of angiotensin.
- Peripheral resistance markedly increases.
- Uric acid is most often elevated: this distinguishes women with preeclampsia from those with chronic hypertension in pregnancy.

Treatment of Hypertension in Pregnancy

For previously untreated patients, consider drug therapy if diastolic blood pressure is ≥100 mm Hg. Methyldopa (most completely studied) is recommended as initial therapy. If this drug is ineffective or not tolerated, consider other drugs. Except for ACE inhibitors, none of the currently available drugs are known to increase perinatal morbidity or mortality. Most of the concern about these drugs is theoretical. There is evidence that β-adrenergic blocking drugs and α-β-blocking drugs are safe and effective for treating chronic hypertension in pregnancy. There is some concern that the use of β-adrenergic blockers early in pregnancy can retard fetal growth and in late pregnancy could slow fetal heart rate.

- For previously untreated patients, use drug therapy if diastolic blood pressure is ≥100 mm Hg.
- Recommended initial therapy: methyldopa.
- ACE inhibitors are contraindicated during pregnancy.

Treatment of Preeclampsia-Eclampsia

Prevention strategies for preeclampsia have limited value. It is important to identify the high-risk patient and monitor her closely to identify preeclampsia early. Low doses of aspirin have received much attention as a possible agent for preventing preeclampsia, but currently its use is investigational. Early recognition of preeclampsia is based primarily on diagnostic blood pressure increases in late second or early third trimester of pregnancy. Proteinuria is an important sign of progression, usually warranting hospitalization. Patients should be kept at rest in bed. Monitor blood pressure, urine output, and fluid retention (estimated by daily weights) daily. Periodically determine platelet count, creatinine level, uric acid level, and urine protein excretion. Evidence of central nervous system involvement (headache, disorientation, visual symptoms) or hepatic distention (abdominal pain, hepatic tenderness) are important findings that suggest progression of preeclampsia. Hepatic rupture is associated with a 65% mortality and can be prevented only by delivery of the fetus. Evidence of progressive preeclampsia after the 30th week of gestation is an indication for delivery. When gestational age is critical (25-30 weeks), delivery is indicated by worsening maternal symptoms, laboratory evidence of end-organ dysfunction, or deterioration of fetal condition. If fetus is immature and preeclampsia is nonprogressive, a period of observation is warranted. Hypertension should be treated with drugs if diastolic blood pressure is >100 mm Hg. Treatment of choice is methyldopa. Calcium channel antagonists, β-adrenergic blockers, or hydralazine are reasonable alternatives.

- Proteinuria is important sign of progression, usually warranting hospitalization.
- Keep patient at bed rest.
- Central nervous system progression or hepatic distention suggests progression of preeclampsia.
- Progressive preeclampsia after 30th week of gestation is indication for delivery.
- Delivery is indicated by worsening maternal symptoms, laboratory evidence of end-organ dysfunction, or deterioration of fetal condition.
- If diastolic blood pressure is >100 mm Hg, treat with drugs.
- Treatment of choice: methyldopa.

Magnesium sulfate is the treatment of choice for impending eclampsia. It can be administered intravenously as 20 mL of 20% solution over 4 minutes. Intermittent doses of a 50% solution given intramuscularly every 4 hours can also be used. Monitor patient's patellar reflex, urine output, and respirations while giving magnesium. Calcium gluconate is the treatment of choice for magnesium toxicity.

- Magnesium sulfate: treatment of choice for impending eclampsia.
- Calcium gluconate: treatment of choice for magnesium toxicity.

Treatment of Hypertensive Crisis

The drug of choice for the treatment of hypertensive crisis during pregnancy is hydralazine administered intravenously. Initially administer a 5-mg bolus. This can be followed by 5-10 mg every 20-30 minutes. Side effects include tachycardia and headache. For hypertension refractory to hydralazine, diazoxide is recommended. Miniboluses (30 mg) should be used. Side effects include

arrest of labor and neonatal hyperglycemia. Labetalol may replace diazoxide as the second-line drug. Calcium antagonists can be used but concomitant use of magnesium sulfate may cause severe hypotension. Diuretics and sodium nitroprusside (cyanide poisoning in the fetus) should be avoided. However, maternal well-being may override these concerns.

- Drug of choice for treating hypertensive crisis: hydralazine given intravenously.
- For hypertension refractory to hydralazine, use diazoxide.
- Avoid diuretics and sodium nitroprusside.

Hypertensive Urgencies and Emergencies

Acute, severe increases in blood pressure are a medical emergency; prompt therapy may be lifesaving.

Definitions

Malignant hypertension is a sudden severe increase in blood pressure associated with acute injury to target organs (brain, heart, kidneys, retina). Parenteral antihypertensive therapy to reduce blood pressure immediately is required. Retinal examination reveals hemorrhages, exudates, and papilledema. Hypertensive encephalopathy may be present; it is cerebral edema due to breakthrough hyperperfusion of the brain caused by severely increased blood pressure. Manifestations include papilledema, headache, confusion, gastrointestinal distress, and seizures. The term "hypertensive emergency" implies malignant hypertension or impending malignant hypertension.

- Malignant hypertension: sudden severe increase in blood pressure associated with acute injury to target organs.
- Parenteral therapy to reduce blood pressure immediately is required.
- Retinal hemorrhages, exudates, and papilledema occur.
- Hypertensive encephalopathy: papilledema, headache, confusion, gastrointestinal distress, seizures.

Accelerated Hypertension

Accelerated hypertension is a sudden increase in blood pressure to less severe levels. It is not associated with acute target organ damage. Retinal examination reveals hemorrhages and exudates but not papilledema. If left untreated, it may progress to malignant hypertension. Blood pressure usually can be reduced to safer levels with oral or parenteral medications over several hours. The term "hypertensive urgency" implies accelerated hypertension or severe elevations in blood pressure without evidence of acute target organ damage occurring in a setting in which it is important to lower blood pressure over several hours.

- Accelerated hypertension: sudden increase in blood pressure to less severe levels.
- Not associated with acute target organ damage.
- Retinal hemorrhages and exudates but not papilledema.
- Can be reduced with oral or parenteral medications.

Causes

Causes of hypertensive urgencies and emergencies include the development of accelerated malignant hypertension on the background of neglected essential hypertension, sudden discontinuation of antihypertensive therapy (especially clonidine and β-blockers), renovascular disease, collagen diseases (especially scleroderma), monoamine oxidase inhibitors and tyramine-containing foods, intracerebral or subarachnoid hemorrhage, acute aortic dissection, pheochromocytoma crisis, acute head injury, and acute stroke.

- Causes of hypertensive urgencies and emergencies: neglected essential hypertension, discontinuation of antihypertensive therapy, renovascular disease, collagen diseases, pheochromocytoma crisis, stroke.

Pathophysiology

Malignant hypertension is a rapidly progressive vasospastic disorder associated with marked increase in peripheral vascular resistance and elevated levels of renin and angiotensin. Locally generated vasoconstricting factors such as endothelin may be important. If not reversed, necrosis of blood vessel walls occurs (fibrinoid necrosis) with severe damage to organs, particularly the brain and kidneys. With progressive increases in blood pressure, autoregulation of cerebral blood flow breaks down. Normally, as blood pressure increases, cerebral blood vessels constrict to maintain constant blood flow. When blood pressure rises to a critical level, cerebral blood vessels suddenly dilate, causing marked hyperperfusion of the brain and leakage of fluid. This leads to cerebral edema and the clinical presentation of hypertensive encephalopathy.

- Malignant hypertension: a rapidly progressive vasospastic disorder.
- Renin and angiotensin levels are increased.

- If not reversed, necrosis of blood vessel walls occurs.

Evaluation and Management

Patients with hypertensive emergencies and evidence of acute organ injury should be hospitalized in an intensive care unit. An arterial catheter should be established to monitor blood pressure closely. Initial studies should include chest radiography, ECG, creatinine or BUN, urinalysis, glucose, sodium, potassium, and hemoglobin. Studies to determine underlying cause should be deferred; however, a spot urine for catecholamines is reasonable. The challenge of treating hypertensive emergencies is to decrease blood pressure promptly without compromising function of vital organs. Blood pressure should be lowered quickly to a diastolic level of approximately 110 mm Hg, after which the patient should be monitored for evidence of worsening cerebral, renal, or cardiac status. Blood pressure is then gradually lowered to a diastolic level of 90-100 mm Hg. Ischemic pancreatitis and intestinal infarction can complicate the picture in some patients.

Generally, sodium nitroprusside is the drug of choice. It must be given in an intensive care setting with an arterial catheter in place. This balanced arterial and venous dilator reduces both preload and afterload. The initial dose is 0.5-10.0 μg/kg per minute. It is titrated to a maximum dose of 500 μg/kg per hour. The infusion must be protected from light. Toxicity is related to the development of cyanide in erythrocytes, and thiocyanate levels should be monitored every 48 hours. Therapy should be discontinued if blood level is >12 mg/dL. Sodium nitrate or hydroxycobalamin can be infused in case of toxicity. Side effects of sodium nitroprusside include nausea, vomiting, agitation, muscular twitching, coarse tremor, and flushing. Frequently, patients with malignant hypertension are volume constricted because of pressure natriuresis. However, as blood pressure decreases, fluid retention occurs and the addition of a loop diuretic is often required.

- Sodium nitroprusside: drug of choice.
- Toxicity is related to development of cyanide in erythrocytes.
- Monitor thiocyanate levels every 48 hours.
- In case of toxicity, infuse sodium nitrate or hydroxycobalamin.
- Sodium nitroprusside side effects: nausea, vomiting, agitation, muscular twitching, coarse tremor, flushing.

Diazoxide is an alternative therapy and should be given by minibolus techniques (50-100-150 mg every 5-10 minutes). This method avoids excessive hypotension with the initial dose. Blood sugar should be monitored in diabetics. Side effects include nausea, hypotension, flushing, tachycardia, and chest pain.

- Diazoxide is an alternative therapy.
- Side effects: nausea, hypotension, flushing, tachycardia, chest pain.

Hydralazine can be used (usually in preeclampsia). It is slower acting than the other agents. Its side effects include tachycardia, flushing, headache, vomiting, and aggravation of angina.

Adrenergic inhibitors include phentolamine and trimethaphan. Phentolamine is administered intravenously in doses of 5-15 mg. Its side effects include tachycardia and flushing. Trimethaphan is administered as an infusion at rate of 0.5-5 mg/minute. Its side effects include paresis of bowel and bladder, orthostatic hypotension, blurred vision, and dry mouth.

- Adrenergic inhibitors: phentolamine and trimethaphan.

- Side effects (trimethaphan): bowel and bladder paresis, orthostatic hypotension, blurred vision, dry mouth.

Labetalol is administered by repetitive intravenous minibolus injections. It has the advantage of being available orally for the ease of conversion. The precautions applying to β-blockers also apply to this drug.

Conditions Requiring Avoidance of Specific Drugs
- Acute myocardial infarction or angina--hydralazine (increases cardiac work), diazoxide (increases cardiac work).
- Dissecting aortic aneurysm--hydralazine (increases cardiac output), diazoxide (increases cardiac output).
- Stroke, head injury, hypertensive encephalopathy--methyldopa (sedation, increases cerebral blood flow), diazoxide (decreases cerebral blood flow).

As soon as possible, initiate regular oral treatment and taper intravenous treatment. After blood pressure is controlled, search for secondary causes of hypertension.

QUESTIONS
(See "Answers" section)

Multiple Choice

1. In a patient with hypertension, which set of laboratory findings is most consistent with the diagnosis of primary aldosteronism?
   a. Na^+, 134 mEq/L; K^+, 3.1 mEq/L; HCO_3, 31 mEq/L; fasting blood glucose, 106 mg/dL
   b. Na^+, 144 mEq/L; K^+, 3.0 mEq/L; HCO_3, 32 mEq/L; 24-hour urinary Na^+, 100 mEq; 24-hour urinary K^+, 40 mEq
   c. Na^+, 143 mEq/L; K^+, 3.4 mEq/L; HCO_3, 32 mEq/L; 24-hour urinary Na^+, 16 mEq; 24-hour urinary K^+, 6.0 mEq
   d. Na^+, 142 mEq/L; K^+, 2.9 mEq/L; HCO_3, 34 mEq/L; 24-hour urinary Na^+, 150 mEq; 24-hour urinary K^+, 10 mEq
   e. Na^+, 140 mEq/L; K^+, 4.0 mEq/L; HCO_3, 29 mEq/L

2. Which of the following drugs is absolutely contraindicated for the treatment of hypertension during pregnancy?
   a. Methyldopa
   b. Labetalol
   c. Lisinopril
   d. Hydralazine
   e. Hydrochlorothiazide

3. Thiazide diuretics are associated with all but one of the following metabolic effects:
   a. Hyponatremia
   b. Hypokalemia

c. Hypercalciuria
d. Alkalosis
e. Elevated fasting blood glucose

4. All the following statements about drugs used for the treatment of hypertension are true except:
   a. Hydralazine may be associated with a lupus-like syndrome
   b. Methyldopa and guanabenz may cause hemolytic anemia
   c. Verapamil may cause an increase in digoxin levels in the blood
   d. Thiazide diuretics may interfere with the elimination of lithium
   e. Furosemide causes an increase in urinary calcium

5. All the following statements about hypertensive crisis are true except:
   a. Rapid decrease in blood pressure may be associated with renal or brain injury
   b. Sodium nitroprusside is the treatment of choice in most situations
   c. Signs of sodium nitroprusside toxicity include nausea, vomiting, tremor, and agitation
   d. Outpatient management with aggressive oral therapy can be attempted in stable patients
   e. Abrupt discontinuation of clonidine may precipitate hypertensive crisis

True/False
6. With regard to pheochromocytoma:
   a. Increase in both plasma and urinary levels of nor-
   epinephrine and epinephrine is highly suggestive of a tumor located in an aberrant site rather than in the adrenal glands
   b. β-Blockers can be safely used as initial therapy for hypertension
   c. von Hippel-Lindau disease and neurofibromatosis may be complicated by pheochromocytoma
   d. A family history of hyperparathyroidism or medullary carcinoma of the thyroid is an indication for screening in a hypertensive person
   e. Labetalol is appropriate initial therapy for hypertension
   f. Hypertension in untreated patients is characterized by volume expansion, increased cardiac output, and increased peripheral vascular resistance

7. With regard to renovascular hypertension, indicate whether the following are true or false:
   a. Fibromuscular dysplasia is often the underlying cause in young females
   b. Laboratory abnormalities include hyperkalemia and rarely polycythemia and nephrotic range proteinuria
   c. The absence of a bruit on physical examination makes the diagnosis unlikely
   d. Patients whose renal function declines with the use of an angiotensin-converting enzyme inhibitor may have bilateral renal artery disease
   e. The longer the duration of hypertension before diagnosis, the greater the likelihood of cure with successful interventional therapy
   f. The captopril radionuclide renal scan is considered the screening method of choice by many

NOTES

CHAPTER 20
INFECTIOUS DISEASES

Douglas R. Osmon, M.D.
William F. Marshall, M.D.

This chapter is not inclusive. Topics that should be common knowledge have been omitted. The emphasis is uncommon manifestations of common infectious diseases and important points covered in the infectious disease literature during the past several years.

SPECIFIC MICROORGANISMS

STREPTOCOCCI

These organisms may be divided into groups (Lancefield) by carbohydrates in cell wall: group A, B, C, etc. Group A may be further divided into types by differences in M proteins--types 1-49+, etc. The M protein is a virulence factor. All streptococci are susceptible to penicillin, except enterococci and penicillin-resistant strains of pneumococci.

● All streptococci are susceptible to penicillin, except enterococci and penicillin-resistant strains of pneumococci.

Group A β-Hemolytic: *Streptococcus pyogenes*

Infections

Impetigo is caused by group A β-hemolytic streptococci (color plate 20-1). If *Staphylococcus aureus* is present, it probably plays no role in the pathology or pathogenesis. Antibiotic therapy shortens duration of infection and prevents suppurative complications but probably does not prevent acute glomerular nephritis.

● Antibiotic probably does not prevent acute glomerular nephritis.

Pharyngitis is a self-limited infection. Antibiotic therapy does not shorten duration of infection. However, antibiotic therapy does prevent acute rheumatic fever. Rapid diagnostic tests for streptococcal pharyngitis are specific but not sensitive (50%-70%). Common complications are otitis media and sinusitis.

● Common complications are otitis media and sinusitis.

Erysipelas usually occurs on the face. It has a sharp border, is violaceous, is painful, and most often occurs in the elderly. It has recently been associated with toxic strep syndrome.

Cellulitis occurs in tissue damaged by trauma, in operative wounds, and in tissue with poor venous and lymphatic drainage (postmastectomy cellulitis of the arm and cellulitis of the leg after saphenous vein harvest for coronary artery bypass grafting may have recurrent episodes). Tinea pedis may also serve as a portal of entry.

Group A streptococcal pneumonia is rare but can be extremely severe. There has been a recent increase in group A streptococcal bacteremia in children and adults. Changes in virulence mechanism may be responsible.

Penicillin is the drug of choice for treatment of group A streptococcal infection. Cephalosporins (first-generation), erythromycin, and vancomycin are alternatives. There are no reports of penicillin resistance to date. There have been reports of an increased prevalence of erythromycin-resistant strains.

● There are no reports of penicillin resistance to date.

Toxins

Group A streptococci produce many toxins. Patients with no previous immunity to erythrogenic toxin may develop scarlet fever. Production of hyaluronidase causes the rapidly advancing margins characteristic of cellulitis due to β-hemolytic streptococci. Exotoxin A is similar to the toxin that causes toxic shock syndrome in patients with *S. aureus* infection (toxic strep syndrome).

Nonsuppurative Complications

There has been a resurgence of acute rheumatic fever among children (urban and rural) and in military recruits. It occurs only after pharyngitis, never after skin infections. Recently, the diagnostic criteria for rheumatic fever were revised (Table 20-1). Treatment is with aspirin and steroids depending on clinical circumstances and the severity of symptoms and organ involvement.

● Resurgence of acute rheumatic fever among children (urban and rural) and in military recruits.

The approach to prophylaxis is controversial. One approach, if a murmur is present, is indefinite prophylaxis with penicillin G, preferably benzathine penicillin 1.2 million units monthly (alternative, oral penicillin V potassium 250 mg twice a day). If the patient is allergic to penicillin, alternatives are sulfonamides and erythromycin. If there is no murmur, prophylactic antibiotics are given until age 25. If there is no murmur, no attack within previous 5 years, and no carditis with previous attack, prophylaxis may be discontinued. Prophylactic antibiotics are used to prevent recurrent acute rheumatic fever, not for prevention of subacute bacterial endocarditis (SBE). SBE prophylaxis differs.

Acute glomerulonephritis may occur after both skin infections and pharyngitis, but it is more common after skin infections (Table 20-2).

● Prophylactic antibiotics are used to prevent recurrent acute rheumatic fever, not for prevention of subacute bacterial endocarditis.
● Acute glomerulonephritis may occur after both skin infections and pharyngitis.

Group B: *Streptococcus agalactiae*

This organism is an important cause of maternal and neonatal bacteremia and neonatal meningitis. It is part of normal flora of the female genital tract and gastrointestinal tract. It is more resistant to penicillin than group A streptococci. Treatment of meningitis is with penicillin or ampicillin plus gentamicin.

Group C

Group C streptococci may be β-hemolytic and may cause pharyngitis; but unlike group A streptococci, they do not cause nonsuppurative complications. Bacteremia may be associated with the presence of malignancy and altered immune systems.

Group D Streptococci and Enterococci

Enterococci are no longer considered group D streptococci. These taxonomy differences are also reflected in the differences in susceptibility to penicillin between enterococci and group D streptococci (Table 20-3). Both cause endocarditis. *Streptococcus bovis* endocarditis and

---

Table 20-1.--Jones Criteria for Diagnosis of Initial Attack of Rheumatic Fever[*] (1992 Update)

Major manifestations
   Carditis
   Polyarthritis
   Chorea
   Erythema marginatum
   Subcutaneous nodules
Minor manifestations
   Clinical findings
      Arthralgia
      Fever
   Laboratory findings
      Elevated acute-phase reactants (erythrocyte sedimentation rate, C-reactive protein)
      Prolonged P-R interval
Supporting evidence of antecedent group A streptococcal infection
   Positive throat culture or rapid diagnostic test
   Elevated or rising streptococcal antibody titer

[*]If supported by evidence of recent group A streptococcal infection, two major, or one major and two minor, criteria are enough for diagnosis. Three exceptions in which Jones criteria do not need to be fulfilled: 1) recurrent rheumatic fever (single major or several minor criteria in patient with a reliable history of previous rheumatic fever if supporting evidence of recent group A streptococcal infection), 2) isolated chorea, and 3) indolent carditis. From Special Writing Group of the Committee on Rheumatic Fever, Endocarditis, and Kawasaki Disease of the Council on Cardiovascular Disease in the Young of the American Heart Association: Guidelines for the diagnosis of rheumatic fever: Jones Criteria, 1992 update. JAMA 268:2069-2073, 1992. By permission of American Medical Association.

Table 20-2.--Differences Between Acute Glomerulonephritis and Acute Rheumatic Fever Caused by Group A Streptococcal Infection

	After infection		Recurrence of disease	Antibiotics prevent disease
	Skin	Pharynx		
AGN	Yes	Yes (<skin)	Rare, if ever	?
ARF	No	Yes	Often	Yes

AGN, acute glomerulonephritis; ARF, acute rheumatic fever.

Table 20-3.--Classification of Group D Streptococci and Enterococci

Group D streptococci	*Enterococcus* (note name change)
S. bovis	*E. faecalis* (80%-90%)
S. equinis (rare)	*E. faecium* (5%-10%)
Penicillin MIC	Penicillin MIC
≤0.1 µg/mL	≥1 µg/mL

MIC, minimal inhibitory concentration.

bacteremia may be associated with carcinoma of the colon or other colonic disease. Consider SBE in anyone with a blood culture positive for group D streptococci or enterococci. SBE often occurs in elderly men (prostatism) and young female patients. Source is the genitourinary tract.

- *S. bovis* endocarditis and bacteremia may be associated with carcinoma of the colon or other colonic disease.

An increasing number of nosocomial bacteremias and urinary tract infections are due to enterococci. Sources are the genitourinary tract, intra-abdominal infection, and intravenous lines. Endocarditis rarely complicates nosocomial enterococcal bacteremia. Nosocomial-acquired strains are more likely to have unusual resistance patterns. Treatment of *S. bovis* and *S. equinis* is with penicillin alone or penicillin plus streptomycin or gentamicin. If the patient is allergic to penicillin, a cephalosporin or vancomycin is used.

- Treatment of *S. bovis* and *S. equinis* is with penicillin alone or penicillin plus streptomycin or gentamicin.

In regard to the in vitro susceptibility of enterococci, they are only inhibited, not killed, by penicillin alone (altered penicillin-binding proteins). They are resistant to all cephalosporins. Increasing numbers of enterococci are resistant to aminoglycosides (aminoglycoside-modifying enzymes), produce β-lactamase, or are resistant to glycopeptides (i.e., vancomycin, particularly among *Enterococcus faecium*) (plasmid-mediated alteration in enzyme that produces peptidoglycan). Nosocomial transmission of these resistant strains has occurred. It is imperative that in vitro susceptibility testing for these drugs be performed on enterococcal isolates causing serious infections.

- Enterococci are resistant to all cephalosporins.

For treatment of SBE, a combination of penicillin (or ampicillin) plus streptomycin or gentamicin must be used for isolates that do not produce β-lactamase and that do not have high-level aminoglycoside resistance. Short-course (2-week) therapy cannot be used for enterococcal endocarditis. If the patient is allergic to penicillin, use vancomycin plus streptomycin or gentamicin. Tobramycin and amikacin are not synergistic with either penicillin or vancomycin. Optimal regimens for isolates resistant to both gentamicin and streptomycin are unknown.

- For SBE, a combination of penicillin (or ampicillin) plus streptomycin or gentamicin must be used for isolates that do not produce β-lactamase.

Urinary tract infections and bacteremia without evidence of endocarditis can usually be treated with penicillin, ampicillin, or vancomycin alone as long as the strains are susceptible in vitro. Options for treatment of uncomplicated urinary tract infection in penicillin-allergic patients are ciprofloxacin, nitrofurantoin, or vancomycin, depending on clinical circumstances.

E. faecium may be relatively resistant to penicillin. In

one study, 35% of *E. faecium* organisms were reported to be resistant. Most effective therapy is vancomycin plus gentamicin. *E. faecium* organisms are resistant to all aminoglycosides except streptomycin and gentamicin. Optimal regimens for vancomycin-resistant strains are unknown.

Group F and Group G

These organisms occasionally cause pharyngitis and bacteremia. They may be β-hemolytic and do not cause nonsuppurative complications. Group G bacteremias have been associated with the presence of malignancy and altered immune systems.

Streptococcus pneumoniae

Complications of pneumococcal pneumonia include empyema and pericarditis from direct extension of infection. Empyema occurs in <1% of patients and should be suspected when there is persistent fever despite appropriate antibiotic therapy. Pericarditis often causes precordial pain and a friction rub.

S. pneumoniae is the most common cause of bacterial meningitis in adults (color plate 10-2). Furthermore, suspect it in any patient with recurrent meningitis. If there is recurrent meningitis, always consider the patient to have a cerebrospinal fluid leak. These patients frequently give a history of previous head trauma. Therapy for pneumococcal meningitis is penicillin; if the patient is allergic, cefotaxime, vancomycin, or chloramphenicol may be used.

- *S. pneumoniae* is the most common cause of bacterial meningitis in adults.
- Always consider patient to have cerebrospinal fluid leak if recurrent *S. pneumoniae* meningitis is present. These patients frequently give a history of previous head trauma.

S. pneumoniae is one of the most common causes of otitis media, especially in children. Spontaneous peritonitis is frequently caused by *S. pneumoniae*, especially in patients with nephrotic syndrome, in the pediatric age group, and in alcoholics. Endocarditis is rare. Acute bacterial arthritis can also occur.

- Spontaneous peritonitis is frequently caused by *S. pneumoniae*, especially in patients with nephrotic syndrome in the pediatric age group and in alcoholics.

Certain patients are at high risk for infection with *S. pneumoniae*. After splenectomy, patients may develop fulminant, usually fatal, pneumococcal bacteremia with disseminated intravascular coagulation and severe bleeding. *S. pneumoniae* infections are more frequent and unusually severe in patients with sickle cell anemia. Patients with multiple myeloma, alcoholism, and hypogammaglobulinemia are also at increased risk.

S. pneumoniae is the leading cause of invasive bacterial respiratory disease in patients with human immunodeficiency virus (HIV) infection. They have a high incidence of pneumonia and bacteremic pneumococcal pneumonia. Diagnosis of pneumococcal bacteremia precedes diagnosis of HIV infection in 50%-80% of cases. Recurrent invasive disease occurs in 8%-25% of cases. Serotypes causing the invasive disease are similar to those causing invasive disease in normal hosts. Clinical presentation and treatment are similar to those in normal hosts. Secondary prophylaxis for recurrent episodes (penicillin) may be necessary. Prophylaxis for *Pneumocystis carinii* pneumonia with trimethoprim-sulfamethoxazole may provide effective primary or secondary prophylaxis.

- After splenectomy, patients may develop fulminant, usually fatal, pneumococcal bacteremia with disseminated intravascular coagulation and severe bleeding.
- *S. pneumoniae* infections are more frequent and unusually severe in patients with sickle cell anemia.
- Patients with multiple myeloma, alcoholism, and hypogammaglobulinemia are also at increased risk of infection.
- *S. pneumoniae* is the leading cause of invasive bacterial respiratory disease in patients with HIV.

Treatment is with penicillin G; if patients are allergic to penicillin, a cephalosporin, vancomycin, or erythromycin may be used. Do not use ciprofloxacin or other fluoroquinolones. From 0.2% to >2% of strains are resistant to penicillin (minimal inhibitory concentration >1 µg/mL). Vancomycin or cefotaxime may be effective. The mechanism of resistance is thought to be alterations in the penicillin-binding proteins. Risk factors for development of penicillin-resistant pneumococci are previous β-lactam antibiotic use, nosocomial acquisition, and multiple previous hospitalizations.

- Do not use ciprofloxacin or other fluoroquinolones to treat pneumococcal disease.

The pneumococcal vaccine is polyvalent. It is used in adults with chronic lung or heart disease and immuno-suppressed patients, especially after splenectomy and in patients with sickle cell disease and hereditary sphero-cytosis. It can be given simultaneously with influenza virus vaccine.

STAPHYLOCOCCI

Staphylococcus aureus

Toxins

Preformed enterotoxins produced by *S. aureus* are a common cause of food poisoning in the United States. The toxin is heat stable; therefore, the toxin is not destroyed by cooking food. An exotoxin, exfoliatin is produced by *S. aureus* belonging to phage group II and produces "scald-ed skin syndrome," an erythematous rash that progress-es to bullous lesions. It should be differentiated from toxic epidermal necrolysis (skin biopsy). It occurs most frequently in pediatric patients and is rare in adults. Therapy is with local skin care and antistaphylococcal antibiotics. Toxic shock syndrome is due to an exotox-in (TSST-1) usually produced by *S. aureus*.

- Preformed enterotoxins produced by *S. aureus* are not destroyed by cooking food.
- Toxic shock syndrome is due to an exotoxin (TSST-1) usually produced by *S. aureus*.

Clinical Syndromes

Superficial infections include folliculitis (infection of hair follicles without involvement of skin or subcuta-neous tissues), furuncle (more extensive follicular infec-tion, often involves subcutaneous tissues and occurs in areas of friction and poor personal hygiene), carbuncle (infection in thick inelastic tissues of the scalp or upper back), and impetigo (much less common than group A β-hemolytic streptococci). Treatment is moist heat to promote drainage. Personal hygiene also needs to be improved. Drainage occasionally is required, as are anti-staphylococcal agents for severe infection.

S. aureus is the most common cause of acute hematoge-nous osteomyelitis in pediatric patients and is a common cause of chronic osteomyelitis in adults. It is the second most common cause of prosthetic joint infection, after coagulase-negative staphylococci.

- *S. aureus* is a common cause of chronic osteomyelitis

in adults.
- It is the second most common cause of prosthetic joint infection.

All cases of community-acquired *S. aureus* bac-teremias must be treated for 4-6 weeks with parenteral antibiotics because of the potential for 1) metastatic abscesses and 2) infective endocarditis. If nosocomial *S. aureus* bacteremias have a removable focus (i.e., intra-venous catheter), it should be removed and treatment given for 14 days. Staphylococcal pneumonia is an infrequent cause of community-acquired disease. It is more frequent after influenza (color plate 20-3). It is a common cause of nosocomial disease in intubated patients, along with hospital-acquired aerobic gram-negative rods. If *S. aureus* is isolated in cases of uri-nary tract infection, consider *S. aureus* bacteremia with seeding of the kidneys.

- All cases of community-acquired *S. aureus* bacteremias must be treated for 4-6 weeks with parenteral antibi-otics.
- Staphylococcal pneumonia is an infrequent cause of community-acquired disease. It is more frequent after influenza.

Mechanisms of Resistance

Mechanisms of resistance for *S. aureus* include β-lac-tamase production for methicillin-susceptible, penicillin-resistant isolates and intrinsic chromosomal resistance that is not plasmid-mediated for methicillin-resistant isolates. This intrinsic resistance is related to a decrease in the affin-ity of β-lactam antibiotics for penicillin-binding proteins.

Treatment

If *S. aureus* is penicillin-susceptible (rare), penicillin G is preferred. Alternatives are cefazolin and vancomycin. If the isolate is methicillin-susceptible, nafcillin, oxacillin, cephalosporins (first-generation), vancomycin, and imipenem are often used.

MRSA Infections

Nosocomial infections caused by methicillin-resistant *S. aureus* (MRSA) are increasing in frequency and are asso-ciated with previous use of multiple antibiotics, intravenous drug abuse, burns, and other hospital-acquired infections. The drug of choice for treatment is vancomycin alone or in combination with gentamicin or rifampin. MRSA may also be susceptible to cotrimoxazole and ciprofloxacin or minocycline with or without rifampin. Emergence of resistance to fluoroquinolone agents is common.

- Nosocomial infections caused by MRSA are increasing in frequency and are associated with previous use of multiple antibiotics, intravenous drug abuse, burns, and other hospital-acquired infections.

MRSA Carrier State

This is a difficult problem in hospitals and long-term-care facilities. The use of mupirocin ointment or other therapies (cotrimoxazole with or without rifampin) is successful for temporarily eradicating the nasal carrier state, but relapse is common.

Coagulase-Negative Staphylococci (*Staphylococcus epidermidis*)

Clinical Syndromes

S. epidermidis is a common cause of prosthetic valve endocarditis, osteomyelitis (usually after joint arthroplasty or other prosthetic implantations), and meningitis after neurosurgical procedures and is associated with wound infection. Treatment often requires removal of the foreign body and administration of appropriate antibiotics. Peritonitis can occur in patients on chronic ambulatory peritoneal dialysis. Bacteremia occurs in patients with infected intravascular devices.

Treatment

For treatment of serious coagulase-negative staphylococcal infection, in vitro susceptibility testing is mandatory. If methicillin resistance is present, the treatment of choice is vancomycin. For treatment of prosthetic valve endocarditis, the regimen should be vancomycin plus rifampin for 6 weeks and gentamicin for at least the first 2 weeks. Ciprofloxacin is also active against most strains, but when used alone emergence of resistance occurs rapidly. The combination of ciprofloxacin and rifampin seems promising.

- If methicillin resistance is present, the treatment of choice is vancomycin.

GRAM-NEGATIVE BACILLI

Escherichia coli Infections

E. coli is part of the normal flora of the gastrointesti-

nal tract. Focal infection is due to ascending infection (urinary tract) or a break in a mucosal barrier (intra-abdominal infection). Bacteremia is often secondary to focal infection elsewhere.

Clinical syndromes associated with *E. coli* include urinary tract infection; it is the most common cause of uncomplicated urinary tract infections in women. Intra-abdominal infections are also associated with *E. coli* and are often a result of perforated appendix, diverticulitis, and cholangitis. These infections are often polymicrobial. *E. coli* is also common in spontaneous bacterial peritonitis. Bacteremia is most commonly a result of pyelonephritis, cholangitis, and intra-abdominal abscess. It can also occur spontaneously in patients with cirrhosis without a portal of entry. *E. coli* gastroenteritis also occurs.

- Bacteremia is most commonly a result of pyelonephritis, cholangitis, and intra-abdominal abscess.

Treatment is surgical drainage when appropriate and antibiotics chosen on the basis of in vitro sensitivity testing. *E. coli* is often susceptible to ampicillin, cephalosporins (including first-generation agents), trimethoprim-sulfamethoxazole, and aminoglycosides.

Proteus, Morganella, Providencia Infections

P. mirabilis is indole-negative and causes 75%-90% of infections. *P. vulgaris* is indole-positive and is a less common cause of infection. *M. morganii* and *P. rettgeri* also cause infection. They are all part of the normal fecal flora and can also be found in soil and water. Urinary tract infections with or without secondary bacteremia are the most common manifestations of these organisms. Urinary tract infections are often associated with an alkaline urine, which enhances production of ammonium-magnesium phosphate stones. Wound infections, sinusitis, corneal ulceration, and peritonitis are much less common clinical infections produced by these organisms.

P. mirabilis is sensitive to ampicillin. The others are not sensitive to ampicillin but are usually susceptible to gentamicin, ticarcillin, mezlocillin, third-generation cephalosporins, imipenem, and ciprofloxacin.

Klebsiella, Enterobacter, Serratia Infections

K. pneumoniae causes both community-acquired and nosocomial pneumonia. It is often associated with alcoholism, diabetes mellitus, and chronic obstructive pulmonary disease. Red current jelly sputum is characteristic. Lung abscess and empyema are more frequent than with other community-acquired pneumonias. *Enterobacter* and *Serratia* are associated with nosocomial infection, including pneumonia and bacteremia.

- Lung abscess and empyema are more frequent than with other community-acquired pneumonias.

Klebsiella is often sensitive to cephalosporins (including first-generation agents), aminoglycosides, trimethoprim-sulfamethoxazole, imipenem, and ciprofloxacin. *Enterobacter* and *Serratia* are usually resistant to first-generation cephalosporins (sensitive to gentamicin and extended-spectrum penicillins, third-generation cephalosporins, imipenem, and ciprofloxacin). The drug of choice depends on results of in vitro sensitivity testing. Recent reports have suggested an increase in resistance to third-generation cephalosporins in certain strains of *Enterobacter*. Third-generation cephalosporins, despite in vitro data suggesting sensitivity, may not be the drug of choice for *Enterobacter* infections because of high rates of emergence of resistance. Quinolones or imipenem may be effective therapy in this setting.

- *Klebsiella* is often sensitive to cephalosporins.
- *Enterobacter* and *Serratia* are usually resistant to first-generation cephalosporins.

Pseudomonas Infections

P. aeruginosa

This organism predominantly causes nosocomial infection. Hospital water supplies are often a source of infection. Any pus described as green should suggest *Pseudomonas* infection. *Pseudomonas*, together with *Staphylococcus aureus*, is most frequent cause of infections complicating massive burns. It is a cause of folliculitis associated with hot tubs, osteomyelitis (particularly in injection drug users or in osteomyelitis complicating a nail puncture wound), and malignant otitis externa in patients with diabetes mellitus. Complicated urinary tract infections are often due to this organism. *P. aeruginosa* is a common cause of nosocomial pneumonia (color plate 20-4). Patients with cystic fibrosis have an especially high frequency of pulmonary infections with *Pseudomonas*. Meningitis caused by *Pseudomonas* can develop after neurosurgical procedures. Patients with neutropenia are also at particularly high risk of infection, especially bacteremia. In neutropenic patients with bacteremia due to *P. aeruginosa,* ecthyma gangrenosum may occur.

- *Pseudomonas*, together with *S. aureus*, is most frequent cause of infections complicating massive burns.
- It is a cause of malignant otitis externa in patients with diabetes mellitus.
- In neutropenic patients with bacteremia due to *P. aeruginosa,* ecthyma gangrenosum may occur.

Extended-spectrum penicillins plus an aminoglycoside are synergistic against most *Pseudomonas* species. Ceftazidime plus an aminoglycoside may be the most effective combination for life-threatening infections. Aztreonam, imipenem, and ciprofloxacin are also active against most strains.

Xanthomonas (Pseudomonas) maltophilia

This organism causes nosocomial infections, pneumonia, and wound infections, most often in patients in intensive-care units. It is associated with person-to-person transmission, especially from failure of adequate hand washing. Multiple drug resistance is common. It may be susceptible to trimethoprim-sulfamethoxazole, ticarcillin/clavulanate, and moxalactam. It is often resistant to aminoglycosides, imipenem, ceftazidime, and ciprofloxacin.

- *X. maltophilia* is associated with person-to-person transmission, especially from failure of adequate hand washing.

Salmonella typhi

S. typhi causes various clinical syndromes, including gastroenteritis, bacteremia with and without suppurative complications, a chronic asymptomatic carrier state, and typhoid fever.

In patients with typhoid fever, findings on physical examination include fever with relative bradycardia and rose spots (50%). The leukocyte count may be decreased. Blood cultures are usually positive within approximately 10 days of symptom onset, whereas stool cultures are positive after 10 days of symptoms. Bone marrow biopsy and culture may also reveal the diagnosis.

- Findings on physical examination include fever with relative bradycardia and rose spots (50%).

The traditional therapy for typhoid fever has been chloramphenicol or ampicillin. Alternatives are cotrimoxazole, third-generation cephalosporins, and ciprofloxacin. There is increasing resistance to chloramphenicol and ampicillin. Once susceptibility results are obtained, appropriate directed therapy can be used.

- The traditional therapy for typhoid fever has been chloramphenicol or ampicillin.

Other *Salmonella* Infections

S. choleraesuis causes chronic bacteremia and mycotic aneurysms. *S. typhimurium* and *S. enteritidis* produce gastroenteritis and occasionally bacteremia.

Haemophilus influenzae

The incidence of disease caused by *H. influenzae* has decreased significantly in children with the institution of the *H. influenzae* vaccine. Adult cases represent approximately 25% of invasive *H. influenzae* disease. Approximately 50% are serotype B. Nontypable strains may be more common in pneumonia, tracheobronchitis, and upper respiratory infection. Bacteremic pneumonia makes up 70% of invasive disease in adults. Other infections include meningitis, obstetrical infections, epiglottitis, and primary bacteremia. Chronic lung disease, pregnancy, human immunodeficiency virus (HIV) infection, splenectomy, and malignancy are risk factors for invasive disease. β-Lactamase production is found in up to 40% of isolates recovered from adults with invasive disease. Overall mortality rate is 28%.

- Adult cases represent approximately 25% of invasive *H. influenzae* disease.
- Chronic lung disease, pregnancy, HIV infection, splenectomy, and malignancy are risk factors for invasive disease.
- β-Lactamase production is found in up to 40% of isolates recovered from adults with invasive disease.

Otitis media, sinusitis, conjunctivitis, and epiglottitis are common in pediatric patients. *H. influenzae* is a common cause of sinusitis in adults. Ampicillin resistance is related to production of β-lactamase. If a strain is β-lactamase negative, ampicillin can be used. *Haemophilus* infections that are β-lactamase positive or negative can be treated with cotrimoxazole, cefuroxime, third-generation cephalosporins, imipenem, ciprofloxacin, aztreonam, or ampicillin/sulbactam.

- *H. influenzae* is a common cause of sinusitis in adults.
- Ampicillin resistance is related to production of β-lactamase.

If *H. influenzae* meningitis occurs in adults, consider hypogammaglobulinemia, asplenia, or cerebrospinal fluid leak. Treatment is based on results of susceptibility testing. Resistance to ampicillin is increasing. A third-generation cephalosporin is the drug of choice. Cefuroxime is not as effective. Alternative treatment is chloramphenicol plus ampicillin until susceptibility results are known. Prophylactic treatment with rifampin is recommended for all household contacts and children in daycare centers.

For epiglottitis, do not use ampicillin as empiric therapy. Therapy is third-generation cephalosporin or ampicillin/sulbactam.

Endocarditis is caused by *H. parainfluenzae* and *H. aphrophilus*. It is often associated with large systemic emboli. Treatment is with ampicillin alone if the organism is susceptible or with third-generation cephalosporin for 3 weeks.

Most cases of pneumonia and tracheal bronchitis are caused by nontypable β-lactamase negative strains of *H. influenzae*. Most are susceptible to ampicillin.

The vaccine is useful for prevention and should be given to all children. It may be useful in patients at increased risk of invasive disease.

Bordetella pertussis

This organism is the cause of whooping cough in children. It may cause severe lymphocytosis (>100,000 lymphocytes/mm^3). The number of reported cases is increasing. There were 27,826 cases in the United States from 1980-1989; 12% were in patients >15 years old. *B. pertussis* is the cause of prolonged bronchitis in older children and adults. Atypical symptoms are common. As many as 50 million adults are now susceptible to infection as a result of waning immunity.

- *B. pertussis* may cause severe lymphocytosis (>100,000 lymphocytes/mm^3).
- It is the cause of prolonged bronchitis in older children and adults.

Diagnosis is made from nasopharyneal culture. Direct fluorescence antibody testing is relatively insensitive. Treatment is with erythromycin and supportive care.

Brucellosis

Brucellosis occurs most frequently in persons exposed to livestock or persons who drink unpasteurized milk. Most cases occur in four states (Texas, California, Virginia,

Florida). It often causes a chronic granulomatous disease, may cause caseating granulomas, and can affect any tissue. It may be a cause of "sterile" pyuria. Chronic brucellosis may cause chronic fever of undetermined origin. Diagnosis is difficult and is one of exclusion. Calcifications in spleen may be an indication of the presence of infection. Serology testing, blood cultures, and bone marrow cultures are helpful in making the diagnosis. Treatment is with tetracycline plus streptomycin or doxycycline plus rifampin. Cotrimoxazole is sometimes also useful.

- Brucellosis is a chronic granulomatous disease and may cause fever of unknown origin.

Legionnaires' Disease

This disease is caused by fastidious gram-negative bacillus (color plate 20-5). A significant amount of sporadic community-acquired legionellosis may be due to contaminated potable water. Most nosocomial legionellosis is also due to contaminated water supplies. Clinical features include weakness, malaise, fever, dry cough progressing to slightly productive cough, diarrhea (a very important part of symptom complex and often precedes other symptoms), pleuritic chest pain, relative bradycardia, diffuse rales bilaterally, and patchy infiltrates on chest radiography, usually bilaterally. Characteristic laboratory features are decreased sodium and phosphorus values, increased leukocyte level, and abnormal liver function tests. The diagnosis must be suspected clinically. The clinical picture of unexplained pneumonitis often accompanied by diarrhea and the other clinical findings described above in association with hyponatremia and decreased serum phosphorus level is sufficient to suspect legionnaires' disease and to begin treatment pending results of serologic and other tests. In suspected cases, do not wait for serologic results before initiating treatment. A fourfold increase or decrease in titer requires 2-6 weeks. A single titer ≥1:256 is suggestive of active infection but not diagnostic. The best means of diagnosis is by culture and a fluorescent antibody test of sputum, bronchoalveolar lavage fluid, or an open lung biopsy specimen.

Treatment includes erythromycin with or without rifampin orally or intravenously for 2-3 weeks. If the patient is allergic to erythromycin, doxycycline or ciprofloxacin can be used.

- In legionnaires' disease, diarrhea is important part of symptom complex and often precedes other symptoms.

- Lab features are decreased sodium and phosphorus values, increased leukocyte level, and abnormal liver function tests.
- The best means of diagnosis is by culture and a fluorescent antibody test of sputum, bronchoalveolar lavage fluid, or open lung biopsy specimen.

Legionella micdadei

This gram-negative bacillus causes infection in hospitalized immunosuppressed patients receiving high-dose corticosteroid therapy. Diagnosis is based on stains and culture of open lung biopsy tissue or bronchoalveolar lavage fluid. Serologic studies may be helpful retrospectively. The organism is moderately resistant to erythromycin, but it is still the drug of choice. Cotrimoxazole plus rifampin may also be effective.

Tularemia

Francisella tularensis is commonly spread by the bite of an arthropod and direct contact with tissues of infected animals. If ulceroglandular fever develops, an ulcer or eschar is usually present at the site of inoculation. Pneumonia can also occur. Treatment is with streptomycin.

- *F. tularensis* is commonly spread by arthropod bite and direct contact with tissues of infected animals.

Plague: *Yersinia pestis*

From 1950-1991, there were 336 cases in the United States; >50% of these occurred after 1980. It is enzootic in the southwestern United States; New Mexico has 56% of cases, and 29% of cases are among American Indians. Rats and fleas are vectors. Clinical presentations include 1) lymphadenopathy with septicemia--the most common form, and 2) the pneumonic form (high case fatality rate). Treatment is with streptomycin.

Pasteurella multocida

A cat bite is the most common mode of acquisition. It causes bacteremia and rarely infective endocarditis. It is sensitive to penicillins and cephalosporins.

Capnocytophaga

These gram-negative bacilli have difficulty growing in routine media. They are found in oral flora in domestic animals and humans. They cause bacteremia in immunosuppressed patients, patients who have had splenectomy, and alcoholics (may be seen on Gram stain of buffy coat). Fulminant sepsis and disseminated intravascular coagulation are also associated with infection. Dog and cat bites are associated with 50% of cases. Treatment includes penicillin or a cephalosporin.

- *Capnocytophaga* organisms cause bacteremia in immunosuppressed patients, patients who have had splenectomy, and alcoholics.

- Dog and cat bites are associated with 50% of cases.

Rochalimaea quintana, R. henselae, and *Afipia felis*

These are small, fastidious, gram-negative rods, recently identified as the etiologic agents of cat scratch disease and bacillary angiomatosis. They are related to *Bartonella bacilliformis*. The characteristics of these two syndromes and their etiologic agents are presented in Table 20-4.

Table 20-4.--Features of Cat Scratch Disease and Bacillary Angiomatosis

Variable	Cat scratch disease	Bacillary angiomatosis
Predominant host	Immunocompetent	Immunosuppressed (AIDS)
Vector	Cats and dogs	Cats
Demonstrated cause	*R. henselae* (majority)	*R. henselae*
	A. felis	*R. quintana*
Pathology	Lymphoid hyperplasia, granulomas, abscess formation	Ectatic capillaries surrounded by neutrophilic infiltrate
Clinical presentation	Papule or pustule at inoculation site, regional lymphadenopathy, fever and malaise in 30%	Cutaneous nodules (do not confuse with Kaposi's sarcoma),visceral peliosis
Natural history	Self-limited (2-4 months)	Progressive
Diagnosis	Histopathology (Warthin-Starry stain), skin test, lymph node culture, serology, analysis of 16S rDNA	Histopathology, blood culture (lysis centrifugation, prolonged incubation), tissue culture, serology
Treatment	Efficacy unclear; rifampin, ciprofloxacin, gentamicin	Doxycycline, erythromycin

From Tompkins DC, Steigbigel RT: *Rochalimaea's* role in cat scratch disease and bacillary angiomatosis. Ann Intern Med 118:388-390, 1993. By permission of American College of Physicians.

GRAM-POSITIVE BACILLI

Anthrax

Bacillus anthracis is an aerobic gram-positive bacillus. Human cases are due to contact with infected animals, bites of contaminated flies, consumption of contaminated meat (rare), and exposure to contaminated animal hides (e.g., imported drums from Haiti, goat hair [yarn]).

- *B. anthracis* due to exposure to contaminated animal hides.

Cutaneous manifestations occur in 95% of cases. The most common presentation is a large, black, chronic skin ulcer, which is frequently a nontender "malignant pustule." Pneumonia ("wool sorter's pneumonia"), bacteremia, meningitis, and gastrointestinal disease are much less common. Treatment is with penicillin G.

Alternatives are erythromycin, tetracycline, and chloramphenicol.

- Cutaneous manifestations occur in 95% of cases.

Listeria monocytogenes

This is a gram-positive, small, motile rod. It causes infection in immunosuppressed (T-cell) patients, neonates, and pregnant women. Epidemics have been associated with consumption of contaminated milk, ice cream, and undercooked hot dogs. Sporadic listeriosis is associated with contaminated food in approximately 34% of cases. Diarrhea is not a feature of epidemic listeriosis.

- *L. monocytogenes* infection in immunosuppressed (T-cell) patients, neonates, and pregnant women.
- Epidemics have been associated with consumption of contaminated milk, ice cream, and undercooked hot dogs.

- Diarrhea is not a feature of epidemic listeriosis.

Meningitis and bacteremia are common clinical manifestations in adults (color plate 20-6).

The approach to treatment is penicillin or ampicillin with or without gentamicin. Cephalosporins are *not* effective. Alternatives are cotrimoxazole and chloramphenicol. Treatment duration is 2-4 weeks.

Corynebacterium diphtheriae

Diphtheria
Clinically, this is usually a focal infection of the respiratory tract (pharynx in 60%-70% of cases, larynx, nasal passages, or tracheobronchial tree). A tightly adherent gray pseudomembrane is the hallmark of the disease, but disease can occur without pseudomembrane formation. Manifestations depend on extent of involvement of upper airway and presence or absence of systemic complications due to toxin. A local complication is respiratory tract obstruction. Toxin-mediated complications include myocarditis (10%-25%), which causes congestive heart failure and dysrhythmias, and polyneuritis (bulbar dysfunction followed by peripheral neuropathy). Respiratory muscles may be paralyzed.

- In diphtheria, toxin-mediated complications include myocarditis (10%-25%), which causes congestive heart failure and dysrhythmias, and polyneuritis.
- Respiratory muscles may be paralyzed.

Diagnosis is definitively established by culture with Löffler's medium. Rapid diagnosis can sometimes be made by methylene blue stain or fluorescent antibody staining of pharyngeal swab specimens. Patients need to be isolated immediately. Antitoxin should be used. Although there is no evidence that antimicrobial agents alter course of disease, they prevent transmission to susceptible hosts. Erythromycin and penicillin G are effective. Close contacts should be evaluated and treated with erythromycin or penicillin G if culture results are positive. The diphtheria-tetanus toxoid should be given.

- Close contacts should be evaluated and treated with erythromycin or penicillin G if culture results are positive.

Cutaneous Diphtheria
This is common in indigent patients and alcoholics. It occurs most often in patients with preexisting dermatologic disease and most often in the lower extremities. Patients can have punched-out lesions with membrane, but they may be indistinguishable from other infected ulcers. Toxin-mediated complications (i.e., myocarditis, neuropathy) are uncommon. Diagnosis is established with methylene blue staining and culture in Löffler's medium.

Erythromycin or penicillin is used for therapy. Antitoxin should also be administered. Immunization series with diphtheria-tetanus toxoid is started.

- Cutaneous diphtheria is common in indigent patients and alcoholics.

Erysipelothrix rhusiopathiae
The nonmotile gram-positive rod is a saprophyte. Infection occurs with traumatic inoculation of organism after a person comes in contact with dead animals and fish. Localized cellulitis around a purple-red papule occurs at the site of inoculation, often a finger or upper extremity in a person who has occupational exposure to these products (veterinarians, fishing industry). This is most common presentation (erysipeloid). If untreated, dissemination with subsequent bacteremia, endocarditis, and septic arthritis can occur. Penicillin G is the drug of choice. Erythromycin is an alternative.

- *E. rhusiopathiae* infection occurs with traumatic inoculation of organism after a person comes in contact with dead animals and fish.

Bacillus Species
These are increasingly recognized as a cause of bacteremia in patients with indwelling catheters or prosthetic devices and in injection drug users. Other syndromes include ocular infections (posttraumatic endophthalmitis) and gastroenteritis. Vancomycin or clindamycin with or without gentamicin is used for therapy.

Rhodococcus equi (Corynebacterium equi)
This organism causes necrotizing pneumonia in immunocompromised hosts (those with AIDS or taking corticosteroids). Mortality rate is 30%. Clinical features include fever, nonproductive cough, and cavity or nodular infiltrates on chest radiography (concomitant brain abscesses have been reported). Bronchoscopy or open lung biopsy is usually required for diagnosis. Treatment is with vancomycin, erythromycin, aminoglycosides, or chloramphenicol.

GRAM-NEGATIVE COCCI

Moraxella catarrhalis (Branhamella catarrhalis) is a respiratory tract pathogen in immunosuppressed, hospitalized patients and those with chronic obstructive pulmonary disease. It causes otitis media, sinusitis, meningitis, bacteremia, and endocarditis in immunosuppressed patients. β-Lactamase production is prevalent. Trimethoprim-sulfamethoxazole, ciprofloxacin, and ampicillin-clavulanate are useful for therapy.

- *M. catarrhalis* causes otitis media, sinusitis, meningitis, bacteremia, and endocarditis in immunosuppressed patients.

ANAEROBIC BACTERIA

Bacteroides Infections

Bacteroides species reside in the oral cavity (*B. melaninogenicus* group) and are also normal colonic flora (*B. fragilis* group). They often are part of a polymicrobial infection. Any pus described as "foul-smelling" is often caused by anaerobic infection. Clinical syndromes commonly associated with *Bacteroides* species include intra-abdominal infection. Abscesses, for example, are associated with disruption of colonic mucosa resulting from appendicitis, cancer, diverticulitis, and other disorders. *Bacteroides* species are also associated with pelvic infections, particularly in females (e.g., septic abortion, tubo-ovarian abscess, endometritis). There are frequently polymicrobial infections. Bacteremia is usually associated with focal infection elsewhere (e.g., intra-abdominal abscess) or with gastrointestinal surgery. *B. fragilis* is the most common isolate. Osteomyelitis usually results from a contiguous source and is often polymicrobial (e.g., diabetic foot ulcer or osteomyelitis of the maxilla or mandible after dental infection). Pleuropulmonary infections include aspiration pneumonia and lung abscess. *B. melaninogenicus* organisms are major pathogens, as are other oral anaerobes. Skin and soft tissue infections caused by anaerobes include diabetic soft tissue infections of the feet, bite wounds, and gangrene.

- *Bacteroides* species are also associated with intra-abdominal and pelvic infections.
- Bacteremia is usually associated with *B. fragilis*.
- Pleuropulmonary infections include aspiration pneumonia and lung abscess.

Many strains of *B. melaninogenicus* and other *Bacteroides* species that are part of the oral flora often produce penicillinase and thus are resistant to penicillin. Because of increased resistance to penicillin of mouth anaerobes, penicillin is no longer drug of choice for treatment of putrid lung abscess. In one study, clindamycin was more effective than penicillin or metronidazole for curing lung abscess.

B. fragilis produces penicillinase and is often resistant to penicillin. Metronidazole, clindamycin (increasing resistance), ampicillin/sulbactam, chloramphenicol, and imipenem are also active. Some cephalosporins (cefoxitin) are active in vitro against some *B. fragilis* organisms but should not be considered the drug of choice. Other third-generation cephalosporins have little activity against *B. fragilis*.

Peptococcus

These anaerobic streptococci are often involved in polymicrobial infection. They are part of normal flora of the oral cavity and colon. They are associated with anaerobic pleuropulmonary infection and intra-abdominal abscess. *Peptostreptococcus* can be a part of the polymicrobial flora of anaerobic cellulitis.

Peptococcus is exquisitely sensitive to penicillin G. In patients allergic to penicillin, the alternatives are clindamycin, chloramphenicol, vancomycin, and cephalosporins. The organism is often resistant to metronidazole.

- *Peptococcus* is exquisitely sensitive to penicillin G.

Tetanus: *Clostridium tetani*

This is a strictly anaerobic gram-positive rod that produces neurotoxin (tetanospasmin). The neurotoxin produced by organisms in contaminated wounds is responsible for the clinical manifestations of disease. Most patients now are women >50 years old (not immunized). Men are usually immunized because of military service and repeated exposure to trauma.

- Most patients with tetanus now are women >50 years old (not immunized).

In generalized tetanus, the first muscles involved are controlled by cranial nerves (trismus, lockjaw, risus sardonicus). Eye muscles (cranial nerves III, IV) are rarely involved. Other muscles are soon involved (generalized rigidity, spasms, opisthotonos). Sympathetic overactivity is common (labile hypertension, hyperpyrexia, arrhythmias). In wound tetanus, manifestations are restricted to muscles near the wound. Diagnosis is based on clinical findings.

- Diagnosis is based on clinical findings.

Treatment includes supportive care, proper wound management, and administration of antiserum (human tetanus immune globulin). Hypersensitivity reactions to tetanus immune globulin are very rare. Penicillin G should be administered to eradicate vegetative organisms in the wound. Metronidazole is an alternative agent. Immunization after recovery should also be provided.

- Penicillin G should be administered to eradicate vegetative organisms in the wound.

Clostridium botulinum

This anaerobic gram-positive rod produces a heat-labile neurotoxin that inhibits acetylcholine release from cholinergic terminals at the motor end plate. Major modes of acquisition in adults include ingestion of contaminated food (home canned products and improperly prepared or handled commercial foods) and wound botulism (contaminated traumatic wounds, injection drug users).

- Neurotoxin of *C. botulinum* inhibits acetylcholine release from cholinergic terminals at the motor end plate.

Clinical manifestations can be mild or severe. The diagnosis is considered in patients with unexplained diplopia; fixed, dilated pupils; dry mouth; and descending flaccid paralysis with normal sensation. Patients are usually alert and oriented and have intact deep tendon reflexes. Fever is rare.

- Diagnosis is considered in patients with unexplained diplopia; fixed, dilated pupils; dry mouth; and descending flaccid paralysis with normal sensation.

For diagnosis, other compatible clinical syndromes need to be ruled out--myasthenia gravis and atypical Guillain-Barré (ascending paralysis, sensory abnormalities). Electromyography may be helpful. One can also check the suspected contaminated food source for toxin.

Treatment is primarily supportive. Equine antitoxin is available, and its use is now recommended by most experts. In food-borne cases, purging the gut with cathartics, enemas, and emetics to remove unabsorbed toxin may also be of value. Antibiotic therapy is not generally recommended.

Other Clostridial Infections

C. perfringens may cause a food-associated illness. *C. difficile* causes antibiotic-associated diarrhea. Among patients with bacteremia caused by *C. septicum* who have no apparent portal of entry, many have occult bowel carcinoma, especially colon or other malignancies. Clostridial bacteremia often is a transient bacteremia unrelated to a typical clinical syndrome (no identifiable genitourinary or gastrointestinal source). These isolates may not require specific therapy. Clostridial bacteremia with an identifiable source or associated with sepsis syndrome does require therapy. *C. perfringens* is most common isolate in either case. Penicillin G is the drug of choice.

- *C. perfringens* may cause a food-associated illness.
- *C. difficile* causes antibiotic-associated diarrhea.
- In patients with *C. septicum* bacteremia, occult bowel carcinoma should be suspected.

MYCOBACTERIAL DISEASES

Mycobacterium tuberculosis

Epidemiology

The number of cases of infection with this organism has been increasing since 1985. In 1990, 25,701 cases were reported to the Centers for Disease Control (increase of 9.4%). The increase is largely due to an increase in cases among persons with human immunodeficiency virus (HIV) and other high-risk groups. Incidence of disease due to drug-resistant strains is also increasing. These strains often are resistant to multiple drugs (i.e., multiple drug-resistant tuberculosis, MDR-TB), including isoniazid (INH), rifampin, and other drugs. In a recent national survey, 14.4% of strains were resistant to one drug and 3.3% were resistant to both INH and rifampin. In the past several years, there have been multiple reports of nosocomial transmission of MDR-TB, resulting in more than 50 deaths among health care workers and a purified protein derivative (PPD) conversion rate of 10%-30%.

- In cases of *M. tuberculosis*, 14.4% of strains were resistant to one drug and 3.3% were resistant to both INH and rifampin.

These outbreaks have been related to delay in diagnosis due to atypical presentations, failure to sterilize secretions because of drug resistance or patient noncompliance, and ineffective isolation practices.

All patients suspected of having tuberculosis should be placed in respiratory isolation when they are hospitalized. These patients include those suspected of having skin lesions due to tuberculosis, because this was recently reported to be a cause of nosocomial transmission of disease.

Transmission is by droplet infection. Infectious droplets are 1-5 μm in diameter. Droplets remain suspended in room atmosphere for 30 minutes-2 hours.

- Transmission is by droplet infection.

Clinical Disease

Most clinically apparent pulmonary and extrapulmonary *M. tuberculosis* infections in adults are due to reactivation, not reinfection (color plate 20-7). Common sites of reactivation (high Po_2 favors reactivation) are apices of lung ($Po_2 = 120$ mm Hg), vertebra ($Po_2 = 100$ mm Hg), and kidney ($Po_2 = 100$ mm Hg). Tuberculosis should be suspected in young persons with an idiopathic pleural effusion. Diagnosis is made by thoracentesis with culture of pleural fluid and pleural biopsy with special stains and culture. Extrapulmonary manifestations are protean. Common sites include spine, kidneys, large joints, and meninges.

- Most pulmonary and extrapulmonary *M. tuberculosis* infections in adults are due to reactivation.
- Tuberculosis should be suspected in young persons with idiopathic pleural effusion.

Screening

An intermediate-strength PPD test should be performed in patients at high risk of infection with *M. tuberculosis*. These groups include those with HIV infection, the foreign born, close contacts (household) of persons known to have or suspected of having tuberculosis, medically underserved, low-income populations (including high-risk minority populations--blacks, Hispanics, Native Americans), the homeless, alcoholics and injection drug users, residents of institutions (e.g., nursing homes, prisons), and persons with medical conditions that predispose to infection with tuberculosis (Table 20-5).

Table 20-5.--Medical Conditions That Predispose Patients to *Mycobacterium tuberculosis* Infection

Silicosis	Immunosuppression (T-cell)
Gastrectomy	Hematologic malignancy
Jejunoileal bypass	Other malignancies
Weight 10% or more below ideal body weight	Person with chest radiograph compatible with old tuberculosis
Chronic renal failure	
Diabetes mellitus	

Prevention

INH prophylaxis reduces the incidence of disease significantly. Lack of compliance is major source of failure. Treatment is with INH 300 mg/day for 1 year (6 months minimum) or 15 mg/kg twice a week under direct supervision. Optimal prophylaxis for INH-resistant strain exposure or exposure to MDR-TB is unknown. An outline for preventive therapy with positive PPD results is given in Table 20-6.

- INH prophylaxis reduces incidence of disease significantly.

Treatment

For persons with pulmonary disease only who do not have HIV infection and the organism is drug-susceptible, 6 months of therapy is as effective as 9 months of therapy. If the 6-month regimen is used, give INH, rifampin, and pyrazinamide for first 2 months only. Add ethambutol to initial drug regimen if patient has history of previous INH therapy or patient is at risk for INH resistance. During last 4 months of treatment, INH and rifampin are used. This regimen can also be adapted to be given under direct supervision (to ensure compliance).

Alternatively, INH and rifampin can be given for 9 months. The 9-month regimen is also effective for renal or skeletal tuberculosis. In INH-resistant cases, use at least two drugs to which the organism is sensitive (rifampin, ethambutol) and treat for 12 months. For MDR-TB (INH-, rifampin-resistant), optimal regimen is unknown. In a recent study of the treatment of MDR-TB in persons without acquired immunodeficiency syndrome (AIDS), therapy consisted of multiple drugs chosen on basis of in vitro susceptibility testing. Minimal duration of therapy is 18-24 months. Initial cure rate

Table 20-6.--Criteria for Determining Need for Preventive Therapy for Persons With Positive Tuberculin Reactions by Category and Age Group

Category	Age	
	<35 yr	≥35 yr
With risk factor[*]	Treat at all ages if PPD ≥10 mm (if PPD >5 mm in HIV positive, recent contact, chest radiographic evidence of old not active TB)	Treat at all ages if PPD ≥10 mm (if PPD >5 mm in HIV positive, recent contact, chest radiographic evidence of old not active TB)
No risk factor (high incidence group)[†]	Treat if PPD ≥10 mm	No treatment
No risk factor (low incidence group)	Treat if PPD ≥15 mm[‡]	No treatment

[*] 1) Persons with HIV infection, or with multiple HIV risk factors, 2) intravenous drug users, 3) recent contact with infected person, 4) recent PPD converters, 5) persons with abnormal chest radiographic finding likely to represent old tuberculosis, 6) persons with certain medical conditions (see Table 20-5).
[†] 1) Foreign-born persons, 2) medically underserved, low-income populations, 3) residents of long-term-care facilities.
[‡] Controversial; some investigators use cutoff of 10 mm. Depends on relative prevalence of cross-reactivity with other mycobacterial organisms in the population.
PPD, purified protein derivative; TB, tuberculosis.
From Centers for Disease Control: Screening for tuberculosis and tuberculous infection in high-risk populations, and The use of preventive therapy for tuberculous infection in the United States. MMWR 39 (no. RR-8):1-12, 1990.

(three consecutive sputum cultures with negative results) was 65%. Among these initial responders, 14% had relapse, most within 2 years. Relapse and treatment failure were associated with a 46% mortality rate. In many of the MDR-TB outbreaks (70%-80% HIV-infected persons), mortality rate has been 70%-80%. Those in whom treatment is unsuccessful but who survive pose major public health problem and must be isolated.

- The 9-month regimen is also effective for renal or skeletal tuberculosis.
- For MDR-TB (INH-, rifampin-resistant), optimal regimen is unknown.
- In many of the MDR-TB outbreaks, mortality rate has been 70%-80%.

Antituberculosis Drugs: Toxicities

Isoniazid

Peripheral neuritis can be prevented with simultaneous use of pyridoxine. Hepatotoxicity is also common and occurs in 1%-2% of patients. The approach for following patients taking INH for possible hepatotoxicity is controversial. It is more likely to occur in older patients. Slow acetylators are more likely to have hepatotoxicity. Most patients will have transient increase in aspartate aminotransferase value.

- With isoniazid, peripheral neuritis can be prevented with simultaneous use of pyridoxine.
- Hepatotoxicity is common.
- Slow acetylators are more likely to have hepatotoxicity.

Risk of hepatotoxicity is 0.3% in patients 20-34 years old, 1.2% in those 35-49 years, 2.3% in those 50-64 years, and 4% in those older than 64 years.

Ethambutol

Toxicity is rare with this agent. If optic neuritis develops, red-green color vision may be lost first.

Rifampin

Toxic effects include neutropenia, thrombocytopenia, and hepatotoxicity. Hepatotoxicity may be identical to that caused by INH. Rifampin is also a hepatic enzyme inducer and thus has interactions with warfarin and birth control pills, among other medications. Fever with flu-like syndrome is also a common toxic manifestation of rifampin. Body fluids are turned orange with administration of rifampin.

Pyrazinamide

Hepatotoxicity is similar to that with INH. Hyperuricemia may also occur.

Mycobacterial Diseases Other Than Tuberculosis (Atypical *Mycobacteria*)

Mycobacterium marinum causes swimming pool granuloma, but now it is most common in people who have aquariums. Infection occurs while cleaning aquariums. It presents with chronic, indurated nodule on finger or hand. Treatment is excision of nodule. Rifampin plus ethambutol, doxycycline, or trimethoprim-sulfamethoxazole may be effective.

- *M. marinum* causes swimming pool granuloma.

Mycobacterium kansasii is indistinguishable from *M. tuberculosis* clinically; it is more resistant to antituberculosis drugs than is *M. tuberculosis*. Standard regimen includes INH, rifampin, and ethambutol. Treatment is for 12-24 months.

- *M. kansasii* is indistinguishable from *M. tuberculosis* clinically.

Mycobacterium avium-intracellulare is an important cause of infection in patients with AIDS. Treatment is usually difficult in patients with AIDS. It is often resistant to the usual antituberculosis agents. Usually 3- to 4-drug regimens are used. Rifampin, ethambutol, clarithromycin, clofazimine, ciprofloxacin, and amikacin, as determined on susceptibility testing, are the most commonly used agents.

- *M. avium-intracellulare* is an important cause of infection in patients with AIDS.
- Usually 3- to 4-drug regimens are used.

M. avium-intracellulare has also been reported in patients without AIDS. Most patients have chronic lung disease. There seem to be four characteristic chest radiographic appearances: multiple discrete nodules (71% of patients), bronchiectasis, upper lobe infiltrates, and diffuse infiltrates. Treament is with INH, rifampin, and ethambutol. Other drugs listed in previous paragraph may also be useful.

Rapid-growing mycobacteria include *Mycobacterium fortuitum* and *Mycobacterium chelonei*. They are associated with subcutaneous abscesses, osteomyelitis, and nosocomial infection (sternal osteomyelitis after cardiac surgery, intramuscular injection). Treatment often requires incision and drainage. They are resistant to antituberculosis drugs. Initial therapy is cefoxitin plus amikacin. Other antimicrobials are used according to results of in vitro susceptibility testing. Clarithromycin may also be useful.

SPIROCHETES

Leptospirosis

Person-to-person transmission does not occur. Humans acquire disease from contact with urine from infected animals (rats, dogs). It is a biphasic disease. The *leptospiremic phase* is characterized by abrupt-onset headache (98%), fever, chills, conjunctivitis, severe muscle aching, gastrointestinal symptoms (50%), changes in sensorium (25%), rash (7%), and hypotension. This phase lasts 3-7 days. Improvement in symptoms coincides with disappearance of *Leptospira* organisms from blood and cerebrospinal fluid. The *second phase* (immune stage) occurs after a relatively asymptomatic period of 1-3 days, when fever and earlier symptoms recur. Meningeal symptoms often develop during this period. The second phase is characterized by appearance of IgM antibodies. Most patients recover after 1-3 days. However, in serious cases, hepatic dysfunction and renal failure may develop. Death in patients with leptospirosis usually occurs in the second phase as a result of hepatic and renal failure. Myocarditis may occur during the second phase.

- In leptospirosis, person-to-person transmission does not occur.
- Humans acquire disease from contact with urine from infected animals (rats, dogs).
- Death usually occurs in the second phase as a result of hepatic and renal failure.

Gastrointestinal complaints, pneumonitis, and aseptic meningitis are common components of leptospirosis and are frequently overlooked. Diagnosis is made with cultures of blood and, rarely, cerebrospinal fluid in first 7-10 days of infection. Urine cultures become positive after the second week of illness. Serologic testing is not helpful until second phase of disease; it must demonstrate fourfold increase in titer for diagnosis to be established. Treatment is with penicillin G. Penicillin is effective *only* if given within the first 3-5 days from onset of symptoms; otherwise, antibiotics are of no help.

- Gastrointestinal complaints, pneumonitis, and aseptic meningitis are common.

Lyme Disease

Epidemiology

Borrelia burgdorferi is the etiologic agent. It is the

most common vector-borne (*Ixodes* ticks) disease reported in the United States. It occurs in summer and fall and is reported in most states. It is most common in coastal Massachusetts, the mid-Atlantic states, Oregon, Northern California, and the Upper Midwest.

- *B. burgdorferi* is etiologic agent of Lyme disease.
- It occurs in summer and fall.

Clinical Syndromes

Stage 1 (early) occurs 3-32 days after the tick bite. It presents with a flu-like illness and erythema migrans (60%). Adenopathy and meningismus may also be present. Rash usually enlarges and resolves over 3-4 weeks.

- *Stage 1* presents with a flu-like illness and erythema migrans.

Stage 2 occurs weeks to months after stage 1. In 10%-15% of cases, neurologic abnormalities develop (facial nerve palsy, lymphocytic meningitis, encephalitis, chorea, myelitis, radiculitis, peripheral neuropathy). Carditis (reversible atrioventricular block) occurs in 10% of patients. Dilated cardiomyopathy has been reported, and conjunctivitis and iritis also occur.

- During stage 2, 10%-15% of cases have neurologic abnormalities.
- Carditis occurs in 10% of patients.

Stage 3 occurs months to years after initial infection. Monoarticular or oligoarticular arthritis occurs in 50% of patients who do not receive effective therapy. It becomes chronic in 10%-20%. Chronic arthritis is related to HLA-DR2 and HLA-DR4. Other manifestations are acrodermatitis chronica atrophicans, progressive, chronic encephalitis, and dementia (diagnosed by presence of locally produced antibodies against *B. burgdorferi* in the spinal fluid); 30%-40% of patients will have arthritis. Most will have positive serum antibodies. Magnetic resonance imaging may show demyelination.

- In stage 3, monoarticular or oligoarticular arthritis occurs in 50%.

Diagnosis

Results of enzyme-linked immunosorbent assay are positive after first 2-6 weeks of illness. Response may be diminished by antimicrobial therapy early in course.

Tests are not standardized. False-positive results occur with infectious mononucleosis, rheumatoid arthritis, systemic lupus erythematosus, echovirus infection, and other spirochetal disease. Western blot test is an adjunct in diagnosis when antibody response is equivocal or when false-positive result is suspected. It is particularly useful in first few months of illness.

Treatment

For stage 1 (early) Lyme disease, agents used are doxycycline (100 mg twice a day for 10-21 days), amoxicillin (500 mg three times a day for 10-21 days), or cefuroxime axetil (500 mg twice a day for 10-21 days). Erythromycin is less effective than doxycycline or amoxicillin. Amoxicillin is used for children and pregnant women.

In Lyme carditis, the outcome is usually favorable. If first-degree atrioventricular block is present or P-R interval is >0.30 second, ceftriaxone, 2 g a day for 14-21 days, or penicillin G, 20 million units a day for 14-21 days, is recommended.

- In Lyme carditis, the outcome is usually favorable.

The outcome in patients with facial palsy is usually favorable; in one study, 105 of 122 patients had complete recovery. Corticosteroids have no role. If only facial nerve palsy is present (no symptoms of meningitis, radiculoneuritis), use oral therapy with doxycycline or amoxicillin. The treatment applied if other neurologic manifestations are present is described below.

- The outcome in patients with facial palsy is usually favorable.

If meningitis is present, ceftriaxone, 2 g a day for 14-21 days, or penicillin G, 20 million units a day for 14-21 days, should be given. Radiculoneuritis and peripheral neuropathy may have a greater tendency for chronicity and often occur with meningitis. Treatment is the same as that for Lyme-associated meningitis. The regimens for encephalopathy and encephalomyelitis are identical to those for meningitis.

- Radiculoneuritis and peripheral neuropathy may have a greater tendency for chronicity and often occur with meningitis.

Optimal regimens for Lyme arthritis (oral vs. intravenous) are not established. Intra-articular corticosteroids may cause treatment failures. Joint rest and aspiration of reaccumulated joint fluid are often needed. Response to antibiotics may be delayed. If no neurologic disease is present, doxycycline is given (100 mg orally twice a day for 30 days). An alternative regimen is amoxicillin and probenecid (500 mg each four times a day for 30 days) or ceftriaxone (2 g per day intravenously for 14 days).

Prevention

Because of risk of vertical transmission, all pregnant women with active Lyme disease should be treated aggressively. Recent cost-benefit analysis suggested that if probability of infection was ≥3.6% after a tick bite, empiric therapy with oral doxycycline was warranted; if probability of infection was ≤1.0%, treatment was not recommended. However, a subsequent placebo-controlled trial showed no difference in the incidence of late manifestations of Lyme disease in treated (amoxicillin) or untreated patients. Furthermore, the risk of late manifestations after a recognized deer tick bite was estimated to be less than 1% in untreated patients. Currently, routine empiric therapy after a tick bite is not recommended. Appropriate use of repellents and protective clothing are recommended.

- All pregnant women with active Lyme disease should be treated aggressively.
- Routine empiric therapy after a tick bite is not recommended.

ACTINOMYCOSIS

This disorder is caused by *Actinomyces israelii*, an anaerobic, gram-positive, branching, filamentous organism. *A. israelii* probably causes infection in only humans and is the only known species to cause human infection. Most frequent preceding event is dental extraction. Infections are associated with any condition that creates an anaerobic environment (e.g., trauma with tissue necrosis, pus). Pathologic characteristic is formation of "sulfur granules," which are clumps of filaments. Lesions often contain pus. Infection is not characterized by granuloma formation.

- In actinomycosis, most frequent preceding event is dental extraction.
- Pathologic characteristic is "sulfur granules" (clumps of filaments).

Manifestations of the disease include "lumpy jaw" caused by a paramandibular infection with a chronic draining sinus, most often after dental extraction. It takes weeks to develop. Pulmonary disease develops from *A. israelii* aspirated from mouth into area of lung with decreased oxygenation (e.g., atelectasis, infection). Chronic suppurative pneumonitis may develop with cavitation, empyema, and, finally, draining sinus through chest wall. It may perforate into esophagus, pericardium, ribs, and vertebrae. There may be spread into bloodstream (e.g., brain), in which case the prognosis is very poor. Gastrointestinal effects probably result from *A. israelii* being swallowed, and infection occurs through small defects in bowel mucosa. Most common site is ileocecal area. Appendicitis may be predisposing factor. Cutaneous fistula (e.g., anorectal or anovaginal) may develop.

- Manifestations include "lumpy jaw" caused by a paramandibular infection with a chronic draining sinus, most often after dental extraction.

Unusual forms of infection include brain abscess, which results from bacteremia (often mixed infection). Bone infection most often involves the mandible or vertebrae. Vertebral infection has a characteristic sieve-like appearance on lateral radiographs because it attacks bodies of vertebrae and not intervertebral spaces; slow progression allows bone to be formed as fast as it is destroyed. Therefore, vertebral collapse is rare; this is an important differentiating characteristic from tuberculosis, malignancy, and other infection. Infection of female pelvic organs may simulate chronic pelvic inflammatory disease and include chronic draining sinuses. It is related to use of intrauterine devices.

- Unusual forms of infection include brain abscess, which results from bacteremia.

Diagnosis involves suspicion of the organism. It must be differentiated from *Nocardia* (which is gram-positive, filamentous, branching organism that is *aerobic* and partially acid-fast). Anaerobic culture is necessary. Organism has special growth requirements, and *Actinomyces* culture must be specifically requested because the organism may not grow on routine anaerobic cultures.

- Anaerobic culture is necessary for diagnosis.

Prognosis is usually good if the infection is recognized

and treated with combined surgical and medical approach. Brain abscess or hematogenous spread is associated with poor prognosis.

Therapy is with penicillin for long periods and surgical management. Treatment may be needed for ≥1 year. If patient is allergic to penicillin, tetracycline or erythromycin is used.

NOCARDIOSIS

Nocardia is an aerobic, gram-positive, filamentous, branching organism that is weakly acid-fast. *N. asteroides* is the cause of most human infections in the United States. *N. brasiliensis* and *N. madurae* cause mycetomas. There is no proof of human-to-human or animal-to-human transmission of *N. asteroides*. Infections are most often opportunistic, occurring in immunosuppressed patients, but they can occur in nonimmunosuppressed patients also.

- In nocardiosis, there is no proof of human-to-human or animal-to-human transmission.
- Infections are most often opportunistic, occurring in immunosuppressed patients.

The respiratory tract is probably the portal of entry. Chronic pneumonitis and lung abscess are the most common findings. Bacteremia may occur. In patients with chronic pneumonia who have neurologic symptoms or signs, *Nocardia* brain abscess should be considered. Any organ may be infected.

- In patients with chronic pneumonia who develop neurologic symptoms, *Nocardia* brain abscess should be considered.

Manifestations are as described in preceding paragraph. Findings depend on the organ involved, but almost all patients have pneumonia; other organs are involved if there is hematogenous spread (±25% of patients). The infection is diagnosed at autopsy in ±40% of cases. The diagnosis depends on a suspicion of the infection and on culture. Cultures of sputum are not very sensitive. Bronchoscopically obtained specimens or open lung biopsy with stains of tissue and culture of pus may be needed to confirm the diagnosis. The disease must be differentiated from other chronic pneumonias (i.e., bacterial, actinomycosis, tuberculosis, fungal infections).

The prognosis is poor in immunosuppressed patients

and very poor in those with brain abscess. If the patient has no underlying disease, prognosis is usually good if there is no hematogenous spread.

Therapy involves drainage and cotrimoxazole (probably drug of choice); imipenem is also effective.

- The infection is diagnosed at autopsy in ±40% of cases.

FUNGAL INFECTIONS

Coccidioidomycosis

Coccidioides immitis is dimorphic; in tissue it is a spherule, and in culture it is mycelial (filamentous) (color plate 20-8). It forms arthrospores that are highly infectious to laboratory personnel. It is endemic in the southwestern United States, especially the San Joaquin Valley of California and central Arizona. Currently, a major epidemic is under way in California. Arthrospores are inhaled. Dissemination is most likely to occur in males (especially Filipino and black) and in pregnant females. Nonpregnant white females seem to be more resistant than white males.

- *C. immitis* is endemic in the southwestern United States.
- Dissemination is most likely to occur in males (especially Filipino and black) and in pregnant females.

Primary infection is pneumonitis. Hilar adenopathy is common; pleural effusion occurs in 12% of cases and cavities in ±5% (typically thin-walled). Solid coin lesions may form. If the infection disseminates, it can affect any organ system. The disease rarely, if ever, reactivates after years (unlike tuberculosis). Caseous necrosis often occurs; on silver stain, spherules can be seen.

- Hilar adenopathy is common; pleural effusion occurs in 12% of cases and cavities in ±5% (typically thin-walled).

Pulmonary disease involves dry cough, fever, and pleural effusion. Erythema nodosum may occur and, if present, is usually a sign of active delayed hypersensitivity and an indication infection will not be disseminated. Erythema nodosum is more common in females and is often associated with arthralgias, especially of knees and ankles. Disseminated disease (1% of cases) is extrapulmonary, and every organ system can be involved. Affected sites are meninges (most severe manifestation), skin (most common), joints (arthritis), and bones (osteomyelitis).

- Erythema nodosum may occur.

Diagnosis is based on suspicion of the disease, positive sputum culture, or biopsy with silver stains. On fungal serology (complement fixation), a titer ≥1:4 indicates the infection. Skin test is of epidemiologic value only.

Amphotericin B is used for therapy (*Coccidioides* is one of more resistant fungi to amphotericin). The acute pulmonary form is usually self-limited and usually requires only symptomatic therapy. It may require therapy if patient is pregnant, has human immunodeficiency virus (HIV) infection, has received a transplant, or has worsening infection without therapy. Ketoconazole is effective for non-life-threatening, nonmeningeal disease in a dosage of 400-800 mg per day for 6 months. If meningitis develops, prognosis is poor and therapy is with fluconazole or intrathecal amphotericin B. The Ommaya reservoir is best means of administering amphotericin. Chronic long-term suppressive therapy is necessary, and there is a high frequency of adhesive arachnoiditis. Fluconazole is effective for long-term suppressive therapy of meningitis.

Histoplasmosis

Histoplasma capsulatum is dimorphic; in tissue it is a small (3 mm in diameter) yeast, and in culture it has a mycelial form. It is especially prevalent in Ohio and Mississippi River valleys. Outbreaks have been associated with cleaning chicken coops and bird nesting areas, where exposure to bird droppings occurs. It is acquired by inhalation of spores; granulomas form which may caseate. Histoplasmosis is only rarely an "opportunistic" infection. It usually occurs in previously normal persons but causes fulminant disease in patients with acquired immunodeficiency syndrome (AIDS).

- Histoplasmosis has been associated with cleaning chicken coops and bird nesting areas, where exposure to bird droppings occurs.
- It usually occurs in previously normal persons.

In endemic areas, the *primary (acute)* form may be indistinguishable from influenza or other upper respiratory tract infections. Multiple small, calcified lesions are found on chest radiography with healing. The *progressive (disseminated)* form is rare. It is most likely to occur

in infants and elderly men. Manifestations may resemble those of lymphoma: e.g., weight loss, fever of undetermined origin, anemia, increased erythrocyte sedimentation rate, and splenomegaly. Gastrointestinal ulcerations, especially in oral cavity, are common. The infection may also cause endocarditis and meningitis. Addison's disease can occur and may be insidious; adrenal function must be checked periodically. The infection occurs in patients with AIDS; the severe form may present as septic shock. *Chronic cavity disease* is indistinguishable from tuberculosis, usually bilateral upper lung involvement.

- *Primary (acute)* form may be indistinguishable from influenza or other upper respiratory tract infections.
- *Chronic cavity disease* is indistinguishable from tuberculosis, usually bilateral upper lung involvement.

Serology is of limited help and plays little role in diagnosis. Biopsy, silver staining, and cultures are best means of diagnosis. Bone marrow stains and cultures and fungal blood cultures are frequently helpful. Biopsy specimens of mouth lesions can be helpful.

The mild, acute forms are usually self-limited and do not require therapy. Amphotericin B in a total dosage of 25-35 mg/kg is drug of choice for all severe, life-threatening cases. Itraconazole is the drug of choice in most nonmeningeal, non-life-threatening cases and has replaced ketoconazole. Dosage is 200-400 mg per day for 6-12 months. Patients with AIDS need chronic maintenance therapy.

Blastomycosis

Blastomyces dermatitidis is dimorphic. In tissue, the yeast forms are thick-walled and have broad-based buds; they are larger than *Histoplasma* organisms (±10 μm diameter). In culture, a mycelial form is found. The means of transmission is unknown. It may be related to contact with soil. The probable entry is through inhalation. Lung infection may be inapparent and may disseminate hematogenously to bone, skin, or prostate. Granulomas occur, but calcification is less frequent than with histoplasmosis or tuberculosis.

Blastomycosis affects lung, skin, bone, and internal genitalia (prostate, epididymis, testis). The pulmonary form has no characteristic findings: pleural effusion is rare, hilar adenopathy develops occasionally, and cavitation is infrequent. It often mimics carcinoma of the lung. The most common clinical form of blastomycosis is cutaneous. Lesions, especially on face, are suggestive of blastomycosis. They are characteristically painless and nonpruritic and have a sharp, spreading border. Chronic, crusty lesions are noted. In bone, vertebral involvement is most common. Infection of internal genitalia manifests as painful swelling of testes and dysuria.

- Blastomycosis affects lungs, skin, bone, and internal genitalia (prostate, epididymis, testis).
- Most common clinical form of blastomycosis is cutaneous.
- In bone, vertebral involvement is most common.

Diagnosis is based on clinical picture, biopsy, stains, and cultures. Serology is of minimal help, and skin testing is of no help. Thick-walled, broad-based budding yeast is found on stains.

- Thick-walled, broad-based budding yeast is found on stains.

Therapy involves amphotericin B (organism is usually susceptible; total dosage is 20-25 mg/kg, and this is used for all severe infections). Itraconazole is also effective (dosage, 200-400 mg per day for 6 months) and is the drug of choice for all non-life-threatening disease in immunocompetent persons; it has replaced ketoconazole.

Aspergillosis

There are many species of *Aspergillus*. *A. fumigatus* is one of the most common pathogens in humans. Pulmonary form of infection is opportunistic in immunosuppressed hosts and is probably acquired by respiratory route. On tissue section, the organisms have large, branching, septate hyphae (phycomycetes are nonseptate) at 45° angle. They may invade blood vessels, producing a striking thrombotic angiitis similar to phycomycosis. Metastatic foci may cause suppurative abscess formation.

- *Aspergillus* organisms may invade blood vessels, producing a striking thrombotic angiitis.

A form of aspergillosis is invasive bronchopulmonary disease, which should be considered in any immunosuppressed (neutropenic) host with acute progressive pneumonitis. It is especially common in patients with acute myelomonocytic leukemia, Hodgkin's disease, and chronic lymphocytic leukemia and in patients who have had organ transplantation. Chronic necrotizing aspergillosis is different from invasive disease in granulocytopenic patients. It occurs in patients with chronic lung disease. The chronic progressive infiltrates of this condition often require invasive techniques for diagnosis. Fungus ball may develop in preexisting lung bullae of immunocompetent or immunosuppressed patients (e.g., ankylosing spondylitis, previous tuberculosis). Fungus ball must be surgically excised because it can erode a pulmonary blood vessel and cause hemorrhage. Disseminated disease can involve any organ. Patients usually die quickly. Kidney and brain are most often involved. In otitis externa, *Aspergillus* is part of usual flora and is opportunistic. Allergic bronchopulmonary aspergillosis presents as asthma with colonization of the respiratory tract. It is characterized by migratory pulmonary infiltrates; thick, brown, tenacious mucous plugs in the sputum; eosinophilia; and positive serology results. Endophthalmitis usually occurs after operation or trauma and often causes blindness. In patients with intact immune defenses, *Aspergillus* is a frequent colonizer of the respiratory tract; therefore, its isolation from sputum culture cannot be relied on as an indication of invasive disease. Cutaneous manifestations of aspergillosis can develop with use of Hickman catheter. Localized black necrotic lesion develops at site of catheter insertion. The catheter is removed and amphotericin B is administered.

- A form of aspergillosis is invasive bronchopulmonary disease, which should be considered in any immunosuppressed (neutropenic) host.
- Chronic necrotizing aspergillosis occurs in patients with chronic lung disease.
- Cutaneous manifestations of aspergillosis can develop with use of Hickman catheter.

Prolonged granulocytopenia is a major risk factor for invasive pulmonary aspergillosis. Serology and skin tests are of no help for diagnosing invasive disease. In patients with granulocytopenia, a positive sputum culture should raise suspicion for the disease, but histologic examination of tissue is necessary to confirm the diagnosis.

- Prolonged granulocytopenia is the major risk factor for invasive pulmonary aspergillosis.

Therapy is with amphotericin B. Combination of flucytosine or rifampin with amphotericin B for severe disease has been suggested but has not yet been proved to be better than amphotericin B alone. Role of itraconazole is still unclear. For fungus ball, excision is standard approach. For allergic bronchopulmonary aspergillosis, amphotericin B is usually of no help; corticosteroids are used in severe cases.

Cryptococcosis

Cryptococcus neoformans is the only species of *Cryptococcus* that is pathogenic for humans. It is a yeast in both tissue and culture, is 4-7 μm in diameter, has thin-walled buds, and a capsule. It is an opportunistic pathogen. Most infections occur in immunosuppressed hosts, especially patients with Hodgkin's disease, hematologic malignancy, organ transplantation, and AIDS. Occasional patients are apparently normal before infections, but they may have some preexisting subtle T-cell dysfunction. Pigeon droppings may play role in transmission. Respiratory tract is probable portal of entry. The infection does not incite much inflammatory reaction, there is little necrosis, and calcification is rare.

- *C. neoformans* is an opportunistic pathogen.
- Pigeon droppings may play role in transmission.

Meningitis is most common form of infection. It may have insidious onset, involve cranial nerves, and cause blindness with involvement of optic nerve. Transient maculopapular rash or subcutaneous masses occur in ±10% of cases.

- Meningitis is most common form of infection.

Isolation of *Cryptococcus* in sputum or bronchial washings in immunosuppressed hosts has high incidence of dissemination. Patients should have cerebrospinal fluid examination and cultures on specimens from other sites, and they should receive antifungal therapy. Normal hosts with isolation of *Cryptococcus* from sputum or bronchial washings usually do not require antifungal therapy. Cryptococcal infection in bone presents as punched-out lesions with little surrounding inflammatory reaction.

Diagnosis is based on demonstration of organism in tissue or cultures. The cryptococcal antigen test is the most helpful of all fungal serologic tests. It measures capsular *antigen*; all other fungal serologic tests measure antibody. If antigen is present in cerebrospinal fluid, consider infection present until proved otherwise. If *C. neoformans* is isolated from any source in a susceptible patient

(e.g., sputum, urine, blood), *always* examine cerebrospinal fluid to detect meningitis.

- If *C. neoformans* is isolated from any source, always examine cerebrospinal fluid to detect meningitis.

Amphotericin B and flucytosine are the preferred therapeutic agents. One successful form of therapy with fewer side effects is flucytosine, 100-150 mg/kg per day, plus amphotericin B, 0.3 mg/kg per day, administered for 6 weeks. However, relapse rates are high in compromised hosts.

Patients with AIDS respond poorly to treatment and usually have persistence of infection despite treatment. (Patients with abnormal mental status, hyponatremia, and *Cryptococcus* found on culture of extraneural site are at increased risk.) Flucytosine has increased hematologic toxicity in patients with AIDS, particularly when levels are not monitored. In a recent study comparing fluconazole (200 mg/day) with amphotericin B for 10 weeks, fluconazole was as effective as amphotericin B (effective is defined as clinical improvement or resolution of symptoms with negative culture results for cerebrospinal fluid), but mortality in the first 2 weeks of therapy was higher with fluconazole (15% vs. 8%). We still recommend initial therapy with amphotericin B with or without flucytosine until culture results of cerebrospinal fluid are negative or there is a need to switch to fluconazole for other reasons. For chronic maintenance, fluconazole is more effective than weekly administration of amphotericin B.

Candidiasis

There are many species of *Candida*. In tissue, it can be either yeast form or mycelial. In culture, it is yeast and mycelial. It is opportunistic and can infect virtually any site in the body.

Cutaneous infection manifests as diaper rash and intertrigo; in the disseminated form maculopapular rash and subcutaneous nodules may be present.

Fungemia develops from infected intravenous catheters, one of most common portals of entry, especially in the immunosuppressed host who is receiving broad-spectrum antimicrobials. It represents 5%-10% of nosocomial bloodstream infections. Risk factors include previous antibacterial therapy, cytotoxic or corticosteroid therapy, and parenteral nutrition. Suspect fungemia in a patient with these risk factors who suddenly becomes febrile while receiving antibacterials. Mouth, gastrointestinal tract, or rectum-anus may be portal of entry. *C. tropicalis* and *C. parapsilosis* most often are found in immunocompromised patients. Endocarditis occurs most often in intravenous drug users. It is often caused by species other than *C. albicans*. Blood culture results are usually positive. Endophthalmitis may occur as long as 1 month after initial fungemia. Therefore, it is necessary to do periodic funduscopic examinations after fungemia occurs.

- Fungemia develops from infected intravenous catheters, especially in the immunosuppressed host.
- Risk factors include previous antibacterial therapy, cytotoxic or corticosteroid therapy, and parenteral nutrition.
- Endocarditis occurs most often in intravenous drug users.
- Endocarditis is often caused by species other than *C. albicans*.

Metastatic abscesses can occur in any site after an episode of *Candida* fungemia. Cystitis and nephritis can occur in patients with chronic indwelling urinary catheters, urinary tract infection, and immunosuppression. Diagnosis is based on positive culture results, symptoms, and absence of other diagnosis. *Candida* pneumonitis is very rare; *Candida* in respiratory secretions almost always is due to asymptomatic colonization. Osteomyelitis and joint infections are rare; they are complications in immunosuppressed patients or after fungemia. Hepatosplenic candidiosis typically occurs in neutropenic patients as the bone marrow recovers and is associated with typical "bull's-eye lesions" on ultrasonography or computed tomography. Diagnosis is made from biopsy of liver. Treatment is at least 2 g amphotericin. Fluconazole or liposomal amphotericin B may also be effective. Esophagitis is common in immunosuppressed patients and those with AIDS. Diagnosis is made with endoscopy. It must be distinguished from cytomegalovirus and herpes simplex virus infection.

- Hepatosplenic candidiasis typically occurs in neutropenic patients as the bone marrow recovers.
- Esophagitis is common in immunosuppressed patients and those with AIDS.

Therapy is described on pages 562 and 563. Need for treating patients with fungemia should be individualized. For central venous catheter-related candidemias, catheter removal followed by amphotericin B (250-500 mg) is indicated. Fluconazole is effective for oral or esophageal candidiasis in patients with AIDS.

Sporotrichosis

Sporothrix schenkii in tissue is round, cigar-shaped yeast. In culture, it is mycelial. It is transmitted through accidental inoculation into skin ("rose gardener's disease") and rarely through inhalation. It manifests as suppurative and granulomatous reaction; occasional giant cells are found.

Cutaneous infection has characteristic, almost diagnostic, crusty, cutaneous lesions ascending the lymphatics in the extremities. Pulmonary infection is possibly acquired through inhalation. It may cause chronic pneumonitis, cavities, and empyema. Joint spaces are rarely involved. Chronic meningitis may also occur.

- In sporotrichosis, crusty, cutaneous lesions ascend the lymphatics in the extremities.
- Pulmonary infection may cause chronic pneumonitis, cavities, and empyema.

Diagnosis is based on suspicion of the infection and on biopsy and culture results. Serology is occasionally helpful.

For cutaneous form, itraconazole or supersaturated solution of potassium iodine is used. For disseminated disease (pulmonary, joint), amphotericin B is used; itraconazole is an alternative agent.

Mucor (*Rhizopus*, **Zygomycetes**)

Rhinocerebral infections are most common. They occur in patients with diabetes who have ketoacidosis and in immunosuppressed patients, especially those with neutropenia. Infection has been reported in patients on hemodialysis who are receiving deferoxamine therapy.

- In mucormycosis, rhinocerebral infections occur in patients with diabetes who have ketoacidosis and in immunosuppressed patients.

Diagnosis is based on findings of typical black necrotic lesions around eye or on soft and hard palates. It is confirmed by biopsy of skin, mucous membrane, lung. It is especially important to consider this diagnosis in patients who are neutropenic. Organism is nonseptate hyphae. *Aspergillus* is *septate* and branches at 45° angle.

● Diagnosis is based on findings of typical black necrotic lesions around eye or on soft and hard palates in the appropriate host.

Treatment usually includes amphotericin B and surgical debridement. Most patients respond very poorly. Only hope for recovery is if neutrophil value increases.

RICKETTSIAL INFECTIONS

Weil-Felix reactions are no longer considered diagnostic for rickettsial infections. All rickettsial infections have insect vector except Q fever (respiratory spread), and all are associated with a rash except Q fever and ehrlichiosis. The rash of Rocky Mountain spotted fever (RMSF) is indistinguishable from that of meningococcal meningitis. RMSF rash begins on extremities and moves centrally. Typhus fever (murine or endemic typhus) rash begins centrally and moves toward the extremities. RMSF is most common in mid-Atlantic states and Oklahoma, not Rocky Mountain states. Pathophysiology of all rickettsial infections includes vasculitis and disseminated intravascular coagulation. Rickettsial pox is a common rickettsial disease in United States. It is usually unrecognized. It is an urban disease and is the only rickettsial disease characterized by vesicular rash. Eschar is present at site of bite on extremities in 95% of patients, but one needs to look for it. Rickettsial pox is spread by bite of mouse mite.

● All rickettsial infections have insect vector except Q fever.
● All are associated with a rash except Q fever and ehrlichiosis.
● RMSF rash begins on extremities and moves centrally.
● RMSF is most common in mid-Atlantic states and Oklahoma, not Rocky Mountain states.

Among persons with Q fever, ±100% have pneumonitis, 15% have hepatitis (granulomatous), and 1% have endocarditis. It is associated with exposure to animal products, especially infected placenta. It can occur in meat packing workers. A mini-epidemic occurred in a group exposed to parturient cats.

● Among persons with Q fever, ±100% have pneumonitis, 15% have hepatitis.
● Can occur in meat packing workers.

Diagnosis is determined with serologic testing. Treatment is with tetracycline or chloramphenicol.

Ehrlichia chafeensis, the etiologic agent of ehrlichiosis, is a tick-borne rickettsia that causes acute infection in humans, mostly in southern states and in spring and summer. The disease was first recognized in humans in 1986. It is a tick-borne zoonosis. The incubation period is 1-3 weeks. The infection is characterized by fever, relative bradycardia, malaise, and headache but *no rash* (spotless RMSF). Patients may have leukopenia (lymphopenia), thrombocytopenia, and increased values on liver function tests (aspartate aminotransferase, alanine aminotransferase).

The diagnosis is made on basis of serologic tests or characteristic inclusions seen on blood smear. The infection is usually self-limited, but deaths have been reported. Treatment with tetracycline seems effective.

Rickettsia conorii infection has been termed Mediterranean spotted fever, boutonneuse fever, Marseilles fever, and South African tick bite fever. The *R. conorii* organism is common in the Far East, Israel, eastern and southern Africa, and the southern Mediterranean. The vector is the tick *Rhipicephalus sanguineus*. The infection occurs in summer months. It has an incubation period of 1 week. It resembles RMSF, except the rash begins on the trunk rather than the extremities. A "tache noire" lesion (cigarette burn) should be sought at site of tick bite. Severe disease occurs in patients with underlying illness. The diagnosis is based on immunofluorescent demonstration of organisms in skin biopsy or serology tests. Treatment is with tetracycline, chloramphenicol, or ciprofloxacin.

MYCOPLASMA PNEUMONIAE

This is one of the smallest microorganisms capable of extracellular replication. It lacks a cell wall; therefore, cell-wall-active antibiotics such as penicillin are not effective in treatment. It is spread by droplet inhalation. It occurs in young, previously healthy persons and presents with sudden onset of headache, dry cough, and fever. Results of physical examination are unremarkable with the possible exception of bullous myringitis. Chest radiography usually shows bilateral patchy pneumonitis. The chest radiographic findings are out of proportion to physical findings. Pleural effusion is present in 15%-20% of cases. Neurologic complications include Guillain-Barré syndrome, cerebellar peripheral neuropathy, aseptic meningitis, and mononeuritis multiplex. Hemolytic anemia may occur late in the illness as a result of circulating cold hemagglutinins. The central nervous system manifestations and hemolytic anemia suggest *Mycoplasma.*

- *M. pneumoniae* is spread by droplet inhalation.
- Chest radiography usually shows bilateral patchy pneumonitis.
- Pleural effusion is present in 15%-20% of cases.
- Neurologic complications include Guillain-Barré syndrome, cerebellar peripheral neuropathy, aseptic meningitis, and mononeuritis multiplex.

Diagnosis is established by specific complement fixation test. Cold agglutinins are nonspecific for *Mycoplasma* infections. Erythromycin is drug of choice for therapy. Tetracycline is an alternative. In a young person with fever, dry cough, patchy pneumonitis, and few physical findings, initial drug of choice is erythromycin, *not* penicillin. Immunity is transient; therefore, reinfection may occur. Clinical relapse of pneumonia occurs in up to 10% of cases of *Mycoplasma* pneumonia.

CHLAMYDIA PNEUMONIAE (TWAR AGENT)

This is a new agent, distinct from *C. trachomatis* and *C. psittaci.* In young adults, it causes 10% of cases of pneumonia and 5% of cases of bronchitis. It has been a cause of community outbreaks, and nosocomial transmission has occurred; 50% of adults are seropositive. Mode of transmission is unknown (not birds). Clinical manifestations are usually mild; the symptoms resemble those caused by *M. pneumoniae.* Pharyngitis may occur 1-3 weeks before onset of pulmonary symptoms, and cough may last for weeks. Diagnosis is based on serologic tests (not routinely available). Treatment is with tetracycline or erythromycin.

- In young adults, *C. pneumoniae* causes 10% of cases of pneumonia and 5% of cases of bronchitis.
- It has been a cause of community outbreaks, and nosocomial transmission has occurred.

VIRAL DISEASES

Influenza

Type A is the most common. Epidemics occur every 2-4 years; pandemics occur every 20-30 years. Epidemics and pandemics are a result of major antigenic shift in the influenza virus. About 80%-90% of deaths due to influenza occur in persons ≥65 years old. Complications include 1) primary influenza pneumonia (interstitial desquamative pneumonia) and 2) secondary bacterial infection, which is usually caused by *Streptococcus pneumoniae* or *Staphylococcus aureus.* A typical history is as follows: an elderly patient, often with chronic obstructive lung disease, develops influenza, which may or may not improve; then, the severity of symptoms increases substantially. with high fever, marked leukocytosis, and often respiratory failure. This is a medical emergency and must be treated as *S. aureus* pneumonia (although pneumococcal pneumonia is more common in this setting). One needs to be alert to the possibility of toxic shock syndrome related to *S. aureus* infection.

- About 80%-90% of deaths due to influenza occur in persons ≥65 years old.
- Secondary infection is usually caused by *Streptococcus pneumoniae* or *Staphylococcus aureus.*

Amantadine is effective against only influenza A virus. Vaccine, together with amantadine, can give ±95% protection against influenza A infection.

Recommendations for prevention of influenza in patients at risk include vaccination each autumn. Vaccine is given as follows: 6-35 months of age, split virus (chemically treated to prevent febrile reaction); 3-12 years of age, split virus; >12 years of age, whole or split virus. The vaccine can be given simultaneously with pneumococcal vaccine (Pneumovax). Reactions include fever, myalgias, and hypersensitivity. Target groups are persons ≥65 years old, residents of chronic care facilities, persons with cardiopulmonary disorders, children 6 months to 18 years old receiving long-term aspirin therapy (Reye's syndrome), health care personnel, employees of chronic care facilities, providers of home health care, and household members of high-risk persons. Amantadine is also used prophylactically: 200 mg/day; if >65 years old, 100 mg/day. The dosage is decreased in patients with impaired renal function (100 mg/day) or seizure disorders (100 mg/day). Toxicity manifests as dizziness, restlessness, and insomnia.

- Vaccine can be given simultaneously with pneumococcal vaccine.
- Target groups are persons ≥65 years old, residents of chronic care facilities, persons with cardiopulmonary disorders, health care personnel, employees of chron-

ic care facilities, providers of home health care, and household members of high-risk persons.

Influenza A is treated with amantadine. It is effective if given within 48 hours after onset of symptoms. After 48 hours, it has no effect.

Poliovirus

There was a recent outbreak in the Netherlands among members of religious groups who were not vaccinated. Centers for Disease Control recommend evaluation of a traveler's immunity before extensive travel in the Netherlands. The frequency and severity of disease are increased during pregnancy. It is most often an asymptomatic infection. Virus affects the nuclei of cranial nerves and anterior motor neurons of spinal cord; therefore, paralysis is flaccid and not spastic. When paralysis develops, it is usually asymmetric.

Rabies

This infection is difficult to diagnose antemortem. Manifestations are hydrophobia and copious salivation. It should be considered in any case of encephalitis or myelitis of unknown cause, especially in persons who have recently traveled outside the United States. The virus spreads along peripheral nerves to central nervous system. The most common sources of exposure are dogs, cats, skunks, foxes, raccoons (Florida, Connecticut), wolves, and bats. Spread by other animals is *very rare*. Rodents rarely, if ever, transmit rabies. From 1980-1989, 9 of 13 cases in the United States were due to exposure to rabid animals outside the country. Rabies has also been reported to occur in patients after corneal transplantation. Aerosol spread is possible; it is most often due to exposure to bats during spelunking or in medical laboratories. The risk of nosocomial transmission is low. Definitive diagnosis is established by the presence of Negri bodies on biopsy of hippocampus. Clinically, serum and cerebrospinal fluid are tested for rabies antibodies. Direct fluorescent antibody testing of skin biopsy specimen from nape of the neck is used to detect rabies antigen.

- Rabies should be considered in any case of encephalitis or myelitis of unknown cause.
- Most common sources of exposure are dogs, cats, skunks, foxes, raccoons, wolves, and bats.
- Definitive diagnosis is established by the presence of Negri bodies on biopsy of hippocampus.

Human diploid vaccine is most effective and least toxic; it has largely replaced duck embryo vaccine. Human rabies immune globulin (HRIG) is widely available now. Do not use horse serum globulin unless human immune globulin is unavailable. HRIG and vaccine are not of benefit after onset of clinical disease.

Slow Viruses

Progressive Multifocal Leukoencephalopathy (PML)

This is associated with acquired immunodeficiency syndrome (AIDS), leukemia, lymphoma, and carcinomatosis. It is caused by a papovavirus (JC virus). Clinically, diffuse or focal central nervous system abnormalities are present. Despite its name, PML usually presents as a solitary lesion on computed tomography or magnetic resonance imaging. Cerebrospinal fluid is normal in most cases. It is now recognized with increased frequency in patients with AIDS. Diagnosis is based on brain biopsy. There is no proven therapy.

- PML is associated with AIDS, leukemia, lymphoma, and carcinomatosis.
- Caused by a papovavirus (JC virus).
- Now recognized with increased frequency in patients with AIDS.

Subacute Sclerosing Panencephalitis (Inclusion Body Encephalitis)

This is a progressively fatal disease of children and adolescents. It is thought to be due to previous measles infection. Patients are <11 years old in 80% of cases. Onset is insidious; mental deterioration is characteristic. Later, myoclonic jerks and diffuse abnormalities occur. Measles antibody levels in sera and cerebrospinal fluid are among highest found in any condition. Brain biopsy is necessary for diagnosis (inclusion body encephalitis). There is no treatment. The disease is uniformly fatal.

Creutzfeldt-Jakob Disease

This is a rare, fatal, degenerative disease of the central nervous system. It occurs equally in both sexes; the median age of patients is in the seventh decade. There are both familial and sporadic forms of the disease. It usually presents as rapidly evolving dementia with myoclonic seizures. Prions (small proteinaceous infectious particles without nucleic acid) are the cause of infection. It has been reported to occur through nosocomial transmission (e.g., corneal transplant recipients, exposure to cerebrospinal fluid). There is no treatment.

- Creutzfeldt-Jakob disease presents as rapidly evolving dementia with myoclonic seizures.

Measles (Rubeola)

There has been a substantial increase in measles cases recently in unvaccinated preschool children and vaccinated high school and college students (1990, 27,786 cases). Prodromal upper respiratory symptoms are prominent. Oral Koplik's spots precede cutaneous rash. The disorder has been associated with temporary cutaneous anergy. *Cases of reactivation of previous Mycobacterium tuberculosis infection have been reported in patients with measles.* Measles vaccine may also cause temporary cutaneous anergy. Therefore, tuberculin skin test should be done before measles vaccinations.

- In measles, oral Koplik's spots precede cutaneous rash.
- Measles vaccine may also cause temporary cutaneous anergy.

Complications of measles include encephalitis and pneumonia. Encephalitis is often severe. It usually occurs after a period of apparent improvement of measles infection. In primary measles pneumonia there are large multinucleated cells (Warthin-Finkeldey cells) found in lung biopsy. Secondary bacterial infection is more common than primary measles pneumonia. *S. aureus* and *Haemophilus influenzae* are the most common bacterial pathogens.

- Complications of measles include encephalitis.
- Secondary bacterial infection is more common than primary measles pneumonia.

Atypical measles occurs in patients vaccinated before 1968. After exposure, atypical rash, fever, arthralgias, and headache (aseptic meningitis) may develop. It can be diagnosed by the presence of high titer of measles antibody in serum.

Rubella

The prodromal symptoms of rubella are mild (unlike those of rubeola). Posterior cervical lymphadenopathy, arthralgia (70% in adults), transient erythematous rash, and fever are characteristic. Infection is subclinical in many cases. Central nervous system complications and thrombocytopenia are rare.

- Characteristics of rubella: posterior cervical lymphadenopathy, arthralgia (70% in adults), transient erythematous rash, and fever.

For a pregnant female exposed to rubella, the serum titer should be checked. If titer indicates immunity, no treatment is needed. If titer indicates non-immunity, the patient should be followed for evidence of clinical rubella. The serum titer should be checked again in 2-3 weeks to determine whether it is increased. If titer is not increased and there is no evidence of clinical rubella, no treatment is needed. In cases of clinical rubella or seroconversion, abortion counseling should be offered, depending on clinical circumstances. Do *not* give gamma globulin to pregnant non-immune female exposed to rubella. It may mask symptoms of rubella but it does not protect the fetus.

- In cases of clinical rubella or seroconversion, consider therapeutic abortion.

From 6%-11% of young adults remain susceptible to rubella after receiving rubella vaccine. Pregnant female should not be given rubella vaccine because it causes congenital abnormalities. Females of childbearing age should be warned not to become pregnant within 2-3 months from time of immunization. Transient arthralgias will develop in 25% of immunized women. They may also develop fever, rash, and lymphadenopathy. Symptoms may occur as long as 2 months after vaccination. They may be confused with other forms of arthritis.

Viral Meningoencephalitis

Viral infections with low cerebrospinal fluid glucose levels may be confused with bacterial, partially treated bacterial, or tuberculous meningitis. Etiologic agents include mumps, enteroviruses, herpes simplex, and, in summer months, the equine encephalitis viruses. Lymphocytic choriomeningitis is acquired by exposure to rodent urine. It causes profound lymphocytosis in the cerebrospinal fluid.

Herpesvirus

There are now seven known types of herpes simplex virus (HSV): type 1, type 2, Epstein-Barr virus (EBV), cytomegalovirus (CMV), varicella-zoster virus (VZV), human herpesvirus 6 (HHV-6), and HHV-7. HHV-6 caused roseola (exanthem subitum) and up to 14% of acute self-limited febrile illnesses in children ≤2 years old who presented to one emergency room. HHV-7 has yet to be associated with disease.

Serologic evidence of infection is common by the time students enter college: HSV-1, 37%; HSV-2, 5%; EBV, 54%; CMV, 25%; VZV, 80%. Rate of infection increases in populations of lower socioeconomic status.

Herpes Simplex

In 75% of cases of genital HSV, infection is caused by HSV-2 and 25% by HSV-1. The reverse is true for oral HSV. Use of sunscreen in patients exposed to significant amounts of sunlight may decrease incidence of recurrence on lips. *Disseminated infection* is most often due to HSV-1 and occurs in immunocompromised hosts with impaired cell-mediated immunity. In cases of herpes simplex encephalitis, patients may mistakenly be thought to be intoxicated. They appear confused and may have seizures. Simultaneous herpes labialis is present in 10%-15%. Antemortem diagnosis is difficult. HSV is rarely cultured from cerebrospinal fluid. Definitive diagnosis is made by brain biopsy. Recently, new techniques such as magnetic resonance imaging and DNA amplification have shown promise. Electroencephalography shows periodic lateralized epileptiform discharges (PLEDs). Abnormalities are located in temporal areas. Poor neurologic status, age >30 years, and encephalitis of more than 4 days in duration are associated with poor outcome.

- In herpes simplex, disseminated infection is most often due to HSV-1 and occurs in immunocompromised hosts.
- In cases of herpes simplex encephalitis, patients may mistakenly be thought to be intoxicated.
- Simultaneous herpes labialis is present in 10%-15%.

HSV pneumonia usually occurs in immunosuppressed patients and is a serious disease. HSV also is associated with mucocutaneous disease (e.g., esophagitis, stomatitis). HSV esophagitis must be distinguished from CMV and *Candida* esophagitis. Diagnosis is made with endoscopic biopsy. *Eczema herpeticum* (Kaposi's varicelliform eruption) occurs in areas of eczema. Large areas of skin are involved. *Herpetic whitlow* is painful infection of finger, often from a contaminated needle. Although nosocomial transmission of HSV-1 is rare, recent reports have stressed the importance of mucous membrane precautions in all patients with HSV, particularly those with respiratory infection who are undergoing invasive procedures.

- *Herpetic whitlow* is painful infection of finger, often from a contaminated needle.

HSV can cause outbreaks among participants in contact sports (wrestlers, herpes gladiatorum). The infection is transmitted by skin-to-skin contact. Lesions appear on head (78%), trunk (28%), and extremities (42%). Rash may be atypical. Large ulcerative lesions can develop in patients with AIDS. Some of the lesions are mistaken for decubitus ulcers. Perianal ulcers can present with pain on defecation or pruritus. Treatment for HSV is outlined in Table 20-7.

- HSV can cause outbreaks among participants in contact sports.
- Large ulcerative lesions can develop in patients with AIDS.

Cytomegalovirus

Primary cytomegalovirus (CMV) infection is usually asymptomatic in immunocompetent patients, although it can cause heterophile-negative mononucleosis syndrome. Perinatal infection occurs in utero, intrapartum, or post partum. It can cause congenital malformations. Children commonly excrete CMV in urine.

- CMV can cause heterophile-negative mononucleosis syndrome.

CMV can be transmitted by blood transfusion; the virus is transmitted by granulocytes, most often in fresh blood. Survival of virus is greatly reduced in stored blood products. Fever and infectious mononucleosis-like picture on peripheral smear are characteristics in postoperative patients who have received blood transfusions. The typical patient has had cardiac bypass 4 weeks previously or has been pregnant and had a large blood loss. Diagnosis is made by detection of seroconversion. CMV causes serious infections (retinitis, pneumonia, gastrointestinal ulcerations, encephalitis, adrenalitis) in patients who have had transplantation (solid organ and bone marrow) and patients with AIDS. Diagnosis is most often established from clinical findings alone (CMV retinitis), by isolation of CMV from sterile body site (blood), or from culture and histopathologic evidence of CMV infection in involved tissue (e.g.,

Table 20-7.--Treatment for Herpes Simplex Virus

Infection	Treatment
Genital herpes	
First episode	Acyclovir, 200 mg orally 5 times/day for 7-10 days
	Acyclovir, 5 mg/kg intravenously every 8 hours for 5 days (severe cases)
Recurrence	Acyclovir, 200 mg orally 5 times/day for 5 days
Frequent recurrence	Acyclovir, 400 mg orally twice a day up to 1 year
Encephalitis	Acyclovir, 10 mg/kg intravenously every 8 hours for 10-14 days (vidarabine [ara-A] is less effective alternative)
Mucocutaneous disease in immunocompromised patient	
Initial episode	Acyclovir, 5 mg/kg intravenously every 8 hours or 200-400 mg orally 5 times/day for 7-10 days
Recurrence	Intravenous or oral acyclovir taken daily prevents recurrence during high-risk periods (immediately after bone marrow transplantation); lesion will likely recur when therapy discontinued
Orolabial disease	
First occurrence	Limited data; acyclovir probably effective, 200 mg orally 5 times/day for 5 days
Frequent recurrence (>6/yr)	Acyclovir, 400 mg twice/day
Acyclovir-resistant strains	Foscarnet, vidarabine

liver, lung, gastrointestinal tract).

- CMV can be transmitted by blood transfusion; the virus is transmitted by granulocytes.
- Fever and infectious mononucleosis-like picture on peripheral smear are characteristics in postoperative patients who have received blood transfusions.
- CMV causes serious infections (retinitis, pneumonia, gastrointestinal ulcerations, encephalitis, adrenalitis) in patients who have had transplantation and patients with AIDS.

Positive blood cultures for CMV in patients with AIDS do not predict subsequent end-organ disease (i.e., low positive predictive value) in the subsequent 6 months of follow-up. This course is in contradistinction to that of patients after solid organ transplantation. Furthermore, only approximately 50% of patients with AIDS and CMV end-organ disease will have positive results of CMV blood culture. In 75% of CMV-negative transplant recipients who receive CMV-positive organs, primary CMV disease will develop. In many of these, end-organ complications will develop. Others will have mononucleosis-like syndrome. This causes enhanced immunosuppression, and patients are more likely to develop other infection (e.g., *Pneumocystis carinii* pneumonia).

CMV retinitis occurs in 20%-30% of patients with advanced AIDS. Diagnosis is based on ophthalmologic examination. CMV esophagitis is third most frequent cause of esophagitis in patients with AIDS. CMV pneumonia is much more common in patients who have had transplantation (bone marrow) than in patients with AIDS. Diagnosis requires tissue confirmation of infection (CMV inclusions in biopsy specimens) because frequently patients can excrete CMV in bronchoalveolar lavage specimens without having active disease. CMV pneumonia can be particularly severe and life-threatening in patients who have had bone marrow transplantation.

- CMV retinitis occurs in 20%-30% of patients with advanced AIDS.
- CMV esophagitis is third most frequent cause of esophagitis in patients with AIDS.
- CMV pneumonia is much more common in patients who have had transplantation (bone marrow) than in patients with AIDS.

Ganciclovir has been the treatment of choice for most

CMV infections. A recent randomized, placebo-controlled trial found that foscarnet and ganciclovir are equally efficacious in halting progression of CMV retinitis in patients with AIDS but that patients taking foscarnet lived longer (12 vs. 8 months). Both drugs are now approved for this indication. The choice of one over the other should be made on an individual basis. All patients with AIDS who have CMV retinitis need chronic suppressive therapy. In patients with CMV pneumonia after bone marrow transplantation, ganciclovir and immunoglobulin containing high titers of CMV antibodies are more effective than ganciclovir alone. Non-immunocompromised patients with CMV do not require treatment.

● Ganciclovir and foscarnet are the treatments of choice for most CMV infections.

Varicella-Zoster

In primary varicella infection (chickenpox), the lesions are in various stages of development in different areas of the body. It differs from smallpox in that lesions are all at the same level of development. Varicella pneumonia occurs in 5%-50% of adults with chickenpox. It occurs 1-6 days after onset of rash and is a serious disease. Pneumonia begins to improve with disappearance of rash, but, in serious cases, pneumonia may persist. Encephalomyelitis is also a serious complication of varicella infection. It occurs predominantly in children. Onset is 3-14 days after appearance of rash.

● Varicella pneumonia occurs in 5%-50% of adults with chickenpox.
● Pneumonia begins to improve with disappearance of rash.

Herpes zoster infection is considered a reactivation of latent varicella infection. It often involves the fifth cranial nerve, especially ophthalmic branch. Nonimmune patients exposed to zoster may develop varicella, but patients exposed to varicella rarely, if ever, develop zoster.

● Herpes zoster infection often involves the fifth cranial nerve, especially ophthalmic branch.

Neurologic complications of herpes zoster include motor paralysis (most common). It usually involves same dermatome and may involve cranial nerves. Encephalitis also occurs. Myelitis is least common neurologic complication.

Varicella immune globulin is indicated for 1) VZV-seronegative immunocompromised hosts who have had close contact with a person with chickenpox and 2) newborns of mothers with varicella infection that occurs 5 days before or 2 days after delivery.

Among mothers with varicella-zoster, 10% transmit the infection to the fetus. During the first trimester, limb hypoplasia, cortical atrophy, and chorioretinitis develop. During the third trimester, multiple visceral involvement develops, including pneumonia. Mortality rate is 31%. Highest risk period is 5 days before and 2 days after delivery.

● Among mothers with varicella-zoster, 10% transmit the infection to the fetus.

Treatment for *varicella (primary varicella-zoster) infection* is based on whether the patient is immunocompetent. Two recent randomized clinical trials showed that acyclovir (800 mg 5 times/day or equivalent) reduced duration of skin lesions and viral shedding in adults and children. Its efficacy for reducing visceral complications (i.e., pneumonia) remains unknown. Early treatment (<24 hours) is necessary. Cost of therapy may limit its usefulness. In immunosuppressed patients, acyclovir or vidarabine reduces complications. Acyclovir is less toxic and so is the preferred therapy. Acyclovir may reduce risk of dissemination and of complications in immunocompromised patients. In immunocompetent patients, acyclovir speeds healing and reduces pain. There is no effect on postherpetic neuralgia. This therapy should always be used for zoster ophthalmicus because treatment reduces the incidence of uveitis and keratitis. For disseminated infections (encephalitis, cranial neuritis), recent controlled trial showed that high-dose intravenous acyclovir was equivalent to vidarabine. Treatment with acyclovir was associated with 3 fewer days of hospitalization than when vidarabine was used. For acyclovir-resistant varicella-zoster infection, intravenous foscarnet is used.

Epstein-Barr Virus (EBV)

Infectious mononucleosis has the clinical triad of fever, pharyngitis, and adenopathy. Pharyngitis is common (±80%). Splenomegaly occurs in 50% of cases. One of the most serious complications is ruptured spleen, in which case the patient has sudden onset of severe abdominal pain. Other serious complications include hemolytic anemia and airway obstruction; encephalitis and transverse myelitis also occur but are uncommon. Corticosteroids may be beneficial in treatment of hemolytic anemia and acute airway obstruction. The infection may be transmitted by blood transfusion. If ampicillin is given, a rash often develops.

- Infectious mononucleosis has the clinical triad of fever, pharyngitis, and adenopathy.
- Pharyngitis is common (±80%).
- Splenomegaly occurs in 50% of cases.
- One of the most serious complications is ruptured spleen.
- If ampicillin is given, a rash often develops.

Uncomplicated cases require symptomatic care only. The patient should not participate in contact sports for several months. Corticosteroids are not indicated for uncomplicated infection. Acyclovir therapy is not effective.

Table 20-8 differentiates EBV from other causes of mononucleosis.

Chronic fatigue syndrome is a vague syndrome characterized by low-grade fever, constitutional symptoms, and fatigue; lymphadenopathy, splenomegaly, and abnormal results of liver function tests may be noted. Studies have shown that elevated titers of antibody to early antigen and viral capsid antigen are no more frequent in cases than in controls. Acyclovir is also not effective. The infection is not caused by EBV.

- Chronic fatigue syndrome is characterized by low-grade fever, constitutional symptoms, and fatigue.
- Lymphadenopathy, splenomegaly, and abnormal results of liver function tests may be noted.

- The infection is not caused by EBV.

EBV infection in males with X-linked lymphoproliferative syndrome is a rare disorder of young boys. Fulminant EBV infections develop; 57% die of the infection. Complications include severe EBV hepatitis with liver failure and hemophagocytic syndrome with bleeding. Survivors develop hypogammaglobulinemia, malignant lymphoma, aplastic anemia, and opportunistic infections. Death occurs by age 40 years in all cases. Acyclovir and corticosteroids do not seem to be beneficial.

In EBV-associated Burkitt's lymphoma and nasopharyngeal carcinoma, patients have high titers of antibody to early antigen. *Polyclonal and monoclonal B-cell lymphoproliferative syndromes* have been associated with EBV in patients who have had organ transplantation and are receiving cyclosporine and in patients with AIDS. Oral hairy leukoplakia in patients with AIDS is associated with EBV infection and responds to acyclovir therapy.

- Polyclonal and monoclonal B-cell lymphoproliferative syndromes have been associated with EBV.

Epidemic Keratoconjunctivitis

This is caused by adenovirus type 8. It is now most common in epidemics occurring in ophthalmology clinics (caused by contaminated fluids or instruments).

Mumps

Orchitis occurs in 20% of males; it is unilateral in approximately 75%. Orchitis is characterized by recrudescence of malaise and appearance of chills, fever, headache, nausea, vomiting, and testicular pain. Sterility is *uncommon* even after bilateral infection.

Mumps meningoencephalitis is one of most common viral meningitides. Patients may have low cerebrospinal

Table 20-8.--Infectious Mononucleosis-Like Syndromes

Disease	Pharyngitis	Adenopathy	Splenomegaly	Atypical lymphocytes	Heterophile	Other test
Infectious mononucleosis	++++	++++	+++	+++	+	Specific EBV antibody + (VCA IgM)
CMV	-	-	+++	++	-	CMV IgM
Toxoplasmosis	-	++++	+++	++	-	Toxoserology

-, absent; +, ++, +++, and ++++, present to varying degrees; VCA, viral capsid antigen.

fluid glucose values. Pancreatitis can occur.

- Mumps meningoencephalitis is one of the most common viral meningitides.

Mumps polyarthritis is most common in men between ages of 20-30 years. Joint symptoms begin 1-2 weeks after subsidence of parotitis. Large joints are involved. It lasts approximately 6 weeks, and complete recovery is usual. This condition may be confused with other forms of arthritis.

- Mumps polyarthritis is most common in men between ages of 20-30 years.
- Large joints are involved.

Deafness is a rare complication of mumps.

Human T-Cell Leukemia Viruses (HTLV)

Infection with these retroviruses is usually asymptomatic. HTLV-I is endemic in parts of Japan, Caribbean basin, Melanesia, and Africa. It may be transmitted by sexual contact, infected blood products, and injection drug use. Vertical transmission (breast feeding) also occurs. HTLV-I is associated with human T-cell leukemia and chronic myelopathy (tropical spastic paraparesis). For HTLV-II, no clinical disease is known. The seroprevalence of HTLV-I or -II is as high as 18% in certain high-risk groups (injection drug users, patients attending sexually transmitted disease clinics) (HTLV-II is 2.5 times more prevalent than HTLV-I). Among voluntary blood donors, seroprevalence in the United States is estimated at 0.016%. The risk of transmission of HTLV-I or -II through blood transfusion with current screening practices is estimated to be 0.0014% (1/70,000 units). Sexual partners of infected persons should be tested for HTLV-I and -II.

- HTLV-I may be transmitted by sexual contact, infected blood products, and injection drug use.
- HTLV-I is associated with human T-cell leukemia and chronic myelopathy.

Parvovirus B19

This is the cause of erythema infectiosum (fifth disease) and transient arthritis. Persistent B19 virus is found in patients with pure red blood cell *aplasia*. This condition has no increase in serum IgG or IgM antibodies and no rash, arthralgias, or other manifestations of fifth disease. Diagnosis is established by demonstration of giant pronor-moblasts in bone marrow or identification of viral protein or DNA of parvovirus in bone marrow. Most patients respond to administration of commercial immunoglobulin infusions for 5-10 days.

- Parvovirus B19 is cause of erythema infectiosum (fifth disease) and transient arthritis.
- B19 virus is found in patients with pure red blood cell aplasia.

PARASITIC DISEASES

Amebic Keratitis

The causative organism is *Acanthamoeba*. This condition should be suspected in patients with keratitis as the result of contamination of contact lens solution or in patients who have been swimming in fresh water while wearing contact lenses. Diagnosis is based on microscopic examination of scrapings of the cornea. Treatment is with topical antifungal agents. Patients often respond poorly to therapy and have progressive corneal destruction.

- In amebic keratitis, causative organism is *Acanthamoeba*.
- Condition is suspected in keratitis caused by contamination of contact lens solution.

Amebic Meningoencephalitis

Causative organism is free-living amebas of the genus *Naegleria*. Many patients have a history of swimming in fresh water lakes, usually in middle Atlantic states or Texas. Presumed portal of entry is through the cribriform plate. Patients have intense hemorrhagic meningoencephalitis. Cerebrospinal fluid findings are like those of bacterial infection--low glucose level, many polymorphonuclear cells, and high erythrocyte count. Motile trophozoites may be found. The infection is almost invariably fatal. Treatment is with amphotericin B (intrathecally and intravenously).

- In amebic meningoencephalitis, portal of entry is through the cribriform plate.

Amebiasias

Sites of involvement, in decreasing order of frequency, are cecum, ascending colon, rectum, and sigmoid. When symptomatic, disease causes diarrhea, abdominal pain, fever in ±50% of cases; bloody diarrhea often occurs.

Trophozoites are found in stool specimens. Trophozoites do *not* spread disease. Treatment is with metronidazole plus diloxanide furoate or paromomycin. In asymptomatic carriers, amebic cysts are excreted in stool specimens. They are contagious and are responsible for spread of disease. Treatment is with diloxanide furoate or paromomycin.

- In amebiasis, sites of involvement, in decreasing order of frequency, are cecum, ascending colon, rectum, and sigmoid.
- Bloody diarrhea often occurs.

Patients with hepatic abscess usually have minimal, if any, diarrhea. They may have low-grade fever. Stool specimens are usually negative. Abscess usually is single and is located in the posterior portion of the right lobe of the liver (because this lobe receives most of the blood draining the right colon--site of most frequent involvement with amebiasis). This anatomic location may result in point tenderness in the posterolateral portion of the lower right intercostal space. Jaundice is uncommon. The anatomic location, the fact that it is usually a single abscess, and the absence of other signs of bacterial infection help to distinguish amebic hepatic abscess from bacterial abscess. Serologic tests (complement fixation) are positive in >90% of patients. Hepatic abscess may rupture through the diaphragm into the right pleural cavity. Rarely, *Entamoeba histolytica* may cause brain abscess. Treatment is with metronidazole plus diloxanide furoate or paromomycin.

- Patients with hepatic abscess usually have minimal, if any, diarrhea.
- Serologic tests (complement fixation) are positive in >90% of patients.

Miscellaneous Parasites

Giardia is most frequently isolated parasite in state laboratories. It characteristically presents with sudden onset of watery diarrhea and malabsorption, bloating, and flatulence. Prolonged disease is particularly common in patients with IgA deficiency. Diagnosis is based on stool examination and duodenal aspirate. Treatment is with metronidazole or quinacrine hydrochloride.

- *Giardia* is most frequently isolated parasite in state laboratories.
- Presents with sudden onset of watery diarrhea and mal-

absorption, bloating, and flatulence. Prolonged disease is particularly common in patients with IgA deficiency.

Toxoplasmosis is acquired from eating undercooked meat or exposure to cat feces. Rash, pneumonitis, and generalized lymphadenopathy are characteristics. Toxoplasmosis causes brain lesions and pneumonia in patients with AIDS. The causative organism may result in infectious mononucleosis-like syndrome. Treatment is with sulfonamide and pyrimethamine.

- Toxoplasmosis is acquired from eating undercooked meat or exposure to cat feces.
- Rash, pneumonitis, and generalized lymphadenopathy are characteristics.
- Causative organism may result in infectious mononucleosis-like syndrome.

Trichinosis is acquired from undercooked meat, especially pork or bear. Features are muscle pain, especially chest and tongue; eosinophilia; and periorbital edema. *Hookworm (Necator americanus)* causes blood loss anemia. Dog or cat hookworms cause cutaneous larval migrans, resulting in severe itching. *Ascariasis* infection produces intestinal obstruction. *Schistosomiasis* is a tropical disease that causes hepatic cirrhosis, hematuria, and carcinoma of the bladder.

- Trichinosis is acquired from undercooked meat, especially pork or bear.
- Features are muscle pain, especially chest and tongue; eosinophilia; and periorbital edema.

The four main species of *malaria* are *Plasmodium vivax, P. falciparum, P. malariae, P. ovale*. Malaria is transmitted by bite of *Anopheles* mosquito. All four species have primary exoerythrocytic (hepatic) stage. *P. vivax* and *P. ovale* have secondary exoerythrocytic (hepatic) stage. *P. falciparum* does not have this secondary exoerythrocytic stage. The asexual erythrocytic cycle requires 36-48 hours for *P. falciparum*, 48 hours for *P. vivax*, and 72 hours for *P. malariae*. The periodicity of febrile paroxysms caused by the different species coincides with the cyclic discharge of organisms from ruptured erythrocytes. Because of the secondary exoerythrocytic period, *P. vivax* and *P. malariae* infections have long (months to years) latent exoerythrocytic periods, and chronic relapses may occur many years after primary infection. These do not occur with *P. falciparum*.

- Malaria is transmitted by bite of *Anopheles* mosquito.

Mosquito-borne malaria occurred in California and Florida in 1990. Self-induced malaria through contaminated blood products, usually in an attempt to cure Lyme disease, has been reported. Cases in military personnel returning from Somalia have been reported.

P. vivax invades only immature erythrocytes, *P. malariae* invades only senescent erythrocytes, and *P. falciparum* invades erythrocytes at any age.

The hallmark of the condition is malarial paroxysm. This occurs regularly in all infections by *P. falciparum*. With *P. vivax*, tertian malaria is most common form. Once synchronization occurs, paroxysms occur on alternate days (48 hours). With *P. malariae*, quartan malaria is most common. Paroxysms occur every third day. *P. malariae* infections may be associated with nephrotic syndrome. With *P. falciparum*, because of the asynchronous cycle of multiplication, the typical paroxysms occur in a minority of patients. *P. falciparum* can multiply in all stages of erythrocyte, so quantity of parasitemia can be large.

Diagnosis of malaria is based on examination of thick and thin blood smear (color plate 20-9).

- Malarial paroxysm occurs regularly in all infections by *P. falciparum*.
- With *P. malariae*, quartan malaria is most common.
- Paroxysms occur every third day.
- Diagnosis of malaria is based on examination of thick and thin blood smear.

Prophylaxis is increasingly difficult because of resistant *P. falciparum*. Personal protection should always be used (e.g., mosquito nets). For travelers to chloroquine-sensitive areas (Central America [north of Panama], Mexico, Haiti, Dominican Republic, and the Middle East), chloroquine phosphate is taken. For travelers to chloroquine-resistant areas, mefloquine, doxycycline, or sulfadoxine-pyrimethamine (Fansidar) is used. Travelers to the mefloquine-resistant areas of the Thai-Myanmar and Thai-Cambodia borders should use doxycycline. Mefloquine should be avoided in patients taking β-blockers. No regimen guarantees 100% prophylaxis. All patients should be advised to seek medical attention if

fever develops within 1 year after return from endemic area. Prophylaxis should begin 2 weeks before travel and continue through 4-6 weeks after leaving an endemic area.

For treatment of known susceptible strains of *P. falciparum* and others, chloroquine is used. In cases of chloroquine resistance, therapy is with quinine and sulfadoxine-pyrimethamine or doxycycline. Primaquine (screen for glucose-6-phosphate dehydrogenase deficiency) is used to eradicate exoerythrocytic phase of *P. ovale* and *P. vivax* infections. Adjunctive therapy may include defuroxamine (iron chelation), which may hasten the clearance of parasitemia and enhance recovery from deep coma in children with cerebral malaria. It also has antimalarial effects in asymptomatic patients with mild parasitemia. Exchange transfusions are used in severe cases with extensive parasitemia.

Pinworms cause anal pruritus. Diagnosis is made by examination of cellophane tape pressed to anus. Stool specimen is *not* helpful in diagnosis.

Cryptosporidiosis is an important cause of diarrhea in AIDS. It may also be a relatively common cause of self-limited diarrhea in otherwise healthy patients. Waterborne outbreaks (Georgia; Milwaukee, Wisconsin) have been reported. They occur most often in late summer or fall; 35% of patients have other pathogen simultaneously, most often *Giardia*. Diagnosis is based on stool examination or acid-fast stain of stool.

- Cryptosporidiosis is an important cause of diarrhea in AIDS.
- 35% of patients have other pathogen simultaneously, most often *Giardia*.

Leishmaniasis has been reported in soldiers returning from Operation Desert Storm. It is a protozoal disease transmitted by sand fly. It causes a visceral syndrome (kala-azar; caused by *Leishmania donovani*). Symptoms are fever, hepatosplenomegaly, hypergammaglobulinemia, cachexia, and pancytopenia. Diagnosis is based on bone marrow aspiration (Giemsa stain). Skin test should not be used. Treatment is with stibogluconate sodium. The cutaneous form is caused by *L. tropica*.

- Leishmaniasis has been reported in soldiers returning from Operation Desert Storm.

Neurocystercercosis is an infection of central nervous system with larval stage of the pork tapeworm (*Taenia solium*). It is endemic in Latin America, Asia, and Africa. It is most common in western United States among foreign-born persons. Recent cases have been reported among household contacts of foreign-born persons (working as domestic employees); the infected persons had not traveled to an endemic area or eaten pork. Common presentations are seizures and computed tomography scan showing cystic brain lesions. Diagnosis is based on serum or cerebrospinal fluid serologic testing or brain biopsy. Treatment is with praziquantel or albendazole with or without steroids. Recent evidence suggests that after medical therapy there is usually remission or marked improvement in the seizure disorder.

- *Neurocystercercosis* is most common in western United States among foreign-born persons.
- Common presentations are seizures and computed tomography scan showing cystic brain lesions.

Babesiosis is a tick-borne (same vector as Lyme disease, *I. dammini*) parasitic disease that affects erythrocytes and causes fever, myalgias, hemolytic anemia, and occasionally splenomegaly. It is a severe disease associated with asplenia. Rash has not been reported. The disease is endemic in the northeastern United States, especially around Nantucket and Cape Cod. Diagnosis is by examination of peripheral blood smear. Treatment is with clindamycin and quinine.

The pathogen of *visceral larva migrans* is common dog and cat roundworm, *Toxocara canis*. Humans (usually children) are infected by ingesting eggs found in soil (pica). Clinical syndrome is due to migration of larva to extraintestinal sites (hematogenous spread). Fever, hepatomegaly, eosinophilia, and hypergammaglobulinemia are common. Pulmonary involvement (asthma, pneumonitis) is rare. Diagnosis is presumptive and based on serologic testing. Course is usually self-limited. For severe cases, treatment is with albendazole or mebendazole with or without steroids.

- The pathogen of *visceral larva migrans* is common dog and cat roundworm, *Toxocara*.
- Humans are infected by ingesting eggs found in soil.
- Fever, hepatomegaly, eosinophilia, and hypergammaglobulinemia are common.

Diagnostic tests for detecting various parasitic diseases are listed in Table 20-9.

Table 20-9.--Preferred Diagnostic Tests for Parasitic Infections

Parasite	Means of diagnosis[*]
Ameba: colonic	Stool O & P
Ameba: extracolonic	Serology
Giardia	Duodenal aspirate
Toxoplasma	Serology
Trichinella	Tissue biopsy
Hookworm	Stool O & P
Ascaris	Stool O & P
Schistosoma	Stool O & P or tissue biopsy
Plasmodium (malaria)	Blood smear
Opisthorchis (clonorchiasis)	Stool O & P
Filaria (filariasis)	Blood smear
Trypanosoma	Tissue biopsy
Tapeworm	Stool O & P
Pinworm	Perianal adhesive tape
Babesia	Blood smear
Pneumocystis	Tissue stain

[*]O & P, ova and parasites.

CLINICAL SYNDROMES

INFECTIVE ENDOCARDITIS

Native Valve Infective Endocarditis

Native valve infective endocarditis is more common in males, and the average age of patients is >50 years. It may present with acute (*Staphylococcus aureus*) or subacute (viridans streptococci) manifestations. In 60%-80% of cases there is a predisposing cardiac lesion. Mitral valve involvement is more common than aortic valve involvement. Congenital heart disease is present in 10%-20% of cases. Risk of infective endocarditis from mitral valve prolapse is low, but the prevalence of mitral valve prolapse makes it the underlying cardiac condition in 20%-25% of cases. Antimicrobial prophylaxis is used in patients with mitral valve prolapse who have murmur or echocardiographic evidence of thickening of mitral valve leaflets and valve redundancy.

- Antimicrobial prophylaxis is used in mitral valve prolapse associated with murmur or thickening of mitral valve leaflets or redundancy.

Microorganisms causing native valve infective endocarditis include viridans streptococci (i.e., *Streptococcus sanguis, S. mutans,* and *S. mitior*), 30%-40% of cases;

enterococci (i.e., *Enterococcus faecalis, E. faecium*), 5%-18%; other streptococci (i.e., *S. bovis, S. pneumoniae*), 15%-25%; *S. aureus*, 10%-27%; coagulase-negative staphylococci, 1%-3%; gram-negative bacilli, 1.5%-13%; fungi, 2%-4%; miscellaneous bacteria, <5%; mixed infections, 1%-2%; and "culture-negative," <5%-24% (data from Scheld WM, Sande MA: Cardiovascular infections. *In* Principles and Practice of Infectious Diseases. Third edition. Edited by GL Mandell, RG Douglas Jr, JE Bennett. New York: Churchill Livingstone, 1990, pp 670-706).

- Organisms most commonly involved in native valve infective endocarditis are viridans streptococci.

Treatment of native valve infective endocarditis includes emphasis on short-course therapy in selected cases (i.e., young patients and patients with uncomplicated left-sided native valve infective endocarditis caused by penicillin-susceptible viridans streptococci or *S. bovis*). For enterococcal endocarditis, combination therapy with penicillin G or ampicillin is recommended. Testing for high-level aminoglycoside resistance (gentamicin, >500 µg/mL; streptomycin, >2,000 µg/mL), β-lactamase production, and vancomycin resistance is mandatory.

Table 20-10 shows the recommended and alternative treatment regimens for native valve infective endocarditis.

Prosthetic Valve Infective Endocarditis

Prosthetic valve endocarditis is more common in males, and the average age of patients is ≥60 years. The aortic valve is affected more often than the mitral valve. Early-onset endocarditis is defined as infection occurring ≤60 days after implantation, and late-onset endocarditis is infection occurring >60 days postoperatively. Early infection tends to have a more acute presentation. Microorganisms that cause infection are outlined in Table 20-11.

Treatment of prosthetic valve infective endocarditis is given in Table 20-12.

Miscellaneous Information About Infective Endocarditis

- Echocardiography is not a screening tool for detecting endocarditis.
- Endocarditis in injection drug users is caused by *S. aureus* (60%), streptococci (16%), gram-negative bacilli (13.5%), polymicrobial organisms (8.1%), and *Corynebacterium* (1.4%). *Candida* endocarditis also occurs in this patient population. *S. aureus* most commonly involves the tricuspid valve.

- Intractable congestive heart failure is the most common indication for surgery.
- Culture-negative endocarditis may be the result of previous use of antibiotics (most common) and endocarditis due to the following organisms: HACEK organisms, nutritionally deficient streptococci, *Brucella*, fungi, *Legionella*, *Coxiella burnetii*, and *Chlamydia psittaci*.

Surgical Therapy

If surgery is needed it should not be delayed to allow additional days of antimicrobial therapy. Surgical treatment is often indicated in cases with refractory congestive heart failure. Other generally accepted indications for surgery include evidence of more than one serious systemic embolic episode, uncontrolled bacteremia despite effective antimicrobial therapy, and inadequate antimicrobial therapy. Other indications include invasive perivalvular infection as manifested by abscess or fistula on echocardiography, new or persistent electrocardiographic changes, persistent unexplained fever, fungal endocarditis, and relapse of appropriately treated prosthetic valve endocarditis due to penicillin-sensitive streptococci.

MENINGITIS

Bacterial Meningitis

The incidence of bacterial meningitis is 4.6-10 cases/100,000 person-years. There are 2,000 deaths per year in the United States, and the case-fatality rate is 14%.

Risk factors for death include age ≥60 years, decreased mental status at admission, and occurrence of seizures within 24 hours of symptom onset. Initial cerebrospinal fluid characteristics include a cell count of 1,000-100,000/µL, a protein value ≥45 mg/dL, and glucose value ≤40 mg/dL. The leukocyte differential is more likely to show a predominance of polymorphonuclear neutrophils. The Gram stain is positive in 75% of untreated cases. Cerebrospinal fluid bacterial cultures are positive in 70%-80% of cases. Countercurrent immunoelectrophoresis or latex agglutination test is useful for *Haemophilus influenzae* type B, *Streptococcus pneumoniae*, and *Neisseria meningitidis* types A, B, C, and Y.

- Risk factors for death in bacterial meningitis: age ≥60 years, decreased mental status at admission, seizures within 24 hours of symptom onset.
- Cerebrospinal fluid bacterial cultures positive in 70%-80% of cases.

Table 20-10.--Treatment of Native Valve Infective Endocarditis

Microorganism	Therapy*	Alternative therapy*
Penicillin-sensitive streptococci		
Streptococcus pyogenes, S. pneumoniae, group B streptococci	Aqueous penicillin G, 20×10^6 U/24 hr i.v. for 4 wk	Vancomycin, 30 mg/kg daily for 4 wk, *or* cefazolin,[†] 1 g i.v. every 8 hr for 4 wk
Viridans streptococci or *S. bovis* (MIC, ≤0.1 µg/mL)	Aqueous penicillin G, 20×10^6 U/24 hr i.v. for 2 wk, *plus* streptomycin,[‡] 7.5 mg/kg i.m. every 12 hr for 2 wk, or gentamicin,[‡] 1 mg/kg i.v. every 8 hr for 2 wk, *or* aqueous penicillin G, 20×10^6 U/24 hr i.v. for 4 wk	Vancomycin, 30 mg/kg daily for 4 wk, *or* cefazolin,[†] 1 g i.v. every 8 hr for 4 wk
Nutritional variant or relatively penicillin-resistant viridans streptococci (MIC, >0.1 µg/mL and <0.5 µg/mL)	Aqueous penicillin G, 20×10^6 U/24 hr i.v. for 4 wk, *plus* streptomycin,[‡] 7.5 mg/kg i.m. every 12 hr for 4 wk, or gentamicin,[‡] 1 mg/kg i.v. every 8 hr for 4 wk	Vancomycin, 30 mg/kg daily for 4 wk, *plus* streptomycin,[‡] 7.5 mg/kg i.m. every 12 hr for 4 wk, or gentamicin,[‡] 1 mg/kg i.v. every 8 hr for 4 wk
Enterococci or streptococci with MIC ≥0.5 µg/mL		
Streptomycin-susceptible (MIC, <2,000 µg/mL); organisms must be penicillin- or vancomycin-susceptible and not have high-level aminoglycoside resistance (streptomycin MIC <2,000 µg/mL and gentamicin MIC <500 µg/mL)	Aqueous penicillin G, 20×10^6 U/24 hr i.v. for 4-6 wk, *plus* streptomycin,[‡] 7.5 mg/kg i.m. every 12 hr for 4-6 wk, or gentamicin,[‡] 1 mg/kg i.v. every 8 hr for 4-6 wk	Vancomycin, 30 mg/kg daily for 4-6 wk, *plus* streptomycin,[‡] 7.5 mg/kg i.m. every 12 hr for 4-6 wk, or gentamicin,[‡] 1 mg/kg i.v. every 8 hr for 4-6 wk
Staphylococcus aureus		
Methicillin-sensitive	Nafcillin, 2.0 g i.v. every 4 hr for 4-6 wk, *plus* gentamicin,[‡] 1 mg/kg every 8 hr for first 5-7 days	Vancomycin, 30 mg/kg daily for 4-6 wk, *or* cefazolin,[†] 2 g i.v. every 8 hr for 4-6 wk, *plus* gentamicin,[‡] 1 mg/kg every 8 hr for first 5-7 days
Methicillin-resistant	Vancomycin, 30 mg/kg daily for 4-6 wk, *plus* gentamicin,[‡] 1 mg/kg i.v. every 8 hr for 5-7 days	Consult infectious diseases specialist
HACEK group	Ampicillin, 1-2 g i.v. every 3 hr for 4 wk or 2nd- or 3rd-generation cephalosporin for 3 wk	Second- or third-generation cephalosporin, 3 wk
Neisseria gonorrhoeae	Ceftriaxone, 1-2 g every 24 hr for 4 wk	Aqueous penicillin G, 20×10^6 U/24 hr i.v. for 4 wk (in β-lactam negative) for penicillin-susceptible isolates
Gram-negative bacilli	Most effective single drug or combination of drugs i.v. for 4-6 wk	
Urgent empiric treatment of culture-negative endocarditis	Vancomycin, 30 mg/kg daily for 6 wk, *plus* gentamicin,[‡] 1.0 mg/kg i.v. every 8 hr for 6 wk	

Table 20-10 (continued)

Microorganism	Therapy*	Alternative therapy*
Fungal endocarditis	Amphotericin B *plus* flucytosine, 37.5 mg/kg p.o. every 6 hr, *plus* cardiac valve replacement (flucytosine levels should be monitored)	

*Dosages suggested are for adults with normal renal and hepatic function.

†Other first-generation cephalosporins or cefuroxime may be substituted for cefazolin in equivalent dosages.

‡Gentamicin and streptomycin doses should not exceed 80 mg and 500 mg, respectively. Serum levels should be monitored and peak streptomycin levels of 20 µg/mL and gentamicin levels of 3 µg/mL are acceptable.

i.m., intramuscularly; i.v., intravenously; MIC, minimal inhibitory concentration; p.o., by mouth.

Modified from Steckelberg JM, Giuliani ER, Wilson WR: Infective endocarditis. *In* Cardiology: Fundamentals and Practice. Vol 2. Second edition. Edited by ER Giuliani, V Fuster, BJ Gersh, MD McGoon, DC McGoon. St. Louis, Mosby Year Book, 1991, pp 1739-1772. By permission of Mayo Foundation.

Table 20-11.--Organisms That Cause Prosthetic Valve Endocarditis

Organism	Onset, %		All, %
	Early	Late	
Coagulase-negative staphylococci	35	12	14
Staphylococcus aureus	17	26	29
Enterococci and group D streptococci	3	9	7
Streptococcus pneumoniae	1	<1	1
Other (i.e., viridans streptococci)	4	25	17
Gram-negative bacilli	16	12	13
Diphtheroids	10	4	7
Other bacteria	1	2	2
Candida	8	4	5
Other fungi	1	<1	1
"Culture negative"	1	4	3

From Threlkeld MG, Cobbs CG: Infectious disorders of prosthetic valves and intravascular devices. *In* Principles and Practice of Infectious Diseases. Third edition. Edited by GL Mandell, RG Douglas Jr, JE Bennett. New York, Churchill Livingstone, 1990, pp 706-715. By permission of the publisher.

Among affected patients, 25% present with a fulminant illness over 24 hours, 50% have been ill for 1-7 days (usually with a respiratory illness), and 25% have had symptoms for 1-3 weeks. Organisms most commonly causing community-acquired infection in adults are *S. pneumoniae, N. meningitidis, H. influenzae, and Listeria monocytogenes.*

- 25% of patients present with fulminant illness over 24 hours.
- Organisms most commonly causing community-acquired infection in adults: *S. pneumoniae, N. meningitidis, H. influenzae, L. monocytogenes.*
- Dexamethasone has decreased incidence of sensorineural hearing loss in children with bacterial meningitis in two controlled trials.
- Dexamethasone treatment in adults remains controversial.

The causative organisms, affected age groups, and predisposing factors in bacterial meningitis are shown in Table 20-13, and treatment is outlined in Table 20-14.

Gram-Negative Meningitis

Gram-negative meningitis that arises spontaneously usually is a result of bacteremia from a focus of infection elsewhere in the body. Gram-negative meningitis also occurs after neurosurgical procedures or head trauma. *Escherichia coli, Klebsiella,* and *Pseudomonas* are the most common pathogens. Treatment often includes a third-generation cephalosporin plus an aminoglycoside. Postoperative gram-negative meningitis is usually the result of a wound infection. It is usually caused by nosocomial bacteria. Multidrug resistance is common.

- Spontaneous gram-negative meningitis usually is result of bacteremia from a focus of infection elsewhere.
- Postoperative gram-negative meningitis is usually result of wound infection.

Table 20-12.--Treatment of Prosthetic Valve Infective Endocarditis

Organism	Therapy*	Therapy for patients allergic to penicillin*
Staphylococcus aureus or *S. epidermidis*		
Penicillin-sensitive (MIC, ≤0.1 μg/mL)	Penicillin G, 20 million U/24 hr i.v. (continuous drip or 6 equal doses) for 4-6 wk	Vancomycin, 30 mg/kg daily for 4-6 wk, *or* cefazolin,[†] 2 g i.v. every 8 hr for 4-6 wk
Penicillin-resistant (MIC, >0.1 μg/mL)	Nafcillin, oxacillin, 2 g i.v. every 4 hr for 4-6 wk	Same as above
Methicillin-resistant	Vancomycin, 30 mg/kg daily, *plus*[‡] rifampin, 300 mg p.o. every 8 hr for 4-6 wk, *plus* gentamicin,[§] 1.5 mg/kg i.v. every 8 hr for first 2 wk of therapy	Consult infectious diseases specialist
Streptococci		
Penicillin-sensitive viridans and non-enterococcal group D (MIC, ≤0.1 μg/mL)	Penicillin G, 20 million U/24 hr i.v. (continuous drip or 6 equal doses) for 4 wk, *plus* streptomycin,[§] 7.5 mg/kg i.m. every 12 hr, *or* gentamicin,[§] 1 mg/kg i.v. every 8 hr for first 14 days	Same as for penicillin-sensitive staphylococci
Enterococci and penicillin-resistant (MIC, >0.1 μg/mL)	Penicillin G, 20 million U/24 hr i.v. (continuous drip or 6 equal doses), *plus* streptomycin,[§] 7.5 mg/kg i.m. every 12 hr, *or* gentamicin,[§] 1 mg/kg i.v. every 8 hr for 4-6 wk	Vancomycin, 30 mg/kg daily, *plus* streptomycin,[§] 7.5 mg/kg i.m. every 12 hr, or gentamicin,[§] 1 mg/kg i.v. every 8 hr for 4-6 wk, *or* desensitize to penicillin
Diphtheroids	Penicillin G, 20 million U/24 hr i.v. (continuous drip or 6 equal doses), *plus* gentamicin,[§] 1 mg/kg i.v. every 8 hr for 4-6 wk	Vancomycin, 30 mg/kg daily for 4-6 wk
Gram-negative bacilli	Most effective and least toxic agent, i.v. for 4-6 wk (selection should be based on results of in vitro MIC, MBC, and synergy tests)	
Fungi	Amphotericin B *plus* flucytosine *plus* cardiac valve replacement (flucytosine levels should be monitored)	

*Dosages suggested are for adults with normal renal and hepatic function.

[†]Other cephalosporins may be used in equivalent dosage, depending on results of in vitro susceptibility studies.

[‡]Vancomycin alone for methicillin-resistant *S. aureus*; combination therapy for methicillin-resistant *S. epidermidis*.

[§]Streptomycin and gentamicin doses should not exceed 500 mg and 120 mg, respectively.

i.m., intramuscularly; i.v., intravenously; MBC, minimal bactericidal concentration; MIC, minimal inhibitory concentration; p.o., by mouth.

Modified from Steckelberg JM, Giuliani ER, Wilson MR: Infective endocarditis. *In* Cardiology: Fundamentals and Practice. Vol 2. Second edition. Edited by ER Giuliani, V Fuster, BJ Gersh, MD McGoon, DC McGoon. St. Louis, Mosby Year Book, 1991, pp 1739-1772. By permission of Mayo Foundation.

Meningococcal Meningitis

Meningitis often occurs in patients who are carriers of meningococci in the nasopharynx. Terminal component complement deficiencies predispose to repeated episodes of infection. Serotypes A, B, C, and Y cause most disease. Meningitis and meningococcemia are the most common presentations. Many patients have a petechial rash. In severe disease, large purpuric areas may develop. Waterhouse-Friderichsen syndrome is not related to adrenal failure; its pathogenesis is probably related to disseminated intravascular coagulation. Treatment is with penicillin G. If patient is allergic to penicillin, chloramphenicol, cefuroxime, or third-generation cephalosporin is used. If the risk of the carrier state is high (household contacts), rifampin or minocycline should be used for prophylaxis. The carrier state is not eliminated by penicillin.

Table 20-13.--Organisms Involved, Affected Age Groups, and Predisposing Factors in Bacterial Meningitis

Organism	Age group	Predisposing factors
Pneumococci	Any age, but often elderly--recurrent meningitis	Cerebrospinal fluid rhinorrhea, alcoholism, splenectomy, multiple myeloma, Hodgkin's disease, HIV
Meningococci	Infants-40 yr	Crowding, military recruits
Haemophilus influenzae	>neonate to 6 yr	Hypogammaglobulinemia in adults, HIV, splenectomy
Escherichia coli, group B streptococci	Neonates	
Listeria monocytogenes	Neonates; immunosuppressed	

HIV, human immunodeficiency virus.

Table 20-14.--Treatment of Bacterial Meningitis

Organism	Therapy	Alternative therapy
Pneumococci	Penicillin (check in vitro susceptibilities)	Cefotaxime, chloramphenicol, ceftriaxone, vancomycin
Meningococci	Penicillin	Same as pneumococci, except do not use vancomycin
Haemophilus influenzae	Cefotaxime, ceftriaxone	Chloramphenicol, ampicillin
Group B streptococci	Penicillin *plus* gentamicin	Same as pneumococci
Listeria	Ampicillin *plus* gentamicin	Cotrimoxazole or chloramphenicol; cephalosporins *not* effective
Gram-negative	Ceftazidime *plus* aminoglycoside	
Empiric therapy to 6 yr	Cefotaxime, ceftriaxone (add ampicillin if *L. monocytogenes* suspected)	

Immunization for certain populations (i.e., military recruits) is also of benefit.

- In meningococcal meningitis, terminal component complement deficiencies predispose to repeated episodes of infection.
- Meningitis and meningococcemia are most common presentations.
- Treatment is with penicillin G.

Aseptic Meningitis

This is a syndrome characterized by an acute onset of meningeal symptoms, fever, cerebrospinal fluid pleocytosis, and negative bacterial cultures from the cerebrospinal fluid. There are many infectious and noninfectious causes, but most often the cause is viral. Viral meningitis is usually a self-limited illness. Common causes include coxsackievirus, echovirus (summer), mumps virus (winter, spring), and others, including arboviruses, lymphocytic choriomeningitis virus, herpes simplex virus types 1 and 2, cytomegalovirus, human immunodeficiency virus, varicella-zoster virus, Epstein-Barr virus, and Colorado tick fever virus.

- Characteristics of aseptic meningitis: meningeal symptoms, fever, cerebrospinal fluid pleocytosis, negative bacterial cultures.
- Cause is often viral.
- Viral meningitis usually self-limited.

SEXUALLY TRANSMITTED DISEASES

Neisseria gonorrhoeae

Uncomplicated infection causes urethritis, cervicitis, and pharyngitis. Symptoms are indistinguishable from those of nongonococcal disease. Gram stain and culture are required for diagnosis. Asymptomatic carrier rate is high in both males and females, and these persons are primarily responsible for continued transmission of the infection. In females, concomitant proctitis is common (rectal cultures should be done in all women). Gonococcal pharyngitis is often asymptomatic. Coexistence of chlamydial infection is common (both conditions should be treated). For diagnosis, Gram stain of urethral exudate showing intracellular diplococci has high sensitivity and specificity. Cervical exudate has sensitivity of only 50% but specificity is high. Definitive diagnosis requires culture on modified Thayer-Martin medium.

- Uncomplicated *N. gonorrhoeae* infection causes urethritis, cervicitis, pharyngitis.
- Asymptomatic carrier rate is high in both males and females.

The prevalence of multiply resistant gonococcal strains is increasing (penicillin and tetracycline resistance). Thus, there have been recent changes in antimicrobial regimens. Primary treatment is ceftriaxone (125 mg intramuscularly) plus doxycycline (100 mg orally twice a day for 7 days). Alternative drugs are cefixime, ciprofloxacin, ofloxacin, and spectinomycin. All alternative agents treat urethral, cervical, rectal, and pharyngeal infection, except spectinomycin. Spectinomycin, cefixime, ciprofloxacin, and ofloxacin may not be active against incubating syphilis. Therapy in pregnant patients involves ceftriaxone (125 mg intramuscularly) plus erythromycin (500 mg orally four times a day for 7 days). If patient is allergic to cephalosporin, treatment is with ciprofloxacin or spectinomycin (2 g intramuscularly) and erythromycin (500 mg orally for 7 days). Follow-up gonococcal cultures need to be performed only if nonstandard regimens are used. All patients with sexually transmitted diseases should be considered at risk for human immunodeficiency virus (HIV) infection and testing should be offered.

- Primary treatment: ceftriaxone (125 mg intramuscularly) plus doxycycline (100 mg orally twice a day for 7 days).

Disseminated gonococcemia is most likely to occur in females during menstruation (sloughing of endometrium allows access to blood supply, enhanced growth of gonococci due to necrotic tissue, and change in pH). There are two distinct phases. Bacteremic phase may manifest by tenosynovitis (±100%), skin lesions (±50%), and polyarthralgias. Joint culture results are usually negative. Nonbacteremic phase may present as monoarticuloarthritis of knee, wrist, and ankle; joint culture results

are positive in ±50%.

- Disseminated gonococcemia most likely to occur in females during menstruation.
- Bacteremic phase may manifest by tenosynovitis (±100%) and skin lesions (±50%); joint cultures usually negative.
- Nonbacteremic phase may present as monoarticuloarthritis of knee, wrist, ankle; joint cultures positive in ±50%.

Treatment is with ceftriaxone (1 g intravenously daily for 7-10 days); alternatives include ceftriaxone (for 3-4 days or until improvement noted) followed by cefixime or ciprofloxacin to complete a course of 7-10 days. If strain is tested and found to be penicillin-susceptible, treatment includes penicillin G (10 million units intravenously daily) for 7-10 days, or it is given for 3-4 days and then oral amoxicillin is used to finish 10-day course. If patient is allergic to cephalosporin, spectinomycin (2 g intramuscularly twice a day for 3 days) is given. Chlamydial infection can coexist with gonococcal infection and should be treated.

- Treatment: ceftriaxone (1 g intravenously daily for 7-10 days).
- Chlamydial infections can coexist with gonococcal infection and should be treated.

For meningitis, treatment includes ceftriaxone (1-2 g intravenously every 12 hours for at least 10-14 days). Alternative drugs are penicillin, if strain is susceptible, or chloramphenicol. For endocarditis, ceftriaxone or penicillin is used for at least 28 days.

Nongonococcal Urethritis and Cervicitis

The most common etiologic agent is *Chlamydia trachomatis*. Doxycycline (100 mg twice a day for 7 days) is standard treatment. Azithromycin as a 1-g single dose and ofloxacin may also be effective. If urethritis does not resolve with a tetracycline, consider tetracycline-resistant *Ureaplasma urealyticum* or *Trichomonas*.

- Nongonococcal urethritis and cervicitis are more commonly caused by *C. trachomatis*.

Herpes Genitalis

For the first episode, therapy with acyclovir (400 mg orally three times a day or 200 mg orally five times a day for 7-10 days) shortens the duration of pain, viral shedding, and systemic symptoms. If symptoms are severe, acyclovir at a dosage of 5 mg/kg intravenously every 8 hours for 5-7 days is used. Topical acyclovir has marginal benefit for decreasing viral shedding and has no effect on symptoms or healing time. For recurrent episodes with severe symptoms, therapy is started at prodrome or within 2 days of onset of symptoms (acyclovir, 400 mg orally three times a day for 5 days). Recurrence after therapy is not related to development of in vitro resistance of herpes simplex to acyclovir. For suppression, in selected patients with more than six recurrences a year, acyclovir, 400 mg twice a day, is used for up to 1 year.

Syphilis

In 1990, the incidence of primary and secondary syphilis was 20/100,000. It is estimated that half of cases are not reported. Incidence has been increasing among heterosexuals since 1985, particularly among inner-city minority populations.

The fluorescent treponemal antibody absorption (FTA-ABS) test is the most helpful serologic test for diagnosis of syphilis (Table 20-15). Results of this test will be positive before those on VDRL testing and thus may be positive without a positive VDRL result in primary syphilis.

- FTA-ABS is most helpful serologic test for diagnosis of syphilis.
- VDRL results may be negative in 30% of patients with primary syphilis.

Table 20-15.--Laboratory Diagnosis of Syphilis

Syphilis	Test, % positive	
	FTA-ABS	VDRL
Primary	85	70
Secondary	100	99
Tertiary	98	1*

*Treated late syphilis.
FTA-ABS, fluorescent treponemal antibody absorption.
Modified from Tramont EC: *Treponema pallidum* (syphilis). *In* Principles and Practice of Infectious Diseases. Third edition. Edited by GL Mandell, RG Douglas Jr, JE Bennett. New York, Churchill Livingstone, 1990, pp 1794-1808. By permission of publisher.

A chancre (clean, indurated ulcer) is the main manifestation of *primary syphilis*. It occurs at the site of inoculation and is usually painless. The incubation period is 3-90 days. It should be distinguished from herpes simplex virus and chancroid (painful exudative ulcer, *Haemophilus ducreyi*). Diagnosis is made by dark field examination.

The manifestations of *secondary syphilis* result from hematogenous dissemination and usually occur 2-8 weeks after appearance of the chancre. Constitutional symptoms occur, in addition to rash, alopecia, condylomata lata, and various other symptoms and signs. Diagnosis is based on the clinical picture and serologic testing. The condition resolves spontaneously without treatment.

Latent syphilis is the asymptomatic stage after symptoms of secondary syphilis subside. Those that occur after 1 year are classified as late. Diagnosis is based on serologic testing.

Tertiary syphilis can involve all body systems (i.e., cardiovascular--aortitis involving ascending aorta, which can cause aneurysms and aortic regurgitation; gummatous osteomyelitis; hepatitis). However, neurosyphilis is the most common manifestation in the United States.

Neurosyphilis is often asymptomatic. Symptomatic disease is divided into several clinical syndromes that may overlap and occur at any time after primary infection. Diagnosis is made by cerebrospinal fluid examination. Abnormalities include mononuclear pleocytosis and elevated protein value. VDRL testing of cerebrospinal fluid is only 30%-70% sensitive. Any cerebrospinal fluid abnormality in a patient who is seropositive for syphilis must be investigated. Syndromes include 1) meningovascular syphilis (occurs 4-7 years after infection and presents with focal central nervous system deficits such as stroke) and 2) parenchymatous syphilis (general paresis or tabes dorsalis). Parenchymatous syphilis occurs decades after infection and may present as general paresis (chronic progressive dementia) or as tabes dorsalis (sensory ataxia, lightning pains, autonomic dysfunction, optic atrophy). A cerebrospinal fluid examination in patients with syphilis is indicated in those with neurologic abnormalities, before re-treatment of relapses, in infants with congenital syphilis, and as baseline study in all patients to be treated with nonpenicillin regimen.

- Neurosyphilis is most common manifestation (in tertiary disease) in United States.
- Diagnosis is made with cerebrospinal fluid examination.
- VDRL testing of cerebrospinal fluid is only 30%-70% sensitive.

Treatment of syphilis is based on whether disease is

early or late. For early syphilis (primary, secondary, or early latent [<1 year]), benzathine penicillin is used-- 2.4 million units intramuscularly; follow-up serologic testing is done. (Some experts recommend a second dose in 7 days in patients with HIV infection.) Alternatives are doxycycline, 100 mg twice a day for 14 days, and erythromycin, 500 mg four times a day for 14 days. Follow-up serologic testing is important. Treatment for late disease (>1 year in duration, cardio-vascular disease, gumma, late latent syphilis) is with benzathine penicillin, 2.4 million units intramuscularly weekly for 3 weeks. Alternatives are doxycycline, 100 mg orally twice a day for 4 weeks. Follow-up serologic tests are recommended.

Treatment for neurosyphilis is with aqueous penicillin G, 12-24 million units intravenously per day for 10-14 days, or procaine penicillin, 2.4 million units intramuscularly per day, plus probenecid, 500 mg four times a day for 10-14 days.

For early and secondary syphilis, follow-up clinical and serologic testing should be performed at 3 and 6 months. Re-treatment with three weekly injections with 2.4 million units of benzathine penicillin G should be given to patients with signs or symptoms that persist or whose VDRL result has a sustained fourfold increase in titer. If VDRL does not decrease fourfold by 3 months, consideration should also be given to re-treatment. Patients with latent syphilis should have follow-up at 6 and 12 months. If titers of VDRL test increase fourfold, if high titer >1:32 fails to decrease fourfold within 12-24 months, of if signs or symptoms attributable to syphilis occur, the patient should be examined for neurosyphilis and re-treated. Follow-up of neurosyphilis should include testing of cerebrospinal fluid every 6 months if cere-brospinal fluid pleocytosis was present initially; this test-ing is done until results are normal. If cell count is not decreased at 6 months or if cerebrospinal fluid is not entirely normal at 2 years, re-treatment should be con-sidered.

Pelvic Inflammatory Disease

In this condition, proximal spread of infection from the endocervix causes endometritis, salpingitis, tubo-ovarian abscess, or pelvic peritonitis in various combi-nations. Organisms responsible are *N. gonorrhoeae, C. trachomatis, Mycoplasma hominis,* and various aerobic gram-negative rods and anaerobes. *Actinomyces israelii* can be a pathogen in setting of intrauterine device. Tuberculosis in older women, including postmenopausal

women, should be considered. Clinical signs and symp-toms include lower abdominal tenderness, adnexal ten-derness, cervical motion tenderness, oral temperature ≥38.3°C, abnormal cervical discharge, increased ery-throcyte sedimentation rate, and evidence of *N. gonor-rhoeae* or *C. trachomatis* infection. Laboratory evidence includes laparoscopic or ultrasound documentation.

- In pelvic inflammatory disease, responsible organisms are *N. gonorrhoeae, C. trachomatis*, and anaerobes.

Treatment for inpatients includes cefoxitin, 2 g intra-venously every 6 hours, cefotetan, 2 g intravenously every 12 hours, or clindamycin and gentamicin plus doxycy-cline, 100 mg intravenously every 12 hours, followed by doxycycline, 100 mg orally twice a day for 14 days. For outpatients, treatment is with ceftriaxone, 250 mg intra-muscularly once, or cefoxitin, 2 g intramuscularly once, plus doxycycline, 100 mg orally twice a day for 14 days. Hospitalization is indicated when diagnosis is uncertain, pelvic abscess or peritonitis is present, patient is preg-nant, patient is adolescent, HIV infection is present, or noncompliance is suspected. Tubo-ovarian abscess may be characterized by adnexal mass on physical examina-tion or radiographic examination or by failure of antimi-crobial therapy. Medical treatment is successful in 50% of cases. Careful follow-up is required.

- Tubo-ovarian abscess characterized by adnexal mass on physical examination or radiographic examination or by failure of antimicrobial therapy.

Trichomonas vaginalis

Infection with this organism produces a yellow, puru-lent discharge in 5%-40% of cases. Dysuria and dys-pareunia occur in 30%-50% of cases. Petechial lesions on cervix are noted with colposcopy (strawberry cervix) in 50% of cases. The vaginal pH is usually ≥4.5. Diagnosis is established by wet mount preparation of vaginal secretion (80% sensitive). Culture is done in dif-ficult cases. Treatment is with metronidazole, 500 mg twice a day for 7 days. All partners should be examined and treated if necessary.

- *T. vaginalis* infection is often characterized by yellow, purulent discharge.
- Diagnosis established with wet mount of vaginal secre-tion.
- Treatment: metronidazole orally.

Gardnerella vaginalis (Bacterial Vaginosis)

This condition is characterized by malodorous "fishy" smell and a grayish discharge that is homogeneous and coats the vaginal walls. Dysuria and pain are relatively uncommon. Other organisms associated with the syndrome are *Mobiluncus* and *Mycoplasma hominis*. The diagnosis is determined by excluding *Candida* and *Trichomonas* infections and other sexually transmitted diseases. The following are characteristics of the vaginal secretion: demonstration of "clue" cells on wet mount examination, pH >4.5 and often ≥6.0, and a "fishy" smell when secretion is mixed with KOH. Metronidazole, 500 mg twice a day, is standard therapy. Topical clindamycin or metronidozole may also be effective. Treatment of asymptomatic carriers is not recommended.

- Diagnosis of *G. vaginalis* established by excluding *Candida, Trichomonas*, other sexually transmitted diseases.
- Vaginal discharge has "clue" cells and a "fishy" smell when mixed with 10% KOH and has pH >4.5.

Vulvovaginal Candidiasis

The predominant symptom of this condition is pruritus. Usually there is no odor, and discharge is scant, watery, and white. "Cottage cheese curds" may adhere to vaginal wall. Diagnosis is made by addition of 10% KOH to discharge to demonstrate pseudohyphae. Culture may detect asymptomatic carrier. Treatment is with topical miconazole, clotrimazole, butoconazole, terconazole, or tioconazole. Oral azoles (ketoconazole, fluconazole) are used only for severe, refractory cases. In severe or recurrent cases, consider HIV infection.

- In vulvovaginal candidiasis, "cottage cheese curds" may adhere to vaginal wall.
- In severe or recurrent cases, consider HIV infection.

Epididymitis

This condition is usually unilateral. It should be distinguished from testicular torsion. In young, sexually active men, *C. trachomatis* and *N. gonorrhoeae* are the common pathogens. In older men, aerobic gram-negative rods and enterococci predominate. Urologic abnormality is more common in this population than in younger men. Doxycycline, 100 mg orally twice a day for 7 days, plus ceftriaxone, 250 mg intramuscularly, is treatment of choice in young males. In older men, treatment is individualized on basis of results of urine Gram stain, results of culture, local susceptibility patterns, and presence of recent instrumentation.

- Epididymitis usually unilateral; should be distinguished from testicular torsion.
- In young, sexually active men, *C. trachomatis* and *N. gonorrhoeae* are the common pathogens.

GASTROINTESTINAL INFECTION

Bacterial Diarrhea

The principal causes of toxigenic diarrhea are listed in Table 20-16, and those of invasive diarrhea are listed in Table 20-17. Fecal leukocytes are usually absent in toxigenic diarrhea. In invasive diarrhea, fecal leukocytes are usually present.

Campylobacter jejuni is being recognized with increasing frequency as a common cause of bacterial diarrhea. Outbreaks are associated with consumption of unpasteurized milk and undercooked poultry. The incidence of disease peaks in summer and early fall. Diarrhea may be bloody. Fever is usually present. Diagnosis is established by isolation of organism from stool; a special medium is required. Treatment is with erythromycin. Alternatives are ciprofloxacin and norfloxacin (emergence of resistance to fluoroquinolones has been reported). Supportive care is also needed.

- Outbreaks of bacterial diarrhea caused by *C. jejuni* are associated with consumption of unpasteurized milk and undercooked poultry.

In bacterial diarrhea caused by *Staphylococcus aureus*, preformed toxin is ingested in contaminated food. Onset is abrupt, with severe vomiting (often predominates), diarrhea, and abdominal cramps. Duration of infection is 8-24 hours. Diagnosis is based on *rapid onset*, absence of fever, and history. Treatment is supportive.

- Bacterial diarrhea caused by *S. aureus* is caused by ingestion of preformed toxin in contaminated food.

Bacterial diarrhea caused by *Clostridium perfringens* is associated with ingestion of bacteria that produce toxin in vivo in precooked foods (meat and poultry products). Food is precooked and toxin is destroyed but spores survive; when food is rewarmed, spores germinate. When food is ingested, toxin is produced. Diarrhea is worse

Table 20-16.--Bacterial Diarrhea: Toxigenic

Organism	Onset after ingestion, hr	Preformed toxin	Fever present	Vomiting predominates
Staphylococcus aureus	2-6	Yes	No	Yes
Clostridium perfringens	8-16	No	No	No
Escherichia coli	12	No	No	No
Vibrio cholerae	12	No	Secondary to dehydration	No
Bacillus cereus				
a.	1-6	Yes	No	Yes
b.	8-16	No	No	No

Table 20-17.--Bacterial Diarrhea: Invasive

Organism	Fever present	Bloody diarrhea present	Antibiotics effective
Shigella species	Yes	Yes	Yes
Salmonella (non-*typhi*)	Yes	No	No
Vibrio parahaemolyticus	Yes	Yes (occasional)	No
Escherichia coli 0157:H7	Yes	Yes	No
Campylobacter	Yes	Yes	Yes
Yersinia	Yes	Yes (occasional)	±

than vomiting, and abdominal cramping is prominent. Onset of symptoms is later than with *S. aureus* infection. Duration of illness is 24 hours. Diagnosis is based on the later onset of symptoms and a typical history. Treatment is supportive.

- In diarrhea caused by *C. perfringens*, ingested bacteria produce toxin in vivo in precooked food.
- Diarrhea worse than vomiting; abdominal cramping prominent.

Two types of food poisoning are associated with *Bacillus cereus* infection. A short incubation period (1-6 hours) is followed by profuse vomiting; this is associated with the ingestion of a preformed toxin (usually in fried rice). A disease with a longer incubation occurs 8-16 hours after consumption; profound diarrhea develops and is usually associated with eating meat or vegetables. Diagnosis is confirmed by isolation of the organism from contaminated food. The illness is self-limited and treatment is supportive.

Diarrhea caused by *Escherichia coli* can be either enterotoxigenic or enterohemorrhagic. Enterotoxigenic

E. coli is the most common etiologic agent in traveler's diarrhea. Treatment consists of fluid and electrolyte replacement along with loperamide plus trimethoprim-sulfamethoxazole, ciprofloxacin, or norfloxacin. Medical evaluation should be sought if fever and bloody diarrhea occur. For prophylaxis, water, fruits, and vegetables need to be chosen carefully. Routine use of trimethoprim-sulfamethoxazole, ciprofloxacin, and doxycycline is not recommended because the risks outweigh the benefits in most travelers. Bismuth subsalicylate reduces the incidence of enterotoxigen *E. coli*-associated diarrhea by up to 60%. Patients who are allergic to salicylates or who are taking therapeutic doses of salicylates or anticoagulants should not use bismuth subsalicylate.

- Enterotoxigenic *E. coli* is the most common etiologic agent in traveler's diarrhea.

A relatively uncommon form of bloody diarrhea is caused by *E. coli* 0157:H7. This agent has been identified as the cause of waterborne illness (Missouri), outbreaks in nursing homes and child-care centers, and sporadic cases. It has also been transmitted by eating undercooked beef. This mode of transmission was recently the cause of an outbreak in patrons of a fast-food restaurant chain in the state of Washington. This enterohemorrhagic illness is characterized by bloody diarrhea, severe abdominal cramps, fever, and profound toxicity. It may resemble ischemic colitis. At extremes of age (old and young), the infection may produce hemolytic-uremic syndrome, thrombocytopenic purpura, and death. This organism should be considered in all patients with hemolytic-uremic syndrome. Antibiotics are not known to be effective.

- *E. coli* 0157:H7 has been identified as cause of waterborne illness, outbreaks in nursing homes and childcare centers, and sporadic cases.
- Also transmitted by eating undercooked beef.
- Characterized by bloody diarrhea, severe abdominal cramps, profound toxicity; may resemble ischemic colitis.
- Organism should be considered in all patients in age group with hemolytic-uremic syndrome.

Vibrio cholerae causes the only toxigenic bacterial diarrheal disease in which antibiotics (tetracycline) clearly shorten the duration of disease. However, fluid replacement therapy is the mainstay of management. It is associated with consumption of undercooked shellfish. Recently, there was an epidemic in Peru and other parts of South America, and cases in the United States have occurred because of this epidemic.

Diarrhea caused by *Shigella* species is often acquired outside the United States. It is often spread by person-to-person transmission but has also been associated with eating contaminated food or water. Recent outbreak was due to contaminated sandwiches on an airliner. Bloody diarrhea is characteristic, bacteremia may occur, and fever is present. Diagnosis is based on results of stool culture and blood culture (occasionally positive). Treatment is with ampicillin; however, *ampicillin-resistant strains are emerging*. Trimethoprim-sulfamethoxazole is also effective, but in some countries increasing resistance is being reported. Norfloxacin and ciprofloxacin are alternatives. The illness may precede onset of Reiter's syndrome. Neurotoxin may cause seizures in pediatric patients.

- Diarrhea caused by *Shigella* species is associated with person-to-person transmission and the consumption of contaminated food or water.
- Bloody diarrhea is characteristic, bacteremia may occur,

and fever is present.
- Illness may precede onset of Reiter's syndrome.

Salmonella (non-*typhi*)-associated illness is most commonly caused by *S. enteritidis* and *S. typhimurium* in the United States. It is associated with consumption of dehydrated foods or poultry products or with exposure to pet turtles, ducklings, and iguanas. *S. javiana* and *S. oranienburg* are found in contaminated cheese. *Salmonella* infection is common cause of severe diarrhea and may cause septicemia in patients with acquired immunodeficiency syndrome (AIDS). Fever is present, and bloody diarrhea is absent (main characteristic distinguishing it from *Shigella* infection). Diagnosis is based on stool culture. Treatment is supportive. Antibiotics only prolong the carrier state and do not affect the course of the disease. Antibiotics are used if blood culture results are positive. This illness may precede onset of Reiter's syndrome.

- *Salmonella* infection is common cause of severe diarrhea.
- May cause septicemia in patients with AIDS.
- Bloody diarrhea is absent (feature distinguishing it from *Shigella* infection).

Vibrio parahaemolyticus infection is acquired through eating undercooked shellfish. It is a common bacterial cause of acute food-borne illness in Japan and is appearing with increasing frequency in the United States (Atlantic Gulf Coast and on cruise ships). Acute onset of explosive watery diarrhea and fever are characteristic. Diagnosis is determined with stool culture. Antibiotic therapy is not required.

- *V. parahaemolyticus* infection is acquired by eating undercooked shellfish.
- Acute onset of watery diarrhea and fever are characteristic.
- Antibiotic therapy is not required.

Clinical syndromes associated with *Vibrio vulnificus* include bacteremia, gastroenteritis, and cellulitis. Most patients with bacteremia have distinctive bullous skin lesions and underlying hepatic disease (cirrhosis). The condition is associated with consumption of raw oysters. The mortality rate is high. Wound infections occur in patients who have had contact with sea water, such as with fishing injuries or contamination of wound with sea water. Affected patients have intense pain and cellulitis in the extremities. Gastrointestinal illness is associated with consumption of raw oysters. The incubation period is 18 hours. Vomiting, diarrhea, and severe abdominal cramps are features. Treatment is with tetracycline or chloramphenicol.

- *V. vulnificus* bacteremia can cause distinctive bullous skin lesions and occur in patients who are immunocompromised or have cirrhosis.
- Associated with consumption of raw oysters.

Yersinia enterocolitica is the etiologic agent of four major clinical syndromes. Acquisition of infection is associated with eating contaminated food products. Pigs are a common reservoir, and the infection may be associated with eating pork. Recently, the illness was associated with transfusion-related bacteremia.

The four syndromes that result from *Y. enterocolitica* infection are as follows.
1. Enterocolitis is the most common, especially in young children. Diarrhea is bloody in 25% of cases. Infection itself is limited. Antibotic therapy is not necessary. 2. Mesenteric adenitis (pseudoappendicitis syndrome) develops in older children and young adults. Antibiotic therapy is not helpful. 3. Postinfectious syndromes usually occur in adults; these include erythema nodosum, polyarthritis, and Reiter's syndrome. Postinfectious syndromes usually begin 1 to 2 weeks after gastrointestinal symptoms. The polyarthritis often includes weight-bearing joints (knees and ankles). Symptoms may last 1 to 4 months or longer. HLA-B27 antigen may be positive in patients with polyarthritis or Reiter's syndrome but is not associated with erythema nodosum. Cultures of synovial fluid are negative. Diagnosis is by stool culture or serologic testing. 4. Bacteremia is associated with contaminated blood products and alcoholism. Many patients have underlying disease such as cirrhosis. Treatment with trimethoprim-sulfamethoxazole, tetracycline, and gentamicin has been effective.

- Adults with *Y. enterocolitica* infection can develop erythema nodosum, polyarthritis, and Reiter's syndrome.

Colitis caused by *Clostridium difficile* should be distinguished from other forms of antibiotic-associated diarrhea (watery stools, no systemic symptoms, negative tests for *C. difficile* toxin). Symptoms often occur 2-4 weeks after stopping use of antibiotics. The illness is associated with antibiotic exposure in 99% of cases (any antibi-

otic can cause it). Nosocomial spread has been documented. Typical features are profuse, watery stools, crampy abdominal pain, constitutional illness, fecal leukocyte value >50%, positive for *C. difficile* toxin. In toxin-negative disease, proctoscopy or flexible sigmoidoscopy can be used to look for pseudomembranes. Disease can be localized to cecum (postoperative patient with ileus) and can present as fever of unknown origin. Treatment consists of vancomycin (125 mg orally four times a day for 7-10 days) or metronidazole (250-500 mg orally three to four times a day for 7-10 days). Cost differences favor metronidazole. Antiperistalsis drugs should not be used. If patient is unable to take drugs orally, intravenous metronidazole (not vancomycin) or vancomycin enemas can be used. Relapse is frequent and requires re-treatment. Treatment of asymptomatic carriers to decrease nosocomial spread of infection or to reduce risk of pseudomembranous colitis is not recommended.

- Colitis caused by *C. difficile* often occurs 2-4 weeks after stopping use of antibiotics.
- Illness is associated with antibiotic exposure in 99% of cases (any antibiotic can cause it).
- Features: profuse watery stools, crampy abdominal pain, constitutional illness, fecal leukocyte >50%, positive for *C. difficile* toxin.
- Treatment: vancomycin (125 mg orally four times a day for 7-10 days) or metronidazole (250-500 mg orally three to four times a day for 7-10 days).
- Relapse is frequent (about 15% of cases).

Viral Diarrhea

Rotavirus infection is the most common cause of sporadic mild diarrhea illness in children. It may be spread from children to adults. It usually occurs during the winter. Vomiting is more common early manifestation than watery diarrhea. Hospitalization for dehydration is common in young children. Diagnosis is made by detection of antigen in stool (enzyme-linked immunosorbent assay). Treatment is symptomatic.

Norwalk virus is a common cause of epidemic diarrhea and "winter vomiting disease" in older children and adults. It occurs in families, communities, and institutions. Outbreaks have been associated with eating shellfish, undercooked fish, cake frosting, and salads and with drinking contaminated water. It is the cause of up to 10% of gastroenteritis outbreaks. Illness is characterized by nausea, vomiting, and watery diarrhea. It is a mild, self-limited (<36 hours) illness. Currently, no diagnostic test is available. Treatment is symptomatic.

- Outbreaks of Norwalk virus are associated with eating shellfish, undercooked fish, cake frosting, and salads and with drinking contaminated water.
- Illness is mild, self-limited (<36 hours).

SEPTIC SHOCK

This clinical syndrome is characterized by impaired tissue perfusion, hypotension, and multiorgan dysfunction in the setting of infection (blood cultures positive in 50%-60% of cases). Causative organism is gram-negative aerobic bacilli in 70% of cases, gram-positive aerobic cocci in 20%-30%, and other organisms in 2%-3% (i.e., *Candida* species). In septic shock, most frequent blood isolates are *Escherichia coli*, *Klebsiella-Enterobacter*, *Proteus*, *Pseudomonas*, *Staphylococcus aureus*, and *Streptococcus pneumoniae*. Frequency of any one organism depends on the host (i.e., neutropenia is associated with *P. aeruginosa*, central lines are associated with coagulase-negative staphylococci, *S. aureus*, and *Candida* species). Overall mortality rate is 20%-30%. Endotoxin activates endogenous mediators of inflammation with catastrophic consequences. Result can be increased vascular permeability, a decrease in peripheral vascular resistance, profound hypotension with progressive lactic acidosis, and death. Management involves maintaining intravascular volume, administering appropriate bactericidal antimicrobials, and correcting any problems that lead to infection (e.g., draining abscesses). Steroids are of no benefit and may be harmful.

- In septic shock, blood cultures positive in 50%-60% of cases.
- Most frequent blood isolates: *E. coli*, *Klebsiella-Enterobacter*, *Proteus*, *Pseudomonas*, *S. aureus*, *S. pneumoniae*.
- Endotoxin activates endogenous mediators of inflammation with catastrophic consequences.

GRANULOCYTOPENIA

This condition is characterized by an absolute polymorphonuclear neutrophil value ≤500/mm^3. If ecthyma gangrenosum is present, *Pseudomonas* infection should be considered. Other gram-negative aerobic rods (i.e., *Escherichia coli*) also cause bacteremia. Aerobic gram-positive cocci (*Staphylococcus aureus*, coagulase-nega-

tive staphylococci, enterococci, viridans streptococci, *C. jeikeium*) are often associated with infection in neutropenic patients with central venous catheters. *Candida* species should be considered in cases associated with nodular skin lesions, fluffy white chorioretinal exudates, and fever unresponsive to empiric antibacterial agents. Anaerobic organisms are uncommon, except in cases of perirectal abscess and gingivitis. Empiric antimicrobial therapy is required. Ceftazidime alone is the preferred initial empiric antibacterial regimen. Alternative therapy is an aminoglycoside plus an antipseudomonal penicillin. There is no need to use vancomycin empirically. If subsequent cultures show presence of staphylococci, vancomycin can be added to regimen. If there is no response after 4-7 days of treatment, amphotericin B therapy is often recommended.

URINARY TRACT INFECTION

In Females

Table 20-18 outlines the categories of acute dysuria.

Because urethritis or cystitis can occur with low colony counts of bacteria, routine urine cultures in young women with dysuria are not recommended. Urinalysis should be done with or without a Gram stain. If pyuria and uncomplicated urinary tract infection (UTI) are present, short-course treatment should be initiated. Only if occult upper tract disease, a complicated UTI, or sexually transmitted disease is suspected should appropriate culture and sensitivity testing be performed. Risk factors for occult infection and complications include emergency room presentation, low socioeconomic status, hospital-acquired infection, pregnancy, use of Foley catheter, recent instrumentation, known urologic abnormality, previous relapse, UTI at age <12 years, acute pyelonephritis or three or more UTIs in 1 year, symptoms ≥7 days, recent antibiotic use, diabetes mellitus, and immunosuppression. Causative organisms include *Escherichia coli* and *Staphylococcus saprophyticus* (susceptible to ampicillin and trimethoprim-sulfamethoxazole).

- Routine urine cultures not recommended in young women with dysuria.
- Associated organisms: *E. coli*, *S. saprophyticus* (susceptible to trimethoprim-sulfamethoxazole).

For first episode of cystitis or urethritis, treatment is given but no investigation is needed. Trimethoprim-sulfamethoxazole is more effective than ampicillin. Short-course treatment (single-dose) has fewer side effects than standard (7-10 days) therapy, but the risk of relapse (due to retention of viable organisms in vaginal or perivaginal area) is higher. Three-day therapy may be associated with relapse rates equal to those with treatment for 7-10 days with less toxicity. If recurrence develops after 3-day therapy, subclinical pyelonephritis is likely and treatment is then given for 14 days. Urologic evaluation is usually not necessary. It should be performed in patients with multiple relapses, painless hematuria, a his-tory of childhood UTI, renal lithiasis, and recurrent pyelo-nephritis.

- For first episode of cystitis or urethritis, trimethoprim-sulfamethoxazole is more effective than ampicillin.
- Short-course treatment (3 days) has fewer side effects than standard (7-10 days) therapy, and risk of relapse of infection may be the same.
- Urologic evaluation should be done in patients with multiple relapses, painless hematuria, history of child-hood UTI, renal lithiasis, and recurrent pyelonephritis.

Table 20-18.--Categorization of Acute Dysuria

Category	Site affected			Colony count	Pyuria present	Antimicrobial treatment effective
	Upper tract	Bladder	Urethra			
Subclinical pyelo-nephritis	Yes	Yes	Yes	>100,000	Yes	Yes
Lower UTI--urethritis or cystitis	No	Yes	Yes	>100	Yes	Yes
Chlamydia, HSV, *Neisseria gonorrhoeae*	No	No	Yes	0-100	Yes	Yes
No recognized pathogen	No	?	Yes	0-100	No	No
Vaginitis	No	No	No	0-100	No	Yes

HSV, herpes simplex virus; UTI, urinary tract infection.

For acute pyelonephritis, 2 weeks of therapy is equal in efficacy to 6 weeks of therapy. Most patients are suf-ficiently ill to require hospitalization. Many are bac-teremic. Unless gram-positive cocci are seen on Gram stain (?enterococci), a third-generation cephalosporin can be used as empiric therapy. If enterococci are suspect-ed, use ampicillin or mezlocillin with or without gen-tamicin. Oral regimens can be quickly substituted as the patient improves. A urine culture is recommended at the completion of therapy. If relapse occurs, treatment is given for 6 weeks and a urologic evaluation is done. For recurrent lower UTI (more than two episodes per year), single-dose therapy, 3-day therapy, or 6-week therapy is used. For treatment failure, chronic suppressive therapy may be used; however, the risk of resistant organisms must be weighed.

- For acute pyelonephritis, 2 weeks of therapy is equal in efficacy to 6 weeks of therapy.
- Urine culture recommended at 2 weeks after therapy.

In Males
UTI is less common in males than females. Urologic abnormalities (e.g., benign prostatic hyperplasia) are com-mon. Symptoms are unreliable for localization. Physical examination should include prostate examination, retrac-tion of foreskin to look for discharge, and palpation of testicle and epididymides. When a UTI is suspected, urine culture and sensitivity testing should always be done. Causative organisms include *E. coli* in 50% of cases, other gram-negative organisms in 25%, entero-cocci in 20%, and others in 5%. If signs and symptoms of epididymitis, acute prostatitis, and pyelonephritis are present, treat accordingly. If uncomplicated lower UTI is present, treat for 10-14 days. If symptoms persist or relapse, repeat the urine culture. If results are positive, treat for a minimum of 6 weeks. If culture results are negative, consider chronic prostatitis or nonbacterial or noninfectious diseases and treat accordingly.

- Causes of UTI in males: *E. coli* in 50%, other gram-negative organisms in 25%, enterococci in 20%, others in 5%.

ANAEROBIC SOFT TISSUE INFECTIONS

These may be caused by various aerobic and anaerobic organisms. Findings and treatments for these are outlined in Table 20-19.

BONE AND JOINT INFECTIONS

Acute Bacterial Arthritis (Nongonococcal)

This is most commonly due to hematogenous spread of bacteria. The hip and knee joints are commonly involved. Bacteria involved are gram-positive aerobic cocci (about 75% of cases): *Staphylococcus aureus* (most common), β-hemolytic streptococci, and *Streptococcus pneumoniae*. Gram-negative aerobic bacilli can also cause infection (about 20% of cases); *Pseudomonas aeruginosa* is a common cause in injection drug users. Anaerobes, fungi, and mycobacteria are unusual causes. Clinical features include involvement usually of monoarticular, large joints. Fever, pain, swelling, and restriction of motion are the most frequent signs and symptoms. Synovial fluid is usually turbid, and leukocyte count is 10,000-300,000/μL (predominantly polymorphonuclear neutrophils). The condition may overlap with other inflammatory arthropathies. Gram stain is 50%-95% sensitive. Culture results are positive unless antibiotics have been used previously or the pathogen is unusual. Blood culture results are often positive. Radiographs are not helpful in routine cases because destructive changes have not had time to occur. Specific antimicrobial therapy is based on results of Gram stain, culture, and sensitivity testing. Duration of therapy is dependent on individual circumstances, such as presence of complicating osteomyelitis. Usually, treatment is given for 2-6 weeks. Empiric therapy should include agents directed against *S. aureus* and gram-negative bacilli. Drainage is essential. Percutaneous, arthroscopic, or open procedures are used. Hip, shoulder, and sternoclavicular joint involvement, development of loculations, and persistently positive culture results (not due to resistant organisms) are standard indications for arthroscopy or open debridement.

- Acute bacterial arthritis (nongonococcal) is most commonly due to hematogenous spread of bacteria.
- Bacteria involved are gram-positive aerobic cocci (about 75% of cases): *S. aureus* is most common.
- Monoarticular, large joints usually involved.
- Fever, pain, swelling, and restriction of motion are frequent.
- Synovial fluid is turbid; leukocyte count is 10,000-300,000/μL.
- Blood culture results positive in 50% of cases.
- Drainage is essential.

Viral Arthritis

This is usually transient, self-limited polyarthritis. It may be caused by rubella (may also occur after vaccination), hepatitis B, mumps, coxsackievirus, adenovirus, and parvovirus B19.

Chronic Monoarticular Arthritis

Organisms involved include *Mycobacteria* (*M. tuber-*

Table 20-19.--Findings and Treatment in Anaerobic Soft Tissue Infections

	Gas gangrene (organism: *Clostridium perfringens*)	Anaerobic cellulitis (polymicrobial)
Clinical finding		
Gas in tissues	1+	4+
Muscle necrosis	Present by definition	Absent by definition
Pain	4+	1+
Appearance	Skin is taut, swollen, edematous, pale; minimal crepitation	4+ crepitation
Treatment	Immediate wide debridement or amputation, antibiotics, ± hyperbaric oxygen treatment	Antibiotics alone, local wound care, incision and drainage

culosis is more common than *M. avium-intercellulare, M. kansasii, M. marinum*), fungi (*Coccidioides immitis* and *Sporothrix schenckii* are more common than *Histoplasma capsulatum*--rare, *Blastomyces dermatitidis*--acute, and *Candida* species--acute), and others (*Brucella, Nocardia*).

- *M. tuberculosis, Coccidioides,* and *Blastomyces* involved in chronic monoarticular arthritis.

Osteomyelitis

Acute hematogenous osteomyelitis is more common in infants and children than adults. Metaphysis of long bones (femur, tibia) is most commonly affected. *S. aureus* is the most common organism. Acute onset of pain and fever are typical features. The illness can present with pain only. Compatible radiographic changes and bone biopsy for culture and pathologic examination are used to establish the diagnosis. Blood culture results may be positive. Specific parenteral antibiotic therapy is used for 3-6 weeks on basis of culture and sensitivity test results. Debridement is usually not necessary unless sequestrum is present.

- *S. aureus* is most common organism in acute hematogenous osteomyelitis.
- Acute onset of pain and fever are typical features.

Chronic osteomyelitis is more common in adults. It results from direct inoculation caused by trauma or adjacent soft tissue infection, for example. Open fractures and diabetic foot ulcers are common predisposing factors. *S. aureus* is the most common organism. Coagulase-negative staphylococci is often a pathogen if a foreign body (e.g., plate, screws) is present. Often, osteomyelitis complicating a foot ulcer is polymicrobial, including aerobic gram-positive and gram-negative organisms and anaerobes. Local pain, tenderness, erythema, and draining sinuses are common. Fever is atypical unless there is concurrent cellulitis. The condition can present with pain only. Compatible radiographic changes (often vague) and bone biopsy for culture and pathologic examination are used to establish the diagnosis. Blood culture results are rarely positive. Adequate debridement, removal of dead space, soft tissue coverage, and fixation of infected fractures are essential. Specific parenteral antibiotic therapy is given for 4-6 weeks on basis of culture and sensitivity test results.

- *S. aureus* is most common organism in chronic osteomyelitis.
- Coagulase-negative staphylococci is a common pathogen if foreign body is present.
- Local pain, tenderness, erythema, and draining sinuses are common.
- Specific parenteral antibiotic therapy is given for 4-6 weeks.

Vertebral Osteomyelitis

This condition often results from hematogenous dissemination from focal source of infection (e.g., urinary tract, pneumonia). *S. aureus* and gram-negative bacilli are the major pathogens. Only 10% of cases have positive blood culture results. Symptoms include pain and local tenderness. Fever may be present. Leukocyte count may be normal or elevated. Sedimentation rate is often increased. Plain radiographs do not show destruction early in the course of disease. Gallium scan is approximately 80% sensitive. Magnetic resonance imaging is diagnostic test of choice because it is sensitive and specific and shows anatomic detail (coexistent epidural abscess). Percutaneous needle biopsy (computed tomography-guided) or open biopsy of bone or disc tissue may be needed. Treatment includes appropriate parenteral antimicrobial therapy for 4-6 weeks. Drainage may be necessary if a concomitant epidural abscess is present.

- In vertebral osteomyelitis, *S. aureus* and gram-negative bacilli are major pathogens.
- Gallium scan is about 80% sensitive; magnetic resonance imaging is diagnostic test of choice.

SINUSITIS IN ADULTS

The physician's overall impression as to presence or absence of sinusitis is the best clinical predictor of disease. Independent clinical predictors of disease are maxillary toothache, poor transillumination, poor response to decongestants, and a history or examination finding of purulent discharge. Pertinent sinus radiographic findings include membrane thickening ≥6 mm (maxillary sinus), opaque sinuses, or air-fluid level. Organisms involved are *Haemophilus influenzae, Streptococcus pneumoniae,* and oral anaerobes. Treatment is with oral trimethoprim-sulfamethoxazole, amoxicillin/clavulanate, or cefuroxime axetil.

- Organisms involved in sinusitis in adults are *H. influenzae, S. pneumoniae,* oral anaerobes.

HEPATIC (BACTERIAL) ABSCESS

Mechanisms of bacterial abscess include portal vein bacteremia resulting from, for example, appendicitis and diverticulitis, bacteremia caused by a primary focus elsewhere in the body, ascending cholangitis, direct extension (subphrenic abscess), or trauma. Fever is common. Right upper quadrant pain, tenderness on percussion, and increased values on liver function tests may or may not be present. Computed tomography and ultrasonography are very helpful in diagnosis. Bacteriology depends on the mechanism of abscess formation. Intra-abdominal infection is often caused by polymicrobial aerobic gram-negative rods, anaerobic streptococci, and *Bacteroides* species. Treatment is individualized and depends on suspected and isolated organisms. Empiric therapy with clindamycin or metronidazole plus third-generation cephalosporin or aminoglycoside is appropriate. If hematogenous route is suspected, antistaphylococcal agent should be used in regimen. Drainage (surgical or percutaneous) is of primary importance.

TOXIC SHOCK SYNDROME

This syndrome is caused by the establishment or growth of a toxin-producing strain of *Staphylococcus aureus* in a non-immune person. Clinical scenarios associated with this syndrome include young menstruating women with prolonged, continuous use of tampons, postoperative and nonoperative wound infections, localized abscesses, and *S. aureus* pneumonia developing after influenza. It is a multisystem disease. Clinical criteria include fever, hypotension, erythroderma (often leads to desquamation, particularly on palms and soles), and involvement in three or more organ systems. Onset is acute; blood culture results are usually negative. Condition is caused by production of staphylococcal toxin (TSST-1). Treatment is supportive; subsequent episodes are treated with β-lactam antibiotic, which decreases frequency and severity of subsequent attacks. Relapse rate may be as high as 30%-40% (menstruation-related disease). Mortality rate is 5%-10%.

- Toxic shock syndrome caused by toxin-producing strain of *S. aureus* in non-immune person.
- Multisystem disease: fever, hypotension, erythroderma (often leads to desquamation, particularly on palms and soles).
- Onset is acute; blood culture results usually negative.
- Condition is caused by production of staphylococcal toxin (TSST-1).

TOXIC STREPTOCOCCAL SYNDROME

This is similar to toxic shock syndrome. Patients have invasive group A streptococcal infections with associated hypotension and two of the following: renal impairment, coagulopathy, liver impairment, adult respiratory distress syndrome, rash (may desquamate), or soft tissue necrosis. It is caused by group A streptococci. Symptoms are caused by production of streptococcal toxin (pyrogenic exotoxin A). Most patients have skin or soft tissue infection, are <50 years old, and are otherwise healthy compared with patients with invasive group A streptococcal infections without the toxic streptococcal syndrome. Most are bacteremic (different from toxic shock syndrome due to *Staphylococcus aureus*). Treatment is with appropriate antibiotics, supportive care, and surgical debridement in some cases. Case-fatality rate is 30%.

- Toxic streptococcal syndrome is caused by group A streptococci.
- Symptoms caused by production of streptococcal toxin.
- Most patients are bacteremic (different from toxic shock syndrome due to *S. aureus*).

INFECTIONS IN SOLID ORGAN TRANSPLANTATION

Spectrum of potential pathogens in patients after solid organ transplantation is diverse. Individual risk of specific infection can be classified according to the following: symptoms and signs of illness at presentation (i.e., meningitis vs. pneumonia), posttransplantation time course, serostatus of recipient and donor for certain infections (e.g., cytomegalovirus, toxoplasmosis), type of organ transplantation, type and duration of immunosuppression, type of antimicrobial prophylaxis patient has received, and travel history and previous exposure to pathogens (e.g., tuberculosis, cocci). The time of occurrence of opportunistic infections in solid organ transplantation is given in Table 20-20.

ANTIMICROBIALS

The mechanisms of action, spectrum of activity, route of excretion, and toxicities of various antimicrobial agents are emphasized. Some of this information is given in Tables 20-21 through 20-25.

Table 20-20.--Opportunistic Infections in Solid Organ Transplantation

Month	Type of infection after transplantation
1	Bacterial infections: related to wound, intravenous lines, urinary tract
	Herpes simplex virus; hepatitis B
1-4	Cytomegalovirus, *Pneumocystic carinii*, *Listeria monocytogenes*, *M. tuberculosis*, *Aspergillus*, *Nocardia*, *Toxoplasma*, hepatitis B, *Legionella*
2-6	Epstein-Barr virus, varicella-zoster virus, hepatitis C, *Legionella*
>6	*Cryptococcus neoformans*, *Legionella*

Table 20-21.--Routes of Excretion of Antimicrobial Agents

Antibiotic	Major route of excretion
Penicillins*	Kidney
Cephalosporins†	Kidney
Aztreonam	Kidney
Imipenem	Kidney
Aminoglycosides	Kidney
Vancomycin	Kidney
Erythromycin	Liver
Clindamycin	Liver
Chloramphenicol	Liver
Tetracycline‡	Kidney
Flucytosine	Kidney
Rifampin	Liver
Cotrimoxazole	Kidney
Metronidazole	Liver
Fluoroquinolones	Kidney

*Nafcillin and oxacillin are excreted by the liver.

†Cefoperazone and ceftriaxone are excreted primarily in bile.

‡Metabolism in liver, excretion by kidneys. Doxycycline is eliminated by the liver.

SPECIFIC ANTIBACTERIAL AGENTS

Penicillins

Natural Penicillins

These *agents* are penicillin G (intravenous, i.v.), penicillin VK (oral), procaine penicillin (intramuscular, i.m.), and benzathine penicillin (i.m., repository formulation).

Their *spectrum of activity* includes nonpenicillinase-producing staphylococci, β-hemolytic streptococci (group A, B, C, G), viridans streptococci, group D streptococci, penicillin-susceptible *Streptococcus pneumoniae*, *Neisseria gonorrhoeae*, *N. meningitidis*, and susceptible anaerobes (*Clostridium* species, oral *Bacteroides* species, *Peptostreptococcus*, and *Fusobacterium*). Enterococci are inhibited but not killed by the natural penicillins. Less common microbes that these agents are active against include *Erysipelothrix*, *Listeria monocytogenes*, *Pasteurella multocida*, *Streptobacillus*, *Spirillum*, *Treponema pallidum*, *Borrelia burgdorferi*, and *Actinomyces israelii*.

Toxicity to these agents includes hypersensitivity reactions. These are the most common adverse reactions (3%-10% of cases). These reactions include maculopapular rash, urticaria, angioedema, serum sickness, and anaphylaxis. True anaphylaxis occurs in 0.004%-0.015% of patients receiving penicillin. Intravenous preparations cause more frequent allergic reactions than oral agents. Skin testing in difficult cases can be used to predict subsequent severe (type I) penicillin allergy but will not predict maculopapular drug eruptions. Patients allergic to one penicillin should be considered allergic to all penicillins. Furthermore, there is a cross-allergenicity rate of 3%-7% with cephalosporin compounds. Cephalosporins should be avoided when possible in patients who have had a severe, immediate penicillin allergy (type I anaphylaxis or urticarial eruption). An intestinal side effect is diarrhea, including *Clostridium difficile* colitis. Hematologic side effects are neutropenia, platelet dysfunction, and hemolytic anemia. Drug fever can also occur. Central nervous system side effects with penicillin G, when given in high doses, may involve tremors, lowered seizure threshold, and neuromuscular irritability.

- With natural penicillins, intravenous preparations cause more frequent allergic reactions than oral agents.
- There is a cross-allergenicity rate of 3%-7% with cephalosporin compounds.

Aminopenicillins

The *agents* are ampicillin and amoxicillin (increased gastrointestinal absorption, decreased incidence of diarrhea, and dosing three times a day are major advantages compared with oral ampicillin).

Their *spectrum of activity* extends the antibacterial spectrum of the natural penicillins to include certain strains of *Escherichia coli*, *Proteus mirabilis*, *Salmonella*, *Shigella* (amoxicillin is less active than ampicillin), and β-lactamase-negative *Haemophilus influenzae* and *Moraxella*

Table 20-22.--Mechanisms of Action of Antibiotics

Cell wall	Protein synthesis	Cell membrane	Cell synthesis	RNA synthesis
Penicillins	Aminoglycosides	Amphotericin B	Naladixic acid	Rifampin
Cephalosporins	Tetracycline	Azoles	Quinolones	
Vancomycin	Clindamycin		Flucytosine	
Imipenem	Chloramphenicol			
Aztreonam	Erythromycin			
	Metronidazole			

Table 20-23.--Antimicrobials and Renal Failure

Antibiotics that do not require reduction of dosage in renal failure
Nafcillin, oxacillin
Cefoperazone, ceftriaxone
Erythromycin*
Clindamycin
Chloramphenicol
Metronidazole
Rifampin
Doxycycline

*May accumulate in patients on hemodialysis and cause reversible deafness.

catarrhalis.

Toxicity is the same as outlined under Natural Penicillins (page 553). Rash is common when these agents are given to patients with infectious mononucleosis.

Penicillinase-Resistant Penicillins

Agents include methicillin (i.v.), oxacillin (i.v.), nafcillin (i.v.), dicloxacillin (oral), and cloxacillin (oral).

Spectrum of activity includes methicillin-susceptible *Staphylococcus aureus.* Treatment of serious infections caused by methicillin-susceptible coagulase-negative staphylococci with these agents is controversial because of the difficulty of detecting resistance in the laboratory. Penicillinase-resistant penicillins have no gram-negative or anaerobic activity but are active against most nonenterococcal streptococci.

Their *toxicities* are the same as outlined under Natural Penicillins (page 553). Nephritis (methicillin), phlebitis (nafcillin), and hepatitis (oxacillin) can occur.

● Penicillinase-resistant penicillins are primarily used for treatment of methicillin-susceptible *S. aureus.*

Carboxypenicillins

Agents include carbenicillin and ticarcillin.

The carboxypenicillins have a broader gram-negative *spectrum of activity* than ampicillin. When used as antipseudomonal agents, they are used in combination with an aminoglycoside to provide synergism and to prevent the emergence of resistant organisms. They have little or no activity against staphylococci, streptococci, enterococci, or *Klebsiella* species. Because ticarcillin has more (2-4 times) antipseudomonal activity in vitro, it is more effective in smaller quantities than carbenicillin against *Pseudomonas aeruginosa*; thus, the adverse effects of large quantities of carbenicillin can be avoided.

Toxicity is the same as described under Natural Penicillins (page 553). Sodium overload, hypokalemia, and platelet dysfunction can occur.

● Carboxypenicillins have little or no activity against staphylococci, streptococci, enterococci, or *Klebsiella* species.

Ureidopenicillins

Agents include mezlocillin, piperacillin, and azlocillin.

These agents have a wide *spectrum of activity* against gram-negative bacteria. Compared with carbenicillin and ticarcillin, they have a lower sodium content per gram, less associated hypokalemia, less platelet inhibition, and greater hepatic excretion. Compared with penicillin G and ampicillin, they are slightly less active against streptococci and enterococci (except mezlocillin), but they are more active against *H. influenzae.* Mezlocillin is more active than carbenicillin and ticarcillin against Enterobacteriaceae, including most strains of *Klebsiella.* It is also more active than ticarcillin against *Bacteroides fragilis.* Its activity against *Pseudomonas* is similar to that of ticarcillin. Azlocillin is more active than ticarcillin against *Pseudomonas* species; however, piperacillin is the most active penicillin against this organism. Like carboxypenicillins, combination therapy with an aminoglycoside may forestall the frequent emergence of resistance by *Pseudomonas* and *Enterobacter* species. Because

Table 20-24.--Cerebrospinal Fluid Penetration of Antibiotics

Excellent without inflammation	Good with inflammation	Fair	Poor or none
Chloramphenicol	Penicillin G	Aminoglycosides	Clindamycin
Flucytosine	Carbenicillin	Amphotericin B	Erythromycin
Rifampin	Nafcillin,	Ketoconazole	Cefazolin
Metronidazole	oxacillin	Itraconazole	
Fluconazole	Ampicillin		
	Cefuroxime		
	Cefotaxime		
	Ceftizoxime		
	Ceftazidime		
	Ceftriaxone		
	Cotrimoxazole		
	(trimethoprim-		
	sulfamethoxazole)		
	Imipenem		
	Ciprofloxacin		

Table 20-25.--Mechanisms of Resistance to Antibiotics

Mechanism	Antibiotic
β-Lactamase production: hydrolyze β-lactam ring so molecule cannot bind to pencillin-binding proteins	Penicillins
	Cephalosporins
	Monobactams
Mutation with altered affinity for penicillin-binding protein (penicillin-resistant pneumococci, methicillin-resistant staphylococci)	Penicillins
	Cephalosporins
	Monobactams
	Carbapenems
Modifying enzymes, plasmid mediated: acetyltransferases, phosphotransferases, adenyltransferases	Aminoglycosides (amikacin and netilmicin resistant to some of these enzymes)
	Chloramphenicol
Alteration ribosomal target site	Streptomycin
Acquired changes in permeability	Aminoglycosides, imipenem
Prevention of binding with ribosomes	Clindamycin
	Erythromycin
Alteration of active transport system	Tetracycline
Single-step mutation	Rifampin
Plasmid-mediated production of enzymes used in folic acid production	Trimethoprim-sulfamethoxazole
Alterations in DNA gyrase	Quinolones

of the cost of ureidopenicillins, the need for frequent dosing, and frequency of primary resistance (20%-40%) among certain Enterobacteriaceae, their use is becoming less common.

Toxicity is the same as detailed under Natural Penicillins (page 553). Other effects are hypokalemia (less common than with carbenicillin and ticarcillin), bleeding (less than with carbenicillin and ticarcillin), and hepatitis (similar to that with carbenicillin and ticarcillin).

β-Lactamase Inhibitors

Agents in this group are amoxicillin/clavulanate, ampicillin/sulbactam, and ticarcillin/clavulanate.

Spectrum of activity is increased by the addition of β-lactamase inhibitors; this results in activity against β-lactamase-producing organisms such as *S. aureus, B. fragilis, Klebsiella pneumoniae, H. influenzae,* and *M. catarrhalis.* These agents are not active against methicillin-resistant *S. aureus* and do not change the activity of the parent compound against most strains of *Pseudomonas.*

Toxicity is the same as discussed under Natural Penicillins (page 553) and the parent compounds. Clavulanate may rarely cause hepatitis.

- β-Lactamase inhibitors are not active against methicillin-resistant *S. aureus.*

Cephalosporins

First-Generation Cephalosporins

Representative agents are cefazolin (long serum half-life allows dosing every 8 hours), cephalothin, and cephalexin.

The *spectrum of activity* of the first-generation agents includes being active against staphylococci, β-hemolytic streptococci, penicillin-susceptible (minimal inhibitory concentration <0.12) pneumococci, and many strains of *Proteus mirabilis, E. coli,* and *Klebsiella* species. They are not active, as are all cephalosporins, against methicillin-resistant staphylococci, enterococci, *L. monocytogenes, Legionella* species, *Chlamydia pneumoniae, Mycoplasma pneumoniae,* and *C. difficile.*

Cephalosporins are usually well tolerated. *Toxicity* can include adverse reactions related to the gastrointestinal tract (e.g., nausea, vomiting, diarrhea); these are the most common. Hypersensitivity reactions, primarily rashes, occur in 1%-3% of patients taking cephalosporins. Anaphylaxis is extremely rare. Cross-allergenicity may occur with penicillins. Other adverse reactions associated with cephalosporins include drug fever and *C. difficile* colitis.

- First-generation cephalosporins are not active against methicillin-resistant staphylococci.

Second-Generation Cephalosporins

Representative agents are cefamandole, cefoxitin, cefuroxime, and cefotetan. *Toxicity* with these agents is similar to that with the first-generation cephalosporins unless specified.

Cefamandole has limited advantage over cefazolin and is more expensive. It has some increase in activity against *E. coli, Klebsiella,* indole-positive *Proteus, Enterobacter,* and non-β-lactamase-producing *H. influenzae.* The methylthiotetrazole (MTT) side chain causes bleeding problems and a disulfiram-like reaction. Dosing is every 4-6 hours.

Cefoxitin has some increase in activity over first-generation agents against *E. coli, Klebsiella,* indole-positive *Proteus,* and *Serratia.* It is less active against *S. aureus* than first-generation cephalosporins. It is active against most strains of *B. fragilis.* It is used for treatment of intra-abdominal infections and pelvic inflammatory disease (in combination with doxycycline). Dosing is every 4-6 hours.

Cefuroxime has good activity against *S. aureus* and β-lactamase-producing *H. influenzae.* It is the only second-generation agent with good penetration of the central nervous system. It is used to treat community-acquired pneumonia and meningitis (except *Listeria*). Dosing is every 8 hours.

Cefotetan is similar to cefoxitin in activity against gram-positive cocci and *B. fragilis,* but it has better activity than cefoxitin against aerobic gram-negative rods. It has the MTT side chain with the associated toxicities described for cefamandole.

Third-Generation Cephalosporins

Representative agents are moxalactam, cefotaxime, ceftizoxime, ceftriaxone, and cefoperazone. Their *toxicity* is similar to that with the first-generation cephalosporins unless specified.

Moxalactam is active against most gram-negative Enterobacteriaceae, many *Pseudomonas* species, anaerobes including *B. fragilis,* and *H. influenzae.* Moxalactam is inactive against enterococci and is less active than first- and second-generation cephalosporins against streptococci and staphylococci. Moxalactam is highly active against *H. influenzae.* It has good cerebrospinal fluid penetration. Moxalactam has the MTT side chain with the associated toxicities described for cefamandole.

Cefotaxime is less active against *Pseudomonas* than ceftazidime or cefoperazone. It has better activity against staphylococci and streptococci than moxalactam, ceftazidime, and cefoperazone. It has good cerebrospinal fluid penetration. It is the drug of choice along with ceftriaxone for community-acquired meningitis (except *Listeria*). It is more effective than cefuroxime in *H. influenzae* meningitis. Desacetyl metabolite may allow dosing every 8 hours except in life-threatening infections.

Ceftizoxime is less active against *P. aeruginosa* than ceftazidime and cefoperazone. Activity against anaerobes is limited. It is essentially the same as cefotaxime.

Ceftriaxone has activity similar to that of other third-generation cephalosporins but is less active against *Pseudomonas* than ceftazidime and cefoperazone. It is less active against *S. aureus* than cefotaxime. One of its advantages is the long half-life (8 hours); thus, it can be given in a single daily dose. It has good cerebrospinal fluid penetration. It has been reported to cause pseudocholelithiasis, cholelithiasis, biliary colic, and cholecystitis as a result of biliary precipitation of ceftriaxone as the calcium salt in up to 2% of cases, especially in children. This effect usually resolves with discontinuation of therapy.

Cefoperazone is more active against *Pseudomonas* than is moxalactam. It is less active against anaerobes than moxalactam. Its activity against other gram-positive cocci is the same as that of moxalactam. Penetration into cerebrospinal fluid is less than that of other available third-generation cephalosporins. Advantages include its excretion primarily in the bile; therefore, there is no change in dose with abnormal renal function. Cefoperazone has the MTT side chain with the associated toxicities described for cefamandole.

In regard to its *spectrum of activity*, ceftazidime is much more active than any other third-generation cephalosporin against *Pseudomonas*. It is less active against *S. aureus* and streptococci than most other third-generation cephalosporins. Pseudomonads may acquire resistance if the drug is used alone. It is often used empirically in patients with neutropenic fever. It penetrates into cerebrospinal fluid as well as cefotaxime and ceftriaxone.

- Ceftazidime is more active than any other third-generation cephalosporin against *Pseudomonas*.

Imipenem

Imipenem is a new, broad-spectrum β-lactam. Its mechanism of action is similar to that of other β-lactam congeners (i.e., inhibition of cell wall synthesis). Bacterial resistance, particularly among *P. aeruginosa*, is increasing and is mediated by various mechanisms. Imipenem is administered intravenously and is hydrolyzed in the kidney by a peptidase located in the brush border of renal tubular cells. Administration with cilastatin, a dihydropeptidase inhibitor, solves this problem.

Imipenem has the broadest antibacterial activity of any antibiotic currently available. Its *spectrum of activity* includes excellent activity against *Pseudomonas*, anaerobes including *B. fragilis*, β-hemolytic streptococci, pneumococci, methicillin-susceptible *S. aureus*, enterococci (inhibited only), Enterobacteriaceae, *H. influenzae*, and *Nocardia*. The agent is not active against methicillin-resistant *S. aureus*, *Enterococcus faecium*, *Legionella*, *Chlamydia* species, *Mycoplasma* species, *Pseudomonas cepacia*, and *Xanthomonas maltophilia*. Toxic effects include nausea and vomiting (particularly during drug infusion) (1% of cases), diarrhea (3%), rash or drug fever (2.7%), and dysgeusia. Seizures occur in 1.5% of patients, particularly those with a history of previous seizure, renal insufficiency, or structural central nervous system defects.

Aztreonam

The monobactam antibacterial agents, of which aztreonam is the only one commercially available, are derivatives of naturally occurring monocyclic β-lactam compounds. The mechanism of action of aztreonam, like that of other β-lactam antimicrobials, is the inhibition of cell wall synthesis. Aztreonam is administered intravenously and is excreted by the kidneys.

Its *spectrum of activity* involves only aerobic gram-negative bacteria, including many *P. aeruginosa*. It has minimal activity against *Acinetobacter*, *Alcaligenes*, *Flavobacterium*, *Pseudomonas fluorescens*, and *X. maltophilia*. Furthermore, it has no activity against gram-positive aerobic or anaerobic bacteria, and it is not synergistic with penicillins against the enterococci, as are gentamicin and streptomycin.

The *toxicity* of aztreonam is similar to that of other β-lactams. Patients with a penicillin allergy may tolerate aztreonam because cross-reactivity is uncommon.

Aminoglycosides

Agents in this group are gentamicin, tobramycin, amikacin, netilmicin, streptomycin, kanamycin, and neomycin.

The *spectrum of activity* of these agents includes aerobic gram-negative bacilli, mycobacteria (*Mycobacterium tuberculosis*, streptomycin; *Mycobacterium avium-intracellulare*, amikacin; *Mycobacterium chelonei*, amikacin), *Brucella* (streptomycin), *Nocardia* (amikacin), *Francisella tularensis* (streptomycin), and *Yersinia pestis* (streptomycin). They are synergistic with certain β-lactams in the treatment of serious infections due to susceptible enterococci (gentamicin, streptomycin), staphylococci, and several aerobic gram-negative species.

The major *adverse reactions* to aminoglycosides include nephrotoxicity and auditory or vestibular toxicity. Neuromuscular blockade, drug fever, and hypersensitivity reactions are much less common. The risk of nephrotoxicity varies among the different aminoglycosides; neomycin is the most nephrotoxic, and streptomycin is the least nephrotoxic. Gentamicin, tobramycin, and amikacin have intermediate nephrotoxicity. Risk factors include old age, hypotension, concomitant use of other nephrotoxic drugs, and liver disease. Aminoglycoside nephrotoxicity is almost always reversible with discontinuation of use of the drug, and it can be minimized or avoided if dosages are adjusted to achieve therapeutic serum concentrations and if renal function is carefully monitored. Nephrotoxicity is potentiated by cisplatin, amphotericin B, vancomycin, and cyclosporine. Ototoxicity is almost always irreversible. Streptomycin, gentamicin, and tobramycin are preferentially toxic to the vestibular system, whereas amikacin and neomycin are toxic to the auditory nerve. Advanced age and concomitant use of ethacrynic acid or furosemide seem to be risk factors for ototoxicity. Because of the imprecision of bedside testing for auditory and vestibular toxicity, routine audiographic and vestibular function evaluation should be considered when prolonged administration is anticipated and in patients predisposed to ototoxicity.

- Major adverse reactions to aminoglycosides are nephrotoxicity and auditory or vestibular toxicity.
- Neomycin is most nephrotoxic, and streptomycin is least nephrotoxic.
- Aminoglycoside nephrotoxicity is almost always reversible with discontinuation of use of drug.
- Ototoxicity is almost always irreversible.

Tetracycline

Agents are short-acting (tetracycline, chlorotetracycline, oxytetracycline), intermediate-acting (demeclocycline, methacycline), and long-acting (doxycycline, minocycline).

These agents are the drugs of choice for *Rickettsia, Chlamydia* species (includes pelvic inflammatory disease), *M. pneumoniae, Vibrio cholerae, Vibrio vulnificus, Brucella* species (with streptomycin or rifampin), *B. burgdorferi* (early stages), and *B. recurrentis*. These agents are also *effective therapy* or *alternatives* for *Actinomyces*, anthrax, *Campylobacter, Pasteurella multocida, Spirillum minus, Streptobacillus moniliformis, Treponema pallidum, F. tularensis*, Whipple's disease, *Y.*

pestis, Nocardia (minocycline), and *Mycobacterium marinum*. Minocycline may be active against methicillin-resistant *S. aureus* (patients who cannot tolerate vancomycin). The tetracyclines are used as *prophylaxis* for traveler's diarrhea and meningococcal disease (minocycline only; rifampin is drug of choice). Although the tetracyclines are active in vitro against many aerobic gram-positive and gram-negative organisms as well as some anaerobes, they are not the drugs of choice to treat the infections caused by these organisms because of the presence or emergence of resistant strains.

Toxicity includes gastrointestinal upset, rash, and photosensitivity. Uremia is increased in patients with renal failure (i.e., catabolic), acute fatty liver of pregnancy, Fanconi's syndrome (old tetracycline), or pseudotumor cerebri. The tetracyclines are not used in pregnant females or in children; they impair bone growth of the fetus and stain teeth of children. Minocycline is associated with vestibular toxicity, and recently cell-mediated hypersensitivity pneumonitis was reported.

Chloramphenicol

The *spectrum of activity* of this agent includes inhibition of most strains of clinically important aerobic and anaerobic bacteria. Exceptions include enterococci, methicillin-resistant *S. aureus*, many *Klebsiella* isolates, *Enterobacter, Serratia*, indole-positive *Proteus*, and *P. aeruginosa*. It is active against *Rickettsia* organisms and has bactericidal activity against *S. pneumoniae, H. influenzae*, and *N. meningitidis*. Major indications are few because of the availability of alternative therapies (severe *Salmonella typhi* infection, bacterial meningitis due to susceptible organisms in patients who cannot tolerate penicillin or cephalosporins, and rickettsial infections in patients who cannot take tetracyclines).

Toxicity includes two types of hematologic manifestations: idiosyncratic aplastic anemia (not dose-related; severe, usually fatal; incidence approximately 1/24,000-1/40,000) and dose-related bone marrow suppression (much more common with a dose >4 g/day). Gray baby syndrome (abdominal distention, cyanosis, vasomotor collapse) occurs in premature infants who cannot conjugate chloramphenicol and who have high serum levels. Rare toxic effects are hemolytic anemia, retrobulbar neuritis, peripheral neuritis, and potentiation action of oral hypoglycemics.

Clindamycin

Clindamycin has an excellent anaerobic *activity*,

although 10%-20% of *B. fragilis* organisms, 10%-20% of non-*Clostridium perfringens* organisms, and 10% of peptostreptococci organisms are resistant to clindamycin. It also is active against many strains of staphylococci and streptococci. However, emergence of resistance by staphylococci is common during treatment. Gram-negative aerobic bacteria and enterococci are resistant to clindamycin.

Toxicity includes antibiotic-associated diarrhea (20%), including *C. difficile* colitis (1%-10%); these are the most common side effects. Minor elevations of transaminase level, reversible neutropenia, thrombocytopenia, and neuromuscular blockade when given concurrently with neuromuscular blocking agents are much less common.

- Emergence of resistance to clindamycin by staphylococci is common during treatment.
- Toxic effects: antibiotic-associated diarrhea (20%), including *C. difficile* colitis (1%-10%).

Metronidazole

Metronidazole has antimicrobial *activity* against most anaerobic microorganisms. The exceptions include some anaerobic gram-positive non-spore-forming bacilli and peptostreptococci, *Actinomyces*, and *Propionibacterium acnes*. The agent is also effective in infections due to *Entamoeba histolytica*, *Giardia lamblia*, and *Gardnerella vaginalis*.

Toxicity includes side effects such as nausea, vomiting, reversible neutropenia, metallic taste, a disulfiram reaction when coadministered with alcohol, and potentiation of the effects of oral anticoagulants. Major adverse reactions are rare; they usually include central nervous system effects (seizure, cerebellar ataxia, peripheral neuropathy).

Macrolides

Erythromycin

Indications for this agent are infections caused by *Legionella* species, *M. pneumoniae*, and *Campylobacter jejuni*. It is an effective or alternative agent for *Chlamydia* species, group A hemolytic streptococci, *S. pneumoniae*, *S. aureus* (methicillin sensitive) (mild skin and soft tissue infections), *N. gonorrhoeae*, and *T. pallidum*. It may eradicate the carrier state of *Corynebacterium diphtheriae* and shorten the duration of *Bordetella pertussis* disease (whooping cough).

Toxicity may include gastrointestinal upset (dose-related), cholestatic jaundice (erythromycin estolate compound), increased theophylline or cyclosporine concen-

tration, increased serum concentrations of terfenadine (may cause ventricular arrhythmias), and transitory deafness, especially with large doses (≥4 g/day).

Clarithromycin

This agent provides excellent *activity* against *S. pneumoniae*, β-hemolytic streptococci, viridans streptococci, *S. aureus* (methicillin-sensitive), *M. catarrhalis*, *Legionella pneumophila*, *M. pneumoniae*, *C. pneumoniae*, *Chlamydia trachomatis*, *B. burgdorferi*, *M. avium-intracellulare*, and *M. chelonei*. It is superior to erythromycin for *S. pneumoniae* and β-hemolytic streptococci. It is moderately effective against *H. influenzae* and *N. gonorrhoeae*. It provides poor activity against *S. aureus* (methicillin-resistant).

In regard to *bioavailability*, excellent concentrations are achieved in many body fluids. The drug penetrates macrophages and polymorphonuclear neutrophils. Food has no effect on absorption. Half-life is 4-6 hours, which allows twice-daily dosing. Excretion is through liver and kidney.

Adverse effects include nausea (3%) and other gastrointestinal complaints; these occur less often than with erythromycin, but they are the most common adverse reactions. As with erythromycin, reversible hearing loss may occur at high dosages. Theophylline and carbamazepine concentrations increase, and levels of terfenadine may increase (cause of arrhythmias).

Clinical uses include mild to moderate upper and lower respiratory tract infection (may not be appropriate initial therapy if *H. influenzae* is expected pathogen). Others are pharyngitis, skin and soft tissue infection, and *M. avium-intracellulare* and other atypical mycobacterial infections.

Azithromycin

The *spectrum of activity* is the same as that of clarithromycin. It is twofold to fourfold less active against streptococci, including pneumococci, than erythromycin. It is more active against *H. influenzae* than clarithromycin.

In regard to *bioavailability*, excellent concentrations are achieved in many body fluids. The agent penetrates macrophages and polymorphonuclear neutrophils. Food decreases absorption. Half-life is 68 hours, which allows once-daily dosing. Excretion is hepatic. *Adverse effects* are the same as those for clarithromycin.

Clinical uses include treatment of mild to moderate upper and lower respiratory tract infection (may not be appropriate initial therapy if *H. influenzae* is expected pathogen), pharyngitis, skin and soft tissue infection, nongonococcal urethritis and cervicitis (single 1-g dose), *M. avium-intracellulare*, other atypical mycobacteria, and *Toxoplasma gondii*.

Vancomycin

Vancomycin, a glycopeptide antibiotic, has a *spectrum of activity* against most aerobic and anaerobic gram-positive organisms, with the exception of certain strains of *Lactobacillus, Leukonostoc, Actinomyces*, and enterococci (vancomycin-resistant strains). Vancomycin is the drug of choice for infections caused by methicillin-resistant *S. aureus*, methicillin-resistant coagulase-negative staphylococci, *Bacillus* species, *Rhodococcus equi*, and other multiply resistant gram-positive organisms such as *Corynebacterium jeikium*. It is also an alternative agent for infections caused by staphylococci, enterococci (synergistic with aminoglycosides), or streptococci in patients intolerant of β-lactam antimicrobials, although recent data suggest that vancomycin may be less effective than antistaphylococcal β-lactams for methicillin-susceptible *S. aureus* infections. Oral vancomycin is not absorbed and is used to treat only *C. difficile* colitis.

Although rare, the major *toxicity* with vancomycin is ototoxicity. This side effect is more common in the elderly and when vancomycin and aminoglycosides are administered concurrently. Infusion-related pruritus and the production of an erythematous rash involving the face, neck, and upper body ("red man" syndrome) are due to nonimmunologic-related release of histamine. Its frequency can be reduced by slowing the rate of infusion and by the administration of antihistamines before vancomycin infusion. Nephrotoxicity is rare with the newer preparations of vancomycin, except when vancomycin and aminoglycosides are administered concurrently. Chemical thrombophlebitis (13%) and reversible neutropenia (2%) are also known side effects.

- Vancomycin is bactericidal against most aerobic and anaerobic gram-positive organisms.
- Vancomycin is drug of choice for infections caused by methicillin-resistant *S. aureus*, methicillin-resistant coagulase-negative staphylococci, *Bacillus* species.
- Major toxic effect is ototoxicity.
- "Red man" syndrome due to nonimmunologic-related release of histamine.

Cotrimoxazole (Trimethoprim-Sulfamethoxazole)

Cotrimoxazole consists of two separate antimicrobials, trimethoprim and sulfamethoxazole, combined in a fixed (1:5) ratio. Both trimethoprim and sulfamethoxazole inhibit microbial folic acid synthesis, and when combined they have a synergistic effect.

The *spectrum of activity* of cotrimoxazole includes a wide variety of aerobic gram-positive cocci and gram-negative bacilli, including *S. aureus* (moderate activity), coagulase-negative staphylococci, *S. pneumoniae, H. influenzae, L. monocytogenes*, and many Enterobacteriaceae. It is not active against anaerobic bacteria and many strains of *Citrobacter freundii, Proteus vulgaris,* and *Providencia*. It is inactive against *P. aeruginosa* and enterococci. It is active against *Pneumocystis carinii, Isospora belli*, and *Nocardia asteroides*.

Toxicity with the agent can include the common adverse reactions of nausea and vomiting (3.2%) and rash (3.4%). Hypersensitivity reactions are common in patients with acquired immunodeficiency syndrome (AIDS; 60%). Diarrhea, nephrotoxicity, neutropenia, drug fever, and cholestatic hepatitis are less common. Its use is contraindicated during the last month of pregnancy and in patients with known glucose-6-phosphatase dehydrogenase deficiency. In 20%-53% of patients with AIDS treated for *Pneumocystis carinii* pneumonia (PCP), hyperkalemia due to trimethoprim component develops. Cotrimoxazole has several known drug interactions, including increasing the activity of oral anticoagulants, increasing plasma phenytoin concentrations, enhancing hypoglycemia in patients on oral hypoglycemics, and contributing to pancytopenia when coadministered with methotrexate.

- With cotrimoxazole, hypersensitivity reactions are common in patients with AIDS.

Fluoroquinolones

Agents are norfloxacin, ciprofloxacin, ofloxacin, lomefloxacin, and enoxacin.

Fluoroquinolones are derivatives of naladixic acid, the first quinolone. They are bactericidal against a wide variety of microorganisms because of their ability to inhibit DNA gyrase, an essential enzyme involved in the supercoiling of bacterial DNA.

Although the *spectrum of activity* of fluoroquinolones varies from drug to drug, they are generally extremely active against selected Enterobacteriaceae (including most strains that cause bacterial gastroenteritis) and *P. aeruginosa. S. aureus* (including methicillin-resistant), coagulase-negative staphylococci, and enterococci (urinary tract isolates only, because of high drug levels achieved in the urine) are less susceptible to all currently available fluoroquinolones, and none of these agents are active against anaerobes. *S. pneumoniae* is generally resistant to quinolones. Bacterial resistance to fluoroquinolones is increasing, particularly among *P. aeruginosa* and staphylococci.

Fluoroquinolones are generally safe. The most common types of *toxicity* are nausea, vomiting, abdominal pain, and diarrhea (1%-5%). *C. difficile* colitis is uncommon. Patients can also experience headache, confusion, restlessness, tremors, and seizures. Patients who have seizures usually have a previous history of a seizure disorder or a central nervous system structural defect. Hypersensitivity reactions, nephrotoxicity, and serum sickness are uncommon. Gastrointestinal absorption of the quinolones may be decreased by coadministration of aluminum- and magnesium-containing antacids, multivitamin preparations that include zinc, oral iron preparations, and high-calcium supplements. Concurrent administration of sucralfate also inhibits ciprofloxacin absorption. Ciprofloxacin increases serum theophylline and caffeine concentrations. Ciprofloxacin can cause erosions in cartilage in animals and thus is not recommended in pregnant women or in patients <18 years old.

- Fluoroquinolones are active against selected Enterobacteriaceae and *P. aeruginosa*.
- Bacterial resistance to fluoroquinolones is increasing, particularly among *P. aeruginosa* and staphylococci.
- *C. difficile* colitis uncommon.
- Gastrointestinal absorption of quinolones may be decreased by coadministration of aluminum- and magnesium-containing antacids and of multivitamin preparations.

Norfloxacin

Excellent concentrations of this agent are achieved in urine, kidney tissue, bile, and feces. Levels are poor in other sites. Food may decrease absorption. It is used for treatment of complicated and uncomplicated urinary tract infection, prostatitis, and bacterial diarrhea. More cost-effective agents are often available. It is also used for bowel decontamination (neutropenic patients).

Ciprofloxacin

Spectrum of activity of this agent is the same as that of other quinolones. In addition, it is active against *N. gonorrhoeae* (including penicillin-resistant strains), *H. influen-*

zae (including penicillin-resistant strains), *M. catarrhalis* (including penicillin-resistant strains), *M. tuberculosis, L. pneumophila,* and *Brucella.* Excellent concentrations are achieved in most body fluids. An adverse effect is more of an increase in theophylline levels than with norfloxacin.

Clinical uses include complicated and uncomplicated urinary tract infection (cure rates are less in infections due to enterococci or in complicated infection) and chronic prostatitis. In many cases, more cost-effective agents are often available. Ciprofloxacin is also used for treatment of infectious diarrhea (recurrence of *Salmonella* and resistance to *C. jejuni* have been reported) and for treatment and prophylaxis of traveler's diarrhea. It may eradicate the *S. typhi* carrier state. When utilized in cases of upper and lower respiratory tract infection, failures against pneumococci have been reported, and it is not drug of choice for empiric therapy of community-acquired pneumonia. Other conditions for which it is used are malignant external otitis due to *P. aeruginosa,* skin and soft tissue infection (avoid in streptococcal cellulitis), bone and joint infection (aerobic gram-negative), *M. avium-intracellulare* and multiple drug-resistant tuberculosis, and uncomplicated gonococcal urethritis or cervicitis; it is also an alternative agent for prophylaxis of meningococci.

Ofloxacin

The *spectrum of activity* is similar to that of ciprofloxacin; it is less active against *P. aeruginosa* and Enterobacteriaceae. This drug increases theophylline levels, but less so than with ciprofloxacin.

Clinical uses are complicated and uncomplicated urinary tract infection (cure rates are lower in infections due to enterococci or in complicated infection) and chronic prostatitis. More cost-effective agents are available in many such cases. Ofloxacin is also used for lower respiratory tract infection (see Ciprofloxacin, this page), skin and soft tissue infection (see Ciprofloxacin, this page), and gonococcal and nongonococcal urethritis and cervicitis.

Lomefloxacin

The *spectrum of activity* of this agent is similar to that of ciprofloxacin. It is not active against *M. tuberculosis, C. trachomatis, C. pneumoniae, L. pneumophila, M. pneumoniae,* or *Brucella.* Theophylline levels are not increased with this drug. Photosensitivity reaction may be more common than with ciprofloxacin.

Clinical uses include complicated and uncomplicated urinary tract infection (cure rates are lower in infections due to enterococci or in complicated infection) and chronic prostatitis. More cost-effective agents are available in many of these cases. It is also used for prophylaxis for transurethral surgical procedures.

Enoxacin

The *spectrum of activity* is similar to that for ciprofloxacin. It is less active against *P. aeruginosa*. It has only moderate activity against staphylococci and enterococci. It is not active against pneumococci, group A streptococci, *M. tuberculosis, C. trachomatis, C. pneumoniae, L. pneumophila, M. pneumoniae*, or *Brucella*. Adverse effects include increased theophylline and caffeine levels (more than with the other quinolones). Ranitidine and other agents may inhibit absorption. Reports from Japan have described convulsions in several patients taking fenbufen (nonsteroidal anti-inflammatory drug) concurrently. Digoxin levels may also increase.

Clinical uses include complicated and uncomplicated urinary tract infection, prostatitis, and gonococcal urethritis and cervicitis.

ANTIFUNGAL THERAPY

Amphotericin B

The *mode of action* of this agent is binding of ergosterol in cell walls and increasing cell wall permeability. Its indications are for most serious or life-threatening fungal infections. Exceptions include *Pseudallescheria boydii* (azoles) and chromoblastomycosis (flucytosine).

Toxicity can include fever, phlebitis, and nephrotoxicity (increased intravascular volume, salt loading may decrease risk of nephrotoxicity). Nephrotoxicity is increased with concomitant use of cyclosporine. In patients with acquired immunodeficiency syndrome (AIDS), acute renal failure has occurred with concomitant use of pentamidine intravenously. Other effects are bone marrow suppression, hypokalemia (may exacerbate digitalis toxicity), hypomagnesemia, and, when given to patients who have had leukocyte transfusion, pulmonary infiltrates.

Flucytosine

The *mode of action* of this agent involves conversion to 5-fluorouracil intracellularly. Resistance develops rapidly when it is used alone. It has *activity* against cryp-

tococci, *Candida* species, and chromoblastomycosis. *Indications* are cryptococcal meningitis (used in combination with amphotericin B), *Candida* meningitis (good cerebrospinal fluid penetration; in combination with amphotericin B), *Candida* cystitis (urinary levels are high), and chromoblastomycosis.

Toxicity is associated with high serum levels. Neutropenia, thrombocytopenia, diarrhea, nausea, gastrointestinal upset, colitis, and hepatotoxicity (idiosyncratic, uncommon) are possible side effects.

Azoles

Pharmacologic properties of the azoles are outlined in Table 20-26.

Ketoconazole

This is a bis-triazole compound that inhibits production of ergosterol, a major constituent of fungal cell membranes, by inhibiting the cytochrome P450 enzyme responsible for conversion of lanosterol to ergosterol. It requires gastric acid for absorption. The presence of low gastric pH should always be determined to ensure the adequate absorption of ketoconazole. Coadministration of isoniazid and rifampin can decrease drug levels. Ketoconazole can elevate cyclosporine levels and potentiate the effect of warfarin.

Ketoconazole is second-line therapy (itraconazole is drug of choice) for nonmeningeal and non-life-threatening *Histoplasmosis* and *Blastomycosis* in immunocompetent patients. It has poor cerebrospinal fluid penetration and should not be used to treat central nervous system fungal infections. The drug is also used for chronic mucocutaneous candidiasis, paracoccidioidomycosis, and *P. boydii*.

The most common *toxic effect* of ketoconazole is dose-related gastrointestinal upset. Decreased synthesis of adrenal corticosteroids, most notably androgenic steroids, has been reported. Patients may have gynecomastia and loss of libido with impotence, especially with higher dosages of ketoconazole. Arterial hypertension has also been reported. Acute hepatitis, which can be fatal, occurs rarely.

- Ketoconazole requires gastric acid for absorption.
- Potentiates the effect of warfarin.
- Gynecomastia is fairly common side effect.

Fluconazole

This is a bis-triazole compound that inhibits ergosterol, a major constituent of fungal cell membranes, by inhibit-

Table 20-26.--Selected Pharmacologic Properties of Azole Drugs

Factor	Ketoconazole	Fluconazole	Itraconazole
Route of administration	Oral	Oral, parenteral	Oral
Requires acid for GI absorption	Yes	No	Yes
Protein binding	99%	12%	99%
CSF concentrations	Nil	≈80%	Nil
Half-life, hr	9	25	15-42
Clearance	Hepatic	Renal	Hepatic
Urinary levels of active drug	Low	High	Low
Dose reduction in renal failure	No	Yes	No

CSF, cerebrospinal fluid; GI, gastrointestinal.

Modified from Terrell CL, Hughes CE: Antifungal agents used for deep-seated mycotic infections. Mayo Clin Proc 67:69-91, 1992. By permission of Mayo Foundation for Medical Education and Research.

ing the cytochrome P450 enzyme responsible for conversion of lanosterol to ergosterol. It has a broad spectrum of antifungal activity in vivo in animal models. Activity has been demonstrated against *Candida, Cryptococcus neoformans, Coccidioides immitis, Histoplasma capsulatum, Blastomyces dermatitidis,* and paracoccidioidomycosis. Food hinders absorption of the drug.

Adverse effects occur in 16% of patients. Discontinuation of therapy is necessary in 1%-2% of patients. Most common effects are gastrointestinal (1.5%-3.5%), rash (1.8%), and headache (1.9%). Fatal hepatic necrosis and exfoliative rash have also been reported. There is no interference with adrenocortical function or synthesis of testosterone, which can occur with ketoconazole.

Fluconazole inhibits metabolism and increases serum levels of phenytoin, oral hyoglycemic agents, carbamazepine, and warfarin. Increases in cyclosporine levels due to fluconazole have been reported. Coadministration with rifampin and isoniazid decreases serum concentrations of fluconazole.

Clinical uses include candidal infection and cryptococcal meningitis. In candidal infection, oropharyngeal and esophageal candidiasis are effectively treated, both in patients with AIDS and in patients with neutropenia. Hepatosplenic candidiasis and vaginitis (topical agents may be more cost-effective) are also treated with fluconazole. For urinary tract infection, no trials have compared the drug with amphotericin B bladder washes. For candidemia, amphotericin B and fluconazole have not

been compared. Failures with fluconazole have been reported. The drug is also used for prophylaxis of candidal infection in neutropenic patients and in patients undergoing bone marrow transplantation. A concern is emergence of resistant fungi (*C. krusei*). Fluconazole is also used as initial therapy for cryptococcal meningitis. A recent randomized study of 194 patients who had AIDS with acute cryptococcal meningitis found no difference in clinical cure or overall survival between groups receiving amphotericin B and fluconazole, but time to cerebrospinal fluid sterilization was less with amphotericin B, and there were more early deaths in the fluconazole group. Most experts still recommend initial therapy with amphotericin B. Maintenance therapy with fluconazole is more efficacious and less toxic than weekly administration of amphotericin B. The role of the drug in treatment of patients without AIDS remains undefined.

Itraconazole

The *mechanism of action* of this drug is similar to that for fluconazole. A major advantage over fluconazole is its greater activity against *Aspergillus, Sporothrix schenckii, H. capsulatum,* and *B. dermatitidis.* Food enhances its absorption.

Minor *side effects* occur in 2%-20% of patients if doses <400 mg/day are used. Most common side effects involve gastrointestinal tract: nausea, 10.6%; vomiting, 5.1%; and abdominal pain, 1.5%. Rash occurs in 8.6% of patients. Hepatitis can occur but is rare. If dose is <400 mg/day, there is no effect on glucocorticoid or testosterone synthesis. At doses >400 mg/day, edema, hypokalemia, nausea, and vomiting can occur.

Itraconazole inhibits metabolism and increases serum levels of cyclosporine, digoxin, and terfenadine. Cyclosporine and digoxin levels should be monitored, and terfenadine should not be administered concurrently because of potentially fatal ventricular arrhythmias. Astemizole coadministration is also contraindicated. Coadministration with rifampin, isoniazid, and H_2 blockers decreases serum concentrations of itraconazole. Failures in therapy have also been reported when phenytoin and carbamazepine have been administered concurrently.

Clinical uses include histoplasmosis: chronic cavitary pulmonary disease and disseminated non-life-threatening, nonmeningeal disease. Itraconazole is also effective maintenance therapy in patients with AIDS. A recent study also demonstrated its effectiveness in pulmonary and nonpulmonary (bone, joint, skin) blastomycosis. It is now the drug of choice for this condition. For coccidioidomycosis (pulmonary, bone and joint), the efficacy rate is 57%-72%. A small number of patients with coccidioidal meningitis have also been effectively treated. When used for sporotrichosis, itraconazole is effective in lymphocutaneous and bone and joint disease, although relapse may occur in disseminated disease. An ongoing trial is comparing fluconazole and itraconazole for treatment of cryptococcal meningitis in patients with AIDS. As therapy for *Aspergillus*, success rates of 44%-77% have been reported for invasive pulmonary and sinus disease. No studies comparing itraconazole with amphotericin B have been reported, and amphotericin B remains the drug of choice for these diseases unless contraindications to its use exist.

ANTIVIRAL AGENTS

Current agents are virustatic and have no activity against nonreplicating or latent viruses.

Acyclovir

This is a nucleoside analog of guanosine. After phosphorylation by virus-specific thymidine kinase to monophosphate and further phosphorylation to triphosphate by cellular enzymes, it inhibits DNA polymerase. In vitro activity and clinical efficacy correlate with the amount of viral-specific thymidine kinase produced (herpes simplex virus type 1 > herpes simplex virus type 2 > varicella-zoster virus > Epstein-Barr virus). Cytomegalovirus does not produce thymidine kinase and is resis-

tant. Oral and intravenous forms are available. Mutations of either viral thymidine kinase or DNA polymerase cause resistance. Most acyclovir-resistant isolates (herpes simplex virus, varicella-zoster virus) have been isolated in patients with AIDS and in recipients of bone marrow transplantation. Drug of choice is then foscarnet.

Acyclovir is generally well tolerated. *Toxicity* includes gastrointestinal distress and headaches (oral form), phlebitis (intravenous form), and crystalline nephropathy (increased risk with high dose, bolus infusion, dehydration, and preexisting renal impairment). Confusion, delirium, lethargy, and seizures can occur (<1% of cases, higher rate with serum concentration >25 µg/mL). Use of the drug is avoided during pregnancy.

Indications for the drug include herpes simplex virus infections. It is effective for treatment of primary and recurrent episodes of herpes genitalis and suppression of frequent recurrences. Topical acyclovir is also effective in primary genital herpes simplex virus infection, but the oral form is more effective. Intravenous therapy should be considered in serious disease. If chronic suppression is used, reassess after 1 year. Oral-labial disease may respond to oral acyclovir, but it is not recommended for routine use. In immunocompromised patients, however, oral or intravenous acyclovir is highly effective in the prophylaxis and treatment of oral-labial disease. Acyclovir is the drug of choice for herpes simplex virus encephalitis; a high dose is used (10 mg/kg every 8 hours). Acyclovir is also used for varicella-zoster virus. Intravenous form in immunocompromised patients halts progression and prevents dissemination of herpes zoster. It is also effective for decreasing viral shedding, decreasing the number of new lesions, and increasing healing in primary varicella in immunocompetent children and adults if it is given within the first 24 hours of rash or in immunocompromised hosts. There is no good evidence that treating primary varicella in immunocompetent adults decreases the risk of visceral dissemination. Oral therapy is effective against herpes zoster ophthalmicus (most effective within 72 hours; 600-800 mg five times a day). Herpes zoster in immunocompetent host responds to acyclovir, 800 mg five times a day (decreased viral shedding, time to healing). There is no effect on postherpetic neuralgia. It should be used only if given within 72 hours after onset of symptoms.

- With acyclovir, crystalline nephropathy increased with high dose, bolus infusion, dehydration, preexisting renal impairment.

- Acyclovir is drug of choice for herpes simplex encephalitis.

Ganciclovir

This agent inhibits DNA polymerase, but it is not dependent on phosphorylation by viral thymidine kinase. Thus, it is active against cytomegalovirus. No oral form is available.

Indications for ganciclovir include treatment of cytomegalovirus retinitis in patients with acquired immunodeficiency syndrome (AIDS). Studies have shown beneficial results in other cytomegalovirus infections (colitis, esophagitis, gastritis, and pneumonia) in patients with AIDS and in immunocompromised hosts. In patients with AIDS, maintenance therapy may be necessary to prevent relapse. Used in combination with hyperimmune globulin, ganciclovir reduces mortality from cytomegalovirus pneumonitis in patients who have had allogeneic bone marrow transplantation. Several recent studies suggest that ganciclovir therapy before the development of cytomegalovirus disease in patients who have had heart or bone marrow transplantation may decrease the incidence of cytomegalovirus infection.

Toxicity may manifest as neutropenia and thrombocytopenia. The incidence of neutropenia is increased when ganciclovir is used in combination with zidovudine in patients with AIDS. Cytopenias are reversible after use of the drug is stopped. It is teratogenic, carcinogenic, and mutagenic in animals. Less common are fever, rash, anemia, and increased values on liver function tests.

Ganciclovir *resistance* is associated with persistent viremia and progressive disease. Mechanism of resistance is postulated to be decreased cellular phosphorylation.

- Ganciclovir, used in combination with hyperimmune globulin, reduces mortality from cytomegalovirus pneumonitis in patients after bone marrow transplantation.
- Incidence of neutropenia is increased when ganciclovir is used in combination with zidovudine in patients with AIDS.

Foscarnet

This is a noncompetitive inhibitor of viral DNA polymerase and reverse transcriptase. It does not require phosphorylation. It has in vitro activity against human immunodeficiency virus (HIV), all human herpes viruses, and hepatitis B.

Indications include cytomegalovirus retinitis, including disease that is due to ganciclovir-resistant strains. It also may be effective in gastrointestinal disease in patients with AIDS. It is more expensive and less well tolerated than ganciclovir. It requires controlled rates of infusions and large volumes of fluid. Controlled trials in patients with AIDS and cytomegalovirus retinitis showed no difference in the progression of the retinitis between foscarnet-treated and ganciclovir-treated patients. However, there was an unexplained increased mortality in the ganciclovir group.

Foscarnet is less well tolerated than ganciclovir. *Toxicity* involves nephrotoxicity, which usually develops during the second week and is reversible. Risk of nephrotoxicity is increased with concurrent use of nephrotoxic drugs (e.g., amphotericin B, aminoglycosides). Hydration may decrease the risk of nephrotoxicity. Electrolyte disturbances, such as hypocalcemia, hyperphosphatemia or hypophosphatemia, hypokalemia, and hypomagnesemia, also occur. Risk of hypocalcemia is increased with concomitant use of pentamidine intravenously. Fever, nausea, vomiting, anemia, fatigue, headache, leukopenia, pancreatitis, and genital ulceration also have been reported.

Resistance has occurred in strains of herpes simplex virus, varicella-zoster virus, and cytomegalovirus, but in vitro resistance has not been correlated with decreased clinical response.

- Foscarnet is effective for cytomegalovirus retinitis, including disease due to ganciclovir-resistant strains.
- With foscarnet, nephrotoxicity may occur; usually develops during second week and is reversible.

Antiretroviral Therapy

Zidovudine (AZT)

This is dideoxynucleoside (thymidine analog) that must be phosphorylated to active triphosphate form by cellular enzymes. Its *mechanism of action* is to inhibit reverse transcriptase and terminate HIV nucleic acid chain elongation. In regard to its *clinical pharmacology*, its rate of absorption is 60%-65%. Central nervous system concentrations are 0.1-1.35 times the serum concentrations. Serum half-life is 1 hour, and intracellular half-life is 3-4 hours. It is eliminated through hepatic metabolism and renal excretion. Elimination is reduced in patients with uremia and cirrhosis (dosing every 8 hours may be appropriate). *Drug interactions* include an increased half-life of AZT when used with probenecid;

ganciclovir and AZT are additive in their myelosuppressive properties.

Clinical indications are HIV infection in adults and children, in which case it is the drug of choice for initial treatment. In patients with AIDS, it decreases frequency of opportunistic infection, increases survival, increases body weight and CD4 cell counts (for 4-6 months), and decreases p24 antigenemia. Studies have shown that 500 mg/day is as effective as 1,500 mg/day in patients with AIDS, but toxicity (neutropenia, anemia) is significantly decreased and survival is prolonged. AZT is effective in the treatment of HIV neurologic disease (1,200-1,500 mg/day) and thrombocytopenia. In asymptomatic HIV infection, AZT delays progression of disease in HIV-infected persons with CD4 counts of 200-500/μL (may or may not increase survival).

Table 20-27 outlines a treatment schedule based on the CD4 cell count.

Adverse effects include anemia and neutropenia, which are dose-limiting toxicities. They are less common with low doses (500-600 mg/day). Granulocyte-macrophage colony-stimulating factor and granulocyte colony-stimulating factor may increase neutrophils, and recombinant erythropoietin in patients with low erythropoietin levels (<500 IU/L) may decrease transfusion requirements. Risk factors for developing anemia include low pretreatment CD4 cell count and hemoglobin value, more advanced HIV disease, and vitamin B_{12} deficiency. Concomitant use of ganciclovir and AZT exacerbates the risk of neutropenia. Asthenia, headache, dizziness, insomnia, anorexia, nausea, vomiting, malaise, and myalgia are common initial events after initiation of therapy, but they usually diminish with continued therapy and seldom require stopping use of the drug. Esophageal ulceration and hyperpigmentation of skin have also been reported. Myopathy occurs in 6%-18% of patients who receive therapy for >6 months. It is difficult to distinguish from HIV-associated myopathy. It occurs 6-12 months after initiation of therapy. Mitochondrial abnormalities are noted on electron microscopy. Most patients (70%-100%) are asymptomatic 6-8 weeks after stopping use of AZT.

Primary infection with AZT-resistant HIV has been reported. The frequency of this finding is unknown. Most reports of in vitro resistance have been in patients treated for at least 6-9 months. Appearance of resistance is related to stage of disease and CD4 cell count. Clinical significance of resistance is unknown. Studies to address this issue are ongoing.

- With AZT, anemia and neutropenia are dose-limiting toxicities.
- Concomitant use of ganciclovir and AZT exacerbates risk of neutropenia.
- Myopathy occurs in 6%-18% of patients who receive AZT for >6 months.

Table 20-27.--Suggested Treatment Schedule for Zidovudine (AZT)

CD4 cells/μL	Treatment
≥500	No AZT, check CD4 value every 3-6 mo
200-500	AZT 500 mg/day
<200	AZT 500 mg/day + PCP prophylaxis

PCP, *Pneumocystis carinii* pneumonia.

Didanosine (ddI)

This dideoxynucleoside is similar to AZT. It also must be phosphorylated to be active. Its *mechanism of action* is identical to that of AZT. In regard to its *clinical pharmacology*, its rate of absorption is 37%, and absorption is decreased with food. Central nervous system concentrations are 0.1-0.85 times the serum concentrations. Serum half-life is 1.4 hours, and intracellular half-life is 8-24 hours. It is eliminated through hepatic metabolism and renal excretion.

Adverse reactions can occur with concomitant use of intravenous pentamidine (pancreatitis). Because ddI tablets contain antacid to enhance absorption, drugs that require gastric acidity (ketoconazole) should be administered 2 hours before ddI. Similarly, quinolones should not be coadministered with ddI.

Clinical indications are advanced HIV infection in patients intolerant of AZT or those in whom AZT is failing. Administration of ddI results in increased CD4 cell count, decreased p24 antigenemia, and decreased symptoms in patients with AIDS.

Toxicity with ddI includes painful peripheral neuropathy. Pancreatitis can develop (7% in one study); risk is increased with high dosage, history of pancreatitis, alcohol abuse, advanced HIV disease, or concomitant use of intravenous pentamidine. Optic neuritis and fulminant hepatitis have also been reported. Anemia and neutropenia significantly less common than in patients administered AZT.

Cross-resistance with AZT has not been reported. Strains resistant to ddI may be resistant to ddC. Patients switched to ddI therapy from AZT therapy may regain AZT sensitivity.

Zalcitabine (ddC)

This is a dideoxynucleoside similar to zidovudine. It also must be phosphorylated to be active. *Mechanism of action* is identical to that of AZT. In regard to its *clinical pharmacology*, its absorption rate is 80%. Absorption is decreased with food. Central nervous system concentrations are 0.1-0.37 times serum concentrations. Serum half-life is 1-3 hours, and intracellular half-life is 8-24 hours. Elimination is through renal excretion. Dose is decreased with renal failure.

Drug interactions occur with concomitant use of drugs that have potential to cause peripheral neuropathy either through direct neurotoxicity or by decreasing renal clearance of ddC. The drug should not be used concomitantly with intravenous pentamidine because of the risk of pancreatitis.

Clinical indications include patients with advanced HIV infection in whom AZT monotherapy is failing; in these cases, ddC is used in combination with AZT. Increased p24 antigenemia, symptoms in patients with AIDS or AIDS-related complex, and CD4 cell counts <300/μL have been cited as indications in small preliminary studies.

Toxicity includes painful distal sensorimotor peripheral neuropathy (17%-31% of cases in monotherapy studies). This is usually reversible with discontinuation of use of the drug. There are no data on use in patients with preexisting neuropathy. Pancreatitis has been reported (<1% of cases) in monotherapy studies. It is assumed that risk factors for pancreatitis due to ddI are also factors with ddC, but no data are available. Esophageal ulcers have been reported. Anemia and neutropenia significantly less common than in patients administered AZT.

Cross-resistance with AZT has not been reported; ddI cross-resistance has been reported.

- AZT should be used in all previously untreated patients with HIV (i.e., first-line therapy), although patients with AZT-resistant strains have been described.
- If clinical failure or toxicity develops with AZT, switching to ddI monotherapy is appropriate if there are no contraindications.
- All patients receiving antiretroviral therapy should be monitored for drug toxicity, which is common and can be life-threatening.

Ribavirin

This is a purine analog. *Indication* for aerosolized rib-

avirin is respiratory syncytial virus bronchiolitis in children, in whom treatment decreases morbidity. *Adverse teratogenic and embryotoxic effects* have been noted in animals. The drug is contraindicated in pregnancy, and precautions must be taken when aerosolized ribavirin is used in the hospital.

IMMUNIZATIONS

Tables 20-28 through 20-31 provide basic information about immunizations.

Table 20-28.--Vaccines Containing Live Viruses

Live viruses
Smallpox
Polio
Yellow fever
Mumps
Rubella
Rubeola

Table 20-29.--Vaccination Schedules in Adults

Vaccine	Age, yr		
	18-24	25-64	≥65
Tetanus, diphtheria	x	x	x
Measles	x	x*	
Mumps	x	x	
Rubella	x	x	
Influenza			x
Pneumococcal			x†

*Indicated for persons born after 1956.

†Persons at high risk of fatal disease (e.g., those who have had transplantation, those with asplenia, those who are nephrotoxic) should be revaccinated after 6 years.

Modified from Centers for Disease Control: Update on adult immunization: recommendations of the Immunization Practices Advisory Committee (ACIP). MMWR 40 (no. RR-12):1-71, 1991.

HUMAN IMMUNODEFICIENCY VIRUS (HIV)

EPIDEMIOLOGY

HIV infection is a global health problem (it is now reported in 150 countries). More than 1 million Americans are now infected with HIV. There are approximately

Table 20-30.--Vaccines Specifically Indicated or Contraindicated, According to Special Health Status or Occupation (United States)

Health status or occupation	Vaccine indicated	Vaccine contraindicated
Pregnant	Tetanus, diphtheria (except first trimester)	Live virus vaccine *Bacille Calmette-Guérin* (BCG), oral typhoid
Immunocompromised	Influenza, pneumococcal, HbCV*	Live virus vaccine *Bacille Calmette-Guérin* (BCG), oral typhoid
Splenic dysfunction	Influenza, pneumococcal, HbCV,* meningococcal	
Hemodialysis/transplant	Hepatitis B, influenza, pneumococcal	
Factor VIII, IX	Hepatitis B†	
Chronic alcoholism	Pneumococcal, influenza	
Nursing home resident, age ≥65 yr, diabetes, CHF, COPD, malignancy, CRF	Pneumococcal, influenza	
Homeless/immigrants	Review all vaccines	
Prison inmates	Hepatitis B	
Health care workers	Hepatitis B, influenza, MMR	

*May be considered.

†May need increased dose.

CHF, congestive heart failure; COPD, chronic obstructive pulmonary disease; CRF, chronic renal failure; HbCV, *Haemophilus influenzae* B conjugate vaccine; MMR, measles, mumps, rubella.

Modified from Centers for Disease Control: Update on adult immunization: recommendations of the Immunization Practices Advisory Committee (ACIP). MMWR 40 (no. RR-12):1-71, 1991.

Table 20-31.--Indicated Vaccines in Human Immunodeficiency Virus (HIV) Infection

Vaccine	Asymptomatic HIV	Symptomatic HIV
DTP/Td	Yes	Yes
OPV	No	No
Enhanced-potency inactivated poliovirus*	Yes	Yes
MMR	Yes	Yes†
HbCV†	Yes	Yes
Pneumococcal	Yes	Yes
Influenza	Yes†	Yes

*For adults ≥18 years of age, use only if indicated.

†Should be considered.

DTP/Td, diphtheria, tetanus, pertussis/tetanus, diphtheria; HbCV, *Haemophilus influenzae* B conjugate vaccine; OPV, oral poliovirus; MMR, measles, mumps, rubella.

Modified from Centers for Disease Control: Update on adult immunization: recommendations of the Immunization Practices Advisory Committee (ACIP). MMWR 40 (no. RR-12):1-71, 1991.

40,000 new cases in the United States each year. As of January 1993, more than 250,000 cases had been reported in the United States.

Transmission

HIV is transmitted perinatally and through blood products, occupational exposure, sexual contact, and, less commonly, transplantation.

HIV infection develops in 16%-30% of infants born to HIV-infected mothers. Infection often occurs in the postnatal period through breast milk.

The risk of acquiring infection through blood transfusion since institution of HIV screening of donors is approximately 0.0017% (1 per 60,000 units transfused), according to a recent study of more than 11,000 patients undergoing cardiovascular operations.

Occupational exposure occurs through needle sticks. About 225,000 HIV-positive patients were admitted to acute-care hospitals in 1990, of which only a third were symptomatic with typical acquired immunodeficiency syndrome (AIDS)-associated illnesses. The seroprevalence of HIV at any one particular hospital varied between 0.2% and 14%. Approximately 0.32% of health care workers will seroconvert if they suffer a needle stick with a sharp that is contaminated with HIV-infected blood. The seroconversion rate depends on the amount of vial inoculum.

With sexual contact (i.e., semen, vaginal secretion), the risk of transmission is increased with traumatic intercourse, genital ulcers, and other sexually transmitted diseases (e.g., syphilis).

The risk of a surgeon transmitting HIV to a patient during an invasive procedure is thought to be between 0.0024% and 0.00024% (1/42,000-1/420,000 procedures). The same probability for transmission of hepatitis B virus infection from surgeon who is positive for hepatitis B antigen to an uninfected patient is between 0.024%-0.24%. The risk of infection through mucous membrane contact is too low to quantitate, but it has occurred.

Demographics

In 1990, 88% of HIV-infected persons were male and 12% were female. By race, 53% were white, 29% were black, 16% were Hispanic, and 0.6% were Asian. The presumed risk factors for infection were as follows: 58%, homosexual contact; 23%, injection drug use; 6%, homosexual contact or injection drug use; 6%, heterosexual transmission; 2%, transfusion; <1%, hemophiliacs; 4%, no identified risk factor.

Recent trends that have been noted have been decreased transmission by transfusion, an increased incidence of disease in injection drug users, heterosexuals, women, children, blacks, and Hispanics; and a decreased number of new cases among homosexuals.

LABORATORY DIAGNOSIS

Routine Tests

The enzyme-linked immunosorbent assay (ELISA) is a screening test that detects specific HIV antibodies (primarily gp41 and p24 antibodies). It is 99% sensitive and specific, but its positive predictive value is low in low-prevalence populations. False-positive results occur because of the presence of cross-reacting antibodies in certain patients (e.g., multiparous women, patients with multiple transfusions). False-negative results are caused by testing patients before seroconversion, patients who have undergone replacement transfusions or bone marrow transplantation, or by poorly manufactured testing equipment.

The Western blot test (confirmatory test) detects antibodies directed against gag (p18, p24, p55), pol (p31, p51, p66), and env (gp41, gp120-160). The Centers for Disease Control guidelines for interpretation of the Western blot are as follows: any 2 of p24, gp41, or gp120-160 = positive, 1 only = indeterminate, and no bands = negative. If results are indeterminate, the clinician should assess risk of HIV infection in the individual patient and retest at 3-6 months. The risk of HIV infection is extremely low in patients with an indeterminate Western blot.

Other Tests

These tests include peripheral blood mononuclear cell co-culture (95%-99% sensitive), HIV p24 antigen test (most prevalent in early and end-stage disease), and polymerase chain reaction (false-positive results can be due to laboratory contamination). These tests may be useful in certain situations (acute infection, indeterminate results of Western blot test, infants of seropositive mothers, prognostic markers). These tests are more expensive than routine tests.

CLINICAL SYNDROMES

Acute Infection

Acute infection is symptomatic in 53%-93% of cases. The incubation period is 2-4 weeks, and clinical illness usually lasts 1-2 weeks. Clinical manifestations are protean (Table 20-32). An atypical lymphocytosis is present in approximately 50% of patients. ELISA results may be negative (usually positive at 6-12 weeks); p24 antigen, HIV culture, or polymerase chain reaction results may be positive. The differential diagnosis includes infection due to Epstein-Barr virus, cytomegalovirus, primary herpes simplex virus, toxoplasmosis, rubella, viral hepatitis, secondary syphilis, and drug reactions. There are few data supporting the concept that antiretroviral therapy hastens resolution of symptoms or prevents development of persistent infection.

Asymptomatic Illness

Asymptomatic illness lasts from months to years. The cumulative incidence of AIDS varies among different patient populations, but in general approximately 50% of patients will develop AIDS (1987 definition) within 7-11 years after seroconversion. It is presumed that immunodeficiency and AIDS will eventually develop in almost all patients. The most reliable clinical predictors of HIV disease progression are development of thrush or unexplained fever, weight loss, or diarrhea. Commonly used laboratory markers for disease progression are listed in Table 20-33. The most experience is with CD4 cells (e.g., the risk of developing *Pneumocystis carinii* pneumonia [PCP] is 4.9-fold more in patients with CD4 cell counts <200/µL, and median survival time is 1 year if CD4 count is <50/µL). CD4 cell counts are also useful for defining when to start antiretroviral therapy and PCP prophylaxis.

AIDS

The diagnosis of AIDS used to require the presence of an HIV-associated opportunistic infection or malignancy as well as documentation of HIV infection. However, the new definition of AIDS by the Centers for Disease Control also includes patients with CD4 cell count ≤200/µL and three new indicator diseases (pulmonary tuberculosis, invasive cervical carcinoma, and

Table 20-32.--Clinical Manifestations of Primary Human Immunodeficiency Virus Infection

General	Neuropathic	Dermatologic	Gastrointestinal
Fever	Headache, retro-orbital pain	Maculopapular rash	Oral candidiasis
Pharyngitis	Meningoencephalitis	Roseola-like rash	Nausea, vomiting
Lymphadenopathy	Peripheral neuropathy	Diffuse urticaria	Diarrhea
Myalgia	Radiculopathy	Desquamation	
Lethargy	Guillain-Barré syndrome	Alopecia	
Anorexia, weight loss	Cognitive impairment	Mucocutaneous ulceration	

From Tindall B, Imrie A, Donovan B, Penny R, Cooper DA: Primary HIV infection. *In* The Medical Management of AIDS. Third edition. Edited by MA Sande, PA Volberding. Philadelphia, WB Saunders Company, 1992, pp 67-86. By permission of publisher.

Table 20-33.--Laboratory Markers of Progression of Human Immunodeficiency Virus (HIV) Disease

Nonspecific markers	Immunologic markers	HIV specific markers
Anemia	Decreased CD4 (or CD4%)	p24 antigenemia
Thrombocytopenia	Decreased CD4:CD8 ratio	Quantitative HIV culture
Elevated erythrocyte sedimentation rate	Elevated β_2-microglobulin	
	Elevated neopterin	
	Absent or decreased anti-p24 antibody	
	Elevated acid labile interferon	

From Clement M, Hollander H: Natural history and management of the seropositive patient. *In* The Medical Management of AIDS. Third edition. Edited by MA Sande, PA Volberding. Philadelphia, WB Saunders Company, 1992, pp 87-96. By permission of publisher.

recurrent [two or more episodes per year] pneumonia). The Centers for Disease Control projected that reported cases of AIDS would increase by 75% in 1993 and 10%-20% in 1994 as a result of the change in the definition of AIDS.

INFECTIONS ASSOCIATED WITH HIV INFECTION

Syndromes associated with HIV, by CD4 cell count, are listed in Table 20-34.

Pneumocystis carinii Pneumonia

PCP is one of the most common opportunistic infections in patients with AIDS (color plate 20-10). It occurs in approximately 80% of patients who do not receive pri-

mary prophylaxis. Onset is insidious with several weeks of fever, weight loss, malaise, and night sweats. The chest radiograph typically shows bilateral interstitial pulmonary infiltrates, but a lobar distribution and spontaneous pneumothoraces may occur. The arterial blood gas analysis usually reveals hypoxia and respiratory alkalosis. A wide A-a gradient (>35 mm Hg) and low Po_2 (<70 mm Hg) are associated with increased mortality. Several methods are used for the diagnosis of PCP. Staining for PCP in hypertonic saline-induced expectorated sputum is 30%-85% sensitive. The sensitivity improves with liquefaction and the use of monoclonal antibody staining, and it decreases with use of PCP prophylaxis. Bronchoalveolar lavage is 85%-90% sensitive. If the patient is receiving PCP prophylaxis, transbronchial lung biopsy may be needed to make diagnosis. Open lung biopsy is rarely needed.

Table 20-34.--General Relationship of Clinical Syndromes to CD4 Cell Count in Human Immunodeficiency Virus-Infected Patients

Clinical syndrome	CD4 cell count			
	>50	200-500	<200	<50
Asymptomatic	x			
Kaposi sarcoma	x			
Fever, sweats, weight loss		x		
Hairy leukoplakia		x		
Oral, esophageal *Candida*		x		
Tuberculosis		x		
PCP			x	
Cryptococcosis			x	
Dementia			x	
Toxoplasmosis				x
MAI				x
CMV				x
Lymphoma				x

CMV, cytomegalovirus; MAI, *Mycobacterium avium-intracellulare*; PCP, *Pneumocystis carinii* pneumonia.

From Shelhamer JH, Toews GB, Masur H, Suffredini AF, Pizzo PA, Walsh TJ, Henderson DK: Respiratory disease in the immunosuppressed patient. Ann Intern Med 117:415-431, 1992. By permission of the American College of Physicians.

The treatment of choice for severe disease is cotrimoxazole, 15-20 mg/kg per day (trimethoprim component) for 21 days. Adverse reactions develop in 76% of cases and include fever, rash, neutropenia, thrombocytopenia, elevated results of liver function tests, and renal dysfunction. Intravenous pentamidine is an alternative to cotrimoxazole (3-4 mg/kg per day for 21 days). The adverse reaction rate is >60%; reactions include hypotension, nephrotoxicity, hypoglycemia, and pancreatitis. If there is no improvement 5-7 days after beginning treatment, switching to or adding an alternative agent should be considered.

For mild to moderate disease, treatment regimens include oral trimethoprim-sulfamethoxazole for 21 days, oral trimethoprim-dapsone (patient should be checked for glucose-6-phosphatase deficiency) for 21 days (mild hyperkalemia and methemoglobinemia can occur), oral primaquine plus clindamycin (methemoglobinemia has been reported with primaquine), aerosolized pentamidine (two studies have found that intravenous administration is more effective than aerosolized pentamidine), trimetrexate plus folinic acid, and atovaquone (for patients intolerant of trimethoprim-sulfamethoxazole).

Controlled studies have shown that adjunctive corticosteroids in patients with moderate to severe disease increase survival in patients with AIDS. Benefit was shown when Pao_2 with patient breathing room air was <70 mm Hg or A-a gradient was >35 mm Hg. Recommended dosages of prednisone are 40 mg orally twice a day on days 1-5, 20 mg orally twice a day on days 6-10, and 20 mg orally each day on days 11-21.

Primary (CD4 cell count <200/μL) and secondary prophylaxis are recommended in patients with AIDS: 1) trimethoprim-sulfamethoxazole is the drug of choice (1 double-strength tablet orally each day or 1 double-strength tablet 3 times per week); 2) aerosolized pentamidine, 300 mg inhaled monthly via Respigard II nebulizer; 3) dapsone, 50 mg orally each day or 100 mg orally twice a week.

Recent trials of trimethoprim-sulfamethoxazole compared with inhaled pentamidine for primary and secondary prophylaxis showed conclusively that trimethoprim-sulfamethoxazole was more effective than inhaled pentamidine. Also, it may add prophylaxis against other infectious agents (*Nocardia, Toxoplasma gondii, Streptococcus pneumoniae, Haemophilus influenzae, Listeria monocytogenes, Isospora belli*) and prevent extrapulmonary pneumocytosis. As expected, there are many more side effects with trimethoprim-sulfamethoxazole.

Mycobacterial Infections

Mycobacterium tuberculosis is increased in frequency in injection drug users, minorities, and foreign-born persons with AIDS. HIV-infected patients have an increased frequency of extrapulmonary disease and atypical chest radiographic appearance. Extrapulmonary disease, however, presents similarly in HIV- and non-HIV-infected patients. HIV-infected patients may have accelerated primary disease if exposed to patients with active disease.

The incidence of multiple drug-resistant (MDR) tuberculosis is increasing. Patients with newly acquired infection may have a fulminant course. Unlike patients with AIDS who are infected with other strains of tuberculosis, patients infected with MDR tuberculosis more commonly have alveolar or reticulonodular infiltrates or cavitation. Mortality rate is 70%-80%. Average duration of survival is 2-3 months.

For treatment of tuberculosis in patients with AIDS,

drugs are the same as used for normal hosts, but drug resistance must be suspected. In initial regimens, if drug resistance is suspected, isoniazid, rifampin, pyrazinamide, and ethambutol are used until drug sensitivity results are available; otherwise, isoniazid, rifampin, and pyrazinamide are used. For drug-susceptible organisms, isoniazid, rifampin, and pyrazinamide are used for 2 months, and isoniazid and rifampin are used for 7 months, or for 6 months after cultures are negative, whichever is longer. For isoniazid-resistant organisms, rifampin and ethambutol with or without pyrazinamide are used for 18 months, or for 12 months after cultures are negative, whichever is longer. Optimal regimens for MDR tuberculosis are unknown. Prophylaxis is used for all patients who are HIV positive with positive results of purified protein derivative testing (≥ 5 mm).

Mycobacterium avium-intracellulare causes infection when immunosuppression is severe (CD4 cell count $<100/\mu L$). Common presentations include low-grade fever, night sweats, weight loss, and diarrhea. Organisms can be isolated from blood, bone marrow, stool, and respiratory tract secretions. The organism is resistant to conventional antimycobacterial agents. Treatment involves multiple drugs with multiple side effects. Some studies have shown an increase in survival with treatment, but symptoms can often be ameliorated. On the basis of in vitro data, three- and four-drug combinations of clofazamine, ciprofloxacin, rifampin, clarithromycin, rifabutin, and ethambutol with or without amikacin are used. Prophylaxis with rifabutin has recently been approved by the Food and Drug Administration.

Treponema pallidum

There are rare reports of seronegative secondary syphilis in patients with AIDS. Neurosyphilis has been reported to occur earlier in patients with AIDS than in HIV-negative patients. Patients with AIDS have also been reported to have unusually severe manifestations of all stages of syphilis. Recent studies, however, suggest that these phenomena are rare. However, because of these concerns, some physicians advocate cerebrospinal fluid examination in patients with primary or secondary syphilis and AIDS before initiating treatment.

Serologic response to standard treatment regimens was the same in HIV-positive and HIV-negative persons in a recent study of 50 injection drug users. However, because of reports of patients with primary, secondary, and latent syphilis failing to respond to intramuscular benzathine or procaine penicillin therapy, some investigators have

suggested treating patients with AIDS and syphilis more aggressively (additional dose of benzathine penicillin or intravenous penicillin therapy for 5-10 days). However, data on the frequency of this problem are not available, and these practices remain controversial.

Ceftriaxone has been advocated as an alternative therapy for patients with AIDS who have neurosyphilis because it attains treponemacidal cerebrospinal fluid levels and is easy to administer. In a recent small study, however, the use of ceftriaxone in patients with latent and presumed latent syphilis (no cerebrospinal fluid examination) and asymptomatic neurosyphilis had a 23% failure rate within 1-2 years of initiation of therapy. For patients with latent or presumed latent disease, the efficacies of the standard penicillin regimen and ceftriaxone were equivalent.

Fungal Infections

Cryptococcus neoformans

Meningitis and disseminated disease occur in 10% of patients with AIDS and are common initial manifestations. Subtle presentations may occur. Meningismus may not be present. Poor prognostic factors include hyponatremia and positive culture results from a source other than cerebrospinal fluid. The diagnosis of cryptococcal disease relies on assays of serum and cerebrospinal fluid cryptococcal antigen and fungal blood and spinal fluid cultures. Initial therapy includes amphotericin B with or without flucytosine. Flucytosine may be associated with increased hematologic toxicity in patients with AIDS, particularly if levels are not measured. Fluconazole is alternative agent in patients with less severe disease. Fluconazole daily is more effective than amphotericin B weekly for chronic suppression. Persistence of infection in prostate may be a cause of relapse of infection.

Dimorphic Fungi (Histoplasma capsulatum, Coccidioides immitis, Blastomyces dermatitidis)

Coccidioidomycosis and histoplasmosis are reported more often than blastomycosis. Disease with all three pathogens usually presents as disseminated infection and can even present as septic shock (histoplasmosis). Localized pulmonary involvement occurs but is much less common, except with blastomycosis (50% of cases). Disseminated disease often involves the central nervous system (blastomycosis, coccidioidomycosis). Organisms may be seen in buffy coat of blood (histoplasmosis) in some cases. Travel history and geographic location are important clues to the diagnosis. Initial therapy is with amphotericin B for all three pathogens. For chronic suppression, itraconazole or amphotericin B is effective for histoplasmosis. For coccidioidomycosis, amphotericin B or fluconazole is used. Treatment of blastomycosis is the same as that of histoplasmosis.

Candida albicans

Mucocutaneous disease (e.g., oral thrush or recurrent vaginitis) is common. Esophagitis is also frequent and is a common cause of dysphagia. Fungemia is rare unless there is a central venous catheter in place. Treatment is with clotrimoxazole troches or nystatin initially for mucocutaneous disease. Fluconazole or ketoconazole is used for treatment of topical treatment failures. In a recent study, fluconazole was more effective than ketoconazole for esophagitis in patients with AIDS. Amphotericin B is used for azole failures.

Aspergillus

Aspergillosis is rare except in the setting of neutropenia.

Viral Infections

Cytomegalovirus retinitis is common cause of blindness (may be asymptomatic; screening eye examinations are necessary). Cytomegalovirus gastrointestinal disease may manifest as abdominal pain, dysphagia, and bloody diarrhea. It most commonly involves the esophagus and colon. Cytomegalovirus can also cause hepatitis, pneumonitis, sclerosing cholangitis, encephalitis, and adrenalitis. Treatment is with ganciclovir or foscarnet.

With herpes simplex virus, severe mucocutaneous ulceration may occur, and the frequency of recurrent oral-labial and genital disease may increase.

Prolonged or severe herpes zoster infection may herald the diagnosis of HIV infection. Central nervous system infection can occur weeks to months after the diagnosis of herpes zoster.

Enteric Infections

Differential diagnoses for various clinical syndromes are outlined in Table 20-35.

Initial evaluation of patients with AIDS who have abdominal pain, large-volume diarrhea, and weight loss should include stool cultures for bacteria, three separate stool specimens for ova and parasites, specific examination for cryptosporidiosis, and *Clostridium difficile* toxin.

Table 20-35.--Differential Diagnoses of Enteric Infections in Association With Human Immunodeficiency Virus

Proctitis	Proctocolitis	Enteritis
Neisseria	*Campylobacter*	*Giardia*
gonorrhoeae	*Shigella*	Cryptosporidiosis
Herpes simplex	*Chlamydia*	*Isospora*
Chlamydia	*Entamoeba*	Microsporidia
Treponema	*histolytica*	
pallidum	*Clostridium*	
Cytomegalovirus	*difficile*	
	Salmonella	
	typhimurium	
	Cytomegalovirus	

In cases of persistent diarrhea despite routine studies, cytomegalovirus or *M. avium-intracellulare* should be considered. If no diagnosis is made, upper and lower gastrointestinal endoscopy and biopsy may yield pathogens that are treatable.

Salmonellosis presents with fever, severe diarrhea, abdominal pain, or typhoidal illness without diarrhea. Bacteremia is common. Ciprofloxacin is used for treatment for 10-14 days. Recurrence is common; maintenance therapy may be needed.

Cryptosporidiosis and *I. belli* infection often cause massive, watery diarrhea, crampy abdominal pain, anorexia, flatulence, and malaise. Fever and bloody diarrhea are uncommon. Malabsorption and dehydration are common. Biliary tract involvement may occur with cryptosporidiosis infection. Acid-fast bacilli smear of stool or cryptosporidium-specific stain of stool is diagnostic. If CD4 cell count is >180/µL, cryptosporidium infection is usually self-limited (<4 weeks); if it is <140/µL, persistent disease will develop in 80%-90%. There is no effective antimicrobial therapy for cryptosporidiosis. For *Isospora*, trimethoprim-sulfamethoxazole is used.

Neurologic Disease

HIV encephalopathy may begin early in the course of HIV disease and is slowly progressive. Subtle cognitive impairment is common; it can progress to severe dementia and marked motor dysfunction. Computed tomography and magnetic resonance imaging show diffuse atrophy. No therapy is proved to be effective. Antiretroviral therapy may be helpful (dosage of zidovudine may need to be increased--1,200 mg/day).

Progressive multifocal leukoencephalopathy is a demyelinating disease caused by papovavirus (JC virus). Symptoms and signs are variable. Magnetic resonance imaging shows characteristic white matter changes. Prognosis is poor, and there is no proven treatment.

The most common symptoms of *Toxoplasma encephalitis* include headache, confusion, and fever. Focal neurologic deficits occur in 69% of cases. Median CD4 cell count at diagnosis is 50/μL. Multiple mass lesions develop in central nervous system in patients with AIDS, typically either toxoplasmosis or lymphoma. Magnetic resonance imaging is more sensitive than computed tomography with contrast (ring-enhancing lesions are characteristic). Single mass lesions are found in up to 40% of patients evaluated by computed tomography and in 20% by magnetic resonance imaging. If serum toxoplasmosis antibody is positive (10%-40% of individuals in United States), treatment should be empiric with pyrimethamine and sulfadiazine plus leucovorin. However, 15%-20% of patients in a recent study were seronegative at presentation. Immunofluorescence assay is less sensitive than enzyme-linked immunosorbent assay. If patient is seronegative, has a single mass lesion, or has no response to empiric therapy (2 weeks), brain biopsy is indicated. Long-term suppressive therapy (secondary prophylaxis) is necessary to prevent relapse, although even with suppressive therapy 20%-25% of patients will have relapse. Primary prophylaxis in seropositive individuals (trimethoprim-sulfamethoxazole) or other regimens is controversial. Alternative therapy is clindamycin and pyrimethamine.

The differential diagnosis of *central nervous system mass lesions* in patients with AIDS includes *Toxoplasma gondii*, neoplasm (lymphoma or Kaposi's sarcoma), *Cryptococcus neoformans, Coccidioides immitis, Candida albicans, Mycobacterium tuberculosis*, and *Nocardia asteroides*, among others.

Neoplastic Diseases

In *Kaposi's sarcoma*, skin, lung, and gastrointestinal tract are the commonly affected organs. Lung involvement may mimic infection. Bloody pleural effusions suggest Kaposi's sarcoma. It is most common in the homosexual population with AIDS. Treatment options include α-interferon therapy, combination chemotherapy, and radiation or cryotherapy.

Non-Hodgkin's lymphoma is a complication of advanced HIV disease. Usually it is B cell in origin. As patients with AIDS live longer, this complication will become more frequent. Central nervous system involvement is common, and it can be the only anatomic site of disease. Treatment options include combination chemotherapy and radiation. Treatment can often improve quality of life, but duration of remission is usually measured in months. Recent reports suggest a link between Hodgkin's disease and HIV, particularly in patients with advanced disease at presentation and with mixed cellular and lymphocyte depletion on pathologic examination.

Miscellaneous Infections and Clinical Syndromes

Idiopathic thrombocytopenic purpura should be suspected in patients with HIV infection in whom purpura or ecchymotic skin lesions develop. Treatment is with antiretroviral therapy; if this fails, prednisone, plasmapheresis, splenic irradiation, or splenectomy can be tried.

Bacillary angiomatosis is a clinical syndrome consisting of constitutional symptoms in conjunction with angiomatous nodules of skin or bone and occasionally peliosis hepatis. Central nervous system mass lesions have also been reported. Diagnosis is established by biopsy, demonstration of organism on Warthin-Starry (Steiner) stain, and cultivation of the causative organisms (*Rochalimaea quintana, R. henselae*). Results of blood culture (lysis centrifugation technique) may also be positive if incubation is prolonged. Treatment is with erythromycin or doxycycline.

Bacterial pneumonia in patients with AIDS may be as common as PCP. In injection drug users, it is particularly common and occurs before and after the onset of HIV infection. Common causes are *S. pneumoniae* and *H. influenzae*. It should be suspected in patients with purulent sputum and lobar infiltrates. Remember that recurrent pneumonia is an AIDS-defining illness.

Endocrine abnormalities in HIV infection can affect the adrenal glands, which are involved by infections, tumor, and medications. Infection is caused by cytomegalovirus, *Mycobacterium tuberculosis* and atypical *Mycobacteria, C. neoformans, H. capsulatum, T. gondii*, and *P. carinii*. Adrenal insufficiency is rare. Noninfectious diseases that involve the adrenal glands include lymphoma, Kaposi's sarcoma, and hemorrhage. Adrenal insufficiency is rare. Hyponatremia should instigate a workup for adrenal insufficiency. Ketoconazole inhibits adrenal steroidogenesis. Rifampin, phenytoin, and opiates accelerate degradation of cortisol.

Most asymptomatic patients have normal thyroid function. Increased thyroxine-binding globulin can cause increased thyroxine level with normal thyroid-stimulating hormone value. Thyroxine and triiodothyronine levels decline with advancing illness. Triiodothyronine level is less than in other chronic illnesses. Persistence of relatively normal triiodothyronine value despite progressive HIV infection may contribute to weight loss. *P. carinii* infection of thyroid has been described.

Common causes of hyponatremia include diarrhea, syndrome of inappropriate secretion of antidiuretic hormone (most common cause if hyponatremia developed while patient hospitalized), and renal insufficiency.

Hypercalcemia can be caused by lymphoma and human T-cell leukemia virus-I coinfection. Hypocalcemia is also caused by ketoconazole and foscarnet.

In regard to gonadal function, testosterone levels are normal in asymptomatic HIV. In advanced disease, gonadal, pituitary, or hypothalamic failure may occur.

Pancreatitis can be caused by cytomegalovirus, trimethoprim-sulfamethoxazole, intravenous pentamidine, didanosine (ddI), and zalcitabine (ddC).

The most common *rheumatologic manifestations* in HIV are Reiter's syndrome, reactive arthritis, polymyositis and polymyalgia, and sicca syndrome. All of these are associated with the onset of active AIDS complications and infections.

Cholangitis and *acalculous cholecystitis* are associated with cytomegalovirus, cryptosporidiosis, and Microsporidia (*Enterocytozoon bieneusi*). Most common syndrome associated with Microsporidia, however, is chronic diarrhea; it can also cause keratoconjunctivitis, hepatitis, and peritonitis.

Renal abnormalities include almost any type of chronic nephropathy, but HIV-associated nephropathy is most common. About 85% of cases have occurred in blacks. Pathologic feature is focal and segmental glomerulosclerosis, which may cause nephrotic syndrome, and this leads rapidly to end-stage renal failure. Peripheral edema and hypertension are usually absent. Renal abnormalities occur in any stage of HIV disease. IgA nephropathy was recently reported.

Common dermatologic diseases that are associated with HIV disease include prurigo xerosis, ichthyosis, seborrheic dermatitis, psoriasis, and neoplasms (Kaposi's sarcoma, lymphoma).

The etiologic agent of *oral hairy leukoplakia* is Epstein-Barr virus. It usually responds to acyclovir therapy.

HIV-2 is a human retrovirus with significant antigenic differences from HIV-1. This infection is prevalent in western Africa. In certain urban centers, 15%-64% of prostitutes are infected. Seroprevalence increases with age; 100% of prostitutes >50 years are infected. By April 1992, 32 cases had been reported in the United States. In all 32 cases, the patient either had lived in western Africa or had sexual partners who had lived there. No cases of transfusion-related disease have been reported. Since June 1992, the blood supply has been screened for HIV-2. Transmission is through sexual contact or blood products. Vertical transmission is less common than with HIV-1. HIV-2 can cause AIDS. Rate of progression to severe immunosuppression and AIDS is 12-13 times slower than with HIV-1. Asymptomatic period is likely much longer. Clinical manifestations of AIDS are similar between HIV-1 and HIV-2. Diagnosis should be considered in patients from endemic areas or patients who have sexual partners who reside in endemic areas. In 80% of HIV-2-infected patients, results of enzyme-linked immunosorbent assay designed to detect HIV-1 will be positive. An HIV-2-specific assay is available. Western blot test results may be indeterminate. The length of seronegative interval after infection is unknown. A polymerase chain reaction test is also available. Antiretroviral therapy is used according to protocols used for HIV-1. However, because of long asymptomatic interval, instituting therapy when the CD4 cell count is beween 200-500/μL is controversial. Treatment strategies for opportunistic infections are identical.

ACKNOWLEDGMENT

The authors gratefully acknowledge the contributions by Walter R. Wilson, M.D., to the earlier versions of this chapter.

NOTES

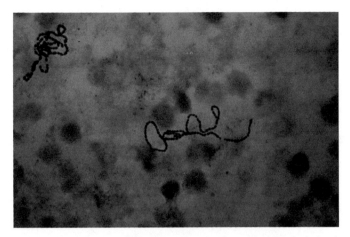

Color plate 20-1. Gram stain showing β-hemolytic streptococci among cellular debris. (From Wood MJ: Skin and soft tissue: bacterial, protozoal and helminth infections. *In* Slide Atlas of Infectious Diseases. Second edition. Edited by WE Farrar, MJ Wood, JA Innes, H Tubbs. London, England, Gower Medical Publishing, 1992, pp 10.1-10.34. By permission of publisher.)

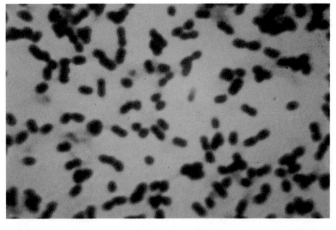

Color plate 20-2. Large numbers of gram-positive diplococci in cerebrospinal fluid of a patient with pneumococcal meningitis. (From Farrar WE: The nervous system. *In* Slide Atlas of Infectious Diseases. Second edition. Edited by WE Farrar, MJ Wood, JA Innes, H Tubbs. London, England, Gower Medical Publishing, 1992, pp 3.1-3.42. By permission of publisher.)

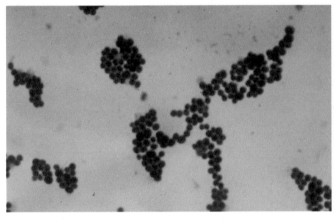

Color plate 20-3. Gram stain of bacterial culture of *Staphylococcus aureus* showing gram-positive cocci in clusters. (From Innes JA: Lower respiratory tract. *In* Slide Atlas of Infectious Diseases. Second edition. Edited by WE Farrar, MJ Wood, JA Innes, H Tubbs. London, England, Gower Medical Publishing, 1992, pp 2.1-2.32. By permission of publisher.)

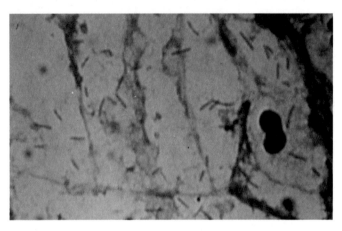

Color plate 20-4. Gram stain of sputum showing gram-negative rods. The bacterial culture revealed *Pseudomonas aeruginosa*. (From Innes JA: Lower respiratory tract. *In* Slide Atlas of Infectious Diseases. Second edition. Edited by WE Farrar, MJ Wood, JA Innes, H Tubbs. London, England, Gower Medical Publishing, 1992, pp 2.1-2.32. By permission of publisher.)

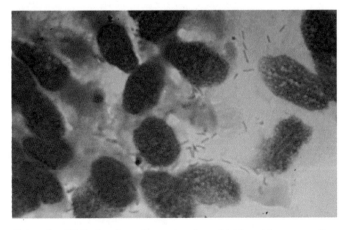

Color plate 20-5. Specimen from a transbronchial lung biopsy revealing *Legionella pneumophila*. (From Innes JA: Lower respiratory tract. *In* Slide Atlas of Infectious Diseases. Second edition. Edited by WE Farrar, MJ Wood, JA Innes, H Tubbs. London, England, Gower Medical Publishing, 1992, pp 2.1-2.32. By permission of publisher.)

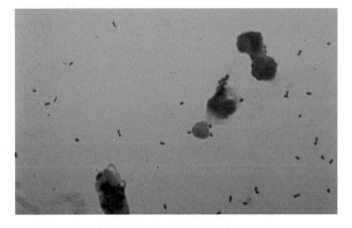

Color plate 20-6. Gram stain of cerebrospinal fluid showing gram-positive rods of *Listeria monocytogenes*. (From Farrar WE: The nervous system. *In* Slide Atlas of Infectious Diseases. Second edition. Edited by WE Farrar, MJ Wood, JA Innes, H Tubbs. London, England, Gower Medical Publishing, 1992, pp 3.1-3.42. By permission of publisher.)

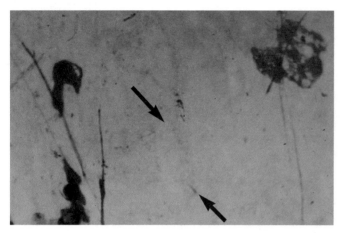

Color plate 20-7. Ziehl-Neelson stain showing large numbers of *Mycobacterium tuberculosis. Arrows*, Acid-fast bacilli. (From Innes JA: Lower respiratory tract. *In* Slide Atlas of Infectious Diseases. Second edition. Edited by WE Farrar, MJ Wood, JA Innes, H Tubbs. London, England, Gower Medical Publishing, 1992, pp 2.1-2.32. By permission of publisher.)

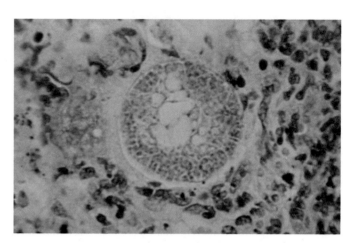

Color plate 20-8. Histopathologic specimen of lung showing spherule of *Coccidioides immitis.* (From Innes JA: Lower respiratory tract. *In* Slide Atlas of Infectious Diseases. Second edition. Edited by WE Farrar, MJ Wood, JA Innes, H Tubbs. London, England, Gower Medical Publishing, 1992, pp 2.1-2.32. By permission of publisher.)

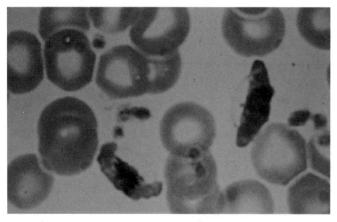

Color plate 20-9. Thin blood smear showing banana-shaped gametocyte of *Plasmodium falciparum.* (From Tubbs H: Systemic infections. *In* Slide Atlas of Infectious Diseases. Second edition. Edited by WE Farrar, MJ Wood, JA Innes, H Tubbs. London, England, Gower Medical Publishing, 1992, pp 13.1-13.26. By permission of publisher.)

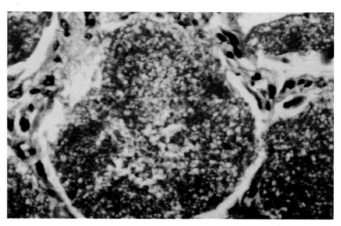

Color plate 20-10. Histopathology of transbronchial lung biopsy showing alveolar spaces filled with *Pneumocystis carinii.* (From Innes JA: Lower respiratory tract. *In* Slide Atlas of Infectious Diseases. Second edition. Edited by WE Farrar, MJ Wood, JA Innes, H Tubbs. London, England, Gower Medical Publishing, 1992, pp 2.1-2.32. By permission of publisher.)

QUESTIONS
(See "Answers" section)

Multiple Choice

1. In January, a 72-year-old female nursing home resident presents to the emergency room with fever, confusion, hypotension, and respiratory failure. Five days earlier she had developed fever and myalgias, which had slowly improved until today. Chest radiograph shows bilateral infiltrates with pneumatoceles. In addition to the usual supportive measures, you begin antibiotic therapy targeted against:
   a. *Pseudomonas aeruginosa*
   b. *Mycobacterium tuberculosis*
   c. *Streptococcus bovis*
   d. *Staphylococcus aureus*
   e. Influenza

2. All of the following antibiotic combinations are bactericidal against most *Enterococcus faecalis* isolates except:
   a. Penicillin and gentamicin
   b. Cefazolin and gentamicin
   c. Ampicillin and streptomycin
   d. Vancomycin and gentamicin
   e. Mezlocillin and gentamicin

3. A 42-year-old man with acute leukemia develops fever and rigors 72 hours after completion of his first course of chemotherapy. On physical examination, the patient is febrile (40°C) and hypotensive. The only other abnormal finding is a 1-cm round, indurated, purple-black area with an ulcerated center in the perirectal area. Laboratory examination is significant for a leukocyte count of 0.2×10^9/L. The organism most likely to be the cause of this patient's infection is:
   a. *Staphylococcus aureus*
   b. *Enterococcus faecalis*
   c. *Escherichia coli*
   d. *Pseudomonas aeruginosa*
   e. *Candida albicans*

4. A 16-year-old previously healthy girl comes to your office complaining of an infected wound. She was bitten by a cat 1 day ago. The wound is now draining pus and surrounded by cellulitis. Gram stain of the pus reveals many gram-negative bacilli. The most likely infecting organism is:

   a. *Francisella tularensis*
   b. *Escherichia coli*
   c. *Staphylococcus epidermidis*
   d. *Pasteurella multocida*
   e. *Pseudomonas aeruginosa*

5. Bacteria cause disease by several mechanisms, including the production of systemically toxic substances without actual tissue invasion by the bacteria. Each of the following organisms can produce such toxins except:
   a. *Staphylococcus aureus*
   b. *Streptococcus pyogenes*
   c. *Clostridium tetani*
   d. *Corynebacterium diphtheriae*
   e. *Streptococcus mitis*

6. Each of the following symptoms can be a manifestation of infection with parvovirus B19 except:
   a. Transient arthralgias
   b. Chronic anemia in individuals infected with human immunodeficiency virus (HIV)
   c. "Slapped face"-appearing rash in children
   d. Chronic fatigue syndrome
   e. Aplastic crisis in sickle cell disease

7. A 32-year-old man with advanced acquired immunodeficiency syndrome (AIDS) is hospitalized because of rapidly deteriorating mental status. Cerebrospinal fluid examination is normal. Computed tomography of the brain shows a 2- by 2-cm, enhancing, white matter lesion in the left parietal area. Biopsy of this lesion reveals progressive multifocal leukoencephalopathy. This is caused by infection with which of the following:
   a. JC virus
   b. Creutzfeld-Jakob agent
   c. *Toxoplasma gondii*
   d. Cytomegalovirus
   e. Human T-cell leukemia virus-1 (HTLV-1)

8. A 54-year-old man from Oklahoma is hospitalized with fever of several days' duration following an insect bite on the leg. He now appears toxic and complains of severe headache. On examination, there is an eschar at the site of injury and inguinal adenopathy on the same side. You initiate antibiotic therapy directed against:
   a. *Borrelia burgdorferi* (Lyme disease)

b. *Rickettsia rickettsii* (Rocky Mountain spotted fever)

c. *Francisella tularensis* (tularemia)

d. Epstein-Barr virus (mononucleosis)

e. *Salmonella typhi* (typhoid fever)

9. Which of the following parasitic infections can be diagnosed by microscopic examination of stool specimens (stool ova and parasites):

a. Babesiosis

b. Trichinosis

c. Ascariasis

d. Trypanosomiasis

e. Leishmaniasis

10. Risk factors for developing toxoplasmosis include all of the following except:

a. Eating raw fish

b. Eating raw meat

c. Receiving a heart transplant

d. Acquired immunodeficiency syndrome (AIDS)

e. Exposure to cat litter boxes

11. A 25-year-old previously healthy white man presents to the emergency room with a 24-hour history of fever (temperature 40°C), chills, and a severe headache. On physical examination, abnormal findings include meningismus and audible crackles in the left lower lung field. Cerebrospinal fluid examination reveals a leukocyte count of 2,000/μL (95% polymorphonuclear neutrophils). The cerebrospinal fluid Gram stain is negative. Chest radiograph reveals a left lower lobe infiltrate. The most likely cause of this case of acute meningitis is:

a. *Haemophilus influenzae*

b. *Neisseria meningitidis*

c. *Streptococcus pneumoniae*

d. *Cryptococcus neoformans*

e. *Mycobacterium tuberculosis*

12. A 35-year-old previously healthy woman is admitted to the hospital with a 2-week history of fever, chills, and malaise. On physical examination, abnormal findings include bilateral conjunctival hemorrhages, splenomegaly, and a 2/6 holosystolic murmur consistent with mitral regurgitation. Three weeks previously she had undergone a routine dental examination. She has no known antimicrobial allergies. Four separate blood cultures 48 hours after admission are positive for *Streptococcus mutans* (penicillin

minimal inhibitory concentration, <0.1 g/mL). The best therapeutic regimen for this patient would be:

a. Aqueous penicillin G intravenously for 2 weeks

b. Aqueous penicillin G intravenously plus gentamicin for 4 weeks

c. Vancomycin intravenously for 4 weeks

d. Aqueous penicillin G intravenously plus gentamicin for 2 weeks

e. Cefazolin intravenously for 2 weeks

13. An 18-year-old single woman presents to the emergency room with a painful left knee. There is no history of tick exposure or family history of rheumatologic disease. On physical examination, her temperature is 38.5°C, the knee is erythematous and warm, and there is marked limitation of motion. A large effusion is also present. Arthrocentesis reveals a synovial leukocyte count of 45,000/μL. The results of Gram stain and bacterial culture are negative. The most likely cause of this acute arthritis is:

a. Rheumatoid arthritis

b. *Staphylococcus aureus*

c. *Borrelia burgdorferi*

d. *Neisseria gonorrhoeae*

e. Coagulase-negative staphylococci

14. The treatment of choice for primary syphilis is:

a. Doxycycline 100 mg orally twice a day for 14 days

b. Benzathine penicillin 2.4 million units intramuscularly, 1 dose

c. Benzathine penicillin 2.4 million units intramuscularly for 3 weeks

d. Erythromycin 500 mg three times a day for 14 days

e. Aqueous penicillin G 12-24 million units intravenously per day for 10 days

15. All of the following organisms are a cause of acute sinusitis in adults except:

a. *Haemophilus influenzae*

b. *Streptococcus pneumoniae*

c. *Peptostreptococcus magnus*

d. *Bacteroides fragilis*

e. *Moraxella catarrhalis*

16. All of the following antimicrobial drugs are excreted primarily by the kidneys except:

a. Penicillin G

b. Ciprofloxacin

c. Nafcillin

d. Cefazolin

e. Gentamicin

17. Fever in the neutropenic patient (absolute neutrophil count 0.5×10^9/L) generally requires empiric antimicrobial therapy before culture results are known. All of the following are acceptable choices for that empiric therapy except:

a. Piperacillin and gentamicin

b. Ceftazidime

c. Ceftazidime and tobramycin

d. Cefoxitin and vancomycin

e. Imipenem

18. A 63-year-old male farmer is hospitalized after 3 days of progressive confusion, lethargy, and a seizure. Because of concern for possible herpes simplex encephalitis, you begin treatment with acyclovir, 10 mg/kg intravenously three times a day. By the fourth hospital day, his creatinine value has increased from 1.5 mg/dL to 3.2 mg/dL. The most likely explanation for the rising creatinine level is:

a. Herpes simplex nephritis

b. Allergic interstitial nephritis caused by acyclovir

c. Precipitation of acyclovir crystals in the renal tubules

d. Acute tubular necrosis

e. Interference of acyclovir with laboratory measurement of serum creatinine

19. Which of the following antibacterial agents is inactive against *Streptococcus pneumoniae* and should never be used to treat pneumococcal infections?

a. Ciprofloxacin

b. Cefazolin

c. Chloramphenicol

d. Erythromycin

e. Penicillin G

20. Which of the following antimicrobial agents is most likely to affect theophylline levels in a 62-year-old woman with asthma?

a. Ampicillin

b. Ganciclovir

c. Amoxicillin/clavulanate

d. Erythromycin

e. Isoniazid

21. A 37-year-old man from Minneapolis with HIV infection (CD4 cell count, 150/μL) is admitted to the hospital with a 10-day history of fever (temperature, 38.3°C) and a dry, nonproductive cough. There is no history of previous tuberculosis or exposure to persons with tuberculosis. His current medications include zidovudine and inhaled pentamidine. Physical examination reveals crackles in the upper lung fields. Chest radiograph reveals bilateral upper lobe infiltrates. Initial results of his induced sputum examination include negative Gram stain, potassium hydroxide and acid-fast smear, and *Pneumocystis carinii* smear. The most likely cause of this man's symptoms is:

a. *Mycobacterium tuberculosis*

b. *Histoplasma capsulatum*

c. *Pneumocystis carinii*

d. Cytomegalovirus

e. *Mycobacterium avium-intracellulare*

22. All of the following organisms cause infections in patients with AIDS which require maintenance antimicrobial therapy to prevent relapse of infection except:

a. *Pneumocystis carinii*

b. *Toxoplasma gondii*

c. *Mycobacterium tuberculosis*

d. *Cryptococcus neoformans*

e. Cytomegalovirus

23. A 40-year-old man with AIDS taking zidovudine and trimethoprim-sulfamethoxazole presents to the emergency room with a seizure. Computed tomography with contrast reveals multiple ring-enhancing mass lesions in the cerebrum. The patient is known to be seronegative for *Toxoplasma gondii*. What is the most appropriate management at this point?

a. Begin empiric chemotherapy for presumed central nervous system lymphoma

b. Perform a lumbar puncture to obtain cerebrospinal fluid for culture

c. Begin empiric amphotericin B therapy

d. Recommend a diagnostic brain biopsy

e. Begin empiric therapy with isoniazid, rifampin, pyrazinamide, and ethambutol

24. A 30-year-old woman who is seropositive for HIV antibody and is taking only zidovudine presents to your office with acute-onset fever, headache, and confusion without focal neurologic signs or symptoms.

Computed tomography with contrast is normal and cerebrospinal fluid examination reveals a leukocyte count of 5,000/μL with 90% lymphocytes, glucose value of 10 mg/dL, and protein level of 250 mg/dL. Gram stain reveals a gram-positive bacillus. Counterimmunoelectrophoresis and cryptococcal antigen are negative. The drug of choice at this point for this infection is:

a. Ampicillin
b. Cefotaxime
c. Cefazolin
d. Trimethoprim-sulfamethoxazole
e. Amphotericin B

25. A 34-year-old foreign-born man who is seropositive for HIV antibody (CD4 cell count, 300/μL) develops pulmonary tuberculosis. The most appropriate *initial* therapy for this patient would be:

a. Isoniazid and rifampin
b. Isoniazid, rifampin, pyrazinamide, and ethambutol
c. Isoniazid and ethambutol
d. Rifampin, ethambutol, and pyrazinamide
e. Isoniazid, rifampin, pyrazinamide, and ciprofloxacin

True/False

26. *Pseudomonas aeruginosa* infection is associated with the following:

a. Spontaneous bacteremia in neutropenic patients
b. Chronic diarrhea
c. Ecthyma gangrenosum
d. Folliculitis associated with hot tubs
e. Nosocomial pneumonias
f. Pneumonia in patients with cystic fibrosis

27. Tuberculosis is increasing in prevalence worldwide. Each of the following identifies a patient group at increased risk for acquiring tuberculosis:

a. Health care personnel
b. Persons with HIV infection
c. Workers in slaughterhouses
d. Persons with silicosis
e. Diabetics
f. Patients who have had previous gastrectomy

28. Each of the following statements describes characteristics of actinomycosis:

a. Most infections are preceded by intestinal perforation

b. Pulmonary infection with *Actinomyces* may drain through the chest wall
c. Therapy with penicillin must often continue for a year or more
d. Animals are a common reservoir for *Actinomyces israelii*
e. When involved in a brain abscess, *Actinomyces* is often present with other organisms
f. *Actinomyces* grows only in anaerobic environments

29. All of the following statements describe characteristics of infections with *Coccidioides immitis* (coccidioidomycosis):

a. Highest incidence is in the Ohio River Valley
b. When associated with erythema nodosum, there is a high incidence of severe disseminated disease
c. Acute pulmonary coccidioidomycosis is usually self-limited and does not require therapy
d. Coccidioidomycosis meningitis is usually cured after a 4-week course of amphotericin B and flucytosine
e. Biopsy of infected tissue reveals angioinvasive hyphae
f. Ketoconazole is effective for treating nonmeningeal coccidioidomycosis

30. True statements concerning toxic shock syndrome (TSS) include:

a. 90% of TSS cases are related to menstruation
b. TSS can occur after an influenza infection
c. Most patients with TSS due to *Staphylococcus aureus* are bacteremic
d. TSS due to *Streptococcus pyogenes* is often associated with tampon use
e. The relapse rate for menstruation-related TSS is as high as 40%
f. The diagnosis of TSS is based on isolation of *S. aureus* or *S. pyogenes* from a normally sterile site

31. Which of the following statements are true regarding infective endocarditis?

a. *Staphylococcus aureus* is the most common cause of early prosthetic valve endocarditis
b. The most important indication for surgical intervention in infective endocarditis is large vegetations found on echocardiography
c. A common cause of culture-negative endocarditis is previous antimicrobial therapy

d. Colonic neoplasms have been associated with *Streptococcus bovis* infective endocarditis

e. The treatment of choice for urgent empiric management of culture-negative endocarditis is imipenem

f. Gram-negative bacilli and *Candida* species are the agents that most commonly cause infective endocarditis in drug addicts

32. Each of the following statements describes an adverse reaction commonly occurring during therapy with amphotericin B:
    a. Hypokalemia
    b. Hypocalcemia
    c. Pancreatitis
    d. Increasing creatinine level
    e. Rigors
    f. Fever

33. β-Lactamase inhibitors such as clavulanate and sulbactam expand the antibacterial spectrum of the penicillins to include each of the following:
    a. *Pseudomonas aeruginosa*
    b. *Bacteroides fragilis*
    c. Methicillin-resistant *Staphylococcus aureus*
    d. Methicillin-susceptible *Staphylococcus aureus*
    e. *Legionella pneumophila*
    f. Ampicillin-resistant *Haemophilus influenzae*

34. Which of the following statements are true concerning infection with *Mycobacterium avium-intracellulare* in patients with AIDS:
    a. It usually presents early in the course of HIV infection when immunosuppression is not severe
    b. It causes low-grade fever, night sweats, and weight loss
    c. It is susceptible to conventional antimycobacterial agents
    d. It is a cause of diarrhea in patients with AIDS
    e. Treatment includes multiple drugs with multiple side effects
    f. It is commonly isolated from the blood of patients with AIDS

35. Which of the following statements are true concerning infection with HIV?
    a. Most patients infected with HIV will seroconvert within 2 weeks of infection
    b. Most patients in whom HIV infection develops are asymptomatic
    c. Aseptic meningitis is the most common presentation of primary HIV infection
    d. HIV infection can cause a self-limited mononucleosis-like syndrome
    e. The enzyme-linked immunosorbent assay (ELISA) for the detection of HIV infection has a high positive predictive value for populations in which the prevalence of HIV infection is low
    f. The mean time to the development of AIDS after an individual is infected with HIV is 5 years

NOTES

CHAPTER 21
NEPHROLOGY

Thomas R. Schwab, M.D.

ACUTE RENAL FAILURE–DEFINITIONS

Three important principles in the clinical evaluation of acute renal failure: 1) It must be determined whether an increase in serum levels of creatinine or urea reflects a *genuine* and *recent* decrease in glomerular filtration rate. Many medications and substances interfere with the measurement of creatinine and urea and its renal handling. 2) If substantial irreversible renal dysfunction is to be avoided, acute renal failure must be recognized early. Remember, an increase in serum creatinine of 0.8 to 1.8 mg/dL reflects as much as a 50% loss of renal function. 3) Appropriate treatment of patients with acute renal failure demands that the cause be pinpointed promptly from the more than 100 potential causes. Acute renal failure is now broadly classified into prerenal, renal, and postrenal types.

- Increase in creatinine levels independently of glomerular filtration rate: ketoacidosis (acetoacetate), cefoxitin, cimetidine, trimethoprim, flucytosine, massive rhabdomyolysis, high intake of meat.
- Increase in urea (BUN) independently of glomerular filtration rate: gastrointestinal tract bleeding, tissue trauma, glucocorticoids, tetracyclines.
- Anuria <50 mL/day (limited differential diagnosis!): rapidly progressive glomerulonephritis, cortical necrosis, bilateral renal artery occlusion (e.g., dissection), but not acute tubular necrosis.
- Oliguria is <400 mL/day or < 20 mL/hour: patients with an inability to concentrate urine may be "oliguric" with 1,000+ mL/day.
- Nonoliguric renal failure is >800 mL/day (most cases are nonoliguric).
- Polyuria is >3,000 mL/day (a clue to partial obstruction).

POSTRENAL FAILURE (OBSTRUCTION)

The pathogenesis of an obstructive uropathy is characterized by early vasoconstriction followed by vasodilatation. Obstruction may be anatomical (e.g., methysergide = retroperitoneal fibrosis) or functional (neurogenic bladder). Wide fluctuations in urine volume may be present with partial obstruction.

- Pathogenesis of obstructive uropathy: early vasoconstriction followed by vasodilatation.
- Obstruction: anatomical or functional.

The most useful clinical test is renal ultrasonography. However, 2% of these studies are falsely negative (usually because of early obstruction or possibly retroperitoneal fibrosis). Up to 26% of ultrasonograms are falsely positive. A combination of renal ultrasonography and abdominal computed tomography (CT) without contrast media is 100% diagnostic for obstruction and can pinpoint the cause of obstruction in 84% of cases. The urinalysis results are usually normal in obstructive uropathy. Hyperchloremic normal anion gap hyperkalemic metabolic acidosis is often a clue to obstruction.

- Renal ultrasonography: 2% of studies are false negative and as many as 26% are false positive.
- Ultrasonography plus CT (no contrast agent): 100% diagnostic; pinpoint cause in 84% of cases.
- Hyperkalemic metabolic acidosis: often a clue to obstruction.

Treatment

Always irrigate and change urinary catheters in evaluating obstructive uropathy. If obstruction is relieved, replace 2/3 of the postobstructive diuresis volume. According to animal studies, treatment instituted within 1 week produces 50% recovery of the glomerular filtration rate; treatment in 2 weeks results in 30% recovery, and treatment after 8 weeks produces little, if any, recovery.

PRERENAL FAILURE

Prerenal failure is defined as a rapidly reversible cause of renal insufficiency due to renal hypoperfusion. It accounts for at least 50% of cases of acute renal failure in hospitalized patients. The urine sediment is benign (hyaline and granular casts). Urinary indices of oliguria are helpful in distinguishing prerenal from renal failure. These diagnostic indices are listed in Table 21-1. It is important in treatment to correct the underlying disorder if known and to replace fluids if hypovolemic.

- Prerenal failure: rapidly reversible renal insufficiency due to renal hypoperfusion.
- Urinary indices of oliguria help to distinguish between prerenal and renal failure.

Table 21-1.--Diagnostic Indices of Oliguria

	Prerenal	Acute tubular necrosis
Urine osmolality, mOsm/L	≥500	≤350
Urine/plasma creatinine ratio	≥40	≤20
BUN/plasma creatinine ratio	>20	<15
Fractional excretion of sodium	<1%	>3%

The fractional excretion of sodium is the most helpful urinary index to distinguish prerenal oliguria from oliguria due to acute intrinsic renal failure. It is an index of the quantity of sodium excreted divided by the quantity of sodium filtered times 100. Normally, this value is <1%; it is also <1% in prerenal insufficiency. Patients with tubular dysfunction have >3% of the sodium filtered eventually excreted. There are causes of acute *intrinsic* renal failure associated with a low fractional excretion of sodium. All these causes have a decrease in renal blood flow. They include renal failure due to nonsteroidal anti-inflammatory drugs, angiotensin-converting enzyme inhibitors, radiocontrast media, hemoglobinomyoglobinuria, early obstruction, acute glomerulonephritis, and hepatorenal failure.

HEPATORENAL SYNDROME

Hepatorenal syndrome is a severe state of prerenal hypoperfusion that occurs in 40%-50% of patients with terminal cirrhosis. It usually occurs in the presence of jaundice, ascites, and stigmata of portal hypertension. This syndrome usually develops in the hospital, triggered by diuretics, gastrointestinal tract bleeding, or paracentesis. Hyponatremia, hypokalemia, and hypoalbuminemia commonly accompany the syndrome. The pathogenesis of this disorder is not well understood. Laboratory findings include urinary sodium <10 mOsm/L, urinary osmolality >500 mOsm/L, and only a transient response to fluids. A transition to acute tubular necrosis is possible, and recovery is only about 10%. Treatment includes liver transplantation, LaVeen shunt, dopamine, and high doses of spironolactone (Aldactone); occasionally, plasma infusions have been beneficial. Other causes of renal failure associated with liver disease include amyloidosis, leptospirosis, methoxyflurane, vasculitis, and acute Wilson's disease.

- Hepatorenal syndrome: severe state of prerenal hypoperfusion.
- Occurs in 40%-50% of patients with terminal cirrhosis.
- Hyponatremia, hypokalemia, and hypoalbuminemia are common.
- Urinary sodium is <10 mOsm/L and urinary osmolality is >500 mOsm/L.
- 10% of patients recover.

ACUTE INTRINSIC RENAL FAILURE

Acute Tubular Necrosis

Most patients (60%) with acute tubular necrosis are not oliguric and carry a better prognosis than oliguric patients (40%). The mean incidence of acute tubular necrosis in hospitals is about 5%. It occurs in 50% of emergency abdominal aortic aneurysm repairs, 10% of elective abdominal aortic aneurysm repairs, and in 20% of patients undergoing heart surgery or operations related to trauma. The pathogenesis of acute tubular necrosis is usually due to ischemia, which may occur without hypotension, as in 50% of postoperative cases. Acute tubular necrosis has more than one cause in 70% of patients. Important toxins that can cause tubular damage include endogenous toxins (calcium, uric acid, hemoglobinuria or myoglobinuria) and exogenous toxins (antibiotics, contrast dye, chemotherapeutic agents, cyclosporin A, and acyclovir).

- Acute tubular necrosis: 60% of patients are not oliguric and 40% are.
- It occurs in 50% of emergency abdominal aortic aneurysm repairs.
- Pathogenesis: usually is ischemia.

Ischemia affects the kidney similar to the way it affects the myocardium. We often think of ischemia being a continuum in the myocardium, going from angina to subendocardial infarction to true transmural infarction. Ischemia can affect the kidney by initially inducing prerenal insufficiency, followed by acute tubular necrosis, and then by cortical necrosis. Studies demonstrate that the redistribution of blood flow, medullary ischemia, backleak of filtrate through damaged tubules, intrarenal obstruction by necrotized tubule casts, and glomerular filter damage all have a role in acute tubular necrosis.

Urinalysis often demonstrates cellular debris, tubular epithelial cell casts, granular casts, and a "muddy brown" appearance. Erythrocyte casts are associated with acute glomerular nephritis and not with acute tubular necrosis. Also, leukocyte casts, leukocytes, and eosinophils accompany acute interstitial nephritis and not acute tubular necrosis.

A stepwise approach to immediate treatment of acute renal failure is outlined in Table 21-2.

Table 21-2.--Stepwise Approach to Immediate Treatment of Acute Renal Failure

1. Exclude postrenal and prerenal causes. Try a volume challenge if indicated.
2. Discontinue use of all nephrotoxic agents.
3. Treat with mannitol (12.5-25 g i.v.) and/or furosemide (20 mg i.v.); 25 g of mannitol increases plasma volume 250 mL. Do not exceed total dose of 50 g in renal failure (mannitol intoxication with hyponatremia, extracellular fluid overload).
4. No response (<60 mL/hr), treat with furosemide (400-500 mg i.v.).
5. Response (>60 mL/hr), 20% mannitol (i.v. infusion; no more than 100 g/24 hr) and furosemide (200 mg) to keep urine output >60 mL/hr. Replace urine 1:1.
6. Other--avoid high doses of furosemide, ethacrynic acid (ototoxicity); use dopamine (2-5 μg).

Urine alkalinization is helpful in acute tubular necrosis induced by uric acid, myoglobin, or methotrexate.

The typical course of acute renal failure includes an oliguric phase, which lasts 1-2 weeks but not usually more than 4 weeks. If the oliguric phase lasts more than 4 weeks, biopsy should be considered to look for causes of acute renal failure other than acute tubular necrosis. The diuretic phase is characterized by increases in urine flow that are not necessarily associated with improvement in creatinine levels early in the disease. Late in the disease, improvement in the creatinine level occurs as the glomerular filtration rate begins to increase. It is during this phase that severe hypercalcemia can occur in rhabdomyolysis-induced renal failure. The third and final phase is the recovery phase of intrinsic renal failure. During this phase, glomerular filtration rate improves over a period of 3-12 months. In general, the condition of 60% of patients stabilizes with reduced glomerular filtration rate, especially if the patients have been oliguric for more than 16 days. Complications of acute renal failure include infection, which is the number one cause of death and occurs in 50%-90% of patients. It is important to note that fever may be absent and that a careful search for pulmonary and urinary tract infections, abscesses, and other sources of infection must be completed. Other complications include gastrointestinal tract bleeding, hypervolemia with congestive heart failure, hyperkalemia, hyponatremia, metabolic acidosis, and uremia.

Management of acute renal failure includes allowing 0.5 lb loss/day for catabolism. Restricting fluid and sodium, in addition to a 100-g carbohydrate diet with limitations of potassium, magnesium, phosphate, and protein, are also recommended. Treatment with thiazide diuretics, magnesium-containing antacids, and nonsteroidal anti-inflammatory agents must stop, and contrast agent must be avoided if possible. It is also important to adjust drug doses, especially of digoxin, antibiotics, antihypertensive agents, and benzodiazepines. Phosphate binders are also helpful in patients taking oral nutrition. Although patients have low serum levels of calcium, this is rarely treated.

Dialysis can be performed with hemodialysis, continuous hemofiltration, or peritoneal dialysis. It is best to anticipate the patients' course and maintain the predialysis BUN <100. Other indications include extracellular fluid volume excess, hyperkalemia, severe acidosis, pericarditis, and the need to make space for parenteral nutrition. Dialysis is often necessary daily in hypercatabolic patients.

Patients with aminoglycoside-induced renal failure are often nonoliguric. The renal failure occurs only after 5-7 days of therapy and correlates with the cumulative dose received. Aminoglycosides are freely filtered and absorbed partially in the proximal tubule: the more amino groups on the aminoglycoside, the more toxic the agent (streptomycin is more toxic than gentamicin, which is as toxic as tobramycin). Magnesium and potassium wasting from tubular dysfunction are common accompaniments, and urine myeloid bodies can sometimes be seen by electron microscopy performed on the urine of affected patients.

- Aminoglycoside-induced renal failure: often non-oliguric.
- Occurs after 5-7 days of therapy.
- Urine myeloid bodies are sometimes seen.

Acute renal dysfunction due to amphotericin B occurs after a 2-3-g dose of treatment and is rare if <600 mg. It is also associated with tubular dysfunction, as are aminoglycosides. Patients also develop nephrogenic diabetes insipidus and a type IV renal tubular acidosis. Some evidence suggests that alkalinizing the urine may be beneficial in these patients.

- Amphotericin-B-induced renal failure: occurs with 2-3-g dose but rarely if dose is <600 mg.

Up to 30% of the patients receiving cisplatin develop renal failure if the cumulative dose is 50-75 mg/m^2. Renal failure can be avoided with adequate hydration and forced diuresis; it is associated with hypomagnesemia and hypokalemia.

- Cisplatin-induced renal failure: occurs in 30% of patients receiving 50-75 mg/m^2.

Methotrexate is a dose-related (>50 mg/kg) cause of renal failure. It precipitates in the renal tubules, as does acyclovir and some sulfas (treatment with an alkaline diuresis has been helpful).

- Methotrexate-induced renal failure: dose related.
- Methotrexate precipitates in the renal tubules.

Contrast dye-induced nephropathy is likely due to vasoconstriction, obstruction, and direct tubular toxicity of contrast agents. Its incidence is probably less than previously believed, but patients who are at risk can be identified, including those with severe renal insufficiency alone or diabetic patients with mild renal insufficiency. Patients who receive multiple exposures to contrast agent are at increased risk, as are patients who receive high doses of contrast agent. The acute renal failure that accompanies radiocontrast dye toxicity is often associated with a low fractional excretion of sodium. The patients usually become oliguric, with dense nephrotomograms on radiography; this reverses within 7 days. Low osmolar, low ionic contrast agents have less allergic reactions and may be helpful in selected patients. Other measures include prevention by hydration, forced diuresis, and decreasing the dose of contrast agent. There is some investigational evidence that calcium channel blockers and atrial natriuretic factor may be helpful in preventing acute contrast-induced nephropathy. Spacing contrast studies for several days is also an important preventive measure. Contrast agent can be removed by dialysis, but this generally is not done clinically.

- Contrast dye-induced renal failure: due to vasoconstriction, obstruction, and direct tubular toxicity.
- Patients at risk: those with severe renal insufficiency and diabetic patients with mild renal insufficiency.
- Prevention: hydration, forced diuresis, low dose of contrast agent.

Heme pigments (Table 21-3) induce renal failure by intrarenal vasoconstriction and obstruction. Rhabdomyolysis can be due to traumatic causes (crush, seizures, alcoholic coma, and ischemia) and to nontraumatic causes (cocaine, clofibrate, lovastatin, heat stroke, sickle cell trait, carbon monoxide poisoning, spider bite, and polydermatomyositis). Hypocalcemia, frequently severe, can often accompany the acute syndrome, followed by severe hypercalcemia in the diuretic phase of recovering renal failure. Treatment includes a forced diuresis and urine alkalinization, with careful attention to the patients' serum levels of calcium and potassium.

- Heme pigment-induced renal failure: due to intrarenal vasoconstriction and obstruction.
- Hypocalcemia can occur in acute phase and hypercalcemia in diuretic phase.

Acute Renovascular Disease

Atheroembolic-induced renal failure is an increasingly recognized cause of renal failure. It generally occurs,

Table 21-3.--Heme Pigments

	Serum color	Haptoglobin	CPK	Heme dipstick	Urine benzidine
Hemoglobin	Red	Decreased	Normal	+	-
Myoglobin	Clear	Normal	Increased	+	+

either spontaneously or after an invasive procedure, in older patients. The patients often have livedo reticularis of the extremities and emboli seen on funduscopic examination. Laboratory studies can demonstrate a high erythrocyte sedimentation rate, low level of complement, eosinophilia, eosinophiluria, and thrombocytopenia. Whereas contrast nephropathy is usually reversible, patients with atheroembolic-induced renal failure often have minimal reversibility. Renal biopsies demonstrate cholesterol emboli in medium-sized arteries with intense tubulointerstitial nephritis. The only treatment is to correct the source of the embolization, looking for atrial fibrillation, cardiac valve disease, endocarditis, etc. Anticoagulation may actually aggravate the tendency for embolization.

- Atheroembolic-induced renal failure: generally in older patients.
- Findings: high erythrocyte sedimentation rate, low levels of complement, eosinophilia, eosinophiluria.

DISORDERS OF WATER BALANCE

The most important principle in understanding disorders of water balance is that the serum level of sodium is the clinical index of total body water. The serum sodium level is not an index of total body sodium. Total body sodium can be determined only by physical examination. The serum sodium level is a useful clinical index to evaluate water balance, not sodium balance disorders. Water balance is regulated by thirst, antidiuretic hormone, and renal medullary concentration of water.

- Total body sodium can be determined only by physical examination.
- Water balance is regulated by thirst, antidiuretic hormone, renal medullary concentration of water.

Hyponatremia

Hyponatremia is the number one electrolyte abnormality in hospitalized patients. Its symptoms are protean, including lethargy, cramps, decreased deep tendon reflexes, and seizures. The diagnosis and management of hyponatremia are shown in Figure 21-1.

- Hyponatremia: number one electrolyte abnormality in hospitalized patients.

Diagnosis

The first step in evaluating patients with hyponatremia is to exclude pseudohyponatremia by measuring serum osmolality. All patients with true hyponatremia have hypotonic hyponatremia. Isotonic hyponatremia may be due to severe hypertriglyceridemia (>1,500, lipemia retinalis is always present), severe hyperproteinemia (>8.0, Waldenström's macroglobulinemia, myeloma), or isotonic infusions of glucose, mannitol, or glycine. Hypertonic hyponatremia is due to severe hyperglycemia (sodium decreases 1.6 for each 100 mg/dL increase in glucose) and to hypertonic infusions of glucose, mannitol, or glycine.

If the patient does not have pseudohyponatremia, the second step is to assess the extracellular fluid volume of the hypotonic hyponatremic patient and determine whether he or she is hypovolemic, euvolemic, or hypervolemic. 1) Hypotonic hypovolemic hyponatremia: check urine osmolality and sodium concentration; common causes are thiazides and adrenal insufficiency. 2) Hypotonic hypervolemic hyponatremia: check urine osmolality and sodium concentration; edematous states and renal failure are common. 3) Hypotonic euvolemic hyponatremia: check cortisol level, thyroid, urine osmolality, hypothyroidism, Addison's disease, reset osmostat, and psychogenic polydipsia.

The syndrome of inappropriate secretion of antidiuretic hormone is a diagnosis of exclusion. Patients must meet the following criteria: 1) hypotonic plasma, 2) urine less than maximally dilute, 3) urine sodium matches intake, 4) absence of hypoadrenocorticism and hypothyroidism, and 5) improvement with water restriction. An important clinical hint is the presence of a low serum level of uric acid. The BUN also tends to be low.

- Syndrome of inappropriate secretion of antidiuretic hormone: serum level of uric acid and BUN are low.

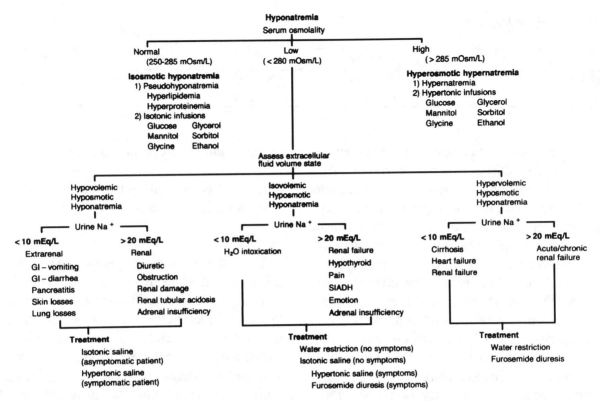

Fig. 21-1. Diagnosis and management of hyponatremia.

Patients with hyponatremia associated with hypovolemia generally respond to infusion of isotonic saline. Hypovolemic patients with hyponatremia should have water intake restricted. They may benefit from loop diuretic administration and, possibly, dialysis. In symptomatic euvolemic patients, isotonic or hypertonic saline administered with loop diuretics is given to increase the serum level of sodium by 1 mEq/L per hour to 120 or 125. In general, hyponatremia should be reversed cautiously to avoid central pontine myelinolysis and should be reversed at the rate at which it developed. In patients with chronic syndrome of inappropriate secretion of antidiuretic hormone, demeclocycline has been of benefit.

Hypernatremia

As in hyponatremia, the symptoms of hypernatremia are often protean, with irritability, hyperreflexia, ataxia, and seizures. All forms of hypernatremia are associated with hypertonicity, so there is no pseudohypernatremia. Cases are categorized as hypovolemic, hypervolemic, and euvolemic hypernatremia. The diagnosis and management of hypernatremia are shown in Figure 21-2.

- Hypovolemic hypernatremia: check urine sodium; may be caused by osmotic diuresis, excess sweating, and diarrhea.

- Hypervolemic hypernatremia: may be caused by sodium poisoning.
- Euvolemic hypernatremia: loss of water; extrarenal (skin, lung) versus renal; diabetes insipidus, central versus nephrogenic water deprivation test.

Patients with hypovolemic hypernatremia often respond to saline followed by hypotonic solution. Patients with hypervolemic hypernatremia respond to diuretics and may or may not need dialysis. Euvolemic patients should receive free water, either orally or intravenously, to correct the serum level of sodium at approximately 1-2 mEq/hr.

DISORDERS OF SODIUM BALANCE

Disorders of sodium balance can be determined only by clinical examination. Orthostatism implies volume depletion and sodium deficiency. Edema implies volume excess and sodium excess.

DISORDERS OF POTASSIUM BALANCE

Potassium is predominantly an intracellular cation. Total body potassium is approximately equal to 4,200 mEq, with only 60 mEq in the total extracellular fluid

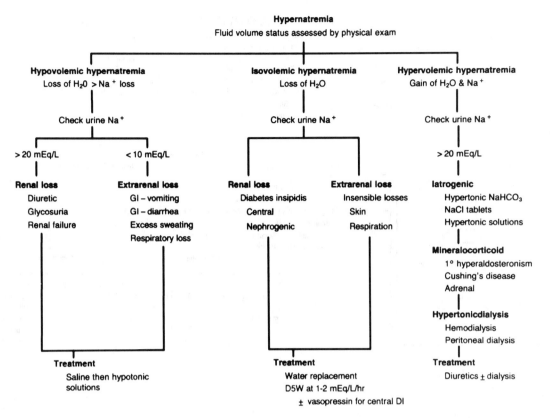

Fig. 21-2. Diagnosis and management of hypernatremia.

volume. Gastric fluid contains 5-10 mEq of potassium/L, and diarrheal fluid contains 10-100 mEq/L. Internal balance of potassium is regulated by endogenous factors such as acidemia, sodium, potassium, ATPase, insulin, catecholamines, and aldosterone. External balance is regulated primarily by potassium excretion, which in large part is regulated by urinary flow rate, aldosterone, antidiuretic hormone, and sodium delivery to the distal tubule.

Hypokalemia

Symptoms of hypokalemia include weakness, ileus, polyuria, and, sometimes, rhabdomyolysis. Hypokalemia also aggravates digoxin toxicity. A stepwise approach to the diagnosis of hypokalemia is given in Table 21-4 and outlined in Figure 21-3.

● Hypokalemia symptoms: weakness, ileus, polyuria.

Therapy. If serum potassium level is <2 mEq/L, total potassium deficit = 1,000 mEq; if serum potassium level is between 2 and 4 mEq/L, then a decrease of 0.3 = 100 to 500 mEq deficit, usually potassium chloride (diabetic ketoacidosis, potassium phosphate; potassium citrate, severe acidosis). Do not exceed 10 mEq/hr i.v. unless using a central catheter and ECG monitoring. Dietary

Table 21-4.--Stepwise Approach to Diagnosis of Hypokalemia

1. Exclude redistribution--β-agonists (albuterol and terbutaline for asthma and ritodrine for labor), acute alkalosis, vitamin B_{12} therapy for pernicious anemia (especially if thrombocytopenic), barium carbonate
2. Determine whether potassium losses are renal or extrarenal--check urine potassium level on high sodium diet, is potassium > or < 20 mEq/day
3. If loss is extrarenal, determine cause (laxative screen)-- usually diarrhea, enemas, laxative abuse, villous adenomas, ureterocolostomy

   If loss is renal, determine if hypertensive or normotensive (diuretic screen)
4. If hypertensive, check plasma renin and aldosterone levels, includes primary aldosteronism or hyperplasia (glycyrrhizic acid in licorice, chewing tobacco), adrenal abnormalities

   If normotensive, check plasma HCO_3 levels and urine chloride, includes renal tubular acidosis, vomiting, diuretic abuse, Bartter's syndrome, magnesium deficiency.

   High doses of penicillin, amphotericin B, cisplatin

   Renal loss and metabolic acidosis--diabetic ketoacidosis, renal tubular acidosis, acetazolamide

   Renal loss and metabolic alkalosis--vomiting, diuretics, Bartter's syndrome, excess aldosterone

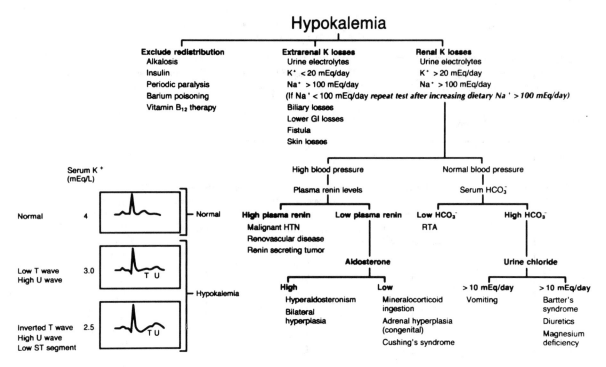

Fig. 21-3. Diagnosis of hypokalemia.

sodium restriction decreases potassium-losing effects of diuretics.

Hyperkalemia

A stepwise approach to the diagnosis of hyperkalemia is given in Table 21-5 and outlined in Figure 21-4.

Therapy: antagonize membrane effects and then redistribute (treat with calcium, then bicarb, then insulin), then resins, and finally dialysis. For chronic therapy, use loop diuretics, $NaHCO_3$, resins, fludrocortisone, dialysis.

Table 21-5.--Stepwise Approach to Diagnosis of Hyperkalemia

1. Exclude pseudohyperkalemia--ECG is normal, heparinized plasma potassium is normal
   Hemolysis of clotted blood (0.3 increase), tourniquet ischemia, severe leukocytosis or thrombocytosis
2. Determine cause based on redistribution or excess total body potassium (see Fig. 21-4)

ACID-BASE DISORDERS

Clinically, it is absolutely critical that a stepwise approach to acid-base disorders be followed. The six steps listed in Table 21-6 should always be followed before interpreting an acid-base disorder.

Metabolic Acidosis

Metabolic acidosis is defined as a primary disturbance in which retention of acid consumes endogenous alkali stores. This is reflected by a decrease in HCO_3. The secondary response is increased ventilation with a decrease in pCO_2. Metabolic acidosis can be caused by overproduction of endogenous acid (e.g., diabetic ketoacidosis), loss of alkali stores (diarrhea, renal tubular acidosis), or failure of renal acid secretion or base resynthesis (renal failure).

- Metabolic acidosis: primary disturbance is retention of acid.
- Secondary response: increased ventilation with pCO_2.

Some of the signs and symptoms of metabolic acidosis include fatigue, dyspnea, abdominal pain, vomiting, Kussmaul's respiration, myocardial depression, hyperkalemia, leukemoid reaction, insulin resistance, and, when pH is <7.2, arteriolar dilatation and hypotension.

Some formulas for the predicted compensation for pure metabolic acidosis (which will take up to 24 hours) are 1) pCO_2 = last two digits of the pH, 2) pCO_2 decreases by 1-1.3 mm Hg for each mEq/L decrease in HCO_3, and 3) $pCO_2 \pm 2 = 1.5 (HCO_3) + 8$ (this is the best formula).

The metabolic acidoses are classified as either normal anion gap or high anion gap. Normal anion gap meta-

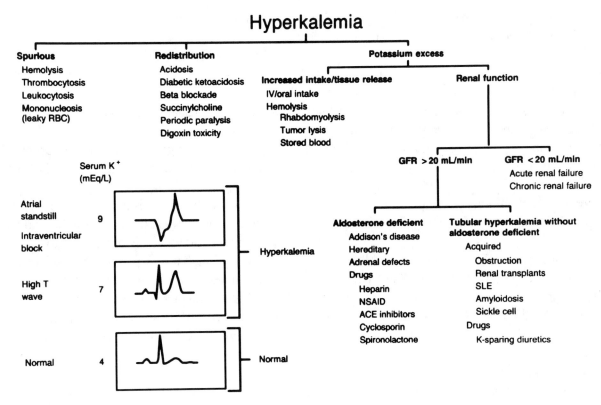

Fig. 21-4. Diagnosis of hyperkalemia.

Table 21-6.--Six Steps for Interpreting Acid-Base Disorder

1. Note the clinical presentation
2. Always check the anion (hidden acidosis) and osmolar gaps if possible
   Normal anion gap Na - (HCO$_3$ + Cl) = 8 to 12
      Cations = Na, gammaglobulins, Ca, Mg, K
      Anions = Cl, HCO$_3$, albumin, PO$_4$, SO$_4$, organic
   High anion gap >12--K-U-S-S-M-A-U-L
   Low anion gap <8--Bromism, paraproteinemia, hypercalcemia/magnesemia, lithium toxicity, severe hypernatremia, severe hypoalbuminemia
   Osmolar gap >10 -OLS--methanol, ethanol, ethylene glycol, isopropyl alcohol, mannitol
3. Use the Henderson equation to check the ABGs validity of the arterial blood gases values:

$$H^+ \text{ (nEq/L)} = \frac{24 \times \text{lungs (pCO}_2)}{\text{kidneys (HCO}_3)}$$

pH	7.00	7.10	7.20	7.30	7.40	7.50	7.60	7.70
H$^+$	100	79	63	50	40	32	25	20

4. Is the pH high or low?
5. Is the primary disturbance metabolic (HCO$_3$) or respiratory (pCO$_2$)?
6. Is it simple or mixed?

bolic acidosis is defined in terms of serum levels of potassium.

Hypokalemic normal anion gap metabolic acidosis can be associated with diarrhea, ureteral diversion, or the use of carbonic anhydrase inhibitors such as acetazolamide. Renal tubular acidosis type I, or classic renal tubular acidosis, is also a cause. This is associated with nephrocalcinosis and osteomalacia. The causes of type I renal tubular acidosis include toluene sniffing, amphotericin B, lithium, Sjögren's syndrome, hypergammaglobulinemia, and sickle cell disease. Type II renal tubular acidosis is also a hypokalemic anion gap metabolic acidosis. In adults, it is often associated with other proximal tubule defects, including glycosuria, uricosuria, phosphaturia, and aminoaciduria (Fanconi's syndrome). Causes of type II renal tubular acidosis include myeloma, cystinosis (not cystinuria), lead, tetracycline, and acetazolamide.

The causes of hyperkalemic normal anion gap metabolic acidosis include acid loads such as NH$_4$Cl, arginine chloride, lysine chloride, cholestyramine, total parenteral nutrition, HCl, oral CaCl$_2$, obstructive uropathy, hypoaldosteronism (Addison's disease), 21-hydoxylase deficiency, sulfur toxicity, and type IV renal tubular acidosis. Type IV renal tubular acidosis is associated with hyporenin and hypoaldosteronism, and it may be caused by diabetes, interstitial nephritis, spironolactone, amiloride, triamterene, or cyclosporin A.

High anion gap metabolic acidosis is due to several causes. In chronic renal failure, the anion gap is usually <25. If anion gaps are >25, one should immediately think of an ingestion of a poison. Isopropyl alcohol increases the osmolar gap but not the anion gap (acetone is not an anion).

- In chronic renal failure, anion gap usually is <25.
- Gap >25 should suggest ingestion of a poison.

Treatment of metabolic acidosis is generally corrected by treating the underlying disorder, but the bicarbonate deficit can be determined by the following formula:

Bicarbonate deficit = 0.2 x body weight (kg) x (normal HCO_3 [i.e., 24] - measured HCO_3)

Metabolic Alkalosis

Metabolic alkalosis is defined as a primary disturbance in which plasma bicarbonate is increased. This can be caused by 1) endogenous alkali, 2) acid loss through gastrointestinal tract or kidney, or 3) loss of nonbicarbonate fluid causing contraction of the remaining fluid around unchanged total body bicarbonate. The kidney must also be stimulated to sustain the high level of plasma bicarbonate. This can occur by 1) extracellular fluid volume contraction, 2) hypercapnia, 3) potassium depletion, 4) steroid excess, 5) hypercalcemia, or 6) hypoparathyroidism. The secondary response is decreased ventilation with an increase in pCO_2. The signs and symptoms of metabolic alkalosis include weakness, muscle cramps, hyperreflexia, alveolar hypoventilation, and dysrhythmias.

- Metabolic alkalosis: primary disturbance is increased plasma bicarbonate.
- Kidney must be stimulated to sustain high level of plasma bicarbonate.
- Secondary response: decreased ventilation with increased pCO_2.

The predicted compensation for pure renal metabolic alkalosis (which will take up to 24 hours) can be calculated by using the following formulas:
1. $pCO_2 \pm 5 = 0.9(HCO_3) + 15$
2. pCO_2 increases 6 mm Hg for each 10 mEq/L increase in HCO_3

Metabolic alkalosis can be classified in terms of the spot urine chloride.

Mixed Acid-Base Disorders

- HCO_3 <15 usually is caused partly by a metabolic acidosis.
- HCO_3 >45 usually is caused partly by a metabolic alkalosis.
- Arterial blood gas values may be normal but a high anion gap indicates a mixed metabolic alkalosis/acidosis.
- In metabolic acidosis and respiratory alkalosis, the pCO_2 is lower than predicted for the acidosis.
- In metabolic alkalosis and respiratory acidosis, the HCO_3 is higher than predicted for acidosis.
- In mixed metabolic and respiratory alkalosis, HCO_3 is higher and pCO_2 lower than expected.
- Triple disorders--diabetic/alcoholic (vomiting) + (keto/lactic acidosis) + (sepsis or liver disease).

CLINICAL MANIFESTATIONS OF GLOMERULAR INJURY

The glomerular basement membrane is an important size barrier (MW, 70,000) and negative charge barrier, repulsing albumin and immune globulins. There is also tubular reabsorption of protein in the range of 500-1,500 mg/24 hours per day by the proximal tubule.

Orthostatic proteinuria is usually benign and remits spontaneously. The diagnosis can be made by obtaining two 12-hour urine collections for protein: one supine and one upright. Significant proteinuria is defined as >75 mg/12 hours. Tubulointerstitial disease is sometimes associated with proteinuria, but it is usually <1,500 g/day. Overflow low molecular weight proteinuria is due to increased light chain or lysozyme excretion without nephrosis.

Renal biopsy is indicated to determine the prognosis and diagnosis of patients with >2 g/day non-nephrotic range proteinuria if it is associated with an abnormal sediment or renal insufficiency. Other indications for biopsy include nephrotic range proteinuria, microscopic hematuria with abnormal urine sediment or renal function, progressive renal insufficiency, acute renal failure lasting >3-4 weeks. Patients with an atypical course of diabetes and undiagnosed systemic disease such as amyloid, systemic lupus erythematosus, and polyarteritis nodosa should undergo biopsy. Renal biopsy is contraindicated in bleeding disorders, uncontrolled hypertension, urinary tract infections, solitary kidneys other than allografts, and uncooperative patients. Complications include microscopic hematuria, gross hematuria (10%-20%), need for nephrectomy, biopsy of other tissue, and death (0.001%).

- Renal biopsy: to determine prognosis and diagnosis of patients with >2 g/day non-nephrotic range proteinuria.
- Other indications: nephrotic range proteinuria, microscopic hematuria, progressive renal insufficiency, acute renal failure lasting >3-4 weeks, atypical course of diabetes, undiagnosed systemic disease.
- Contraindications: bleeding disorders, uncontrolled hypertension, urinary tract infections, solitary kidneys other than allografts, uncooperative patients.

Nephrotic Syndrome

Nephrotic syndrome is defined by the presence of urinary protein >3.5 g/1.73 m^2 per day, hypoalbuminemia (<3.0 g/dL), peripheral edema, and hypercholesterolemia (total >200 mg/dL). Urinalysis demonstrates waxy casts, free fat, oval fat bodies, and lipiduria. Other associations include hypogammaglobulinemia (increases infection risk), vitamin D deficiency due to loss of vitamin D-binding protein, and iron deficiency anemia due to hypotransferrinemia. Renal vein thrombosis may occur because of an increased thromboembolic tendency (increased factor V, VIII, fibrinogen, platelets, decreased antithrombin III and antiplasmin). Management includes controlling blood pressure and limiting sodium and lipid intake.

- Nephrotic syndrome: urinary protein >3.5 g/1.73 m^2 daily.
- Hypoalbuminemia, <3 g/dL.
- Peripheral edema.
- Hypercholesterolemia, total >200 mg/dL.

Nephritic Syndrome

Nephritic syndrome is characterized by the presence of erythrocyte casts with variable amounts of proteinuria. Because of methemoglobin formation in acid urine, it has a Coca-Cola or smokey appearance.

- Nephritic syndrome: erythrocyte casts with variable amounts of proteinuria.
- Urine: Coca-Cola or smokey appearance.

GLOMERULAR DISEASE WITH ACUTE REVERSIBLE RENAL FAILURE

Poststreptococcal Glomerulonephritis

Poststreptococcal glomerulonephritis is usually caused by group A β-hemolytic streptococcal infections. The latent period is 6-21 days (type 12 pharyngeal infection) or 14-28 days (type 49 skin infection). The urine sediment is active, with usually <3 g proteinuria/24 hours, and a fractional excretion of sodium <1%. Because of activation of the alternative complement pathway, total and C3 complements are low but only up to 8 weeks. Antistreptolysin-O is present in pharyngeal infections and anti-DNase B in skin infections. In renal biopsy specimens, light microscopy demonstrates many polymorphonuclear neutrophils, with proliferation and subepithelial deposits or humps. Immunofluorescence demonstrates a granular "lumpy-bumpy" pattern with IgG and C3. Treatment is supportive alone, with control of blood pressure and edema. Penicillin therapy for patient and contacts may prevent new cases. The course and prognosis are excellent in children and adults unless crescents or persistent proteinuria is present.

- Poststreptococcal glomerulonephritis: usually due to group A β-hemolytic streptococcal infections.
- Urine sediment: active, <3 g proteinuria/24 hours and fractional excretion of sodium is <1%.
- Total and C3 complement are low.
- Immunofluorescence: granular "lumpy-bumpy" pattern with IgG and C3.

Other forms of postinfectious glomerulonephritis include bacterial endocarditis and infected ventriculoatrial shunts.

CRESCENTIC GLOMERULAR DISEASE WITH PROGRESSIVE RENAL FAILURE

Rapidly progressive glomerulonephritis is defined as an acute (days to weeks to months) deterioration of renal function associated with active urinary sediment and crescentic glomerulonephritis. Usually, adults (mean age, 55 years) are affected. The pulmonary-renal syndrome is frequent, and oliguria is not uncommon. On light microscopy, there is fibrinoid necrosis and >50% crescents. Immunofluorescence demonstrates three patterns: type I, linear IgG (Goodpasture's syndrome or anti-GBM mediated); type II, granular immune complexes (D-penicillamine); and type III, negative immunofluorescence. Treatment of rapidly progressive glomerulonephritis: pulse methylprednisolone sodium succinate (SoluMedrol), 1 g for 3 days, with or without cytotoxic agents. Plasmapheresis is helpful if there is pulmonary hemorrhage in Goodpasture's syndrome. Prognosis: 35% develop end-stage renal disease with 25% mortality and 40% progress to chronic renal insufficiency. Oliguria, a high creatinine level (>7), and old age are poor prognostic signs.

- Rapidly progressive glomerulonephritis: subacute deterioration of renal function.
- Crescentic glomerulonephritis.
- Pulmonary-renal syndrome is common; oliguria is not uncommon.
- 25% mortality.
- 40% progress to chronic renal insufficiency.

GLOMERULAR DISEASE WITH HEMATURIA AND VARIABLE PROTEINURIA AND FUNCTION

IgA Nephropathy

IgA nephropathy is the commonest glomerulopathy worldwide. Patients present with synpharyngitic hematuria (microscopic with or without macroscopic hematuria), often with erythrocyte casts. Urine sediment activity may be exacerbated by an upper respiratory tract infection. Pathogenesis may be due partly to exaggerated IgA mucosal production. Secondary causes include advanced chronic liver disease, sprue, dermatitis herpetiformis, and ankylosing spondylitis. Poor prognostic signs are heavy proteinuria, hypertension, and renal insufficiency. Plasma IgA is increased in only 50% of the patients. Skin biopsy for IgA is not helpful. Renal biopsy in IgA demonstrates mesangial proliferation on light microscopy. The immunofluorescence studies are diagnostic and demonstrate IgA within the mesangium. There is no known therapy for IgA nephropathy, but the prognosis is generally good; however, 20% of cases may reach end-stage renal disease in 20 years. This disorder often recurs in renal transplant recipients but often is not clinically significant. Poor prognostic signs are diminished renal function, heavy proteinuria, and hypertension.

- IgA nephropathy: commonest glomerulopathy worldwide.

- Presents with synpharyngitic hematuria, often with erythrocyte casts.
- Pathogenesis: exaggerated IgA mucosal production or regulation.
- Secondary causes: advanced chronic liver disease, sprue, dermatitis herpetiformis, ankylosing spondylitis.
- Plasma IgA increased in only 50% of patients.
- Prognosis: generally good.

Henoch-Schönlein Purpura

Patients with Henoch-Schönlein purpura present with microscopic and/or macrohematuria along with erythrocyte casts, purpura, and abdominal pain. Renal biopsy findings are similar to those of IgA nephropathy with or without vasculitis. The prognosis for children generally is good and variable for adults. Treatment is supportive only.

Membranoproliferative Glomerulonephritis

Patients with membranoproliferative glomerulonephritis present with nephrotic syndrome (50% of patients), non-nephrotic range proteinuria (30%), or nephritic sediment (20%). Complement values are persistently low (>8 weeks). Antistreptolysin-O may be present, and a C3 nephritic factor is present in many cases. It is an autoantibody to alternative pathway C3 convertase, resulting in persistent C3 breakdown. Secondary causes include chronic infections, "shunt nephritis," malaria, hepatitis B, systemic lupus erythematosus, congenital complement deficiency (C2, C3), mixed cryoglobulinemia, sickle cell disease, partial lipodystrophy (only type II), and α_1-antitrypsin deficiency. The two idiopathic forms are type I and type II (dense-deposit disease).

- Membranoproliferative glomerulonephritis: presents with nephrotic syndrome in 50% of patients, non-nephrotic range proteinuria in 30%, and nephritic sediment in 20%.
- Complements are persistently low.
- C3 nephritic factor is often present.
- Secondary causes: chronic infections, "shunt nephritis," hepatitis B, systemic lupus erythematosus, sickle cell disease.

In biopsy samples of membranoproliferative glomerulonephritis, light microscopy demonstrates duplication or splitting, tramtracking, or double contouring of the glomerular basement membrane. This proliferation within the glomerulus and capillary loop thickening results in a lobular appearance of the glomeruli. Immunofluorescence demonstrates complex deposition in the mesangium and capillary walls. Electron microscopy demonstrates a distinctive ribboning or sausaging of dense material in type II membranoproliferative glomerulonephritis. Generally, adults receive supportive care; steroids have been helpful in some children. Dipyridamole (225 mg/day) and aspirin (975 mg/day) have been used to slow the progression of adult membranoproliferative glomerulonephritis. The prognosis is worse with hypertension, poor renal function, and heavy proteinuria. This disorder tends to recur in transplants (type I, 30%; type II, 90%).

- Prognosis: worse with hypertension, poor renal function, heavy proteinuria.

GLOMERULAR DISEASE WITH HEAVY PROTEINURIA AND VARIABLE RENAL FAILURE

Minimal Change Nephropathy

Patients with minimal change nephropathy present with abrupt nephrotic syndrome with normal renal function (exceptions, hypovolemia and nonsteroidal anti-inflammatory drugs). This is the number one cause of nephrotic syndrome in children and the cause of 20% of adult cases of idiopathic nephrotic syndrome. Pathogenesis may be due to an attack on the glomerular epithelial cells by T-cell lymphokines, resulting in fusion of the foot processes. The heparin sulfate basement membrane negative charge barrier is lost. Secondary causes include Hodgkin's disease and nonsteroidal anti-inflammatory drugs (with interstitial nephritis). Light microscopic and immunofluorescence findings on renal biopsy specimens in minimal change nephropathy are normal. Electron microscopy shows fusion of the foot processes. A relapsing course is common (60% of cases). Patients are generally responsive and 90% have complete remission within 4 weeks. Generally, therapy is continued for 4 weeks after remission. Although 80% of adults respond to steroid therapy, 60% have repeated relapses. Cyclophosphamide can prolong remission and may decrease steroid dependence after 8 weeks of therapy; 50% of these patients have prolonged remissions. If patients are unresponsive, another biopsy is indicated to exclude focal segmental glomerulosclerosis.

- Minimal change nephropathy: abrupt nephrotic syndrome with normal renal function.
- Number one cause of nephrotic syndrome in children and cause of 20% of adult cases of idiopathic nephrotic syndrome.
- Secondary causes: Hodgkin's disease, nonsteroidal anti-inflammatory drugs (with interstitial nephritis).
- 80% of adults respond to steroid therapy; 60% have repeated relapses.

Focal Glomerular Sclerosis

Focal glomerular sclerosis accounts for 10% of cases of adult nephrotic syndrome. Mean age at disease onset is 21 years. Patients present with hypertension, renal insufficiency, proteinuria, and gross or microscopic hematuria. Secondary causes include AIDS (more frequent in drug abusers than in homosexuals), heroin abuse, reflux nephropathy, and massive obesity. Light microscopic results of renal biopsy samples demonstrate focal and segmental sclerosis without proliferation. Foam cells are often seen. Immunofluorescence shows IgM and C3 and deposits within the mesangium. Electron microscopy demonstrates fusion of foot processes in all glomeruli. Generally, therapy is supportive, although <10% of patients may respond to a course of steroid treatment. In selected patients with heavy proteinuria, meclofenamate has decreased complications due to the proteinuria. This disorder can recur in renal transplant recipients, and its prognosis is poor if proteinuria is >10 g/day.

- Focal glomerular sclerosis: 10% of cases of adult nephrotic syndrome.
- Mean age is 21 years.
- Presents with hypertension, renal insufficiency, proteinuria, gross or microscopic hematuria.
- Secondary causes: AIDS, heroin abuse, reflux nephropathy, massive obesity.
- Steroid therapy: <10% of patients respond.
- Prognosis is poor if proteinuria is >10 g/day.

Membranous Glomerulopathy

Membranous glomerulopathy is the primary cause of idiopathic nephrotic syndrome in adults (50% of cases). Mean age at disease onset is 35 years. However, 25% of the patients do not have nephrotic range proteinuria. Patients are often hypertensive (40%), with some renal insufficiency. Pathogenesis is due to in situ deposition of cationic antigens in the subepithelial space. Renal vein thrombosis (25%-50%) of cases may cause sudden loss of renal function. Secondary causes include infections (hepatitis B, quartan malaria, syphilis), multisystem disease (systemic lupus erythematosus, Sjögren's syndrome, sarcoid), and neoplasms (1.5% of cases, including carcinoma [lung, colon, stomach, breast] and lymphoma). Medications that cause membranous glomerulopathy are gold, D-penicillamine, captopril, and probenecid. Hereditary and metabolic causes include sickle cell disease. Renal biopsy demonstrates "spike and dome" epithelial deposits with thickened capillary loops seen on light microscopy. Granular IgG and C3 are seen on immunofluorescence. Therapy for membranous nephropathy is generally supportive, although 8 weeks of alternate-day steroids are often recommended. Other measures include the necessity to control hypertension and to treat any underlying disorders. Nearly 25% of the patients have spontaneous complete remission and 50% have partial remission. Approximately 20% of these patients progress to end-stage renal disease; the prognosis is related to the degree of proteinuria.

- Membranous glomerulopathy: primary cause of idiopathic nephrotic syndrome in adults.
- Mean age is 35 years.
- Pathogenesis: in situ deposition of cationic antigens in subepithelial space.
- Renal vein thrombosis causes sudden loss of renal function in 25%-50% of cases.
- Secondary causes: infections, multisystem disease, neoplasms, medications.
- Complete remission in 25% and partial remission in 50%.

OTHER GLOMERULAR DISORDERS

Diabetes Mellitus

From 2%-4% of U.S. citizens have diabetes. Diabetic nephropathy occurs in both insulin-dependent (30%-40%) and noninsulin-dependent (20%-30%) diabetics. More than 30% of patients hospitalized with end-stage renal disease have diabetic nephropathy, the single most common cause of end-stage renal disease in the U.S. Pathogenesis is secondary to glycosylation, renal hemodynamic changes, and hypertension. Microalbuminuria is the primary predictor of renal disease. The stages of diabetic nephropathy are listed in Table 21-7.

- Diabetic nephropathy occurs in insulin-dependent

(30%-40%) and noninsulin-dependent (20%-30%) diabetics.
- Diabetes is single most common cause of end-stage renal disease in U.S.
- Microalbuminuria is the primary predictor of renal disease.

Table 21-7.--Stages of Diabetic Nephropathy

Stage I	Hyperfiltration, glomerular filtration rate is 20%-50% above normal, microalbuminuria (>300 mg/24 hours)
Stage II	Normalization of glomerular filtration rate with early structural damage
Stage III	Early hypertension
Stage IV	Progression to proteinuria >0.5 g/day, hypertension, declining glomerular filtration rate (lasts 10-15 years)
Stage V	Progression to end-stage renal disease (5-7 years), heavy proteinuria persists even to end-stage disease

Renal biopsy of diabetic involvement of the kidney demonstrates a nodular and diffuse glomerular scarring or sclerosis. Capsular drop lesions and fibrin cap lesions are also pathognomonic. There is thickening of all basement membranes, with arteriolar hyalinosis and arteriosclerosis. Interstitial fibrosis and tubular atrophy may also be present. Other manifestations of diabetic urinary tract disease include papillary necrosis, perinephric abscess, acute pyelonephritis, neurogenic bladder and hydronephrosis with functional obstruction, bacteriuria, cystitis, and hypertension. Although tight glucose control by all current means available does not reverse diabetic nephropathy, it does tend to slow development of the disease. Patients with end-stage renal disease due to diabetes are kidney transplant candidates. Hemodialysis and continuous ambulatory peritoneal dialysis are also alternatives. Whether combined kidney/pancreas transplantation will prevent diabetic nephropathy is not clear. However, it is clear that aggressive control of blood pressure and glycemia definitely slows the progression of diabetic nephropathy.

- Other manifestations of diabetic urinary tract disease: papillary necrosis, perinephric abscess, acute pyelonephritis, neurogenic bladder and hydronephrosis with functional obstruction, bacteriuria, cystitis, hypertension.

- Aggressive control of blood pressure and glycemia slows progression.

Lupus

Of patients with lupus, 50% have renal disease at presentation and 90% have renal disease at sometime. If renal involvement occurs with lupus, it usually presents early in the course of the disease. The presenting histologic renal lesion is fairly stable except that a focal proliferative lesion progresses to diffuse proliferative lesion in 20% of cases. An active diffuse proliferative lesion is treatable with steroids with or without cytotoxic agents. Membranous systemic lupus erythematosus is usually not treatable with immunosuppressive agents. Kidney biopsy is indicated for active urinary sediment with or without decreased glomerular function to define the renal lesion in lupus. The five classes of renal disease that may be present are listed in Table 21-8.

- Lupus: 50% of patients present with renal disease and 90% have renal disease sometime during the course of lupus.
- Active diffuse proliferative lesion is treatable with steroids with or without cytotoxic agents.
- Membranous systemic lupus erythematosus usually is not treatable with immunosuppressive agents.

Table 21-8.--Five Classes of Renal Diseases
Present With Lupus

Class I	Normal
Class II	Mild mesangial change (no clinical findings of renal disease in 50% of patients)
Class III	Focal and segmental proliferative glomerulonephritis (20% nephritic with or without nephrotic syndrome)
Class IV	Diffuse proliferative glomerulonephritis (70% nephritic with or without nephrotic syndrome), "wire loop"
Class V	Membranous glomerulonephritis (nephrotic but not active sediment)

Other manifestations of lupus include acute and chronic tubulointerstital nephritis and vasculitis. Chronic changes include glomerular scarring, tubular atrophy, and interstitial fibrosis, all of which are untreatable. Therapy for lupus nephritis is often limited to treatment of prolif-

erative nephritis. Patients with acute proliferative nephritis and acute renal failure should receive high doses of steroids with or without cytotoxic agents. Diffuse proliferative glomerulonephritis without azotemia is also treated with high doses of steroids for 6-8 weeks. Cyclophosphamide can be added to the therapy if necessary. Aside from proteinuria, membranous lupus involvement often is characterized by weakly positive or negative antinuclear antibody without red cell casts. Generally, therapy is supportive only. It is important to remember that drug-induced lupus rarely involves the kidney. Pregnancy should be delayed until after lupus is inactive for 6 months; 25%-45% of lupus patients have exacerbations usually 8 weeks after delivery. Lupus "burns out" with end-stage renal disease and generally does not recur in transplant recipients.

- Drug-induced lupus rarely involves kidney.
- Pregnancy should be delayed until after lupus is inactive for 6 months.
- Lupus "burns out" with end-stage renal disease and generally does not occur in transplant recipients.

Vasculitis

The types of vasculitis are listed in Table 21-9.

Microscopic polyarteritis nodosa presents with hypertension, weight loss, arthralgias, myalgias, mononeuritis multiplex, epididymitis, subcutaneous nodules, gastrointestinal tract bleeding, active urine sediment, and proteinuria. Anemia, azotemia, normal levels of complement, perinuclear ANCA, and erythrocyte sedimentation rate >100 mm/hour are common. Renal biopsy and not angiography is best to determine diagnosis in patients with abnormal urinalysis. Light microscopy of biopsy sample demonstrates a segmental necrotizing glomerulonephritis with or without crescents. Renal granulomas are rarely seen in Wegener's granulomatosis. Prednisone with a slow taper over 6-12 months is often prescribed for therapy. Dialysis-dependent patients have regained renal function after treatment. Remissions are common but vasculitis may recur. Patients with Wegener's granulomatosis often have positive cytoplasmic ANCA and respond to steroids and cyclophosphamide (Cytoxan) given orally.

- Microscopic polyarteritis nodosa: presentation includes hypertension, weight loss, arthralgias, myalgias, mononeuritis multiplex, epididymitis, subcutaneous nodules, gastrointestinal tract bleeding, active urine sediment, proteinuria.

- Common features: anemia, azotemia, normal levels of complement, perinuclear ANCA, erythrocyte sedimentation rate >100 mm/hour.
- Renal biopsy and not angiography is best for determining diagnosis.

Table 21-9.--Types of Vasculitis

Microscopic polyarteritis nodosa--overlap (most common form of vasculitis) (p-ANCA)

Wegener's granulomatosis c-ANCA

Classic polyarteritis nodosa

Allergic granulomatosis (Churg-Strauss syndrome)

Hypersensitivity vasculitis

Essential mixed cryoglobulinemia

Rheumatoid arthritis, systemic lupus erythematosus-associated vasculitis

Giant cell arteritis (no renal involvement?)

MONOCLONAL GAMMOPATHIES

Amyloidosis, multiple myeloma, light chain nephropathy, and immunotactoid nephropathy are renal manifestations of monoclonal gammopathies. Renal manifestations include proteinuria (λ light chains: amyloid; κ light chains: light chain nephropathy; λ and κ light chains: myeloma), nephrotic syndrome, hematuria, nephritic syndrome, acute renal failure, and tubulointerstitial disease. Patients may also have renal manifestations of myeloma, including normal- or large-sized kidneys, pseudohyponatremia, low anion gap, hypercalcemia, Fanconi's syndrome (low phosphorous, urate, potassium; glycosuria; aminoaciduria; type II and renal tubular acidosis), and Bence Jones proteinuria.

Renal biopsy: diagnostic stains for amyloid are Congo red, thioflavin T, methyl violet. Light chain nephropathy demonstrates κ light chain deposition and the nodular glomerulosclerosis often mimics diabetes. Immunofluorescence generally demonstrates λ light chains in amyloid and κ light chains in light chain nephropathy. Electron microscopy is helpful in further differentiating the type of light chain fibrils. Renal biopsy findings correlate poorly with the clinical course and renal function in patients with monoclonal gammopathies. Treatment is often supportive, but melphalan and prednisone have had some beneficial effect in selected patients. In secondary causes of this disorder, it is necessary to treat the underlying disorder. Colchicine is helpful in the treatment of familial Mediterranean fever.

CRYOGLOBULINEMIAS

Patients with cryoglobulinemia often present with palpable purpura and are either nephritic or nephrotic (Table 21-10). Acute renal failure can occur if the cryocrit is >1 g/dL. Renal biopsy demonstrates characteristic fibrin thrombi within glomeruli. Prednisone, cytotoxic agents, and plasmapheresis are used with variable results in cryoglobulinemia.

HEMOLYTIC UREMIC SYNDROME AND THROMBOCYTOPENIC PURPURA

Patients present with severe hypertension, proteinuria, active sediment, and renal failure. Both hemolytic uremic syndrome and thrombocytopenic purpura are associated with a microhemangiopathic hemolytic anemia and thrombocytopenia. Endothelial cell injury and subendothelial deposits are present on biopsy, "endotheliosis." The glomerular lesion is also seen in malignant hypertension, scleroderma, and postpartum acute renal failure. Secondary causes include mitomycin C, bleomycin,

Table 21-10.--Cryoglobulins and Associated Diseases

Cryoglobulin type	Ig class	Associated disease
I, monoclonal immunoglobulins	M>G>A>BJP	Myeloma, Waldenström's macroglobulinemia
II, mixed cryoglobulins with monoclonal immunoglobulins	M/G>>G/G	Sjögren's syndrome, Waldenström's macroglobulinemia, lymphoma
		Essential cryoglobulinemia
III, mixed polyclonal immunoglobulins	M/G	Infection, systemic lupus erythematosus, vasculitis, neoplasia
		Essential cryoglobulinemia

cyclosporin A, *E. coli* 0157, and radiation. Children with hemolytic uremia syndrome have a good prognosis (90% recover renal function), but adults have a poor prognosis. Thrombocytopenic purpura includes fever, neurologic signs, and purpura in addition to the above. Therapy is plasma infusion and plasmapheresis with or without antiplatelet therapy. For scleroderma, the therapy includes treating hypertension with angiotensin-converting enzyme inhibitors.

- Presentation: severe hypertension, proteinuria, active sediment, renal failure.
- Associated with: microhemangiopathic hemolytic anemia and thrombocytopenia.
- Glomerular lesion also seen in malignant hypertension, scleroderma, postpartum acute renal failure.
- Therapy: plasma infusion plus plasmapheresis with or without antiplatelet therapy.

ALPORT'S SYNDROME AND THIN GLOMERULAR BASEMENT MEMBRANE DISEASE--DISEASES WITH GLOMERULAR BASEMENT MEMBRANE ABNORMALITIES

Patients present with hematuria, proteinuria, and nephrosis (end-stage renal disease by age 16-30). High-frequency hearing loss and ocular abnormalities (anterior lenticonus and cataracts) are present. Inheritance is X-linked dominant (males have a worse prognosis). Transplant recipients may develop anti-glomerular basement membrane-mediated renal disease. In Alport's syndrome, the lack of the domain of noncollagenous type IV collagen and the absence of Goodpasture's antigen mean that anti-glomerular basement membrane antibodies cannot be bound.

In thin glomerular basement membrane disease, the glomerular basement membrane is 200-nm thick. Patients present with hematuria.

CLINICAL MANIFESTATIONS OF TUBULOINTERSTITIAL RENAL DISEASE

Acute and chronic acute interstitial disease preferentially involves renal tubules. Some of the patterns of renal tubular injury are 1) tubular proteinuria, <1.5-2 g/day; 2) proximal tubule dysfunction (hypokalemia, hypouricemia, hypophosphatemia, acidosis, glycosuria, aminoaciduria); 3) distal tubule dysfunction (hyperchloremic acidosis, hyperkalemia or hypokalemia, salt wasting); 4) medullary concentration dysfunction, nephrogenic diabetes insipidus with decreased urine concentrating ability; 5) urine sediment (pyuria, leukocyte casts, eosinophilia, hematuria); and 6) azotemia, renal insufficiency.

- Tubular proteinuria, <1.5-2 g/day.
- Proximal tubule dysfunction and distal tubule dysfunction.
- Medullary concentration dysfunction.

ACUTE INTERSTITIAL NEPHRITIS

Patients with acute tubulointerstitial nephritis present with fever of mean onset of 15 days (90% of patients), rash (25%), arthralgias (25%), pyuria (100%), eosinophilia (50%), proteinuria (75%), hematuria (95%), and renal insufficiency (60%). Diagnosis sometimes requires renal biopsy. Gallium or indium scans can also be helpful.

- Acute tubulointerstitial nephritis: 90% have fever; 25%, arthralgias; 100%, pyuria; 50%, eosinophilia; 60%, renal insufficiency.

Drug-induced acute tubulointerstitial nephritis can be due to several agents:
1. Antibiotics--penicillin, methicillin (anti-tubular basement membrane antibodies), ampicillin, rifampin, sulfa drugs, ciprofloxacin, pentamidine
2. Nonsteroidal anti-inflammatory drugs--tubulointerstitial nephritis with nephrotic syndrome and renal insufficiency may have a latent period, not dose-dependent, recurs, possibly T-cell mediated, allergic signs and symptoms are absent
3. Diuretics--thiazides, furosemide, bumetanide (sulfa derivatives)
4. Cimetidine
5. Allopurinol, phenytoin, phenindione--exfoliative dermatitis, hepatitis, and acute tubulointerstitial nephritis
6. Cyclosporin A--acute renal vasoconstriction

Treatment is to discontinue use of the drug and possibly to prescribe a short course of prednisone (60 mg every other day).

- Methicillin (anti-tubular basement membrane antibodies).
- Nonsteroidal anti-inflammatory drugs: tubulointerstitial nephritis with nephrotic syndrome and renal insufficiency.

- Sulfa derivatives.
- Cimetidine.

Acute interstitial nephritis can be caused by infection (streptococcosis, leptospirosis, Rocky Mountain spotted fever, legionnaires' disease, Epstein-Barr virus, cytomegalovirus), lymphoma, leukemic infiltration, lupus, renal transplant rejection, toxic radiation, and acute pyelonephritis.

ANALGESIC CHRONIC INTERSTITIAL NEPHRITIS

Analgesic nephropathy is a good example of chronic interstitial nephritis and is responsible for 20% of cases of tubulointerstitial nephritis, with 3%-10% of patients entering end-stage renal disease. Patients have a chronic pain problem. Other features: headache (80% of patients), arthritis and muscular aches, female (85%), anemia (85%), history of peptic ulcer (40%), urinary tract infection with history of dysuria (25%), history of obstruction (10%), hypertension (40%), and premature aging. Patients generally do not admit to analgesic abuse. Findings include sterile pyuria, normal excretory urogram (10%), small kidneys (50%), and papillary necrosis (30%). Phenacetin and its metabolites are concentrated in the renal papillae. Renal hydroperoxidases react with these metabolites and produce reactive intermediates that damage the papilla by lipid peroxidation. Aspirin diminishes local renal blood flow and lowers the concentration of glutathione, which normally inactivates phenacetin metabolites. The result is papillary ischemia and eventually necrosis. Amount necessary to cause analgesic nephropathy: total intake of 3 kg of phenacetin or 1 g/day for 3 years. Aspirin or acetaminophen alone do *not* cause this disorder but nonsteroidal anti-inflammatory drugs may. Patients with a history of analgesic ingestion may even continue ingestion after kidney transplantation. Multicentric transitional cell carcinomas of the collecting system, although rare, are more common in patients with analgesic nephropathy. Evidence suggests that these patients have accelerated arteriosclerosis. Papillary necrosis is a common accompaniment of analgesic nephropathy. Other causes of papillary necrosis can be remembered by the mnemonic P-O-S-T C-A-R-D (pyelonephritis, obstruction, sickle cell disease or trait, tuberculosis, chronic alcoholism with cirrhosis, analgesics, renal vein thrombosis, and diabetes mellitus).

- Analgesic nephropathy: responsible for 20% of cases of chronic tubulointerstitial nephritis (3%-10% have end-stage renal disease).
- Chronic pain problem, headache (80%), arthritis and muscular aches, female (80%), history of peptic ulcer (40%).
- Patients generally do not admit to analgesic abuse.
- Findings: sterile pyuria, normal excretory urogram (10%), small kidneys (50%), papillary necrosis (30%).
- Phenacetin and its metabolites are concentrated in the renal papillae.
- Amount necessary to cause analgesic nephropathy: total intake of 3 kg of phenacetin or 1 g/day for 3 years.

OTHER RENAL DISEASE PRESENTING WITH INTERSTITIAL NEPHRITIS

Other renal diseases presenting with interstitial nephritis are glomerular injury (lupus, mixed cryoglobulinemia, hypertension, diabetes, Sjögren's syndrome, Alport's syndrome, myeloma), Balkan nephropathy (as with analgesic nephropathy, increased incidence of uroepithelial cancers), granulomatous nephropathy (tuberculosis, sarcoid), and sickle cell trait/disease.

ELECTROLYTE- AND TOXIN-INDUCED INTERSTITIAL NEPHRITIS

Acute uric acid nephropathy is associated with the tumor lysis syndrome after chemotherapy, myeloproliferative disorders, heat stroke, status epilepticus, and Lesch-Nyhan syndrome. In this disorder, intraluminal crystals cause intrarenal obstruction, and serum uric acid is often >15 mg and 24-hour urinary uric acid is >1,000 mg. The spot urinary uric acid divided by spot urinary creatinine is often >1.0. Prevention requires alkaline diuresis, allopurinol, and, sometimes, hemodialysis. This disorder generally is completely reversible. Chronic uric acid nephropathy due to saturnine gout (lead from "moonshine" or paint) or chronic tophaceous gout is due to interstitial crystal formation, microtophi present in the renal parenchyma. It has only limited reversibility. Remember that de novo gout in renal failure is rare; in this setting, it should be assumed that the patient has lead nephropathy until proved otherwise.

- Acute uric acid nephropathy associated with tumor lysis syndrome and myeloproliferative disorders.
- Serum uric acid is >15 mg and 24-hour urinary uric

acid is >1,000 mg.
- Prevention: alkaline diuresis and allopurinol.

Early on, hypercalcemia results in mitochondrial deposits of calcium in the proximal and distal tubules as well as in the collecting duct. Later, tubular degeneration with calcium deposition and obstruction occurs. Calcium inhibits sodium transport, induces nephrogenic diabetes insipidus, and causes intrarenal vasoconstriction. It also stimulates the release of renin and catecholamines, producing increased blood pressure.

Hypokalemia has been associated with vascularization of the proximal and distal tubules and possibly chronic interstitial fibrosis. Nephrogenic diabetes insipidus is also associated with chronic hypokalemia.

Oxalate deposition from primary hyperoxaluria causes renal and extrarenal oxalate deposition. Extrarenal sites include the eye, heart, bone, joint, and vascular system. Oxalate deposition from secondary causes can be due to ethylene glycol, methoxyflurane, high doses of ascorbic acid, vitamin B_6 deficiency, and enteric hyperoxaluria.

Lithium induces a nephrogenic diabetes insipidus and microcystic changes in the renal tubules. Interstitial fibrosis may be present.

Heavy metals such as cadmium, pigments, glass, plastic, metal alloys, electrical equipment manufacturing, and some cigarettes induce a proximal renal tubular acidosis and tubulointerstitial nephritis. Lead intoxication can cause lead nephropathy, as mentioned above. The organic salt of mercury can induce chronic tubulointerstitial nephritis and membranous nephritis or acute tubulonecrosis.

CYSTIC RENAL DISEASE

Autosomal-dominant polycystic kidney disease is the cause of renal failure in 10% of all patients who reach end-stage renal failure. Of chromosome abnormalities found thus far, the best recognized is a mutation of the short arm of chromosome 16. Patients with polycystic kidney disease have cysts that grow from birth and are present in all nephron segments. By age 25, the cysts are usually seen on ultrasonography or CT. Other cysts can form in the liver, spleen, and pancreas. Urinary tract infections are common in polycystic kidney disease and can be localized by CT, gallium or indium scans, or MRI. Lipid-soluble antibiotics tend to penetrate the cysts well. Hematuria may also be seen, with hemorrhage into a cyst, a stone, or, sometimes, a malignancy. Uric acid

and calcium oxalate stones are common. Other associations with adult autosomal-dominant polycystic kidney include diverticulosis, cardiac valve myxomatous degeneration, and cerebral aneurysms. Also, the hematocrit may be higher than expected because of production of renal erythropoietin.

- Autosomal-dominant polycystic kidney disease: cause of 10% of cases of end-stage renal failure.
- By age 25, cysts usually seen with ultrasonography or CT.
- Other cysts in liver, spleen, pancreas.
- Other associations: diverticulosis, cardiac valve myxomatous degeneration, cerebral aneurysms.

Medullary sponge kidney is due to dilated collecting ducts, seen on excretory urography, and may be unilateral, bilateral, or involve a single papilla. There is no known pattern of inheritance of this disorder, which is associated with nephrolithiasis and some renotubular abnormalities.

Acquired renal cystic disease can affect up to 50% of long-term dialysis patients and may present with hematuria and an increasing hematocrit. Although these cysts sometimes have neoplastic potential, they rarely metastasize.

UROLITHIASIS

The prevalence of urolithiasis is about 5% in the U.S. (there is an increased incidence of urolithiasis in the southeastern U.S.). The annual incidence is about 0.1%. Of patients with urolithiasis who are untreated, 50%-75% have recurrence within 7 years. Urolithiasis is strongly familial and related to diet and urine volume. Most patients have a metabolic disorder that can be demonstrated with further testing, but conservative treatment with diet and increased fluid intake eliminates the stone-forming tendency in 70% of patients. For those who fail conservative therapy, medications are curative in another 25%.

- Prevalence of urolithiasis in the U.S., about 5%.
- It is strongly familial and related to diet and urine volume.

Urine pH is important in the pathogenesis of some renal stones. Struvite and calcium phosphate stones tend to form in alkaline urine; uric acid and cystine stones form in acid urine. Some anatomical factors predisposing to urolithiasis include medullary sponge kidney, polycystic kidney disease, and chronic obstruction.

- Struvite and calcium phosphate stones form in alkaline urine.
- Cystine stones and uric acid form in acid urine.

An evaluation of patients with urolithiasis is important to classify the patient's activity. Surgical activity: indicated by hydronephrosis, unrelieved pain, decreasing function (stones <5 mm should pass). Metabolic activity: formation of new stone or growth of an existing stone within 1 year. Historical factors include fluid intake, dietary intake, urinary tract infection history, drugs, family history, and other illnesses. Laboratory studies should include reviewing earlier radiographic findings; excretory urography; stone analysis; serum calcium and phosphorus; fasting urinalysis; urine culture; 24-hour urinary volume; and calcium, phosphorus, citrate, creatinine, oxalate, and cystine analysis with usual diet.

Calcium Stones

From 75%-85% of all renal stones contain calcium. Patients may develop calcium oxalate and calcium phosphate stones or, rarely, pure calcium phosphate stones. Causes include idiopathic hypercalciuria, other hypercalciuric states, hypouricosuria, hyperoxaluria, and reduced inhibitor excretion (see below). Conservative treatment includes correcting dietary stresses and increasing urine volume >2.5 L/day. Medications include neutral sodium phosphate for idiopathic calcium urolithiasis (2 g/day, but not in cases of urinary tract infection or renal insufficiency), thiazides for patients with hypercalciuria (sodium must be restricted for urine calcium to decrease 50%), and allopurinol for patients with hyperuricosuria.

Pure Uric Acid Stones

Patients with uric acid urolithiasis often have normal plasma and urinary uric acid. They often have very acidic urine. Of patients with primary gout, 25% form renal stones. Dietary protein excess also can predispose to uric acid stones, as can colectomy and ileostomy, because of decreased intestinal ureolysis. Uric acid urolithiasis is treated with preventative measures such as increased intake of fluid and decreased protein intake. Alkalinizing the urine to pH 6.5 not only helps prevent uric acid urolithiasis but dissolves renal stones. Although allopurinol is not as effective as alkalinizing the urine, it can be helpful

in patients with hyperuricosuria.

- Renal stones form in 25% of patients with primary gout.
- Colectomy and ileostomy predispose to stones because of decreased intestinal ureolysis.

Struvite Stones

All patients with magnesium ammonium phosphate stones are infected with urease-producing bacteria, which can include *Proteus*, *Staphylococcus*, *Klebsiella*, *Pseudomonas*, and *E. coli*. The urine pH of these patients is alkaline, sometimes >7.8. Also, most of the patients have an underlying stone-forming tendency. Staghorn stones are not uncommon, and 50% are bilateral. Treatment includes antibiotics given preoperatively and then surgical removal of all stone material followed by an attempt to identify the underlying stone-forming tendency and treatment of this followed by bactericidal antibiotics for 6-12 months for suppression.

- All patients with magnesium ammonium phosphate stones are infected with urease-producing bacteria.
- Urine pH is very alkaline.
- 50% of staghorn stones are bilateral.
- Treatment: bactericidal antibiotics for 6-12 months for suppression.

Urolithiasis and Bowel Disease

Hyperoxaluria: patients must have an intact colon to absorb free oxalate. Free oxalate is malabsorbed when free fatty acids complex calcium and magnesium (the usual oxalate complexers). Fatty acids and bile acids also increase the colonic permeability to oxalate. Other factors that increase hyperoxaluria and malabsorption include decreased water absorption, decreased bicarbonate absorption, and decreased absorption of magnesium, phosphate, and pyrophosphate (inhibitors). Treatment of this disorder includes correcting the underlying problem, increasing dietary calcium, decreasing dietary oxalate and fat, considering cholestyramine to bind bile acids, and chelating oxalate.

- Absorption of free oxalate requires an intact colon.

Patients with bowel disease may also develop uric acid urolithiasis. Ileostomy patients are frequently susceptible to these stones because of the loss of alkali and water. Treatment includes alkali, fluids, and allopurinol.

Renal Tubular Disorders

Renal tubular disorders associated with urolithiasis include distal renal tubular acidosis type I. These patients can often make pure calcium phosphate stones. They also have nephrocalcinosis, a urine pH that is always >5.3, and a hyperchloremic hypokalemic normal anion gap acidosis with decreased urinary citrate (a stone inhibitor) and high level of urinary calcium. Treatment is to correct the acidosis with alkali and to monitor urinary citrate excretion.

Cystinuria is an autosomal recessive disorder in which homozygotes develop urolithiasis. Cystine crystalluria in routine urine is diagnostic, as are positive findings on the nitroprusside test. These patients have a defect in the renal and intestinal absorption of cystine, ornithine, lysine, and arginine ("COLA"). The stones can be dissolved with urinary alkalinization and high intake of fluid; however, urinary alkalinization must be very intense, with urine pH maintained at about 7. D-Penicillamine is useful in decreasing the solubility of the increased cystine excretion. Remember that D-penicillamine can be associated with blood dyscrasias, gastrointestinal tract upset, membranous glomerulopathy, and a Goodpasture-like syndrome. Patients with cystinuria often receive pyridoxine (25 mg/day) in addition to the above.

Some medications that increase the tendency for stone formation are listed in Table 21-11.

Table 21-11.--Medications Increasing the Tendency for Stone Formation

Acetazolamide for glaucoma (calcium phosphate stones)
Calcium carbonate (milk alkali)
Allopurinol (xanthine or oxypurinol stones)
Triamterene
Methoxyflurane (oxalate)
Vitamin D, nonthiazide diuretics, steroids (hypercalciuria)
Chemotherapy (increased urate load)

Enzyme Disorders

Several enzyme disorders can be associated with increased stone formation.

Primary hyperoxaluria is the most aggressive stone disease. Type I, glycolic and oxalic aciduria (glyoxylate carboxylase deficiency); type II, L-glyceric and oxalic aciduria (D-glyceric dehydrogenase deficiency). Treatment includes fluids, pyridoxine (alters glycine metabolism, an oxalate precursor), orthophosphates, and liver trans-

plantation.

Xanthinuria, caused by xanthine oxidase deficiency, is characterized by low serum and urinary levels of uric acid. Xanthine stones are radiolucent. Treatment: fluids, alkalinization of urine, and allopurinol.

2,8-Dihydroxyadenuria is caused by deficient adenine phosphoribosyl transferase. The stones resemble urate stones. Treatment is with allopurinol.

CHRONIC RENAL FAILURE

Chronic renal failure is defined as a decrease in glomerular filtration rate to <25-33 mL/min. End-stage renal failure is generally defined as glomerular filtration rate <8-10 mL/min. Often, patients with chronic renal failure have small kidneys (<10 cm), as seen on KUB with tomograms. The renal size is often preserved in end-stage renal disease in diabetes, amyloidosis, myeloma, and polycystic kidney disease. Chronic renal insufficiency tends to be progressive because of the persistence of the underlying disorder and possible hyperfiltration by the remaining nephrons. The causes of end-stage renal disease include chronic glomerulonephritis (33%), chronic tubulointerstitial disease (21%), polycystic kidney disease (10%), diabetes (20%), hypertension (33% blacks, 10% whites), analgesics (5%), familial (5%), and unknown (5%). One should approach chronic renal failure by first excluding any reversible cause such as heart failure, hypertension, infection, hypothyroidism, hypoadrenalism, obstruction, hypercalcemia, medications, and volume loss in salt wasters. After excluding reversible causes, management includes control of blood pressure and early treatment of metabolic acidosis and use of phosphate binders. Late treatment and management includes the use of erythropoietin, fluid, sodium, potassium, and protein restrictions; treatment of acidosis; calcium and vitamin D supplements; and use of loop diuretics.

- Chronic renal failure: glomerular filtration rate <25-33 mL/min.
- End-stage renal failure: glomerular filtration rate <8-10 mL/min.
- Small kidneys, <10 cm.
- Kidney size preserved in diabetes, amyloidosis, myeloma, polycystic kidney disease.

UREMIC SIGNS AND SYMPTOMS

Anemia of chronic renal failure is normochromic, normocytic, and multifactorial, i.e., decreased erythropoietin production, hemolysis, and blood loss.

The metabolic acidosis of chronic renal failure is first a normal then a high anion gap due to decreased ammonium secretion, followed by retention of phosphates and sulfates. Always check the anion gap in chronic renal failure; it is rarely >25.

Hypertension is common and is associated with extracellular fluid excess and, in some cases, with excess renin production. Multiple agents are often necessary to control hypertension.

Heart failure is common in chronic renal failure. Thus, use caution with digoxin, long-acting calcium channel blockers, and angiotensin-converting enzyme inhibitors.

Pericarditis frequently occurs in two patterns: pattern I is a hemorrhagic pericarditis that often occurs predialysis and for which dialysis is helpful. Pattern II is sometimes hemorrhagic, occasionally with tamponade, and can occur in well-dialyzed patients. Intrapericardial steroids are often necessary. Pattern II may be due to viral pericarditis.

Hyperkalemia occurs in two patterns: pattern I is associated with a glomerular filtration rate of <20 mL/min and oliguria. Pattern II occurs when the glomerular filtration rate is >20 mL/min and often is associated with type IV renal tubular acidosis due to aldosterone deficiency, particularly in diabetics. Other causes of hyperkalemia include nonsteroidal anti-inflammatory agents, β-blockers, angiotensin-converting enzyme inhibitors, and potassium-sparing diuretics. Emergent treatment of hyperkalemia includes the use of calcium infusion to protect the myocardium, followed by bicarbonate and then insulin to redistribute the potassium, then resins and dialysis are used to eliminate potassium.

Bleeding tendency is common in chronic renal failure due to a platelet defect. Thus, use of antiplatelet drugs should be avoided. Treatment with desamino-D-arginine vasopressin is helpful in reversing the bleeding tendency acutely.

Renal osteodystrophy has four components: 1) osteitis fibrosa cystica: hyperparathyroidism, osteoclastic overactivity; 2) osteomalacia due to 1,25-vitamin D deficiency, in which case there is increased osteoid formation within bone; 3) osteoporosis; and 4) growth retardation. Renal disease leads to phosphate retention, which decreases urinary calcium and stimulates parathyroid hormone excretion. Bone is often poorly responsive to parathyroid hormone in chronic renal failure. Also, the 1,25-vitamin D deficiency leads to a vicious cycle of steadily increasing

phosphorus and parathyroid hormone. Treatment is to bind phosphorus enterically by giving calcium-containing antacids such as calcium carbonate and calcium acetate to decrease the serum level of phosphorus and to increase calcium. Vitamin D supplements are often necessary. Selected patients who have received aluminum-containing salts for many years become hypercalcemic with low serum levels of parathyroid hormone and 1,25-vitamin D. These patients often have microcytic anemia and frequent fractures and need to have an iliac crest bone biopsy for diagnosis. Aluminum osteodystrophy is treated with deferoxamine chelation.

Endocrine abnormalities in chronic renal failure include low levels of total thyroxine and high levels of growth hormone, luteinizing hormone, and prolactin despite thyroid, adrenal, and pituitary function usually being normal. Hypergastrinemia is present, but peptic ulcer disease is not more common in these patients. Impaired fertility and sexual function and amenorrhea are common. Pregnancy is rare if the creatinine level is >2.0 μg/dL. There is increased resistance to insulin but also decreased insulin degradation associated with an impaired carbohydrate tolerance.

Hyperlipidemia and accelerated atherosclerosis are common. Gastritis, not peptic ulcer disease, is common and usually drug-induced. Constipation is common and aggravated by phosphate binders that contain aluminum. Pseudogout and periarthritis are due to hydroxyapatite deposited in joint spaces.

In peripheral neuropathy of chronic renal failure, sensory fibers are affected more than motor fibers and the lower extremities are involved more than the upper extremities. It is often associated with asterixis and seizures.

DIALYSIS

Indications for dialysis include uremia, pericarditis, neuropathy, hyperkalemia, and intractable metabolic acidosis.

Complications

Hepatitis B--Patients may have mild or no symptoms and may go on to carrier state (also cytomegalovirus, Epstein-Barr virus, non-A non-B hepatitis, methyldopa, anabolic steroids, azathioprine). Treatment is with vaccine and hepatitis B immune globulin. Hepatitis C is the type of hepatitis that is most common in dialysis patients. Neurologic complications include dialysis disequilibrium (brain edema and osmolar shifts), subdural hema-

um (brain edema and osmolar shifts), subdural hematomas, and dialysis dementia (dyspraxia, myoclonus, and gait disturbance due to aluminum overload). Infections: vascular access, peritonitis, tuberculosis (10x the frequency of that in the normal population).

Continuous Ambulatory Peritoneal Dialysis

Indications for continuous ambulatory peritoneal dialysis are cardiovascular instability, poor hemodialysis access, and patient preference. Recent abdominal surgery, colostomy, nephrostomy, and adhesions are contraindications. Complications include peritonitis, catheter leak, hyperlipidemia, obesity, hyperglycemia, and protein malnutrition.

Continuous Arteriovenous Hemofiltration or Slow Continuous Ultrafiltration

The indications for these techniques are cardiogenic shock and pulmonary edema, diuretic unresponsive congestive heart failure, and acute renal failure with hemodynamic instability.

Dialysis and Overdoses

Dialysis can be used to treat overdoses of methanol, aspirin, ethylene glycol, lithium, sodium, mannitol, theophylline. Dialysis is not used for overdoses of tricyclics, benzodiazepines, digoxin, dilantin, phenothiazines.

Medications in Dialysis

Of the antibiotics, ampicillin and cephalosporins are helpful. **AVOID** using tetracyclines, nitrofurantoin, probenecid, neomycin, bacitracin, methenamine, nalidixic acid, clofibrate, lovastatin, magnesium, oral hypoglycemic agents, and antiplatelet drugs. Be careful when using angiotensin-converting enzyme inhibitors, other potassium-sparing agents, metoclopramide, nonsteroidal anti-inflammatory drugs, acyclovir, long-acting calcium channel blockers, and renal-excreted β-blockers.

TRANSPLANTATION

Transplantation is the treatment of choice of eligible patients with end-stage renal disease. Since the time of the first kidney transplantation (performed in 1955), more than 100,000 of these procedures have been performed; 10,000 are performed annually (8,000 cadaveric and 2,000 living related). The main limitation is the limited number of donor kidneys. Lifetime immunosuppression is required. Recipients are from <1 to >50 years old. The recipients must not have cancer; infections (e.g., teeth, sinuses, bladder) have to be eradicated, and cholecystectomy for gallstones has to be performed. Living-related donors must be >18 years old and without systemic or renal disease. Cadaveric donors must be >6 months old and be without infection or malignancy (except for nonmetastasizing brain cancer).

- Transplantation is the treatment of choice for eligible patients with end-stage renal disease.
- Lifetime immunosuppression is required.

Recurrent Allograft Renal Disease

Causes of recurrent allograft renal disease include type II membranoproliferative glomerulonephritis, focal glomerulosclerosis, diabetes, primary hyperoxaluria, hemolytic-uremic syndrome, and IgA (not clinically significant).

Immunosuppression

Agents for immunosuppression include the following: 1) prednisone, which blocks interleukin-1 production by macrophages and cytokine production (complications include cataracts, psychoses, peptic ulcer disease, infection, diverticulitis, aseptic necrosis); 2) azathioprine, which inhibits proliferation of activated T cells (marrow suppression, cholestasis, infection; never treat with allopurinol); 3) cyclosporine A, which inhibits helper T cell activation and interleukin-2,#-3,#-4, and -5 production; it is hydrophobic and lipophilic, requiring bile acids for absorption.

Cyclosporine A levels are increased or decreased by the following agents: increased levels with ketoconazole, cimetidine, ranitidine, verapamil, diltiazem, and erythromycin and decreased levels with phenytoin, phenobarbital, ethambutol, sulfamethoxazole, ethanol, and cholestyramine.

Toxicity effects of immunosuppression include gum hyperplasia, hyperkalemia, hypertension, hemolytic-uremic syndrome, and thrombotic thrombocytopenic purpura.

Graft Failure (Chronic Rejection Most Commonly)

Graft failure commonly is due to chronic rejection. Acute tubular necrosis occurs after transplantation in 20%-50% of cases. The stages of rejection are hyperacute (hours), acute (days to years), and chronic (months-years). Treat only acute stages of rejection. Recurrent disease occurs in 1% of cases. Surgical complications include renal artery stenosis, ureteral obstruction-leak, and lymphocele.

Medical complications--Opportunistic infections are the number one cause of death. *Anything is possible.* Cardiovascular problems are the number two cause. Other complications are hyperlipidemia; suicide (9% of patients); cancer (1%, including skin, sarcomas, lymphomas [Epstein-Barr virus-associated], solid tumors); polycythemia; proximal/distal renal tubular acidosis; and kidney stones (1%).

PREGNANCY AND THE KIDNEY

Anatomical changes associated with pregnancy are renal enlargement (1 cm) and dilatation of the calyces, renal pelvis, and ureters. Physiologic changes include 1) a 30%-50% increase in glomerular filtration rate and renal blood flow; 2) mean creatinine level of 0.5 µg/dL and mean urea of 18 (limits: creatinine of 0.8 and urea of 26); 3) intermittent glycosuria independent of plasma glucose (<1 g/day); 4) proteinuria but <300 mg/day (sometimes postural); 5) aminoaciduria <2 g/day (most but not all amino acids); 6) increased uric acid excretion; 7) increased total body water (6-8 L) with osmostat resetting; 8) 50% increases in plasma volume and cardiac output; and 9) increased ureteral peristalsis. Bacterial growth in urine is promoted by the intermittent glycosuria and amino-aciduria. Hormonal effects are 1) increased levels of renin, angiotensin II, aldosterone, cortisol, estrogens, prostaglandins (E_2, I_2), and progesterone; 2) insensitivity to pressor effects of norepinephrine and angiotensin II; and 3) progesterone counteracting the kaliuretic effects of aldosterone.

Urinary Tract Infections

The prevalence of asymptomatic bacteriuria among pregnant women is similar to that among nonpregnant women, except it is higher in those with diabetes and sickle cell trait. Asymptomatic urinary tract infections progress to pyelonephritis or cystitis in 40% of pregnant women. Screen for asymptomatic bacteriuria monthly, and treat asymptomatic bacteriuria (10-14 days). Symptomatic urinary tract infections relapse and reinfect frequently. Pyelonephritis occurs in 1%-2% of cases. Treat symptomatic urinary tract infection aggressively with antibiotics (ampicillin, cephalosporins) for 6 weeks.

Perform follow-up cultures every 2 weeks. Avoid use of sulfa drugs near term and tetracyclines (because of fetal bone and teeth development and maternal liver failure).

Acute Renal Failure in Pregnancy

Conditions predisposing to acute renal failure in pregnancy are sepsis, severe eclampsia, abruptio placenta, intrauterine fetal death, uterine hemorrhage, and nephrotoxins. Cortical necrosis--10%-30% of cases of gestational acute renal failure. Patients become anuric. Although they may have partial recovery, they can have progression to end-stage renal disease years later. Idiopathic postpartum renal failure (retained placenta?) presents at 3-6 weeks post partum. It is characterized by acute oliguria, uremia, severe hypertension, and microhemangiopathic hemolytic anemia. There are disseminated intravascular coagulation and Schwartzman reaction, as in thrombotic thrombocytopenic purpura. Therapy includes dilatation and curettage, support, antiplatelet therapy(?), plasma infusion. Acute renal failure and acute fatty liver of pregnancy (similar to hepatorenal syndrome) are caused by tetracyclines and possibly disseminated intravascular coagulation. Progressive hepatic failure has a mortality rate of 75%.

Parenchymal Renal Disease in Pregnancy

Lupus--Outcome depends on clinical status prepartum. If the disease is quiescent 6 months before birth, 90% have live births. If the disease is active prepartum, 50% exacerbation and 35% fetal loss. If disease is stable prepartum, 30% have reversible exacerbations. Congenital heart block may occur in the newborn. Glucocorticoids and cytotoxic agents have been used without teratogenicity.

Diabetes--It is associated with increased asymptomatic and symptomatic bacteriuria and increased preeclampsia. Proteinuria and hypertension may worsen, but renal function usually is stable.

Renal transplant recipients--These women should postpone pregnancy for 2 years after transplantation. Increased preeclampsia, infection, and adrenal insufficiency occur. It is usually uncomplicated if the creatinine level is <1.5, blood pressure is normal, and patient is taking a low dose of immunosuppressive agent. Preeclampsia occurs in 25% of cases, prematurity in 7%, and loss of renal function in 7%. Nonobstetrical abdominal pain indicates allograft stone or

EVALUATION OF KIDNEY FUNCTION

Urinalysis

Causes of urine discoloration are listed in Table 21-12.

Urinary sediment: dysmorphic erythrocytes (>80%) indicate upper urinary tract bleeding. Hansel's stain: urine eosinophils.

Osmolality and pH--Urine osmolality is 40-1,200 mOsm/kg and pH is 4-7.5. pH <5.5 excludes renal tubular acidosis type I. pH >7:? infection. Acid urine is indicative of high protein diet, acidosis, and potassium depletion. Alkaline urine is associated with a vegetarian diet, alkalosis (unless potassium depleted), and urease-producing bacteria.

Glucose--Glycosuria in the absence of hyperglycemia suggests proximal tubule dysfunction.

Renal blood flow--Clearance of p-aminohippurate is a measure of renal blood flow. Ortho-iodohippurate is used in renal scans.

Glomerular filtration rate--Clearance of inulin, iothalamate, DTPA, and creatinine are measures of glomerular filtration rate. The Cockgroft-Gault Estimate formula for males is

$$GFR = \frac{(140 - \text{age in years}) \times (\text{lean body weight in kg})}{S_{Cr} \times 72}$$

in which GFR is glomerular filtration rate and S_{Cr} is serum level of creatinine. For females, the formula is males x 0.85. Creatinine levels are increased independently of the glomerular filtration rate with ketoacidosis (acetoacetate), cefoxitin, cimetidine, trimethoprim, flucytosine, massive rhabdomyolysis, high meat intake, and probenecid. Urea (BUN) levels are increased independently of glomerular filtration rate with gastrointestinal tract bleeding, tissue trauma, glucocorticoids, and tetracyclines.

Renal Imaging

1. KUB-plain films magnify kidneys 30%. Normal renal size is 3.5 x height of vertebra L-2 (>11 cm). The left kidney is up to 1.5 cm longer than the right one. An enlarged kidney indicates obstruction, infiltration (amyloid, leukemia, diabetes), acute glomerulonephritis, acute tubulointerstitial nephropathy, renal vein thrombosis, and polycystic kidney disease. Calcifications are associated with stone, tuberculosis, aneurysms, and papillary tip necrosis.

Table 21-12.--Causes of Urine Discoloration

Color	Cause
Dark yellow, brown	Bilirubin
Brown-black	Homogentisic acid (ochronosis)
	Melanin (melanoma)
	Metronidazole
	Methyldopa/levodopa
	Phenothiazine
Red	Beets
	Rifampin
	Porphyria
	Hemoglobinuria/myoglobinuria
	Phenazopyridine hydrochloride (Pyridium)
	Urates
Blue-green	Indomethacin
	Amitriptyline
Turbid white	Pyuria
	Chylous fistula
	Crystalluria

2. Excretory urography provides a detailed definition of the collecting system and can be used to assess renal size and contour and to detect and locate calculi. It is also used to assess qualitative renal function. Poor screen for renovascular hypertension--rapid sequence excretory urography. Complications: large osmotic load (congestive heart failure), reactions (5%). Premedicate with antihistamines/glucocorticoids, iodine load (hyperthyroidism).

3. Ultrasonography is used to measure renal size (>9 cm) and to screen for obstruction, but the results may be negative early. Ultrasonography can be used to characterize mass lesions (angiomyolipoma, solid versus cystic) and to screen for polycystic kidney disease. Use it to assess for renal vein thrombosis, i.e., presence or absence of blood flow. It is not a screen for renal artery stenosis.

4. Computed tomography shows calcification patterns. It is used to stage neoplasms and as an adjunct to determining the cause of obstruction (no contrast). Computed tomography assesses cysts, abscesses, and hematomas.

5. Magnetic resonance imaging can be used to identify adrenal hemorrhage and to assess a mass in patients sensitive to contrast dyes. Magnetic resonance imaging angiography is a promising screen for renal artery stenosis.

6. Arteriography and venography are used in cases of

arterial stenosis, aneurysm, fistulae, vasculitis, and mass lesions and to assess living-related donor transplants.

7. Gallium/indium scans are used in cases of acute interstitial nephritis, abscess, pyelonephritis, lymphoma, and leukemia.

8. DTPA/hippuran renal scan is used to assess post-transplant kidney, obstruction (pre- and post-furosemide), and infarct (presence or absence of blood flow).

QUESTIONS
(See "Answers" section)

Multiple Choice

1. Acute renal failure due to rhabdomyolysis is associated with all the following except:
   a. Acute hypocalcemia
   b. Carbon monoxide poisoning
   c. Negative findings on urine benzidine dipstick test
   d. Normal appearance of serum
   e. Cocaine overdose

2. Which of the following increases serum creatinine levels independently of decreases in glomerular filtration rate?
   a. Penicillin
   b. Gentamicin
   c. Acetoacetate
   d. Ranitidine
   e. Cefazolin

3. Diagnostic criteria for syndrome of inappropriate antidiuretic hormone include all the following except:
   a. Hypotonicity of plasma
   b. Urine is not maximally dilute
   c. Water restriction hyponatremia
   d. Urine sodium excretion exceeds intake
   e. Absence of hypocortisol and hypothyroidism

4. The osmolar gap is *not* increased due to the ingestion of:
   a. Isopropyl alcohol
   b. Methanol
   c. Aspirin
   d. Ethanol
   e. Ethylene glycol

5. A low urine chloride level is common in which of the following causes of hypokalemia?
   a. Vomiting
   b. Bartter's syndrome
   c. Loop diuretic abuse
   d. Magnesium deficiency
   e. Primary hyperaldosteronism

6. A high anion gap metabolic acidosis is associated with all of the following ingestions except:
   a. Isopropyl alcohol
   b. Ethanol
   c. Methanol
   d. Ethylene glycol
   e. Aspirin

7. The number one predictor of eventual diabetic nephropathy is:
   a. Hypertension
   b. Family history
   c. Microalbuminuria
   d. Glycosylated hemoglobin >12%
   e. Diabetic retinopathy

8. Focal glomerulosclerosis has been associated with all the following except:
   a. HIV infection
   b. Reflux nephropathy
   c. Heroin use
   d. Massive obesity
   e. Hodgkin's disease

9. Red blood cell casts may be seen in each of the following except:
   a. Amyloidosis
   b. Poststreptococcal glomerulonephritis
   c. IgA nephropathy
   d. Polyarteritis nodosa
   e. Goodpasture's syndrome

10. All the following may respond to corticosteroid therapy except:
    a. Proliferative lupus nephritis
    b. Wegener's granulomatosis
    c. Rapidly progressive glomerulonephritis
    d. Hemolytic uremic syndrome
    e. Minimal change nephropathy

11. Each of the following associations with tubulointerstitial nephritis is correct except:
    a. Nephrogenic diabetes insipidus--lithium
    b. Acute renal failure--ethylene glycol ingestion
    c. Gout--lead nephropathy
    d. Low urine uric acid-to-urine creatinine ratio--tumor lysis syndrome
    e. Nephrogenic diabetes insipidus--hypercalcemia

12. Polycystic kidney disease is associated with which of the following:
    a. X-linked dominant inheritance
    b. Invariable end-stage renal disease
    c. Deafness
    d. Relative excess of erythropoietin production
    e. 1% of all end-stage renal disease patients in the U.S.

13. The renal stone likely to form in acid urine is:
    a. Struvite
    b. Calcium oxalate
    c. Calcium phosphate
    d. Calcium carbonate
    e. Uric acid

14. Treatment of struvite stones includes:
    a. Long-term antibiotic suppressive therapy
    b. Surgical removal
    c. Identification of underlying stone-forming tendency
    d. All the above
    e. None of the above

15. Stone formers with idiopathic hypercalciuria should be treated with:
    a. Thiazide diuretics
    b. Aluminum hydroxide
    c. Loop diuretics
    d. Calcium carbonate
    e. Citrate

16. All the following are components of renal osteodystrophy except:
    a. Osteitis fibrosa cystica
    b. Osteomalacia
    c. Osteoporosis
    d. Growth retardation
    e. Hypophosphatemia

17. Abnormal endocrine disturbances in hemodialysis patients include all the following except:
    a. Low total thyroxine
    b. Increased level of growth hormone
    c. Hypergastrinemia
    d. Impaired fertility
    e. Low level of prolactin

18. Initial treatment for renal osteodystrophy is best accomplished with:
    a. Calcium carbonate
    b. Calcium phosphate
    c. Calcium acetate
    d. 1,25 vitamin D
    e. Dietary phosphorus restriction

19. Metabolic acidosis due to early chronic renal failure is:
    a. A type of IV renal tubular acidosis
    b. Secondary to decreased ammonia production
    c. A high anion-gap acidosis
    d. Associated with hyperkalemia
    e. A triple acid-base disorder

20. Preserved kidney size is a feature of chronic renal failure due to:
    a. Hypertension
    b. Polycystic kidney disease
    c. Diabetes
    d. Analgesics
    e. IgA nephropathy

True/False

21. Indicate whether the following statements about acute

renal failure are true or false.
a. Oliguria in acute tubular necrosis commonly lasts 8 weeks
b. Maintaining the BUN <100 is associated with improved outcome
c. Hypocalcemia is common and requires treatment
d. Ethylene glycol poisoning is a cause of acute renal failure
e. Atheroembolic renal failure is associated with eosinophilia

22. Which of the following diuretics are paired correctly with their site of action?
a. Proximal tubule--thiazides
b. Proximal tubule--acetazolamide
c. Loop of Henle--ethacrynic acid
d. Distal convoluted tubule--furosemide
e. Collecting duct--spironolactone

23. Multiple myeloma with renal involvement can be associated with:
a. Pseudohyponatremia
b. Low anion gap
c. Hypercalcemia
d. Type II renal tubular acidosis
e. Nephrotic syndrome

24. Which of the following are associated with hypocomplementemia?
a. Lupus nephritis
b. Poststreptococcal glomerulonephritis
c. Membranoproliferative glomerulonephritis, type II
d. Polyarteritis nodosa
e. Wegener's granulomatosis

25. Analgesic nephropathy has been associated with:
a. Aspirin use alone
b. Multicentric transitional cell carcinomas
c. Hypertension
d. Anemia
e. Acetaminophen use alone

26. Inherited forms of cystic renal disease include:
a. Medullary cystic disease
b. Medullary sponge kidney
c. Parapelvic renal cysts
d. Simple renal cysts
e. Long-term dialysis cystic disease

27. Which of the following medications require dose adjustments in chronic renal failure?
a. Angiotensin-converting enzyme inhibitors
b. Magnesium
c. Digoxin
d. Acyclovir
e. Long-acting calcium channel blockers

28. Erythropoietin therapy is associated with which of the following?
a. Allergic reactions
b. Hypertension
c. Improved appetite
d. Decreased hemodialysis efficiency
e. Reticulocytosis

CHAPTER 22
NEUROLOGY

Frank A. Rubino, M.D.

PART I
GENERAL PRINCIPLES OF THE NEUROLOGICAL EXAMINATION

INTRODUCTION

Neurologic disorders are commonly seen in general clinical practice. In decreasing frequency, disorders that neurologists see are headache, spinal column pain and radiculopathies, cerebrovascular disease, head and spinal cord injury, seizure disorders, dementias, developmental disorders including mental retardation, Parkinson's disease, multiple sclerosis, acquired peripheral neuropathies, genetically determined degenerative disorders, brain tumors, neurologic complications of malignancy, and neurologic complications of HIV infection. Because of increasing number of older people throughout the world, cerebrovascular disorders, dementias, and Parkinson's disease are assuming increasing importance. Continued spread of HIV infection, development of AIDS in those already infected, and improved methods for achieving longer survival increase the number of HIV-positive patients presenting with encephalopathies, infections, lymphomas, and other neurologic manifestations of AIDS.

- About 10% of patients of primary care physicians in U.S.A. have nervous system disorders.
- About 25% of inpatients have nervous system disorder as a primary or secondary problem.

NEUROLOGIC ASSESSMENT

The best approach to neurologic patients is a thorough history and physical examination. Correlation of clinical examination findings with abnormalities seen on diagnostic testing is important. This is especially important in elderly patients because most healthy elderly people have spondylitic abnormalities on plain cervical and lumbar radiographs and on magnetic resonance imaging (MRI) and computed tomography (CT) of same areas, white matter changes on head MRI, mild focal slowing on electroencephalography (EEG), slowing of nerve conduction velocities on electrophysiologic testing, etc.

- Most healthy elderly people have spondylitic abnormalities on plain cervical and lumbar radiographs.

Complete neurologic examination includes description of the items in Table 22-1. Accurately describe neurologic history and examination in everyday terms. Carefully interpret the signs and symptoms, deciding what is normal and what is abnormal. Signs and symptoms may be bilateral and symmetrical, as in myopathies and certain polyneuropathies. Asymmetrical findings may be a clue to cause (e.g., mononeuropathy multiplex in connective tissue disease). Look for asymmetries on the two sides of the body to detect subtle neurologic abnormalities (e.g., unilateral asterixis in focal cerebral disease vs. bilateral asterixis in diffuse systemic encephalopathies).

Next, make as accurate an anatomical diagnosis as possible in terms of general principles of practical neuroanatomy. In many cases, you should be able to state that the problem is on one side or other and in cerebral hemisphere, brain stem, spinal cord, peripheral nerve, muscle, myoneuronal junction, etc. Finally, make etiologic diagnosis and fairly uncomplicated differential diagnosis consisting of a few logical choices. If neurologic problems are approached this way, you can make an accurate assessment and plan, including diagnostic procedures, therapeutic options, and patient education.

Table 22-1.--Neurologic Examination

Mental status and state of consciousness evaluation
Gait and station evaluation
Cranial nerve evaluation
Sensory evaluation
    Primary sensations
    Cortical sensations
Motor evaluation
    Strength
    Muscle bulk
    Muscle tone
Evaluation of reflexes
    Muscle stretch reflexes (deep tendon reflexes)
    Abnormal reflexes (Babinski's sign, grasping of hand and
        feet)*
    Superficial reflexes (abdominal and cremasteric reflexes)
Evaluation of coordination
    Finger-to-nose and heel-to-knee tests
    Observation of abnormal movements or tremor

*Note that unusual reflexes such as snouting, sucking, and palmomental reflexes are common in elderly patients and usually are *not* pathologic. However, grasping reflexes and paratonic rigidity (Gegenhalten) in *awake* patients are pathologic.

GENERAL PRINCIPLES FROM LEVEL OF CEREBRAL CORTEX THROUGH NEURAXIS TO MUSCLE

Consciousness and Cognition

Consciousness has two dimensions: arousal and cognitive content. Arousal is vegetative function maintained by brain stem/medial diencephalic structures. Cognitive content--learning, memory, self-awareness, and adaptive behavior--depends on functional integrity of cerebral cortex and associated subcortical nuclei.

Coma or unconsciousness results from either bilateral dysfunction of cerebral cortex or dysfunction of reticular activating system in upper brain stem (above midpons).

- Brain death is absence of cerebral cortex and brain stem function.
- Persistent vegetative state is absence of cerebral cortex function with normal brain stem function (deafferentated state).
- "Locked-in" syndrome is normal cerebral cortex function with absence of brain stem function (lesion usually in pons, causing quadriplegia and inability to speak, swallow, and move eyes horizontally--de-efferenated

state).
- Acute confusional state is malfunction of cerebral cortex and reticular activating system.
- Dementia is malfunction of cerebral cortex but normal function of brain stem.

Dementia

Diagnosis of dementia is considered in patients with impaired intellect together with impaired memory, orientation, and judgment and changes in personality and behavior. Dementia is not a disease but an entity with various causes, which can be categorized as follows:
1. Primary generalized brain disease--Alzheimer's disease, Pick's disease, Huntington's disease, Creutzfeldt-Jakob disease, etc.
2. Focal brain disease that mimics generalized disease--subfrontal meningioma.
3. Systemic disease secondarily affecting entire brain--hypothyroidism, B_{12} deficiency.
4. Pseudodementia--not a dementia but psychologic disorder such as depression which mimics dementia.

- Dementia is not a disease.

Acute Confusional States

Acute confusional states are abrupt, of recent onset, and often associated with fluctuations in state of awareness and cognition. They are manifested by confusion, inattention, disorientation, and delirium. Thus, patients may be inattentive, dazed, stuporous, restless, agitated, or excited and may have marked autonomic dysfunction and visual and tactile hallucinations. Abnormal motor manifestations are common, including paratonia, asterixis, tremor, and myoclonus. Usual etiologic factors of acute confusional states are toxic, metabolic, traumatic, infectious, organ failure of any sort, or ictal or postictal encephalopathies. Three large categories of general causes are systemic causes, neurologic causes, and psychophysiologic causes.

- Three large categories of causes of acute confusional states are systemic, neurologic, and psychophysiologic causes.

Stupor and Coma

For one to stay awake, the cerebral hemispheres and reticular activating system must be intact. Patients with dysfunction of only one cerebral hemisphere have focal neurologic deficit but are awake. Most common, important, potentially reversible causes of stupor and coma are toxic, metabolic, and infectious problems affecting both cerebral hemispheres diffusely. Thus, most patients in stupor and coma have underlying systemic problem.

- Most common reversible causes of stupor and coma are toxic, metabolic, and infectious causes.

Patients with systemic encephalopathies have changes in mental status and awareness before going into stupor and coma, but they have no focal signs. Their corneal reflexes are lost early but pupillary reflexes remain. Also, ocular motility tested by doll's eye maneuver (oculocephalic reflexes) and cold caloric response (oculovestibular reflex) are fully intact, at least early in the disease.

- Patients with systemic encephalopathies have no focal signs.
- Their corneal reflexes are lost early but pupillary reflexes remain.

Patients with large unilateral cerebral lesion may go into stupor and coma if lesion causes shifting and pressure changes in other parts of the brain such as opposite hemisphere or brain stem. These patients have focal neurologic signs. Patients with brain stem lesions affecting ascending reticular activating system directly are in coma but have focal signs. Finally, people who feign coma have no focal signs, no abnormal reflexes, normal caloric responses, and normal EEG. They are a small percentage of patients seen in stupor and coma.

- Large unilateral cerebral lesions causing shift and pressure changes in other hemisphere or brain stem produce focal neurologic signs together with coma.
- Brain stem lesions causing coma also produce focal signs.
- People feigning coma have no focal signs, no abnormal reflexes, normal caloric response, and normal EEG.

Headache and Facial Pain

Headache
Headache may indicate intracranial or systemic disease, personality or situational problem, or combination of these. Some headaches have readily identified organic cause. Classical migraine and cluster headaches form distinctive, easily recognized clinical entities but pathophysiology is not understood. The major challenge is that often neither location nor intensity of the pain is reliable clue to nature of the problem. Episodic tension headache and migraine can be difficult to distinguish.

- Neither location nor intensity of headache pain is reliable clue to nature of problem.

Vascular theory of migraine and muscle contraction theory of tension headaches are no longer tenable. Headache pain may be generated centrally and involve serotonergic and adrenergic pain-modulating systems. Neurogenically mediated inflammation may account for some migraine pain (sterile inflammation).

Conditions that alert physicians a headache may have a serious cause are listed in Table 22-2. Chronic recurrent headaches are rarely, if ever, caused by eye strain, chronic sinusitis, dental problems, food allergies, high blood pressure, or temporal mandibular joint syndrome. Headache without other neurologic signs or symptoms is rarely caused by brain tumor. Serious causes of headache in which neuroimaging findings may be negative and lead to false sense of security are listed in Table 22-3.

- "Worst or first headache of my life" is serious.
- Headache with abnormal neurologic findings, papilledema, obscuration of vision, or diplopia is serious.
- Most of the signs and symptoms in Table 22-2 can occur with chronic benign headache (tension-migraine headache).
- Headache without other neurologic signs/symptoms is rarely caused by brain tumor.

Trigeminal Neuralgia
Characteristically trigeminal neuralgia is always on same side and usually in second or third division of trigeminal nerve. Idiopathic variety occurs in middle-aged and elderly patients and is heralded by sharp, lancinating pain that usually has a trigger point. Chewing often precipitates trigeminal neuralgia pain, whereas swallowing often precipitates glossopharyngeal neuralgia pain.

The pain in glossopharyngeal neuralgia is similar to that in trigeminal neuralgia but is in throat and neck and often radiates to ear.

In elderly, trigeminal neuralgia may be due to enlarged artery (rarely a vein) compressing trigeminal nerve. Importantly, in idiopathic trigeminal neuralgia, results of

Table 22-2.--Conditions Indicating Headache May
Have a Serious Cause

"Worst or first headache of my life"

Headache in person not prone to headache, especially middle-aged and elderly patients

Headache associated with abnormal neurologic findings, papilledema, obscurations of vision, or diplopia

Headaches that change with different positions or increase with exertion, coughing, or sneezing

Changes in headache patterns--character, frequency, severity--in someone who has had chronic recurring headaches previously

Headaches that awaken one from sound sleep

Most of above signs and symptoms may occur in chronic benign headache (e.g., tension migraine)

Table 22-3.--Serious Causes of Headache in Which
Neuroimaging Findings May Be Negative

Cranial arteritis

Glaucoma

Trigeminal and glossopharyngeal neuralgia

Lesions around sella turcica

Warning leak of aneurysm

Inflammation, infection, or neoplastic invasion of leptomeninges

Cervical spondylosis

Pseudotumor cerebri

Low intracranial pressure syndromes (cerebrospinal fluid leaks)

---

examining sensory and motor functions of trigeminal nerve should be normal when patient is examined during asymptomatic period. If there are signs or symptoms except pain, look for other compressive lesions, e.g., neoplasm. Consider possibility of multiple sclerosis if trigeminal neuralgia is in young person and pain is unilateral, bilateral, or switches from side to side.

- Chewing often precipitates pain in trigeminal neuralgia, as does swallowing in glossopharyngeal neuralgia.
- In idiopathic trigeminal neuralgia, there should be no other signs/symptoms when patient is examined in asymptomatic period.
- Consider multiple sclerosis if trigeminal neuralgia is in young person and pain is unilateral or bilateral or

switches sides.

- Glossopharyngeal pain is in throat and neck, radiating to ear.

Intracranial Lesions

Leptomeningeal Lesions

Inflammation, infection, or neoplastic invasion of the leptomeninges may present with similar signs and symptoms, as follows:

1. Cerebral--headache, seizures, focal neurologic signs.
2. Cranial nerve--any cranial nerve (CN) can be affected, especially CN III, IV, VI, and VII (the latter is often affected in Lyme disease).
3. Radicular (radiculoneuropathy or radiculomyelopathy)--neck and back pain as well as radicular pain and spinal cord signs.

- CN VII is often affected in Lyme disease.

Parasagittal Lesions

Because leg area and cortical control for urinary bladder are located in interhemispheric area, parasagittal lesions can cause spastic paraparesis with urinary problems. Meningioma is common lesion in this area and may also be manifested by seizures and headache.

- Parasagittal lesions may cause paraparesis with urinary problems.
- Meningioma may also be manifested by seizures and headache.

Cortical Lesions

Cortical lesions lead to focal signs. If in the dominant hemisphere, they cause language dysfunction, including reading, writing, and speaking. Cortical lesions can also impair higher cortical function, producing apraxias, agnosias, and denial of illness or body parts, and impair cortical sensation. Dense loss of primary sensation (e.g., pinprick and touch) occurs with thalamic lesions.

- Cortical lesions may produce apraxia and agnosia.
- Thalamic lesions cause loss of primary sensation (e.g., touch).

Hydrocephalus

Combination of signs and symptoms--impaired mental status, gait disturbance, urinary problems--suggest hydrocephalus. If it is the obstructive type, signs of increased intracranial pressure may be present, including lethargy, nausea, vomiting and headache, and obscurations of vision often associated with changes in position.

The following are types of hydrocephalus:

1. Hydrocephalus ex vacuo--due to loss of parenchyma, either gray or white matter, and not associated with the signs listed above (normal examination results if hydrocephalus due to aging and dementia if due to Alzheimer's disease).
2. Normal-pressure hydrocephalus--due to decreased reabsorption of cerebrospinal fluid (CSF).
3. Hydrocephalus due to overproduction of CSF--rare and controversial; supposedly occurs with choroid plexus lesions.
4. Types 1-3 above are called communicating hydrocephalus.
5. Obstructive (noncommunicating) hydrocephalus --due to obstructive lesion anywhere in ventricular system.

- Hydrocephalus ex vacuo is due to loss of parenchyma and is not necessarily associated with impaired mental status, gait disturbance, and urinary problems.

Brain Stem Lesions

Brain stem lesions can produce crossed syndromes; impairment of ocular motility; medial longitudinal fasciculus (MLF) syndrome (internuclear ophthalmoplegia); rotary, horizontal, and vertical nystagmus (downbeat nystagmus is highly suggestive of lesion at cervical-medullary junction); ataxia; dysarthria; diplopia; and dysphagia. Cranial nerve signs are ipsilateral to lesion, but long-tract signs are usually contralateral (crossed syndrome).

- Downbeat nystagmus is highly suggestive of lesion at cervical-medullary junction.
- Cranial nerve signs are ipsilateral to lesion.
- Long-tract signs are usually contralateral to lesion.

Cerebellar Lesions

Problems with equilibrium and coordination suggest cerebellar lesion. Cerebellar hemisphere lesions usually produce ipsilateral ataxia of arm and leg. Lesions restricted to anterior superior vermis, as in alcoholism, usually cause ataxia of gait, i.e., wide-based gait and heel-to-shin ataxia with relative sparing of arms, speech, and ocular motility. Lesions of flocculonodular lobe cause marked difficulty with equilibrium and walking but not much difficulty with finger-to-nose and heel-to-shin tests if patient is lying down.

Spinal Cord Lesions

Sensory levels, signs of anterior horn cell involvement (atrophy and fasciculations), and long-tract signs in the posterior columns, corticospinal tract, and spinothalamic tract suggest spinal cord lesion. Extramedullary cord lesions usually heralded by radicular pain. Intramedullary cord lesions are usually painless but may have an ill-described nonlocalizable pain and sensory dissociation and sacral sparing. Conus medullaris lesions often indicated by "saddle anesthesia" and early involvement of urinary bladder.

- Extramedullary lesions heralded by radicular pain.
- Intramedullary lesions are usually painless.
- Conus medullaris lesions are indicated by saddle anesthesia and early bladder involvement.

Radiculopathy

Nerve root lesions are usually indicated by root pain that is often sharp and lancinating, follows dermatomal pattern, and is increased by increasing intraspinal pressure (e.g., sneezing and coughing) or by stretching nerve root. Pain often follows myotomal (e.g., C-5, 6 root pain in deltoid and biceps muscles) rather than dermatomal pattern, with paresthesias in dermatomal pattern. Findings are in root distribution and include weakness, sensory impairment, and decreased muscle stretch reflexes. Radiculopathies have many causes, including compressive lesions (osteophytes, ruptured disks, and neoplasms) and noncompressive ones (postinfectious and inflammatory radiculopathies and metabolic radiculopathies as in diabetes).

- Nerve root lesions are indicated by sharp, lancinating root pain with dermatomal pattern.
- Pain is increased by sneezing and coughing.
- Pain often has myotomal rather than dermatomal pattern.
- Findings are weakness, sensory impairment, and decreased muscle stretch reflexes.
- Radiculopathies have many causes.

Neuropathy

Peripheral neuropathies are usually indicated by distal weakness and distal sensory changes, usually symmetrical, more often in legs than arms and often accompanied by loss of or impaired distal muscle stretch reflexes.

Neuropathy has many causes, and extensive search usually uncovers cause in 70%-80% of cases. High percentage of cases of "idiopathic neuropathy" referred to specialty centers are in fact hereditary neuropathies.

The pattern of the neuropathy might suggest its cause. Mononeuropathy (impairment of single nerve) is usually due to compression, as in compressive ulnar neuropathy at elbow, compressive median neuropathy in carpal tunnel, and compression of peroneal nerve as it winds around the fibula. Mononeuropathy multiplex (asymmetrical involvement of several nerves) suggests such causes as diabetes, vasculitis, leprosy, sarcoidosis, or Tangier disease. Neuropathy with autonomic dysfunction (e.g., orthostatic hypertension, urinary bladder and bowel dysfunction, and impotency) suggests amyloidosis, diabetes, Guillain-Barré syndrome, porphyria, or familial neuropathy.

Predominantly motor polyneuropathy suggests acute or chronic inflammatory demyelinating polyneuropathy (AIDP or CIDP), hereditary neuropathy, osteosclerotic myeloma, porphyria, lead or organophosphate poisoning, or hypoglycemia. Predominantly sensory polyneuropathy suggests diabetes, cancer, Sjögren's syndrome, dysproteinemias, AIDS, vitamin B_{12} deficiency, cisplatin toxicity, vitamin B_6 excess, or hereditary neuropathy. Most neuropathies are distal, but occasionally there is predominant proximal weakness, which suggests AIDP, CIPD, porphyria, or diabetic proximal motor neuropathy.

Diabetes causes CN III neuropathy usually including sudden diplopia, eye pain, impairment of muscles supplied by CN III, and relative sparing of pupil. With compressive CN III lesions, pupil usually is involved early.

- Peripheral neuropathy: distal weakness and sensory changes more in legs than arms, usually symmetrical, absent or impaired distal muscle stretch reflexes.
- Cause of peripheral neuropathy usually found in 70%-80% of cases.
- Pattern of neuropathy suggests cause.
- Mononeuropathy multiplex: diabetes, vasculitis, leprosy, sarcoidosis, Tangier disease.
- Neuropathy with autonomic dysfunction: amyloidosis, diabetes, Guillain-Barré syndrome, porphyria, familial neuropathy.
- Motor polyneuropathy: inflammatory demyelinating polyneuropathy, hereditary neuropathy, osteosclerotic myeloma, porphyria, lead poisoning, organophosphate toxicity, hypoglycemia.

- Sensory polyneuropathy: diabetes, cancer, Sjögren's syndrome, dysproteinemias, AIDS, vitamin B_{12} deficiency, cisplatin toxicity, vitamin B_6 excess, hereditary neuropathy.
- Diabetes causes CN III neuropathy.
- Pupil involved early in compression of CN III.

Myoneural Junction Lesions

Myoneural junction lesions are often missed clinically. Drugs may cause problems at myoneural junction, e.g., penicillamine can cause syndrome that looks like myasthenia gravis. Three major clinical syndromes of the myoneural junction are the following:

1. Botulism. This should be suspected when more than one person has syndrome that looks like myasthenia gravis or when single person has abdominal and gastrointestinal symptoms preceding a syndrome that looks like myasthenia gravis.
2. Myasthenia gravis. This is usually seen in young women and older men and is often heralded by such cranial nerve findings as diplopia, dysarthria, dysphagia, dyspnea, and also fatigability. However, muscle stretch reflexes, sensation, mentation, and sphincter function are normal. Because of remissions and exacerbations in this disease, patients often are considered "hysterical."
3. Myasthenic syndrome, or the Lambert-Eaton syndrome. There is often proximal weakness in legs and decreased or absent muscle stretch reflexes (sometimes, reflexes elicited after brief exercise). This syndrome is usually seen in middle-aged men, who often have such vague complaints as diplopia, impotency, urinary dysfunction, paresthesias, mouth dryness, and other autonomic dysfunctions (orthostatic hypotension). Lambert-Eaton syndrome is often associated with lung small cell carcinoma.

- Myoneural junction lesions are often missed clinically.
- Drugs (penicillamine) cause myoneural junction problem.
- Botulism: suspect it if more than one person develops syndrome that looks like myasthenia.
- Myasthenia gravis usually in young women, older men.
- Onset of myasthenia gravis: diplopia, dysarthria, dysphagia, dyspnea, fatigability.
- Patients with myasthenia gravis are often considered hysterical.

- In myasthenic syndrome, proximal weakness of legs and decreased/absent muscle stretch reflexes.
- Myasthenic syndrome occurs in middle-age men, who have vague complaints of diplopia, impotency, urinary dysfunction, dry mouth.
- Myasthenic syndrome is often associated with small cell carcinoma.

Muscle Disease

Muscle disease is usually indicated by symmetrical proximal weakness (legs more than arms) and weakness of neck flexors and occasionally of smooth and cardiac muscle. Other neurologic findings are normal.

Muscle stretch reflexes are usually normal early in muscle disease.

Muscle disease may be acquired disease or progressive hereditary disease. "Myopathy" is general term for muscle disease. If the disease is progressive and familial, it is called "dystrophy."

Two exceptions to proximal weakness in myopathy are:

1. Unusual distal myopathy, called "distal myopathy," occurs mainly in Scandinavian countries.
2. Myotonic dystrophy is more common and seen everywhere. Atrophy and weakness begin distally and in face and especially in sternocleidomastoid muscles. Interesting feature of this dystrophy is myotonia, which is normal contraction of muscle with slow relaxation. Test for myotonia by striking thenar eminence with reflex hammer. Test the myotonia by shaking patient's hand and noting patient cannot let go quickly.

In evaluating acquired myopathy such as inflammatory myopathy, look for underlying cause, but often it is not found in adults. There probably is increased incidence of occult carcinomas in patients with dermatomyositis. Other important underlying causes of myopathies include collagen vascular disease, endocrinopathies (especially thyroid disease), sarcoidosis, or remote nonmetastatic effects of cancer.

- In early muscle disease, stretch reflexes are normal.
- Muscle disease is "myopathy."
- If the disease is progressive and familial, "dystrophy."
- Distal myopathy is unusual and mainly in Scandinavia.
- Myotonic dystrophy--atrophy and weakness in face and sternocleidomastoid muscles.
- Myotonia (normal contraction, slow relaxation) feature of myotonic dystrophy.

- With myotonia, patient cannot let go quickly after handshake.
- Acquired myopathy: no underlying cause in most adults.
- Increased incidence of occult carcinomas in patients with dermatomyositis.
- Causes of myopathies: collagen vascular disease, endocrinopathy, sarcoidosis, remote nonmetastatic effects of cancer.

Classification of myopathies is given in Table 22-4.

Table 22-4.--Classification of Myopathies

Dystrophies
Nonprogressive or relatively nonprogressive congenital myopathies
Inflammatory myopathies
Infectious--toxoplasmosis, trichinosis
Granulomatous--sarcoidosis
Idiopathic--polymyositis, dermatomyositis
With collagen vascular disease
Metabolic myopathies
Glycogenoses
Endocrine
Periodic paralyses
Toxic--emetine, chloroquine, vincristine
Paroxysmal rhabdomyolysis
Miscellaneous

Acute Muscular Weakness

Physicians may overlook serious underlying diseases in patients with chief or only complaint of weakness, especially if there are few or no obvious clinical signs. Delayed or missed diagnosis can lead to life-threatening complications such as respiratory failure, irreversible spinal cord dysfunction, and acute renal failure. Respiratory muscles may be affected, although strength in extremities is relatively normal. Patients with early Guillain-Barré syndrome may have distal paresthesias and increased respiratory effort and be given diagnosis of hysterical hyperventilation.

- Missed diagnosis can lead to life-threatening complications: respiratory failure, irreversible spinal cord function, acute renal failure.
- Early Guillain-Barré syndrome may be misdiagnosed as hysterical hyperventilation.

Acute muscle weakness can be classified into four groups: disease of spinal cord, peripheral nerve, myoneural junction, muscle.

Spinal Cord Disease

Compressive or noncompressive cord lesion may cause muscle weakness.

Most common noncompressive lesion is transverse myelitis, usually of unknown cause. Some patients have history of vaccination or symptoms suggestive of viral disease, usually preceding neurologic symptoms by few days to 1-2 weeks.

Compressive myelopathy is commonly due to metastatic epidural neoplasm. Most patients present with local vertebral column pain at level of spinal cord lesion. This symptom is present for weeks to months before gross neurologic deficits, although bony pain occasionally may antedate other symptoms by only a few hours.

- Weakness is due to compressive or noncompressive lesion.
- Transverse myelitis is most common noncompressive lesion.

Peripheral Nerve Disease

1. Guillain-Barré syndrome. About 50% of patients typically have mild respiratory or gastrointestinal infection 1-3 weeks before neurologic symptoms. In the others, syndrome may be preceded by surgery, viral exanthems, or vaccinations. Also, syndrome may develop in patients with autoimmune disease or lymphoreticular malignancies. Syndrome has no particular seasonal, age, or sex predilection.
2. Acute intermittent porphyria. Patients are prone to have severe, rapidly progressive, symmetrical polyneuropathy with or without psychosis, delirium, confusion, and convulsions. In most cases, weakness is most pronounced in proximal muscles.
3. Tick paralysis. This is rapid, progressive ascending motor weakness caused by neurotoxin injected by female wood tick. It occurs endemically in southeastern and northwestern U.S.A. After asymptomatic period (about 1 week), symptoms develop, usually with leg weakness.
4. Diabetic neuropathy. Acute or subacute muscle weakness can occur in various forms of diabetic neuropathy. Weakness, atrophy, and pain affect pelvic girdle and thigh muscles (asymmetrical or unilateral--diabetic amyotrophy). In second form, elderly diabetics have bilateral proximal and pelvic girdle weakness, wasting, weight loss, and autonomic dysfunction.

- 50% of Guillain-Barré patients have mild respiratory or gastrointestinal infection 1-3 weeks previously.
- Surgery, viral exanthems, vaccinations may precede Guillain-Barré syndrome.
- Guillain-Barré syndrome may develop in autoimmune disease or lymphoreticular malignancy.
- No predilection for season, age, sex in Guillain-Barré.
- Severe, rapidly progressive, symmetrical polyneuropathy with pronounced proximal muscle weakness develops in acute intermittent porphyria.
- Tick paralysis, endemic in southeast and northwest U.S.A., caused by female wood tick neurotoxin.
- Asymptomatic for about 1 week after neurotoxin injected.
- In diabetic neuropathy: weakness, atrophy, and pain of pelvic girdle and thigh muscles.
- In elderly diabetics: bilateral proximal and pelvic girdle weakness, wasting, weight loss, autonomic dysfunction.

Myoneural Junction Disease

1. Botulism. Occurs after ingestion of improperly canned vegetables, fruit, meat, or fish contaminated by exotoxin of *C. botulinum*. Paralysis caused by toxin-mediated inhibition of acetylcholine release from terminals at myoneural junction.
2. Organophosphate toxicity. This causes characteristic combination of miosis, excessive bodily secretions, and fasciculations. Key pathophysiologic factor is reduced acetylcholinesterase activity causing excessive acetylcholine at myoneural junction. Onset of symptoms varies from 5 minutes to 12 hours after exposure. Treatment is atropine.

- Ingestion of exotoxin of *C. botulinum* causes botulism.
- Acetylcholine release inhibited at myoneural junction.
- In organophosphate toxicity, reduced acetylcholinesterase activity causes excessive acetylcholine at myoneural junction.
- Atropine is treatment.

Muscle Disease

1. Polymyalgia rheumatica. It affects elderly patients with aching or pain and stiffness in neck, upper back, shoulders, upper arms, and hip girdle. Systemic symptoms include various degrees of fever, anorexia, weight

loss, apathy, and depression. True muscle weakness is not present except when attributed to pain. This syndrome is sometimes associated with cranial arteritis.

2. Acute alcoholic myopathy. There is acute pain, swelling, tenderness, and weakness of mainly proximal muscles. Gross myoglobinuria may cause renal failure.

3. Electrolyte imbalance. Severe hypokalemia (<2.5 mEq/L) or hyperkalemia (>7 mEq/L) produces muscle weakness, as do hyper- and hypocalcemia and hypophosphatemia. Familial periodic paralysis of hypo-, hyper-, or normokalemic type-episodes of acute paralysis last 2-24 hours and can be precipitated by large carbohydrate meal or strenuous exercise; cranial or respiratory muscle paralysis is rare.

4. Endocrine diseases: hyper- and hypothyroidism, hyper- and hypoadrenalism, acromegaly, and primary and secondary hyperparathyroidism cause muscle weakness.

Causes of acute muscle weakness are summarized in Table 22-5.

- Polymyalgia rheumatica: elderly patient with aching/pain and stiffness of neck, upper back, shoulders, upper arms, and hip girdle.
- No true muscle weakness, but fever, anorexia, weight loss.
- Gross myoglobinuria often in acute alcoholic myopathy.

GENERAL PRINCIPLES FOR INTERPRETING NEUROLOGIC SYMPTOMS

Neurologic symptoms can be subdivided into four general categories.
1. Ill-defined, nonspecific, nonanatomical, and nonphysiologic regional or generalized symptoms.
2. Diffuse cerebral symptoms.
3. Positive focal symptoms (hyperactivity).
4. Negative focal symptoms (loss of function).

Ill-Defined Symptoms

These include such things as ill-defined dizziness, diffuse or unusual regional pain, diffuse and unusual numbness, vague memory problems, and unusual gait. Generally, no serious underlying problem is found, especially if symptoms are long-standing. Many cases have serious underlying psychopathology, but patient often either does not recognize or denies this fact. However, be

Table 22-5.--Important Causes of Acute Muscle Weakness

Spinal cord disease
   Transverse myelitis
   Epidural abscess
   Extradural tumor
   Epidural hematoma
   Herniated intervertebral disk
   Spinal cord tumor
Peripheral nerve disease
   Guillain-Barré syndrome
   Acute intermittent porphyria
   Arsenic poisoning
   Toxic neuropathies
   Tick paralysis
Myoneural junction disease
   Myasthenia gravis
   Botulism
   Organophosphate poisoning
Muscle disease
   Polymyositis
   Rhabdomyolysis-myoglobinuria
   Acute alcoholic myopathy
   Electrolyte imbalances
   Endocrine disease

From Karkal SS: Rapid accurate appraisal of acute muscular weakness. Updates Neurology 1991; pp 31-39. By permission of American Health Consultants.

careful in making a psychiatric diagnosis, which should be made on basis of positive psychologic factors and not only because physical examination findings and laboratory studies are normal.

- With ill-defined symptoms, no serious underlying problem in most cases.
- Many have underlying psychopathology.
- Make psychiatric diagnosis based on positive psychologic factors, not because of normal physical exam/lab findings.

Diffuse Cerebral Symptoms

Diffuse cognitive problems occur in dementia and acute confusional states. However, a common diffuse symptom is syncope or presyncope, which usually implies diffuse and *not* focal cerebral ischemia. Vasovagal syncope is the major culprit, especially in the young. Syncope is *not* a transient ischemic attack (TIA). Most causes of syncope are systemic, *not* neurologic, problems. In primary autonomic dysfunction, other neurologic signs and symptoms usually help make diagnosis (e.g., Shy-Drager syndrome, diabetic and amyloid autonomic neuropathy).

- Diffuse cerebral symptoms imply diffuse, not focal, cerebral ischemia.
- Syncope is not TIA.
- Systemic, not neurologic, problems usually cause syncope.

Positive Phenomena

Example of positive sensory phenomenon is marching paresthesia and of positive motor phenomenon, tonic or clonic movement. Lights, flashes, sparkles, and formed images are examples of positive visual phenomena. Example of positive language phenomenon is unusual vocalization. Positive central phenomena usually indicate seizures or migraine accompaniments. Positive peripheral phenomena occur with nerve damage and repair.

Negative Phenomena

They usually indicate damage to specific central or peripheral area. TIAs and strokes usually produce negative phenomena; if there is more than one symptom, all symptoms tend to appear at same time. Migraine syndromes may have positive and negative phenomena; if more than one symptom, symptoms tend to come on one after another and "build up."

- TIAs and strokes produce negative phenomena.
- Migraine syndromes have positive and negative phenomena.

GENERAL PRINCIPLES OF NEUROLOGIC DIAGNOSTIC TESTING

CT and MRI Imaging

CT is good initial test in evaluating suspected TIA or stroke and is superior to MRI in identifying acute hemorrhage in brain parenchyma or subarachnoid space. Subacute and chronic intracerebral hemorrhages are better defined by MRI, which is usually first neuroimaging test to reveal abnormalities during evolution of ischemic cerebral infarct. CT (even with contrast enhancement) often gives equivocal or negative results in first 24-48 hours of ischemic cerebral infarct. In subacute and chronic stages of ischemic cerebral infarct, MRI and CT give equivalent information.

- For acute hemorrhage in brain and subarachnoid space, CT is better than MRI.
- During evolving ischemic cerebral infarct, MRI is best.
- CT scan with contrast not useful in first 24-48 hours after ischemic cerebral infarct.
- For subacute and chronic stages of ischemic cerebral infarct, CT and MRI are equivalent.

Trauma

MRI is competitive with but not comparable to CT for assessing brain after craniocerebral trauma. During first 1-3 days after injury, CT is preferable because examination time is shorter and hemorrhage at this time is more reliably demonstrated by CT. Standard radiographic examination or CT is necessary to evaluate skull fractures because bone cortex not visualized by MRI.

CT highly dependable for subdural hematomas, which are also visualized by MRI. Coronal MRI sections usually best for size, shape, location, and extent of subdural hematomas.

- For first 1-3 days after trauma, CT is best because more reliable for hemorrhage.
- Radiography and CT needed to evaluate skull fractures.
- CT very dependable for showing subdural hematomas.

Vasculitic Lesions or Microinfarcts

These lesions, as in such diseases as systemic lupus erythematosus, often seen on MRI but missed on CT.

Intracranial Tumors

Wide spectrum of intracranial tumors visualized by MRI and CT. MRI often shows more extensive involvement than CT, especially in low-grade gliomas. CT is superior to MRI in detecting meningiomas. MRI is far superior to CT for identifying all types of posterior fossa tumors. It is study of choice for identifying brain stem gliomas.

- MRI superior to CT for posterior fossa tumors and brain stem gliomas.

White Matter Lesions

MRI is superior to CT in detecting abnormalities in white matter. MRI is far superior to CT for identifying multiple sclerosis lesions and assessing patients with isolated optic neuritis. MRI shows that Binswanger's disease may be common cause of adult-onset dementia (along with multi-infarct dementia). White matter changes in elderly must be interpreted carefully because most of them have white matter changes on MRI.

- Most normal elderly people have white matter changes on MRI.

Cervical Cord

Wide spectrum of lesions at the cervical-medullary junction and the cervical spinal cord can be clearly seen with MRI because of the ability to make direct sagittal and coronal sections. MRI is the study of choice for assessing cervical-medullary and cervical spinal cord regions. Generally, MRI is best for identifying intramedullary and extramedullary lesions of spinal cord.

- MRI is best for assessing cervical-medullary and cervical spinal cord regions and intra- and extramedullary cord tumors.

Dementia

In assessing dementia, either CT or MRI can be used to demonstrate remedial lesions. MRI shows more lesions than CT in multi-infarct dementia. MRI has *not* exceeded CT in assessing dementia.

- For dementia, CT and MRI are equivalent.
- In multi-infarct dementia, MRI shows more lesions.

Disk Disease

Protruding disks are seen well on MRI sagittal sections, showing relationship to spine and nerve roots. MRI is equal to CT myelography in evaluating herniated disks at cervical and thoracic levels, but at lumbar level, MRI is better than/equal to CT. In spinal stenosis, MRI and CT are roughly equal and less invasive than myelography.

CT myelography has greatest diagnostic accuracy for cervical radiculopathy due to hypertrophic degenerative changes. Bony spicules impinging on nerve roots are not directly shown by MRI, which may replace myelography for cervical and lumbar disease. Often CT myelography is needed in defining surgical problems.

- MRI sagittal sections show protruding disks.
- For cervical and thoracic herniated disks, MRI is same as CT myelography.
- CT myelography is best for cervical radiculopathy due to hypertrophic degenerative change.
- CT myelography needed for defining surgical problems.

Additional Comments

Magnetic resonance angiography (MRA) is not invasive but not yet ready to replace regular angiography.

MRI is best for evaluating seizure disorders.

ELECTROMYOGRAPHIC (EMG) NERVE CONDUCTION VELOCITY STUDIES

EMG studies should be performed by experts familiar with intricacies of procedure and who know its value and limitations. EMG tests are excellent for eliciting motor unit problems and thus are valuable in diseases of anterior horn cell, nerve root, peripheral nerve, myoneural junction, and muscle. These tests are extension of neurologic examination, helping to localize and better define further diagnostic studies.

- EMG--performed by experts.
- EMG valuable for motor unit problems--anterior horn cell, nerve root, myoneural junction, muscle.

ELECTROENCEPHALOGRAPHY (EEG)

Main use of EEG is study of seizure disorders. But EEG is specific in only a few forms of epilepsy such as petit mal epilepsy. Seizure disorder is clinical diagnosis and *not* an EEG diagnosis, and normal EEG does *not* rule out seizure disorder. EEG has many nonspecific patterns that should not be over-interpreted.

Ambulatory EEG is available for detecting frequent unusual spells. Telemetered EEG with videomonitoring is good for defining epileptic surgical candidates, nonepileptic spells (pseudoseizures), and unusual seizures. EEG is imperative in diagnosing nonconvulsive status epilepticus.

- EEG specific in only few forms of epilepsy.
- Seizure disorder is clinical, not EEG, diagnosis.
- Normal EEG does not rule out seizure disorder.
- Telemetered EEG good for defining epileptic surgical candidates, nonepileptic spells, unusual seizures.

EEG is valuable for evaluating various encephalopathies. Many drugs cause unusual fast pattern, and most metabolic encephalopathies cause diffuse slow or triphasic pattern. Diffuse slow patterns also seen in diffuse cerebral disease (Alzheimer's disease). Unusual high-amplitude slow and spike activity helps define Creutzfeldt-Jakob disease and subacute sclerosing panencephalitis. EEG is often valuable in infectious encephalopathies (herpes simplex encephalitis).

EEG is essential for diagnosing various sleep disorders and is *adjuvant* tool in diagnosing brain death. Remember, brain death is a clinical diagnosis. EEG is monitoring device in surgery (during carotid endarterectomy).

EEG at 6 hours or more after hypoxic insult indicates likelihood of neurologic recovery. Poor outcome is seen with "alpha" coma, burst suppression, periodic patterns, and electrocerebral silence.

- EEG is valuable in infectious encephalopathies (herpes simplex encephalitis).
- EEG is adjuvant tool in diagnosing brain death.
- Brain death is a clinical diagnosis.

EVOKED POTENTIALS

Evoked potentials indicate intactness of various pathways: visual evoked potentials, somatosensory evoked potentials, brain stem auditory evoked potentials, motor evoked potentials. Generally, these tests are not practical clinical tool. They are excellent monitoring devices for spinal surgery and posterior fossa surgery (monitoring cranial nerve function intraoperatively). Also, they may help substantiate nonorganic disease, e.g., hysterical paraplegia or hysterical blindness.

- Evoked potentials help substantiate nonorganic disease (hysterical paraplegia, hysterical blindness).

ANTICONVULSANT BLOOD LEVELS

Anticonvulsant blood levels are readily available and help attain best seizure control. It is extremely important to remember that therapeutic levels represent an average bell-shaped curve and that patients with well-controlled seizures are included under the bell-shaped curve. Many patients with levels below or above therapeutic levels do well. Anticonvulsant dose should *never* be changed based on blood levels alone. Remember, toxicity is a clinical, *not* a laboratory, phenomenon.

- Therapeutic levels represent average bell-shaped curve.
- Anticonvulsant dose should never be changed based on blood levels alone.
- Toxicity is a clinical, not a laboratory, phenomenon.

LUMBAR PUNCTURE AND CSF ANALYSIS

Perform lumbar puncture only after thorough clinical evaluation and serious consideration of potential value versus hazards of procedure.

Indications for Lumbar Puncture

Urgent lumbar puncture performed for suspected acute meningitis, encephalitis, or subarachnoid hemorrhage (unless preceding CT indicates otherwise) and for fever (even without meningeal signs) in infancy, acute confusional states, and immunocompromised patients. Another indication for lumbar puncture is unexplained dementia.

Multiple sclerosis is indication for lumbar puncture. If cell count is >100, look for another disease (e.g., sarcoid). Although IgG synthesis is increased, this is nonspecific. Demonstration of oligoclonal bands is useful, but they occur in other inflammatory diseases of central nervous system. Myelin basic protein is not clinically useful.

Lumbar puncture is used to record CSF pressure. High pressure is seen in pseudotumor cerebri. Low pressure is seen in positional headache and CSF leak.

Lumbar puncture indicated in infectious disease: AIDS, Lyme disease, and any suspected acute, subacute, or chronic infection (viral, bacterial, fungal). It is also indicated in paraneoplastic syndromes: 1) Hu and Yo antibodies to cerebellar Purkinje cells in paraneoplastic cerebellar degeneration, 2) neuronal antinuclear antibodies in subacute sensory neuronopathy and sensory neuropathy, and 3) retinal antibodies in paraneoplastic retinopathy.

Other indications for lumbar puncture are meningeal carcinomatosis, certain neuropathies (Guillain-Barré syndrome, AIDP, and CIDP), and gliomatosis cerebri.

Contraindications for Lumbar Puncture

Suppuration in the skin and deeper tissues overlying the spinal canal and anticoagulation therapy or bleeding diathesis are contraindications. Minimum of 1-2 hours should elapse after lumbar puncture before beginning heparin therapy. If platelet count <20,000, transfuse platelets before procedure.

Increased intracranial pressure is contraindication. Lumbar puncture is dangerous when papilledema is due to intracranial mass, but it is safe (and has been used therapeutically) in pseudotumor cerebri. In complete spinal block, lumbar puncture may aggravate signs of spinal cord disease.

- Perform lumbar puncture only after thorough clinical

evaluation.

- Increased IgG synthesis is nonspecific.
- High CSF pressure in pseudotumor cerebri.
- Low CSF pressure in positional headache and CSF leak.
- In paraneoplastic cerebellar degeneration, Hu and Yo antibodies to cerebellar Purkinje cells.
- In paraneoplastic retinopathy, retinal antibodies.
- Lumbar puncture is dangerous when intracranial mass causes papilledema.
- Lumbar puncture is safe in pseudotumor cerebri.
- Lumbar puncture aggravates signs of cord disease in complete spinal block.

PART II
SPECIFIC ENTITIES

SEIZURE DISORDERS

- "Seizures" refer to electroclinical events, and "epilepsy" indicates tendency for recurrent seizures.

Classification of seizures is given in Table 22-6.

Causes

Seizures occur at any age but 70%-90% of all epileptic patients have first seizure before age 20. Both cause and type of epilepsy are related to age at onset. However, the cause may not be found in many patients. Neonatal seizures are often due to congenital defects or prenatal injury, and head trauma is often cause of focal seizures in young adults. Brain tumors and vascular disease are major known causes of seizures in later life. Seizures often occur during withdrawal from alcohol, barbiturates, and benzodiazepines in young and old adults. Also, seizures occur during acute use of such drugs as cocaine, usually in young adults. Metabolic derangements (e.g., hypoglycemia, hypocalcemia, hypo- and hypernatremia, etc.) can occur at any age, as can infections (e.g., meningitis, encephalitis).

Pseudoseizures (psychogenic, nonepileptic) are sudden changes in behavior or mentation not associated with any physiologic cause or abnormal paroxysmal discharge of electrical activity from brain. They are often the cause in so-called intractable seizures.

- 70%-90% of epileptics have first seizure before age 20.

Table 22-6.--Classification of Seizures

Partial (focal) seizures
Simple partial seizures
Partial simple sensory
Partial simple motor
Partial simple special sensory (unusual smells or tastes)
Speech arrest or unusual vocalizations
Complex partial seizures
Consciousness impaired at onset
Simple partial onset followed by impaired consciousness
Evolving to generalized tonic/clonic convulsions (secondary generalized tonic/clonic seizures)
Simple evolving to generalized tonic/clonic
Complex evolving to generalized tonic/clonic (including those with simple partial onset)
True auras--are actually simple partial seizures
Generalized seizures--convulsive or nonconvulsive (primary generalized seizures--generalized from onset)
Absence and atypical absence
Myoclonic
Clonic
Tonic
Tonic/clonic
Atonic
Unclassified epileptic seizures (includes some neonatal seizures)

- Cause and type of epilepsy related to age at onset.
- Head trauma is cause of focal seizures in young adults.
- Brain tumors and vascular disease major causes of seizure in older people.
- Seizures occur with withdrawal from alcohol, barbiturates, and benzodiazepines.
- Seizures occur during acute use of cocaine (young adults).
- Pseudoseizures are often basis for so-called intractable seizures.

Status Epilepticus

This is a medical emergency and life-threatening condition. Seizure is prolonged, lasting >15-30 minutes, or there are repetitive seizures without recovery in between. Follow ABCs of cardiopulmonary resuscitation or trauma: airway, breathing, circulation. Draw blood sample for glucose, electrolytes, BUN, etc. Give 50 mL of 50% dextrose with 100 mg thiamine intravenously. Slow intravenous administration of diazepam or lorazepam can be initiated. You can begin with a loading dose of phenytoin or phenobarbital. If starting with benzodiazepine, then have to go to long-acting anticonvulsant, e.g., phenytoin or phenobarbital. Give them intravenously: phenytoin, 18-20 mg/kg (50 mg/minute), phenobarbital, 10-20 mg/kg (100 mg/minute). Consider general anesthesia or barbiturate coma if these fail.

Medications for status epilepticus are outlined in Table 22-7.

- Status epilepticus is life threatening and medical emergency.
- Seizure lasting >15-30 minutes or repetitive seizures without recovery.
- Give 50 mL of 50% dextrose with 100 mg thiamine intravenously.
- Slow intravenous diazepam or lorazepam.
- Loading dose of phenytoin or phenobarbital.

Anticonvulsant Therapy

Monotherapy is the treatment of choice, increasing the drug as high as necessary and as much as can be tolerated. Coadministration of antiepileptic drugs has *not* been proved to have more antiseizure efficacy than one drug without concurrently increasing toxicity. For a large population, one drug may be shown more efficacious and less toxic, but for a given patient an alternate drug may be more effective or have fewer side effects. With enzyme-inducing antiepileptic drugs (e.g., carbamazepine, phenobarbital, phenytoin, primidone), oral contraceptives may be less effective in preventing pregnancy. Valproate does not cause enzyme induction and may be optimal for women using oral contraceptives.

Phenytoin, carbamazepine, primidone, and phenobarbital can cause developmental fetal abnormalities. In general, multiple drugs at high doses are associated with greater frequency of anomalies. Lowest dosage possible should be given as monotherapy to minimize teratogenic risks, regardless of antiepileptic drug used. Valproate (and probably carbamazepine) can cause failure of midline structures to close (neural tube defects).

Anticonvulsants are outlined in Table 22-8.

- Treatment of choice is monotherapy.
- Enzyme-inducing drugs may render oral contraceptives ineffective.
- Valproate may be best for women taking oral contraceptives.

- Phenytoin, carbamazepine, primidone, and phenobarbital can cause developmental abnormalities.
- Valproate may cause neural tube defects.

If an epileptic patient under treatment has breakthrough seizures, consider the following: 1) compliance; 2) excessive use of alcohol and other "recreational drugs"; 3) psychologic and physiologic stress (lack of sleep, anxiety, etc.); 4) combination of 1) - 3); 5) systemic disease of any type, organ failure of any type, or systemic infection; 6) new cause of seizures (neoplasm); 7) newly prescribed medication, including other anticonvulsants (polypharmacy) and over-the-counter drugs; 8) toxic levels of anticonvulsants (with definite clinical toxicity); 9) pseudoseizures; 10) progressive CNS lesion not seen previously on neuroimaginig or lumbar puncture; 11) no cause found--at this point, must readjust anticonvulsants or replace one with another.

Surgery for Epilepsy

With improved technology, site of seizure origin is more accurately identified; surgical advances have made operative management safer. Of the 150,000 patients who develop epilepsy each year, 10%-20% have "medically intractable epilepsy." Brain surgery is an alternative therapy if antiepileptic drugs fail. However, before seizures are deemed intractable, ascertain that correct drugs have been used in correct amounts. Anterior temporal lobe operations and other cortical resections involve removal of epileptic region and are done for complex partial seizures. Corpus callosotomy, severing connections between right and left sides of the brain, is used for some types of generalized epilepsy.

- If antiepileptic drugs fail, brain surgery is alternative.
- Anterior temporal lobe and other cortical resections remove epileptic region.
- Resection operations are for complex partial seizures.
- Corpus callosotomy severs connections between left and right sides of brain and is used for generalized epilepsy.

HEADACHE

Cluster Headache

Cluster headache, unlike migraine, predominantly affects men. Onset usually is in late 20s but may occur at any age. Main feature of cluster headache is periodicity.

Table 22-7.--Medications for Status Epilepticus

Name	Common dose (route of administration)	Effectiveness	Advantages	Disadvantages
Benzodiazepines				
Diazepam (Valium)	5-20 mg (iv)	5-15 min	Rapid acting	Short effective half-life
Lorazepam (Ativan)	2-8 mg (iv)	2-8 hr	Rapid acting Longer duration of action than diazepam	May depress CNS function for hours
Midazolam (Versed)	1-10 mg (iv, im)	Min	Rapid acting May be given im	Short effective half-life Not FDA-approved for status epilepticus
Phenytoin (Dilantin)	500-1,000 mg (18 mg/kg) (iv)	24 hr	No CNS or respiratory depression	May be ineffective in status from nonidiopathic causes Hypotension and arrhythmias at high infusion rates Takes 20-40 min to administer
Barbiturates				
Phenobarbital (Luminal)	500-1,000 mg (iv, im)	Min	Long-lasting	Long-lasting depression of CNS function
Thiopental (Pentothal)	250-500 mg (iv)			Short effective half-life Respiratory depression Respiratory arrest Hypotension Myocardial depression
Pentobarbital (Nembutal)	250-500 mg (iv)			

CNS, central nervous system; im, intramuscularly; iv, intravenously.
From Slovis CM: ED management of unstable patients with status epilepticus. Updates Neurology 1991; pp 23-30. By permission of America Health Consultants.

Table 22-8.--Anticonvulsant Medications

Drug	Indication	Maintenance dose (range of dose), mg/kg daily	Half-life, hr	Therapeutic serum levels (range of levels), µg/mL	Minimum no. daily doses
Phenytoin	GTC, P	3-5 (4-8)	18-24	10-20	1
Phenobarbital	GTC, P	2-3 (2-5)	48-120	15-45 (10-40)	1
Primidone	GTC, P	10-25 (5-20)	6-12	5-12 (5-15)	3
Carbamazepine	GTC, P	10-20 (5-25)	12-18	4-8 (4-12)	2
Valproic acid	GTC, A, M	20-60 (10-60)	6-18	40-100 (40-100)	3
Ethosuximide	A	20-35	24-36	40-100	2
Clonazepam	A, M	0.05-0.2	20-40	20-80 (mg/mL)	2

A, absence; GTC, generalized tonic/clonic; M, myoclonic; P, simple or complex partial.

The cluster period lasts on average 2-3 months and typically occurs every 1-2 years. Attacks occur at frequency of 1-3 times daily and tend to be nocturnal in more than 50% of patients. Average period of remission is about 2 years. Cluster is not associated with an aura. Pain reaches peak in about 10-15 minutes and lasts 45-60 minutes. It is excruciating, penetrating, usually nonthrobbing, and maximal behind eye and in region of the supraorbital nerve and temples. Attacks of pain are typically unilateral. Autonomic features are both sympathetic paresis and parasympathetic overreaction. They may include 1) ipsilateral lacrimation, injection of conjunctiva, and nasal stuffiness or rhinorrhea, 2) ptosis and miosis (ptosis may become permanent), periorbital swelling, and bradycardia. Scalp, face, and carotid artery may be tender.

Abortive Therapy

Abortive therapy includes 1) oxygen inhalation, 5-8 L/min for 10 minutes; 2) ergotamine, especially inhalation or suppositories; 3) dihydroergotamine (DHE); 4) sumatriptan, 5-HT$_1$ agonist; 5) corticosteroids (e.g., 8 mg dexamethasone); 6) local anesthesia (intranasal 4% lidocaine); and 7) capsaicin in ipsilateral nostril. Surgical intervention may be indicated under certain circumstances for *chronic* cluster headache but never for episodic headache.

Prophylactic Treatment

Prophylactic treatment is mainstay of cluster headache treatment. Calcium channel blockers (verapamil) are widely used. Usual dose of lithium is 600-900 mg in divided doses. Its effectiveness is known within 1 week. Methysergide (Sansert) is most effective in early course of disease and least effective in later years. Ergotamine at bedtime is particularly beneficial for nocturnal attacks. Corticosteroids are helpful for short-term use, especially in patients resistant to above drugs or combination of above. Usual dose is 40 mg prednisone tapered over 3 weeks. Most effective treatment for *chronic* cluster headache is combination of verapamil and lithium. Valproate may also be useful.

- Cluster headache affects men.
- Onset is in late 20s.
- Periodicity is main feature.
- Cluster period lasts 2-3 months.
- Average remission is 2 years.
- Cluster not associated with aura.
- Pain peaks in 10-15 minutes and lasts 45-60 minutes.

- Pain is typically unilateral, excruciating, penetrating, nonthrobbing, and maximal behind eye.
- In >50% cases, pain is nocturnal.
- Autonomic features are present.
- Tenderness of scalp, face, and carotid artery.
- Prophylactic treatment is mainstay.
- Calcium channel blockers are widely used.
- Methysergide is effective early in disease.
- Ergotamine is effective for nocturnal attacks.
- Corticosteroids are helpful short-term.
- Combination of verapamil and lithium best for chronic condition.

Migraine and Tension Headache

Psychologic and physical therapy and pharmacotherapy are components of systemic approach to treating headache. Abortive headache medications may range from simple analgesics to anxiolytics, nonsteroidal anti-inflammatory drugs, ergots, and steroids to major tranquilizers and narcotics. Prophylactic medication should not be used when attacks occur no more than 2-3 times per month unless the attacks are incapacitating, associated with focal neurologic signs, or of prolonged duration. When prophylactic medication is indicated, the following should be observed:

1. Begin with low dose and increase it slowly.
2. Perform an adequate trial of medication (1-2 months).
3. Ensure that patient is not taking drugs that might interact with headache agent (vasodilator, estrogens, oral contraceptives).
4. Determine that female patient is not pregnant and that she is using effective contraception.
5. Attempt to taper and discontinue prophylactic medication after headaches are well-controlled.
6. Avoid polypharmacy.
7. Establish strong doctor-patient relationship; emphasize that management of headache is often team effort with patient playing an equal role.
8. Best medication is *no* medication.

Drugs used for prophylaxis include antiserotoninergic agents, β-blockers, calcium channel blockers, and antiprostaglandins. The antiserotoninergic agents are methysergide (Sansert), cyproheptadine (Periactin), and amitriptyline (Elavil). Most widely used β-blocker is propranolol (Inderal); others are atenolol, metoprolol, and timolol. Most useful calcium channel blocker is verapamil. Naproxen (Naprosyn and Anaprox) is most useful antiprostaglandin medication.

Nonsteroidal anti-inflammatory drugs produce analgesia through alternate pathways that do not appear to induce dependence. They may be useful in 1) migraine, both for acute attacks and prophylaxis; 2) menstrual migraine (especially naproxen); 3) benign exertional migraine and sex-induced headache (especially indomethacin [Indocin]); 4) cluster variants (chronic paroxysmal hemicrania, episodic paroxysmal hemicrania, and hemicrania continua); 5) idiopathic stabbing headache, jabs and jolts, needle-in-the-eye, and ice-pick headaches (indomethacin often useful); 6) muscle contraction headaches; 7) mixed headaches; and 8) ergotamine-induced headache.

- Begin with low dose.
- Give adequate trial, 1-2 months.
- Avoid polypharmacy.
- Best medication is no medication.
- Use nonsteroidal anti-inflammatory drugs for acute attacks and prophylaxis.

Transformation/Withdrawal Syndrome

Chronic daily headache is often accompanied by sleep disturbances, depression, anxiety, and overuse of analgesics; 90% of patients with this disorder have family history of headache. Episodic migraine and other episodic benign headaches can evolve into a daily refractory intense headache. This syndrome is usually due to the overuse (>2 days/week) of ergotamine tartrate, analgesics, especially combination analgesics and narcotics, and perhaps even benzodiazepines. Discontinuation of these medications is necessary to control the headache. Two points have to be stressed: 1) overuse of these medications causes daily headache, and 2) daily use of these medications prevents other useful medications from working effectively.

Treatment of daily refractory headaches usually requires hospitalization and withdrawal of overused medication with repetitive intravenous administration of dihydroergotamine.

Nonsteroidal anti-inflammatory drugs, β-blocker drugs, calcium channel blocker drugs, and tricyclic antidepressants do *not* cause transformation/withdrawal syndrome. Also, nonheadache patients who take large amounts of analgesics for other conditions, e.g., arthritis, do *not* develop analgesic/rebound headache. Simple withdrawal from analgesics produces significant improvement in patients with chronic daily headache. Nonprescription medication can be withdrawn abruptly. However, prescription medications (ergotamine tartrate, narcotics, barbiturates) have to be withdrawn gradually. When narcotics or com-

pounds containing codeine and ergotamine tartrate are withdrawn, clonidine may be helpful in repressing withdrawal symptoms. Some think even simple analgesics (aspirin, acetaminophen [Tylenol]) used >2 days/week can cause daily headache syndrome.

- Associated with daily headache are sleep disturbances, depression, anxiety, and analgesic overuse.
- 90% have family history of headache.
- Migraine and other headaches can become refractory intense headache.
- Overuse of medications causes daily headache and prevents effective action of other drugs.
- Hospitalization and withdrawal of overused drugs usually required.
- Nonsteroidal anti-inflammatory drugs, β-blockers, calcium channel blockers, and tricyclic antidepressants do *not* cause transformation/withdrawal syndrome.
- Significant improvement with withdrawal of analgesics.

VERTIGO AND DIZZINESS

Accurate visual, vestibular, proprioceptive, tactile, and auditory perceptions are necessary for normal spatial orientation. These inputs are integrated in the brain stem and cerebral hemispheres. Outputs are motor systems, extrapyramidal system, and cerebellar system. Impairments of any of these functions or of their input, integration, or output cause complaint of "dizziness" (a sensation of altered orientation or space). Dizziness, vertigo, and disequilibrium are common complaints. Results of diagnostic tests are often normal. Diagnosis depends mainly on history, with physical examination findings in some cases. Vestibular tests rarely provide an exact diagnosis. Types of dizziness are listed in Table 22-9.

Vertigo

Vertigo is an illusion of movement, usually that of rotation, and feeling of vertical or horizontal rotation of either the person or the environment. Most patients report this as "spinning" or "rotational" feelings. Others mainly experience staggering sensation. In contrast to vertigo, disequilibrium is feeling of unsteadiness or insecurity about the environment without a rotatory sensation. Vertigo occurs when there is imbalance, especially acute, between left and right vestibular systems. Sudden unilateral loss of vestibular function is dramatic; patient complains of severe vertigo and nausea and vomiting and is pale and diaphoretic. With acute vertigo, patient also has prob-

Table 22-9.--Types of Dizziness

Vertigo
    Peripheral
    Central
Presyncopal light-headedness
    Orthostatic hypotension
    Vasovagal attacks
    Impaired cardiac output
    Hyperventilation
Psychophysiologic dizziness
    Acute anxiety
    Agoraphobia (fear and avoidance of being in public
        places)
    Chronic anxiety
Disequilibrium
    Lesions of basal ganglia, frontal lobes, and white matter
    Hydrocephalus
    Cerebellar dysfunction
Ocular dizziness
    High magnification and lens implant
    Imbalance in extraocular muscles
    Oscillopsia
Multisensory dizziness
Physiologic dizziness
    Motion sickness
    Space sickness
    Height vertigo

lems with equilibrium and vision, often described as "blurred vision," or diplopia. Autonomic symptoms are common--sweating, pallor, nausea, vomiting--and can cause vasovagal syncope.

Fluctuating hearing loss and tinnitus are characteristic of Meniere's syndrome. Abrupt complete unilateral deafness and vertigo occur with viral involvement of labyrinth and/or CN VIII, and with vascular occlusion of inner ear. Patients who slowly lose vestibular function bilaterally, as with ototoxic drugs, often do not complain of vertigo but have oscillopsia with head movements and instability with walking. Even with unilateral vestibular loss, if it is slow (acoustic neuroma), patients usually do not complain of vertigo; they typically present with unilateral hearing loss and tinnitus. Vertigo invariably occurs in episodes. Common vestibular disorders with a genetic predisposition include migraine, Meniere's syndrome, otosclerosis, neurofibromatosis, and spinocerebellar degeneration.

Benign positional vertigo is single most common cause of vertigo. No cause is found in about half of patients. For other half, most common causes are post-traumatic and postviral neurolabyrinthitis. Brief episodes of vertigo usually last <30 seconds with positional change, e.g.,

turning over in bed, getting in or out of bed, bending over and straightening up, extending neck to look up.

Typically, bouts of benign positional vertigo are intermixed with variable periods of remission. Periods of vertigo rarely last >1 minute, although after flurry of episodes, patients may complain of more prolonged nonspecific dizziness lasting hours to days (light-headedness, swimming sensation associated with nausea). Management includes reassurance and positional exercises (vestibular exercises). Drugs are not very useful, but meclizine and phenergan may help with nausea and nonspecific dizziness. Rarely, surgical treatment (section of ampullary nerve) may be undertaken in intractable cases.

Vertigo of CNS origin caused by acute cerebellar lesions (hemorrhages or infarcts) or acute brain stem lesions (especially, lateral medullary [Wallenberg's] syndrome). Basilar-vertebral artery disease is also a cause, but vertigo by itself is never a TIA. Other symptoms are necessary to make diagnosis of basilar-vertebral insufficiency--dysarthria, dysphagia, diplopia, facial numbness, crossed syndromes, hemiparesis or alternating hemiparesis, ataxia, visual field defects, etc.

Presyncopal Light-Headedness

This is best described as "sensation of impending faint." It results from pancerebral ischemia. Presyncopal light-headedness is not symptom of focal occlusive cerebrovascular disease but may indicate orthostatic hypotension usually due to reduced blood volume, chronic use of hypotensive drugs, or autonomic dysfunction. Symptoms of vasovagal attacks are induced when such emotions as fear and anxiety activate medullary vasodepressor centers. Vasodepressor episodes can also be precipitated by acute visceral pain or sudden severe attacks of vertigo. Impaired cardiac output causes presyncopal light-headedness, as does hyperventilation. Chronic anxiety with associated hyperventilation is commonest cause of persistent presyncopal light-headedness in young patients. In most subjects, only moderate increase in respiratory rate can drop the $PaCO_2$ level to ≤ 25 mm Hg in few minutes.

Five types of syncopal attacks especially common in the elderly are:
1. Orthostatic--multiple causes.
2. Autonomic dysfunction due to peripheral (postganglionic) or central (preganglionic) involvement.
3. Reflex--such as carotid sinus syncope or cough or micturition syncope.
4. Vasovagal syncope--occurs less frequently in elderly

than in young; however, prognosis is worse in elderly, with about 16% of them having major morbidity and mortality in following 6 months compared with <1% of patients <30 years; common precipitating events in elderly include emotional stress, prolonged bed rest, prolonged standing, and painful stimuli.

5. Cardiac syncope.

- Sensation of impending faint.
- Is not common symptom of occlusive cerebrovascular disease.
- Vasovagal attacks occur less frequently in the elderly.
- In young, common cause of persistent presyncopal light-headedness is chronic anxiety with hyperventilation.
- Worse prognosis for elderly; 16% have major morbidity/mortality within 6 months.
- In elderly, precipitated by emotional stress, bed rest, prolonged standing, pain.

Psychophysiologic Dizziness

Patients usually describe this as "floating," "swimming," or "giddiness." They also may report feeling of imbalance, rocking or falling sensation, or a spinning inside the head. Symptoms not associated with illusion of movement or movement of environment or with nystagmus. Commonly associated symptoms include tension headache, heart palpitations, gastric distress, urinary frequency, backache, and generalized feeling of weakness and fatigue. Psychophysiologic dizziness can also be associated with panic attacks.

Disequilibrium

Patients who slowly lose vestibular function on one side, as with an acoustic neuroma, usually do not have vertigo but often describe vague feeling of imbalance and unsteadiness on their feet. Disequilibrium may be presenting symptom of lesions involving motor centers of basal ganglia and frontal lobe, e.g., Parkinson's disease, hydrocephalus, and multiple lacunar infarction syndrome. Broad-based ataxic gait of cerebellar disorders is readily distinguished from milder gait disorders seen with vestibular or sensory loss or with senile gait.

- Disequilibrium may be presenting symptom of basal ganglia or frontal lobe lesions.

Multisensory Dizziness

This is commonly seen in elderly and especially patients with such systemic disorders as diabetes. A typical combination includes such things as mild peripheral neuropathy causing diminished touch and proprioceptive input, decreased visual acuity, impaired hearing, and decreased baroreceptor function. In such patients, an added vestibular impairment as from ototoxic drug can be devastating.

Resulting sensation of dizziness is usually present only when patient walks or moves and not present when supine or seated. There is feeling of insecurity of gait and motion. Patient is usually helped by walking close to wall, using cane, or holding on to another person. Drugs should *not* be used for this disorder. Instead, use of cane or walker is important to improve support and increase somatosensory signals.

- Multisensory dizziness common in elderly diabetics.
- Added vestibular impairment can be devastating.
- Do not use drugs for this disorder.

NEUROLOGIC DISEASE IN PATIENTS WITH SYSTEMIC CANCER

Incidence of neurologic complications from systemic cancer may be increasing because of improved survival in patients with cancer. Neurologic problems are frequent reason for admitting patients with systemic cancer to hospital. These problems include pain, headache, and other complications.

Common metastatic causes of neck and back pain are epidural tumor (usually extends from vertebral body metastasis), isolated bone metastasis, radiculopathy from paravertebral tumor, tumor plexopathy, and leptomeningeal metastasis. Commonest nonmetastatic cause of back or neck pain is degenerative arthritis of spine. Other causes are epidural abscess, vertebral compressive fracture of osteoporosis, referred pain (as from hepatic metastasis), subcutaneous hematoma, etc.

- Degenerative arthritis of spine is commonest cause of neck/back pain.

No structural cause found in many cases of headache, which is tension-migraine type. Some identified causes are fever, side effects of therapy and post-lumbar puncture headache, metastasis (cerebral, leptomeningeal, base of skull), and intracranial hemorrhage (thrombocytopenia, hemorrhage due to intracranial metastasis).

Another neurologic complication in systemic cancer is altered mental status. Commonest cause is metabolic encephalopathy. Others are intracranial metastatic disease (parenchymal and meningeal), intracranial hemorrhage, primary dementia, cerebral infarction, psychiatric disorder, new primary brain tumor, bacterial meningitis, and transient global amnesia.

General Comments

The most common neurologic complication of systemic cancer is metastatic disease of which cerebral metastasis is the commonest. Local nonradicular pain is usually related to bone metastasis. However, MRI or myelography sometimes shows epidural extension of tumor. Leptomeningeal metastasis is as common as tumor plexopathy.

Most common nonmetastatic manifestation of cancer is metabolic encephalopathy and commonest symptom is headache, which may or may not be directly related to the cancer.

Cancers commonly causing neurologic problems are those of lung and breast, leukemia, lymphoma, and colorectal cancer. Breast, lung, and prostate cancer are commonly associated with bony metastasis and epidural metastasis. Most common brain metastasis is from lung. Meningeal metastases are common in lung and breast cancers, melanoma, leukemia, and lymphoma. Colorectal cancer causes local pelvic metastasis and is most frequent cause of tumor plexopathy. Head and neck cancer are most frequent cause of base of skull metastasis. Proportionally, melanoma causes the most nervous system involvement. Gastrointestinal tract tumors (stomach, esophagus, pancreas) have least number of neurologic complications.

Back pain in patients with cancer is symptom requiring urgent attention. Metabolic encephalopathy is commonest cause of altered mental status in patients with systemic cancer. This encephalopathy rarely has single cause; the often multiple factors include vital organ failure, electrolyte imbalance (including hypercalcemia), treatment side effects, analgesic medication, and infection. Metabolic factors are also common reasons for seizures in patients with cancer.

Many neurologic problems in patients with cancer can be diagnosed on basis of history and findings on neurologic examination and require knowledge of both nonmetastatic- and noncancer-related neurologic illness. In general, neurologic complications of systemic cancer can be divided into following categories:

1. Metastatic--parenchymal, leptomeningeal, epidural, subdural, brachial and lumbosacral plexuses, and nerve infiltration. This is *common*.

2. Infectious--unusual CNS infections because of immunosuppression.
3. Complications of systemic metastases--hepatic encephalopathy.
4. Vascular complications--cerebral infarction from hypercoagulable states, nonbacterial thrombotic endocarditis, radiation damage to carotid arteries, etc.; cerebral hemorrhage from such entities as thrombocytopenia and hemorrhagic metastases.
5. Systemic encephalopathies--usually from multiple causes, hypercalcemia, syndrome of inappropriate secretion of antidiuretic hormone (SIADH), medications, systemic infections, etc.
6. Complications of treatment--radiation, chemotherapy, surgery: radiation necrosis of brain, radiation myelopathy, radiation plexopathy, fibrosis of carotid arteries, neuropathies, encephalopathies, cerebellar ataxia.
7. Nonmetastatic "remote" effect--syndromes have been described from cerebral cortex through central and peripheral neuraxes to muscle; they are rare.
8. Miscellaneous--various systemic and neurologic illnesses having nothing to do with the cancer.

- Cerebral metastasis is commonest neurologic complication of systemic cancer.
- Metabolic encephalopathy is commonest nonmetastatic manifestation of cancer.
- Commonest symptom is headache.
- Cancers commonly causing neurologic problems are lung, breast, and colorectal cancers, leukemia, and lymphoma.
- Commonest brain metastasis is from lung and breast cancers, melanoma, leukemia, and lymphoma.
- Most frequent cause of tumor plexopathy is colorectal cancer.
- Proportionally, melanoma causes most nervous system involvement.
- Parenchymal, leptomeningeal, epidural, subdural, brachial and lumbosacral plexuses, and nerve infiltration are common metastatic sites.
- Syndromes of nonmetastatic remote effects are rare.

MOVEMENT DISORDERS

Essential Tremor

Essential tremor is commonest movement disorder. It is often misdiagnosed and inappropriately treated. It is monosymptomatic condition manifested as rhythmic oscillations of various body parts. Middle-aged and older people are most commonly affected, and there is often genetic component. Hands are most affected, with the tremor present in postural position and often having kinetic component. Head and voice are often affected. Head tremor can be either horizontal (no-no) or vertical (yes-yes). It almost never occurs in Parkinson's disease, but parkinsonian patients may have tremor of mouth, lips, tongue, and jaw. Legs and trunk (orthostatic tremor) are affected less frequently in essential tremor.

Essential tremor is slowly progressive condition with unknown pathophysiology. It may be due to "central pacemaker" located in cerebellum, motor nuclei of thalamus, or inferior olivary nucleus.

Agent most effective in reducing essential tremor is alcohol. Alcoholic drinks substantially reduce tremor for 45-60 minutes. Rate of alcoholism in patients with essential tremor is no different from that in general population. Propranolol (80-320 mg daily) and other β-blockers and primidone (25-250 mg at bedtime) are effective. Stereotaxic thalamotomy can be effective in patients with severe functional disability who are unresponsive to drug therapy; surgery is probably underused.

- Movement disorders mostly in middle-aged and older people.
- Often genetic component.
- Hands are affected most.
- Head tremor almost never seen in Parkinson's disease.

Parkinson's Disease

Sinemet CR

A major problem in long-term management of Parkinson's disease is motor fluctuations and unpredictable periods of levodopa unresponsiveness. Fluctuations can be eliminated by continuous intravenous and intraintestinal levodopa infusions.

Controlled released Sinemet may give more stable blood levels. Sinemet CR contains 50 mg of carbidopa and 200 mg of levodopa. Its peak antiparkinsonian effect is expected to occur later and last longer than that of regular Sinemet. Regular Sinemet produces peak plasma level within 30-60 minutes and falls to baseline by 2-3 hours. Sinemet CR takes longer to achieve peak concentrations but lasts 4-6 hours. Bioavailability of Sinemet CR relative to standard Sinemet is about 70%-75%. Splitting Sinemet CR in half increases bioavailability. However, crushing or chewing the tablets disables controlled release function. Dyskinesias may be *increased*

with Sinemet CR. Usual equivalent dose of Sinemet CR is roughly 20%-30% more per day than regular Sinemet. Sinemet CR is also used in nonfluctuating or new parkinsonian patients.

- Sinemet CR may increase dyskinesias.

Selegiline Hydrochloride (Deprenyl, Eldepryl)

This is a monoamine oxidase (MAO) type B inhibitor that potentiates effects of levodopa. Selegiline alone may have mild antiparkinsonian effects. The main mechanism, however, is related to blockade of exogenous dopamine metabolism or to blockade of dopamine reuptake. Selegiline is more effective added to levodopa in patients with less advanced disease. When given to newly diagnosed parkinsonian patient, selegiline delays need for levodopa. It is also useful in patients with "wearing off" phenomena, less useful in those with "on-off" phenomena, and not useful in those with "freezing spells."

- Selegiline potentiates levodopa effects.
- Selegiline alone may have antiparkinsonian effect.
- In new Parkinson's patient, selegiline delays need for levodopa.

NEUROLOGY OF SEPSIS

Nervous system is commonly affected in sepsis syndrome. Reversible encephalopathy occurs early in course.

Neuropathy and failure to wean from ventilator occur as the encephalopathy is lessening or there may be overlap. First to clear is encephalopathy, then respiratory failure, and last, neuropathy. In mild cases encephalopathy may be brief. Clinically significant peripheral nervous complications are usually features of severe sepsis.

- Early in sepsis is reversible encephalopathy.
- Encephalopathy is always first to clear.

Septic Encephalopathy

Septic encephalopathy is brain dysfunction in association with systemic infection *without* overt infection of brain or meninges. Early encephalopathy often begins before failure of other organs and is not secondary to single or multiple organ failure. Endotoxin does not cross blood-brain barrier and so probably does not directly affect adult brain. Cytokines, important components of sepsis syndrome, may contribute to encephalopathy. Gegenhalten or paratonic rigidity occurs in >50% of cases and tremor, asterixis, and multifocal myoclonus in about

25%. Seizures and focal neurologic signs are rare.

EEG is sensitive indicator of encephalopathy. Mildest abnormality is diffuse excessive theta low-voltage activity (4-7 Hz). Next level of severity is intermittent rhythmic delta activity (<4 Hz). Worsening leads to delta becoming arrhythmic and continuous. Typical triphasic waves occur in severe cases.

Adult respiratory distress syndrome is common in severe but not mild encephalopathic cases.

- Brain dysfunction associated with systemic infection.
- Encephalopathy precedes failure of other organs.
- Cytokines important part of sepsis syndrome.
- In >50% of cases, paratonic rigidity.
- In 25% of cases, tremor, asterixis, and multifocal myoclonus.
- EEG is sensitive indicator.

Critical Illness Polyneuropathy

This occurs in 70% of patients with sepsis and multiple organ failure. There is often unexplained difficulty in weaning from mechanical ventilation. Nerve biopsy shows primary axonal degeneration of motor and sensory fibers without inflammation. Recovery from polyneuropathy is satisfactory if patient survives sepsis and multiple organ failure.

- Nerve biopsy shows primary axonal degeneration of motor and sensory fibers without inflammation.
- Satisfactory recovery from polyneuropathy.

Septic Myopathy

Septic myopathy is difficult to demonstrate because of concurrent polyneuropathy. Muscle biopsies show denervation atrophy, but there may be scattered necrotic muscle fibers. EMG may have myopathic appearance.

Cachexia

Muscle wasting in sepsis may contribute to muscle weakness. If this alone occurs CK level is not elevated and EMG is normal. Muscle biopsy shows type II atrophy.

Panfascicular Muscle Necrosis

This is rare reaction of skeletal muscles to infection or trauma. Severe muscle weakness appears suddenly, with marked elevation of CK. Myoglobinuria often occurs and may require hemodialysis. Recovery can be rapid and is usually complete.

ISCHEMIC CEREBROVASCULAR DISEASE

Pathophysiologic Mechanisms

Pathophysiologic mechanisms of ischemic cerebrovascular disease include artery-to-artery emboli (e.g., extracranial carotid bifurcation to branch of middle cerebral artery), cardiac embolic stroke, and lacunar infarction (small vessel disease). Other causes are hematologic disorders and states of altered coagulability (polycythemia, sickle cell anemia, thrombocytosis, severe leukocytosis, abnormalities of cellular constituents of blood such as serologic factors like homocystinuria, deficiencies of antithrombin III, protein C, protein S, anticardiolipin antibodies, lupus anticoagulant, and mucin produced by adenocarcinomas which can cause hypercoagulable state). Still other causes are nonarteriosclerotic vasculopathies (fibromuscular hyperplasia, granulomatous angiitis, congophilic angiopathy, systemic lupus erythematosus, etc.), dissection of carotid or vertebral arteries, hemodynamic crisis with impairment of distal flow, mechanical compression of arteries, steal syndromes, and AIDS. "Recreational drugs" are a major risk factor for stroke in young adults.

- Pathophysiologic mechanisms include cardiac embolic stroke, hematologic disorders, vasculopathies, and AIDS.
- In young, "recreational drugs" are major risk factor for stroke.

Risk Factors

Risk factors are similar to those predisposing to coronary artery disease: hypertension, male gender, advanced age, cigarette smoking, diabetes mellitus, hypercholesterolemia, and oral contraceptives. Emboli from intracardiac mural thrombi are also important cause of TIA and cerebral infarct. Major cardiac risk factors include left-sided chamber enlargement or aneurysm, congestive heart failure, atrial fibrillation, transmural myocardial infarction, mitral valve disease, septic emboli, paradoxical emboli, and atrial myxoma.

TIAs

TIAs place patients at high risk for subsequent cerebral infarctions; estimates are from 4%-10% within 1 year to 33% within patient's lifetime. Most TIAs are fleeting, usually lasting <10-15 minutes; 88% resolve within 1 hour. Infarcts, hemorrhages, and mass lesions can present like TIAs.

Amaurosis fugax is temporary, partial, or complete

monocular blindness and is classic symptom of carotid artery TIA. It can be mimicked by glaucoma, vitreous hemorrhage, retinal detachment, papilledema, migrainous aura, temporal arteritis, and even ectopic floaters.

Long-term prognosis for patient with TIA generally follows the rules of 3s: 1/3 go on to have cerebral infarctions, 1/3 have at least one more TIA, 1/3 have no further TIAs.

- With TIAs, high risk for subsequent cerebral infarction.
- 1/3 will have cerebral infarction, 1/3 will have one more TIA, 1/3 will have no more TIAs.
- Most TIAs last <10-15 minutes.
- Infarcts, hemorrhages, and mass lesions can present like TIA.
- Amaurosis fugax is classic symptom of carotid artery TIA.

Cerebral Infarction

Myocardial ischemia and cardiac arrhythmias cause about 50% of deaths in patients with acute cerebral infarction, and about 5% of deaths are related to herniation. Most of other deaths are consequence of pulmonary complications, e.g., aspiration pneumonia or pulmonary embolism.

- In cerebral infarction, 5% of deaths related to herniation.
- Other deaths due to pulmonary complications.

Cerebral Embolism

Embolic infarction often has apoplectic onset associated with rapid loss of consciousness followed by maximum deficit and occurring in about 80% of cases of cardiogenic emboli.

Small percentage of patients have stepwise or progressive course during first 24-48 hours caused by distal migration of embolus.

Stroke Syndromes in Young Patients

Strokes in patients <40 years old are commonly caused by rheumatic heart disease, migraine, and oral contraceptive use. Cocaine abuse is also important cause. Abuse of other toxic drugs implicated in cerebral infarcts includes sympathomimetic agents, e.g., amphetamines and over-the-counter diet pills. Spontaneous dissection of carotid or vertebral arteries is another important cause. Incidence of HIV infections presenting with stroke-like features is increasing.

- Cocaine abuse important cause of stroke.
- HIV infections present with stroke-like features.

Carotid Endarterectomy

This operation is useful in symptomatic patients with high-grade stenosis (70%-99%). Symptoms must be those of carotid territory TIA or stroke with good recovery and must be of recent onset (<3 months). Surgery should be by surgeons with low rates of perioperative morbidity and mortality, and patient should be good surgical risk. Asymptomatic patients with high-grade stenoses may benefit from surgery, but this is still to be decided.

- Carotid endarterectomy is useful in symptomatic patients.
- Symptoms must be of recent onset.

"Recreational Drugs"

Mechanisms for stroke are thrombosis (vasculitis, vasospasm), embolism (endocarditis), subarachnoid hemorrhage (aneurysm), and intracerebral hemorrhage (vasculitis, vascular malformation, mycotic aneurysm). Main drugs involved in acute stroke, especially in the young, are amphetamines and particularly cocaine.

Cocaine hydrochloride is more commonly associated with hemorrhagic stroke. Hemorrhagic stroke occurs twice as often as ischemic stroke in intranasal users and is only kind that occurs with intravenous use. Alkaloidal cocaine ("freebase") is associated with ischemic and hemorrhagic cerebrovascular disease.

Cocaine is associated with infarction at all levels of CNS, including spinal cord and retina. Hemorrhagic strokes are intraparenchymal, intraventricular, or subarachnoid. Cocaine hydrochloride is more often associated with intracranial hemorrhage--about half the time from ruptured, preexisting cerebral saccular aneurysms or vascular malformations. Cocaine rarely causes frank vasculitis but does cause cardiovascular effects including acute hypertension, which can lead to hemorrhagic stroke, and cardiac arrhythmias and cardiomyopathies, which can lead to ischemic infarction from cardiogenic emboli. Cocaine also directly causes cerebral vasoconstriction, which can cause stroke. Concomitant use of alcohol could potentiate cerebrovascular spasm and rupture. Magnesium may help reverse cocaine-induced cerebrovasospasm.

Cocaine enhances platelet response to arachidonic acid, possibly leading to increased thromboxane production and platelet aggregation.

- Cocaine most commonly associated with hemorrhagic stroke.

- Hemorrhagic stroke is twice as frequent as ischemic stroke in intranasal users.
- In intravenous use, only hemorrhagic stroke.
- With cocaine, infarction at all levels of CNS.
- Cocaine associated with intracranial hemorrhage.
- Cocaine causes cerebral vasoconstriction.

Amphetamines cause inflammatory vasculopathy with vessel wall necrosis, leading to vessel wall rupture and hemorrhage.

Stroke Risks With Nonvalvular Atrial Fibrillation

Atrial fibrillation is associated with up to 24% of ischemic strokes and 50% of embolic strokes. Stroke rate for entire cohort of patients with chronic atrial fibrillation generally is about 5% per year. However, patients < 60 with "lone atrial fibrillation" have lower risk of stroke than other patients with atrial fibrillation. Stroke risk factors with atrial fibrillation include history of hypertension, recent congestive heart failure, previous thromboembolism including TIAs, left ventricular dysfunction identified on two-dimensional echocardiograms, and size of left atrium identified on M-mode echocardiograms. Patients with atrial fibrillation who have one or more risk factors should receive anticoagulation therapy (low intensity anticoagulation is recommended) and those at low risk should receive aspirin.

- Atrial fibrillation associated with 24% of ischemic strokes and 50% of embolic strokes.
- Stroke rate is about 5% per year.
- Patients with "lone atrial fibrillation" have lower risk of stroke.

Ticlopidine Hydrochloride (Ticlid)

This is a platelet aggregation inhibitor. It interferes with platelet membrane function by inhibiting ADP-induced platelet/fibrinogen binding and subsequent platelet/platelet interactions. The effect on platelet function is irreversible for life of the platelet. It also increases bleeding time, improves red blood cell deformability, and reduces blood viscosity. Cyclooxygenase is not inhibited. Ticlopidine may be useful in both sexes for completed stroke, TIA, minor stroke, or reversible ischemic neurologic deficit and probably should be second-line choice for prevention of thrombotic stroke and be reserved for patients intolerant of aspirin. Also, it may be useful in women, patients who have had vertebral-basilar symptoms, patients with cerebral ischemic symptoms while taking aspirin or receiving anticoagulant therapy, and patients with diffuse atherosclerotic disease rather than high-grade carotid stenosis.

Neutropenia occurred in 2.4% of patients and was severe (<450 neutrophils/mL) in 0.8%. Severe episodes of neutropenia occur during the first 3 months of treatment and are reversible when the drug is stopped. Onset of neutropenia is 3 weeks-3 months after beginning therapy, with recovery occurring 1-3 weeks after discontinuing therapy. Complete blood cell count and differential must be done as baseline and repeated every 2 weeks from the second week to the end of the third month of therapy.

- Ticlopidine increases bleeding time and reduces blood viscosity.
- It does not inhibit cyclooxygenase.
- It is second-line choice for preventing thrombotic stroke.
- Can cause neutropenia.
- Baseline complete blood cell count and differential must be done.

HEMORRHAGIC CEREBROVASCULAR DISEASE

Hypertension commonly affects deep penetrating cerebral vessels, especially ones supplying basal ganglia, cerebral white matter, thalamus, pons, and cerebellum. Common old *misconcepts* of intracerebral hemorrhage are 1) onset is generally sudden and catastrophic, 2) hypertension is invariably severe, 3) headache is always present, 4) reduced consciousness or frank coma is usually present, 5) CSF is always bloody, and 6) prognosis is poor and mortality high. None of these may be present, and prognosis depends on size and location of hemorrhage.

- Prognosis depends on size and site of hemorrhage.

Cerebellar Hemorrhage

It is important to recognize this because drainage may be lifesaving. Important clinical findings are vomiting and inability to walk. Long tract signs are usually *not* present. Patient may have ipsilateral gaze palsy, ipsilateral CN VI palsy, or ipsilateral nuclear type CN VII palsy and may or may not have headache, vertigo, and lethargy. Cerebellar hemorrhage may cause obstructive hydrocephalus.

- Vomiting and inability to walk are important findings in cerebellar hemorrhage.
- Long tract signs not present.
- May cause obstructive hydrocephalus.

Subarachnoid Hemorrhage

Subarachnoid hemorrhage accounts for about 10% of strokes, including about half of those in patients <45 years old, with peak age range between 35 and 65. In up to 50% of cases, alert patient with aneurysm may have small sentinel bleed with warning headache, or aneurysmal expansion may cause focal neurologic signs or symptoms, e.g., an incomplete CN III palsy. Prognosis is directly related to state of consciousness at time of intervention. The headache is characteristically sudden in onset and, although 1/3 occur during exertion, 1/3 also occur during rest, and 1/3 during sleep. Peak incidence of vasospasm associated with subarachnoid hemorrhage occurs between days 4 and 12 after initial hemorrhage. Other complications include hemorrhagic infiltration into brain, ventricles, and even subdural space, which requires evacuation; hyponatremia associated with diabetes insipidus or syndrome of inappropriate secretion of antidiuretic hormone; and communicating hydrocephalus.

Outpouring of catecholamines may cause myocardial damage with accompanying ECG abnormalities, pulmonary edema, and arrhythmias. Arrhythmias can be both supraventricular and ventricular and are most likely during initial hours or days after moderate to severe subarachnoid hemorrhage.

- About 10% of strokes are subarachnoid hemorrhage.
- In 50% of cases, alert patient with aneurysm may have small sentinel bleed.
- Prognosis is related directly to state of consciousness at time of intervention.
- Characteristically, headache has sudden onset.

Hemorrhagic cerebrovascular disease is outlined in Table 22-10.

The physical signs associated with hemorrhages in different loci are outlined in Table 22-11.

LYME DISEASE--MULTISYSTEM DISORDER

Stage I disease begins with bite of infected tick. Any body area may be bitten, but thigh, groin, and axilla are common sites. Patient often cannot recall tick bite.

Stage II disease begins weeks to months after initial

Table 22-10.--Hemorrhagic Cerebrovascular Disease

Hemorrhage into parenchyma
    Hypertensive intracerebral
    Due to trauma--primarily frontal and temporal
    Hemorrhagic infarction
    Secondary to brain tumors (primary and secondary neoplasms)
    Secondary to inflammatory diseases of vasculature
    Related to disorders of blood-forming organs (blood dyscrasia, especially leukemia and thrombocytopenic purpura)
    Related to anticoagulant therapy
    Secondary to increased intracranial pressure (brain stem) (Duret hemorrhages)
    Secondary to aneurysms and congenital anomalies of blood vessels
    Early-life carotid occlusion
    Postsurgical
    Fat embolism (petechial)
    Hemorrhagic encephalitis (petechial)
    Undetermined cause (normal blood pressure, no other recognizable disorder)
    Amyloid angiopathy

Hemorrhage into arachnoid (subarachnoid hemorrhage)
    Trauma
    Due to aneurysm
        Saccular ("berry," "congenital")
        Fusiform (arteriosclerotic)--rarely causes hemorrhage
        Mycotic
    Due to vascular malformation
    Many of same causes as for parenchyma above

Subdural and epidural hemorrhage (hematoma)
    Mainly traumatic
    Many of same causes as for parenchyma above

Hemorrhage into pituitary (pituitary apoplexy)

infection and is characterized by neurologic, cardiac, and ophthalmic involvement. Approximately 15% of patients in U.S.A. have neurologic involvement, usually meningoencephalitis, cranial neuritis, or radiculoneuropathy. Cranial neuropathies are common, most frequently CN VII (bilaterally in 1/3 of cases). Thus, bilateral CN VII palsies in patient from endemic area are almost diagnostic of Lyme disease. Peripheral nervous system involvement can include spinal roots, plexuses, and peripheral nerves.

Stage III disease marks chronic phase and begins months to years after initial infection. This stage is her-

Table 22-11.--Physical Signs With Hemorrhages in Different Loci

Locus	Motor sign	Extraocular eye movement	Pupils
Putamen	Hemiplegia	Conjugate gaze paresis to side of hemiparesis	Normal
Hemisphere	Unilateral paresis (may be absent)	Normal or conjugate gaze paresis to side of hemiparesis	Normal
Thalamus	Hemiparesis	Conjugate gaze defect to either side, upward-gaze palsy, skewing, eyes down and in, CN VI pseudopalsy	Small, poorly reactive to light
Pons	Quadriparesis	Horizontal gaze paresis to both sides; preserved reflex vertical gaze	Small, reactive to light
Cerebellum	Ataxia but no lateralized weakness	CN VI or gaze palsy to side of hemorrhage	Small or normal size and reactive to light

alded by arthritic and neurologic symptoms. Any CNS symptom is possible, and there may be psychiatric symptoms and cognitive impairment. Severe fatigue is particularly prominent feature. Rarely, a multiple sclerosis-like demyelinating illness featuring gait disturbance, urinary bladder dysfunction, spastic paraparesis, and dysarthria may develop. These symptoms may undergo exacerbations and remissions; MRI and CT reveal multifocal white matter lesions.

- Lyme disease is multisystem disorder.
- Patients often do not recall tick bite.
- In U.S.A., 15% of patients have neurologic involvement.
- Cranial neuropathies, especially CN VII, are common.
- Bilateral CN VII palsies in endemic area are diagnostic of Lyme disease.
- In stage III, severe fatigue is prominent.

NEUROLOGIC COMPLICATIONS OF AIDS

General Considerations

Nervous system is affected clinically in up to 40% of HIV patients, and pathologic changes in nervous system are found at autopsy in up to 90%. Neurologic features may be presenting manifestation of illness in 5%-10%. Neurologic spectrum encompasses all levels of neuraxis. Most opportunistic nervous system disease occurs with CD4 counts <200. Multiple nervous system lesions may occur. Most radiologic patterns are nonspecific, and accurate diagnosis of CNS lesions often requires biopsy.

- Nervous system affected in 40% of HIV patients.
- At autopsy, 90% of cases show neuropathologic changes.
- Neurologic features are presenting manifestation in 5%-10%.

Meningitis

Aseptic meningitis is common in HIV-1 infected patients with or without neurologic symptoms. Symptomatic meningitis may occur with seroconversion and include headache, meningismus, cranial neuropathies, encephalopathy, and isolated cases of myelitis or neuritis. CSF findings include mild-to-moderate lymphocytic pleocytosis, mild-to-moderate elevation of protein with increased gamma globulin, and increased IgG synthesis. HIV-1 can be cultured from CSF in up to 60% of cases, but CSF may be normal. HIV-1 serology may be negative on initial testing at presentation of aseptic meningitis.

- CSF findings in meningitis are lymphocytic pleocytosis and increased IgG synthesis.
- HIV-1 cultured in 60% of cases.

Cryptococcal meningitis is commonest opportunistic meningitis in HIV-1 patients. Clinical symptoms may be subtle or absent--80% of patients may have fever and headaches, <50% have meningismus, and 20% have encephalopathy. CSF is often atypical, and cell count, protein, and glucose can be normal or only mildly abnormal. India ink is positive in 65%-80% of the cases; cryptococcal antigen is usually positive but can be negative; and cultures are almost always positive. Relapse rate is high.

Leptomeningeal lymphomas are usually diffuse and

of high-grade B-cell type. There is frequent spread to CNS in up to 50% of cases, and clinical features are similar to those of symptomatic aseptic meningitis. Diagnosis is by CSF cytology. Neurosyphilis is a relatively common complication of AIDS.

Encephalopathy

HIV-1-associated dementia complex is commonest neurologic complication in AIDS and characterized by cognitive, motor, and behavioral symptoms. Memory, attention, and concentration impairment progress to global dementia. Pyramidal tract signs, weakness, extrapyramidal signs, tremor, loss of fine motor coordination, incontinence, myoclonus, and seizures may occur. There is often apathy, social withdrawal but occasional agitation and psychosis.

Encephalopathy most often occurs in setting of other systemic features of AIDS and with immunosuppression. Occasionally, it can be presenting or sole manifestation of HIV-1 infection and is now considered an AIDS-defining condition. HIV-1 can be recovered from brain tissue and CSF. MRI findings may be normal, show cerebral atrophy, punctate or confluence white matter changes, but they usually are nonspecific. AZT is helpful initially but long-term benefit is uncertain.

- Encephalopathy commonest neurologic problem in AIDS.
- Is characterized by cognitive, motor, and sensory symptoms.
- Occurs in setting of systemic features of AIDS.
- MRI findings may be normal.

The course of CNS toxoplasmosis is usually subacute and progressive over days to weeks, with headache, fever, and later focal or multifocal neurologic signs or a diffuse encephalopathy. CT scan usually shows multiple lesions with thick, irregular ring enhancement or nodular enhancement. Up to 19% of cases may have single lesions. MRI may show lesions not seen on CT; however, imaging patterns are not pathognomonic. There is predilection for basal ganglia and junction of gray and white matter of cerebral hemispheres. Therapeutic response is rapid and can be used as diagnostic test, and CT scan improvement may lag clinical response. Therapy for CNS toxoplasmosis is with pyrimethamine; life-long therapy is required to prevent relapse.

- CT shows thick, irregular ring enhancement or nodular enhancement.

- Predilection for basal ganglia and junction of gray and white matter of cerebral hemispheres.
- Treat with pyrimethamine.
- Rapid therapeutic response.

Primary CNS lymphoma affects 2%-5% of AIDS patients. Clinical features include progressive focal and multifocal signs or diffuse encephalopathy, headache, hemiparesis, seizures, and confusion. There is predilection for basal ganglia, thalamus, cerebellar vermis, periventricular white matter, and corpus callosum. Imaging patterns are not pathognomonic and difficult to distinguish from toxoplasmosis. Treatment for the lymphoma is radiation therapy.

- Progressive focal and multifocal signs with CNS lymphoma.
- Predilection for basal ganglia, thalamus, cerebellar vermis, periventricular white matter, and corpus callosum.
- Treat with radiation therapy.

Progressive, multifocal leukoencephalopathy is a latent viral infection occurring in 1%-4% of AIDS patients. Clinical features include progressive neurologic deficit over weeks to months, with cognitive changes, ataxia, visual impairment, seizures, and headache. MRI is more sensitive than CT in showing white matter lesions, which essentially are white matter lesions without mass effect. Biopsy is required to establish diagnosis. No treatment of established benefit is available. Occasionally, there is spontaneous remission, but usual course is relentless progression.

- Latent viral infection.
- Occurs in 1%-4% of AIDS patients.
- White matter lesions seen better with MRI than CT.
- Biopsy needed for diagnosis.
- No treatment is available.

Tuberculosis is more common in intravenous drug abusers and Haitians and resembles disease in non-HIV-1-infected patients but may be more aggressive.

Myelopathy

Vacuolar myelopathy is noninflammatory and occurs in about 20% of AIDS patients. It is considered part of HIV-1-associated dementia complex. Clinical features include progressive spastic paraparesis, sensory ataxia, and urinary incontinence. Diagnosis is by exclusion.

Acute myelopathy with seroconversion is rare and

manifested clinically by acute spastic paraparesis with clinical improvement.

- Myelopathy occurs in 20% of AIDS cases.
- Diagnosis is by exclusion.

Neuropathy

HIV-1-associated acute inflammatory demyelinating polyneuropathy tends to occur early in course of HIV-1 infection. Clinical features (identical to those of non-HIV-1 infected patients) are progressive motor weakness, areflexia, and mild sensory symptoms. It may be presenting symptom of HIV infection. Prognosis is good; spontaneous resolution may occur or the neuropathy may be treated with plasmapheresis or prednisone.

HIV-1-associated predominantly sensory polyneuropathy characterized by painful burning dysesthesias in feet. There are distal sensory and sometimes mild motor signs such as decreased ankle jerks.

- Acute inflammatory demyelinating polyneuropathy may be presenting symptom of HIV infection.
- Prognosis is good.

In mononeuropathies, there may be cranial and isolated peripheral nerve involvement. Symptoms are variable, as is course.

- Course of mononeuropathies varies.

Polyradiculomyelopathy is manifested by progressive lumbosacral radicular symptoms, with weakness, areflexia, and sensory loss in legs. Usual cause is cytomegalovirus infection. Disorders that must be excluded are compressive myelopathies, conus or cauda equina syndrome from lymphoma, toxoplasmosis, and zoster myelitis. Therapy is with ganciclovir.

- Polyradiculomyelopathy usually caused by cytomegalovirus.
- Treat with ganciclovir.

Myopathy

HIV-1-associated myopathy is slowly progressive proximal muscle weakness with elevated serum CK levels and electrophysiologic features of typical myopathy.

AZT myopathy typically appears after about 6 months of therapy. Serum CK is elevated, and electrophysiologic features typical of myopathy. Biopsy reveals ragged red fibers and abnormal mitochondria. AZT myopathy is often reversible with discontinuation of AZT.

- AZT myopathy appears after 6 months of therapy.
- Serum CK is elevated.
- AZT myopathy is often reversible.

Polymyositis, typical lymphocytic inflammatory infiltrate, may respond to steroid therapy.

QUESTIONS
(See "Answers" section)

Multiple Choice

1. Which of the following is not seen in normal healthy elderly people?
   a. Impairment of upward gaze
   b. Wasting of the small muscles of the hands
   c. Snouting and palmomental reflexes
   d. Grasping reflexes of the hands and feet
   e. Impairment of vibratory sensation in the legs

2. All the following are characteristic of dementia except:
   a. Impairment of intellect
   b. Impairment of memory
   c. Changes in personality and behavior
   d. Impairment of orientation and judgment
   e. Impairment of consciousness

3. A lumbar puncture with CSF analysis is useful in all

the following except:

a. Cerebral abscess
b. Neoplastic invasion of the leptomeninges
c. Idiopathic intracranial hypertension (pseudotumor cerebri)
d. Acute confusional states in immunocompromised patients
e. Unexplained dementia

4. All the following are characteristic of cluster headaches except:

a. Unilateral pulsatile headache
b. Nocturnal attacks
c. Horner's syndrome
d. More common in males than females
e. Scalp and face tenderness

5. A 76-year-old diabetic complains of a feeling of insecurity when walking (dizziness). On examination, there is mild decrease in visual acuity and moderate hearing impairment. There are also signs of a mild sensorimotor neuropathy. Otherwise, the results of the neurologic examination are normal for his age. The most appropriate initial procedure would be:

a. MRI scan of the brain
b. Treatment with meclizine (Antivert)
c. Gait training and use of a cane

d. Electromyographic studies
e. MRI scan of the cervical spine

True/False

6. The following signs and symptoms can be seen in acute confusional states:

a. Fluctuations in states of awareness and cognition
b. Anomia, alexia, agraphia
c. Unsteadiness in gait
d. Blepharospasm
e. Hemifacial spasm
f. Paratonic rigidity

7. With regard to seizures, indicate whether the following are true or false:

a. It is important to measure frequent anticonvulsant blood levels
b. Coadministration of two antiepileptic drugs is often more effective than monotherapy
c. Epilepsy surgery is under-used
d. Status epilepticus is best treated with monotherapy using a benzodiazepine (diazepam or lorazepam)
e. The seizures that usually occur with metabolic encephalopathy are partial simple or partial complex seizures
f. Pseudoseizures (psychogenic seizures) are a common cause of so-called intractable epilepsy

NOTES

CHAPTER 23
ONCOLOGY

Lynn C. Hartmann, M.D.

BREAST CANCER

Magnitude of the Problem

Breast cancer is the most common life-threatening malignancy in North American women (it represents one-third of all serious cancers). It will develop in approximately one in nine American women who achieve a normal life expectancy. In 1993, 180,000 new cases will be diagnosed in the United States. The incidence is increasing, but this is a complex issue. Much of the increase is due to earlier detection. Breast cancer is the second most common cause of death due to cancer in American women (lung cancer is the most common). There are 45,000 deaths due to breast cancer in this country annually.

- Breast cancer will develop in one in nine American women.
- Incidence is increasing (largely due to screening).
- It is second most common cause of death from cancer in American women.

Risk Factors

The risk factors for breast cancer are outlined in Table 23–1.

Table 23-1.--Risk Factors for Breast Cancer[*]

High risk: relative risk >4.0	Moderate risk: relative risk 2-4	Low risk: relative risk 1-2
Older age	Any first-degree relative with breast cancer	Menarche before age 12 years
Personal history of breast cancer		Menopause after age 55 years
Family history of premenopausal bilateral breast cancer or familial cancer syndrome	Personal history of ovarian or endometrial cancer	White race
		Moderate alcohol intake
Breast biopsy showing proliferative disease with atypia	Age at first full-term pregnancy >30 years	Long-duration (≥15 years) estrogen replacement therapy
	Nulliparous	
	Obesity in postmenopausal women	
	Upper socioeconomic class	

[*]Numerous studies have failed to quantify a clear relationship between use of oral contraceptives and subsequent breast cancer risk. Of note, the American Cancer Society estimates that 75% of cases of breast cancer occur in women with no known high-risk factors.

Screening

Controlled trials performed during the past 30 years have shown that screening for breast cancer can reduce mortality from this disease. Both mammography and physical examination of the breasts by skilled examiners have been shown to contribute to this decrease in mortality (note that breast self-examination has not been appropriately evaluated in a screening study). The Health Insurance Plan (HIP) study of greater New York was the first randomized controlled trial to evaluate screening for any type of cancer.

- Screening for breast cancer can reduce mortality.
- Mammography and physical exam of breasts contribute to decreased mortality.

In 1964, 64,000 women aged 40-64 years were enrolled. Screening with annual mammography and clinical breast examination over 4 consecutive years was offered to 32,000 women. The randomization group included 32,000 women (controls) who received their usual medical care. At 18 years from study entry, there were 22% fewer deaths from breast cancer in the screened group than the control group. One-third of the breast cancers detected in the screened group were found by mammography alone. Most of the benefit was derived from the physical examination, but mammography was in its infancy at that time. The reduction in mortality was noted in all age groups.

Clinical examination of the breast (i.e., by physician or nurse practitioner) and mammography are the basic screening methods; both are necessary to achieve maximal detection rates.

There is general consensus that women ≥50 years old should be screened with annual clinical examination and mammography. However, the timing for initiation of screening is controversial. Specifically, there is disagreement regarding the value of screening women aged 40-50 years. Certainly, in women deemed at high risk for breast cancer (for example, on the basis of family history), screening measures should be instituted at an appropriately earlier age, generally taken as 5 years before the earliest diagnosis of breast cancer in the family.

- Clinical exam of breast and mammography are basic detection methods.
- Women ≥50 years old need annual exam and mammography.
- Disagreement about screening women 40-50 years old.

Mammography is currently regarded as the most important screening test. About 10% of breast cancers detectable on physical examination are missed by mammography. Thus, biopsy of a suspicious palpable lump should be done despite a negative mammogram.

- Mammography is most important screening test.
- 10% of breast cancers found on physical exam are missed by mammography.
- Need biopsy for suspicious palpable lump, even if mammogram negative.

Pathology

Breast cancers are classified as ductal or lobular, corresponding to the ducts and lobules of the normal breast (Fig. 23-1). Infiltrating ductal carcinoma is the most common histologic type (70% of breast cancers). Lobular disease is more frequently multifocal and bilateral. Carcinoma in situ (CIS) refers to disease confined within the lumen of the ducts or lobules. It may be called ductal CIS (or intraductal carcinoma) or lobular CIS. This is noninvasive disease (i.e., the basement membrane is preserved); that is, there has been no invasion of malignant cells into the stroma of the breast. Thus, there has been no access to the vasculature and no potential for spread of disease. Thus, CIS of the breast is treated with local measures only.

- Infiltrating ductal carcinoma is most common histologic type.
- Lobular disease is more frequently multifocal and bilateral.
- Carcinoma in situ is noninvasive disease (basement membrane preserved) and needs local therapy only.

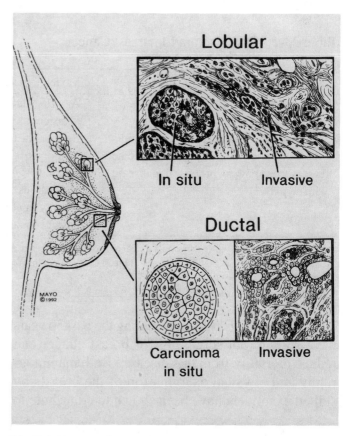

Fig. 23-1. Breast carcinomas: ductal vs. lobular, in situ vs. invasive.

Staging

The staging system of the American Joint Committee on Cancer is shown in Table 23-2.

Initial staging studies include 1) history and physical examination; 2) complete blood cell count; 3) chemistry panel; 4) chest radiography; 5) bilateral mammography; 6) bone scanning (stages II-IV); and 7) other imaging studies as clinically indicated.

Table 23-2.--Staging of Breast Cancer

Primary tumor (T)
TIS	Carcinoma in situ	
T1	T = ≤2 cm	
T2	T = 2.1-5 cm	
T3	T = >5 cm	
T4	T of any size with direct extension to chest wall or skin	

Regional nodes (N)
- N0 No involved nodes
- N1 Movable ipsilateral axillary nodes
- N2 Matted or fixed nodes

Distant metastasis (M)
- M0 None detected
- M1 Distant metastasis present (includes ipsilateral supraclavicular nodes)

Stage grouping

Stage I	T1 N0	
Stage IIA	T1 N1	
	T2 N0	= Operable disease
Stage IIB	T2 N1	
	T3 N0	
Stage IIIA	T1 N2	
	T2 N2	
	T3 N1,N2	= Locally advanced disease
Stage IIIB	T4, Any N	
Stage IV	Any T Any N M1	= Advanced or metastatic

Data from American Joint Committee on Cancer: Breast. *In* Manual for Staging of Cancer. Fourth edition. Edited by OH Beahrs, DE Henson, RVP Hutter, BJ Kennedy. Philadelphia, JB Lippincott Company, 1992, pp 149-154.

Natural History and Prognostic Factors

Nodal Status

The number of involved axillary nodes remains the single best predictor of outcome (Fig. 23-2).

Tumor Size

After nodal status, tumor size is generally the most important prognostic factor (Table 23-3).

Hormone Receptor Status

In general, patients with estrogen-receptor-positive tumors have a better prognosis. However, the difference in recurrence rates at 5 years is only 8%-10%.

Grade

Most breast cancers are high-grade. Patients with low-grade tumors have fewer recurrences and longer survival.

- Number of involved axillary nodes is best predictor of outcome.
- After nodal status, tumor size is most important prognostic factor.
- Patients with receptor-positive tumors have better prognosis.
- Patients with low-grade tumors have better prognosis.

Treatment

Primary or Local-Regional Therapy

Primary therapy is that treatment applied to the involved breast after biopsy confirmation of breast carcinoma. The approach has changed significantly during the past 15 years. Radical surgical procedures have been replaced by lesser surgical procedures that can conserve the breast. This latter approach is combined with breast irradiation.

- Radical surgical procedures now replaced with lesser operations.

Breast Conservation Versus Mastectomy

Several randomized controlled clinical trials have compared breast conservation (lumpectomy + axillary dissection + radiation) with mastectomy for the treatment of invasive breast cancer. All of these trials have demonstrated the therapeutic equivalence of these two options. The National Cancer Institute conducted a Consensus Conference on Early-Stage Breast Cancer in June 1990. The conclusion was that "Breast conservation treatment

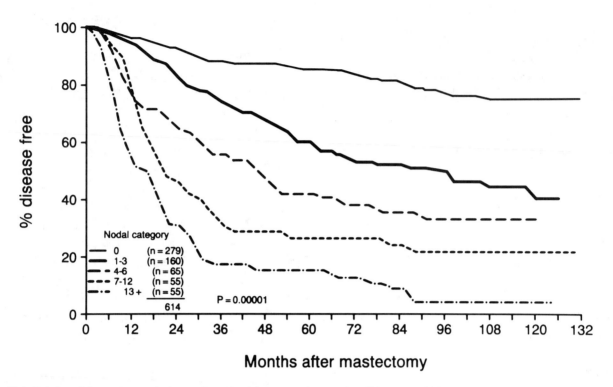

Fig. 23-2. Relation of disease-free survival to numbers of nodal metastases in more than 600 women with breast cancer treated with radical mastectomy alone in the early 1970s. (From Fisher ER, Sass R, Fisher B, and Collaborating NSABP Investigators: Pathologic findings from the National Surgical Adjuvant Project for Breast Cancers [protocol no. 4]. X. Discriminants for tenth year treatment failure. Cancer 53:712-723, 1984. By permission of American Cancer Society.)

Table 23-3.--Long-Term Results[*] in Patients With Node-Negative Breast Cancer Treated Surgically

Tumor size, cm	No. of patients	% free of recurrence	% dead of disease
<1	171	88	10
1.1-2.0	303	74	24
2.1-3.0	188	72	24
3.1-5.0	105	61	36

[*]Median duration of follow-up was 18 years.
Data from Rosen PP, Groshen S, Kinne DW: Survival and prognostic factors in node-negative breast cancer: results of long-term follow-up studies. Monogr Natl Cancer Inst 11:159-162, 1992.

is an appropriate method of primary therapy for the majority of women with stage I and II breast cancer and is preferable because it provides survival rates equivalent to those of total mastectomy and axillary dissection while preserving the breast."

- Numerous trials have demonstrated therapeutic equivalence of breast conservation and mastectomy.
- Breast conservation is suitable primary therapy for

most women with stage I or II breast cancer and is preferable.

Breast conservation is therapeutically equivalent to mastectomy for the primary therapy of breast cancer because the disease-free survival and overall survival rates with these two treatments have been shown to be identical. They are equivalent because the ultimate outcome of patients with breast cancer does not depend on the disease in the breast; rather, outcome depends on the presence of distant microscopic metastatic disease, which will eventually develop into clinically significant recurrent disease and death. Primary therapy does not affect distant disease.

- Distant microscopic metastatic disease determines outcome in patients with breast cancer and is not affected by the choice of primary therapy.

Recommendations for Lumpectomy and Radiation Therapy

It is appropriate to excise the primary lesion with a normal tissue margin of approximately 1 cm. When margins are grossly involved with tumor, further resection, to achieve negative margins, is indicated. An axillary dissection is needed for all patients, whether lumpectomy or mastectomy is done. This procedure provides vital prognostic information. Megavoltage radiation therapy to the whole breast to a dose of 4,500-5,000 cGy should be used. (Lumpectomy alone, without radiation therapy, leads to a high rate of recurrences in the breast, on the order of 40%.) Axillary nodal irradiation after an axillary dissection is not routinely indicated and, in fact, can result in unacceptable lymphedema.

- Axillary dissection needed for all patients.
- Megavoltage radiation therapy to whole breast should be used.
- Axillary node irradiation after axillary dissection is not routinely indicated.

There are no data suggesting an increased risk of secondary malignancies, including contralateral breast cancer, resulting from breast irradiation. Certain women are not candidates for breast conservation. These include 1) women with multicentric breast malignancies, including those with more than one mass, or diffuse microcalcifications on mammography; and 2) women in whom an unacceptable cosmetic result would be predicted. This includes those whose tumors are large relative to breast size and those with certain collagen vascular diseases, in whom excessive fibrosis can result after breast irradiation. Breast reconstruction is an option for interested women who have a mastectomy.

- Certain women are not candidates for breast conservation: those with 1) multicentric breast malignancies or diffuse microcalcifications on mammography or 2) predictable unacceptable cosmetic result.
- Breast reconstruction is option after mastectomy.

Systemic Therapy

This consists of either hormonal therapy or combination chemotherapy. It may be administered in the adjuvant setting (see this page) or for advanced disease (see page 648).

Hormonal Agents

Tamoxifen is the most widely used hormonal agent in the treatment of patients with breast cancer. Tamoxifen is a nonsteroidal compound with both anti-estrogen and estrogen-like (agonist) activity. Its beneficial effects include 1) its recognized antitumor effects on breast can-

cer cells, 2) a decrease in new, contralateral breast cancers in women taking adjuvant tamoxifen, 3) a favorable effect on bone density (estrogen-like effect), and 4) a favorable effect on lipid profiles (estrogen-like effect). Its side effects include hot flashes, vaginal dryness, nausea, thromboembolic events (1%-2% of patients), irregular menses in premenopausal women, and an increase in the incidence of endometrial cancer (possibly due to the estrogen-like effect on endometrial tissue).

- Tamoxifen has both anti-estrogen and estrogen-like (agonist) activity.
- Beneficial effects of tamoxifen: 1) decrease in new, contralateral breast cancer in women taking adjuvant tamoxifen; 2) favorable effect on bone density.
- Side effects of tamoxifen: 1) hot flashes, vaginal dryness, nausea, thromboembolic events; 2) increase in endometrial cancer.

Megestrol acetate is a progestational agent. Its side effects include appetite stimulation, weight gain, and fluid retention. *Fluoxymesterone* is an androgen. Side effects are those of virilization with hirsutism, male pattern baldness, deepening of the voice, and clitoromegaly. *Aminoglutethimide* suppresses adrenal steroid synthesis. Thus, addisonian symptoms are usually prevented by also giving glucocorticoid replacement. Side effects, besides adrenal insufficiency, include nausea and anorexia.

Chemotherapy

Active drugs include doxorubicin (Adriamycin, A), cyclophosphamide (C), methotrexate (M), 5-fluorouracil (F), vincristine/vinblastine, mitomycin-C, VP-16, cisplatin, and paclitaxel. Among the most commonly used combinations are CMF and CAF. Side effects of chemotherapy include reversible lowering of the blood cell counts and reversible hair loss. Severe gastrointestinal side effects are unusual. After 20 years of follow-up, no increase in second malignancies has been noted in patients who have received adjuvant chemotherapy for breast cancer.

Adjuvant Therapy

Adjuvant therapy is that administered in addition to primary localized treatment. It usually refers to systemic therapy.

In patients with *positive nodes*, the following recommendations were put forward by a 1985 National Institutes of Health Consensus Conference on Adjuvant

Chemotherapy and Endocrine Therapy for Breast Cancer. Premenopausal patients with positive nodes receive chemotherapy regardless of their estrogen-receptor status (Table 23-4).

- Node-positive premenopausal patients receive chemotherapy regardless of their estrogen-receptor status.

Table 23-4.--Adjuvant Therapy: Node-Positive Breast Cancer

| | Estrogen-receptor status | |
	Positive	Negative
Premenopausal	Chemo	Chemo
Postmenopausal	Tamoxifen	Consider chemo

Chemo, combination chemotherapy.

In patients with *negative nodes*, recommendations for adjuvant therapy are less defined. Most of these women are cured with local-regional therapy alone. Nevertheless, recurrent disease develops in approximately 25%-30% of these patients, and thus adjuvant trials have been conducted in this population to attempt to reduce disease recurrences. Several randomized trials comparing adjuvant treatment with no adjuvant treatment have been performed in node-negative breast cancer, and in general the risk of recurrence has been reduced by one-third in the treated patients. Thus, current practice has evolved to treat more and more patients who have node-negative disease. In patients with tumors ≤1 cm in diameter, however, the recurrence rate is so low that adjuvant therapy is generally not recommended.

- Most patients with node-negative breast cancer are cured with local-regional therapy alone.
- About 25%-30% of such patients develop recurrent disease.
- Risk of recurrence in patients with node-negative disease is reduced by a third with adjuvant treatment.
- Adjuvant therapy not recommended in patients with node-negative disease whose tumors are ≤1 cm in diameter.

Table 23-5 lists general guidelines for adjuvant therapy in patients with negative nodes. These are based on

clinical trials that have shown improvement in disease-free survival in treated patients compared with controls; overall survival differences, however, have not been shown with the use of adjuvant treatment in all of these subgroups.

Table 23-5.--Adjuvant Therapy: Node-Negative Breast Cancer[*]

Tumor size	Management	
≤1 cm	Observe	
>1 cm		
	Estrogen-receptor status	
	Positive	Negative
Premenopausal	Tamoxifen or chemotherapy	Chemotherapy
Postmenopausal	Tamoxifen	Consider chemotherapy

[*]Most oncologists treat node-negative tumors ≥2 cm in size; treatment is individualized for tumors of 1-2 cm in size.

In no subset of patients, either node-positive or node-negative, is combined chemotherapy and endocrine therapy routinely recommended. This issue is being actively studied in several settings.

Therapy for Advanced Disease

We currently lack curative therapy for recurrent breast cancer. The median duration of survival in patients with recurrence is approximately 2.5 years from the time of diagnosis of recurrent disease; there is tremendous variability with this disease, however. Survival is longer with bone or soft tissue recurrence than with visceral recurrence. Hormone therapy is generally the initial systemic treatment for patients with estrogen-receptor-positive advanced disease; tamoxifen is usually the first choice, and other agents include megestrol acetate, fluoxymesterone, and aminoglutethimide. Chemotherapy is used in estrogen-receptor-negative disease, rapidly progressive or life-threatening situations, or hormonally refractory disease. Radiation therapy is used for symptomatic localized disease.

- Survival with recurrent breast cancer is about 2.5 years from diagnosis of recurrence.
- Tamoxifen is usually first choice of therapy for estrogen-receptor-positive advanced disease.
- Radiation is used for symptomatic localized disease.

LUNG CANCER

Magnitude of the Problem

Approximately 170,000 new cases of lung cancer are diagnosed in the United States annually, resulting in 150,000 deaths. Thus, only approximately 10% of patients diagnosed with lung cancer survive their disease. Lung cancer is the leading cause of cancer mortality in American men and women.

Risk Factors

About 95% of lung cancers in men and about 80% of lung cancers in women result from cigarette smoking. Men who smoke 1-2 packs per day have up to a 25-fold increase in lung cancer compared with those who have never smoked. The risk of lung cancer in an ex-smoker declines with time. Passive smoking may be associated with an increased risk of lung cancer. Certain occupations (smelter workers, iron workers), chemicals (arsenic, methyl ethyl ether), and exposure to radioactive agents (radon, uranium) have been associated with increased risks for development of lung cancer. Diets high in fruit (possibly due to high β-carotene levels) may offer some protection.

- 95% of lung cancers in men and 80% in women result from cigarette smoking.
- Men who smoke 1-2 packs a day have 25-fold increase in lung cancer compared with those who never smoked.
- Passive smoking may be associated with increased risk of lung cancer.

Screening

The only readily available tools for early detection are chest radiography and sputum cytology. Data from the Mayo Lung Project concluded that "results do not justify recommending large-scale radiologic or cytologic screening for early lung cancer at this time" (Cancer 67:1155-1164, 1991). Prospective population-based studies have shown no improvement in survival by screening with chest radiography or sputum cytology. Contrary positions hold that yearly chest radiography in smokers >50 years increases the detection rate of stage I disease and improves 5-year survival rate compared with the general population (Semin. Oncol. 18:87-98, 1991).

- Only readily available tools for early detection of lung cancer are chest radiography and sputum cytology.
- In prospective population-based studies, survival not improved with screening.
- In smokers >50 years, yearly chest radiography increases detection of stage I disease.

Histologic Types and Characteristics

Adenocarcinoma typically has a peripheral location. It represents the most frequent histologic subtype found in nonsmokers. It is also called "scar carcinoma." Squamous cell cancers are found centrally. They are associated with hypercalcemia (via paraneoplastic parathyroid-hormone-like peptide). They may cavitate. Small cell carcinomas also occur centrally. They are characterized by prominent adenopathy; the primary tumor may be small. Syndrome of inappropriate antidiuretic hormone secretion and various neurologic abnormalities can occur as associated paraneoplastic syndromes with small cell carcinomas. Large cell carcinomas may be found peripherally. They are large lesions that may also cavitate.

Staging

The "classic *Tumor-Node-Metastasis*" system is simplified in Table 23-6.

Table 23-6.--Staging of Lung Cancer

Stage I	Node negative
Stage II	Hilar nodes positive
Stage III	Mediastinal or supraclavicular nodes positive or tumor extends directly into chest wall or mediastinal structures
Stage IV	Distant disease

Simplified staging system for small cell lung cancer	
Limited	Stages I-III (one hemithorax) or disease can be encompassed within one radiation port
Extensive	Metastases

Natural History

The natural history of lung cancer, by stage, is shown in Figure 23-3.

Treatment

Non-Small-Cell Lung Cancer

The treatment of choice is surgical. Resection, presuming reasonably normal cardiac, pulmonary, and other major organ function, is safe. Preoperative irradiation

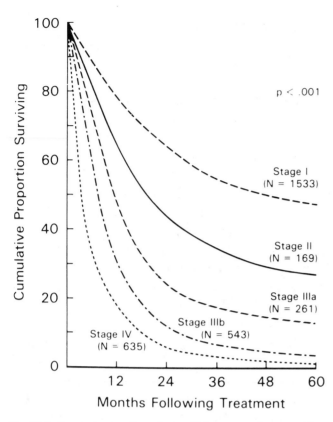

Fig. 23-3. Survival curves for patients with lung cancer by stage. (From Mountain CF: A new international staging system for lung cancer. Chest 89:225S-233S, 1986. By permission of American College of Chest Physicians.)

has shown no survival benefit in two large prospective trials, although the percentage of patients who had resection was increased. Postoperative radiation therapy has not improved survival over operation alone in any prospective trial. It definitely has no role in node-negative disease. In a prospective trial of patients with node-positive disease who had resection of squamous cell cancers, postoperative irradiation did not improve survival, even though it did significantly decrease the local recurrence rate. Postoperative adjuvant chemotherapy has not consistently improved survival in prospective trials. For nonresectable, localized, non-small-cell lung cancer, the treatment of choice is less certain. The "best" 5-year survival rates are 5%-7% for radiation alone and 10%-15% for radiation and chemotherapy. Many physicians advocate radiation therapy for patients with pain, cough, and hemoptysis; some physicians use chemotherapy or supportive care only.

- For early-stage non-small-cell lung cancer, treatment of choice is surgical.
- Preoperative irradiation has shown no survival benefit.

- Postoperative irradiation has not improved survival.
- Postoperative adjuvant chemotherapy has not consistently improved survival.

Small-Cell Lung Cancer

Treatment of limited-stage small-cell lung cancer consists of both chemotherapy and chest irradiation. The specific drugs, radiation schedules, doses, and timing are still the subjects of investigation. For patients who have a complete response to chemotherapy and chest radiation therapy, prophylactic cranial irradiation is generally used to decrease the frequency of failure in the central nervous system. However, cranial radiation therapy has been associated with brain damage in a third or more of patients so treated. For limited-stage small cell disease, the median duration of survival is approximately 18 months; 30%-40% of patients survive 2 years, and 10%-20% survive 5 years.

- For small-cell lung cancer, treatment of limited-stage disease is both chemotherapy and chest irradiation.
- If prophylactic cranial irradiation is used, a third or more of patients have associated brain damage.
- Median survival is 18 months.

Treatment of extensive stage (stage IV) small-cell lung cancer is with chemotherapy. Combination chemotherapy is favored over single-agent therapy. Active drugs include etoposide, cisplatin, cyclophosphamide, doxorubicin, and vincristine. High-dose chemotherapy with or without autologous bone marrow transplantation or marrow colony-stimulating factors has not yet been proved superior, on a consistent basis, to standard chemotherapy. The median duration of survival is approximately 10 months; about 10% of patients survive 2 years, and ≤1% survive 5 years.

- For extensive stage small-cell lung cancer, treatment is chemotherapy.
- High-dose chemotherapy not yet proved superior to standard.
- Median survival is 10 months.

COLORECTAL CANCER

Background

Colorectal cancer is diagnosed in approximately 150,000 Americans each year and causes 60,000 deaths.

Colorectal cancer is most common in North America and Europe. It is associated with high-fat, low-fiber diets. Population screening with fecal occult blood testing remains problematic. Although one recent study showed a reduction in mortality from colorectal cancer with fecal occult blood screening (N. Engl. J. Med. 328:1365-1371, 1993), it should be noted that any participants who had positive results went on to have colonoscopy. Another recent study showed that fecal occult blood tests failed to detect 70% of colorectal cancers and 80% of large (≥2 cm) polyps (JAMA 269:1262-1267, 1993). For high-risk patients, such as those with a family history of colorectal cancer or a prior colorectal cancer, structural studies of the entire large bowel, such as colonoscopy or proctoscopy plus barium enema, should be performed at appropriate intervals (e.g., every 1-3 years).

- Colorectal cancer associated with high-fat, low-fiber diets.
- For colorectal cancer, fecal occult blood testing was shown to decrease mortality in one study.
- For high-risk patients, entire large bowel should be studied at appropriate intervals.

Risk Factors

High-risk groups include persons with 1) familial polyposis syndromes (familial adenomatous polyposis--gene recently identified on chromosome 5--and Gardner's syndrome--gut polyps plus desmoid tumors, lipomas, sebaceous cysts, and other abnormalities); 2) familial cancer syndromes without polyps (hereditary nonpolyposis coli or Lynch syndromes, which are marked by colon cancer with or without endometrial, breast, and other cancers); and 3) inflammatory bowel disease.

- High-risk factors are familial polyposis syndromes, including Gardner's syndrome (gut polyps, desmoid tumors, lipomas, sebaceous cysts, other abnormalities); select familial cancer syndromes; and inflammatory bowel disease.

Treatment

Surgery

Surgical resection is the preferred method of curative treatment for carcinomas of the colon or rectum. The probability of cure is highly related to stage of disease (Table 23-7), which is determined by the depth of penetration through the bowel wall and the involvement of regional nodes (Table 23-8). Cancers of the rectum tend to have a worse prognosis than cancers of the colon, stage for stage.

- Preferred treatment for colorectal cancer is surgical resection.
- Cure rate related to stage.
- Cancer of rectum has worse prognosis than cancer of colon.

Table 23-7.--Survival Rates in Colorectal Cancer, by Stage

5-year survival (surgery only), %	AJCC stage	Dukes stage
90	I	A
60-80	II	B
30-60	III	C

AJCC, American Joint Committee on Cancer.

Table 23-8.--Staging of Colorectal Cancer, by Depth of Penetration

Depth of penetration	Node	Modified Dukes stage
Mucosa	Negative	A
Into or through bowel wall	Negative	B
	Positive	C

Adjuvant Therapy

For *rectal cancer*, adjuvant pelvic irradiation and 5-fluorouracil are recommended for deeply invasive or node-positive lesions. For *colon cancer*, adjuvant 5-fluorouracil and levamisole are recommended for node-positive disease. Levamisole is an antihelminthic drug that has immunomodulatory activity, and it may also potentiate the cytotoxicity of 5-fluorouracil.

- For rectal cancer, adjuvant therapy includes pelvic irradiation and 5-fluorouracil.
- For colon cancer, adjuvant therapy includes 5-fluorouracil and levamisole.

Metastatic Disease

Select patients with minimal advanced or stage IV colorectal cancer may be candidates for an attempt at curative resection of their metastatic disease. Of carefully selected patients with limited metastatic disease to the liver or occasionally the lung, 25% will survive beyond 5 years without further evidence of disease recurrence.

The vast majority of patients with advanced or metastatic colorectal cancer are incurable with present techniques but are candidates for palliative chemotherapy. The use of leucovorin, a modulator of 5-fluorouracil, along with 5-fluorouracil is a standard approach. This yields tumor response rates ranging from 30%-40% and a 4- to 5-month longer median survival than in patients who receive 5-fluorouracil alone. The median survival is 6 months for patients treated with 5-fluorouracil alone and 10-12 months for those treated with 5-fluorouracil and leucovorin. Patients with indolent metastatic colon cancer who are asymptomatic may be observed without treatment, occasionally for prolonged periods.

- Select patients with limited disease may be candidates for curative resection.
- For patients with colorectal cancer who have metastatic disease, the vast majority are incurable.
- 5-Fluorouracil plus leucovorin is standard therapy.

Carcinoembyronic Antigen (CEA)

Determination of the CEA concentration is the best currently available noninvasive technique to detect recurrent colorectal cancer. Unfortunately, the vast majority of patients with elevated postoperative CEA values have diffuse metastatic disease beyond surgical cure.

PROSTATE CANCER

Background

There are 130,000 new cases of prostate cancer annually in the United States. It is the most common cancer in men in the United States and is the second leading cause of death from cancer in men in the United States. The American Cancer Society recommends a digital rectal examination in men aged 40 years or older and determination of the prostate-specific antigen (PSA) value in men 50 years or older. Use of the PSA value for prostate cancer screening is a controversial issue and has not been shown to reduce mortality.

- Prostate cancer is most common cancer in men in United States.

- Second leading cause of death from cancer in men in United States.

Prognostic factors include stage of disease and grade of malignancy. The Gleason scoring system is used for grading: grading ranges from 1 (better differentiated, better prognosis) to 5 (less differentiated, worse prognosis). More than one pattern of differentiation may be present in a surgical specimen. The pathologist grades the two predominant ones individually and adds them to yield a final Gleason grade (e.g., $3 + 5 = 8$). Gleason grades 2-6 are associated with a better prognosis.

- Prognostic factors for prostate cancer are stage and grade.
- Gleason grades 2-6 have better prognosis.

Management

Management of Specific Stages

Figure 23-4 summarizes therapy of prostate cancer by stage. For stage C disease (locally advanced), x-ray therapy is usually used. Some centers use androgen deprivation, and other centers use an aggressive surgical approach.

For stage D1 disease (positive pelvic nodes), the management is controversial. Divergent approaches include androgen deprivation alone, x-ray therapy with or without androgen deprivation, close observation with androgen deprivation at progression, or prostatectomy with androgen deprivation.

For advanced (D2) disease, bone is the most frequent site of metastatic disease. Hormonal therapy, although it is very effective and produces a response in most patients, is noncurative. The average duration of response to initial hormonal maneuver is 18 months. The average duration of survival is 2 to 3 years. Once the disease progresses after the initial hormonal maneuver, it is typically very refractory to secondary treatment attempts (e.g., hormonal or chemotherapy).

- Bone is most frequent site of metastatic disease from prostate.
- Hormonal therapy effective and produces response, but is noncurative.
- Average duration of survival with advanced prostatic cancer is 2-3 years.

Prostatectomy

This is reserved for patients with localized disease. The 15-year disease-specific survival rate after prosta-

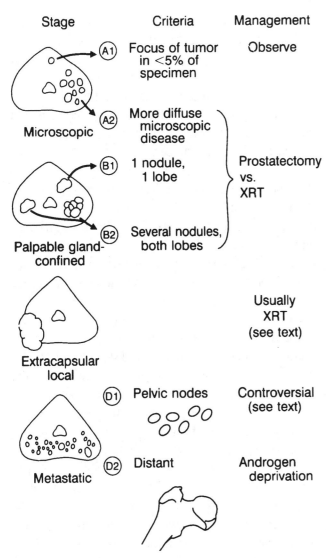

Stage	Criteria	Management
Microscopic	(A1) Focus of tumor in <5% of specimen	Observe
	(A2) More diffuse microscopic disease	Prostatectomy vs. XRT
Palpable gland-confined	(B1) 1 nodule, 1 lobe	
	(B2) Several nodules, both lobes	
Extracapsular local		Usually XRT (see text)
Metastatic	(D1) Pelvic nodes	Controversial (see text)
	(D2) Distant	Androgen deprivation

Fig. 23-4. Therapy for prostate cancer, by stage of disease. XRT, x-ray therapy.

tectomy is 85%-90% for stage A2 or B disease. Impotence occurs in most patients, especially older individuals. Urinary incontinence is rare (<2% of patients).

- Prostatectomy used for localized disease.
- 15-year survival rate is 85%-90% for stage A2 or B disease.

Radiation Therapy

External beam radiotherapy is considered the equivalent of prostatectomy. It is preferred for stage C disease at most centers. Impotence can occur, but less often than with prostatectomy. A concern related to radiotherapy is that repeat biopsies after treatment have shown apparently viable tumor in >35% of patients. The clinical importance of this residual tumor is unclear, but there may be a correlation with the subsequent appearance of distant metastasis.

- External beam radiotherapy considered equivalent of prostatectomy at most centers.
- Impotence less frequent with radiotherapy than prostatectomy.

Androgen Deprivation

The two sources of androgens in men are the testes (testosterone, 95%) and adrenal glands (5%). Androgen deprivation can be accomplished surgically with orchiectomy or medically. Potental agents include luteinizing hormone-releasing hormone (LHRH) agonists such as leuprolide, buserelin, and goserelin. They decrease androgen levels through continuous binding of the LHRH receptor and subsequent decrease of LH and thus testosterone. They are administered as a monthly injection of a depot preparation. LHRH agonists, on initial binding of the LHRH receptor, transiently stimulate LH release and thus cause an initial rise in testosterone level. This explains the transient flare of prostate cancer that can occur in men with advanced disease when therapy with an LHRH agonist is first started. This possibility must be considered in patients with impending spinal cord compression or urinary obstruction.

- Androgen deprivation accomplished with orchiectomy or medically.
- Luteinizing hormone-releasing hormone agonists depress androgen levels.
- These agonists initially stimulate release of luteinizing hormone and testosterone.

Antiandrogens compete with androgens at the receptor level. Examples include cyproterone and flutamide. To effect total androgen blockade, an antiandrogen is added to therapy in patients who have had orchiectomy or who are receiving an LHRH agonist (these block testicular testosterone production but do not block adrenal androgen production). A prospective U.S. study combining an LHRH analog with flutamide versus placebo suggested an advantage for the addition of flutamide. However, other studies of total blockade have failed to show an advantage. Studies comparing orchiectomy alone with orchiectomy plus flutamide are under way in the United States. One advantage of flutamide is that it blocks the "flare" induced by LHRH agonists.

- Some physicians believe flutamide should be used in

combination with orchiectomy or LHRH agonist.
- Flutamide blocks "flare" induced by LHRH agonists.

Prostate-Specific Antigen (PSA)

PSA is produced by normal and neoplastic prostatic ductal epithelium. Its concentration is proportional to the total prostatic mass. PSA's inability to differentiate benign prostatic hyperplasia from carcinoma renders it inadequate as the sole screening method for prostate cancer. PSA is useful for monitoring response to therapy in cases of known prostate cancer, particularly after radical prostatectomy.

- Concentration of PSA is proportional to total prostatic mass.
- PSA test inadequate as sole screening test for prostate cancer.
- PSA useful for monitoring response to therapy.

OVARIAN CANCER

This disease is diagnosed annually in 20,000 American women. It is the leading cause of death due to gynecologic cancer. There are no early warning signs; most patients present with vague gastrointestinal complaints such as bloating. Most patients (75%) present with advanced disease (i.e., stages III and IV, disease spread beyond the pelvis). The term "ovarian cancer" encompasses tumors derived from the ovarian surface epithelium, not germ cell tumors.

Staging

Stage I is confined to the ovary, stage II is confined to the pelvis, stage III includes spread to upper abdomen, and stage IV includes spread to distant sites.

- Ovarian cancer is leading cause of death due to gynecologic cancer.
- There are no early warning signs.
- Most patients (75%) present with advanced disease.

Screening

The tools evaluated thus far, namely, pelvic ultrasonography and determination of serum cancer antigen (CA)-125 are inadequate for screening the general female population. Screening for this disease is difficult for several reasons. The incidence of ovarian cancer is relatively low, and there are no recognized pre-invasive lesions. Moreover, pelvic ultrasonography and CA-125 lack suf-

ficient sensitivity and specificity. However, it seems reasonable to apply these techniques on a periodic basis to women at particularly high risk of ovarian cancer, for example, those with a family history of the disease. The cause of epithelial ovarian cancer is unknown. A small subset of patients (<5%) has an inherited predisposition to this disease. Generally, this occurs in families with both breast and ovarian cancer.

- Population screening for ovarian cancer is not generally recommended.
- Pelvic ultrasonography and CA-125 lack sufficient sensitivity and specificity.
- A small subset (<5%) of patients have an inherited predisposition to ovarian cancer and should be screened.

Treatment

The initial management of patients with epithelial ovarian cancer includes a thorough surgical staging and debulking procedure. Outcome in this disease depends on the amount of tumor tissue removed at initial operation. Subsequently, patients are treated with at least six cycles of platinum-based chemotherapy. The tumor antigen, CA-125, is expressed by approximately 85% of epithelial ovarian tumors and released into the circulation. The highest serum levels of CA-125 are found in patients with ovarian cancer, but the serum CA-125 level may also be increased in other malignancies, as well as in pregnancy, endometriosis, and menstruation. CA-125 is clearly of value for monitoring the course of ovarian cancer.

- Management of ovarian cancer includes thorough surgical staging and debulking followed by chemotherapy.
- Outcome depends on amount of tumor tissue removed at initial operation.
- CA-125 expressed by about 85% of epithelial ovarian tumors.
- CA-125 level may also be increased in other malignancies and in pregnancy, endometriosis, menstruation.
- CA-125 useful for monitoring course of disease.

TESTICULAR CANCER

Background

This cancer is diagnosed in 6,000 to 7,000 men annually. It is the most common carcinoma in males aged 15 to 35 years. It is highly curable, even when metastatic. At high risk are males with cryptorchid testes (40-fold relative risk) or Klinefelter's syndrome (also increased risk of breast cancer). Two broad categories are seminomas (40%) and nonseminomas. Types of nonseminomas include embryonal carcinoma, mature and immature teratoma, choriocarcinoma, yolk sac, and endodermal sinus tumors. There is often an admixture of several cell types within nonseminomas. Any nonseminomatous component plus seminoma is treated as a nonseminoma.

- Testicular cancer is the most common carcinoma in males 15-35 years old.
- Testicular cancer highly curable, even when metastatic.
- High-risk factors: cryptorchid testes, Klinefelter's syndrome.
- Two categories: seminomas (40%) and nonseminomas.

Evaluation of metastatic disease includes determination of β-human chorionic gonadotropin (hCG) and α-fetoprotein values and computed tomography of the abdomen (retroperitoneal nodes) and chest (mediastinal nodes or pulmonary nodules).

Staging

Stage I disease is confined to the testis, stage II includes infradiaphragmatic nodal metastases, stage III includes supradiaphragmatic nodal metastases, and stage IV includes extranodal metastases. About 85% of nonseminomas have elevated β-hCG or α-fetoprotein values. Approximately 10% of seminomas have increased β-hCG level. α-Fetoprotein value is never increased in pure seminoma; if present, tumor is nonseminoma and should be treated as such.

- 85% of nonseminomas have elevated β-hCG or α-fetoprotein.
- 10% of seminomas have increased β-hCG.
- α-Fetoprotein never increased in pure seminoma.

Management

Radical (inguinal) orchiectomy is the definitive procedure for both pathologic diagnosis and local control. Scrotal orchiectomy or biopsy is associated with a high incidence of local recurrence or spread to inguinal nodes. Following orchiectomy, the management depends on cell type (Table 23-9). Seminomas are radiosensitive. For stage I and nonbulky stage II seminoma, infradiaphrag-

matic lymphatic irradiation is used. The 5-year disease-free survival rate is >95%. For bulky stage II disease and stages III and IV, platinum-based chemotherapy is used. Approximately 85% of patients are cured. For stage I nonseminoma, close follow-up is often used rather than immediate retroperitoneal node dissection (a controversial approach). For stages II through IV, platinum-based chemotherapy is given. Cure rates are >95% for minimal metastatic disease, 90% for moderate bulk disease, and about 50% for bulky disease (multiple pulmonary metastases, bulky abdominal masses, liver, bone, or central nervous system metastases).

- Radical orchiectomy is definitive initial procedure for testicular cancer.
- Early-stage seminoma is treated with x-ray therapy.
- Stage I nonseminoma may require no treatment after orchiectomy.
- Platinum-based chemotherapy is used for all other patients and results in high cure rates.

Table 23-9.--Management of Testicular Cancer

Stage	Treatment, by cell type	
	Seminona	Nonseminoma
I	XRT	? Observe
II	XRT	Chemo
III	Chemo	Chemo
IV	Chemo	Chemo

Chemo, chemotherapy; XRT, x-ray therapy.

Extragonadal Germ Cell Tumor

This is uncommon. Patients present with elevated hCG or α-fetoprotein values with midline mass lesions (retroperitoneum, mediastinum, or pineal gland). No gonadal primary tumor is identifiable on examination or ultrasonography. Cisplatin-based chemotherapy is frequently curative.

MELANOMA

Background

Malignant melanoma is increasing at a rapid rate. If current trends continue, by the year 2,000 approximately 1% of Americans will have a malignant melanoma. Fortunately, the 5-year survival rate has doubled from approximately 40% in the 1940s to approximately 80%

now, a change attributed to earlier detection. This disease is far more common in populations living at high altitudes and those living close to the equator. Its incidence is higher in fair-skinned persons.

- Incidence of malignant melanoma increasing rapidly.
- 5-year survival rate has doubled as result of earlier detection.
- Disease is related to sunlight exposure.

Diagnosis: "ABCD"

Keys to the diagnosis include the following:

A: Asymmetry, especially a changing lesion
B: Borders are irregular
C: Color is variable, especially with blues, blacks, and tans dispersed throughout the lesion
D: Diameter ≥ 6 mm

Excisional biopsy is recommended. The thickness (i.e., depth of penetration of the tumor from the epidermis into the dermis/subcutis) of a malignant melanoma is the best independent predictor of survival (Table 23-10).

Table 23-10.--Ten-Year Survival in Melanoma, by Depth of Tumor

Depth, mm	% alive
<0.85	96
0.85-1.69	87
1.7-3.6	66.5
>3.6	46

Data from Friedman RJ, Rigel DS, Silverman MK, Kopf AW, Vossaert KA: Malignant melanoma in the 1990s: the continued importance of early detection and the role of physician examination and self-examination of the skin. CA Cancer J Clin 41:201-226, July/Aug 1991.

Management

Surgical excision remains the principal treatment for primary malignant melanoma. The preferred approach is wide local excision to achieve a 1- to 3-cm margin. In the absence of palpable adenopathy, a lymph node dissection is not routinely performed. However, with palpable nodes, a node dissection is standard practice. Metastatic melanoma is incurable with current approaches.

PARANEOPLASTIC SYNDROMES

General

These syndromes are defined as the effects of a cancer occurring at a distance from the tumor; they are called "remote effects." They do not indicate metastatic disease. The syndromes and associated tumor types are listed in Table 23-11.

Carcinoid Syndrome

This is caused by peptide mediators secreted by carcinoid tumors of the small intestine which have metastasized extensively to the liver. It is less frequent with primary carcinoids arising from other sites such as lung, thymus, or ovary. Most common symptoms are episodic flushing and diarrhea; bronchospasm may occur. Flushing and diarrhea may occur spontaneously or be precipitated by emotional factors or ingestion of food or alcohol. Carcinoid heart disease (right-sided valvular disease) is a potential late complication.

Lambert-Eaton Syndrome

This consists of muscle weakness (proximal) and gait disturbance. Strength is increased with exercise. It is associated with small-cell lung cancer.

Dermatomyositis

The female:male ratio is 2:1. Findings include muscle weakness (proximal), inflammatory myopathy, and increased creatine kinase values. Skin changes are variable and include heliotrope rash, periorbital edema, and Gottron's papules. Underlying malignancy (lung, breast, gastrointestinal) is common in patients >50 years old.

CHEMOTHERAPY

Basic Concepts

Currently, approximately 40 cytotoxic agents are available for use in North America. Taken generally, chemotherapeutic agents impair the process of cell division. Their selectivity for tumor cells is based primarily on a higher replicative rate in neoplastic cells. This selectivity for rapidly dividing cells explains the typical patterns of toxicity that occur with chemotherapy (i.e., bone marrow, gastrointestinal mucosa, and hair follicles). The general classes and mechanisms of chemotherapeutics are shown in Figure 23-5.

Applications

The settings in which chemotherapy is used are 1) advanced disease, 2) as adjuvant therapy after definitive local treatment, and 3) as primary or "neo-adjuvant" therapy. The last application refers to situations in which

Table 23-11.--Classification of Paraneoplastic Syndromes

Syndrome	Mediator	Tumor type
Endocrine		
Cushing's syndrome[*]	ACTH	Small-cell lung cancer
SIADH[*]	ADH	Lung, especially small cell
Hypercalcemia[*]	PTH-like peptide	Lung, especially squamous; breast; myeloma
Carcinoid syndrome	? serotonin ? substance P	Gut neuroendocrine tumors
Hypoglycemia	Insulin Insulin-like growth factors	Gut neuroendocrine tumors; other
Neuromuscular		
Cerebellar degeneration	Anti-Purkinje cell antibodies	Lung, especially small cell; ovarian; breast
Dementia	?	Lung
Peripheral neuropathy[*]	Autoantibodies	Lung, gastrointestinal, breast
Lambert-Eaton	Antibodies to cholinergic receptor	Small-cell lung cancer
Dermatomyositis	?	Lung, breast
Skin		
Dermatomyositis	?	Lung, breast
Acanthosis nigricans	? TGF-α	Intra-abdominal cancer, usually gastric
Hematologic		
Venous thrombosis[*]	Activators of clotting cascade and platelets	Various adenocarcinomas, especially pancreatic and gastric
Nonbacterial thrombotic endocarditis	Activators of clotting cascade and platelets	Various adenocarcinomas, especially pancreatic and gastric

[*]Most common types.
ACTH, adrenocorticotropic hormone; ADH, antidiuretic hormone; PTH, parathyroid hormone; SIADH, syndrome of inappropriate secretion of antidiuretic hormone; TGF-α, transforming growth factor-α.

patients present with a locally advanced malignancy and initial tumor reduction is needed before a primary treatment (i.e., surgery or radiation) can be applied.

Solid Tumors Sensitive to Chemotherapy

Germ cell tumors of the testis and ovary, choriocarcinomas, breast cancer, ovarian cancer, and small-cell lung cancer are in this category. In recent years, combination chemotherapy regimens have also produced impressive tumor reductions in transitional cell carcinomas of the bladder, head and neck cancer, and cervical cancer.

Why Chemotherapy Fails to Cure Most Advanced Solid Tumors

The reasons for failure are 1) tumor cell heterogeneity, including populations of cells resistant to cytotoxic agents; 2) large numbers of noncycling or resting cells; and 3) pharmacologic sanctuaries--blood-tissue barriers and blood supply-tumor barriers.

Side Effects

The most common side effects of various chemotherapeutic agents are outlined in Table 23-12.

Mechanisms of Tumor Cell Drug Resistance

The mechanisms include decreased drug uptake, increased drug efflux, decreased drug activation, increased drug inactivation, and increased production of a target enzyme.

Tumor cells may be resistant to a specific drug or they can have broad cross-resistance to structurally dissimilar drugs. This latter phenomenon is referred to as "multidrug resistance." This seems to be mediated by a large plasma membrane glycoprotein, termed the "p-glycoprotein," that functions as an energy-dependent drug-efflux pump.

- Tumor cells may be resistant to structurally dissimilar chemotherapy drugs ("multidrug resistance").

CHEMOTHERAPY

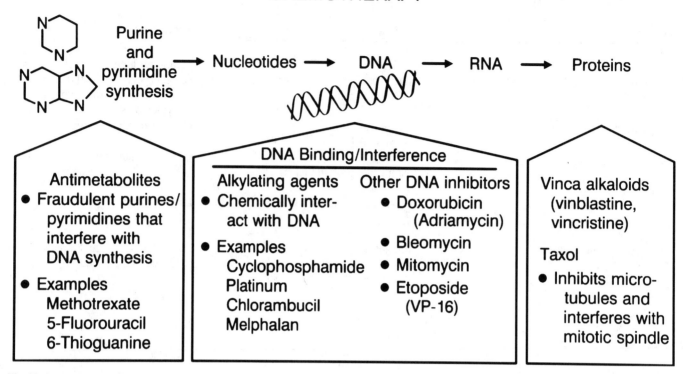

Fig. 23-5. General classes of chemotherapeutic agents.

Table 23-12.--Side Effects of Chemotherapy

Class or agent	Side effects	
	Acute	Chronic
Alkylating agents	Nausea, vomiting	Marrow: secondary leukemias
	Marrow	Pulmonary
		Gonads: decreased fertility, premature menopause
Cisplatin	Nausea, vomiting	
	Renal: ↓ GFR; tubular damage leads to electrolyte losses, especially cations	Renal: ↓ GFR; tubular damage and electrolyte losses, especially cations
	Peripheral neuropathy	Peripheral neuropathy
	Tinnitus, hearing loss	Tinnitus, hearing loss
Doxorubicin	Nausea, vomiting	Cardiac
	Marrow	Congestive heart failure
	Cardiac	Cumulative, dose-dependent, occurs in
	Pump or conduction	1%-10% of patients receiving 550 mg/m^2
	Stomatitis	
Bleomycin	Pulmonary	Pulmonary (may be aggravated by high FIO$_2$, as
	Skin (hyperpigmentation)	in perioperative period)
	Fever	
Antimetabolites	Mucositis/diarrhea	
	Marrow	
Microtubule inhibitors	Neuropathy	Neuropathy
Vincristine	Cardiac (taxol): conduction	
Taxol		

FIO$_2$, fraction of inspired oxygen; GFR, glomerular filtration rate.

Colony-Stimulating Factors

In recent years, bone marrow colony-stimulating factors have been isolated and are now available for clinical use. These naturally occurring glycoproteins stimulate the proliferation, differentiation, and function of specific cells in the bone marrow. They may act at the level of the earliest stem cell or at later mature functional cells. They differ in their specificity.

Granulocyte colony-stimulating factor (G-CSF), for example, acts fairly specifically to stimulate the production of mature neutrophils; granulocyte-macrophage CSF (GM-CSF) acts more generally, stimulating several cell lineages, including monocytes, eosinophils, and neutrophils. Both G-CSF and GM-CSF have been used to stimulate the marrow to recover after chemotherapy-induced myelosuppression. As a general rule, CSFs do not affect the depth of the leukocyte nadir but shorten the duration of neutropenia. Unfortunately, no currently available CSF reliably protects against thrombocytopenia.

ONCOLOGIC COMPLICATIONS AND EMERGENCIES

Hypercalcemia

The most common underlying causes are malignancies and primary hyperparathyroidism. Patients with primary hyperparathyroidism have elevated serum parathyroid hormone values, but parathyroid hormone (PTH) is suppressed in cancer-associated hypercalcemia. Cancer-related hypercalcemia is often mediated by a PTH-related protein secreted by the tumor. This PTH-related protein can be detected with current assays. Tumors can also cause hypercalcemia by secreting other bone-resorbing substances or by enhancing conversion of 25-hydroxyvitamin D to 1,25-dihydroxyvitamin D. Another mechanism is due to the local effects of osteolytic bone metastases.

Effects on bone and kidney contribute to hypercalcemia. Accelerated bone resorption is due to activation of osteoclasts by various mediators, primarily the PTH-like peptide. The same factors that induce osteoclast-mediated bone resorption also stimulate renal tubular reabsorption of calcium. The hypercalcemic state interferes with renal resorption of sodium and water, leading to polyuria and eventual depletion of extracellular fluid volume. This reduces glomerular filtration rate, further increasing serum calcium level. Immobilization tips the balance toward bone resorption, worsening the hypercalcemia.

- PTH suppressed in cancer-associated hypercalcemia.
- This disease often mediated by PTH-related protein secreted by tumor.
- Bone and kidney pathophysiology lead to elevated calcium level.

Symptoms of hypercalcemia include gastrointestinal (anorexia, nausea, vomiting, constipation), renal (polyuria, polydipsia, dehydration), central nervous system (cognitive difficulties, apathy, somnolence, or even coma), and cardiovascular (hypertension, shortened QT, enhanced sensitivity to digitalis).

Cancers associated with hypercalcemia include lung (squamous cell), renal, myeloma, lymphoma, breast, and head and neck. Patients with breast cancer and those with myeloma are more likely to have bony involvement with their disease.

For treatment of hypercalcemia, the magnitude of the hypercalcemia and the degree of symptoms are key considerations. Generally, patients with a serum calcium value >14 mg/dL should be hospitalized for immediate treatment. The serum calcium value should be adjusted if the serum albumin value is abnormal. The conversion formula is 0.8 mg/dL of serum total calcium for every 1 g of serum albumin more or less than 4 g/dL. If the serum albumin value is elevated (as with dehydration), the total calcium value should be adjusted downward; if the serum albumin value is reduced (as in chronic illness), the total calcium value should be adjusted upward.

For hydration, intravenously administered normal saline (200-400 mL/hr) is initially given. Loop diuretics are used after volume expansion. Furosemide facilitates urinary excretion of calcium by inhibiting calcium resorption in the thick ascending loop of Henle. A loop diuretic will help correct for volume overload once the patient has been rehydrated. Specific agents are listed below:

1. Bisphosphonates (pamidronate or etidronate) are given intravenously (gastrointestinal absorption is poor). They bind to hydroxyapatite and inhibit osteoclasts.
2. Gallium nitrate (200 mg/m^2 per day) is given as continuous intravenous infusion for 5 days (unless normocalcemia is achieved earlier). It is a highly effective inhibitor of bone resorption.
3. Mithramycin (25 μg/kg) is given intravenously over 4 hours; this treatment can be repeated if necessary.

Maximal hypocalcemic effect is reached at 48-72 hours. It is associated with hepatic and renal side effects.

4. Glucocorticoids have an antitumor effect on neoplastic lymphoid tissue.

5. Calcitonin is given subcutaneously or intramuscularly. It has a rapid onset of action; thus, it is useful in immediate life-threatening situations. It is a relatively weak agent with short-lived effect. Allergic reactions to salmon calcitonin are unusual, but an initial skin test with 1 unit is recommended before a full dose is given.

- Volume expansion must precede administration of furosemide.
- Furosemide inhibits calcium resorption in thick ascending loop of Henle.
- Bisphosphonates bind to hydroxyapatite and inhibit osteoclasts.
- Mithramycin has hepatic and renal side effects.
- Calcitonin relatively weak agent with rapid, short-lived effect.

Tumor Lysis Syndrome

This syndrome occurs as a result of the overwhelming release of tumor cell contents into the bloodstream such that concentrations of certain substances become life-threatening. It most commonly occurs in cancers with large tumor burdens and high proliferation rates which are exquisitely sensitive to chemotherapy. Examples include high-grade lymphomas, leukemia, and, much less commonly, solid tumors. The syndrome is characterized by increased uric acid, which leads to renal complications; acidosis; increased potassium, which can cause lethal cardiac arrhythmias; increased phosphate, which leads to acute renal failure; and decreased calcium, which causes muscle cramps, cardiac arrhythmias, and tetany. The syndrome can be prevented with adequate hydration, alkalinization, and administration of allopurinol before chemotherapy.

- Tumor lysis syndrome is result of overwhelming release of tumor cell contents into bloodstream.
- Most common in cancers with large tumor burdens and high proliferation rates exquisitely sensitive to chemotherapy.
- Characterized by increased uric acid, increased potassium, increased phosphate, acidosis, and decreased calcium.

Febrile Neutropenia

This is defined as temperature $\geq38.5°C$ on one occasion or three episodes $\geq38.0°C$ plus an absolute neutrophil count $\leq500 \times 10^9/L$ (or leukocyte count $\leq1,000 \times 10^9/L$). Management involves immediate hospitalization and institution of parenteral, broad-spectrum antibiotics. Patients usually have no infection documented, but appropriate cultures should be rapidly obtained before antibiotics are given. Use of colony-stimulating factors at the time of documentation of febrile neutropenia is controversial.

Spinal Cord Compression

Acute cord compression is a neurologic emergency. It results most commonly from epidural compression by metastatic tumor (lung, breast, prostate, myeloma, kidney). Occasionally, compression can occur from neighboring nodal involvement and tumor infiltration through intervertebral foramina (lymphoma). The locations are cervical in 10% of cases, thoracic in 70%, and lumbar in 20%. Multiple noncontiguous levels are involved in 10%-40%.

More than 90% of patients present with pain. Cervical pain may radiate down the arm. Thoracic pain radiates around the rib cage or abdominal wall; it may be described as a compressing band bilaterally around chest or abdomen. Lumbar pain may radiate into the groin or down the leg. Pain may be aggravated by coughing, sneezing, or straight-leg raising. Focal neurologic signs depend on the level affected. Paresthesias (tingling, numbness), weakness, and altered reflexes also can be present (Table 23-13). Tenderness over the spine may help localize the level. Autonomic changes of urinary or fecal retention or incontinence may be present.

Table 23-13.--Reflexes and Their Corresponding Roots and Muscles

Reflex	Root(s)	Muscle
Biceps	C5-6	Biceps
Triceps	C7-8	Triceps
Knee jerk	L2-4	Quadriceps
Ankle jerk	S1	Gastrocnemius

Imaging studies include bone scanning or plain radiography, which reveal vertebral metastases in approximately 85% of patients with epidural compression.

Myelography or magnetic resonance imaging of entire spine is generally recommended

Treatment usually includes an initial bolus of 10-100 mg of dexamethasone intravenously, depending on the severity of block. Thereafter, dexamethasone is given (4 mg four times a day), although some physicians favor higher doses for a few days followed by a rapid taper. Radiation therapy is applied to involved area(s). Surgery is used in select circumstances: if no previous diagnosis of malignancy, spine instability, prior radiation to cord tolerance, and progressive neurologic decline despite radiation.

Outcome depends on the patient's neurologic function at presentation (Table 23-14).

Table 23-14.--Outcome of Patients With Spinal Cord Compression, by Neurologic Status

Status at presentation	% ambulatory after radiation
Ambulatory	>80
Paraparetic	<50
Paraplegic	<10

PALLIATIVE CARE

Background

More than 70% of patients with cancer have significant pain during the course of their disease. Evaluation should include 1) a history regarding onset, quality, severity, and location of pain; exacerbating and relieving factors; associated symptoms; and 2) physical examination, which should include a complete neurologic examination. Diagnostic studies are determined by the results of the history and physical examination.

Treatment

Three-Tiered Approach

Step 1: For mild pain, administer acetaminophen or a nonsteroidal anti-inflammatory drug around-the-clock. Step 2: When step 1 fails to provide adequate analgesia, or for moderate pain, add codeine or oxycodone. Step 3: For severe pain or adequate pain relief with steps 1 and 2, agents include morphine, hydromorphone, levorphanol, methadone, and fentanyl (Table 23-15).

General Principles

Choose the appropriate drug and route. Generally, the oral route is preferred. Orally administered immediate-release morphine is the usual first-line drug selected for severe pain from cancer. Begin with a low dose. Titrate the dose until analgesia is achieved or side effects occur. There is no "standard dose"; therapy must be individualized. Use around-the-clock dosing with "rescue" doses available to the patient for breakthrough pain. The fentanyl patch (a transdermal formulation) delivers drug continuously over 72 hours. It is especially useful for patients with poor tolerance of orally administered opioids or those unable to take medications orally. Adverse effects of opioids include sedation, nausea, constipation, respiratory depression, and myoclonus. No narcotic is more or less likely to result in a particular side effect profile. However, one narcotic may produce an adverse effect in a patient whereas another will not. Thus, sequential trials of different opioids may be needed to determine the one best suited for a patient.

Table 23-15.--Doses of Narcotics That Provide Equal Analgesia

Drug	Doses of equal analgesia	Half-life, hr	Peak effect, hr	Duration of effect, hr
Morphine	10 mg i.m./i.v.	2-4	0.5-1	4-6
	20-60 mg p.o.*	2-4	2	4-6
Slow-release morphine	20-60 mg p.o.*	3-4	4-6	8-12
Hydromorphone	1.5 mg i.m	2-3	0.5-1	4-6
	7.5 mg p.o.	2-3	1-2	4-6
Levorphanol	2.0 mg i.m.	12-16	0.5-1	4-6
	4.0 mg p.o.	12-16	1	4-6
Methadone	10 mg i.m.	15-150+	0.5-1.5	4-6
	20 mg p.o.	15-150+	0.5-1.5	4-6
Codeine	130 mg i.m.	2-4	1	4-6
	200 mg p.o.	2-4	1-2	4-6
Oxycodone	30 mg p.o.	2-3	1	3-6
Meperidine	75 mg i.m.	3-4	0.5-1	3-5
	300 mg p.o.	3-4	1-2	4-6
Fentanyl	0.1 mg i.v.	3-4	0.25	0.5-2
	Transdermal patch	See text	See text	72

*Relative potency of intramuscular:oral morphine changes from 1:6 to 1:2-3 with chronic dosing.
i.m., intramuscular; i.v., intravenous; p.o., oral dose.
Modified from Foley KM: The treatment of cancer pain. N. Engl. J. Med. 313:84-95, 1985. By permission of the journal.

QUESTIONS
(See "Answers" section)

Multiple Choice

1. A 60-year-old woman found a new abnormality in her left breast. Her local physician concurred that there was a suspicious nodule in the left breast at the 3-o'clock position. A mammogram was normal. What would you recommend?
   a. One month of oral contraceptives and repeat examination
   b. Wire localization biopsy
   c. Mastectomy
   d. Excisional biopsy
   e. Repeat mammogram in 3 months

2. Which of the following would not be expected as a long-term consequence of tamoxifen use?
   a. Decrease in recurrence of breast cancer in postmenopausal patients with node-positive disease
   b. Loss of bone density
   c. Hot flashes
   d. Endometrial hyperplasia
   e. Thromboembolic events

3. A 40-year-old woman presents with a newly detected 1-cm nodule in the tail of her left breast. An excisional biopsy shows the presence of an infiltrating ductal adenocarcinoma. Axillary node dissection reveals tumor involvement in 2 of 21 nodes. The estrogen receptor is positive at 31 fmol/mg and the progesterone receptor is positive at 60 fmol/mg. A mastectomy is performed. The patient is still menstruating regularly. The most appropriate course of

action is:
a. Postoperative irradiation to the ipsilateral chest wall and nodal areas
b. Close follow-up every 3 months for 3 years and every 6 months for 2 additional years
c. Six cycles of adjuvant cyclophosphamide, methotrexate, and 5-fluorouracil
d. Five years of adjuvant tamoxifen
e. Two years of adjuvant tamoxifen

4. Which of the following is not an established risk factor for breast cancer?
a. First-degree relative with breast cancer in her 30s
b. Use of oral contraceptives
c. Previous breast biopsy showing atypical hyperplasia
d. Late menopause
e. Nulliparity

5. A 60-year-old woman has made several visits to her physician during the last several months with gastrointestinal complaints. Currently, she complains of abdominal bloating and early satiety. An abdominal examination is unrevealing, but a pelvic examination discloses a large mass. The patient undergoes operation, and extensive abdominal carcinomatosis is detected, apparently resulting from a large right ovarian papillary serous carcinoma. The most appropriate management strategy would begin with:
a. Whole abdominal radiation therapy
b. Symptomatic and supportive care
c. Cisplatin-based combination chemotherapy
d. Hysterectomy, bilateral salpingo-oophorectomy, omentectomy, and debulking
e. Leuprolide

6. Which of the following factors is the best predictor of outcome in patients with malignant melanoma?
a. Age of patient
b. Lifetime sunlight exposure
c. Thickness of the primary lesion
d. Use of adjuvant irradiation
e. Performance of a node dissection

7. Small cell carcinoma of the lung is associated with all except which of the following paraneoplastic syndromes?
a. Syndrome of inappropriate secretion of antidiuretic hormone

b. Cerebellar degeneration due to anti-Purkinje cell antibodies
c. Lambert-Eaton syndrome
d. Right-sided heart failure with prominent tricuspid regurgitation
e. Cushing's syndrome

8. What cancer is most likely to be associated with ectopic adrenocorticotropic hormone production?
a. Squamous cell carcinoma of the lung
b. Small cell carcinoma of the lung
c. Adrenal carcinoma
d. Pituitoma
e. Prostate cancer

9. Cigarette smoking has been linked with all except which of the following cancers?
a. Lung
b. Esophagus
c. Bladder
d. Oral cavity
e. Breast

10. A 63-year-old nun with metastatic breast cancer to bone presents with a 1- to 2-week history of fatigue, anorexia, nausea, vomiting, and constipation. She is lethargic on examination; the neurologic examination is nonfocal. Blood evaluation reveals a calcium value of 15 mg/dL and a creatinine value of 2.0 mg/dL. The most appropriate first step in management is:
a. Oral phosphate
b. Intravenous furosemide
c. Mithramycin
d. Normal saline
e. Tamoxifen

True/False

11. Which of the following are true concerning serum tumor markers of testicular carcinoma?
a. α-Fetoprotein value is increased only in patients with nonseminomatous germ cell malignancies
b. β-Human chorionic gonadotropin value is increased in 50% of patients with seminoma
c. In the absence of radiographic or examination evidence of malignancy, increasing levels of α-fetoprotein or β-chorionic gonadotropin are of no clinical significance
d. Most patients with nonseminomatous germ cell tumors have elevated values of tumor markers

12. A 38-year-old man presents with a 6-week history of increasing retrosternal fullness and dyspnea. Physical examination is totally normal. Chest radiography reveals a large (18-cm) anterior mediastinal mass. Abdominal computed tomography is negative. Tests for the following should be ordered:
    a. Carcinoembryonic antigen
    b. CA-125
    c. Prostate-specific antigen
    d. α-Fetoprotein

13. A 68-year-old woman presents with a 3-cm mass in the right breast. Mammography confirms the presence of an abnormality and reveals no other lesions. A biopsy reveals an infiltrating ductal carcinoma. Which of the following statements are true?
    a. Node dissection is indicated only if there is palpable adenopathy
    b. If the patient chooses lumpectomy, axillary dissection is not necessary
    c. Lumpectomy followed by close observation is an option
    d. For this patient, either mastectomy or breast conservation is an option
    e. Given the size of the lesion, a modified radical mastectomy is indicated
    f. Neoadjuvant chemotherapy provides the best chance for long-term disease-free status

14. Resistance to chemotherapy is complex. The following mechanisms are thought to mediate drug resistance:
    a. Presence of noncycling or resting tumor cells
    b. Decreased drug uptake
    c. Increased drug efflux
    d. Increased drug activation
    e. Enhanced DNA repair
    f. Increased production of a target enzyme

CHAPTER 24
PREVENTIVE MEDICINE

Philip T. Hagen, M.D.

DEFINITIONS

Preventive medicine is the practice of medicine that detects and alters or ameliorates 1) host susceptibility in a premorbid state (e.g., immunization), 2) risk factors for disease in a predisease state (e.g., elevated cholesterol level), and 3) disease in the presymptomatic state (e.g., in situ cervical cancer). Not all disease is preventable because 1) not all risk factors (or all individuals at risk) are known, 2) the cost of screening everyone is not feasible, 3) barriers to medical access exist, 4) interval disease occurs, 5) characteristics of the target disease vary, 6) screening tests are imperfect, and 7) treatments are imperfect.

Primary prevention is the prevention of disease occurrence (e.g., immunization to prevent infection and blood pressure control to prevent stroke). *Secondary prevention* is the detection and amelioration of disease in a presymptomatic or preclinical stage (e.g., mammography detects small foci of cancer and Pap smear detects in situ cancer). *Tertiary prevention* is the prevention of future negative health effects of existing clinical disease (e.g., use of aspirin and β-blockers after myocardial infarction to prevent recurrence).

Efficacy is the potential or maximum benefit derived from applying a test or procedure under ideal circumstances (e.g., research studies with compliant patients, with ideal testing conditions, techniques, etc.). *Effectiveness* is the actual benefit that is derived from a test or procedure that is applied under usual--less than ideal--circumstances. Randomized trials in which results are analyzed by the "intention to treat" principle, i.e., all members of a group are included in the analysis whether they complied or not, gives a measure of effectiveness in a population. *Cost effectiveness* is the unit of cost incurred to achieve a given level of effectiveness. It is often expressed as the dollars spent per year of life saved. Often, the most cost-effective method of testing is not the most effective. For example, performing Pap smears every 5 or 10 years is more cost-effective, but performing them every year is more effective.

- Cost effectiveness: cost incurred to achieve a given level of effectiveness.
- The most cost-effective test may not be the most effective test or treatment.

Years of potential life lost is one measure of the relative impact of a disease on society. This term usually refers to the years lost due to death from a disease before age 65 (or sometimes 70). For example, colon cancer kills approximately 57,000 men and women annually and breast cancer kills approximately 46,000 women. However, on average, breast cancer kills at a younger age and so has nearly 3x as many "years of potential life lost."

- Years of potential life lost: the years lost due to death from a disease before age 65 (or sometimes 70).

Incidence (rate) refers to the number of new events (deaths, diagnoses) that occur in a population in a given time (e.g., 140 cancer deaths per 100,000 people in the U.S. annually). *Prevalence* refers to the number of cases of a condition existing at a point in time in a population (e.g., currently, 1,200,000 people in the U.S. are infected with the HIV virus).

PRINCIPLES OF SCREENING FOR DISEASE

The term *mass screening* is generally applied to the relatively indiscriminate testing of a population with the intent to improve the aggregate health of the population but not necessarily of every person in the population. An example is blood pressure or cholesterol testing in a public setting such as a shopping mall.

- Mass screening: indiscriminate testing of a population to improve the aggregate health of the population.

Case finding is the technical term often used for screening conducted in the office setting. The intent is to detect asymptomatic disease and to improve the health of the individual. In this setting, the dictum of "first do no harm" is important because testing is applied to asymptomatic persons.

- Case finding: screening conducted in the office setting to detect asymptomatic disease and to improve the health of an individual.

Desirable Screening

1. Disease characteristics: the diseases screened should be common, cause significant morbidity and mortality, have a long preclinical phase (which is curable/modifiable), have an effective treatment that is available to those screened, and have an acceptable treatment (i.e., one that is not excessively painful or disfiguring).
2. Test characteristics: the tests should be inexpensive, safe, acceptable, easy to administer, technically easy to perform, highly sensitive, and have a complementary, highly specific confirmatory test.
3. Host characteristics: the person be at risk, have access to testing, be likely to comply with follow-up testing, and have adequate overall life expectancy/functional life expectancy.

Burden of U.S. Disease

Diseases that cause the most morbidity and mortality in the U.S. may or may not be amenable to screening or case finding. Heart disease and cancer are clearly the leading causes of death in the U.S. (Tables 24-1 and 24-2). The most recent year for which actual statistics exist is 1989.

Table 24-1.--Mortality for Leading Causes of Death in The U. S., 1989

	No. of deaths	Death rate per 100,000 population[*]	% of total deaths
Heart diseases	733,867	231.5	34.1
Cancer	496,152	171.3	23.1
Cerebrovascular diseases	145,551	44.3	6.8
Accidents	95,028	35.0	4.4
Chronic obstructive lung diseases	84,344	27.5	3.9

[*]Age-adjusted to the 1970 U.S. standard population.
From Boring CC, Squires TS, Tong T: Cancer statistics, 1993. CA Cancer J Clin 43:7-26, Jan/Feb, 1993. By permission of American Cancer Society.

Cancer Screening

Lung Cancer

Lung cancer is a highly lethal/virulent form of cancer (it kills most of the people it afflicts) and is the leading cause of cancer death for men and women. Burden of disease (1993 estimates from the American Cancer Society): 170,000 new cases, 149,000 deaths. Peak incidence is 470/100,000 in 75-year-old men and 155/100,000 in 70-year-old women. Risk factors include 1) smoking--10x increased risk over nonsmoker and 2.5x increase over population average incidence rates; 2) age--70 year old, 10x greater risk than for 40 year old; 3) sex--male-to-female ratio is 3:1 and is primarily related to duration and intensity of smoking; 4) industrial, occupational, environmental exposure--asbestos, hydrocarbons, uranium, radon. Tests include chest radiography and sputum cytology. Screening probably is not effective. Although the Mayo Clinic Lung Project detected more cancers, mortality was not altered in approximately 12 years of follow-up study. This may have been because of "overdiagnosis" of clinically irrelevant lesions or lead-time bias. Annual chest radiography (or sputum cytology) solely to look for treatable stage lung cancer should not

Table 24-2.--Cancer Mortality for Women and Men, 1989 (U.S. Vital Statistics)

Age, yr					
35-54		55-74		≥75	
Women					
Breast	8,983	Lung	28,925	Colon and rectum	15,650
Lung	5,226	Breast	20,164	Lung	13,820
Uterus	1,883	Colon and rectum	11,447	Breast	13,027
Colon and rectum	1,881	Ovary	6,537	Pancreas	6,044
Ovary	1,676	Pancreas	5,755	Non-Hodgkin's lymphomas	4,080
Men					
Lung	8,875	Lung	55,339	Lung	24,673
Colon and rectum	2,278	Colon and rectum	14,409	Prostate	18,391
Non-Hodgkin's lymphoma	1,458	Prostate	11,798	Colon and rectum	11,368
Brain and CNS	1,368	Pancreas	6,707	Pancreas	4,026
Skin	1,265	Esophagus	4,438	Bladder	3,588

From Boring CC, Squires TS, Tong T: Cancer statistics, 1993. CA Cancer J Clin 43:7-26, Jan/Feb, 1993. By permission of American Cancer Society.

be performed. Smoking is the leading preventable cause of cancer in the U.S. (and a leading cause of heart disease and stroke).

- Lung cancer: the leading cause of cancer death for men and women.
- Risk factors for lung cancer: smoking, age, sex (3:1 male-to-female ratio), environmental exposure.
- Annual chest radiography (or sputum cytology) solely to look for treatable stage lung cancer should not be performed.
- Smoking is the leading preventable cause of cancer in the U.S.
- Physician advice to quit smoking and referral to smoke cessation counseling are probably the most cost-effective preventive measures available.

Breast Cancer

Breast cancer is the second leading cause of cancer death for women. The lifetime risk is estimated at 1 in 9 women. Burden of disease (1993 estimates from the American Cancer Society): 182,000 new cases and 46,000 deaths. Thus, breast cancer is moderately lethal/virulent (it kills many but not most of the people it afflicts). The risk factors include 1) age--the risk increases throughout life, and the risk for an 80-year-old woman is 12x that for a 30-year-old woman; 2) family history--one first-degree relative with breast cancer, 2x-4x risk and two first-degree relatives, 3x-8x risk (if no first-degree relatives, slight-

ly reduced risk); 3) socioeconomic status--high, increases risk 2x-4x; 4) nulliparity or age at first full-term pregnancy--if >30 years old, risk is increased 2x-4x; 5) history of benign proliferative disease--dysplastic mammographic parenchymal patterns, history of breast cancer, and high-dose radiation all increase risk approximately 2x. Risk factor analysis can define a subgroup that concentrates 85% of breast cancer in 40% of women, a relative risk of approximately 2x for the high-risk group and 0.25x for the low-risk group.

- Breast cancer: the second leading cause of cancer death for women.
- Lifetime risk: 1 in 9 women.
- One first-degree relative with breast cancer, 2x-4x risk; two first-degree relatives, 3x-8x risk.

Screening procedures include:
1. Breast self-examination: recommended to the patient but not of demonstrated effectiveness.
2. Clinical breast examination: has a sensitivity of about 50%-70% and a specificity >90% and costs about $25.
3. Screen film mammography: has a sensitivity of 80%-95% for women ≥50 years old and 60%-80% for women younger than 50. Specificity is 95%-99%. Positive predictive values (PPV) are about 5%-10%, with 20%-50% of biopsies revealing cancer, depending on age (higher percentages in older

women). The cost is about $100.

4. Randomized control trials worldwide have examined the effectiveness of mammography. They showed an approximate 30% decrease in mortality, but only two showed statistical significance. Data are conflicting or inconclusive in women younger than 50 years or older than 70.

- Breast physical examination has a sensitivity of 50%-70% and a specificity of >90%.
- Mammography has a sensitivity of 80%-95% and a specificity of 95%-99%.
- Studies are inconclusive about the benefit of mammography for women younger than 50 and older than 70 years.

Screening risks--Radiation is estimated to produce 60 additional breast cancers in 1,000,000 women screened compared with the 93,000 cases expected to be detected. Breast cancer detection and demonstration project showed that 2% of women were referred for surgical evaluation/aspiration, and of those referred for biopsy, half were cancer in 50 to 65-year old women. About 3% of women 40-49 years old were referred for biopsy, with a smaller percentage yielding cancer.

- Radiation: 60 additional breast cancers in 1,000,000 women screened.
- Approximately 2% of screened women 50-65 years old will have biopsy and 3% of women 40-49 years old.

Cost effectiveness: if 25% of women 40-75 years old in the U.S. were screened annually, 11,000,000/year would be screened at a cost of $1.3 billion annually for physical examination and mammography. The cost of screening and the work-up would be 100x as expensive as the costs saved by reduced treatment. Cost per year of life saved ranges from about $9,000 to $12,000, with the lower costs in the 50-year-old group and higher costs in the older age group.

- Cost of screening and work-up would be 100x as expensive as the costs saved by reduced treatment.
- Cost per year of life saved is $9,000-$12,000.

Recommendations:
1. General agreement--clinical breast examination yearly after age 40, clinical breast examination and mammography yearly for women 50-65 years old. Otherwise, recommendations vary.
2. American Cancer Society and several other groups--Clinical breast examination yearly for women ≥40 years old and mammography every 1-2 years. For women ≥50 years old, annual clinical breast examination and mammography.
3. United States Preventive Services Task Force (USPSTF)--Annual clinical breast examination for women 40-49 years old and annual clinical breast examination and mammography every 1-2 years for women ≥50 years old. Screening may begin sooner for women at high risk.
4. American College of Physicians and American Academy of Family Practice--Annual clinical breast examination for women ≥40 years old and annual mammography for women ≥50 years old (sooner if at high risk).

Colon and Rectal Cancer

Colon cancer is the second leading cause of cancer death in the U.S. Burden of disease (1993 estimates from the American Cancer Society): 152,000 new cases of colorectal cancer and 57,000 deaths due to colorectal cancer. The lifetime risk of developing colon cancer is approximately 6%. Less than 2% of colon cancers occur in people <40 years old and 90% occur in those >50 years old. The risk of developing colon cancer is approximately 2.5x greater than the risk of dying of it (which reflects potential survivability of colon cancer and the age of the population involved, i.e., there are competing causes of mortality). Colon cancer is now the second cancer for which randomized controlled trial evidence has demonstrated decreased mortality due to screening.

- Colon cancer is the second leading cause of cancer death.
- Lifetime risk is 6%.
- 90% of colon cancers are in people older than 50 years.

Natural history: cancers may develop de novo in the colon, but most of them probably develop from adenomatous polyps. The risk of a polyp becoming malignant appears to be related to time and size. Clinically significant polyps are those larger than 7 mm. The average time from formation to malignant transformation for a polyp is 7-10 years. Ten-year survival for Dukes' A or B cancer is 74%, 36% for Dukes' C, and 5% for Dukes' D.

- The risk of a polyp becoming malignant appears to be related to time and size.
- Clinically significant polyps: ones larger than 7 mm.
- The time from polyp formation to malignant transformation is 7-10 years.

The risk factors include 1) age--risk doubles every 7 years over age 50; 2) sex--risk for males is slightly greater than for females; 3) family history--if a first-degree relative has disease, the risk increases 2x-3x; 4) previous adenomatous polyps increase risk 2x-3x; 5) history of endometrial, ovarian, or breast cancer increases risk 2x; 6) familial polyposis, Gardner's syndrome--approximately 100% risk by age 40; 7) ulcerative colitis--approximately 50% risk with a 30-year history of disease; and 8) cancer family syndrome (adenocarcinoma at various locations at an early age in multiple sibs)--approximately a 50% risk.

- Risk for colon/rectal cancer doubles every 7 years over age 50.
- If first-degree relative has colon/rectal cancer, risk increases 2x-3x.
- Previous adenomatous polyps, risk increases 2x-3x.
- History of endometrial, ovarian, or breast cancer, risk increases 2x.
- Familial polyposis (Gardner's syndrome), risk is nearly 100% by age 40.
- Ulcerative colitis, about a 50% risk with a 30-year history of disease.

Tests: 1) fecal occult blood testing is 20%-30% sensitive and does not detect polyps well; 2) proctoscopy is more than 90% sensitive for the bowel visualized and could detect about 30% of cancers; 3) flexible sigmoidoscopy is also more than 90% sensitive for the bowel visualized and could detect about 60% of cancers; 4) barium enema and colonoscopy usually visualize the entire colon and are 85%-95% sensitive.

- Fecal occult blood testing is 20%-30% sensitive.
- Proctoscopy and flexible sigmoidoscopy are more than 90% sensitive for the area of the colon visualized.
- Barium enema and colonoscopy visualize the entire colon and are 85%-95% sensitive.

Recommendations--Randomized control trial data that are available show about a 30% decrease in mortality with annual fecal occult blood testing. Yet, there is little consensus about whether to screen and how to screen for colorectal cancer. Mathematical modeling suggests that annual screening with barium enema or colonoscopy might reduce mortality by 85%, but the cost would be prohibitive. The American Cancer Society recommends digital rectal examination (for prostate examination) yearly for men >40 years old and yearly for women (as part of pelvic examination) >40. Fecal occult blood testing--yearly over age 50, and sigmoidoscopy every 3-5 years over age 50. Before the recent study supporting annual fecal occult blood testing, the USPSTF concluded that the evidence was insufficient and so made no recommendation for average risk population. It recommended against colonoscopy except for family history of two or more first-degree relatives or existence of high-risk conditions. Updated recommendations are under review. The American College of Physicians recommends fecal occult blood testing annually over age 50 and over age 40 for those at high risk. Sigmoidoscopy--every 3-5 years over age 50 or substitution of barium enema every 5 years for sigmoidoscopy. The College recommends against colonoscopy except for persons with high-risk conditions or a family history of colon cancer in a first-degree relative. The recommendations for these people is colonoscopy over age 40 every 3-5 years (air-contrast barium enema is an acceptable alternative).

- Fecal occult blood screening annually decreases mortality by 30%.
- Annual screening with barium enema or colonoscopy might reduce mortality by 85%, but the cost would be prohibitive.

Prostate Cancer

For the purposes of screening, prostate cancer is a troublesome disease, primarily because of the great difference between the "burden" of prevalent disease and the "burden" of clinical disease. The 1993 estimates from the American Cancer Society are 165,000 new cases of prostate cancer and 35,000 deaths due to it. Pathologic studies show that a small focus of prostate cancer can be found in 30%-40% of 60-year-old men. Yet in only 8%-9% of the men will prostate cancer be diagnosed, with many cases diagnosed incidentally at transurethral resection of the prostate. Currently, 80% of diagnoses are made in men older than 65 years. Very few men with prostate cancer die of the disease, only 2%-3% of U.S. men.

- 8%-9% of U.S. males in their lifetime will have the diagnosis of prostate cancer.
- 2%-3% of U.S. males die of prostate cancer.
- 80% of the diagnoses are made in men older than 65 years.

Natural history--Prostate cancer is a hormonally induced cancer that is generally slow growing. In most host males, it does not alter the life span or lifestyle. Growth of a tiny nidus of cancerous cells into a clinically important cancer takes 10-15 years. In elderly hosts, this process is usually halted by intervening causes of mortality. Aggressiveness and morbidity are related to size, grade, and ploidy. TA1 NxMO: Usually follow age-based mortality curve, normal survival. Mortality due to prostatic cancer is <5%. TA2 NxMO: near normal 10-year survival. TB2 or 3 NxMO: 5-year survival is about 50%.

- Prostate cancer is a hormonally induced cancer.
- It does not alter the life span or lifestyle of most host males.
- Growth into a clinically important cancer takes 10-15 years.

The risk factors include: 1) age--the risk increases exponentially after age 50; 2) race--blacks have 2x the risk of whites, and whites have 2x the risk of Asians; 3) family history--a first-degree relative increases the risk 3x, a brother with cancer before age 63 increases the risk 4x, and a sister with breast cancer increases the risk 2x.

- For prostate cancer in the U.S., blacks have twice the risk of whites, who have twice the risk of Asians.

Tests: 1) digital rectal examination has a PPV of 6.5%; 2) transrectal ultrasonography has a PPV of about 20% (values vary depending on population and prior screening); and 3) prostate-specific antigen (PSA) has a PPV of about 25% (values vary depending on population and prior screening). Note: because there is much undetected disease, PPV values do not have the usual meaning.

Recommendations: no good data are available from randomized controlled trials on the impact of early detection and treatment on survival. There is little agreement on recommendations for screening. Aggressive screening for prostate cancer will uncover many new cases (causing a surge in incidence) and result in many additional treatments. However, because of the natural his-

tory of the disease, screening may have minimal effect in decreasing mortality, the desired benefit. The American Cancer Society recommends digital rectal examination yearly for men >40 years old and this examination plus PSA for men ≥50 years and for men ≥40 years old at high risk. The American College of Physicians and USPSTF make no recommendations.

- There is little agreement on recommendations for screening for prostate cancer.

Several authorities have recommended *against* any form of screening--rectal examination, ultrasonography, or PSA--primarily because of concern that the impact on survival will be minimal and that the costs in detection and follow-up treatment and in deaths due to treatment (perioperative deaths) will be significant. The risk that the harm outweighs the good from detection of early stage disease exists. Screening, if performed, should be done in men likely to have a 10-year survival (the average life expectancy for a 50-year-old man is about 25 years and >10 years for a 70-year-old man).

Cervical Cancer

The 1993 estimates from the American Cancer Society are for 13,500 new cases (the same number as for 1992) of cervical cancer and 4,400 deaths. Cervical cancer has a bimodal risk curve divided between in situ carcinoma and invasive carcinoma. This cancer has a long preclinical phase, and progression from dysplasia to invasive cancer may take 10 to 15 or more years. A strong association exists between human papillomavirus (types 16, 18, and others) and cervical cancer. Cervical cancer may be largely a sexually transmitted disease.

- Cervical cancer: bimodal risk curve divided between in situ carcinoma and invasive carcinoma.
- It has a long preclinical phase.
- Cervical cancer is strongly associated with human papillomavirus.

The risk factors include: 1) age--the risk of invasive carcinoma increases throughout life; 2) sexual activity--early age at onset; 3) multiple sexual partners; 4) a history of sexually transmitted disease; and 5) smoking.

- Cervical cancer risk factors: early age at onset of sexual activity, multiple sexual partners, a history of sexually transmitted disease, smoking.

Test: Pap smear has a sensitivity of 55%-80% and a specificity of 90%-99%. Experienced cytologists and pathologists and clinician sampling technique are important to test effectiveness.

- Pap smear has a 55%-80% sensitivity and a 90%-99% specificity.

Screening effectiveness--No randomized controlled trial of screening has been conducted in a general population. However, a significant body of evidence from case control studies and observational studies suggests effectiveness. Estimated overall effect of Pap smear: every 10 years, 64% reduction in invasive cancer; every 5 years, 84% reduction; every 3 years, 91% reduction; every 2 years, 92.5% reduction; and every year 93.5% reduction.

Recommendations--The general agreement is to recommend screening at the onset of sexual activity and every 1-3 years thereafter, depending on risk. The American Cancer Society recommends screening every 1-3 years for women >18 years, depending on risk factors. The American College of Physicians recommends screening every 3 years for women between 20 and 65 years old and every 2 years if they are at increased risk; for women >65 years, every 3 years if not screened within 10 years before current examination. USPSTF recommends screening every 1-3 years for women 18-65, depending on risk factors, and every 1-3 years if >65 years and if no regular screening was performed in the 10 years previously.

- General recommendation: screen at the onset of sexual activity and every 1-3 years thereafter, depending on risk.

Ovarian Cancer

Ovarian cancer is the fourth leading cause of cancer death in women. Burden of disease (1993 estimates from the American Cancer Society): 22,000 new cases of ovarian cancer and 13,300 deaths. Ovarian cancer is the leading cause of gynecologic cancer death. Age-adjusted death rates have been increasing slowly in the last 25 years.

- Ovarian cancer is the fourth leading cause of cancer death in women.
- Age-adjusted death rates have been increasing slowly.

Risk factors: 1) Lower risk--history of at least one term pregnancy has a relative risk of 0.64. The use of oral contraceptives for <1 year has the relative risk of 0.97, if used >3 years, the relative risk is 0.40. Estimated 12% decrease in risk per year of use of oral contraceptive pill up to 7 years. 2) Higher risk--family history as a risk is not well quantified, but it is an important factor if first-degree relative has disease (only 1%-5% of ovarian cancers are familial). High-fat diet, long duration of ovulatory years (i.e., late menopause), and coffee intake are possible risk factors.

- 12% decrease in risk per year with use of oral contraceptive pill up to 7 years.
- 1%-5% of ovarian cancers are familial.

Screening tests: 1) bimanual examination is insensitive; 2) ultrasonography, transvaginal or transabdominal, is more sensitive than bimanual examination but has a poor PPV; 3) CA 125 (blood test) is more sensitive than bimanual examination but also has a poor PPV. Ultrasonography or CA 125 has a significant false-positive rate. No study has been done on the impact of screening on mortality. It is estimated that 10-60 abdominal operations would have to be performed for every one cancer detected, at a cost of more than $13 billion annually to screen the 43 million woman >45 years old. An adequate study of efficacy, even with a highly sensitive and specific test, would require tens of thousands of participants.

- For ovarian cancer, bimanual examination is insensitive.
- Ultrasonography and CA 125 both are more sensitive than bimanual examination but both have a poor PPV.
- For every one ovarian cancer detected, 10-60 abdominal operations would have to be performed.

Recommendations: no randomized controlled trial screening data exist to guide recommendations. The American Cancer Society recommends bimanual palpation every 1-3 years for women age 20-40 and every year for women >40. USPSTF recommends against screening for ovarian cancer.

Tuberculosis Prevention

Burden of disease: the worldwide prevalence of tuberculosis (TB) infection (past or active) is greater than 1 billion cases, with an annual incidence rate of about 8 million. Approximately 3,000,000 people worldwide die annually of TB. The U.S. incidence is approximately 25,000 cases per year, with a mortality of 2,000 cases. The incidence decreased from 1953 to 1985, but since then TB has made a resurgence, probably because of immigration from endemic areas, HIV infection, and increased use of immunosuppressive drugs.

- TB: the U.S. incidence is approximately 25,000 cases and 2,000 deaths annually.

Natural history: infection occurs through inhalation of *Mycobacterium tuberculosis*-bearing droplets. After being infected, healthy persons are usually asymptomatic. However, it is believed that the tubercle bacillus remains viable in granulomata for many years. The risk of reactivation after asymptomatic infection (PPD conversion) is 2%/year for the first 2-3 years. A second reactivation peak occurs in the elderly, with debility and disease.

- The tubercle bacillus remains viable in granulomata for many years.
- The risk of reactivation (PPD conversion) is 2%/year for first 2-3 years after infection.
- A second reactivation peak occurs in the elderly with debility and disease.

Risk factors include: 1) foreign-born, with recent immigration; 2) institutionalization, e.g., in nursing home, 5x-30x increased risk; 3) prisoners (10x increased risk); and 4) HIV/AIDS infection. If a person is HIV-positive and has a positive PPD, the 2-year risk is 15%. If TB occurs in a young person, check their HIV status.

- If a person is HIV-positive and has a positive PPD, the 2-year risk is 15%.
- If TB occurs in a young person, check his or her HIV status.

Test: the PPD (Mantoux) skin test--5-tuberculin units intradermal skin test. Measure the area of induration (not erythema) at 48-72 hours. In low-risk persons, consider the reaction positive if it is >15 mm (10 mm if the person is in a high-risk group). If there has been recent contact with an infected person, 5 mm is considered positive. HIV-infected persons may be anergic and 5 mm may be considered positive. Elderly persons may be relatively anergic but can be boosted by repeating the same dose of testing. Previous BCG vaccine will produce skin

reactivity, but induration >15 mm should be treated as a positive reaction in an adult vaccinated as a child. Recent MMR vaccination (6 weeks) may diminish skin reactivity, and testing should be avoided during this interval. Chest radiography and sputum are not useful screening tests for conversion but may detect active disease in high-risk persons.

- Chest radiography and sputum are not useful screening tests for TB.

Preventive measures: 1) Primary prevention is with BCG vaccine, an attenuated species of *Mycobacterium bovus*. It may be as much as 80% effective when used properly. It is indicated in high-risk areas because it is inexpensive, requires a single shot, and has a low risk (only 100 fatalities in 2 billion administrations). BCG vaccine is not indicated in low-prevalence areas because it confuses interpretation of PPD response. Another primary preventive measure is environmental controls, especially in health-care environment, with respiratory isolation and either a high-efficiency filter or a special venting of rooms/wards with TB cases.

- BCG vaccine is 80% effective when used properly.
- Its use is not indicated in low-prevalence areas.

2) Secondary prevention is with isoniazid (INH) treatment. Its use is indicated for recent converters (<2 years), contacts of infected persons with >5 mm PPD, history of TB with inadequate treatment, positive skin tests with abnormal but stable chest radiograph, and positive PPD (of any duration) if <35 years old. The dosage is 5-10 mg/kg daily, up to a maximum of 300 mg daily (the usual adult dose) in a single oral dose. Treatment should continue for 6-12 months (the longer the treatment, the greater the efficacy). Primary side effects are liver toxicity and peripheral neuropathy. Peak toxicity is in persons >50 years old (2%-3%). Side-effect monitoring is generally through symptoms only, except in older persons (because of higher risk for toxicity) in whom AST or ALT (liver function testing) every 6 weeks may be used.

- Isoniazid: 5-10 mg/kg daily up to maximum of 300 mg daily.
- Treatment should continue for 6-12 months.
- Peak toxicity is in persons older than 50 years (2%-3%).

IMMUNIZATIONS

One of the greatest successes of modern medicine for preventing disease and for extending life has been immunization. Adults have continuing immunization needs throughout life. Physicians who administer vaccines are required by law to keep permanent vaccine records (National Childhood Vaccine Act of 1986) and to report adverse events through the vaccine adverse event reporting system (VAERS). Service in the military may be considered verification of vaccination to measles, rubella, tetanus, diphtheria, and polio. Providers are now required to give patients "vaccine information pamphlets" before vaccination as a mechanism for informed consent.

Immunity may be of two types. Passive immunity--preformed antibodies are provided in large quantities to prevent or diminish the impact of infection or associated toxins (e.g., tetanus immunoglobulin [TIG] and hepatitis B immunoglobulin [HBIG]). Passive immunity lasts for up to 3 months. Active immunity--an antigen is presented to the host immune system that in turn develops antibodies (e.g., hepatitis or tetanus) or specific immune cells (e.g., BCG). Active immunity generally lasts from years to a lifetime. Active immunity may be induced by live virus vaccines (e.g., measles), killed virus vaccines (e.g., influenza), or refined antigen vaccines (e.g., pneumococcal).

Live virus vaccines are important primarily for *who should not receive them*. In general, pregnant women, people with immune-deficiency diseases, leukemia, lymphoma, generalized malignancy, or those who are immune-suppressed because of therapy with corticosteroids, alkalating drugs, antimetabolites, or radiation should *not* be given live virus vaccines. HIV-infected persons who are immune-competent and leukemia patients who have been in remission for ≥3 months after chemotherapy may generally be vaccinated with live virus vaccines. Live virus vaccines include measles, mumps, rubella, smallpox, varicella zoster, yellow fever, and polio.

Inactivated virus vaccines include enhanced inactivated polio (eIPV), hepatitis B, influenza, and rabies. Inactivated bacterial vaccines include cholera, hemophilus influenza B, meningococcal, plague, and pneumococcal.

Diphtheria--Diphtheria is a rare disease primarily because of vaccination. However, up to 40% of adults lack protective antibody levels. Recommendation: vaccination in combination with tetanus toxoid (see tetanus), as Td.

Tetanus--Approximately 50 cases of tetanus are reported each year; most are in adults who are either unvacci-

nated or inadequately vaccinated. Vaccination is nearly 100% effective. Recommendations: primary series, a three-dose series, should be completed before adulthood, usually in early childhood. Primary series consists of Td followed in 4 weeks or more by Td followed in 6-12 months or more by another Td. The last childhood dose is usually a booster at age 15. For adults who have had a primary series, vaccinate every 10 years (e.g., mid-decade is easy to remember; if last childhood dose at 15, vaccinate at ages 25, 35, 45, etc.). Clean, minor wounds received in the 10-year interval require no further vaccination. However, for a contaminated wound, the patient should get a booster if it has been more than 5 years since the last booster. If immune status is unknown or lacking (specifically, no primary series) both toxoid and TIG should be given, 250 units i.m. Td is the preferred toxoid in an emergency setting as well as for routine vaccination. Td and TIG when given in the emergency setting should be given in separate syringes at separate locations, but they may be given at the same time.

- Tetanus vaccination: the primary series is a three-dose series.
- Adults who have had a primary series should receive a booster every 10 years.
- For a contaminated wound, the patient should get a booster if it has been more than 5 years since the last booster.

Side effects: Td may be given in pregnancy, although it is desirable to wait until the second trimester. Maternal antibodies are passed to infant transplacentally and confer passive immunity for a few months after birth.

- Maternal antibodies are passed to infant transplacentally.

A history of neurologic reaction, urticaria, anaphylaxis, or other severe hypersensitivity reaction is a contraindication to the readministration of toxoids. Skin testing may be performed if necessary. In the emergency setting, if other than a clean minor wound is sustained, TIG may be used when T or Td is contraindicated. Arthus-type hypersensitivity, a severe local reaction occurring 2-8 hours after injection and often with fever and malaise, may occur in persons who have received multiple boosters. These people have very high levels of antitoxin and do not need boosters, even in the emergency room setting, more frequently than every 10 years.

Measles--Vaccination has reduced the number of cases of measles from 500,000 yearly (with 500 deaths) to 3,600 cases yearly in the mid-1980s. A disease resurgence has occurred, and in 1990, there were 27,000 cases. The risk of encephalitis with measles infection in an adult is approximately 1 in 1,000. Infection in pregnancy may induce abortion, premature labor, and low birth weight. Malformation does not appear to be as much of a problem as with rubella.

- A resurgence in measles has occurred.
- The risk of encephalitis with measles infection in an adult is approximately 1 in 1,000.

Target: Adults born after 1956 who have no medical contraindication and who have no dated documentation of at least one dose of live measles vaccination on or after their first birthday, physician-documented disease, or documented immune titers should receive vaccination. Persons with expected exposure to measles should consider revaccination or titer measurement because 10% of persons born before 1957 are not immune. Persons at risk include travelers to endemic areas, those in school settings, and health-care workers. They should have documented two doses of measles vaccine on or after their first birthday. MMR is the preferred vaccine. If they have never been vaccinated, they should receive two doses given at least 1 month apart.

Exposure precautions: If the person exposed is unvaccinated, vaccinate within 72 hours if possible and give immunoglobulin if the person is not a vaccine candidate (0.5 mL/kg i.m., up to 15 mL). Health-care workers should remain away from work for days 5-21 after exposure if they are not immune.

Side effects: 1) fever, temperature >103°F usually occurs on day 5-12 in 5%-15% of those vaccinated; 2) rash occurs in 5%; 3) encephalitis is rare, if it occurs at all; 4) a local reaction occurs especially in those having received killed vaccine. No apparent increase in side effects occurs with a second vaccination. Contraindications are immunoglobulin or blood products given within the previous 3 months, pregnancy, egg or neomycin allergy, and others as noted above for live virus vaccines.

Mumps--A highly effective vaccination program has reduced the number of cases of mumps from approximately 200,000 yearly to 3,000-5,000 yearly. Side effects of rash, pruritus, and purpura are uncommon, and central nervous system problems and parotitis are rare. There is no increased risk with revaccination. The contraindications are the same as for measles.

Rubella--Infection with rubella in the first trimester results in congenital rubella syndrome in up to 80% of infected fetuses. The goal of vaccination is to prevent the occurrence of this disease. Vaccination is highly effective, and there is no evidence of transmission of vaccine virus to close household contacts. The target population includes all women of childbearing age, all health-care workers, and travelers to endemic areas. The side effects include: arthralgias in 25% and transient arthritis in 10%, usually 1-3 weeks postvaccination. Vaccination rarely causes chronic joint problems, certainly much less frequently than natural infection. Contraindications are immunoglobulin given within the previous 3 months (but not blood products, e.g., $Rh_o(D)$ immune globulin [RhoGAM]), pregnant women or women likely to become pregnant within 3 months (although there are no documented cases of congenital rubella syndrome in vaccinated pregnant women), and allergy to neomycin but not to egg (as prepared in a diploid cell culture).

Influenza--Since 1957, 19 influenza epidemics, with more than 10,000 excess deaths each, have occurred, and 80%-90% of the deaths occurred in persons ≥65 years old. Peak incidences occur in mid to late winter (i.e., after December). Influenza A is classified by two surface antigens: hemagglutinin (subtypes H1, H2, H3) and neuraminidase (subtypes N1, N2). Because of differing subtypes and antigenic drift, infection or vaccination more than 1 year previously may not give protection the following year. Influenza B is antigenically more stable but still has moderate drift. Control is with vaccination (both influenza A and B) and/or chemoprophylaxis (for influenza A only).

The vaccine is an inactivated (killed) virus vaccine (virus grown in egg culture). Each year it contains three viruses, two A-type viruses and one B-type virus. Vaccines may contain whole virus, subvarion, or purified surface antigen. Subvarion and purified antigen are used in children to decrease febrile reaction. All forms may be used in adults. Ideally, vaccination should be given in October and November.

The side effects include 1) local soreness (occurs in <1/3); 2) fever, malaise, myalgia (occurs 6-12 hours postvaccination and may last 1-2 days); and 3) anaphylactic reaction (probably due to egg protein). The target population includes 1) persons ≥65 years old who reside in a nursing home or chronic care facility; 2) persons with chronic pulmonary or cardiovascular disease, including asthma, chronic metabolic diseases such as diabetes mellitus, renal dysfunction, immunosuppression; and 3) health-care workers. Consideration may be given to persons in vital roles, institutional settings, or who travel to the southern hemisphere between April and September. Contraindications are 1) first trimester of pregnancy, except for those at high risk because of underlying disease, and 2) egg allergy.

Chemoprophylaxis is with amantadine hydrochloride (for influenza A only). This drug interferes with the replication cycle of influenza A. In healthy populations, it is given daily throughout the epidemic and is 70%-90% effective at preventing disease. For treatment of disease, it decreases fever and other symptoms if given within 48 hours of disease onset. Amantadine is used to control influenza outbreaks, usually in institutions, and is given to all unvaccinated workers and residents. It may be given regardless of vaccine status to individuals at high risk. Workers should continue it until 2 weeks after vaccination or indefinitely if the vaccine is contraindicated. The dose is 200 mg daily.

- Amantadine is used for influenza A only.
- It is 70%-90% effective.
- It is used to control influenza outbreaks, usually in institutions, and is given to all unvaccinated workers and residents.

The side effects are usually minor, occurring in 5%-10%, and may abate with continued use. Central nervous system side effects are nervousness, anxiety, insomnia, and decreased concentration, and those of the gastrointestinal system include anorexia and nausea. Serious side effects are seizure and confusion, usually seen in the elderly or in those with renal disease. In this group, the dose may be decreased to 100 mg daily, which appears to be nearly as effective as the higher dose.

Hepatitis B--The lifetime risk of acquiring hepatitis B is 5% for the general population; 300,000 cases occur annually in the U.S., resulting in 10,000 hospitalizations and 250 deaths. Of the patients affected, 90% are ≥20 years old; 5%-10% become carriers, and one-quarter of these have chronic active hepatitis. Annually, 4,000 die of hepatitis B virus-related cirrhosis and 800 die of hepatitis B virus-related liver cancer.

- The lifetime risk of acquiring hepatitis B is 5% for the general population.
- 5%-10% become carriers.

- Annually, 4,000 die of hepatitis B virus-related cirrhosis and 800 die of hepatitis B virus-related liver cancer.

The current vaccine is yeast recombinant, developed from the insertion of a plasmid into *Sacchromyces cerevisiae*, which produces the copies of the surface antigen. Human-purified vaccine is no longer made. The target population includes 1) adults at increased risk, i.e., homosexual males, i.v. drug users, heterosexual persons with multiple sexual partners, and those with a history of other sexually transmitted diseases; 2) household and sexual contacts of hepatitis B virus carriers; 3) workers in health-related and public safety occupations involving exposure to blood or body fluids; 4) hemodialysis patients; 5) recipients of concentrates of clotting factors VIII and IX; 6) morticians and their assistants; and 7) travelers who will be living for extended periods in high-prevalence areas or who are likely to have sexual contacts or contact with blood in the endemic areas (especially in eastern Asia and sub-Sahara Africa).

Vaccination--Normally, vaccination consists of three doses at 0, 1 month, and 6 months. An alternative dosing schedule to induce immunity more rapidly, e.g., after exposure, involves 4 doses, the first three given 1 month apart and a fourth dose at 12 months. Postexposure prophylaxis consists of HBIG given in a single dose of 0.06 mL/kg or 5 mL for adults. It should be administered along with the vaccine in separate syringes at separate sites, but they may be administered at the same time. Current evidence suggests that for most vaccinees the vaccination has a duration of ≥7 years. Currently, revaccination is not routinely recommended. For persons who receive the vaccine in the buttock or whose management depends on knowledge of immune status (e.g., surgeons or venipuncturists), periodic serologic testing may be valuable. Those with titers <10 mIU should be revaccinated. Revaccination with a single dose is usually effective.

- Currently, revaccination is not routinely recommended.

The most common side effect is localized soreness. Guillain-Barré syndrome (0.5 per 100,000) was associated with human-derived hepatitis B vaccines. Comparable information is not available for the recombinant vaccination. Vaccination in pregnancy is considered advisable for women who are at risk for hepatitis B infection.

The risk of hepatitis B virus infection in pregnancy far outweighs the risk of vaccine-associated problems.

- Guillain-Barré syndrome (0.5 per 100,000) was associated with human-derived hepatitis B vaccines.

Pneumococcal vaccine--Two-thirds of people with serious pneumococcal disease have been hospitalized in the previous 5 years (a missed opportunity to vaccinate). The risk of bacteremia for persons ≥65 years old is 50 per 100,000. The current vaccine is a purified capsular material of 23 different serotypes of streptococcus pneumonia. In most healthy adults, titers persist for ≥5 years. Persons who have received a 14-valent vaccine need not be routinely revaccinated. However, persons at highest risk for pneumococcal infections, such as asplenic patients, should be revaccinated with the 23-valent vaccine if it has been >6 years since the previous dose. Patients with nephrotic syndrome and renal failure and transplant patients should be revaccinated every 3-5 years because of waning immunity.

The target population is persons ≥65 years old, adults with chronic disease states such as cardiovascular or pulmonary disease, or persons at higher risk for pneumococcal infection, e.g., because of alcoholism or cerebrospinal fluid leak. The target population also includes immunocompromised persons (such as those who are asplenic) and patients with Hodgkin's disease, lymphoma, multiple myeloma, chronic renal failure, nephrotic syndrome, HIV infection, or organ transplant. Side effects are erythema (50% of cases) and fever, myalgia, and local reaction (<1%). Five per 1,000,000 of those vaccinated develop anaphylaxis. Revaccination within approximately 1 year is associated with increased local reaction.

- The target population is persons ≥65 years old or adults with chronic disease.

Smallpox (vaccinia)--In May 1980, WHO declared the world free of smallpox. Vaccination is no longer indicated except for persons working directly with the orthopoxviruses.

- Smallpox vaccination is no longer indicated except for persons working directly with the orthopoxviruses.

Polio--Polio is a low-risk disease in the U.S. There are OPV (live virus) and eIPV (killed virus) vaccinations. A primary series with either one has >95% effectiveness. Polio vaccination is not recommended for persons >18 years old unless they plan to travel to an endemic area and have no history of a previous primary series. For these persons, use eIPV because of the slightly lower risk of paralysis. The primary series consists of eIPV followed in 4-8 weeks by eIPV, followed in 6-12 months by eIPV. If it is <4 weeks before travel, give a single dose of either OPV or eIPV. If the primary series is incomplete, complete it despite the interval since the previous dose. If the person previously received IPV, give one dose of OPV or eIPV. For OPV, the risk of paralysis is approximately 1 in 1,000,000 after the first dose, and for susceptible household contacts, it is approximately 1 in 2,000,000.

- Polio vaccination is not recommended for persons >18 years old unless they plan to travel to an endemic area.

Rabies--Preexposure prophylaxis is recommended for animal handlers, lab workers, persons traveling to endemic areas for >1 month, or those with vocations/avocations with exposure to skunks, raccoons, and bats as well as other animals. The reservoir of infection includes carniverous animals, particularly skunks, raccoons, foxes, and bats in the U.S. Except for woodchucks, rodents are rarely infected.

QUESTIONS
(See "Answers" section)

Multiple Choice

1. Secondary prevention refers to detection and elimination or amelioration of:
   a. Risk factors for disease
   b. Recurrent disease such as tamoxifen treatment after breast cancer
   c. Individual characteristics that may place a person in a risk category
   d. Disease in a presymptomatic (preclinical) stage
   e. Need for immunization updates

2. Incidence rate refers to:
   a. The number of new events (deaths, diagnoses) that occur in a given population in a specified period of time
   b. The number of cancer deaths or diagnoses that occur in the U.S. population
   c. The number of cases of a specific condition that exists in a population at a point in time
   d. Fatal accidents that occur at a given highway speed
   e. An estimate of the impact on society of a disease in terms of lost life and productivity

3. A desirable screening characteristic of a disease is:
   a. The disease is rare
   b. The disease is virulent and rapidly progresses to fatality
   c. The disease occurs late in life, often near the end of productive years
   d. The disease has a long preclinical phase
   e. The natural history of the disease is not well understood

4. Lung cancer is the leading cause of cancer death for both men and women. Screening tests for lung cancer should include:
   a. Chest radiography
   b. Sputum cytology
   c. Bronchoscopy
   d. Routine screening tests for lung cancer are not indicated
   e. Pulmonary function testing

5. All the major policy setting groups with respect to breast cancer agree that:
   a. Women should receive a baseline mammogram between ages 35 and 40
   b. Mammography should be used in conjunction with breast physical examination for women between the ages of 50 and 65
   c. The seven major trials of mammography show benefit in 40- to 49-year-old women
   d. Annual clinic breast examination should be performed between the ages of 20 and 50 in women and mammography should be added to the screening program at the age of 50.
   e. There is no significant agreement among groups making recommendations

True/False

6. A 52-year-old woman with a family history of colon cancer in her 60-year-old brother and a 45 pack-year history of smoking comes for a general physical examination. She feels well but has not seen a physician for more than 10 years and thought she was due for a checkup. Preventive maneuvers that you should recommend for her include:
   a. A tetanus booster (Td). She had completed a primary series as a child and had a booster in her 30s
   b. Measles, mumps, rubella vaccination
   c. Chest radiography for lung cancer screening
   d. Mammography (findings on physical examination are normal)
   e. Fecal occult blood testing
   f. CA125 assay for ovarian cancer screening

7. Live virus vaccines include:
   a. Measles
   b. Oral polio virus (OPV)
   c. Human-derived hepatitis B vaccine
   d. Influenza vaccine
   e. Rubella vaccine
   f. Pneumococcal vaccine

8. A 43-year-old farmer sustains a sizable gash in his leg from the blade of his plow. You are examining him in the emergency room and have completed cleaning and dressing the wound. While he reaches for his pack of cigarettes, he indicates to you that he has never been to a doctor before, even as a child. Appropriate preventive measures include:
   a. Recommendation for contrast barium enema for colon cancer screening
   b. Injection with tetanus immune globulin (TIG)

c. Injection with tetanus/diphtheria vaccine (Td)
d. A brief discussion about smoking cessation
e. Recommendation for the primary series for oral polio virus
f. Request for direct payment because he may not be seen for another 40 years

CHAPTER 25
PSYCHIATRY

Deborah C. Newman, M.D.

Many psychiatric symptoms are as nonspecific as fever. Some signify problems of severe magnitude, whereas others are much less significant. Generally, the symptoms can be and should be investigated further before simply recommending symptomatic relief. The current paradigm of psychiatric assessment is the biopsychosocial model in which the biologic, psychologic, and social factors contributing to the patient's clinical presentation are evaluated.

Psychiatric disorders are divided into major diagnostic groups. A simplified way to conceptualize these groups is to look at the major symptomatic features of the patient's presentation: 1) mood--depression or mania; 2) anxiety--situational stress, panic disorder, generalized anxiety, others; 3) thought--psychotic process; acute (drug induced, metabolic/toxic) versus chronic (schizophrenic process).

Any of the above diagnostic groups can be altered by alcohol or substance abuse/dependence or organic mental disorders such as delirium or dementia. The common psychiatric disorders seen by general physicians in outpatient settings are anxiety disorders, mood disorders, substance abuse, psychophysiologic disorders, and adjustment disorders. In the general hospital setting, the common psychiatric groups are mood disorders, adjustment disorders, substance abuse, and organic mental disorders, primarily delirium and dementia. The descriptions of the psychiatric disorders in this syllabus are based on the criteria described in *The Diagnostic and Statistical Manual (DSM III R) of the American Psychiatric Association 1987.*

- Common psychiatric disorders seen by general physicians in outpatient setting: anxiety disorders, mood disorders, substance abuse, psychophysiologic disorders, adjustment disorders.
- Common psychiatric groups in general hospital setting: mood disorders, adjustment disorders, substance abuse, and organic mental disorders, primarily delirium and dementia.

MOOD DISORDERS

The prevalence of mood disorders in the general population of the U.S. is estimated at 5%-8%; however, in the general medical setting, the rate may be as high as 5%-15%.

Although the essential feature of mood disorders is a disturbance of mood, it is accompanied by related cognitive, psychomotor, vegetative (sleep, appetite, etc.), and interpersonal difficulties. Fluctuations in mood are a normal occurrence. It is only when the frequency and/or intensity of these changes is extreme and accompanied by the other features described that a formal mood disorder is diagnosed. The five major groups of mood disorders cover the range from mild to severe depression to the opposite extreme of mania. Three groups relate to depression: adjustment disorder with depressed mood, dysthymia, and major depression. Two groups relate to problems with mood fluctuations between various degrees of depression and mania: cyclothymia and bipolar disorder. Each of these five major groups has several subgroups. Another important group is organic mood disorders, which refers to cases in which the disturbance of mood, either depression or mania, is attributable to an organic factor such as a metabolic or toxic cause or some other medical or neurologic condition. The clinical phenomenology is similar to that of a manic or depressive episode.

- Mood disorders: essential feature is disturbance of mood.
- They are accompanied by related cognitive, psychomotor, vegetative, interpersonal difficulties.
- Organic mood disorder: disturbance of mood, either depression or mania.

Adjustment Disorder With Depressed Mood

Adjustment disorder with depressed mood is a reaction that develops in response to an identifiable psychosocial stressor(s), e.g., divorce, job loss, family or marital problems. It can occur any time in anyone if the psychosocial stressors are severe. The severity of the adjustment disorder (degree of impairment) does not always parallel the intensity of the precipitating event. The critical factor appears to be the relevance of the event or stressor to the individual and his or her ability to cope with the stress. In general, these reactions are relatively transient. Although they generally can be managed by an empathic primary care physician, the development of extreme withdrawal, suicidal ideation, or failure to improve as the circumstances improve may prompt psychiatric referral. Treatment includes supportive psychotherapy, psychosocial interventions, and, sometimes, use of antidepressant agents.

Dysthymia

Dysthymia is a form of chronic depression that may have either an early or late onset, as defined by onset before or after, respectively, age 21. It can be disabling for the person because the depressed mood is present most of the time during at least a 2-year period. Many of the patients have some associated vegetative signs such as disturbance of sleep and appetite, but they also often feel inadequate, have low self-esteem, and struggle with interpersonal relationships. If onset is in late adolescence, the dysthymia may become intertwined with the person's personality, behavior, and general attitude toward life. Treatment is usually a combination of psychotherapy (insight-oriented, cognitive, or interpersonal), behavioral therapy, and pharmacotherapy. Psychopharmacotherapy may be particularly useful in patients with a positive family history of mood disorders or in those who have the early onset form of dysthymia. Patients with dysthymia may develop major depressive episodes. Also, some are prone to turn to alcohol or other substance abuse to "treat" their dysphoria.

- Dysthymia: a form of chronic depression.

- Depressed mood is present most of the time during at least a 2-year period.
- Treatment is usually a combination of psychotherapy and pharmacotherapy.
- Patients with dysthymia may develop major depressive episodes.

Major Depression

Major depression is a serious psychiatric disorder that is set apart from adjustment disorder and dysthymia by the severity of the mood and cognitive disturbances and the presence of significant somatic symptoms. The primary symptoms of major depression include: depressed mood, diminished interest or pleasure in all or almost all activities, significant weight loss or weight gain (>5% of body weight in a month), decrease or increase in appetite, insomnia or hypersomnia, psychomotor agitation or retardation, fatigue or loss of energy, feelings of worthlessness or of excessive or inappropriate guilt, diminished ability to concentrate, recurrent thoughts of death or suicidal ideation, or a suicide attempt. If delusions or hallucinations are also present, then it would be classified as "major depression with psychotic features." Another severe form of major depression is the melancholic type. In addition to the symptoms listed above, this form is also characterized by the lack of reactivity to pleasurable stimuli (does not feel better even temporarily if involved in what is usually a pleasurable activity), diurnal mood variation (depression regularly worse in the morning), and early morning awakening (at least 2 hours before usual time of awakening).

- Major depression: symptoms are depressed mood, diminished interest or pleasure in all or almost all activities, significant weight loss or weight gain.
- Melancholic type: characterized by lack of reactivity to pleasurable stimuli, diurnal mood variation, early morning awakening.

Every year about 10 million Americans have a depressive episode, but about only 20% of people usually seek treatment. Of those that seek treatment from a physician, as many as one-third are not diagnosed or are sometimes misdiagnosed because they often present with somatic complaints. As our population ages and more elderly patients seek medical care, diagnosing and treating their mood disorders is becoming more complicated because these patients often have overlapping medical and neurologic problems. Sometimes they present with the combination of a dementing process and depression, which if treated can help manage some of the other problems. The prevalence of depression in women is twice as high as in men. The peak age of onset of depression in women is 33-45 years and in men, >55 years.

- Of persons seeking treatment for major depression, as many as one-third are not diagnosed or are misdiagnosed.
- In elderly patients, diagnosing and treating mood disorders is becoming more complicated.
- Prevalence of depression in women is twice as high as in men.

Seasonal Affective Disorder

Seasonal affective disorder is a form of depression usually characterized by the onset of depression between the beginning of October and the end of November, disappearing from mid-February to mid-April. It occurs twice as commonly in women as in men and is associated with psychomotor retardation, hypersomnia, overeating (carbohydrate craving), and weight gain. To make the diagnosis, this has to be a recurrent pattern for 2-3 consecutive years. The treatment has relied primarily on phototherapy, using a full-spectrum light source 2,500 lux for 2 hours/day at a distance of 30 inches from the eyes or 10,000 lux sources, which can be used for 30 minutes/day. Newer sources of lights are being investigated, as are more specific details about the cause of this disorder. It appears that the antidepressant agents that selectively block serotonin reuptake (fluoxetine) may also be helpful in treating this disorder.

- Seasonal affective disorder: onset of depression between beginning of October and end of November.
- It is twice as common in women as in men.
- It is associated with psychomotor retardation, hypersomnia, overeating.
- Treatment: primarily phototherapy.

Depressions are heterogeneous in their clinical presentation and so probably do not have a single etiologic agent. It appears that depression is more related to alterations of several neurotransmitter systems and neuropeptides, effects on presynaptic and postsynaptic receptors, neurohormonal alterations, and, in general, an alteration in the overall balance of these systems that are so interdependent on one another.

Treatment of Depression

There are four major groups of treatment modalities for depression: psychotherapy, pharmacotherapy, electroconvulsive therapy, and circadian rhythm manipulation such as sleep deprivation or phototherapy. Generally, they are used in some combination.

Psychotherapy: There are multiple forms of psychotherapy, many of which can be used in the treatment of depression. However, the two forms that have been used extensively for treating depression are cognitive therapy and interpersonal therapy. Cognitive therapy strives to help patients have a better integration of cognitions (thoughts), emotions, and behaviors. This therapy is based on the premise that our thoughts have a profound impact on our emotions, which have an impact on our behaviors. If we can learn more adaptive ways of thinking, it may improve our general outlook and ultimately our behavior, with an increase in a sense of worth and improved self-esteem. Interpersonal therapy focuses on current interpersonal functioning. It is based on the concept that depression is associated with impaired social relationships that either precipitate or perpetuate the disorder.

- Cognitive therapy: to help patients have a better integration of cognitions (thoughts), emotions, and behaviors.
- Interpersonal therapy: focuses on current interpersonal functioning.

Pharmacotherapy: The selection of medication is based on the side-effect profile of the medication and the clinical profile of the patient. Dose--Start slowly and titrate to a therapeutic dose based on clinical judgment and blood levels (when available). Duration of treatment--Usually a minimum of 6 months, counting from the time the patient attained significant improvement. Often patients may benefit from extended use of antidepressant agents, especially if they have had multiple episodes of depression. Antidepressant agents should generally be tapered when discontinued rather than abruptly stopping their use. If the response to the first antidepressant agent is minimal or none, consider the addition of lithium carbonate or synthetic thyroid (T_3 or T_4), change to a different class of drug, or use electroconvulsive therapy, which is still probably the most consistently effective treatment for severe depression.

Cyclothymia

Cyclothymia can be thought of as a less severe form of bipolar disorder. By definition, it is a chronic disorder that usually appears in the late teens or early twenties and involves multiple hypomanic and depressive episodes that are not severe enough to meet criteria for mania or depression and do not generally cause significant impairment of occupational or social functioning. About 20% of patients with cyclothymia have a family history of bipolar disorder. About half of the patients report improvement while taking lithium.

- Cyclothymia: a less severe form of bipolar disorder.
- It is a chronic disorder that usually appears in the late teens to early twenties.
- It generally does not cause significant impairment of occupational or social functioning.

Mania and Bipolar Disorder

The essential features of a manic episode are the presence of an abnormally euphoric, expansive, or irritable mood associated with some of the following: inflated self-esteem or grandiosity, decreased need for sleep, pressured speech, flight of ideas, distractibility, increase in goal-directed activity or psychomotor agitation, and excessive involvement in pleasurable activities that have a high potential for painful consequences (e.g., unrestrained buying sprees, sexual indiscretions, or inappropriate financial investments). To make the diagnosis of a bipolar disorder, the patient must have had episodes of both depression and mania.

- Mania: essential feature is an abnormally euphoric, expansive, or irritable mood.
- The prevalence of bipolar disorder is estimated to be about 1%.
- Bipolar disorder seems to occur at about the same frequency in women and men.
- The usual age of onset is from the teens to age 30.
- Patients generally have a positive family history for bipolar or other mood disorder.

Treatment is aimed at mood stabilization and improved social and occupational functioning. The primary pharmacologic treatment is lithium carbonate (see below). Other agents that are helpful include carbamazepine and valproic acid. Lithium may take up to 5-10 days to be effective. During this waiting period, the judicious use of antipsychotic agents or clonazepam is helpful in controlling the acute symptoms.

- Treatment of mania and bipolar disorder: aimed at

mood stabilization and improved social and occupational functioning.
- Primary pharmacologic treatment: lithium carbonate.

Organic Mood Disorders

The essential feature of organic mood disorders is a disturbance of mood that is attributable to a specific organic factor. Many medical conditions and medications can induce mood changes. Medications that have been implicated in inducing these disorders include steroids, reserpine, methyldopa, propranolol, carbonic anhydrase inhibitors, stimulants, hallucinogens, chronic use and abuse of alcohol, sedative-hypnotics, benzodiazepines, and narcotics. Medical conditions that may present as mood disorders include endocrinopathies (Cushing's syndrome, Addison's disease, hypothyroidism, and hypocalcemia or hypercalcemia), malignancy (occult cancers, lymphomas, pancreatic carcinoma, gliomas), and infections (hepatitis, encephalitis, mononucleosis, HIV).

- Organic mood disorders: essential feature is a disturbance of mood attributable to a specific organic factor.
- Many medical conditions and medications induce mood changes.

PSYCHOTIC DISORDERS

"Psychosis" is a generic term used to describe behavior marked by a break from reality. Psychotic symptoms can occur in various medical, neurologic, and psychiatric disorders. Many psychotic reactions seen in medical settings are associated with the use of recreational or prescription drugs (Table 25-1). Some of these drug-induced psychotic reactions are nearly indistinguishable from schizophrenia (e.g., amphetamine and phencyclidine [PCP] psychoses). Other reactions may manifest as more nonspecific psychotic syndromes. Many brain regions may be involved with the production of psychotic symptoms, but abnormalities in the frontal, temporal, and limbic regions are more likely than others to produce psychotic features.

- Psychosis: a generic term describing behavior marked by a break from reality.
- Many psychotic reactions may be associated with use of recreational or prescription drugs.
- Some drug-induced psychotic reactions are nearly indistinguishable from schizophrenia.

Table 25-1.--Classes of Drugs That Can Produce
Psychiatric Symptoms

Stimulants
Hallucinogens
Phencyclidine (PCP)
Catecholaminergic drugs
Anticholinergic drugs
Central nervous system depressants
Glucocorticoids
Heavy metals (lead, mercury, manganese, arsenic, thallium)
Others (digitalis, disulfiram, cimetidine, bromide)

There are disorders throughout the lifespan that may be associated with schizophrenia-like psychoses. These include genetic abnormalities, intrauterine events, neonatal brain injury, childhood neurologic insults, adolescent neuroendocrine changes, adult neurologic disorders, medical and metabolic diseases (e.g., infections, inflammatory disorders, endocrinopathies, nutritional deficiencies, uremia, hepatic encephalopathy), drug abuse, and psychologic stressors.

Schizophrenia in particular may also have a multifactorial cause. Current diagnostic criteria are divided into inclusion and exclusion criteria. Inclusion criteria include 1) presence of delusions and hallucinations; 2) marked decrement in functional level in areas such as work, school, social relations, and self-care; and 3) continuous signs of the disturbance for at least 6 months. Exclusion criteria include 1) absence of a consistent mood disorder component and 2) lack of evidence of an organic factor that produces the symptoms.

- Schizophrenia may have a multifactorial cause.

The five subtypes of schizophrenia are catatonic, disorganized, paranoid, undifferentiated, and residual.

ANXIETY DISORDERS

This group of disorders includes some of the ones seen most frequently in the outpatient setting. Anxiety symptoms may be misinterpreted as those of medical illness because many of the symptoms overlap, e.g., tachycardia, diaphoresis, tremor, shortness of breath, nausea, abdominal pain, and chest pain. Autonomic arousal and anxious agitation in a medically ill patient can also be quickly attributed to stress or anxiety when it may represent pulmonary embolus or cardiac arrhythmia. Common

sources of anxiety in the medical setting relate to fears of death, abandonment, loss of function, loss of a body part, pain, dependency, and loss of control. When to treat or to seek psychiatric consultation depends on the assessment of the degree of anxiety--is it at a level "expected" under the circumstances or is it unrealistic.

- Anxiety symptoms may be misinterpreted as those of medical illness.
- Common sources of anxiety in the medical setting relate to fears of death, abandonment, loss of function, loss of a body part, etc.

Adjustment Disorder With Anxious Mood

Adjustment disorder with anxious mood is a maladaptive reaction to an identifiable environmental or psychosocial stress, accompanied primarily by symptoms of anxiety that interfere with the patient's usual functioning. Treatment may include supportive counseling and help with identifying the stressor. However, in some cases the anxiety may be so severe as to require short-term use of anxiolytic agents. However, they should be used with caution to avoid problems of long-term use and possible dependence.

- Adjustment disorder with anxious mood: a maladaptive reaction to an identifiable environmental or psychosocial stress accompanied by symptoms of stress.
- It may require short-term use of anxiolytic agents.

Panic Disorder With or Without Agoraphobia

Panic disorder is recurrent, discrete episodes of extreme anxiety accompanied by various somatic symptoms such as dyspnea, unsteady feelings, palpitations, paresthesias, hyperventilation, trembling, diaphoresis, chest pain or discomfort, or abdominal distress. Agoraphobia refers to extreme fear of being in places or situations from which escape may be difficult (or embarrassing). This may lead to avoidance of such situations as driving, travel in general, being in a crowded place, and many other situations, ultimately causing severe limitations in daily functioning for the person. Panic disorder is more common in women than in men; the usual age of onset is from the late teens to the early thirties. A history of childhood separation anxiety is reported in 20%-50% of patients. The incidence is higher in first- and second-degree relatives. Most patients (78%) describe their first panic attack as spontaneous. They generally go to an emergency room after the first attack, believing they are having a heart attack or some severe medical problem.

- Panic disorder: recurrent, discrete episodes of extreme anxiety accompanied by various somatic symptoms.
- Agoraphobia: extreme fear of being in places or situations from which escape may be difficult.
- Agoraphobia is more common in women than in men.
- Patients generally go to an emergency room after first panic attack, believing they are having a heart attack or some severe medical problem.

Some medical diagnostic groups to consider are 1) endocrine disturbances: hyperthyroidism, pheochromocytoma, and hypoglycemia; 2) gastrointestinal disturbances: colitis and irritable bowel syndrome; 3) cardiopulmonary disturbances: pulmonary embolism, exacerbation of chronic obstructive pulmonary disease, and acute allergic reactions; and 4) neurologic conditions: those associated with paresthesias, faintness, or dizziness. Patients with panic attacks may also be prone to major episodes of depression. Alcohol use may temporarily reduce some of the distress of the panic attack and the interim anticipatory anxiety but soon may yield to rebound symptoms and potentially lead to alcohol overuse. Benzodiazepines may similarly be abused.

- Patients with panic attacks may be prone to episodes of major depression.
- Alcohol: may reduce distress of panic attacks but symptoms may rebound, potentially leading to alcohol abuse.
- Benzodiazepines may similarly be abused.

Post-Traumatic Stress Disorder

Post-traumatic stress disorder can be a brief reaction that soon follows an extremely traumatic, overwhelming, or catastrophic experience or it may be a chronic condition that produces severe disability. The syndrome is characterized by intrusive memories, flashbacks, nightmares, avoidance of reminders of the event, and often a restricted range of affect. It may occur in children. There is increased comorbidity with substance abuse, depression, and other anxiety disorders. Patients may be more prone to impulsivity, including suicide. As for other anxiety disorders, treatment is usually a combination of behavioral, psychotherapeutic, and, if necessary, pharmacologic interventions.

- Post-traumatic stress disorder: may be a brief reac-

tion or a chronic condition that produces severe disability.
- Patients may be prone to impulsivity, including suicide.

Generalized Anxiety Disorder

Generalized anxiety disorder is characterized by chronic excessive anxiety and apprehension about life circumstances accompanied by somatic symptoms of anxiety, such as trembling, restlessness, autonomic hyperactivity, and hypervigilance. Treatment is usually a mixture of behavioral, progressive muscle relaxation, psychotherapeutic, and adjunctive psychopharmacologic modalities.

SOMATOFORM DISORDERS, FACTITIOUS DISORDERS, AND MALINGERING

Each of these disorders represents illness behaviors but differ with regard to whether the symptoms and motivations for their persistence are conscious or unconscious.

Somatoform Disorders

These include somatization disorder, conversion disorder, hypochondriasis, somatoform pain disorder (chronic pain syndromes), and body dysmorphic disorder.

Somatization Disorder

Somatization disorder is a polysymptomatic disorder that begins in early life and is characterized by recurrent multiple somatic complaints and an overwhelmingly positive review of symptoms. It mostly affects women. This disorder is often best managed with collaborative work with an empathic primary care physician and mental health professional. Regularly scheduled appointments with the primary care physician seem to lessen "doctor shopping" and frequent emergency room visits.

- Somatization disorder: begins in early life; characterized by recurrent multiple somatic complaints.
- It mostly affects women.
- "Doctor shopping" and frequent emergency room visits.

Conversion Disorder

Conversion disorder is a loss or alteration of physical functioning suggestive of a medical/neurologic disorder, but it cannot be explained on the basis of known physiologic mechanisms. The person is not conscious of intentially producing the symptom. The disorder is not limited to pain or sexual dysfunction. It most often is seen in the outpatient setting. Patients frequently respond to any of several therapeutic modalities which suggest hope of a cure. If it becomes more of a chronic conversion disorder, it carries a poorer prognosis and is difficult to treat. Treatment focuses on management of the symptom rather than cure, much as in somatization or somatoform pain disorders.

- Conversion disorder: loss or alteration of physical functioning.
- It cannot be explained by known physiologic mechanisms.
- It is usually seen in the outpatient setting.
- Treatment focuses on management of the symptoms.

Somatoform Pain Disorder

Somatoform pain disorder (chronic pain syndromes) may occur at any age but most often starts in the 30s or 40s. It is diagnosed twice as often in women as in men and is characterized by preoccupation with pain for at least 6 months. No organic pathology is found to account for the pain, or if there is a related organic lesion, the complaint of pain or resulting interference with usual life activities is in excess of what would be expected from the physical findings. Treatment is usually multidisciplinary and focused on helping the patient manage or live with the pain rather than continuing with the expectation of "cure." Avoidance of long-term dependence on addictive substances is a general goal.

- Somatoform pain disorder: chronic pain syndromes that occur at any age but usually start in the 30s or 40s.
- It is diagnosed twice as often in women as in men.
- It is characterized by preoccupation with pain for at least 6 months.
- Treatment: usually multidisciplinary.

Hypochondriasis

Hypochondriasis is an intense preoccupation with the fear of having or the belief that one has a serious disease despite the lack of physical evidence to support the concern. It tends to be a chronic problem for the patient.

Factitious Disorders

Factitious disorders are characterized by the voluntary production of signs or symptoms of disease. The diagnosis of these disorders requires that the physician be highly suspicious. The most extreme form of the disorder is Münchausen syndrome, which is characterized by the triad of simulating disease, pathologic lying, and wandering. These cases have frequently involved men of lower socioeconomic class who have had a lifelong pattern of poor social adjustment. However, the common form generally occurs among "socially conforming young women of a higher socioeconomic class who are intelligent, educated, and frequently employed in a medically related field." The possibility of a coexisting medical disorder or intercurrent illness needs to be appreciated in the diagnostic and therapeutic management of these difficult cases. Factitious disorders are often found in patients with a history of childhood emotional traumas. These patients through their illness may be seeking to compensate for childhood traumas and secondarily to escape from and make up for stressful life situations.

- Factitious disorders: voluntary production of signs or symptoms of disease in order to assume the sick role.
- Münchausen syndrome: most extreme form of factitious disorder; characteristic triad of simulating disease, pathologic lying, wandering.
- Common form: occurs among socially conforming young women of a higher socioeconomic class.
- Factitious disorders: often in patients with a history of childhood emotional traumas.

Malingering

The essential feature of malingering is the intentional production of false or exaggerated physical or psychologic symptoms. It is motivated by external incentives such as avoiding military service or work, obtaining financial compensation or drugs, evading criminal prosecution, or securing better living conditions. Malingering should be suspected in cases in which 1) a medicolegal context overshadows the clinical presentation, 2) a marked discrepancy exists between the person's claimed stress or disability and the objective findings, 3) there is lack of cooperation during the diagnostic evaluation and in compliance with prescribed treatments, and 4) there is presence of an antisocial personality disorder. The person who is malingering is much less likely to present his or her symptoms in the context of emotional conflict, and the presenting symptoms are less likely to be symbolically related to an underlying emotional conflict.

- Malingering: intentional production of false or exaggerated physical or psychologic symptoms.
- It is motivated by external incentives.

DELIRIUM AND DEMENTIA

The primary distinguishing feature between dementia and delirium is the retention and stability of alertness in dementia.

Delirium

Delirium is characterized by a fluctuating course of an altered state of awareness and consciousness. Although the onset usually is abrupt, it may occasionally be insidious. It may be accompanied by hallucinations (tactile, auditory, visual, or olfactory), illusions (misperceptions of sensory stimuli), delusions, emotional lability, paranoia, alterations in the sleep-wake cycle, and psychomotor slowing or hyperactivity. Delirium is usually reversible with correction of the underlying cause. It often is related to an external toxic agent, medication side effect, metabolic abnormalities, CNS abnormality, or withdrawal of a medication or drug. Delirium is relatively common in medical/surgical inpatients older than 65 years (range, 10%-30%). The diagnosis is primarily made by clinical assessment and changes in the patient's mental status examination. High-risk groups include 1) elderly patients with medical illnesses (especially congestive heart failure, urinary tract infections, hyperkalemia, hyponatremia, malnutrition, dehydration, strokes); 2) postcardiotomy patients; 3) patients with brain damage; 4) patients in drug withdrawal; 5) burn patients; and 6) patients with AIDS.

- Delirium: fluctuating course of an altered state of awareness and consciousness.
- It is usually reversible with correction of the underlying cause.
- It is often related to: external toxic agent, medication side effect, metabolic abnormalities, CNS abnormality, or withdrawal of a medication or drug.
- Delirium is relatively common in medical/surgical patients older than 65.

The commonest cause of delirium in the elderly probably is intoxication with psychotropic drugs, especially drugs with sedative and anticholinergic side effects. Treatment initially can be separated by whether the cause is known. If it is, treating the underlying cause is most beneficial. If the cause is unknown and the patient's behavior interferes with his or her safety and medical care, several categories of intervention can be considered. Management aspects include 1) medical: monitor vital signs, electrolytes, fluid balance, etc.; 2) pharmacologic:

neuroleptic agents in parenteral form are helpful, such as haloperidol given intravenously; 3) environmental supports: to help with orientation, use calendars, clock, windows (family and others with orientation information are also helpful); 4) psychosocial supports: family or other care providers can be helpful.

- Commonest cause of delirium in the elderly: intoxication with psychotropic drugs.

Dementia

Dementia is a syndrome of acquired persistent impairment of mental function involving at least three of the following five domains: memory, language, visuospatial skills, personality or mood, and cognition (including abstraction, judgment, calculations, and executive function). Some of the more common types of dementia are the following:

1. Cortical dementia--The common form is Alzheimer's disease; other types include Pick's disease and Creutzfeldt-Jakob disease. The overall prevalence is estimated at 2%-10% of the population over 65 and 15%-20% of those older than 85.
2. Subcortical dementia--Patients with this type of dementia often have an associated gait disturbance. The common type is multi-infarct dementia; other forms include normal-pressure hydrocephalus, Huntington's disease, and Parkinson's disease.
3. HIV-related dementia.
4. Dementias associated with multiple sclerosis, amyotrophic lateral sclerosis, vitamin B_{12} deficiency, hypothyroidism, and Wilson's disease.

- Cortical dementia: the common form is Alzheimer's type.
- Subcortical dementia: the common type is multi-infarct dementia.

Dementia is distinguished from delirium by intact arousal, more preserved attention, and persistence of the cognitive changes. Some forms may be reversible, as in dementia related to hypothyroidism, and some may be "treatable" without reversing the intellectual deficits, e.g., preventing further ischemic injury in patients with vascular dementia. The dementia may be a chronic progressive form in which treatment is generally related to improved control of the behavioral disturbances.

PSYCHOLOGIC ASPECTS OF AIDS

From the early to the terminal phases of AIDS and its sequelae, many psychiatric symptoms and complications are possible. The organic mental disorders associated with this process can be primary (directly induced by HIV infection), secondary (related to the effects of the HIV infection leading to immunodeficiency and opportunistic infections or tumors systemically or within the CNS), or iatrogenic (resulting from the treatment of HIV or its sequelae). The delirium of AIDS often has a multifactorial cause, similar to delirium in general, i.e., electrolyte imbalance, encephalopathy from intracranial or systemic infections, hypoxemia, or medication side effects. HIV itself causes encephalopathy. The dementia of AIDS can result from the chronic sequelae of most of the causes of delirium. However, direct cerebral infection with HIV probably causes much of the dementia. Other psychiatric symptoms are more nonspecific, such as anger, depression, mania, psychosis, and the general problems of dealing with a terminal illness. Also, all of these might be complicated by undiagnosed and, thus, untreated alcohol or drug dependence, especially in the early phases of the disease.

- AIDS: many possible psychiatric symptoms and complications.
- Organic mental disorders can be primary (due to HIV infection), secondary (due to immunodeficiency and opportunistic infections), or iatrogenic.
- Delirium in AIDS is multifactorial.
- Dementia in AIDS: can result from chronic sequelae of most of the causes of delirium.

THE SUICIDAL PATIENT

Suicide is not an uncommon consequence of mental illness. It occurs in all psychiatric diagnostic categories. Emergency medicine physicians are often the first to deal with patients who have either completed suicide, attempted suicide, or have suicidal ideation. The recognition of risk factors for suicide and the acute medical management of the patient are important. Although the person who overdoses with a benzodiazepine may be more serious about the intent, the person who overdoses on aspirin may be at more risk for serious medical complications.

- Suicide: occurs in all psychiatric diagnostic categories.
- Recognition of the risk factors for suicide is important.

Recognition of a suicidal gesture is important in evaluating a patient in an emergency room. Although drug overdoses are the commonest form, alcohol intoxication, single vehicle accidents, and falls from heights at times merit further investigation. Many suicidal patients saw a physician the week before the attempt. Some of the risk factors to be aware of include: older divorced or widowed men, Caucasians, unemployment, poor physical health, past suicide attempts, family history of suicide (especially if parent), psychosis, alcoholism or drug abuse, chronic painful disease, sudden life changes, living alone, anniversary of significant loss. Almost without exception, patients who come to an emergency room with intense suicidal ideation or gestures should not be sent home alone.

- In evaluating patients in an emergency room, recognition of a suicidal gesture is important.
- Many suicidal patients saw a physician the week before the attempt.
- Patients who come to an emergency room with intense suicidal ideation or gestures should not be sent home alone.

EATING DISORDERS

The two common eating disorders are anorexia nervosa and bulimia. Both are more prevalent in women than in men. The onset is usually in the teenage or young adult years but can start prepubertally or after age 40. These disorders are now found across all income, racial, and ethnic groups. Both disorders have a primary symptom of preoccupation with weight and a desire to be thinner. The disorders are not mutually exclusive, and about 50% of patients with anorexia nervosa also have bulimia. Many patients with bulimia previously had at least a subclinical case of anorexia nervosa.

- The two common eating disorders: anorexia nervosa and bulimia.
- They are more prevalent in women than in men.
- Primary symptom: preoccupation with weight and a desire to be thinner.

Anorexia Nervosa

To meet the diagnostic criteria of anorexia nervosa, weight loss must be 15% below that expected for age and height. However, weight loss of 30%-40% below normal is not uncommon and leads to medical complications of starvation, such as depletion of fat, muscle wasting (including cardiac muscle in severe cases), bradycardia and other arrhythmias, ventricular tachycardia and sudden death, constipation, abdominal pain, leukopenia, hypercortisolemia, osteoporosis, and, in extreme cases, development of lanugo, and metabolic alterations to conserve energy (thyroid--low levels of T_3, cold intolerance, and difficulty maintaining core body temperature; reproductive--marked decrease or cessation of LH and FSH secretion and secondary amenorrhea).

Bulimia

The patients always feel as though their eating is out of control; many patients may have a concurrent depressive or anxiety disorder. Physical complications of the binge-purge cycle may include fluid and electrolyte abnormalities, hypochloremic-hypokalemic alkalosis, esophageal and gastric irritation and bleeding, large bowel abnormalities due to laxative abuse, marked erosion of dental enamel with associated decay, parotid and salivary gland hypertrophy, and hyperamylasemia (25%-40% more than normal). If bulimia is untreated, it often becomes chronic. Some patients have a gradual spontaneous remission of some symptoms.

- Patients with bulimia may have a concurrent depressive or anxiety disorder.
- The binge-purge cycle causes physical complications.

ALCOHOLISM AND SUBSTANCE ABUSE DISORDERS

Alcoholism and substance abuse disorders are a major concern in all age groups and across all ethnic, socioeconomic, and racial groups. Despite national and international efforts to curb the problem and to make treatment more readily available, many people go undiagnosed and fewer than 10% of addicted people are involved in some form of treatment, either self-help groups or with professional supervision. The lifetime incidence of alcohol and drug abuse approaches 20% of the population. These disorders have devastating effects on families and significant others and contribute to other social problems such as motor vehicle accidents and fatalities, domestic violence, suicide, and increasing health care costs. Untreated alcoholics have been estimated to generate twice the general health care costs of nonalcoholics. Patients with addictive disorders are a heterogeneous group. They may present in many different ways. What

may be most critical is improvement in the diagnostic skills in recognizing addictive disorders. The current definition of alcoholism approved by the National Council on Alcoholism and Drug Dependence may also be applicable to other drugs of abuse: alcoholism is a primary, chronic disease with genetic, psychosocial, and environmental factors influencing its development and manifestations. The disease is often progressive and fatal. It is characterized by continuous or periodic impaired control over drinking, preoccupation with the drug alcohol, use despite adverse consequences, and distortions in thinking, most notably denial.

- Fewer than 10% of addicted people are involved in some form of treatment.
- Lifetime incidence of alcohol and drug abuse approaches 20% of the population.
- Untreated alcoholics generate twice the general health care costs of nonalcoholics.
- Patients with addictive disorders are a heterogeneous group.

The adverse consequences of alcoholism and substance abuse disorders cross over into several domains:
1. Physical health--Alcohol withdrawal syndromes, liver disease, gastritis, anemia, and neurologic disorders.
2. Psychologic functioning--Impairment in cognition and changes in mood and behavior.
3. Interpersonal functioning--Marital problems and child abuse and impaired social relationships.
4. Occupational functioning--Scholastic or job problems.
5. Legal, financial, and spiritual problems.

The substance abuse disorders are divided into ten major groups: alcohol; amphetamine; cannabis; cocaine; hallucinogens; inhalants; nicotine; opioids; phencyclidine; and benzodiazepines, sedative hypnotics, and anxiolytics. Some things are specific to each of these groups, but what may be surprising is that they probably have more similarities than differences when it comes to diagnosing a problem of abuse and/or dependence. In Table 25-2, these drugs are grouped according to their perceived effects. The descriptive titles of the groups give an idea of the physiologic and psychologic activity of the drug when taken. If one thinks of the converse of these states, the withdrawal states can partly be determined. As an example, if in the group of "downers," heart rate, blood pressure, and general autonomic functions slow down when they are used, the opposite reaction would be expected with withdrawal from the substance. Another significant point is that within the group of "downers" there is considerable potential for crossover addictions.

● Within the group of "downers," there is considerable potential for crossover addictions.

Table 25-2.--Drugs Grouped According to Their Perceived Effects

Uppers	Downers	"All arounders"
Cocaine	Alcohol	Cannabis
Amphetamine	Opioids	Hallucinogens
Caffeine	Benzodiazepines	Inhalants
Nicotine	Sedative-hypnotics	Phencyclidine
	Barbiturates	

Alcoholism

Alcoholism is defined above. Medical data from physical examination and laboratory tests can be helpful. However, most of the pertinent findings are not apparent until after several years (often up to 5 years) of alcohol use and so are more reflective of middle-to-late stages of the disease. Two of the earlier detectable signs are increases of serum γ–glutamyltransferase and increased mean corpuscular volume. In both men and women, the combination of increased γ-glutamyltransferase levels and mean corpuscular volume can identify up to 90% of alcoholics. Other lab abnormalities include elevated levels of alkaline phosphatase, bilirubin, uric acid, and triglycerides. However, because of the number of false-negative results, it is not practical to rely on lab data alone for the diagnosis of alcoholism. Alcohol withdrawal can range from mild to quite severe, with the occurrence of withdrawal seizures and/or delirium tremens. The medical complications of alcoholism can affect nearly every organ system, but the CNS, liver, gastrointestinal tract, pancreas, and cardiovascular system are particularly sensitive to the effects of alcohol.

● Increased γ-glutamyltransferase levels and mean corpuscular volume can identify up to 90% of alcoholics.
● It is not practical to rely on lab data alone to make the diagnosis of alcoholism.
● Medical complications of alcoholism can affect nearly every organ system.

Benzodiazepines, Sedative-Hypnotics, and Anxiolytics

In contrast to many of the other groups, benzodiazepines, sedative-hypnotics, and anxiolytics are widely used in many areas of medicine, so that the addictions that are often seen are iatrogenic. However, five characteristics may help distinguish medical use from nonmedical use: 1) Intent--What is the purpose of the use? 2) Effect--What is the effect on the user's life? 3) Control--Is the use controlled by only the user or does a physician share in the control? 4) Legality--Is the use of the drug legal or illegal? Medical drug use is legal. 5) Pattern--In what settings is the drug used?

These same characteristics can also be used to distinguish medical from nonmedical use of opioids. Withdrawal from use of benzodiazepines and barbiturates, in particular, can be serious because of the increased risk of withdrawal seizures.

● Withdrawal of use of benzodiazepines and barbiturates, in particular, can be serious because of the increased risk of withdrawal seizures

PSYCHOPHARMACOLOGY

The use of a pharmacologic treatment for a psychiatric disorder or the use of psychoactive medications in other disorders is a decision that generally is made after considering multiple factors in the case. Medication alone is rarely the sole treatment for a psychiatric disorder but rather a component of a broader treatment plan. Because psychoactive medications are used in various circumstances for many different indications, the major groups of these medications--antidepressants, antipsychotics, antimanic agents, anxiolytics, and sedative drugs--are discussed below in general terms rather than for treatment of specific disorders. The choice of a medication generally is based on its side-effect profile and the clinical profile of the patient. There are many effective drugs in each of the major groups, but they differ in terms of pharmacokinetics, side effects, and available routes of administration.

● Medication alone is rarely the sole treatment for a psychiatric disorder.
● The choice of a medication generally is based on its side-effect profile and the clinical profile of the patient.

Antipsychotic Agents

The several classes of antipsychotic agents can be categorized by chemical structure: phenothiazines (including their derivatives and peperidines and piperazines), thioxanthenes, butyrophenones, dibenzoxazepine, indole derivatives, pimozide, and dibenzodiazepine (Clozaril). The choice of medication is based on the patient's clinical situation, side-effect profile of the chosen agent, history of previous response, and issues related to compliance. The prevailing theory about the mechanism of action of these agents is that they cause blockade of dopamine postsynaptic receptors. This relates to both the antipsychotic activity and other side effects, depending on which dopamine pathways in the brain are affected and which of the several types of dopamine receptor is preferentially affected. If the nigrostriatal dopaminergic system (involved with motor activity) is affected, extrapyramidal symptoms may result. Blockade of the dopamine pathways in the pituitary and hypothalamus causes increased prolactin release and changes in appetite and temperature regulation. The effects of these drugs on the limbic system, midbrain tegmentum, septal nuclei, and mesocortical dopaminergic projections are thought to be responsible for their antipsychotic action.

- The theory about the mechanism of action of antipsychotic agents is that they cause blockade of dopamine postsynaptic receptors.
- The antipsychotic effects of these agents are due to their action on the limbic system, midbrain tegmentum, septal nuclei, and mesocortical dopaminergic projections.

Potency relates to the milligram equivalents of the drugs and not to their relative efficacy. By convention, the potency of antipsychotic drugs is compared with a standard 100-mg dose of chlorpromazine (Thorazine). For example, 2 mg haloperidol = 100 mg chlorpromazine and 12 mg haloperidol = 600 mg chlorpromazine.

- The **low-potency** drugs (chlorpromazine and thioridazine) have *low* extrapyramidal side effects and relatively high anticholinergic and orthostatic hypotensive side effects.
- The **high-potency** drugs (haloperidol and fluphenazine) have a *high* propensity for extrapyramidal side effects and low anticholinergic and orthostatic hypotensive effects.
- Intermediate potency drugs (5- to 40-mg equivalents) have side effects at an intermediate level.

Side Effects: Extrapyramidal Reactions

Acute dystonic reactions occur within hours or days after initiating treatment with antipsychotic drugs. These reactions are characterized by uncontrollable tightening of the face and neck muscles with spasms. The effect on the eyes may cause an oculogyric crisis, and the effect on the laryngeal muscles may cause respiratory or ventilatory difficulties. Treatment is usually with intravenous or intramuscular administration of an anticholinergic agent, followed by the use of an oral anticholinergic agent for a few days (antipsychotic agents have long half-lives).

- Acute dystonic reactions: occur within hours or days after initiating treatment with antipsychotic drugs.
- Reactions: uncontrollable tightening of the face and neck muscles with spasms.
- Treatment: i.v. or i.m. administration of an anticholinergic agent.

1. Parkinsonian syndrome has a more gradual onset and can be treated with oral anticholinergic agents and/or decreased doses of the antipsychotic agent.
2. Akathisia is an unpleasant feeling of restlessness and the inability to sit still. It often occurs within days of initiating therapy with antipsychotic agents. Akathisia is sometimes mistaken for exacerbation of the psychosis. Treatment, if possible, is to decrease the dose of the antipsychotic agent or to try using a β-adrenergic blocking agent such as propranolol, if not contraindicated.
3. Akinesia is characterized by diminished spontaneity, few gestures, and apathy. It may be mistaken for a depressive reaction. This condition usually can be treated with an anticholinergic agent.

- Akathisia: unpleasant feeling of restlessness and the inability to sit still.

Tardive dyskinesia consists of involuntary movements of the face, trunk, or extremities. The most consistent risk factor for its development is older age. Prevention is the most important aspect of management, because no reliable treatment is available. It is best if treatment with the antipsychotic agent can be discontinued, although there may be a temporary increase in the symptoms of tardive dyskinesia.

- Tardive dyskinesia: involuntary movements of the face, trunk, or extremities.
- Prevention: the most important aspect of management.

Neuroleptic malignant syndrome is a potentially life-threatening disorder that may occur after the use of any antipsychotic agent, although it is generally more common with the high-potency antipsychotics. Its clinical presentation is characterized by severe rigidity, fever, leukocytosis, tachycardia, tachypnea, diaphoresis, blood pressure fluctuations, and marked increase in CPK levels due to muscle breakdown. The treatment consists of discontinuing the use of the antipsychotic agent and providing life-support measures (ventilation, cooling, etc.). Pharmacologic interventions may include the use of dantrolene sodium, which is a direct-acting muscle relaxant, and/or bromocriptine, which is a centrally acting dopamine agonist. Often, one of the most effective treatments is electroconvulsive therapy.

- Neuroleptic malignant syndrome: potentially life-threatening.
- It may occur after the use of any antipsychotic agent.
- Characteristics: severe rigidity, fever, leukocytosis, tachycardia, tachypnea, diaphoresis, blood pressure fluctuations, marked increase in CPK levels (muscle breakdown).

Other, non-extrapyramidal side effects of antipsychotic agents are listed in Table 25-3.

Table 25-3.--Side Effects of Antipsychotic Agents Aside From Extrapyramidal Effects

Anticholinergic
Orthostatic hypotension--related to α-adrenergic receptor blockade
Hyperprolactinemia--gynecomastia possible in men and women, galactorrhea (rare), amenorrhea, weight gain, breast tenderness, decreased libido
Sexual dysfunction
Dermatologic--pigmentary changes in the skin and photosensitivity
Decreased seizure threshold--caused by most antipsychotic agents

Clozapine

Clozapine is a newer antipsychotic agent with different dopamine receptor-blocking activity and fewer extrapyramidal side effects. It does not increase prolactin levels, but it has a 2% risk of producing agranulocytosis, which is reversible if the medication is withdrawn.

Because of this serious potential side effect, there is a specific requirement for performing weekly blood cell counts.

Antianxiety Medications

These drugs most appropriately are used to treat time-limited anxiety or insomnia related to an identifiable stress or change in sleep cycle. If used for a long term (>2-3 months), benzodiazepines and related substances should be tapered rather than abruptly discontinued to avoid any of the three "discontinuation syndromes."

1. Relapse--Return of the original anxiety symptoms, often after weeks to months.
2. Rebound--Intensification of the original symptoms; it usually lasts several days and appears within hours to days of abrupt cessation of drug use.
3. Withdrawal--May be mild to severe and includes autonomic and CNS symptoms that are different from the original presenting symptoms of the disorder.

Benzodiazepines are well-absorbed orally but have unpredictable availability with intramuscular use, except for lorazepam. There is great variability among the benzodiazepines in terms of their pharmacokinetics. Many of these drugs have metabolites with very long half-lives. Therefore, much smaller doses need to be used in the elderly, in patients with brain damage, and in children--all these patient groups are prone to the paradoxical reactions (anxiety, irritability, aggression, agitation, insomnia), especially patients with known brain damage.

- Benzodiazepines: great variability in terms of their pharmacokinetics.

Buspirone is a non-benzodiazepine anxiolytic drug whose mechanism of action is not known. However, the drug has effects on many neurotransmitter systems, especially the serotonergic and dopaminergic systems. Cross-tolerance does not exist between the benzodiazepines and buspirone. It generally takes 2-3 weeks for the drug to become effective.

- Buspirone: a non-benzodiazepine anxiolytic drug.
- It takes 2-3 weeks for the drug to become effective.

Antidepressant Agents

The several classes of antidepressant agents differ in their chemical structure, site of action, side-effect profiles, and other variables. These groups include:

1. Tricyclics--Tertiary amines, including imipramine, amitriptyline, doxepin, and trimipramine, and secondary amines, including desipramine, nortriptyline, and protriptyline.
2. Other cyclic antidepressants--Maprotiline, amoxapine, trazodone, bupropion, fluoxetine, and sertraline.
3. Monoamine oxidase inhibitors--Phenelzine, isocarboxazid, tranylcypromine, and pargyline.

The mechanism of action is their effect on the catecholaminergic and serotonergic systems of the CNS. The various cyclic antidepressant agents block the reuptake of norepinephrine and/or serotonin, increasing the amount of these neurotransmitters at the synapse. Monoamine oxidase inhibitors block the catabolism of several biogenic amines (norepinephrine, serotonin, tyramine, phenylephrine, and dopamine), thereby increasing the amount of these neurotransmitters available for synaptic release.

- Antidepressant agents affect the catecholaminergic and serotonergic systems of the CNS.
- Monoamine oxidase inhibitors block the catabolism of several biogenic amines.

Antidepressant agents are primarily approved for use in the treatment of depression. However, they are useful in several other disorders, including panic disorder, obsessive compulsive disorder, enuresis, chronic pain, migraine headache, bulimia, and attention deficit disorder. Because they are so widely used, familiarity with the basics of their use, side effects, and drug interactions may be helpful. The choice of which antidepressant agent to use is often based on the side-effect profile of the drug and the clinical presentation of the patient. The side effects of the major groups of antidepressant agents are listed in Table 25-4.

A complete trial of antidepressant medication consists of 6 weeks of therapeutic doses before considering refractoriness. If some improvement has occurred with the initial trial but the condition is not yet back to baseline, it may be worthwhile to try augmenting therapy with lithium carbonate before changing the medication to another class of antidepressant. Another alternative is a trial of thyroid hormone (T_3) supplementation before switching use of antidepressant medications. After clinical improvement is noted, the medication may need to be maintained for an extended period of time.

- A complete trial of antidepressant medication: 6 weeks of therapeutic doses.
- Augmenting therapy with lithium carbonate may be worthwhile before changing the medication to another class of antidepressant.

Table 25-4.--Side Effects of the Major Groups of Antidepressant Agents

Orthostatic hypotension--The cardiovascular side effect that most commonly results in serious morbidity, especially in the elderly

Anticholinergic effects--Dry mouth, blurred vision, urinary retention, etc.; beware of these side effects in patients with prostatic hypertrophy and narrow-angle glaucoma. Drugs with more anticholinergic side effects also seem to be the more sedating, e.g., tertiary amine tricyclics

Cardiac conduction effects--Most of the tricyclics prolong PR and QRS intervals. Therefore, these drugs need to be used with caution in patients with preexisting heart block, such as second-degree heart block or markedly prolonged QRS and QT intervals. The tricyclics are potent antiarrhythmic agents because of their quinidine-like effect. Newer generation antidepressants such as trazadone, fluoxetine, and sertraline have far fewer cardiac interactions.

Sedating types--Tertiary amine tricyclics and trazadone

Potentially more stimulating types--Secondary amine tricyclics, bupropion, fluoxetine, and sertraline

Monoamine Oxidase Inhibitors

Most clinical concerns about the use of monoamine oxidase inhibitors relate to reactions from the ingestion of tyramine, which is not metabolized because of the inhibition of intestinal monoamine oxidase. Tyramine may act as a false transmitter and displace norepinephrine from synaptic vesicles. Patients should be instructed in a tyramine-restricted diet, especially to avoid aged cheeses, smoked meats, pickled herring, beer and red wine (generally all alcohol should be restricted), yeast extracts, fava beans, and overripe bananas and avocadoes. Certain general anesthetics and drugs with sympathomimetic activity should be avoided; especially beware of over-the-counter cough and cold preparations, decongestants, and appetite suppressants. Meperidine (Demerol) is absolutely contraindicated because of its potentially lethal interaction with monoamine oxidase inhibitors.

- Clinical concerns about monoamine oxidase inhibitors: reactions due to ingestion of tyramine, which is not metabolized.

- Tyramine: a false neurotransmitter that displaces norepinephrine from synaptic vesicles.
- Meperidine (Demerol): absolutely contraindicated because of its potentially lethal interaction with monoamine oxidase inhibitors.

Treatment of hypertensive reactions relies on administering drugs with α-adrenergic blocking properties, such as intravenous administration of phentolamine. This should be done in an emergency room. Patients may take nifedipine (10 mg sublingually) before reaching an emergency room if they have moderate-to-severe occipital headache while taking a monoamine oxidase inhibitor.

ANTIMANIC DRUGS

Lithium carbonate is the drug of choice for treating bipolar disorders. It can also be effective in patients with recurrent unipolar depressions and as an adjunct for maintenance of remission of depression after electroconvulsive therapy. Acute manic symptoms usually respond to treatment with lithium within 7-10 days. While waiting for this effect, the adjunctive use of antipsychotic agents may be helpful. Lithium is well absorbed from the gastrointestinal tract, with peak levels in 1-2 hours. Its half-life is about 24 hours. Levels are generally checked 10-12 hours after the last dose. Relatively common side effects include fine hand tremor, diarrhea, polyuria, polydipsia, thirst, and nausea, which is often improved by taking the medication on a full stomach. Lithium is contraindicated in the first trimester of pregnancy, because of its potential for causing defects in the developing cardiac system. Renal effects generally can be reversed with discontinuation of treatment with lithium. The most noticeable renal effect is the vasopressin-resistant effect leading to impaired concentrating ability and nephrogenic diabetes insipidus with polyuria and polydipsia. Most patients who take lithium develop some polyuria but not all develop more severe manifestations of nephrogenic diabetes insipidus. Renal function should be followed in all patients receiving maintenance lithium therapy. However, whether lithium has significant nephrotoxic effects is a matter of controversy. A hematologic side effect is a benign leukocytosis. Hypothyroidism may occur in as many as 20% of patients taking lithium, because of the direct inhibitory effects on thyroid hormone production or increased antithyroid antibodies.

- Lithium carbonate: drug of choice for treating bipolar

disorders.
- Common side effects: hand tremor, diarrhea, polyuria, polydipsia, thirst, nausea.
- Renal effects generally can be reversed with discontinuation of treatment with lithium.
- Most noticeable renal effect: impaired concentrating ability.
- Hypothyroidism occurs in as many as 20% of patients receiving lithium.

Because the range between the therapeutic and toxic levels of lithium in the plasma is narrow, patients and physicians should be familiar with conditions that may increase or decrease lithium levels and with the signs and symptoms of lithium toxicity so it can be recognized and treated promptly (Tables 25-5 and 25-6).

Other Antimanic Agents

Carbamazepine appears to be effective for controlling acute manic attacks and for prophylactic maintenance therapy. It is used in doses similar to those used for seizure disorders. Carbamazepine is similar in chemical structure to the tricyclic antidepressant agents and has a quinidine-like effect. Other antimanic drugs being investigated include valproic acid, clonazepam, and verapamil.

ELECTROCONVULSIVE THERAPY

Electroconvulsive therapy is the most effective treatment for severely depressed patients, especially those with psychotic features. It is also helpful in treating catatonia and mania and may be used in children and adults. Also, electroconvulsive therapy can be administered to pregnant women. It may be effective in patients with overlapping depression and Parkinson's disease and/or dementia. Electroconvulsive therapy is administered with the patient under barbiturate anesthesia, with succinylcholine or a similar muscle relaxant to minimize peripheral manifestations of the seizure. An anticholinergic agent such as atropine is generally given to decrease secretions and to prevent bradycardia caused by central stimulation of the vagus nerve. A usual course of treatment is 6-12 sessions given over a 2-4 week period. Therapy is often initiated with unilateral, nondominant electrode placement to minimize memory loss. If satisfactory results cannot be obtained with this method, bilateral electrode placement is used.

- Electroconvulsive therapy: most effective treatment

Table 25-5.--Conditions That Increase or Decrease Lithium Levels in the Plasma

Increase levels	Decrease levels
Dehydration	Increased caffeine consumption
Overheating and increased perspiration with exercise and/or hot weather	Theophylline
Nonsteroidal anti-inflammatory drugs	
Thiazide diuretics	
Angiotensin-converting enzyme inhibitors	
Certain antibiotics--tetracycline, spectinomycin, and metronidazole	

Table 25-6.--Signs and Symptoms of Lithium Toxicity

Mild-to-moderate toxicity (plasma levels, 1.5-2.0 mEq/L)	Moderate-to-severe toxicity (plasma levels, 2.0-2.5 mEq/L)	Severe toxicity (plasma levels, >2.5 mEq/L)
Vomiting	Persistent nausea and vomiting	Generalized seizures
Abdominal pain	Anorexia	Oliguria and renal failure
Dry mouth	Blurred vision	Death
Ataxia	Muscle fasciculations	
Slurred speech	Hyperactive deep tendon reflexes	
Nystagmus	Delirium	
Muscle weakness	Convulsions	
	Electroencephalographic changes	
	Stupor and coma	
	Circulatory system failure	
	Lowered blood pressure	
	Cardiac arrhythmias	
	Conduction abnormalities	

Modified from Silver JM, Hales RE, Yudofsky SC: Biological therapies for mental disorders. *In* Clinical Psychiatry for Medical Students. Edited by A Stoudemire. Philadelphia, JB Lippincott Company, 1990, pp 459-496. By permission of publisher.

for severely depressed patients, especially those with psychotic features.

- It is also helpful in treating catatonia and mania.
- It can be given to pregnant women.
- It may be helpful in cases of overlapping depression and Parkinson's disease and/or dementia.

Mechanism of action--Electroconvulsive therapy induces changes in several transmitter-receptor systems, particularly acetylcholine, norepinephrine, dopamine, and serotonin. It downregulates β-adrenergic receptors and may decrease calcium levels in the cerebrospinal fluid. It may also affect neuropeptides and electrical conduction systems (similar to those studied by cardiac electrophysiologists).

- Electroconvulsive therapy induces changes in acetylcholine, norepinephrine, dopamine, and serotonin transmitter-receptor systems.

- It downregulates β-adrenergic receptors.
- It may decrease calcium levels in the cerebrospinal fluid.

No longer are there any absolute contraindications to electroconvulsive therapy, although there are several relative contraindications. Previously, the only absolute contraindication was the presence of an intracranial space-occupying lesion and increased intracranial pressure. Serious complications or mortality is generally reported as less than 1 per 10,000, which makes this therapy one of the safest interventions that uses general anesthesia. Morbidity and mortality usually are due to cardiovascular complications, such as arrhythmia, myocardial infarction, or hypotension. The major risks are those associated with the brief general anesthesia. Medical evaluations performed before giving the therapy should pay particular attention to cardiovascular function, pulmonary function (because positive pressure respiration is used during anesthesia), electrolyte balance, and the patient's previous experiences with anesthesia.

- Electroconvulsive therapy: no longer any absolute contraindications.
- There are several relative contraindications.
- Morbidity and mortality are usually due to cardiovascular complications.

QUESTIONS
(See "Answers" section)

Multiple Choice

1. Major depression may be manifested by all the following except:
   a. Increased or decreased appetite
   b. Insomnia
   c. Markedly diminished interest or pleasure in all or almost all activities
   d. Confabulation
   e. Diminished ability to concentrate

2. You are asked to see a 77-year-old woman who has been living in a nursing home for the last 3 months. The nursing home staff report that she uses foul language. Her sleep is restless and her eating patterns are erratic; she eats only small amounts when strongly encouraged by the staff. Differential diagnoses would include all the following except:
   a. Progressive dementing process
   b. Depressive disorder
   c. Subdural hematoma
   d. Anorexia nervosa
   e. Heavy metal toxicity

3. Patients with a high risk for developing delirium include all the following except:
   a. Postcardiotomy patients
   b. Patients with schizophrenia
   c. Elderly patients
   d. Patients in acute alcohol or drug withdrawal
   e. AIDS patients

4. The common cause of psychosis in hospitalized medical or surgical patients is:
   a. Schizophrenia
   b. Reaction to stress
   c. Personality disorders
   d. Depression
   e. Drug-induced psychosis

5. Alternatives to long-term use of benzodiazepines in patients with anxiety disorders include all the following except:
   a. Psychotherapy
   b. Behavioral therapy
   c. Trial of antidepressant agents
   d. Electroconvulsive therapy
   e. Progressive muscle relaxation

True/False

6. The diagnosis of alcoholism is based on the following factors:
   a. Preoccupation with using or obtaining alcohol interferes with important social, occupational, and recreational activities
   b. Continued use despite social, medical, or psychologic consequences
   c. Previous attempts to cut down or control alcohol use
   d. Specific variables of quantity and frequency of alcohol use per week
   e. Use of denial to reduce awareness of alcohol being a cause of many of the patient's problems rather than the solution
   f. Drinking larger quantities for longer periods of

time than the person intended

7. Indicate whether or not the following cause increased lithium levels in the plasma, potentially leading to lithium toxicity:
   a. Caffeine
   b. Thiazide diuretics
   c. Angiotensin-converting enzyme inhibitor antihypertensive agents
   d. Low sodium diet
   e. Theophylline
   f. Nonsteroidal anti-inflammatory drugs

CHAPTER 26

PULMONARY DISEASES

Udaya B. S. Prakash, M.D.

SYMPTOMS AND SIGNS

Cough

Cough can be voluntary or reflex. The afferent arm of the reflex consists of the sensory branches of the trigeminal, glossopharyngeal, superior laryngeal, and vagus nerves. The efferent limb includes the recurrent laryngeal and spinal nerves. Lesions in the following organs can cause cough: nose, ears, pharynx, larynx, bronchi, lungs, pleura, and abdominal viscera. Types of cough: brassy (tracheal involvement), barking (epiglottitis), wheezy (asthma), nocturnal (reflux), and positional (abscess, tumors).

- Lesion (inflammatory, mechanical, chemical, or thermal) in any afferent limb of the reflex can cause cough.
- Cough can be the presenting or only manifestation of asthma.
- Positional cough occurs with lung abscess, obstructing lesions (tumors), nocturnal reflux.

Chronic cough is defined as cough lasting ≥3 weeks without an obvious cause. Evaluation should include ear-nose-throat examination, esophagography and/or acid reflux test, and methacholine inhalation challenge to exclude asthma. Nonpulmonary diseases (temporal arteritis, rheumatoid bronchiolitis, Sjögren's syndrome, and reflux esophagitis) may present with cough. Bronchoscopy in the absence of chest radiographic abnormalities carries a low diagnostic yield.

- Most common causes of chronic cough: postnasal drip, asthma, reflux, and postinfectious.
- Complications of cough: cough syncope, rib fractures, pneumothorax.

- Cough syncope: hard cough produces increased intrathoracic pressure, which causes decreased cardiac output and cerebral perfusion.
- Bronchoscopy has a low diagnostic yield if chest radiographic findings are normal.
- Nonpulmonary diseases can present with cough.
- Nearly 6% of patients taking angiotensin-converting enzyme (ACE) inhibitors develop cough as a complication. Cross reactivity is present among different ACE inhibitors.

Sputum

Purulent sputum occurs in bronchiectasis and lung abscess. Frothy pink sputum is seen in pulmonary edema. Expectoration of bronchial casts, mucous plugs, or thin strings occurs in asthma, bronchopulmonary aspergillosis, and mucoid impaction syndrome, and expectoration of stone (lithoptysis) occurs in broncholithiasis. Bronchorrhea (expectoration of thin serous fluid >100 mL/day) is seen in 20% of patients with diffuse alveolar cell carcinoma. Expectoration of worms is found in parasitic infections (*Ascaris*).

- Bronchorrhea occurs in diffuse alveolar cell carcinoma.
- Sputum microscopy for eosinophils, Charcot-Leyden crystals, Curschmann's spirals in asthmatics.

Hemoptysis

Hemoptysis is the expectoration of blood or blood-streaked sputum. Bleeding from bronchial circulation is seen in chronic bronchitis, bronchiectasis, malignancies, broncholithiasis, and foreign bodies. Bleeding from pulmonary arterial circulation is seen in pulmonary arteriovenous malformations, fungus ball, tumors, vas-

697

culitis, pulmonary hypertension, and lung abscess. Bleeding from pulmonary alveolar-capillary location occurs in mitral stenosis, left ventricular failure, pulmonary infarction, vasculitis, Goodpasture's syndrome, and idiopathic pulmonary hemosiderosis. A fistula between airways and blood vessels (tracheoinnominate) can cause massive hemoptysis. Massive hemoptysis ≥200 mL/24 hours, but the underlying lung dysfunction determines outcome.

- Hemoptysis must be differentiated from pseudohemoptysis (expectoration of blood previously aspirated into airways or lungs from the gastrointestinal tract, nose, or supraglottic areas).
- History, examination, and chest radiography are important in the diagnosis.
- Commonest cause of streaky hemoptysis is chronic bronchitis or postinfectious.
- Almost all patients with hemoptysis should have bronchoscopy.
- Cause of death in massive hemoptysis is asphyxiation, not exsanguination.

Dyspnea

Dyspnea is the symptom (or awareness) of breathlessness. The causes include disorders of the pulmonary, cardiac, skeletal (kyphoscoliosis, etc.), endocrine, metabolic, neurologic, and hematologic systems. Other causes are physiologic dyspnea of pregnancy, drugs, psychogenic, deconditioning, and obesity. Severity is clinically assessed by grading: grade 0, no dyspnea except with strenuous exercise; grade 1, slight dyspnea on hurrying on a level surface or walking up a hill; grade 2, dyspnea while walking on a level surface and being unable to keep up with peers and having to stop to catch breath; grade 3, dyspnea on walking 100 yards or after a few minutes and the need to stop for breath; grade 4, dyspnea on dressing or undressing or minimal exertion; and grade 5, dyspnea at rest.

- Each organ system is a potential source for the cause of dyspnea.
- Cardiopulmonary diseases are the most common causes.
- Initial clinical grading of dyspnea is helpful in planning further tests.

In most cases, dyspnea is the result of increased work of breathing. Other mechanisms include abnormal activation of respiratory centers, voluntary hyperventila-tion, and Cheyne-Stokes breathing. Clinical history, physical examination, chest radiography, and cardiopulmonary physiologic testing are important. Orthopnea: dyspnea in the supine posture (associated with congestive heart failure, bilateral diaphragmatic paralysis, severe chronic obstructive pulmonary disease [COPD], asthma, sleep apnea, and severe reflux). Paroxysmal nocturnal dyspnea: nocturnal episodes of dyspnea resulting in frequent waking up (associated with left ventricular failure, asthma).

- Tachypnea >20 breaths/min and bradypnea <10 breaths/min.
- Trepopnea: dyspnea in left or right lateral decubitus position (associated with heart disease, tumors of mainstem bronchi, unilateral pleural effusion, postpneumonectomy).
- Platypnea: dyspnea in upright posture (due to increased right-to-left shunt in lung bases; seen in liver disease, severe lung fibrosis, and after pneumonectomy).
- Orthodeoxia: oxygen desaturation in upright position (seen with platypnea).

Chest Pain

Pulmonary causes of chest pain are often difficult to distinguish from cardiac and other causes. Tightness of chest and dyspnea are also described as chest pain by patients. Pleuritic pain encountered in pleuritis, pleuropericarditis, pericarditis, pneumothorax, pleural effusion, mediastinitis, pulmonary embolism/infarction, esophageal diseases, aortic dissection, and chest wall trauma. Subdiaphragmatic diseases that produce chest pain include pancreatitis, cholecystitis, and colonic distension.

Cyanosis

Cyanosis is the bluish discoloration of the skin and mucous membranes that occurs when the capillary content of reduced hemoglobin is >5 mg/dL. Clinically, it may be difficult to detect. Cyanosis may occur when arterial hemoglobin is unsaturated or when tissue extraction is high. Causes of central cyanosis: severe hypoxia (PaO_2 is usually <55 mm Hg); anatomical shunts, mild hypoxia with polycythemia, shock, abnormal hemoglobin, methemoglobinemia, and sulfhemoglobinemia. Anemia, even when severe, does not cause cyanosis unless reduced hemoglobin is >5 g/dL. Peripheral cyanosis results from decreased peripheral perfusion with increased O_2 extraction.

- Cyanosis occurs when reduced hemoglobin is >5 mg/dL.
- Important to distinguish central from peripheral cyanosis.
- Cherry-red flush (not cyanosis) is caused by carboxy-hemoglobinemia.
- Polycythemia vera causes "red cyanosis."
- Argyria (from silver nitrate) and hemochromatosis may cause "pseudocyanosis."

Clubbing

Clubbing is the bulbous enlargement of the distal segment of a digit (fingers or toes) caused by increased soft tissue mass. Mechanisms include neurogenic, humoral/hormonal, hereditary, and idiopathic. It can be the presenting manifestation of lung cancer, mesothelioma, and infective endocarditis. Causes of CLUBBING include **C** (cyanotic heart diseases), **L** (lung cancer, lung abscess, lung fibrosis), **U** (ulcerative colitis), **B** (bronchiectasis), **B** (benign mesothelioma), **I** (infective endocarditis, idiopathic, inherited), **N** (neurogenic tumors), **G** (gastrointestinal diseases, e.g., cirrhosis, regional enteritis).

- Clubbing may precede the onset of lung cancer.
- Common causes of clubbing include pulmonary fibrosis, congenital heart disease with right-to-left shunt, cystic fibrosis, and idiopathic.
- Differential diagnosis includes items in the mnemonic "CLUBBING" and hypertrophic pulmonary osteoarthropathy.

Hypertrophic Pulmonary Osteoarthropathy

Hypertrophic pulmonary osteoarthropathy consists of clubbing, painful periosteal hypertrophy of long bones, and symmetrical arthralgias of large joints (usually knees, elbows, and wrists). Other manifestations include gynecomastia, fever, and an increased erythrocyte sedimentation rate (ESR). Mechanisms of hypertrophic pulmonary osteoarthropathy include neurogenic (vagal afferents), hormonal, and idiopathic. The commonest cause is bronchogenic carcinoma, usually adenocarcinoma or large cell carcinoma. Radiographs of long bones reveal thickened and raised periosteum. Bone scans show increased uptake of radionuclide by the affected periosteum. If resection of the tumor does not relieve the hypertrophic pulmonary osteoarthropathy, ipsilateral vagotomy is performed.

- Hypertrophic pulmonary osteoarthropathy: adenocarcinoma and large cell carcinoma of the lung are the common causes.
- Radionuclide bone scans show characteristic changes.
- Perform ipsilateral vagotomy if resection of primary tumor does not resolve the condition.

Horner's Syndrome

Horner's syndrome encompasses ipsilateral miosis, anhidrosis, and ptosis on the side of the lesion. It is seen as a complication of superior sulcus tumor (Pancoast's tumor) of the lung and is most frequently caused by squamous cell carcinoma.

- Horner's syndrome: ipsilateral miosis, anhidrosis, and ptosis.
- Superior sulcus tumor (Pancoast's tumor).

Superior Vena Cava Syndrome

Superior vena cava syndrome is caused by obstruction of blood flow through the superior vena cava. Common causes include lung cancer (particularly small cell cancer), Hodgkin's lymphoma, and other tumors. Mediastinal fibrosis, radiation fibrosis, and large tumors in the upper anterior mediastinum are other causes. Facial edema, fullness of the head, and prominent venous channels over the chest are often noted.

Other Signs and Symptoms

Conjunctival suffusion is seen in severe hypercarbia, superior vena cava syndrome, and conjunctival sarcoid. Asterixis is seen in severe acute or subacute hypercarbia. Telangiectasia of the skin and mucous membranes occurs in patients with pulmonary arteriovenous malformation. Skin lesions of various types can be seen in patients with pulmonary involvement by eosinophilic granuloma (histiocytosis X), tuberous sclerosis, sarcoidosis, and lung cancer.

HISTORY AND EXAMINATION

An approach to history taking and physical examination in patients with pulmonary disease is outlined in Table 26-1.

Percussion and auscultation findings associated with various pulmonary conditions are listed in Table 26-2.

Table 26-1.--History and Physical Examination in Patients
With Pulmonary Disease

History
  Smoking
  Occupational exposure
  Exposure to infected persons or animals
  Hobbies and pets
  Family history of diseases of lung and other organs
  Past malignancy
  Systemic (nonpulmonary) diseases
  Immune status (suppressed, receiving chemotherapy, etc.)
  History of trauma
  Previous chest radiography
Examination
  Inspection
    Respiratory rate
    Respiratory rhythm (apneustic, Biot's, Cheyne-Stokes,
      Kussmaul's, parkinsonian)
    Accessory muscles of respiration in action (FEV_1 <30%)
    Postural dyspnea (orthopnea, platypnea, trepopnea)
    Intercostal retraction
    Paradoxical motions of abdomen/diaphragm
    Cough (type, sputum, blood)
    Wheeze (audible with or without stethoscope)
    Pursed lip breathing/glottic wheeze (patients with
      chronic obstructive pulmonary disease)
    Cyanosis
    Conjunctival suffusion (CO_2 retention)
    Clubbing
    Thoracic cage (anteroposterior diameter, kyphoscoliosis,
      pectus, etc.)
    Trachea, deviation
    Superior vena cava syndrome
    Asterixis, central nervous system status
    Cardiac impulse, jugular venous pressure, pedal edema
      (signs of cor pulmonale)
  Palpation
    Clubbing
    Tibial tenderness (hypertrophic pulmonary
     osteoarthropathy)
    Motion of thoracic cage (hand or tape measure)
    Chest wall tenderness (costochondritis, rib fracture,
      pulmonary embolism)
    Tracheal deviation, tenderness
    Tactile (vocal) fremitus
    Subcutaneous emphysema
    Succussion splash (effusion, air-fluid level in thorax)
  Percussion
    Thoracic cage (dullness, resonance)
    Diaphragmatic motion (normal, 5-7 cm)
    Upper abdomen (liver)

  Auscultation
    Tracheal auscultation
    Normal breath sounds
    Bronchial breath sounds
    Expiratory slowing (time it in seconds)
    Crackles (describe)
    Wheezes (describe)
    Pleural rub
    Mediastinal noises (mediastinal crunch)
    Heart sounds
    Miscellaneous (muscle tremor, etc.; see section on Other
      Signs and Symptoms)

DIAGNOSTIC TESTS

Radiography

Chest radiography, plain tomography, computed tomography (CT) of chest, magnetic resonance imaging (MRI), bronchography, pulmonary angiography, and bronchial arteriography scan are among the tests used in the diagnosis of chest diseases.

Plain Chest Radiography

The interpretation of chest radiographs is discussed in Chapter 7. Lesions that can be easily missed are pneumothorax, solitary pulmonary nodule, lesions behind the ribs and clavicles, apical lesions, lesions behind diaphragm and heart, and hilar and mediastinal lesions. Decubitus chest radiography is important for evaluating free pleural effusion.

Tomography

Tomography is used in evaluating solitary lung nodule. Calcification, location of the lesion, margins of the nodule, cavitation within the nodule, and presence of adjacent tiny nodules (satellite lesions) can be discerned with tomography. Overall, tomography is less expensive than CT.

● Simple tomography is useful in evaluating solitary pulmonary nodule.

Fluoroscopy

Fluoroscopy is useful in localizing lesions during biopsy and aspiration procedures. It is also valuable in assessing diaphragmatic motion and in diagnosing diaphragmatic paralysis by sniff test.

Table 26-2.--Percussion and Auscultation Findings

	Chest expansion	Fremitus	Resonance	Breath sounds	Egophony	Bronchophony
Pleural effusion	Decreased	Reduced	Reduced	Decreased	Absent>>present	Absent>>present
Consolidation	Decreased	Increased	Reduced	Bronchial	Present	Present
Atelectasis	Decreased	Reduced	Reduced	Decreased	Absent>present	Absent>present
Pneumothorax	Variable	Reduced	Increased	Decreased	Absent	Absent

Note: Trachea is shifted ipsilaterally in atelectasis and contralaterally in effusion. Whispered pectoriloquy is present in consolidation.

Computed Tomography

CT is useful in the staging of lung cancer and in assessing mediastinal and hilar lesions, diffuse lung disease, and pleural processes. It has become valuable in diagnosing diffuse lung diseases. High-resolution CT (HRCT) is capable of revealing greater details of pulmonary parenchyma. Characteristic HRCT findings are found in pulmonary eosinophilic granuloma (cystic spaces in the upper lung fields), lymphangioleiomyomatosis (nodular cystic spaces in the upper lung zones), idiopathic pulmonary fibrosis (subpleural honeycombing), and lymphangitic pulmonary metastasis (interlobular septal enlargement and nodularity).

- Characteristic CT findings in pulmonary eosinophilic granuloma (histiocytosis X), lymphangioleiomyomatosis, idiopathic pulmonary fibrosis, lymphangitic pulmonary metastasis.
- CT is helpful in the staging of lung cancer.
- CT is useful in evaluating presence of multiple lung nodules (metastatic), calcification in the nodule.
- HRCT is good for assessing pulmonary parenchyma but not entire chest.

Conventional CT and HRCT are required for the overall assessment of the thorax. Abnormal signs that indicate diffuse lung disease include abnormal interfaces, thickened interlobular septa, nodules, airspace opacification ("ground-glass"). HRCT findings in pulmonary fibrotic diseases are >90% accurate. Honeycombing is seen in 90% of patients as compared with 30% on chest radiography. Other diseases in which HRCT is suggestive of the underlying pulmonary process are certain cases of asbestosis, sarcoidosis, pulmonary alveolar phospholipoproteinosis, chronic eosinophilic pneumonia, and bronchiolitis obliterans.

- Clinical correlation with HRCT finding is very important.
- HRCT is excellent for diagnosing bronchiectasis.

Magnetic Resonance Imaging

MRI is considered the procedure of choice in the evaluation of chest wall invasion with cancer and for cases in which iodinated agents are contraindicated. MRI may be superior to CT in evaluating superior sulcus tumors, brachial plexus lesions, occult mediastinal neoplasms, pulmonary sequestration, arteriovenous malformation, and tumor recurrence in patients with total pneumonectomy. It is also useful in imaging the vascular structures within the thorax.

Bronchography

Bronchography is used infrequently because of the ability of HRCT in detecting bronchiectasis. Bronchography is indicated 1) if HRCT findings are doubtful in the presence of clinical features of bronchiectasis, 2) if better mapping of bronchiectatic areas is needed before lung resection for the disease, 3) in certain cases of bronchial strictures, and 4) in very young children in whom HRCT scan is not possible.

- HRCT has almost replaced bronchography for diagnosing bronchiectasis.

Pulmonary Angiography

The main indication for pulmonary angiography is to detect pulmonary emboli. Although the accuracy of detecting emboli in the major vessels is good, peripheral pulmonary embolism may not be seen. Anticoagulation is not a contraindication to the test. Pulmonary angiography is useful in the diagnosis of pulmonary arteriovenous fistula and malformations, and it is a prerequisite if embolotherapy is planned.

- Pulmonary angiography: main indication is pulmonary thromboembolism.
- Pulmonary angiography may not detect peripheral or tiny pulmonary embolism.
- It is helpful in detecting pulmonary arteriovenous malformations and fistula.

Bronchial Angiography

Bronchial angiography is used to determine whether the bronchial arteries are causing massive pulmonary hemorrhage or massive hemoptysis. It is a prerequisite if bronchial arterial embolotherapy is planned. Complications include neurologic deficits if the spinal artery, a branch of the bronchial artery, is accidentally embolized.

- Complication of bronchial arterial embolotherapy includes spinal artery embolization resulting in neurologic defects.
- Both pulmonary and bronchial angiography may be needed for some patients with massive hemoptysis.

Radionuclide Lung Scan

Ventilation-perfusion ($\dot{V}$/Q) scan, quantitative $\dot{V}$/Q scan, and gallium lung scan are used in diagnosing various lung diseases.

$\dot{V}$/Q Scan

The $\dot{V}$/Q scan is commonly used in diagnosing pulmonary embolism. The likelihood of pulmonary embolism in a scan that shows "high probability" and a scan that shows "low probability" is >90% and <5%, respectively. An "intermediate probability" scan usually requires documentation of pulmonary embolism by pulmonary angiography.

Quantitative $\dot{V}$/Q Scan

The quantitative $\dot{V}$/Q scan is used to assess unilateral and regional pulmonary function by measuring $\dot{V}$/Q relationships. It is indicated in patients who are poor surgical candidates for lung resection because of their underlying pulmonary dysfunction. If the lung region to be resected shows minimal or no lung function by the quantitative $\dot{V}$/Q scan, the resection is unlikely to impair further the patient's pulmonary reserve.

Gallium Scan

[67]Gallium citrate is of minimal or no use in clinical practice. The test lacks specificity and is expensive. Although earlier reports claimed that gallium scan was helpful in identifying the activity of diffuse lung disease such as idiopathic pulmonary fibrosis and sarcoidosis, it currently is seldom used clinically. Correlation of bronchoalveolar lavage findings and gallium citrate is not well established and both of these tests are of little help in noninfectious diffuse lung disease. For the purposes of the American Board of Internal Medicine examination and in clinical practice, neither of these tests is recommended in evaluating a noninfectious diffuse pulmonary process (see below).

- Low or intermediate probability results of $\dot{V}$/Q scan may require further clinical evaluation and tests.
- Quantitative $\dot{V}$/Q scan to assess unilateral or regional pulmonary function; useful in assessing lung resectability in patients with poor lung function.
- Gallium scan has no clinical role in the diagnosis of diffuse lung disease.

Sputum

Simple microscopy using "wet" slide preparation is important in evaluating sputum eosinophilia and Charcot-Leyden crystals, particularly in asthmatics. Gram's staining of sputum should be used to evaluate bacterial infections. Routine examination with Gram's stain is unnecessary in all patients with COPD who present with acute exacerbations. Induced sputum is helpful in identifying mycobacteria, fungi, *Pneumocystis carinii*, and malignant cells. Gastric washings are used to identify mycobacteria and fungi.

- Simple microscopy using "wet" slide preparation is an inexpensive method to evaluate sputum eosinophilia and to identify Charcot-Leyden crystals.
- Hemosiderin-laden macrophages in sputum indicates blood ingested by alveolar macrophages.
- Smokers have a significant number of hemosiderin-laden macrophages.
- Induced sputum is excellent for identification of *Pneumocystis carinii*.

Blood and Serologic Tests

Differential leukocyte count, assessment of eosinophilia, measurement of serum angiotensin-converting enzyme (SACE), antineutrophilic antibodies (ANCA), and other tests (antinuclear antibody [ANA], rheumatoid factor, gamma globulins) are used in diagnosing various pulmonary diseases. Serology is performed in patients suspected to have fungal lung infections, hypersensitivity pneumonitides, and certain occupational lung diseases (these are discussed under appropriate diseases). The role of SACE is discussed here. ANCA is discussed under Wegener's granulomatosis.

SACE

SACE levels are applicable only to adults (>20 years), because children and teenagers have high and widely variable levels. Nearly 80% of patients with active sarcoidosis have increased levels of SACE, 70% with type I disease, 80% with type II, and 90% with type III. SACE levels are increased in 5% of normal subjects. Changes in levels may correspond to the activity of sarcoid. Some physicians use SACE levels to monitor disease activity, but the clinical usefulness of this practice is questionable. Increased SACE levels are not diagnostic of sarcoid, because the level can be elevated in several conditions, including primary biliary cirrhosis, Gaucher's disease, leprosy, atypical mycobacteriosis, miliary tuberculosis, acute histoplasmosis, silicosis, hyperparathyroidism, and histiocytic lymphoma.

- SACE levels are elevated in 70%-80% of patients with sarcoidosis.
- Increased SACE levels do not establish the diagnosis of sarcoidosis.
- SACE levels are also increased in mycobacterioses, mycoses, Gaucher's disease, and hyperparathyroidism.

Physiology

Physiology of COPD

Decreased flow rates are characteristic of COPD. Lung compliance is increased in emphysema, and elastic recoil is decreased. Diffusing capacity for carbon monoxide is diminished in emphysema. Reversibility on pulmonary function tests suggests a bronchospastic component. Hyperexpansion is manifested by increased total lung capacity and residual volume. Retention of CO_2 is more common in bronchitic patients. Normal lung compliance = 0.2 L/cm H_2O. Compliance is increased in emphysema and decreased in fibrosis and restrictive lung diseases.

Pulmonary Function Tests

The major indication for pulmonary function tests is dyspnea. These tests do not diagnose lung disease. They assess the mechanical function of the respiratory system and quantitate the loss of lung function. These tests are used to separate obstructive from restrictive phenomena and to detect bronchospastic component by using methacholine inhalation challenge.

- Obstructive disease usually indicates obstruction to outflow of air from the lungs because of airway narrowing during expiration. Flow rates and volumes are affected.
- Inflow and outflow of air are limited in asthma because

of bronchoconstriction throughout respiration.
- Methacholine inhalation test is helpful in detecting presence or absence of bronchospastic disease (see below).
- Increase in flow rates after bronchodilator therapy suggests reversible airway disease.
- Restrictive disease indicates limitation to full expansion of lungs because of disease in the lung parenchyma, chest wall, or diaphragm. Volumes are diminished but flow rates are normal.
- A combination of obstructive and restrictive patterns is also possible (e.g., COPD with pulmonary fibrosis).
- Results of previous pulmonary function tests are helpful in following the course of lung disease.
- Spirometry can measure lung volumes and flows.

Provocation Inhalation Challenge Tests

Provocation inhalation challenge tests are performed by inhalation challenge of methacholine, carbachol, histamine, industrial irritants suspected of causing occupational asthma, exercise, isocapneic hyperventilation, or cold air. The results define the level of nonspecific airway hyperreactivity in those suspected to have asthma. A 20% reduction in forced expiratory volume in 1 second (FEV_1) from baseline is considered a positive test. These tests are useful when the diagnosis of asthma or hyperactive airway disease is uncertain. Many normal subjects exhibit positive inhalational challenge without symptoms of asthma.

Interpretation of Pulmonary Function Tests

A step-by-step approach is helpful:
1. Evaluate volumes and flows as separate groups.
2. Total lung capacity, functional residual capacity, and residual volume indicate volumes. Total lung capacity is equal to vital capacity plus residual volume (i.e., TLC = VC + RV). Increases in total lung capacity and residual volume generally suggest hyperinflation, as in COPD and bullae. If volumes (total lung capacity, vital capacity, and reserve capacity) are decreased, consider restrictive lung disease (e.g., fibrosis) or loss of lung volume (e.g., surgery, diaphragmatic paralysis, skeletal problems).
3. The vital capacity measured during a slow--not forced--expiration is not affected by airway collapse in COPD. Forced vital capacity may be low with forced expiration because of airway collapse. In normal subjects, vital capacity equals forced vital capacity (i.e., VC = FVC).

4. FEV_1 and forced expiratory flow between 25%-75% of vital capacity indicate flows. Flows are characteristically diminished in COPD, but smaller decreases in flows can be seen in the presence of low lung volumes. When FEV_1 expressed as a percentage of the forced vital capacity is low, it indicates obstructive pulmonary disease.

5. Maximal voluntary ventilation test involves rapid inspiratory and expiratory maneuvers and thus tests airflow through major airways and muscle strength. Patients with severe COPD may have low maximal voluntary ventilation, whereas those with restrictive lung diseases have normal maximal voluntary ventilation (because there is no obstruction to airflow). Maximal voluntary ventilation also tests muscle strength. Neuromuscular diseases may lead to decreased maximal voluntary ventilation.

- Normally, maximal voluntary ventilation is decreased in obstructive disease (i.e., $MVV = FEV_1$ x 33).
- If maximal voluntary ventilation is low and flow rates are normal (i.e., no airway obstruction), consider weakness of the respiratory muscles, especially the diaphragm.
- A good clinical estimate of respiratory muscle strength is obtained by measuring maximal inspiratory and expiratory pressures.
- Flow rates are normal or near normal in pure restrictive lung disease.

- Clinical features (symptoms and signs) should be correlated with the results of pulmonary function tests.

6. Diffusing capacity (DLCO) is dependent on thickness of alveolocapillary membrane (DM), hemoglobin level (θ), and pulmonary capillary volume (Vc) ($\frac{1}{DLCO} = \frac{1}{DM} + \frac{1}{\theta Vc}$). Diffusing capacity is low in anatomical emphysema ($\downarrow$Vc), anemia ($\downarrow\theta$), restrictive lung diseases ($\uparrow$DM), pneumonectomy ($\downarrow$Vc), pulmonary hypertension and recurrent pulmonary emboli ($\downarrow$Vc). Diffusing capacity is increased in supine posture ($\uparrow$Vc), after exercise ($\uparrow$Vc), polycythemia ($\uparrow\theta$), obesity ($\uparrow$Vc), left-to-right shunt ($\uparrow$Vc), and in some asthmatics. Isolated low diffusing capacity (with normal results on pulmonary function tests) is seen in pulmonary hypertension, multiple pulmonary emboli, and anemia.

- Diffusing capacity is reduced in anatomical emphysema but not in bronchitis or asthma.
- Isolated (meaning normal volumes and flows) reduction in diffusing capacity is seen in pulmonary hypertension, multiple pulmonary emboli, and severe anemia.
- Decrease in hemoglobin by 1 g diminishes the diffusing capacity by 7%.
- Flow-volume curves are helpful in separating intrathoracic from extrathoracic obstructive lesions in the major airways.

Table 26-3.--Try to Interpret These Results of Pulmonary Function Tests Before Reading the Explanations*

Patient	1	2	3	4	5	6	7	8	9	10
Age (yr) and sex	73 M	43 M	53 F	43 M	50 M	20 M	58 F	40 M	28 F	44 M
Weight, kg	52	53	50	63	73	80	59	75	52	148
Tobacco	63PY	NS	NS	NS	20PY	NS	NS	NS	NS	NS
Total lung capacity, %	140	128	84	118	110	100	56	68	108	90
Vital capacity, %	52	75	86	78	82	95	62	58	106	86
Residual volume, %	160	140	90	110	112	90	65	80	98	90
FEV_1, %	35	38	82	48	80	90	85	42	112	96
FEV_1/FVC, %	40	34	80	40	60	85	88	50	85	78
FEF_{25-75}	18	14	80	35	75	88	82	24	102	88
Maximal voluntary ventilation, %	62	48	40	60	105	120	108	62	88	90
Diffusing capacity	9	10	20	28	26	32	8	8	6	40
(normal)	(22)	(28)	(20)	(28)	(27)	(34)	(26)	(28)	(32)	(28)

*Values of 80%-120% of predicted are considered normal.

FEF_{25-75}, forced expiratory flow between 25%-75% of vital capacity; FEV_1, forced expiratory volume in 1 second; FVC, forced vital capacity; NS, nonsmoker; PY, pack-years of smoking.

Explanations of Table 26-3

Patient 1. The typical features of hyperinflation are indicated by high values for total lung capacity and residual volume. Vital capacity is low because of high residual volume (total lung capacity minus residual volume equals vital capacity). Flow rates are extremely low and maximal voluntary ventilation is moderately reduced. The very low diffusing capacity suggests parenchymal damage. Without knowing the response of spirometric variables to inhalation of bronchodilator, it is not possible to tell whether the patient has a bronchospastic component. Diagnosis: moderately severe obstructive disease with severe anatomical emphysema.

Patient 2. Young nonsmoker with features of hyperinflation (high total lung capacity and residual volume). Flow rates and maximal voluntary ventilation are also severely decreased. These features suggest obstructive lung disease. The low diffusing capacity suggests parenchymal damage (emphysema). Diagnosis: severe COPD (emphysema) caused by familial deficiency of alpha$_1$-antitrypsin.

Patient 3. Airflows and lung volumes are slightly reduced but within normal limits. Note the severely reduced maximal voluntary ventilation (this test requires rapid inspiratory and expiratory movements by the patient). In this patient, maximal inspiratory and expiratory values were severely reduced, suggesting muscle weakness. Diagnosis: severe thyrotoxicosis with proximal muscle weakness (thyrotoxic myopathy). This pattern of results on pulmonary function tests can be seen in neuromuscular diseases such as amyotrophic lateral sclerosis and myasthenia gravis.

Patient 4. A young nonsmoker with slightly increased but normal total lung capacity and slightly diminished vital capacity. Flow rates, however, are moderately reduced. This patient has mild-to-moderate obstructive phenomenon. Normal diffusing capacity excludes anatomical emphysema or other parenchymal problems. Bronchodilator testing showed improvement in lung volumes and flow rates. Diagnosis: typical asthma.

Patient 5. A middle-aged patient and 20-pack-year smoker with mild hyperinflation (increased total lung volume and residual volume). Because these are within normal limits (80%-120% of predicted), true hyperinflation is not present. Flow rates show slight reductions, and maximal voluntary ventilation and diffusing capacity are normal. Bronchodilator inhalation showed no improvement. Note the slightly diminished

FEV$_1$/FVC ratio. This together with slightly diminished FEF$_{25-75}$ suggests a mild obstructive lung disease of a nonasthmatic type. Because of normal diffusing capacity, significant anatomical emphysema can be excluded. Diagnosis: nonasthmatic bronchitis.

Patient 6. A 20-year-old nonsmoker with normal lung volumes and flows (80%-120% of predicted normal). This patient used to be a "super athlete" and recently noted cough and chest tightness after exertion. No previous pulmonary function tests. Important points from this example are as follows: 1) in a young, otherwise healthy patient, the lung volumes and flows are usually "supernormal," more so in an athlete. 2) This patient may have had very high volumes and flows in the past, but without previous pulmonary function testing, no comparison can be made (if earlier pulmonary function test results were available, the present results might represent severe reduction in pulmonary function). 3) The medical history suggests the possibility of exercise-induced asthma, and spirometry after a treadmill exercise test showed 28% reduction in flow rates 5-10 min after termination of exercise. 4) Note the relatively high diffusing capacity in this patient. Asthmatic patients, for some unknown reason (some believe as a result of increased V̇/Q distribution in the lungs), show increased diffusing capacity. Diagnosis: exercise-induced asthma.

Patient 7. A middle-aged nonsmoker with moderately severe decrease in lung volumes and normal flow rates. Maximal voluntary ventilation is within normal limits, but diffusing capacity is severely diminished. These suggest severe restrictive lung disease with significant parenchymal disease. The slightly diminished flow rates are a secondary phenomenon related to decreased lung volumes. Diagnosis: biopsy-proved idiopathic pulmonary fibrosis. Classic example of restrictive lung disease. Note that FEV$_1$/FVC ratio is usually higher in true restrictive lung disease. Patients who have had lung resection also have diminished lung volumes and decreased diffusing capacity.

Patient 8. A relatively young man with moderately decreased lung volumes. Flow rates are also diminished more than expected from the decreases in lung volumes. Reduction in FEV$_1$/FVC ratio suggests the presence of obstructive lung disease. Maximal voluntary ventilation is also reduced, and diffusing capacity is severely reduced. Compared with patient 7, this patient has obstructive disease in addition to severe restrictive lung disease. Very low diffusing capacity suggests parenchymal disease. Chest radiography disclosed bilaterally diffuse nodular interstitial changes, especially in the upper two-thirds of the lungs. Bronchoscopic examination revealed extensive endobronchial sarcoid granulomas. Diagnosis: severe restrictive lung disease from pulmonary parenchymal sarcoidosis and obstructive airway disease secondary to endobronchial sarcoidosis.

Patient 9. A young woman with normal lung volumes and flow rates. Maximal voluntary ventilation is slightly reduced but within normal limits. Diffusing capacity is very low. PaO_2 was 56 mm Hg. Diagnosis: primary pulmonary hypertension.

Patient 10. A relatively young man with normal lung volumes and flow rates. Previous pulmonary function test results were not available for comparison. Diffusing capacity is abnormally high. This patient was extremely obese and all the abnormal results on pulmonary function tests can be explained on the basis of this. Obese patients show diminished lung volumes because of poor effort made during testing. Abnormally high diffusing capacity is reported to be a result of increased pulmonary capillary volume. In an otherwise healthy but obese person, slightly diminished or diminished diffusing capacity should suggest a primary pulmonary problem rather than obesity-related pulmonary dysfunction. Diagnosis: obesity-related pulmonary dysfunction.

Preoperative Evaluation of Lung Functions

Every pneumonectomy patient should be evaluated with pulmonary function tests. A patient can tolerate pneumonectomy if FEV_1 is >50% of predicted, maximal voluntary ventilation is >50% of predicted, residual volume to total lung capacity ratio is 50% of predicted, and diffusing capacity is >50% of predicted value. If values are worse than any of the above, use split ventilatory functions and/or quantitative differential perfusion-ventilation scan. Pulmonary preparation will decrease the rate of postoperative pulmonary complications. Increased morbidity and mortality are associated with severe COPD, $PaCO_2$ >45 mm Hg (hypoxemia is not a reliable indicator), and if pulmonary artery pressure (intraoperatively) is >30 mm Hg with temporary unilateral occlusion of a pulmonary artery. Upper abdominal operations (gallbladder, abdominal aortic aneurysm repair) carry higher rates of pulmonary complications.

Exercise Test

Exercise testing can assess cardiopulmonary function. Indications for exercise testing include unexplained dyspnea or effort intolerance, ability/disability evaluation, quantitation of severity of pulmonary dysfunction, separation of cardiac from pulmonary causes of disability, evaluation of progression of a given disease process, estimation of operative risks before cardiopulmonary surgery, and evaluation of need for supplemental oxygen. Special equipment and expertise are required to perform properly an exercise study.

Blood Gases and Oximetry

Interpretation of blood gas abnormalities is discussed in Chapter 3.

Bronchoscopy

Most common diagnostic indications for bronchoscopy include persistent cough, hemoptysis, suspected cancer, lung nodule, atelectasis, diffuse lung disease, and lung infections. Therapeutic indications include atelectasis, retained secretions, tracheobronchial foreign bodies, airway stenosis (dilatation), and obstructing lesions (laser therapy, stent placement). Bronchoscopy is valuable in the staging of lung cancer. Complications from bronchoscopy are minimal and include bleeding from biopsy, pneumothorax (from lung biopsy), and hypoxemia. The risk of bleeding is increased in patients with renal failure, thrombocytopenia, and other bleeding diatheses.

- Bronchoscopy: low diagnostic yield in chronic cough if chest radiograph is normal or unchanged.
- Low diagnostic yield in pleural effusion without other chest radiographic findings.
- Bronchoscopy is valuable in the diagnosis and staging of lung cancer.
- Bronchoscopy carries a low risk of complications.

Bronchoalveolar Lavage

Bronchoalveolar lavage is performed by wedging a flexible bronchoscope into a segmental bronchus and instilling 100-150 mL of normal saline into the distal (abnormal) segments of the lung. The instilled saline is aspirated back via the bronchoscope and can be analyzed for cell counts, morphology, and typing. Protein and constituents can be measured in the lavage. The cells seen in the fluid are thought to represent the cells in the alveoli. Bronchoalveolar lavage from normal subjects shows pulmonary alveolar macrophages (93% ± 3%) and lymphocytes (7% ± 1%). Other types of leukocytes are rarely found in normal nonsmokers. Because several of the diffuse lung diseases are reported to result from the inflammatory and immune cells, the presence of these cells may help in understanding the pathogenesis.

- Bronchoalveolar lavage can quantify and identify cell morphology at the alveolar level.
- Normal subjects show macrophages (93%), lymphocytes (7%), and neutrophils (<1%).

Increased numbers of neutrophils with normal lymphocytes are reported in idiopathic pulmonary fibrosis, familial pulmonary fibrosis, and asbestosis. Increased numbers of lymphocytes without neutrophilia have been noted in sarcoidosis and hypersensitivity pneumonitis. Variable cell counts are seen in other diffuse lung diseases. Bronchoalveolar lavage should be considered a research tool to study the pathogenesis of lung diseases, but it currently has no value in the diagnosis of sarcoid or idiopathic pulmonary fibrosis. However, it may be helpful in diagnosing alveolar proteinosis, some infections, histiocytosis X, and lymphangitic pulmonary metastasis.

- Bronchoalveolar lavage has a limited role in the diagnosis of sarcoid, hypersensitivity lung disease, and idiopathic pulmonary fibrosis.
- Bronchoalveolar lavage is valuable in diagnosing histiocytosis X and alveolar proteinosis.
- It is diagnostic of malignancy in 60% of patients with lymphangitic carcinomatosis of the lungs.
- Bronchoalveolar lavage is helpful in diagnosing opportunistic lung infections.

Lung Biopsy

Lung biopsy can be obtained via bronchoscopy, thoracoscopy, or thoracotomy. The indications for lung biopsy in diffuse lung disease should be based on the clinical features, treatment planned, and risks from biopsy and risk from treatment without a pathologic diagnosis. Bronchoscopic lung biopsy provides a higher diagnostic yield in sarcoidosis, histiocytosis X, eosinophilic pneumonitis, lymphangioleiomyomatosis, infections, pulmonary alveolar proteinosis, lymphangitic carcinomatosis, drug-induced lung disease, and hypersensitivity pneumonitis.

OBSTRUCTIVE LUNG DISEASES

A common pathophysiologic feature of obstructive lung diseases is the obstruction to outflow of air as a result of intrinsic (asthma, bronchitis, bronchiolitis, bronchiectasis, cystic fibrosis, strictures), luminal (bronchitis, bronchiolitis, cystic fibrosis, strictures and stenoses), or extrinsic (emphysema, bullous lung disease, extraluminal compression from masses, vascular lesions) diseases of the airways. Under this heading are discussed emphysema, bronchitis, asthma, bronchiectasis, cystic fibrosis, bronchiolitis, bullous lung disease, and strictures and stenoses. Obstructive sleep apnea is also included in this section.

- Emphysema is defined as a condition characterized by the enlargement of airspaces distal to terminal bronchioles, accompanied by destruction of the alveolar walls. The definition implies histologic documentation, but this is impractical in clinical practice.
- Chronic bronchitis is a disorder characterized by excessive mucous production in the bronchial tree and manifested by chronic or recurrent cough that is present on most days for a minimum of 3 months in the year and for no less than 2 successive years.
- Asthma is an acute or chronic disease characterized by recurrent episodes of reversible bronchospasm leading to paroxysmal obstruction of the airways.
- Bronchiectasis is the irreversible and pathologic dilatation of bronchi.

Bronchiectasis in allergic bronchopulmonary aspergillosis, some cases of bronchitis, and other infections is reversible.

Chronic Obstructive Pulmonary Disease

Definition

The term *COPD* is applied to describe the common obstructive lung diseases, namely emphysema, bronchitis, and asthma. It is often difficult to clearly separate these entities from one another. Nearly 80% of patients with COPD have features of all three diseases. However, it is better to describe the type of COPD in each patient.

Etiology

Tobacco smoking is the major cause of COPD. Smokers have 10x the risk of nonsmokers of dying of chronic bronchitis and emphysema. Pipe and cigar smokers have between 1.5x and 3x the risk of nonsmokers. Smoking increases the risk of developing COPD in people with alpha$_1$-antitrypsin deficiency. Smokers have increased incidence of COPD, lung carcinoma, atherosclerosis, carcinoma of pancreas, and skeletal chest pains. Decline in FEV$_1$ is proportional to the number of pack years of smoking.

- Other diseases associated with or aggravated by smoking: asthma, pulmonary fibrosis, carcinoma of bladder, esophagus, larynx, and pancreas, calcification of pleural plaques in asbestosis, pulmonary alveolar phospholipoproteinosis, pulmonary eosinophilic granuloma, and alveolar hemorrhage in Goodpasture's syndrome.

Air pollution caused by oxidants, oxides of nitrogen, hydrocarbons, and sulphur dioxide has a significant role in exacerbations of COPD. Occupational exposures, heredity (alpha$_1$-antitrypsin deficiency), infections, allergy (in asthma), and other factors are also involved in the cause of COPD.

Pathophysiology

The main problem in COPD is reduced airflow caused by the narrowing of the airways, particularly during expiration. In asthma, the narrowing is caused by bronchoconstriction, increased mucous secretion, mucosal inflammation, and mucous gland hypertrophy during inspiration and expiration. In emphysema, the lack of radial traction (due to loss of lung parenchyma and lung recoil) on the bronchi causes airway collapse during inspiration. In bronchitis, the abnormality underlying airflow obstruction is mucosal inflammation, increased mucous secretions, and mucous gland hypertrophy. In bullous lung disease, large bullae compress the airways. In emphysema, the premature expiratory closure of airways results in air-trapping, causing the lungs to become hyperinflated. Elastic recoil (retractive force) is lost in emphysema. Histologically, centrilobular emphysema is the commonest type and usually starts in upper lobes; most patients with bronchitis-related COPD have this. The panlobular type usually starts in the lower lobes. It is seen in classic anatomical emphysema and in patients with alpha$_1$-antitrypsin deficiency.

- The compliance (volume/pressure) is increased in emphysema. Compliance in the normal human lung is 200 mL/cm H$_2$O.

Chronic Bronchitis

Chronic bronchitis, as defined above, is a common problem. Most patients with this condition have chronic productive cough. Cigarette smoking is the commonest cause of chronic bronchitis. Occupational exposure and air pollution also contribute to the exacerbations. The patients exhibit productive cough, have a tendency to retain CO$_2$, have lower PaO$_2$, have a tendency toward cyanosis, and tend to be slightly overweight. Hence, these patients are described as "blue bloaters."

- Blue bloaters retain CO$_2$, cough, and develop cor pulmonale sooner than pink puffers do.

Emphysema

Pure anatomical emphysema is not as common as chronic bronchitis. Most patients with COPD have a combination of chronic bronchitis and emphysema. Emphysematous patients are thin, maintain near normal PaO$_2$ by increasing the work of breathing, and look adequately oxygenated. Hence, they are known as "pink puffers." A relatively common finding is severe weight loss in some patients. Carbon dioxide retention is not seen until late in the disease.

- Pink puffers have emphysema, lose weight, do not retain CO$_2$, and develop cor pulmonale late in the disease.

Bullous Lung Disease

Small apical bullae are present in many normal persons. Bullous lung disease can be congenital or acquired. Lack of communication with bronchi may cause air-trapping. Complications include pneumothorax, COPD, infection with lung abscess, bleeding into bulla, and compression of adjacent normal lung. Surgical therapy may improve lung function by 5%-10% in 10%-15% of patients.

- Panlobular emphysema may look like a bulla.
- Bullous changes are seen in Marfan and Ehlers-Danlos syndromes, burnt-out sarcoid, and cadmium exposure.

Alpha$_1$-Antitrypsin Deficiency

Synthesis of alpha$_1$-antitrypsin, a secretory glycoprotein, by hepatocytes is determined by the alpha$_1$-antitrypsin gene on chromosome 14. Alpha$_1$-antitrypsin inhibits many proteolytic enzymes and, thus, protects the lungs from destructive emphysema. It is autosomal recessive. Phenotypes and levels = normals (M) >250 mg%, heterozygote (MZ) 150 mg%, and homozygote (Z) <50 mg%. From 5% to 10% of patients with alpha$_1$-antitrypsin deficiency do not have emphysema. Evidence for the association of MZ heterozygote and emphysema is not as convincing as for the Z homozygote. Smoking hastens the onset of emphysema. Z phenotypes may have hepatocytic globules that take up PAS stain. Signs and symptoms appear during 3rd or 4th decade of life.

- Alpha$_1$-antitrypsin deficiency in neonatal and liver disease (hepatitis, cryptogenic cirrhosis, periportal fibrosis), respiratory distress syndrome, and in certain hemorrhagic syndromes (platelet dysfunction, disseminated intravascular coagulation, and clotting disturbances in infants).
- Alpha$_1$-antitrypsin (Prolastin) derived from human plasma is available for replacement therapy, but there are no data to show that this prevents disease progression. Treatment is expensive.
- Chest radiography shows basal emphysema, lung scan shows no perfusion to bases, absence of alpha-1 globulin on protein electrophoresis, patient with COPD and a strong family history of COPD.
- Phenotyping is better than measurement of level of alpha$_1$-antitrypsin.
- In the case of a young patient with clinical features of COPD: consider asthma, alpha$_1$-antitrypsin deficiency, cystic fibrosis, ciliary dyskinesia, obstructive azoospermia (Young's syndrome), and congenital or acquired immunoglobulin deficiency.

Asthma

More detailed discussion can be found in Chapter 2. However, several important points require reiteration. Currently, the clinical impression is that asthma is primarily an inflammatory disease. Therefore, inhaled corticosteroids are now considered the first line of therapy in mild asthma. Controversy remains regarding the purported increase in mortality rate in asthmatics. Cough can be the only presenting symptom of bronchial asthma. Exercise-induced asthma is more common in younger people and presents as chest tightness or cough after termination of exercise. Patients have normal findings on pulmonary function tests and may require methacholine inhalation challenge to document the presence of hyperreactive airway disease. Reduction in flow rates to 20% or below that of baseline is considered a positive methacholine test. Although wheezing may not be heard after methacholine, a good response is seen to treatment with bronchodilators. Simple microscopy with wet sputum preparation can be used to detect sputum eosinophilia, Charcot-Leyden crystals, and Curschmann's spirals.

- All that wheezes is not asthma and not all asthmatics wheeze.
- Nonasthmatic causes of wheezing: drug-induced that induces bronchospasm (β-blockers), prostaglandin inhibitors (acetylsalicylic acid, indomethacin), ultrasonic nebulizers, acetylcysteine, ascaris antigen, and occupational exposures (platinum dust, detergent enzymes, baker's flour; toluene diisocyanate, byssinosis, bagassosis, grain dust, etc.).
- Methacholine inhalation challenge to detect airway reactivity.

Complications and Causes for Exacerbation of COPD

The complications and causes for exacerbation of COPD include respiratory infections (*Haemophilus influenzae, Moraxella catarrhalis, Streptococcus pneumoniae*), cor pulmonale, myocardial infarction, cardiac arrhythmias, pneumothorax, pulmonary emboli, bronchogenic carcinoma, environmental exposure, over-sedation, neglect of therapy, excessive oxygen use (suppression of hypoxemic drive), and excessive use of β$_2$-agonist (tachyphylaxis). Nocturnal oxygen desaturation is common in blue bloaters, as are premature ventricular contractions and episodic pulmonary hypertension. Decrease in SaO$_2$ correlates with increase in pulmonary artery pressure. Severe weight loss, sometimes >50 kg, is noted in 30% of patients with severe COPD.

- Infections in COPD caused by *H. influenzae, M. catarrhalis, S. pneumoniae*.
- Nocturnal oxygen desaturation is common in blue bloaters.
- Decrease in SaO$_2$ correlates with increase in pulmonary artery pressure.

Treatment of COPD

Treatment includes education, cessation of smoking, hydration, immunization against influenza and *S. pneumoniae*, inhaled and oral bronchodilators, supplemental oxygen, treatment of complications, and rehabilitation. Systemic corticosteroids improve lung functions in <10% of nonasthmatic COPD patients. Inhaled corticosteroids are the main agents used in asthma. Knowledge of bronchodilators and their mode of action is important.

- Inhaled corticosteroids are the main agents used in asthma.
- Systemic corticosteroids improve lung functions in <10% of nonasthmatic COPD patients.

Theophylline acts by preventing the breakdown of cyclic AMP (cyclic AMP is important for maintenance of bronchodilatation) by intracellular phosphodiesterase. Tobacco smoke decreases the efficacy of theophylline action. The loading dose is 6 mg/kg (range, 5 to 7 mg); maintenance dose is 0.5 mg/kg per hour or 1.15 g/24 hours; and average dose is 250 mg 4 times daily. Longer-acting preparations may be given in single doses of 300-600 mg. The dosage should be decreased by 50% if the patient has received theophylline in the previous 24 hours or has heart failure, severe hypoxemia, hepatic insufficiency, or seizures. The dosage should be increased by 50% if the effect is suboptimal and in smokers who tolerate the drug. Increase each dose by 50-100 mg if the effect is suboptimal in patients with increased clearance rate (smokers). Decrease each dose by 50-100 mg if toxic effects develop or if progressive cardiac or liver failure develops. The maintenance dose for children is larger because they tolerate the drugs better than adults.

- Theophylline inhibits phosphodiesterase and, thus, increases cyclic AMP(questionable mechanism).
- Tobacco smoking decreases the half-life of theophylline.
- Recommended blood level is 10-15 μL/mL.
- Frequent measuring of serum theophylline level is unnecessary in clinical practice.

Recent publications have questioned the role of theophylline in COPD and asthma. Overall, its use has diminished, and beta agonists are being used more often in its place. Theophylline decreases respiratory muscle contractility in a dose-related fashion. Its clearance is decreased by the concomitant use of erythromycin, cimetidine, allopurinol, oral contraceptives, and caffeine and is increased by phenobarbital, phenytoin, and tobacco smoke.

- Theophylline clearance is decreased by concomitant use of erythromycin, cimetidine, oral contraceptives, and caffeine.
- Theophylline clearance is increased by phenobarbital, phenytoin, and tobacco smoke.

β_2-Agonists (isoetharine, albuterol, terbutaline, metaproterenol, pirbuterol, salmeterol, etc.) stimulate cyclic AMP production through activation of adenyl cyclase in the cell membrane. Main side effects include tremor, aggravation of prostatism, tachycardia, and arrhythmias. Cromolyn sodium stabilizes the cell membrane by coating it externally and blocking the release of slow-reacting substance of anaphylaxis, eosinophilic chemotactic factor, serotonin, histamine, and other bronchoconstrictor mediators. Cromolyn sodium is a preventive drug and not a therapeutic agent to be used in a full-blown asthmatic episode. It is a good drug for exercise-induced asthma and for asthmatics with known allergen. Anticholinergic agents (ipratropium, atropine, etc.) are indicated in patients with excessive sputum production. The FDA has not recommended its use for asthmatics, although many patients benefit from ipratropium. The mechanism of action of steroids (inhaled and systemic) is unclear. Corticosteroid aerosols have none of the side effects of systemic steroid therapy. The commonest side effect is oral candidiasis.

- β_2-Agonists stimulate cyclic AMP production.
- Side effects of β_2-agonists include tremor, aggravation of prostatism, tachycardia, and arrhythmias.
- Cromolyn sodium should be used to prevent asthma.
- Anticholinergic agents are indicated for patients with excessive sputum production.

Oxygen

Nocturnal low-flow O_2 (<2 L/min) therapy is recommended when PaO_2 is <55 mm Hg. The lack of CO_2 retention should be ascertained before recommending oxygen. Continuous oxygen therapy is indicated for patients with persistent polycythemia, recurrent episodes of cor pulmonale, severe hypoxemia, and central nervous system symptoms induced by hypoxemia. For each liter of oxygen administered, the fraction of inhaled oxygen (FIO_2) increases by 3%. Nocturnal oxygen therapy is indicated for patients with PaO_2 <55 mm Hg and in the presence of severe cor pulmonale, increased pulmonary vascular resistance, serious arrhythmias, personality changes from oxygen desaturation, and marked polycythemia. Exercise therapy improves exercise tolerance and maximal oxygen uptake and may diminish desaturation, but exercise does not improve performance on pulmonary function tests.

- Oxygen therapy is recommended if PaO_2 is <55 mm Hg and/or SaO_2 is <88%.
- FIO_2 increases by 3% for each liter of supplemental oxygen.
- Exercise program does not improve results of pulmonary function tests.

Other Topics in COPD

Nicotine gum and patch help maintain nicotine blood levels while the smoker tries to cope with the psychologic and other aspects of addiction. Nicotine from gum is absorbed more slowly from the buccal mucosa and stomach than from the airways with inhaled smoke. Side effects include mucosal burning, light-headedness, nausea, stomachache, and hiccups. The patch causes rash in a significant number of patients. Use of the nicotine patch with continued smoking aggravates cardiac problems. Intermittent positive pressure breathing in COPD has no advantage over compressed nebulizer therapy. Furthermore, it is more expensive than simple nebulizer or compressed nebulizer. Intermittent positive pressure breathing may be helpful in selected situations such as postoperative atelectasis, cystic fibrosis, and bronchiectasis. Pneumovax is now recommended every 10 years for patients with COPD.

Cystic Fibrosis

Cystic fibrosis is the commonest lethal autosomal recessive disease among Caucasians in the U.S. The locus of the responsible gene is on the long arm of chromosome 7. Cystic fibrosis develops in 1 in 2,000 to 3,500 live births among Caucasians; about 1 in 20 Caucasians is a heterozygous carrier. There is no sex predominance. Occurrence in blacks is 1 in 17,000 and 1 in 90,000 in Orientals. Parents of a child with cystic fibrosis must both be heterozygotes; siblings of such a child have a 50%-65% chance of being heterozygotes. The pathogenesis of cystic fibrosis is unknown, although all exocrine glands seem affected. The diagnosis is made in 80% of patients before the age of 10 years; in 10%, the diagnosis is not made until adolescent years. Obstruction of exocrine glands, with the exception of sweat glands, by viscous secretions causes almost all clinical manifestations. Mucociliary clearance is normal in the patients with minimal pulmonary dysfunction and is decreased in those with obstructive phenomena. Secretion of mucous glycoproteins is increased in cystic fibrosis and is responsible for forming viscoelastic gels.

- Cystic fibrosis: the commonest lethal autosomal recessive disease among Caucasians.
- In 10% of patients, the diagnosis is not made until adolescent years.
- Parents of a child with cystic fibrosis must both be heterozygotes.
- Siblings of children with cystic fibrosis have 50%-65% chance of being heterozygotes.
- All exocrine glands, except for sweat glands, are affected.

Patients with cystic fibrosis and heterozygous carriers demonstrate nonspecific airway responses similar to those in asthmatics. This may be secondary to diminished β-adrenergic responsiveness, presumably related to defective cyclic AMP-mediated mechanisms. Patients with cystic fibrosis have an increased susceptibility to asthma and atopy, and many of them exhibit type I and type III hypersensitivity reactions to an assortment of antigens. Positive serology to *Aspergillus* species and *Candida albicans* occurs with higher frequency in cystic fibrosis patients than in asthmatics. Allergic bronchopulmonary aspergillosis has been noted in 10% of cystic fibrosis patients.

- Patients with cystic fibrosis and carriers exhibit increased airway response.
- Patients have increased susceptibility to develop asthma and atopy.
- Allergic bronchopulmonary aspergillosis in 10% of patients with cystic fibrosis.

There is no evidence for a primary defect in sodium transport. However, there is indication that epithelial cells in cystic fibrosis patients are poorly permeable to chloride ions. A discrete chloride channel has not been identified. The potential difference across a membrane is normally negative but becomes more negative (due to chloride impermeability) in cystic fibrosis. This phenomenon may indeed represent the genetic defect in cystic fibrosis.

- No evidence for a primary defect in sodium transport in cystic fibrosis.
- Epithelial cells in cystic fibrosis patients are poorly permeable to chloride ions.
- Marked increase in the electrical potential difference across the nasal and tracheobronchial epithelium in comparison with normal subjects and heterozygote relatives.

Quantitative pilocarpine iontophoresis is helpful in diagnosis; abnormal results on at least two tests are necessary for the diagnosis. Other conditions that are associated with high levels of sweat sodium/chloride include smoking, chronic bronchitis, malnutrition, hereditary nephrogenic diabetes mellitus, adrenal insufficiency, and ectodermal dysplasia. The concentration of sweat sodium/chloride increases with age. Heterozygotes may have normal sweat sodium/chloride values. False-negative test results are common in edematous state. Abnormal sweat chloride: adult, >80 mEq/L; child, >60 mEq/L.

- Diagnosis in adults depends on three or more of the following: clinical features of cystic fibrosis, positive family history, sweat chloride ≥80 mEq/L, and pancreatic insufficiency.
- Respiratory manifestations include sinusitis, nasal polyps, purulent sputum, atelectasis, hemoptysis, and pneumothorax. Azoospermia occurs in 80%-90%.
- Progressive bronchiectasis (cystic type).
- *Pseudomonas aeruginosa* is the dominant organism; despite aggressive antipseudomonadal therapy, it is impossible to eradicate it.
- Increased incidence of *Pseudomonas cepacia* in the respiratory secretions of cystic fibrosis patients; the presence of *P. cepacia* is associated with rapid deterioration.

Cystic fibrosis is the commonest cause of COPD and pancreatic deficiency in the first three decades of life in the U.S. Males constitute 55% of the adult patients with cystic fibrosis. The diagnosis is made after the age of 15 years in 17%-25%. In adults (≥17 years), COPD is the major cause of morbidity and mortality. Adults with cystic fibrosis show a higher incidence of minor hemoptysis (60%), major hemoptysis (71%), pneumothorax (16%), and sinusitis and nasal polyposis (48%). Pancreatic insufficiency is present in 95%, but it is seldom symptomatic. Intussusception and fecal impaction (similar to meconium ileus) are more frequent (21%) in adults than in children. Hyperinflation of lungs on chest radiography and lobar atelectasis are both less frequent in adults than in children. Mean age at onset of massive hemoptysis is 19 years, and median survival from the initial episode of hemoptysis is about 3.5 years. Mean age of occurrence of pneumothorax in adults is 22 years. Azoospermia is seen in 95%.

- COPD is present in 97% of adults with cystic fibrosis

and is the major cause of morbidity and mortality.
- In adults with cystic fibrosis: minor hemoptysis (60%), major hemoptysis (71%), pneumothorax (16%), and sinusitis and nasal polyposis (48%).
- Pancreatic insufficiency in 95%; it is seldom symptomatic.

Treatment of cystic fibrosis includes management of obstructive lung disease, chest physiotherapy, postural drainage, immunization against influenza, hydration, and aggressive antibiotic therapy. Newer antibiotics are effective against *P. aeruginosa*. Intravenous administration of antibiotics at home is now an accepted method. Lung transplant is an option for advanced cases. Controversial issues: nebulized antibiotic therapy, domiciliary long-term intravenous antibiotic therapy, systemic corticosteroids, repeated sputum culture, hospitalization for acute exacerbation, and frequent bronchoscopy to clear airways.

- Poor prognostic factors: hemoptysis, recurrent bacterial infections, presence of *P. cepacia*, and systemic complications.
- Overall survival rate for cystic fibrosis patients older than 17 years is closer to 50%.

Bronchiectasis

Bronchiectasis is ectasia or dilatation of bronchi due to the irreversible destruction of bronchial walls. The reversible type of bronchiectasis is seen in patients with severe bronchitis, acute pneumonia, and allergic bronchopulmonary aspergillosis. Bronchiectasis most commonly occurs in lower lung fields. Mild cylindrical bronchiectasis seen in many heavy smokers with chronic bronchitis may be diffuse. Distal bronchial segments are involved in most cases of bronchiectasis. An exception to this is the proximal bronchial involvement in allergic bronchopulmonary aspergillosis. In most cases of bronchiectasis, second- to fourth-order bronchi are involved. Disease is bilateral in 30% of all bronchiectatic cases.

- Reversible bronchiectasis in allergic bronchopulmonary aspergillosis, acute pneumonia, and chronic bronchitis.
- Upper lobe involvement in cystic fibrosis, allergic bronchopulmonary aspergillosis, and chronic mycotic and mycobacterial infections.

Most cases are diagnosed on clinical grounds (chronic cough productive of purulent sputum). Some cases with "dry bronchiectasis" caused by tuberculosis do not have productive cough but may develop episodes of significant hemoptysis. Many mildly symptomatic or asymptomatic patients with atelectatic segments of right middle lobe and lingular segments of left upper lobe have minor degrees of bronchiectasis. Chest radiographs show increased markings in bases, crowding of bronchi, segmental atelectasis, honeycombing with cystic spaces measuring <2.0 cm, loss of lung volume, and air-fluid levels (if cystic bronchiectasis is present). Chest HRCT findings include signet-ring shadows (thickened bronchi with bronchial artery forming the "stone"), bronchial wall thickening, dilated bronchi extending to the periphery, bronchial obstruction due to inspissated purulent secretions, loss of volume, and air-fluid levels if cystic or saccular changes are present. Bronchography should be considered if surgical resection is planned. Bronchography is still the most accurate diagnostic test to map out bronchiectasis.

- Nonpulmonary symptoms include fetor oris, anorexia, weight loss, arthralgia, clubbing, and hypertrophic pulmonary osteoarthropathy.
- HRCT of chest is helpful in making the diagnosis.
- No studies have documented superiority of chest CT over conventional bronchography.
- Pulmonary function tests usually show obstructive phenomena; restrictive pattern is seen in patients with large areas of atelectasis.

Causes and Associations of Bronchiectasis

Bronchiectasis has many causes and associations. It is important to identify the cause or association in each patient.

Infections

Most cases of bronchiectasis in adults are related to viral (adenovirus types 7 and 21) and/or bacterial infections (measles, influenza, or pertussis) in childhood. Tuberculosis is a common cause of bronchiectasis, particularly in the upper lobes.

- "Dry bronchiectasis" with episodes of significant hemoptysis without sputum is usually due to bronchiectasis in an area of old tuberculous damage.
- Bronchiectasis may result from chronic mycoses.

Ciliary Dyskinesia (Immotile Cilia) Syndrome

Cilia are seen in the following locations (clinical problems associated with ciliary dysfunction are mentioned in parentheses): nasal mucosa (nasal polyps), paranasal sinuses (chronic sinusitis), eustachian tubes (inner ear infection, deafness), tracheobronchial tree (chronic bronchitis, bronchiectasis), olfactory receptor cells (reduced olfactory function), vestibular sensory nerves (unknown), fallopian tubes (infertility?), ependymal lining of spinal cord and brain ventricles (recurrent headaches and depression), corneal inner surface (corneal deformities), vas efferens (infertility?), sperm tails (immotile sperm), and visceral primordial cells (situs inversus). Many types of ciliary abnormalities (loss of radial spokes, eccentric tubules, absent tubules, adhesion of multiple cilia, etc.) are described. Even though the term "immotile cilia" is commonly used, the cilia do move, but the motion is abnormal and dyssynchronous.

- Many ciliary abnormalities have been described.
- Ciliary dyskinesia, rather than ciliary immotility, is the major abnormality.

The immotile cilia syndrome (Kartagener's syndrome) is an autosomal recessive disorder. Loss of the dynein arm--the fundamental defect--is an inherited abnormality involving a single protein. The prevalence of the disorder is 1 in 20,000 to 40,000 persons. Nearly 50% of patients have the triad of situs inversus, sinusitis, and bronchiectasis or at least bronchitis. Loss of the dynein arm results in sinusitis and otitis (less common in adults), nasal polyposis, bronchiectasis (in 75% of adults), situs inversus, and infertility in males. Infertility is not a universal phenomenon and, in fact, women with immotile cilia syndrome are often fertile. Kartagener's syndrome accounts for 0.5% of the cases of bronchiectases and 15% of dextrocardia.

- Ciliary dyskinesia (Kartagener's syndrome) is an autosomal recessive disorder.
- Loss of dynein arm is the fundamental defect.
- Situs inversus, sinusitis, and bronchiectasis seen in 50% of cases.

Deficiency of radial spokes may result in sinusitis, nasal polyposis, otitis, mastoiditis, recurrent bronchitis, and infertility in both sexes. The diagnosis depends on clinical features and documentation of ciliary abnormalities by electron microscopic examination of nasal mucosa, bronchial mucosa, or semen. At least 20 types of axonemal defects have been described. Ciliary defects are not always inherited; acquired forms of ciliary dyskinesia are seen in smokers and patients with bronchitis, viral infections, or other pulmonary diseases.

- Ciliary defects are not always inherited.
- Acquired ciliary defects seen in smokers, in patients with bronchitis, and after viral infections.

Hypogammaglobulinemia

Congenital (or Bruton's X-linked) agammaglobulinemia predisposes to recurrent bacterial infections and bronchiectasis. Bacteria isolated in these patients include *H. influenzae, S. aureus*, and *S. pneumoniae*. Acquired agammaglobulinemia (common variable) may be manifested as sinopulmonary infections in the second or third decades. Despite the inability to form antibody, most patients have a normal number of circulating B cells, which fail to dedifferentiate into plasma cells that make immunoglobulins. Unusual bacteria (*M. catarrhalis*) may be isolated from some patients.

- Overall incidence of bronchiectasis in hypo/agammaglobulinemia is about 10%.
- Selective IgA deficiency is the commonest immunoglobulin deficiency; most of these patients are asymptomatic.
- IgA deficiency is frequently associated with IgG subclass (IgG2 and IgG4) deficiency.
- Hypogammaglobulinemic patients develop lymphocytic interstitial pneumonitis, thymoma, asthmatic bronchitis (low IgE levels), squamous cell carcinoma of the lung, and non-Hodgkin's lymphoma.

Right Middle Lobe Syndrome

Right middle lobe syndrome is recurrent atelectasis of the right middle lobe in the absence of endobronchial obstruction. Isolated bronchiectasis is limited to segments of the right middle lobe. Mechanisms include compression of the middle lobe bronchus by lymph nodes, acute angulation of the origin, narrow opening of the bronchus, lengthy bronchus, and lack of collateral ventilation. Chest radiography usually points to the diagnosis, although many patients remain asymptomatic.

- Chest radiography shows chronic atelectasis and loss of volume in right middle lobe (look for blurring of right cardiac border).
- Diagnosis made on incidental chest radiographic finding.
- Most patients are asymptomatic.

Allergic Bronchopulmonary Aspergillosis

More than 95% of patients with allergic bronchopulmonary aspergillosis have extrinsic asthma, and 10% of patients with extrinsic asthma develop this condition. Overall prevalence is 6%. The mechanism is unknown but is thought to be hypersensitivity to presence of *Aspergillus* in the bronchial wall. Type I (bronchospasm), type III (pulmonary destructive changes), and type IV (parenchymal granuloma and mononuclear cell infiltrates) reactions are involved. Asthma previously under control that becomes refractory to treatment with nonsteroidal bronchodilators, expectoration of brownish mucus plugs, segmental atelectasis, and increasing eosinophilia and serum IgE are indicators of allergic bronchopulmonary aspergillosis. Major criteria: asthma, blood esosinophilia >1,000/mm³, immediate skin reactivity (type I reaction--IgE dependent) to *Aspergillus fumigatus*, precipitating antibodies (type III reaction) against *Aspergillus fumigatus*, high IgE (>1,000 ng/mL), transient or fixed pulmonary infiltrates, and central bronchiectasis. Minor criteria: presence of *Aspergillus fumigatus* in sputum, expectoration of brownish mucus plugs, and Arthus reactivity to *Aspergillus* antigen. Chest radiography: fleeting infiltrates in 85% of cases, mucoid impaction in 15%-40%, ring shadows, tram-track lines, toothpaste shadows, atelectasis, and central bronchiectasis.

- Allergic bronchopulmonary aspergillosis: almost always in patients with extrinsic asthma; upper lobe central bronchiectasis.
- Types I, III, and IV immune reactions may be involved.
- Asthma refractory to nonsteroidal bronchodilator therapy.
- Presence of *A. fumigatus* is only a minor criterion for the diagnosis.
- Systemic steroid therapy for >6 months required in most cases.

Yellow Nail Syndrome

Triad of yellow to yellow-green discoloration of nails with thickened and curved appearance in all extremities, lymphedema of lower extremities, and pleural effusion. Bronchiectasis is seen in about 20% of patients. Lymphedema may affect the breasts. Raynaud's phenomenon is noted in some. The cause is unknown, but lymphangiography has revealed lymphatic hypoplasia and atresia. Patients may present with chronic and insidious edema of the extremities.

Pleural effusions occur in 35%-40% of patients, and in about one-third, recurrent pleural effusions are noted. Pleural effusions may appear years after the nail changes and tend to be bilateral and small-to-moderate in amount. Exudates and transudates both are described.

Obstructive Azoospermia (Young's Syndrome)

Obstructive azoospermia denotes primary infertility in males who have normal spermatozoa in the epididymis but none in the ejaculate. This is different from the ciliary dysmotility syndromes and cystic fibrosis. The following pulmonary abnormalities have been noted: grossly abnormal sinus radiograph (59% of patients), sinusitis (56%), repeated otitis media (32%), chronic bronchitis (35%), abnormal chest radiographic findings (53%), and bronchiectasis (29%). The reason for the relationship between obstructive azoospermia and lung disease is unknown.

- Obstructive azoospermia and bronchiectasis.
- Pulmonary and ENT symptoms in 30% of patients.

Unilateral Hyperlucent Lung Syndrome (Swyer-James or Macleod Syndrome)

Normally, unilateral hyperlucent lung syndrome is a radiographic diagnosis (incidental in most cases). Hyperlucency and hyperinflation of the lung (usually left) is found in conjunction with a small pulmonary artery. Bronchiectasis is seen in 25% of patients but most are asymptomatic. The cause is unknown, but congenital atresia of the pulmonary artery or acquired bronchiolitis soon after birth is postulated. Panacinar emphysema is found in the affected lung.

- Unilateral hyperlucent lung syndrome: unilateral hyperlucency of the lung with small ipsilateral pulmonary artery.
- Bronchiectasis in 25%; most patients are asymptomatic.

Miscellaneous Causes and Associations

Nearly 10% of bronchiectatic patients may demonstrate an abnormal alpha$_1$-antitrypsin phenotype with serum levels <66% of normal. Other entities include rheumatoid arthritis (Felty's syndrome), toxic chemicals, recurrent aspiration, heroin, inflammatory bowel disease, foreign body, sequestrated lung, relapsing polychondritis, chronic tracheoesophageal fistula, heart-lung transplantation, chronic granulomatous disease of childhood, and postobstructive (tumors, long-standing foreign body, stenosis, etc.).

- Uncommon causes of bronchiectasis include alpha$_1$-antitrypsin deficiency, Felty's syndrome, toxic inhalation, chronic tracheobronchial stenosis.

Complications of Bronchiectasis

Complications include hemoptysis (in 50% of patients), progressive respiratory failure with hypoxemia and cor pulmonale, and secondary infections by fungi and noninfectious mycobacterioses. Presence of these organisms usually represents a saprophytic state, but active infection has to be excluded. The most commonly isolated bacterium in bronchiectasis is *P. aeruginosa*. As in cystic fibrosis, it is impossible to eradicate this bacterium. Routine culture of respiratory secretions is not warranted in all patients.

- Source of bleeding in bronchiectasis is the bronchial (systemic) circulation and, hence, can be brisk.
- Presence of mycobacteria and fungi may represent saprophytic growth.

Treatment

Treatment of bronchiectasis is aimed at controlling the symptoms and preventing complications. Predisposing conditions should be sought and treated aggressively (gamma globulin injections, removal of foreign body or tumor, control of aspiration, treatment of infections of paranasal sinuses, gums, and teeth). Postural drainage, chest physiotherapy, humidification, bronchodilators, and cyclic antibiotic therapy are effective in many patients. Surgical treatment is reserved for patients with troublesome symptoms, localized disease, and severe hemoptysis.

Bronchiolitis Obliterans With Organizing Pneumonia (BOOP)

Bronchiolitis obliterans with organizing pneumonia is a nonspecific diagnosis. It is a pathologic diagnosis. The main abnormality is the presence of intraluminal fibrosis within the distal airways, alveolar ducts, and perialveolar spaces. This condition is seen in patients with rheumatoid arthritis, systemic lupus erythematosus, polymyositis-dermatomyositis, mixed connective tissue disease, and silo filler's lung and after exposure to noxious gases, bleomycin, amiodarone, cytomegalovirus, influenza virus, bacteria (*Legionella, Nocardia*), *Mycoplasma*, *Cryptococcus*, and *Pneumocystis carinii*. Bronchiolitis obliterans with organizing pneumonia also occurs after heart and bone marrow transplants and in chronic eosinophilic pneumonia and is observed as a secondary phenomenon in Wegener's granulomatosis, infarcts, granulomas, and neoplasms. Chest radiography usually shows a patchy and diffuse ground glass infiltrate or features similar to idiopathic pulmonary fibrosis and chronic eosinophilic pneumonia (peripheral alveolar infiltrate). Diagnosis of idiopathic bronchiolitis obliterans with organizing pneumonia is one of exclusion. Treatment consists of excluding offending agents and high doses of systemic corticosteroids.

Sleep Apnea

In normal subjects, two types of sleep are observed: rapid eye movement (REM) and non-REM. Most sleep is non-REM and is characterized by parasympathetic dominance. Its clinically notable aspects include a decrease in respiratory rate, heart rate, and blood pressure. REM sleep is dominated by sympathetic discharges and is manifested by increase in heart rate, respiratory rate, and blood pressure. Dreams are common. Stages 1-4 of non-REM sleep last for 90 minutes, followed by REM sleep for 10-20 minutes. There are 4-5 episodes of REM sleep nightly.

- Non-REM sleep is characterized by parasympathetic dominance.
- REM sleep is dominated by sympathetic discharges.

Apnea is defined as cessation of all airflow at the nose and mouth for at least 10 seconds. Sleep apnea syndrome is present if, during a 7-hour sleep, there are at least 30 episodes of apnea. The three main forms of sleep apnea are 1) obstructive, 2) central, and 3) mixed. Although most patients have a predominantly obstructive pattern, the mixed type is the commonest form. Although the patients are usually obese, this is not a necessary criterion for making the diagnosis.

- Apnea: cessation of all airflow at the nose and mouth for at least 10 seconds.
- Sleep apnea is present if, during a 7-hour sleep, there are at least 30 episodes of apnea.
- Of the three main forms of sleep apnea (obstructive, central, and mixed), the mixed form is the commonest.

- Obstructive sleep apnea is present in 1%-2% of the population.

Clinical features of obstructive sleep apnea: sonorous snoring, abnormal motor behavior during sleep, daytime somnolence, personality changes, intellectual deterioration, systemic hypertension, sexual dysfunction, abnormal behavioral outbursts, morning headaches, nightmares, hypnogogic hallucinations/automatic behavior, and nocturnal enuresis. It is important to obtain a sleep history from spouse or relatives. Polysomnography (Fig. 26-1) establishes the diagnosis. In obstructive apnea, there is apnea, but contraction by thoracoabdominal muscles is seen. In central apnea, in addition to apnea, there is no contraction by respiratory muscles. Patients develop severe oxygen desaturation during sleep (clinically significant desaturation is a decrease of ≥4% from the baseline). Sinus arrhythmia is seen in 90% of patients. Other forms of cardiac rhythm problems include second-degree block, premature ventricular contractions, and ventricular tachycardia.

- Clinical features: sonorous snoring, apneic episodes, abnormal motor behavior during sleep.
- Important to obtain a sleep history from sleep observer.
- Polysomnography is helpful in making the diagnosis and in identifying different types of sleep disorders.

Pulmonary hypertension is episodic in the early stages of significant sleep apnea but can remain sustained later on. The site of airway obstruction in obstructive sleep apnea is the oropharynx; here, the tone of the genioglossus muscle and pharyngeal abductors (geniohyoid) decreases, and the resulting pharyngeal collapse produces obstruction. Before polysomnography is performed, patients should have an ENT examination, thyroid function testing, and pulmonary function tests, because similar symptoms are seen in patients with myxedema, ENT abnormalities, and COPD. Sleep apnea is also seen in "bird-like facies syndrome," cordotomy, poliomyelitis, Shy-Drager syndrome, sudden infant death syndrome, adenotonsillar hypertrophy, and severe altitude-related polycythemia. During REM sleep in COPD, diminished tone of the intercostal muscles, decreased function reserve capacity, increased $\dot{V}/Q$ mismatch, increased right-to-left intrapulmonary shunts, and prolonged desaturation have been demonstrated.

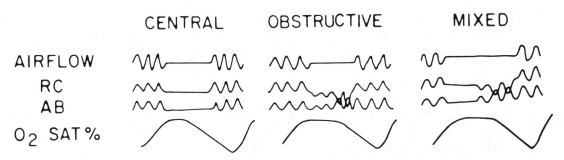

Fig. 26-1. Polysomnography in sleep apnea; airflow is absent in all forms of sleep apnea. Rib cage (RC) and abdominal (AB) movements are absent in central apnea but present in obstructive apnea. (From Strohl KP, Cherniack NS, Gothe B: Physiologic basis of therapy for sleep apnea. Am Rev Respir Dis 134:791-802, 1986. By permission of American Lung Association.)

- Site of airway obstruction in obstructive sleep apnea is the oropharynx.
- Exclude hypothyroidism, ENT causes, narcolepsy, severe COPD before performing polysomnography.
- COPD can produce disordered breathing, apnea, hypopnea, and periodic breathing.

Treatment of obstructive sleep apnea includes weight loss (in obese patients), nasal continuous positive airway pressure, tracheostomy, and uvulopalatopharyngoplasty. In patients with predominantly central sleep apnea, respiratory stimulants such as medroxyprogesterone acetate have been tried. Other treatments used are methylphenidate (Ritalin), etc. The response to these medications is variable. Treatment in severe cases of obstructive apnea with congestive heart failure, polycythemia, bizarre behavior, and cardiac arrhythmias should include weight loss, treatment of the congestive heart failure, oxygen therapy, and consideration of tracheostomy.

- Treatment of obstructive sleep apnea: weight loss, avoidance of alcohol and tobacco, nasal continuous positive airway pressure, tracheostomy.
- Respiratory stimulants for central sleep apnea.

Pickwickian Syndrome

The pickwickian syndrome constitutes only 5% of all sleep apnea cases. Patients usually are morbidly obese, hypersomnolent, cyanotic, plethoric, and polycythemic. In late stages, right ventricular failure is followed by left ventricular failure. Hypoxemia and hypercarbia are common. The efficiency of respiratory muscles is reduced to 60%-70% of normal.

DIFFUSE LUNG DISEASES

Diffuse lung disease usually refers to an infiltrative process affecting most of the segments of both lungs. The term "diffuse lung disease" is not generally used to describe infectious or neoplastic diseases. The term usually implies interstitial and/or alveolar filling defects. Diffuse lung disease is the result of injury to structures in alveolar space, interstitial space, or both. The interstitial space is located between the alveolar lining cells and the capillary endothelium. The interstitium contains reticular and elastic fibers, alveolar interstitial cells (alveolar cells and histiocytes), small lymphocytes, arterioles, and a capillary network.

Pathology

Alveolar cell injury is often associated with altered permeability and resultant alveolar exudation followed by invasion of various cell types into the alveolar spaces. This produces an "alveolar" infiltrate on chest radiographs. Infiltration of interstitial spaces by mononuclear cells, neutrophils, and other cells increases the thickness of the pulmonary interstitium. In chronic cases, deposition of fibrous tissue in the interstitium contributes to the interstitial infiltrate seen on radiographs. Capillary damage causes increased permeability and edema formation within interstitial spaces or alveolar spaces or both.

Physiology

Lung volumes are generally decreased in most diffuse lung diseases. Total lung capacity, vital capacity, and residual volume decrease with disease progression. This is commonly referred to as a "restrictive defect." The loss of lung volumes is best correlated with interstitial fibrosis, although it can be marked in some alveolar diseases. Early in the disease, lung volumes may be normal. Airflow rates are usually normal until late in the course of the disease, when marked reduction in the volumes can be associated with mild-to-moderately reduced flow rates. The static compliance is decreased, but airway resistance is normal. The "stiff lung" increases the work of breathing, and patients typically exhibit rapid, shallow breathing. Gas-exchange abnormality is the earliest change to occur in interstitial lung disease. Hypoxemia on exercise and a decrease in diffusing capacity are seen fairly early. Carbon dioxide retention is not a feature, unless the patient develops "respiratory exhaustion" resulting in muscle weakness.

- Decreased lung volumes (restrictive pattern).
- Flow rates are near normal.
- Lung compliance is decreased and elastic recoil is increased; lungs are stiff.
- Diffusing capacity is decreased early in the course.
- Exercise-induced hypoxemia.
- Hypocarbia in most patients (from hyperventilation); hypercarbia in late disease.

Radiology

Typical CT findings in diffuse lung diseases are described above. The main abnormalities seen on chest radiographs in diffuse lung diseases can be classified into alveolar (air space) and interstitial patterns. Many diseases demonstrate both patterns. The alveolar pattern is limited to a smaller number of diseases, i.e., pulmonary edema (cardiogenic and noncardiogenic), alveolar sarcoidosis, uremic lung, intra-alveolar hemorrhage, aspiration pneumonia, pulmonary alveolar (phospholipo)proteinosis, certain bacterial pneumonias, desquamative pneumonia, certain viral and protozoal pneumonias, diffuse alveolar cell carcinoma, and diffuse pulmonary lymphoma.

- Alveolar pattern is seen in most diseases that begin with the word "alveolar."
- Pulmonary edema is the commonest cause of alveolar pattern seen on chest radiographs.

Because the interstitial pattern includes many diseases, it is convenient to group them into the following categories: idiopathic pulmonary fibrosis, systemic diseases (e.g., rheumatologic diseases), occupational lung diseases (including pneumoconioses and toxic exposures), drug-induced lung diseases (including radiation pneumonitis), granulomatous lung diseases (sarcoid, etc.), lymphan-

gitic pulmonary metastasis, chronic mycotic and mycobacterial infections, unusual diseases (histiocytosis X, lymphangioleiomyomatosis, tuberous sclerosis), and others (chronic bronchiectasis, cystic fibrosis, etc.).

- Grouping of interstitial pattern is helpful in considering differential diagnosis in diffuse interstitial lung diseases.
- Lymphangitic lung metastasis is an important cause of interstitial lung disease.

The combination of alveolar-interstitial patterns and diffuse micronodular changes is also common. The anatomical distribution of the infiltrates is an important clinical consideration because certain diseases predominantly affect upper lung zones. Other diseases may involve lower zones. These entities may produce an interstitial, alveolar, or a combination of alveolar-interstitial pattern on chest radiographs.

- Bilateral upper lobe process: silicosis, coal workers' pneumoconiosis, sarcoidosis, mycoses, mycobacterioses, cystic fibrosis, pulmonary eosinophilic granuloma (histiocytosis X), and pulmonary lymphangioleiomyomatosis.
- Alveolar infiltrates are seen in: pulmonary edema, hematogenous metastases, acute respiratory distress syndrome, noxious gas exposure, alveolar hemorrhage syndromes, diffuse alveolar cell carcinoma, pulmonary alveolar phospholipoproteinosis, desquamative interstitial pneumonitis, early rheumatoid lung disease, amyloidosis, and alveolar microlithiasis.

Classification of Diffuse Pulmonary Diseases

Many of the diffuse pulmonary processes are classified on the basis of morphologic features. The number of abbreviations used to describe these (see below) has resulted in significant confusion for the practicing physician; the abbreviations are listed in Table 26-4.

Idiopathic Pulmonary Fibrosis

Idiopathic pulmonary fibrosis is the commonest cause of chronic diffuse interstitial lung disease. The diagnosis is based on clinical features, which include gradually progressive interstitial process (chest radiography typically shows a bibasilar interstitial process that eventually spreads upward), progressive dyspnea, clubbing (>70%), Velcro crackles, positive rheumatoid factor (30%), antinuclear antibody (35%), or polyclonal gammopathy

Table 26-4.--Abbreviations Used in the Literature to Describe Diffuse Pulmonary Diseases

BIP	Bronchiolitis-interstitial pneumonitis (a form of bronchiolitis obliterans with organizing pneumonia)
BOOP*	Bronchiolitis obliterans with organizing pneumonia
CIPF	Classic interstitial pneumonitis-fibrosis
DAD*	Diffuse alveolar damage (as in adult respiratory distress syndrome)
DIP	Desquamative interstitial pneumonitis (thought to predispose to idiopathic pulmonary fibrosis)
GIP	Giant cell interstitial pneumonitis (very rare)
HRS	Hamman-Rich syndrome
IAF	Idiopathic alveolar fibrosis (same as idiopathic pulmonary fibrosis)
IPF*	Idiopathic pulmonary fibrosis
LIP*	Lymphocytic interstitial pneumonitis (many causes)
PIP	Plasma cell interstitial pneumonitis (uncommon)
RAD	Regional alveolar damage
UIP	Usual interstitial pneumonitis (an earlier term for idiopathic pulmonary fibrosis)

*For clinical purposes (as well as for the examination), these entities are important because they constitute >90% of all of the above.

(>60%). HRCT shows subpleural honeycombing and an interstitial process in the basal areas. Pulmonary function tests show restrictive pulmonary dysfunction, low diffusing capacity, hypoxemia worsened by exercise, and hypocapnia. Other causes (see below) of interstitial process should be excluded. Lung biopsy shows nonspecific interstitial fibrosis without granuloma formation. Response is poor to steroids (<20% show measurable improvement) and immunosuppressive drugs. Hypoxemic patients benefit from supplemental oxygen. Gradual progression leads to cor pulmonale. Five-year survival is <30%.

- Clubbing, Velcro crackles, and abnormal immunologic findings (rheumatoid factor, antinuclear antibody).
- Restrictive lung dysfunction.
- Hypoxemia, low diffusing capacity, and hypocapnia.
- Poor response to steroids and other agents.

Differential Diagnosis of Idiopathic Pulmonary Fibrosis

Many disease entities can produce nonspecific lung fibrosis, and at times, it is difficult to differentiate idiopathic pulmonary fibrosis from these diseases. Important ones to consider in this group are rheumatoid lung, scleroderma lung, late stages of sarcoidosis, certain drug-induced lung diseases (e.g., nitrofurantoin), radiation pneumonitis, end-stage hypersensitivity pneumonitis, certain pneumoconioses (asbestos), noxious gases, paraquat, recurrent pulmonary edema, end-stage histiocytosis X, end-stage cystic fibrosis and bronchiectasis, chronic aspiration pneumonia, and recurrent intra-alveolar hemorrhage (e.g., mitral stenosis, pulmonary hemosiderosis, and Goodpasture's syndrome).

- Rheumatoid lung and scleroderma lung can mimic idiopathic pulmonary fibrosis.
- Any end-stage diffuse lung disease can mimic idiopathic pulmonary fibrosis.

Lymphocytic Interstitial Pneumonitis

The diagnosis of lymphocytic interstitial pneumonitis is based on lung biopsy demonstration of diffuse interstitial infiltration by lymphocytes. Lymphocytic interstitial pneumonitis may result from Hodgkin's lymphoma, non-Hodgkin's lymphoma, early lymphomatoid granulomatosis, chronic lymphocytic leukemia, Waldenström's macroglobulinemia, angioimmunoblastic lymphadenopathy, Sézary syndrome, pseudolymphoma, acquired immune deficiency syndrome (AIDS), graft-versus-host disease, and congenital agammaglobulinemia. Idiopathic lymphocytic interstitial pneumonitis is a diagnosis of exclusion, although current understanding is that almost all cases of the disease indeed represent low-grade B-cell lymphoma.

- Most lymphoproliferative diseases can produce lymphocytic interstitial pneumonitis.
- Most cases of lymphocytic interstitial pneumonitis represent low-grade B-cell lymphoma.
- Lymphocytic interstitial pneumonitis is a pulmonary complication in AIDS and graft-versus-host disease.

Sarcoidosis

Sarcoidosis is a multisystemic granulomatous disease of unknown cause. It affects persons in the 25-45 year age group. Sarcoidosis is characterized by widespread noncaseous epithelioid cell granulomas, depression of delayed type hypersensitivity and decreased number of T lymphocytes, proliferation of B lymphocytes, and frequently positive Kveim skin test (rarely used).

- Sarcoidosis: multisystemic disease.

- Diminished number of T lymphocytes and increased number of B lymphocytes.
- Presence of noncaseous granuloma is not diagnostic of sarcoid.
- Other granulomatous diseases with noncaseous granulomas: mycobacterioses (noncaseous in early stages), leprosy, mycoses, syphilis, mononucleosis, carcinoma, silicosis, hypersensitivity pneumonitis, zirconium, berylliosis, talcosis, Bakelite exposure, Crohn's ileitis, primary biliary cirrhosis, cat-scratch disease, foreign-body granulomas, hypogammaglobulinemia, and granulomatous arteritis.

Clinical Staging

Clinical staging of sarcoidosis is based on chest radiographic findings rather than clinical severity, even though the radiographic changes roughly parallel the clinical disease. Five types (formerly known as stages) of disease are seen. 1) Type 0: normal radiographic findings, with noncaseous granulomas in other sites (e.g., conjunctival, hepatic, lymphoid tissue, etc.). 2) Type I: bilateral hilar and paratracheal lymphadenopathy (40%-50% of all cases, erythema nodosum in 3%-30%, iridocyclitis in 5%-8%). 3) Type II: bilateral hilar and paratracheal lymphadenopathy with pulmonary parenchymal involvement (40%-50% of cases). 4) Type III: diffuse pulmonary parenchymal disease without lymphadenopathy (14%-16% of cases). 5) Type IV: end-stage pulmonary fibrosis with bullous changes (<5% of cases).

- Note that bilateral hilar lymphadenopathy is seen in sarcoidosis, Hodgkin's and non-Hodgkin's lymphoma, metastatic carcinoma, histoplasmosis, coccidioidomycosis, tuberculosis, berylliosis, etc.
- Most diseases that produce noncaseous granulomas also produce hilar lymphadenopathy.

Clinical Features of Sarcoidosis

Intrathoracic disease is present in 90% of patients, but almost all organs can be involved. Generalized lymphadenopathy occurs in 25% of patients, skin (lupus pernio, nodules) excluding nodosum in 25%, eyes (lacrimal enlargement, corneal band opacities, iridocyclitis, glaucoma, and choroidoretinitis) in 25%, liver involvement in 25%, splenomegaly in 14%, endobronchial involvement in 11%, central nervous system involvement (paralysis of seventh cranial nerve, chronic meningitis, hypopituitarism) in 7%, bone cysts in 6%, and kidney involvement in 5%. Other manifestations include salivary gland involvement (uveoparotid fever or Heerfordt's syndrome) in 6%, nasal mucosal lesions, keloid in areas of surgical scars, diffuse arthralgias of small joints, heart (arrhythmias) in 5%, persistent violaceous skin plaques, transient vesicular eruptions on fingers, and persistent scars of old trauma on the knees. Initial complaints are lymphadenopathy (8%-70% of patients), cough (30%), dyspnea (28%), weight loss (20%-28%), fatigue (20%-27%), skin lesions (14%-25%), visual complaints (10%-21%), and fever (10%-15%). Asymptomatic disease is seen in 12%-34% of the patients.

- Almost any organ can be affected by sarcoid.
- Band keratopathy, lupus pernio.
- Cystic bone lesions in terminal phalanges.
- Cranial nerve VII involvement.

Laboratory Tests

Complete or partial anergy to skin tests (PPD and others) is seen in 60% of patients, positive Kveim test (not used anymore) in 95%, increased CD4/CD8 ratio, high serum antibodies to mycoplasma viruses (Epstein-Barr virus, rubella, parainfluenza, herpes simplex), autoantibodies to rheumatoid factor, antinuclear antibody, and T cells. Hypercalcemia results from increased sensitivity to vitamin D and increased gastrointestinal absorption of calcium (15% of patients), hypercalciuria in 40%, and increased IgG (50%), IgA (25%), IgM (12%), and alkaline phosphatase (15%).

- Negative PPD in 60% of patients (due to suppressed T lymphocytes).
- Increased antibodies to viruses and hyperglobulinemia (due to increased B lymphocytes).
- Increased sensitivity to vitamin D.
- Increased serum levels of angiotensin-converting enzyme in 70%-80%.

Biopsy

Noncaseous granulomas can be identified in nearly 100% of biopsies from epitrochlear nodes, mediastinal nodes, lung, nasal mucosal lesions, and subcutaneous nodules. Diagnostic rates of 80%-90% can be obtained from biopsies of skin lesions, palpable scalene nodes, bronchial lesions, conjunctival lesions, and liver. Diagnostic accuracy falls to less than 65% with biopsies of bone marrow, scalene fat pad, and normal-appearing bronchial mucosa.

- Biopsy of involved organs provides high-diagnostic rate.
- Common areas biopsied: mediastinal nodes, lung, tracheobronchial mucosa.
- Noncaseous granuloma is not diagnostic of sarcoidosis.
- Important to obtain culture of biopsy specimens to exclude infectious causes of noncaseous granuloma.

Treatment

Systemic corticosteroids are indicated in progressive or symptomatic type II and type III disease, ocular sarcoid, persistent hypercalcemia or calciuria, progressive or disfiguring skin lesions, neurosarcoid, myocardial sarcoid, and progressive systemic disease. Phenylbutazone and antimalarial drugs have been tried in sarcoid refractory to treatment with steroids.

- Systemic corticosteroids in progressive or symptomatic type II and type III disease.
- Avoid vitamin D and calcium supplements.

Pulmonary Infiltrate With Eosinophilia

Pulmonary infiltrate with eosinophilia refers to pulmonary infiltrates on chest radiography in conjunction with peripheral (blood) eosinophilia. The following conditions belong to this group of disorders.

1. Asthma: commonest cause of pulmonary infiltrate with eosinophilia. The pulmonary infiltrate is usually caused by lung infection, and the eosinophilia results from exacerbation of asthma. The eosinophil count is usually 15%-20%. Appropriate therapy of infection and asthma produces full resolution.
2. Allergic bronchopulmonary aspergillosis: difficult to separate from the above, but the eosinophilia is more severe (30%) and longer lasting. Therapy consists of long-term systemic corticosteroids.
3. Chronic eosinophilic pneumonia: more common in asthmatics. May present with severe respiratory distress, fever, and very high peripheral (>40%) and tissue eosinophilia. Chest radiography usually shows peripheral alveolar infiltrates in lower two-thirds of lung fields. The pathologic features include tissue eosinophilia and bronchiolitis obliterans with organizing pneumonia. Biopsy is not required in most patients. Therapy consists of high doses of systemic corticosteroids for months to years.
4. Churg-Strauss syndrome: uncommon disease. Most patients have significant asthma. Eosinophil count is very high (>50%). Diffuse feathery type of infil-

trates are described on chest radiographs. Prognosis is poor in those who respond poorly to high doses of systemic corticosteroids. This entity is discussed further below.

5. Tropical eosinophilia: the cause is unclear, although parasitic infestation was thought to be responsible. Eosinophil count ranges from 20% to 50%. Many patients develop asthma-like illness. Response to systemic corticosteroids is variable but that to diethylcarbamazine citrate (hetrazan) is better.
6. Drug-induced: many drugs can induce pulmonary infiltrate with eosinophilia. Nitrofurantoin, aspirin, and other drugs can produce pulmonary infiltrates and peripheral eosinophilia.
7. Neoplasms: pulmonary neoplasms (adenocarcinoma, lymphoma, and other tumors) are associated with peripheral eosinophilia. The mechanism is unknown, although eosinophilic chemotactic factor secreted by tumors is thought to be responsible.
8. Parasites: tropical parasites (*Ascaris, Wuchereria*) produce peripheral eosinophilia and pulmonary infiltrates during the pulmonary passage of parasites.

- Drug-induced (nitrofurantoin) pulmonary infiltrate with eosinophilia is important to remember.
- Allergic bronchopulmonary aspergillosis is a common cause of pulmonary infiltrate with eosinophilia in the western hemisphere.
- Chronic eosinophilic pneumonia can present with respiratory distress, fever, and high erythrocyte sedimentation rate.
- Almost all syndromes of pulmonary infiltrate with eosinophilia (except parasitic variety) require long-term systemic corticosteroid therapy.

Pulmonary Eosinophilic Granuloma

Pulmonary eosinophilic granuloma belongs to the reticuloendothelioses, a group of diseases of unknown cause in which an abnormal proliferation of histiocytes occurs without association of any known infectious agent or abnormality of lipid metabolism. Three clinical entities comprise this disease group: eosinophilic granuloma, Hand-Schüller-Christian disease, and Letterer-Siwe disease. Histologic features consist of proliferation of histiocytes in sheet-like masses with numerous eosinophils interspersed.

- Pulmonary eosinophilic granuloma: also known as histiocytosis X, Langerhans' cell granuloma, and reticuloendotheliosis.

- Pulmonary eosinophilic granuloma is more common in adults.
- More than 95% of the patients are smokers.
- It is commonly limited to the lungs or bones or both.

Pulmonary eosinophilic granuloma is uncommon. Approximately 1,500 cases are reported. It is more frequent in Caucasians and rare in blacks. Nearly 30% of the patients have nonspecific symptoms: fatigue, fever, and weight loss. Dyspnea is observed in 40% of patients and may result from a spontaneous pneumothorax or an osteolytic rib lesion. Physical findings are unhelpful in diagnosis. Pulmonary function tests show a restrictive type of defect, with decreased lung volumes, normal flow rates, and decreased diffusing capacity. It is usual to see good results on pulmonary function testing in patients with pulmonary eosinophilic granuloma, even when chest radiography reveals extensive abnormalities. As the disease progresses, fibrosis replaces the granulomatous process, with formation of characteristic honeycomb cysts. Pulmonary function testing at this stage may show obstructive changes. Typically, the involvement is diffuse, bilateral, and most pronounced in the upper two-thirds of the lung fields. Treatment with corticosteroids and *Vinca* alkaloid derivatives is of varying efficacy.

- Spontaneous pneumothorax is common (25%) and may be the first indicator of pulmonary eosinophilic granuloma.
- Young patient with spontaneous pneumothorax and honeycomb changes on chest radiography.
- The clinical course is usually benign, despite the persistence of severe abnormalities on chest radiography.

Pulmonary Alveolar Phospholipoproteinosis

Pulmonary alveolar phospholipoproteinosis, a rare disease of unknown cause, affects mostly young adults. The male-to-female ratio is 3:1. An initial febrile episode is followed (after an interval) by progressive dyspnea with productive cough, low-grade fever, chest pain, and weight loss. Chest radiography shows alveolar filling defect in the lower two-thirds of the lung field. The alveoli contain a granular eosinophilic material that is strongly PAS-positive. Similar pathologic features are found in silica exposure, mycobacterial infections, fungal infections, tuberculosis, leukemia, and pneumocystis. Infections by *Nocardia* are reported to occur with a higher frequency. The alveolar material contains large amounts of dipalmytoil lecithin (surfactant). Laminated bodies and birefringent crystals can be demonstrated. The pathogenesis is likely related to excessive production of surfactant and/or diminished clearance of surfactant by alveolar macrophages. Restrictive pattern seen on pulmonary function testing in combination with decreased diffusing capacity is typical. Lung biopsy may be needed to make the diagnosis. The chest radiographs resemble those of pulmonary edema.

- Most patients are smokers.
- Alveolar infiltrates in lower one-third of lung fields.
- PAS-positive intra-alveolar material in biopsy specimen.
- Treatment: therapeutic alveolar lavage.

Pulmonary Alveolar Microlithiasis

Pulmonary alveolar microlithiasis is a rare, often familial (autosomal recessive) disorder of unknown cause. It is characterized radiographically by fine, sand-like mottling uniformly distributed through both lungs and extensive intra-alveolar deposition of calcium bodies. This disease is relatively asymptomatic, but cor pulmonale may be seen in progressive cases. Most patients are between 30 and 50 years old, with an equal male-to-female ratio. Siblings are commonly affected. The lungs are solid and sink in water, and "onion-skin" bodies in alveoli and fibrosis are seen on sectioning. Dyspnea is a major complaint in advanced cases, but most patients are asymptomatic. There is no known therapy.

- Fine, well-defined, sand-like infiltrates on chest radiographs.
- No known cause or treatment.

Lymphangiomyomatosis

Lymphangiomyomatosis is an uncommon progressive disorder of women of childbearing age. It is characterized by nodular and diffuse interstitial proliferation of the smooth muscle in lungs, lymph nodes, and thoracic duct. Dyspnea, hemoptysis, and spontaneous pneumothorax are common. Two-thirds of the patients have chylous pleural effusion and a few have chylous ascites, a result of obstruction of the thoracic duct. Radiographic features: diffuse nodular-interstitial infiltrates with multiple small bullae at bases. Pulmonary function tests: obstructive features and decreased diffusing capacity. This condition is thought to be a forme fruste of tuberous sclerosis, a rare disease that exhibits identical pathologic and clinical features. Treatment has included hormonal therapy, oophorectomy, and lung transplantation.

- Lymphangiomyomatosis: women of childbearing age with recurrent pneumothorax, chylous effusion, doughy abdomen, and hemoptysis.
- Obstructive pattern on pulmonary function testing, with low diffusing capacity, hypoxemia.
- Hyperinflated lungs with reticulonodular/nodular infiltrates.

Tuberous Sclerosis

Tuberous sclerosis, an inherited disease of mesodermal development, is characterized by epilepsy, mental retardation, congenital tumors, and malformations of the brain, skin, and viscera. Pulmonary involvement occurs in a small number ($\leq 8\%$) of patients, most of whom are women. Onset of the respiratory symptoms is between the ages of 18 and 34 years. Pathologic features of the lungs are similar to those in lymphangiomyomatosis: multiple cysts measuring a few millimeters in diameter, with walls formed of smooth muscle cells (pulmonary myomatosis). Chest radiography shows diffuse interstitial infiltrates. Reticulonodular changes and pleural effusions are found in the early stages. Spontaneous pneumothorax is common. Pulmonary function tests reveal increased lung volumes. Pulmonary tuberous sclerosis is usually accompanied by involvement of other organs.

- Tuberous sclerosis is identical to lymphangiomyomatosis with regard to chest radiography, lung abnormalities, and findings on pulmonary function tests.
- Several diseases reveal diffuse interstitial/alveolar/nodular changes on chest radiography, but pulmonary function testing shows an obstructive instead of a restrictive pattern. Examples: pulmonary lymphangioleiomyomatosis, histiocytosis X, tuberous sclerosis, cystic fibrosis, bronchiectasis, sarcoidosis with endobronchial involvement, and rheumatoid lung.

Neurofibromatosis of von Recklinghausen

Neurofibromatosis is a relatively common disease of dominant inheritance. It is manifested clinically by café-au-lait spots, freckling, and neurofibromas of skin and internal organs. Pulmonary fibrosis is seen in $\leq 10\%$ of the patients. The interstitial fibrosis is usually seen in the basal areas of the lungs, whereas the bullous lesions occur in the apical areas. Clinical manifestations are mild, usually consisting only of exertional dyspnea, but a restrictive pattern on pulmonary function testing and decreased diffusing capacity are often observed. Intrathoracic neurofibromas and meningoceles may occur. Pulmonary manifestations become evident in adulthood.

- Neurofibromatosis of von Recklinghausen: common disease of dominant inheritance.
- Features: pulmonary fibrosis, bullous lung disease, and intrathoracic meningiomas.

Hereditary Hemorrhagic Telangiectasia (Osler-Weber-Rendu Disease)

Hereditary hemorrhagic telangiectasia is an inherited disorder characterized by telangiectasia of the skin and mucous membranes and intermittent bleeding from vascular abnormalities. About 20% of the patients have pulmonary arteriovenous malformations/fistulas, which are located in the lower lobes and are multiple in one-third of the patients. On chest radiographs, the arteriovenous malformations appear as oval or round homogeneous nodular lesions, from a few millimeters to several centimeters in diameter. Tomograms of the lesion usually disclose an artery entering the fistula and a vein leaving it. Angiographic examination confirms the diagnosis in virtually all cases. Symptoms depend on the degree of shunting. Paradoxical embolism is a potential complication. Central nervous system symptoms related to paradoxical embolic phenomenon are common. Most arteriovenous malformations are diagnosed in the third and fourth decades of life; the male-to-female ratio is 1:2. Dyspnea is present in nearly 60% of cases, but hemoptysis is the most common presenting symptom. Physical examination reveals cyanosis, clubbing of nails, and a bruit or a continuous murmur over the site of the arteriovenous malformation. Catheterization studies: decreased PaO_2 and SaO_2 but normal pulmonary artery pressure. In most cases, embolization or surgical resection of the malformation is recommended.

- Hereditary hemorrhagic telangiectasia: pulmonary arteriovenous malformation is seen in 20% of patients and is multiple in 35%.
- Symptoms depend on the degree of right-to-left shunt.
- Central nervous system complications secondary to paradoxical embolism are common.
- Embolotherapy or surgical resection is indicated in most cases.

Marfan Syndrome

Marfan syndrome is a heritable, generalized disorder of connective tissue. Pulmonary abnormalities seen in about 10% of the patients in the form of emphysema, bullous disease, generalized honeycombing, spontaneous pneumothorax (most common, seen in 5%), and bronchiectasis. Spontaneous pneumothorax and bullae are causally related to Marfan syndrome. Upper lobe fibrosis is also described in this syndrome.

- Marfan syndrome: bullous lung disease.
- Spontaneous pneumothorax in 5% of patients.

OCCUPATIONAL LUNG DISEASES

Among the occupational lung diseases, the following are important: asbestos-induced lung diseases, silicosis, coal workers' pneumoconiosis, hypersensitivity pneumonitis, and gaseous inhalational diseases due to toluene diisocyanate and oxides of nitrogen.

Asbestos

Prolonged exposure to asbestos fibers may cause parietal pleural plaques, pleural thickening, pleural effusions, pulmonary fibrosis (asbestosis), malignant mesothelioma (both pleural and peritoneal), gastrointestinal cancer, and laryngeal carcinoma. The interval between exposure and increase in the number of deaths is 15-35 years for bronchogenic carcinoma, and 30-40 years for malignant mesothelioma. The annual death rate from malignant mesothelioma is 1,200 (smoking has no effect on death rate in this group) and 100 deaths from asbestosis (smokers have 3x higher death rates).

- Majority of asbestos-related deaths are due to bronchogenic carcinoma.
- Prolonged exposure is necessary to develop asbestos-induced mesothelioma.

Pleural Plaque (Hyalinosis Simplex)

The commonest asbestos-related disorder is pleural plaque. It usually represents exposure that occurred more than 20 years earlier. It is neither harmful nor precancerous, but it tends to progress and to calcify over a long period (with 20-30 years' exposure, 10% of patients have calcification and with >40 years, 60% have calcification). The disease is bilateral and symmetrical, and in a third of patients, it is associated with asbestosis.

- Pleural plaque is the commonest asbestos-related disorder.
- Not precancerous.
- Calcified diaphragmatic pleura on chest radiography is almost always diagnostic of asbestos (other causes include ankylosing spondylitis and old tuberculous pleurisy).

Thickened Pleura (Hyalinosis Complicata)

Thickened pleura is an uncommon complication. Progressive calcification involves both visceral and parietal pleurae, lung apices, and pericardium. A recurrent acute inflammatory phase is associated with fever and exudative pleural effusion. Restrictive disease can lead to cor pulmonale.

Pleural Effusion

Pleural effusion is seen in association with asbestosis, pleural thickening, and malignant mesothelioma. It is always an exudate, unilateral or bilateral, or recurrent, and in 70% of patients, it is bloody, with red blood cells exceeding 100,000/dL.

- Bloody effusion, recurrent, unilateral or bilateral.
- Difficult to differentiate from malignant mesothelioma.

Asbestosis

Asbestosis represents pulmonary fibrosis as well as fibrosis of visceral pleura; progressive fibrosis and honeycombing can lead to cor pulmonale. Progressive massive fibrosis is a complication. The pathogenesis is unknown, but many patients are positive for rheumatoid factor and antinuclear antibody. Early massive exposure produces severe disease. Asbestosis is clinically similar to idiopathic pulmonary fibrosis.

- Asbestosis: similar to idiopathic pulmonary fibrosis.
- Positive findings on antinuclear antibody and rheumatoid factor (presumed immune mechanism) tests.

Bronchogenic Carcinoma

Nearly 2.5% of all lung carcinomas may be asbestos related. Carcinogenicity is not well understood. Lower lobes to upper lobes ratio is 2:1. Tumors are peripheral and frequently involve the pleura. Adenocarcinoma is more common than squamous cell carcinoma.

- Peripheral adenocarcinoma in lower lobes.

Malignant Mesothelioma

Malignant mesothelioma is not always related to asbestos, but all types of asbestos fibers have been implicated. There is no correlation with smoking. Initial exposure: more than 40 years before tumor is diagnosed; incidence: 60 million/year. It is more common in patients >70 years. Insulation workers are at greatest risk. Common symptoms are chest pain and dyspnea. Effusions are always exudative. Metastatic lesions in the liver may calcify.

- Malignant mesothelioma: not always related to asbestos exposure.
- Not related to smoking.
- Seen many years (>40 years) after exposure to asbestos.

Silicosis

Silicon dioxide exposure occurs in mines, quarries, sandblasting areas, road building, stone finishing, foundry, ceramics, etc. There is no increase in the risk of malignancy after silica exposure. Four clinical problems can be seen.

1. Acute silicosis: rare, progressively fatal course in months to years. Ceramic workers, silica fluoro/soap workers, and tunneling operators are at risk. Chest radiography shows ground glass or alveolar (upper lung fields) or fibrotic-appearing infiltrates. The pathologic features are sometimes akin to pulmonary proteinosis (silicoproteinosis).
2. Chronic simple silicosis: silicotic nodules of varying sizes (from millimeters to <1.5 cm) occur predominantly in upper lung zones. The nodules may enlarge and coalesce and produce mass-like changes (progressive massive fibrosis). The number and size of nodules increase with increased exposure. Eggshell calcification of hilar nodes is common. Findings on pulmonary function tests are normal or minimally abnormal.
3. Complicated silicosis or progressive massive fibrosis: progressive massive fibrosis, less common than in coal workers' pneumoconiosis, is disabling and life-threatening. It starts as simple silicosis and gradually produces bilateral symmetrical pulmonary masses (>1 cm) in the upper lung fields. Compensatory emphysema with both obstructive and restrictive lung functions produces hypoxemia, which in turn causes cor pulmonale. An autoimmune mechanism is postulated because of the high prevalence of abnormal immunologic laboratory data (antinuclear antibody, rheumatoid factor, etc.). Caplan's syndrome may be a more benign form of progressive massive fibrosis.
4. Silicotuberculosis: silica is toxic to pulmonary alveolar macrophages, which therefore are unable to ingest and kill mycobacteria. The risk of tuberculosis is 4x-6x higher in those with silicosis. Radiographic features: it is difficult to differentiate tuberculosis changes from silicosis-induced changes. The relapse rate of tuberculosis is high, and longer-than-usual antituberculous therapy may be needed.

- Silicosis does not increase the risk of developing lung cancer.
- Acute silicosis (rare) produces changes similar to those of alveolar proteinosis (silicoproteinosis).
- Eggshell calcification of hilar lymph nodes is seen in silicosis and sarcoidosis.
- High prevalence of positive rheumatoid factor and antinuclear antibody in progressive massive fibrosis.
- In a patient with silicosis and fever with or without weight loss, consider silicotuberculosis.
- In a silicotic subject with positive PPD, consider isoniazid treatment.

Coal Workers' Pneumoconiosis

Because of increased mechanization of coal extraction, coal workers' pneumoconiosis is becoming less common. Coal macule is usually <4 mm in size and is made of macrophages, fibroblasts, and reticulin and collagen fibers. Collections of these macules around small airways cause bronchiolar dilatation and focal spongy emphysema. Chest radiography shows tiny nodular infiltrates in the upper lung zones; these may become profuse and lead to progressive massive fibrosis. Unless smoking is present, the results of pulmonary function tests are normal. Slight decrease in FEV_1 may be related to centrilobular emphysema.

- Pulmonary function test abnormalities are usually caused by smoking.
- Coal workers' pneumoconiosis does not increase risk of malignancy or tuberculosis.

Hypersensitivity Pneumonitis

Hypersensitivity pneumonitis is also known as "extrinsic allergic alveolitis." Many fungal precipitins are known to cause this condition. Acute (classic) and chronic forms of hypersensitivity pneumonitis are well described. Acute farmer's lung is the prototype of the acute form. Precipitins in *Mycopolyspora faeni* and *Thermoactinomyces vulgaris* are usually responsible. Symptoms appear 4-6 hours after exposure and include fever, chills, sweats, dry cough, and dyspnea. On examination, tachypnea and basal crackles without wheezing are the findings. Leukocytosis, hyperglobulinemia, and precipitating antibody can be demonstrated. Symptoms resolve rapidly (within 18-24 hours) and recur on reexposure. Chest radiography may show increased bronchovascular markings and fine reticular and nodular defects. Biopsy (rarely indicated) may show bronchiolitis obliterans with organizing pneumonia.

- Symptoms in classic farmer's lung start 6-8 hours after exposure to causative precipitin; some show biphasic (immediate and late) reaction.
- Respiratory distress of varying intensity; wheezing is not a feature.
- Symptoms resolve within 18-24 hours; recur on reexposure.

Chronic farmer's lung results with repeated exposure to precipitins. Symptoms are insidious in onset, eventually resulting in progressive fibrosis. Decrease in lung volumes, compliance, and diffusing capacity and exercise-induced hypoxemia are typical in late stages. This disease is clinically identical to idiopathic pulmonary fibrosis. Lung biopsy usually reveals granulomatous reaction with round cell infiltrates, epithelioid cells, and septal swelling with lymphocytic and plasma cells. In pigeon breeder's lung disease, the histologic features consist of foamy macrophages along with interstitial granulomas. Positive serology is not diagnostic because 20% of asymptomatic farmers have positive precipitins, 10% of symptomatic farmers have negative precipitins, and 40% of asymptomatic pigeon breeders have positive precipitins. The treatment for symptomatic patients is to avoid exposure to causative precipitins and use of steroids.

- Obtaining a good history is very important in making the diagnosis of chronic hypersensitivity pneumonitis.
- Majority of cases of hypersensitivity pneumonitis are due to fungal precipitins.
- Pigeon breeder's lung disease is due to proteins.
- Typically restrictive lung dysfunction.

The points to remember about occupational lung diseases are summarized in Table 26-5.

DRUG-INDUCED LUNG DISEASE

Mechanisms of drug-induced lung disease include hypersensitivity, direct damage from toxic metabolites and oxygen radicals, alkylation of pulmonary tissue macromolecules, antigen-antibody reaction (type III), and type-I immune reactions. Table 26-6 lists different types of pulmonary problems caused by various drugs.

Drug-Induced Systemic Lupus Erythematosus

Older Caucasians are more prone to drug-induced systemic lupus erythematosus. Clinical features include arthralgias and arthritis (90% of patients) and fever and malaise (40%). Abnormal test results for antinuclear antibody (100% of patients), lupus erythematosus cell clot (75%), rheumatoid factor (33%), and low complement level (70%). It is caused by cardiac drugs (procainamide, quinidine, and practolol), antibiotics (nitrofurantoin, penicillin, griseofulvin, sulpha, tetracycline), anticonvulsant agents (phenytoin, mephenytoin, carbamazepine), antihypertensive drugs (hydralazine, methyldopa, L-dopa), antituberculous drugs (isoniazid, streptomycin, para-aminosalicylic acid), phenothiazines (chlorpromazine, promethazine), and miscellaneous agents (D-penicillamine, methysergide, oral contraceptives, phenylbutazone, propylthiouracil, tolazamide, etc.).

- Drug-induced systemic lupus erythematosus: pleural effusion in 50%, pulmonary infiltrates in 30%.
- Procainamide, nitrofurantoin, phenytoin, hydralazine, isoniazid.

Narcotic Abuse

Heroin, morphine, methadone, and propoxyphene cause pulmonary edema, adult respiratory distress syndrome, pneumonia (in 30% of heroin addicts), bronchiectasis, and talc granulomas. Pulmonary edema is the commonest complication of heroin and morphine overdose; it is usually seen within hours and resolves within 24-48 hours. Capillary endothelial damage is the most likely cause of narcotic-associated pulmonary edema. Pneumonia may be secondary to aspiration of gastric contents and septic emboli from endocarditis. Methadone produces similar pulmonary problems. Talc granuloma is the result of intravenous use of crushed analgesic tablets, talc contamination, and cotton fibers used as filters.

Table 26-5.--Pulmonary Diseases: Causes and Associations

Pulmonary disease	Causes and associations
Progressive massive fibrosis	Silicosis, coal, hematite, kaolin, graphite, asbestosis
Autoimmune mechanism	Silicosis, asbestosis, berylliosis
Monday morning sickness	Byssinosis, bagassosis, metal fume fever
Metals and fumes producing asthma	Bakers' asthma, meat wrappers' asthma, printers' asthma, nickel, platinum, toluene diisocyanate, cigarette cutters' asthma
Increased incidence of tuberculosis	Silicosis, hematite lung
Increased incidence of carcinoma	Asbestos, hematite, arsenic, nickel, uranium, chromate
Welder's lung	Siderosis, pulmonary edema, bronchitis, emphysema
Centrilobar emphysema	Coal, hematite
Generalized emphysema	Cadmium
Silo filler's lung	Nitrogen dioxide
Farmer's lung	*Thermoactinomyces, Micropolyspora*
Asbestos exposure	Mesothelioma, bronchogenic cancer, gastrointestinal tract cancer
Eggshell calcification	Silicosis, sarcoid
Sarcoid-like disease	Berylliosis
Diaphragmatic calcification	Asbestosis (also ankylosing spondylitis)
Nonfibrogenic pneumoconioses	Tin, emery, antimony, titanium, barium
Minimal abnormality in lungs	Siderosis, baritosis, stannosis
Bullous emphysema	Bauxite lung
Occupational asthma	Toluene diisocyanate, laboratory animals, grain dust, biologic enzymes, gum acacia, tragacanth, silkworm, anhydrides, wood dust, platinum, nickel, formaldehyde, Freon, drugs

Cornstarch (used as adulterant) also causes granulomas.

- Noncardiogenic pulmonary edema is due to capillary damage.
- Narcotic abuse: adult respiratory distress syndrome, pneumonia, endocarditis, talc granulomas.

Nitrofurantoin

Nitrofurantoin is the drug most commonly reported to produce pulmonary abnormalities. Acute reaction (from 3 hours to 3 months) includes dyspnea (90% of patients), cough (66%), fever (70%), crackles (65%), wheezes (40%), eosinophilia (30%), patchy process (30%), and effusions (10%-20%). Chronic cases (6 months to 7 years) are uncommon but show similar features, although diffuse process is more common (50%). Average dose, 150 mg/day. Pulmonary functions in acute reactions may reveal obstructive phenomena, whereas chronic cases usually show restrictive type of pulmonary dysfunction. Most patients recover after drug is withdrawn from use.

- Acute reaction within 3 hours to 3 months; average dose 150 mg.

- Cough, wheeze, pleural effusion, eosinophilia.

Chemotherapeutic Agents

The mechanism of pulmonary reaction to chemotherapeutic agents is not clear. Many chemotherapeutic drugs produce cytotoxic changes characterized by "bizarre-appearing" type II pneumocytes. Nonspecific changes are common. Symptoms include cough, dyspnea, and fever. Fever is present in most patients and may precede the onset of dyspnea or radiographic abnormalities. Pulmonary function tests reveal a restrictive pattern. Arterial oxygen desaturation is common. Busulfan (Myleran) causes "busulfan lung" in about 8% of patients. Findings on pulmonary function tests may be abnormal without clinical or radiographic evidence of disease. Pulmonary reaction is usually seen after 6 months of therapy. Chest radiography shows diffuse interstitial and alveolar infiltrates. Death may occur despite stopping the use of the drug and using steroids. Cyclophosphamide (Cytoxan) produces (but less commonly) similar reactions. However, changes are seen earlier than with busulfan. Bleomycin has a 10% incidence of pulmonary toxicity, which increases with increasing age (>70 years) and

Table 26-6.--Drug-Induced Pulmonary Diseases

Interstitial pneumonitis/fibrosis

    Chemotherapeutic agents
    Nitrofurantoin (chronic)
    Drug-induced systemic lupus erythematosus
    Gold
    Talc (intravenous use)
    Aspirated oil
    D-Penicillamine
    Pituitary snuff
    Radiation
    Oxygen
    Sulfasalazine (Azulfidine)
    Cromolyn sodium
    Methysergide
    Hexamethonium, pentolinium, mecamylamine

Noncardiac pulmonary edema

    Heroin, methadone, morphine
    Acetylsalicylic acid
    Nitrofurantoin (acute)
    Chlordiazepoxide (Librium)
    Ethchlorvynol (Placidyl)

Pleural effusion

    Nitrofurantoin (acute)
    Methysergide (chronic)
    Drug-induced systemic lupus erythematosus
    Chemotherapeutic drugs
    Radiation
    Dantrolene

Drug-induced pulmonary infiltrate with eosinophilia

    Sulfonamides
    Sulfasalazine (Azulfidine)
    Penicillin
    Isoniazid
    Aminosalicylate
    Nitrofurantoin

    Leukoagglutinin
    Methotrexate
    Procarbazine
    Carbamazepine (Tegretol)
    Imipramine (Tofranil)
    Salicylates
    Cromolyn sodium
    Methylphenidate (Ritalin)
    Dantrolene

Drug-induced hilar and mediastinal widening

    Corticosteroids
    Methotrexate
    Phenytoin (Dilantin)

Bronchospasm

    Propranolol, other β-blockers
    Acetylsalicylic acid
    Indomethacin
    Fenoprofen
    Mefenamate
    Isuprel
    Drugs that produce pulmonary infiltrate with
      eosinophilia
    Nebulized medications

Pulmonary hypertension

    Oral contraceptives
    Aminorex
    15-methyl-prostaglandin-F_2

Pulmonary granulomas

    Talc
    Mineral oil
    Methotrexate
    Cromolyn sodium
    Cotton fibers (intravenous drug use)

---

increasing dosage (>450 units). Acute hypersensitivity reaction with eosinophilia has been reported in some patients. Chlorambucil (uncommonly) produces complications similar to those caused by busulfan, cyclophosphamide, and bleomycin. Carmustine produces pulmonary reactions in 1% of patients within 8 months, sim-

ilar to those seen with other chemotherapeutic agents. A higher incidence of pneumothorax has been noted. Methotrexate is the only antimetabolite known to produce pulmonary disease that is self-limiting and is frequently associated with peripheral eosinophilia. Most pulmonary reactions reported have been in children treated for acute lymphatic leukemia. Chest radiography shows diffuse fine interstitial infiltrates, hilar adenopathy, or pleural effusion in 10% of patients. Symptoms begin within a few days to several weeks after initiation of therapy.

- Cough, dyspnea, fever, patchy lung infiltrates.
- Bizarre type II pneumocytes in most cases except in those treated with methotrexate.
- "Busulfan lung" occurs in 8%-10% of patients, usually after 6 months of therapy.
- Bleomycin lung toxicity occurs in 10% of patients; dose- (>450 units) and age- (>70 yr) related.
- Methotrexate produces eosinophilia, hilar adenopathy, and pleural effusion.
- The treatment is discontinuation of the drug; corticosteroids may be tried.

Radiation

Type II pneumocytes and pulmonary capillary endothelial cells are initially affected by radiation. Radiation effects may be cumulative; the rate at which it is given is most important. A second or third course of radiation to the lung is more likely to result in a pneumonitis that can occur earlier and be devastating. Underlying lung disease has no role in the pathologic process. During the acute phase, type II pneumocyte changes and an inflammatory process can be seen. In the chronic stage, nonspecific fibrosis is common. Symptoms of radiation pneumonitis begin insidiously 1-3 months after completion of radiation. Cough, fever, and dyspnea may precede the onset of radiographic changes. The late phase begins after 6 months of radiation therapy. Dyspnea is usually out of proportion to the radiographic changes. Steroid therapy has varying response.

- Capillary endothelial damage has a major role in radiation-induced lung disease.
- Radiation pneumonitis is not dependent on the dose, rate, or the volume of lung radiated.
- Concomitant use of bleomycin and cyclophosphamide, and withdrawal of steroid therapy increase the risk of radiation pneumonitis.
- Acute phase occurs about 1-2 months after radiation, and the chronic phase is seen after 9 months.
- The earlier the onset, the worse the prognosis.

Corticosteroids

Patients receiving high doses (>1 mg/kg per day) of corticosteroids are more likely to develop opportunistic infections from *Nocardia asteroides,* cytomegalovirus, *Mycobacterium tuberculosis, Aspergillus fumigatus, Candida albicans,* and *Cryptococcus neoformans.* Mediastinal lipomatosis in the mid and anterior mediastinum results from excessive deposition of fat in these areas. CT of the mediastinum is diagnostic. Rapid withdrawal of steroid therapy may enhance the onset of radiation pneumonitis.

- Mediastinal lipomatosis is diagnosed with CT.

Analgesic Agents

Salicylates produce bronchospasm in aspirin-sensitive patients, pulmonary infiltrates with eosinophilia, and noncardiogenic and pulmonary edema (when blood level is >50 mg/dL). Pulmonary edema occurs within 1-2 hours after ingestion; radiographic changes may persist for a week or longer. Gold sodium thiomalate and aurothioglucose produce pulmonary toxicity in 3%-5% of patients. Chest radiography shows diffuse interstitial process. Symptoms include cough, fever, and dyspnea. Histologic features are lymphocytic and plasma cell infiltrates. Pulmonary reactions to use of other analgesics include bronchospasm (naproxen, indomethacin, ibuprofen, and mefenamate) and pulmonary edema (phenylbutazone and oxyphenbutazone).

- Bronchospasm occurs with acetylsalicylic acid but not with all salicylates.
- Respiratory alkalosis is followed by metabolic acidosis in salicylate overdose.
- With gold therapy, lung reaction can be acute or insidious and is usually dose-related, with most patients having received >300 mg.

Oxygen

Oxygen toxicity can be avoided if the FIO_2 is kept below 0.5. If the duration of FIO_2 of 1.0 exceeds 24 hours or if FIO_2 of 0.6 exceeds 72 hours, the risk of pulmonary damage increases. Oxygen-induced adult respiratory distress syndrome is not amenable to any treatment, and the patients usually succumb to lung failure. Histologic features include an early exudative phase followed by an irreversible proliferative and fibrotic phase.

Oil Aspiration

With the aspiration of oil, abnormalities range from solitary nodules to various types of infiltrates, especially in the dependent lower lung fields. Mineral oil for softening stools, oily nose drops, ophthalmic drops, and other oily preparations are used frequently. Bronchographic medium has the potential to induce bronchospasm and transient changes in pulmonary functions.

- Aspiration of oil: common but frequently overlooked cause of pulmonary infiltrates.
- Important to obtain the history of use of these agents.

Inhaled Medications

Inhaled medications cause bronchospasm, irritation of the upper airways, and cough in some patients. Cromolyn sodium, used in asthmatics, can produce bronchospasm, pulmonary infiltrates with eosinophilia, and nonspecific upper airway irritation.

- Cromolyn can produce bronchospasm, eosinophilia, and lung infiltrates.
- Ultrafine nebulized aerosols can cause cough and bronchospasm.

Blood Products

Leukoagglutinins in the blood may produce acute pulmonary edema. The exact mechanism is unknown, but a hypersensitivity reaction has been postulated. There is acute onset of fever, chills, cough, and dyspnea. Pulmonary infiltrates may persist for several days. Eosinophilia is seen in some patients. Radiography shows varying picture of pulmonary edema. HIV transmission from transfusion of blood or blood products.

- Blood products: pulmonary edema, eosinophilia, lung infiltrates, HIV transmission.

Miscellaneous

β-Blockers (propranolol, metoprolol, nadolol, and timolol) may aggravate asthma; amiodarone causes interstitial pneumonitis in 1%-4% of patients. Lung pathologic reaction is dose-related and is seen usually with a dose exceeding 400 mg/day. Dyspnea and cough are noted 2-3 months after starting therapy with the drug. ACE inhibitors cause cough in 6%. D-Penicillamine provokes four types of pulmonary reaction: bronchiolitis obliterans, a Goodpasture's syndrome-like illness, diffuse alveolitis, and drug-induced systemic lupus erythematosus. Paraquat is a potent weed killer; most cases of illness induced by it are due to accidental ingestion. Bronchiolitis, adult respiratory distress syndrome, and severe pulmonary fibrosis are common. Lung changes can be acute. L-Tryptophan-induced eosinophilia-myalgia syndrome is related to a contaminant in the manufacturing process. The result is myalgia, eosinophilia, pulmonary infiltrates, pleural effusion, and pulmonary hypertension. Iodized contrast media produce pulmonary infiltrates, restrictive dysfunction, and low diffusing capacity. "Stippling" type of radiographic changes are seen with lymphangiographic examinations. Methysergide (Sansert) may cause insidious onset of pleuropulmonary fibrosis; pleural effusion is seen in nearly 50% of patients with pleuropulmonary fibrosis.

- β-Blockers aggravate asthma and COPD.
- Amiodarone causes diffuse lung infiltrates; dose usually >400 mg/day.
- ACE inhibitors cause cough in 4%-6% of patients.
- Penicillamine can cause bronchiolitis and drug-induced systemic lupus erythematosus.

EFFECTS OF ALTITUDE, DIVING, AND DROWNING

High-Altitude Sickness

Acute exposure to hypoxia increases minute ventilation and reduces $PaCO_2$. This reaction is mediated by peripheral chemoreceptors. It can be reversed rapidly by oxygen inhalation. Similar changes occur acutely at high altitudes, but after 5-10 days, there is a further increase in ventilation and a greater decrease in $PaCO_2$, which an ambient PO_2 fails to correct. Highlanders ventilate less than acclimatized lowlanders and maintain a higher $PaCO_2$ and a lower PaO_2. This is due to a marked insensitivity to hypoxia, which is a permanent characteristic resulting from low ambient PO_2 during the first 2 years of life. It is clinically manifested by polycythemia (due to increased erythropoietin), decreased oxygen affinity (shift of the oxygen-hemoglobin curve to the right and increased 2,3-diphosphoglycerate [DPG]), cardiac output and stroke volume during exercise, and pulmonary hypertension.

Acute mountain sickness affects lowlanders 6-90 hours after ascent, producing lethargy, insomnia, headache, nausea, vomiting, and dyspnea. Cyanosis and signs of cerebral edema can occur. Prophylactic diuretic therapy (before ascent) prevents acute mountain sickness.

- Acute mountain sickness affects lowlanders 6-90 hours after ascent; diuretics before ascent are recommended.

High-altitude pulmonary edema commonly occurs in high-altitude natives returning to altitude after several weeks at sea level. A time lag from 9 to 36 hours is common. Clinically, high-altitude pulmonary edema is similar to acute pulmonary edema from other causes, but left ventricular failure is not a feature. Chest radiography shows patchy inhalation infiltrates. These disappear 6-48 hours after return to sea level or with oxygen. The pathogenesis is not fully understood.

- High-altitude pulmonary edema occurs commonly in high-altitude natives returning to high altitude after several weeks at sea level; cold weather and exertion contribute to this condition.

Chronic mountain sickness is the result of progressive loss of acclimatization to high altitude. Highlanders develop chronic malaise, headache, dizziness, easy fatigability, paresthesias, somnolence, and diminished mental activity. Marked cyanosis, clubbing of the fingers, polycythemia, oxygen desaturation, and cardiac enlargement occur, but the lung fields appear normal. The respiratory drive is lost and patients develop primary alveolar hypoventilation. Pulmonary arterial pressure is twice as high as that of the healthy dweller at altitude. After 2 months at sea level, reduction in pulmonary hypertension is seen.

- Chronic mountain sickness is the result of progressive loss of acclimatization to high altitude.

Diving and Near Drowning

Most drowning accidents occur in the pediatric age group and in fresh water. The greatest risk factor for drowning in adults and teenagers is alcohol consumption. Arterial gas embolism is an important cause of death among scuba divers. Although hypothermia by itself is rarely the actual cause of death, it can have a significant effect on the prognosis of near-drowning victims. Aspiration occurs in about 85% of drowning or near-drowning victims; the other 15% develop laryngospasm and, thus, do not have signs of aspiration. The duration of hypoxemia caused by drowning is far more important in predicting the mortality rather than fresh water versus salt water drowning or the electrolyte imbalance. Pulmonary complications such as adult respiratory distress syndrome and aspiration pneumonia are more common in those who aspirate.

- Alcohol consumption is a major risk factor for drowning in adults.
- Pulmonary complications are more common in those with aspiration.

Barotrauma is more common in divers and is caused by the contraction or expansion of gas that occurs because of changes in barometric pressure after a descent or ascent. Pulmonary complications that result from overdistension include mild hemoptysis, chest pain, interstitial emphysema, pneumothorax, and arterial gas embolism. Interstitial emphysema and pneumomediastinum may remain asymptomatic. Arterial gas embolization produces sudden and dramatic loss of consciousness, blindness, seizures, hemiparesis, and other neurologic signs.

- Interstitial emphysema is more common than pneumothorax in deep sea divers.

PULMONARY NEOPLASMS

Solitary Pulmonary Nodule

A solitary pulmonary nodule is defined as a solitary lesion seen on plain chest radiographs. It is <4 cm and is round, ovoid, or slightly lobulated. The lesion is located in lung parenchyma, is at least moderately circumscribed, and uncalcified on plain radiographs. It is not associated with satellite lesions or other abnormalities on plain chest radiographs. Common causes include carcinoma of the lung (15%-50% of patients), mycoses (5%-50%), tuberculosis, unidentified granulomas, resolving pneumonia, hamartoma, and metastatic lesions. Uncommon causes include carcinoid, bronchogenic cyst, resolving infarction, rheumatoid and vasculitic nodules, and arteriovenous malformation.

- Solitary pulmonary nodule: pleural, skin, and other extrapulmonary lesions should be excluded.
- Granulomas and hamartomas make up 40%-60% of all solitary pulmonary nodules and 90% of nonmalignant solitary pulmonary nodules.
- Hamartomas alone comprise <10% of nonmalignant nodules.

History

The following aspects are important in the evaluation of solitary pulmonary nodules: age of the patient, availability of previous chest radiographs, smoking history, previous malignancy, exposure to tuberculous patients, travel to areas endemic for mycoses, recent respiratory infection, recent pulmonary infarction, recent trauma to chest, asthma, mucoid impaction, systemic diseases (congestive heart failure, rheumatoid arthritis, etc.), ENT symptoms (Wegener's vasculitis), mineral oil, oily nose drops, immune defense mechanisms, and family history (arteriovenous malformation).

- History: old chest radiographs, age, smoking history, previous malignancy, and exposure history are important.

Diagnosis

Physical examination, routine complete blood cell count, chemistry group, and the exclusion of obvious causes (congestive heart failure, vasculitis, rheumatoid arthritis, etc.) are important for making the diagnosis. Obtain earlier chest radiographs for comparison. Sputum cytology, skin tests, serologies, and cultures on a routine basis are generally unrewarding in asymptomatic patients. Localized tomograms identify the location of a solitary pulmonary nodule, calcification, cavitation, satellite lesions, and margins. Chest CT is helpful in assessing calcification, density, multiple nodules (particularly in evaluating metastatic malignancy), and staging of lung cancer.

- In asymptomatic patients with single pulmonary nodule, extensive studies (gastrointestinal tract series, intravenous pyelography, scans of bone, brain, liver, bone marrow, etc.) are not indicated because of the low diagnostic yield (<3%).
- CT detects 30% more nodules than chest radiography, but the role of CT in separating benign from malignant lesions is not established.
- Bronchoscopic brush and biopsy has about a 60% diagnostic yield in cancer.
- Transthoracic needle aspiration (CT- or fluoroscopy-guided) has an 85% diagnostic yield in cancer; 20% risk of pneumothorax.

Decision Making

General guidelines for decision making are given in Table 26-7. If benign etiology cannot be firmly established after complete clinical, imaging, culture, and biopsy evaluations, the following two decisions advocate surgical resection: 1) the solitary pulmonary nodule is probably malignant, because little or no other clinical information is available to indicate a benign diagnosis or 2) the nodule may be benign but must be resected now because the benign nature cannot be established. If the clinical information firmly indicates a benign cause, follow-up chest radiography is recommended.

- If there is no change in the size or shape of the solitary pulmonary nodule for over 2 years, repeat chest radiography every 6-12 months.
- If the patient is a poor surgical risk or if surgeon or patient refuses the operation, repeat chest radiography every 3 months (enlargement of lesion may convince patient/surgeon to consider resection).

Table 26-7.--Likelihood of Benign or Malignant Single Pulmonary Nodule According to Clinical and Radiographic Variables

Clinical factor, radiographic result	More likely benign	More likely malignant
Age	<35 yr	>35 yr
Sex	Female	Male
Smoking	No	Yes
Symptoms	No	Yes
Exposure to tuberculosis, cocci, etc.	Yes	No
Previous malignancy	No	Yes
Nodule size	<2.0 cm	>2.0 cm
Nodule age	>2 yr	<2 yr
Doubling time	<30 days	>30 days
Nodule margins	Smooth	Irregular
Calcification	Yes	No
Satellite lesions	Yes	No

Primary Lung Cancer

Lung cancer is the commonest malignant disease and the commonest cause of cancer death in the U.S. The estimated incidence of lung cancer for the 1990s is 20% (of all cancers) for men (prostate, 20%; colon and rectum, 15%) and 11% for women (breast, 29%; colon and rectum, 15%). The estimated cancer death from lung cancer for the 1990s is 34% for men (11% for colon cancer) and 21% for women (18% for breast and 13% for colon). The male-to-female ratio is 2:1. More than 150,000 new cases of cancer and >110,000 lung cancer deaths per year are predicted for the next several years. The risk factors include cigarette smoking, other carcinogens, cocarcinogens, radon daughters (uranium mining), arsenic (glass workers, smelters, pesticides), asbestos (insulation, textile, asbestos mining), coal dust (coke oven, road work, roofer), chromium (leather, ceramic, metal), vinyl chloride (plastic), chloromethyl methyl ether (chemical), and chronic lung injury (idiopathic pulmonary fibrosis, COPD).

The WHO classification of pathologic types of pulmonary neoplasms is given in Table 26-8 and the TNM classification for staging of non-small-cell lung cancer, in Table 26-9.

Small cell cancer is staged as follows:
1. Limited: single hemithorax, mediastinum, ipsilateral supraclavicular nodes.
2. Extensive: anything beyond limited stage.

Table 26-8.--WHO Classification of Pulmonary Neoplasms

Type	
I	Squamous cell carcinoma
II	Small cell carcinoma
	Oat cell carcinoma
	Intermediate cell carcinoma
	Combined oat cell carcinoma
III	Adenocarcinoma
	Acinar adenocarcinoma
	Papillary adenocarcinoma
	Bronchoalveolar carcinoma
	Solid carcinoma with mucus formation
IV	Large cell carcinoma
	Giant cell carcinoma
	Clear cell carcinoma
V	Combined cell types
VI	Carcinoid tumors
VII	Bronchial gland tumors
	Cylindroma
	Mucoepidermoid
VIII	Papillary tumors

Overall Survival

Occult and in situ cancers have >70% overall survival. Overall survival for other stages is as follows: stage I, 50%; stage II, <20%; and stage III, <10%. One-year survival for stage I cancer is >80%. In small cell cancer, the median survival is <12 months; 5-year survival for limited stage cancer is 15%-20% and for extensive disease, 1%-5%.

Cell Types and Clinical Features

Most patients are >50 years old. The presentation is highly variable and depends on cell type, location, rate of growth, paraneoplastic syndromes, systemic symptoms, and other factors. Cough is the most frequent symptom and is more likely in squamous and small cell cancers. Hemoptysis occurs in 35%-50% of patients and is more common with squamous, small cell, and endobronchial metastases. Wheezing is due to intraluminal tumor or extrinsic compression. Dyspnea depends on the extensiveness of the tumor, COPD, degree of bronchial obstruction, etc. Persistent chest pain may suggest rib metastasis, local extension, or pleural involvement. Superior vena cava syndrome may suggest small cell carcinoma, lymphoma, squamous cell carcinoma, or Pancoast's tumor. Horner's syndrome is indicative of Pancoast's tumor. Fever, postobstructive pneumonitis, nonthoracic skeletal pains, central nervous system symptoms, and abdominal pain/discomfort and hepatomegaly are indicative of possible distant metastases. Central nervous system metastasis is found in 15% of patients with squamous cell carcinoma, in 25% with adenocarcinoma, in 28% with large cell carcinoma, and in 30% with small cell carcinoma.

- Cough and hemoptysis are more common in squamous cell carcinoma and carcinoid.
- Chest pain may indicate pleural effusion or pleural metastasis.
- Nonpulmonary symptoms may indicate distant metastases.
- Paraneoplastic syndromes are more common in patients with lung cancers.
- Central nervous system metastasis is more common with small cell carcinoma.

Squamous Cell Carcinoma

Most squamous cell carcinomas arise in the proximal tracheobronchial tree (first four subdivisions). They also may arise in the upper airway and esophagus. Symptoms appear early in the course of the disease because of proximal bronchial involvement and consist of cough, hemoptysis, and lobar/segmental collapse with postobstructive pneumonia. Chest radiography shows perihilar/peripheral mass with or without lobar/segmental obstruction. One-third of cases present as peripheral masses. Sputum cytology and bronchoscopy are indicated for almost all patients. One-third of squamous cell carcinomas have thick-walled irregular cavities. Treatment is with resec-

Table 26-9.--Staging of Lung Cancer: TNM Classification

T, primary tumor

T0	No evidence of primary tumor
TX	Cancer cells in respiratory secretions; no tumor on chest radiographs or at bronchoscopy
Tis	Carcinoma in situ
T1	Tumor ≤3 cm in greatest dimension, surrounded by lung tissue; no bronchoscopic evidence of tumor proximal to lobar bronchus
T2	Tumor >3 cm in diameter, or tumor of any size that involves visceral pleura, or associated with atelectasis extending to hilum (but not involving entire lung); must be ≥2 cm from main carina
T3	Tumor involves chest wall, diaphragm, mediastinal pleura, or pericardium, or is <2 cm from main carina (but does not involve it)
T4	Tumor involves main carina or trachea, or invades mediastinum, heart, great vessels, esophagus, or vertebra, or malignant pleural effusion

N, nodal involvement

N0	No demonstrable lymph node involvement
N1	Ipsilateral peribronchial or hilar lymph nodes involved
N2	Metastasis to ipsilateral mediastinal lymph nodes, or to subcarinal lymph nodes
N3	Metastasis to contralateral mediastinal and/or hilar lymph nodes, or to scalene and/or supraclavicular lymph nodes

M, metastasis

M0	No known distant metastasis
M1	Distant metastasis present (specify site or sites)

TNM subsets for staging lung cancer

Stage 0	Tis
Stage I	T1 N0 M0
	T2 N0 M0
Stage II	T1 N1 M0
	T2 N1 M0
Stage IIIa	T3 N0 M0
	T3 N1 M0
	T1-3 N2 M0
Stage IIIb	Any T N3 M0
	T4 Any N M0
Stage IV	Any T Any N M1

---

tion, radiation, and chemotherapy. Laser bronchoscopy and endobronchial brachytherapy are palliative measures.

- Squamous cell carcinoma: proximal airway disease in 66%; peripheral mass in 33%.
- Sputum cytology and bronchoscopy are important tests.
- One-third of the masses show cavitation.

Adenocarcinoma

Most adenocarcinomas arise in the periphery and, thus, remain undetected until they have spread locally or distally. Adenocarcinoma is the commonest type of peripheral primary lung cancer. It may not produce pulmonary symptoms early in the course of the disease because of peripheral location. This means the chance of dissemination to extrapulmonary sites is higher for these tumors. Sputum cytology has a low yield in those without pulmonary symptoms. Advanced stages are more common in symptomatic patients; however, incidentally detected peripheral carcinomas tend to be in an early stage. The commonest presentation is as a solitary peripheral nodule. A small number cavitate. Clubbing and hypertrophic pulmonary osteoarthropathy are more common than in other kinds of primary lung cancer. The response to radiation and chemotherapy is generally poor.

- Adenocarcinoma: most of them arise as a solitary pulmonary nodule in the periphery and, hence, are usually asymptomatic.
- Symptomatic stage usually denotes advanced disease.
- Sputum cytology has low diagnostic yield in the absence of cough and hemoptysis.
- Clubbing and hypertrophic pulmonary osteoarthropathy are more common than in squamous cell carcinoma.

Bronchoalveolar Cell Carcinoma

Bronchoalveolar carcinoma is thought to arise from alveolar type 2 pneumocytes and/or Clara cells. The tumor presents in two forms: as a localized solitary nodular lesion and as a diffuse alveolar process. The solitary form has the best prognosis of all types of lung cancer, with a 1-year survival rate of >80%. The diffuse variety has a mean survival rate of <6 months. Bronchorrhea (>100 mL of thin serous mucus secretion/24 hours) is seen in 20% of patients. Chest radiography shows a solitary nodule, localized infiltrate with vacuoles on tomography, pneumonic lesions. Both forms of bronchoalveolar cell carcinoma can mimic ordinary pneumonia. The chronic course of the disease because of slow growth may suggest a benign process; thus, close surveillance is imperative. Treatment for a solitary lesion is resection. The response to radiation and chemotherapy is poor, although bronchorrhea seems to respond to radiation in some patients.

- Bronchoalveolar cell carcinoma: unrelated to tobacco smoking.
- The solitary form has slow growth; may mimic benign pulmonary nodule.
- Solitary (localized) form has >80% 1-year survival rate after resection.
- The diffuse form has a mean survival rate of <6 months.
- Bronchorrhea occurs in 20% of patients (usually diffuse form).

Large Cell Carcinoma

Large cells are seen on histologic examination, and radiography shows large masses. Large cell carcinoma grows more rapidly than adenocarcinoma. Cavitation is seen in 20%-25% of patients. Clubbing and hypertrophic pulmonary osteoarthropathy are more common than in other tumors except for adenocarcinoma. Treatment is surgical. The response to radiation and chemotherapy is poor.

- Large cell carcinoma: large, rapidly growing lung mass; cavitation in 25% of patients.
- Clubbing and hypertrophic pulmonary osteoarthropathy are common.

Small Cell Carcinoma

Small cell carcinoma, which accounts for 25% of all bronchogenic carcinomas, is also called "oat cell (ovoid cells) carcinoma." The tumor originates from neuroendocrine cells (Kulchitsky cells). The tumor invades the tracheobronchial tree and spreads submucosally. Later, it breaks through the mucosa and produces changes similar to those seen in squamous cell carcinoma. Chest radiography shows a unilateral, rapidly enlarging hilar or perihilar mass or widening of the hila/mediastinum. Less than 20% of these tumors are peripheral. Bronchoscopy may show heaped-up or thickened mucosa. This tumor responds better to radiation and chemotherapy than do other lung tumors. Prophylactic brain radiation is standard at many medical centers; this decreases the frequency of brain metastasis but does not prolong survival. Peripheral nodules that are found to be small cell carcinoma after resection should be treated as any small cell carcinoma.

- Small cell carcinoma: smokers and uranium miners are more prone.
- Positive antineuronal antibody in blood.
- Small cell carcinoma may be associated with many paraneoplastic syndromes: syndrome of inappropriate antidiuretic hormone, ACTH production, myasthenic syndrome.
- Surgical treatment is not a standard therapeutic option; radiation and chemotherapy are.

Carcinoid

Carcinoid arises from the same cells as small cell carcinoma, but its clinical behavior is different. Typically, carcinoid presents with cough, with or without hemoptysis, in young adults. Chest radiography may show a solitary nodule or segmental atelectasis. Paraneoplastic syndromes develop from hormonal secretion (ACTH, PTH). Treatment is surgical resection of the tumor without lung resection. The diagnosis of malignant carcinoid is based on the extent of spread noted at resection or clinical behavior.

- Carcinoid: young adult with cough and hemoptysis.
- Symptoms may be related to production of ACTH

(Cushing's syndrome, hypertension) and PTH (hypercalcemia).

- Carcinoid "syndrome" is rare, occurring in <1% of patients with bronchial carcinoid.

Bronchial Gland Tumors

Cylindroma and mucoepidermoid tumors are usually located centrally and cause cough, hemoptysis, and obstructive pneumonia. Distant metastasis is unusual. Surgical treatment is used for major airway obstructive lesions. The response to radiation and chemotherapy is poor.

- Cylindroma arising in salivary glands can metastasize to the lungs after many years.

Mesenchymal Tumors

This group of tumors includes lymphoma, lymphosarcoma, carcinosarcoma, fibrosarcoma, mesothelioma (discussed above), and soft tissue sarcomas. Many of these present as large peripheral masses, homogeneous densities, and cavitated lesions.

Lymphoma

Pulmonary involvement occurs in 65% and 45% of patients with Hodgkin's and non-Hodgkin's lymphoma, respectively. Radiographic findings include bilateral hilar adenopathy, chylous pleural effusion, segmental atelectasis from endobronchial lesions, diffuse nodular process, fluffy infiltrates, and diffuse interstitial/alveolar infiltrates. Pseudolymphoma is a collection of abnormal lymphocytes and presents as a slow-growing lung mass; currently, it is considered a low-grade malignancy. Similarly, many of the patients thought to have lymphocytic interstitial pneumonitis currently are considered to have low-grade lymphomas that have a good response to chemotherapy. These tumors originate from the mucosa-associated lymphoid tissue.

- Intrathoracic involvement is common in Hodgkin's lymphoma.
- Bilateral hilar lymphadenopathy and chylous pleural effusion occur in young adults.
- Hodgkin's lymphoma can produce any type of radiographic abnormality.

Diagnostic Tests

The results of sputum cytology are positive in 60% of patients with squamous cell carcinomas, in 21% with small cell carcinoma, in 16% with adenocarcinoma, and in 13% with large cell carcinoma. Radiography is used to diagnose more tumors than sputum cytology but is not recommended as a surveillance tool for all patients. Bronchoscopy is helpful in diagnosing the cell type, in assessing staging and resectability, in using laser treatment for large airway tumors, and in brachytherapy. Transthoracic needle aspiration has an 85%-90% yield, but the incidence of pneumothorax is 25%, with most patients requiring chest tube drainage. CT scan is helpful in assessing the number of nodules in patients with pulmonary metastasis and in examination of the hila and mediastinum. Positive results on pleural fluid cytology establish stage III disease. Mediastinoscopy and mediastinotomy (Chamberlain procedure) are staging procedures that are often used before thoracotomy is performed.

- Chest radiography helps diagnose more lung tumors than sputum cytology.
- Sputum cytology findings are positive in 60% of patients with squamous cell cancer.
- Routine surveillance of all susceptible persons (heavy smokers) with radiography and sputum cytology is not recommended.

Paraneoplastic Syndromes

As a group, primary lung tumors are the commonest cause of paraneoplastic syndromes. The presence of a paraneoplastic syndrome does not indicate metastatic spread of lung cancer. The mechanism for the production of these syndromes varies. In clinical practice, it is more helpful to consider paraneoplastic manifestations based on each organ system, as described below.

- Primary lung tumors cause most of the paraneoplastic manifestations.
- Paraneoplastic syndrome does not indicate metastatic spread of lung cancer.

Endocrine

Small cell carcinoma is associated with syndrome of inappropriate antidiuretic hormone and ACTH production. Hypokalemia, muscle weakness, and radiographic abnormality should suggest ACTH production. Note that these patients do not live long enough to develop typical Cushing's syndrome. The ACTH levels are very high and are not suppressed by dexamethasone. The overall frequency of hypercalcemia is 13%, with squamous cell cancer causing it in 25% of patients, large cell carcinoma in 13%, and adenocarcinoma in 3%. Hypercalcemia is not associated with small cell carcinoma. Bony metastasis can also cause hypercalcemia. Hyperpigmentation from MSH occurs in small cell carcinoma. Calcitonin is secreted in 70% of patients with small cell carcinoma and in adenocarcinoma. Syndrome of inappropriate antidiuretic hormone is also seen in some patients with alveolar cell carcinoma and adenocarcinoma. Hypoglycemia with insulin-like polypeptide is found in patients with squamous cell carcinoma and mesothelioma. The hCG, LH, and FSH secreted by adenocarcinoma and large cell carcinoma may be responsible for gynecomastia.

- Abnormal radiographic findings in hyponatremia: small cell carcinoma (syndrome of inappropriate antidiuretic hormone).
- Abnormal radiographic findings, hypokalemia, and muscle weakness: small cell carcinoma (ACTH).
- ACTH is also produced by bronchial carcinoid.
- Hypercalcemia: squamous cell carcinoma and carcinoid.
- Calcitonin: small cell carcinoma and adenocarcinoma.
- Gynecomastia: adenocarcinoma or large cell carcinoma (FSH).

Central Nervous System

The mechanism for encephalopathy, myelopathy, sensory-motor neuropathies, and polymyositis is unknown but may include toxic, nutritional, autoimmune, and infectious causes. Cerebellar ataxia is similar to alcohol-induced ataxia and is more common with squamous cell carcinoma. Myasthenic syndrome (Lambert-Eaton syndrome) is closely associated with small cell carcinoma; there is initial weakness in the proximal muscles, but strength returns to normal with repeated stimulation. Focal neurologic signs should suggest central nervous system metastasis. Acute and rapidly progressive lower extremity signs should indicate spinal cord compression by tumor.

- Myasthenic syndrome may precede clinical detection of small cell carcinoma.
- Cerebellar ataxia (similar to alcohol-induced ataxia) is more common in squamous cell carcinoma.

- Focal neurologic signs should indicate central nervous system metastasis.

Skeletal

Hypertrophic pulmonary oestoarthropathy indicates periosteal bone formation and is associated with clubbing and symmetrical arthralgias. Other features include fever, gynecomastia, and increased erythrocyte sedimentation rate. Proposed mechanisms: neural (vagal afferents), hormonal, and others. Hypertrophic pulmonary osteoarthropathy is more common in adenocarcinoma and large cell carcinoma and may precede the tumor by months. Clubbing alone can be the only feature. Removal of the tumor relieves the hypertrophic pulmonary osteoarthropathy.

- Hypertrophic pulmonary osteoarthropathy is more common in adenocarcinoma and large cell carcinoma.
- Ipsilateral vagotomy is indicated if the hypertrophic pulmonary osteoarthropathy persists after resection of tumor.

Others

Other paraneoplastic manifestations include: malignant cachexia, marantic endocarditis, increased incidence of thrombophlebitis, fever, erythrocytosis, leukocytosis, lymphocytopenia, eosinophilia, thrombocytosis, leukemoid reaction, disseminated intravascular coagulation, dysproteinemia, fever, acanthosis nigricans (adenocarcinoma), epidermolysis bullosa (squamous cell carcinoma), and nephrotic syndrome.

Pulmonary Metastases

Nearly 30% of all cases of malignant disease from extrapulmonary sites metastasize to the lung. More than 75% present with multiple lesions and the rest may present as a solitary pulmonary nodule, diffuse process, lymphangitic spread (breast, stomach, thyroid, pancreas, lung itself), and endobronchial metastases (kidney, colon, Hodgkin's lymphoma, breast). Solitary metastases are more common with carcinoma of the colon, sarcoma, kidneys, testis, breast, and melanoma. The estimated occurrence of pulmonary metastasis by primary tumor is as follows: choriocarcinoma, 80%; osteosarcoma, 75%; kidney, 70%; thyroid, 65%; melanoma, 60%; breast, 55%; prostate, 45%; nasopharyngeal, 20%; gastrointestinal malignancies, 20%; and gynecologic malignancies, 20%.

MEDIASTINUM

Mediastinal Lesions

Clinically, it is useful to divide mediastinal lesions into their location, namely, anterior, middle, and posterior mediastinum. The anterior compartment contains the thymus, ascending aorta, innominate artery and vein, superior vena cava, fat, and lymph nodes. More than 50% of mediastinal tumors are located in this compartment, and 60% of them are thymic tumors, lymphomas, and germ cell tumors. The middle mediastinum contains the cardiac chambers, pericardium, aortic arch and its branches, trachea and bronchi, esophagus, and mediastinal nodes. Most of the tumors in this compartment are cystic and 25% are metastatic malignancies. The posterior compartment contains the lower esophagus, descending aorta, sympathetic chain, and intercostal nerves. Nearly 25% of all mediastinal tumors are in the posterior compartment, and 70% of them are neurogenic tumors.

- Nearly 30% of mediastinal masses are malignant.
- Anterior mediastinum: the "6 Ts"--**T**hymoma, **T**eratoma, **T**umor (lymphoma and carcinomas), **T**horacic aortic aneurysm, **T**rauma (hematoma, aneurysm), **T**hyroid.
- Posterior mediastinum: neurogenic tumors make up 70% of the tumors.
- Middle mediastinum: one-fourth are metastatic tumors.

Thymoma is the commonest tumor in the anterior mediastinum and is associated with myasthenia gravis, red cell aplasia, and collagenoses. Neurilemmoma and neurofibroma are the most common tumors in the posterior mediastinum. In adults, <4% of these tumors are malignant. Up to 40% of patients with neurofibromas have von Recklinghausen's disease. MRI may be required to exclude intraspinal extension of a mediastinal neurogenic tumor.

- Thymoma: 15%-45% of them are associated with myasthenia gravis.
- 10%-15% of patients with myasthenia gravis have thymoma.
- Thymoma is also associated with red cell aplasia, hypogammaglobulinemia, Cushing's syndrome (ACTH from thymic carcinoid).
- Malignant changes are uncommon in posterior mediastinal tumors in adults.

PLEURA

Pleural Effusion

Fluid collects in the pleural space when fluid collection exceeds removal by normal mechanisms. Hydrostatic, oncotic, and intrapleural pressures regulate fluid movement in the pleural space. Any of the following mechanisms can produce pleural effusion: changes in capillary permeability (inflammation), increased hydrostatic pressure, decreased plasma oncotic pressure, impaired lymphatic drainage, increased negative intrapleural pressure, and movement of fluid (through diaphragmatic pores, lymphatic vessels) from the peritoneum. The principal causes of pleural effusion are listed in Table 26-10.

Transudate Versus Exudate

The effusion is a transudate if the protein content is <3 g, specific gravity is <1,016, and fluid lactic dehydrogenase is <60% of serum (fluid/serum <0.6). It is an exudate if the protein content is >3 g, fluid/serum protein is >0.5, specific gravity is >1,016, and fluid lactic dehydrogenase is >60% of serum lactic dehydrogenase or fluid lactic dehydrogenase is >200 units. Increased lactic dehydrogenase in fluid is nonspecific, but it is increased in pulmonary embolism, rheumatoid effusion, and most exudative effusions.

- It is not necessary to perform all the above tests to differentiate a transudate from an exudate.
- Clinically, it is more useful to classify cause by considering the source (organ system) of the fluid (see Table 26-10).
- Classification of pleural fluid into transudates and exudates will not permit consideration of all causes.
- Commonest cause of transudate is congestive heart failure.
- Commonest cause of exudate is pneumonia (parapneumonic effusion).

Glucose and pH

Pleural fluid hypoglycemia (<60 mg/dL or fluid/plasma glucose <0.6) is seen in rheumatoid effusion, malignant mesothelioma, empyema, systemic lupus erythematosus, esophageal rupture, and yellow nail syndrome. The pH of pleural fluid is <7.20 in empyema, esophageal rupture, rheumatoid effusion, tuberculosis, carcinoma, and trauma. If the pH is low (<7.20) and clinical suspicion is high for infection, drainage with a chest tube should be considered.

Table 26-10.--Principal Causes of Pleural Effusion

Osmotic-hydraulic*
   Congestive cardiac failure
   Superior vena caval obstruction
   Constrictive pericarditis
   Cirrhosis with ascites
   Hypoalbuminemia
   Salt-retaining syndromes
   Peritoneal dialysis
   Hydronephrosis
   Nephrotic syndrome
Infections†
   Parapneumonic (bacterial) effusions
   Bacterial empyema
   Tuberculosis
   Fungi
   Parasites
   Viruses and mycoplasma
Neoplasms†
   Primary and metastatic lung tumors
   Lymphoma and leukemia
   Benign and malignant tumors of pleura
   Intra-abdominal tumors with ascites
Vascular disease†
   Pulmonary embolism
   Wegener's granulomatosis
Intra-abdominal diseases†
   Pancreatitis and pancreatic pseudocyst
   Subdiaphragmatic abscess
   Malignancy with ascites
   Meigs' syndrome*
   Hepatic cirrhosis with ascites*
Trauma†
   Hemothorax
   Chylothorax
   Esophageal rupture
   Intra-abdominal surgery
Miscellaneous
   Drug-induced effusions†
   Uremic pleuritis†
   Myxedema*
   Yellow nail syndrome†
   Dressler's syndrome†
   Familial Mediterranean fever†

*Usually a transudate.
†Usually an exudate.

- Pleural fluid glucose concentration and pH usually go together (i.e., if glucose is low, so is pH).
- Low glucose levels in rheumatoid effusion, malignant mesothelioma, and empyema.
- Empyema caused by *Proteus* species produces pH >7.8 (because of ammonia production).

Amylase

Pleural fluid amylase concentration increases in pancreatitis, pseudocyst of pancreas, rupture of abdominal viscera, and esophageal rupture. The amylase level in the fluid remains higher for longer periods than that in the serum.

- Increased concentration of pleural fluid amylase in esophageal rupture is due to leakage of salivary amylase.
- In any unexplained left-sided effusion, consider pancreatitis and measure the amylase level in the pleural fluid.

Chylous Effusion

Chylous effusion cannot be diagnosed on the basis of the color or appearance of the fluid. More than 90% of true chylous effusions contain triglyceride levels >100 mg/dL, and a triglyceride level <50 mg/dL is less likely to be chylous. Make sure that the serum level of triglyceride is normal. Cholesterol effusions (fluid cholesterol >250 mg/dL) are not true chylous effusions. They are seen in old tuberculous effusions and rheumatoid effusions and in some cases of nephrotic syndrome.

- Chylous effusion seen in the "5 Ts," i.e., **T**horacic duct **T**rauma, **T**umor (lymphoma), **T**uberculosis, **T**uberous sclerosis (lymphangiomyomatosis).
- True chylous effusion contains chylomicrons.
- Cholesterol effusions are not true chylous effusions.

Complement

Total, C3, and C4 components in the pleural fluid are decreased in systemic lupus erythematosus (80% of patients), rheumatoid arthritis (40%-60% of patients), carcinoma, pneumonia, and tuberculosis.

- Low complement level in pleural fluid in systemic lupus erythematosus (included in drug-induced form).
- Presence of lupus erythematosus cells in pleural fluid is diagnostic of systemic lupus erythematosus.

Blood Cell Counts

A red blood cell count >100,000/dL in the pleural fluid produces a "bloody effusion." This is seen in trauma, tumor, asbestos effusion, pancreatitis (60%), pulmonary embolism with infarctions, etc. A white blood cell count >20,000/dL is seen in parapneumonic effusions, empyema, and leukemic effusions (rare). Pleural fluid eosinophilia is nonspecific and occurs in trauma, pulmonary infarction, psittacosis, drug-induced effusion, pulmonary infiltrate with eosinophilia-associated effusions, and pneumothorax. Pleural fluid lymphocytosis occurs in tuberculosis, chronic effusions, lymphoma, and some collagenoses.

- Bloody effusion, even if cytology is negative, in the presence of lung tumor usually denotes pleural metastasis.
- Eosinophilia in pleural fluid is nonspecific.
- Differential leukocyte count in pleural fluid is generally unhelpful.

Cytology

Cytologic examination should be conducted on most effusions in adults if the clinical features do not suggest an obvious benign cause. Cytologic findings are positive in 60% of all malignant effusions. Pleural biopsy results are positive in <50% of all malignant effusions. Cytologic examination and biopsy give a slightly higher yield than either one does alone. Cytologic examination is less helpful in malignant mesothelioma, and an open biopsy is often necessary. Positive fluid cytologic findings in primary lung carcinoma mean unresectability (stage III).

- Cytologic examination is an important test in most adults with an "unknown" effusion.
- Overall yield from cytologic examination is 60%; less in cases of mesothelioma and lymphoma.

Cultures

Tuberculous effusions (fluid alone) yield positive cultures in <15% of cases. Pleural biopsy (histology and culture) has a higher (>70%) diagnostic yield. Culture is of value in effusions secondary to actinomycosis and nocardia, but it is less helpful in other mycoses. Cultures for viruses (influenza A, ornithosis, coxsackievirus B, and mycoplasma) are often negative. Paragonimiasis causes pleural effusion.

- Important to culture pleural biopsy in tuberculosis.
- Poor yield in viral infections.

Miscellaneous

At least 350-400 mL of fluid should be present to be seen on radiography. Look for subpulmonic effusions, for elevated hemidiaphragms, and blunting of the costophrenic angle. When in doubt, obtain a lateral decubitus radiograph. Ultrasonography is helpful in tapping small amounts of fluid and loculated fluid collections. Look for signs of trauma (rib fracture), abdominal surgery, acute abdomen, pancreatitis, cirrhosis, etc. Asbestos-induced effusions are notorious and frequently mimic malignant pleural mesothelioma, with pain, bloody fluid, and recurrence. Mesothelioma should be excluded by repeated thoracentesis, pleural biopsy, or thoracotomy.

- Small effusions are common after abdominal operations and normal labor; almost all resolve spontaneously.
- Drug-induced pleural effusion: nitrofurantoin, methysergide, drug-induced systemic lupus erythematosus, and busulfan.
- Nearly 20% of all effusions are undiagnosed despite extensive studies, including open pleural biopsy.

Complications

Complications of thoracentesis include pneumothorax, hemothorax, pulmonary edema, intrapulmonary hemorrhage, hemoptysis, vagal inhibition, air embolism, subcutaneous emphysema, bronchopleural fistula, empyema, and puncture of liver or spleen.

Pneumothorax

Spontaneous pneumothorax occurs more commonly in young, previously healthy adults. It is caused by the rupture of apical bullae. Spontaneous pneumothorax occurs in histiocytosis X, asthma, emphysema, bullous lung disease, lung tumors, end-stage fibrosis and honeycombing of the lungs, Marfan's disease, and during the menses in young females (catamenial pneumothorax). Secondary pneumothorax occurs after thoracentesis, trauma, esophageal rupture, tracheal fracture, subclavian needle sticks, high positive end-expiratory pressure, transtracheal aspiration, severe Valsalva maneuver, and secondary to pneumoperitoneum. Treatment of spontaneous pneumothorax includes chest tube drainage, chemical pleurodesis (tetracycline or other chemicals), talc pleurodesis, and surgical decortication.

- Spontaneous pneumothorax occurs in histiocytosis X, peripheral lung tumors, lymphangioleiomyomatosis, bullous lung disease, COPD.

- In females with pleuritic chest pain during menses, consider catamenial pneumothorax.
- Chest radiograph made after full expiration is better for identifying a small pneumothorax.

Empyema

Empyema is the collection of pus in the pleural space. It is caused by: bacterial pneumonia in >50% of cases, bacteremia in <10%, compromised host in <10%, trauma in 5%-15%, thoracic surgery in 10%-25%, and by esophageal perforation, lung abscess, and infarction. Bacteria that commonly are isolated are *S. aureus* (25%-35% of cases), anaerobes (15%-35%), gram-negative bacilli (15%-30%), and *S. pneumoniae* and other streptococci (12%-15%). In one-third of the cases of anaerobic empyema, cultures of the fluid are positive, whereas <5% of parapneumonic effusion due to *S. pneumoniae* is positive on culture. Treatment consists of systemic antibiotics, chest tube drainage, thoracostomy, and decortication. Mortality is higher in older patients and in those with multiple bacterial isolates, gram-negative bacilli, serious illnesses, and hospital-acquired empyema.

VASCULAR DISEASES

Deep Vein Thrombosis

Deep vein thrombosis is detected in 40% of all cases of pulmonary embolisms. The commonest site of these thromboses is the venous plexus in the soleus muscles. From 5%-15% of the deep vein thromboses from the calves propagate to the thigh and iliac veins. Nearly 45% of femoral and iliac deep vein thromboses embolize, and 5%-15% of superficial thrombophlebitis is associated with deep vein thrombosis. Factors predisposing to deep vein thrombosis include congestive heart failure, shock, estrogens, dysproteinemias, neoplasms, surgical procedures, prolonged immobilization, obesity, trauma, varicose veins, previous deep vein thrombosis, pregnancy, deficiencies of antithrombin III, protein S and C, and the presence of lupus anticoagulant (antiphospholipid antibodies).

- Deep vein thrombosis is detected in 40% of all pulmonary embolisms.
- 20%-40% increased risk of deep vein thrombosis in patients with history of these thromboses.
- Among predisposing factors for deep vein thrombosis and pulmonary embolism, consider deficiencies of

antithrombin III, protein S and C, and presence of lupus anticoagulant.

Deep vein thrombosis is diagnosed in only 50% of clinical cases. A diagnosis based on physical examination findings is unreliable. Homans' sign is elicited in <40% of cases of deep vein thrombosis, and a false-positive Homans' sign occurs in 30% of high-risk patients. Impedance plethysmography and duplex ultrasonography together are the most commonly used tests and have a diagnostic accuracy of 90%-95% in detecting iliac and femoral deep vein thromboses. Furthermore, they are noninvasive methods and can be performed at the bedside. Serial impedance plethysmographic studies are useful in detecting extension of calf vein thrombi. Impedance plethysmography and duplex ultrasonography are excellent for diagnosing proximal thrombi.

- Impedance plethysmography and duplex ultrasonographic examinations have a diagnostic accuracy of >90%.
- Venography is the best test for diagnosing deep vein thrombosis.
- In patients in whom recurrent deep vein thrombosis is questioned, venography may help differentiate a new thrombosis from an old one.
- Incidence of deep vein thrombosis with various circumstances: major abdominal surgery, 14%-33%; thoracic surgery, 25%-60%; gynecologic surgery, 15%-20%; hip surgery, 50%-75%; post-myocardial infarction, 20%-40%; stroke with paralysis, 50%; and post-partum, 3%.

Pulmonary Embolism (PE)

Pulmonary embolism is one of the most underdiagnosed problems and is the major cause of death in 15% of patients dying in general hospitals. It is detected in 25%-30% of routine autopsy cases. Nearly 200,000 deaths/year are said to be the result of pulmonary embolism. Antemortem diagnosis is made in <30% of patients. Most pulmonary embolisms result from deep vein thrombosis in the lower extremities.

Pulmonary embolism has no typical clinical symptoms and signs. Tachypnea and tachycardia are observed in nearly all patients. Other symptoms include dyspnea in 80% of patients, pleuritic pain in up to 75%, hemoptysis in <25%, pleural friction rub in 20%, and wheezing in 15%. Nonspecific ECG changes are found in 80% of patients, ST and T changes in 65%, T inversion in 40%,

S_1Q_3 pattern in 15%, right bundle branch block in 12%, and lactic acid dehydrogenase in 12%. Chest radiography may show diaphragmatic elevation in 60% of patients, infiltrates in 30%, focal oligemia in 10%-50%, effusion in 20%, enlarged pulmonary artery in 20%, and normal radiographic findings in 30%.

- No typical symptoms and signs for diagnosing pulmonary embolism.
- Dyspnea, tachypnea, and pleuritic pain are common.
- Radiographic findings are normal in 30%; ECG shows S_1Q_3 pattern in <20%.
- PaO_2 may be normal but $(A-a)O_2$ gradient is widened.

Perfusion scan is excellent in the absence of COPD; a normal or low-probability perfusion scan rules out pulmonary embolism in more than 95% of cases. Matched segmental defects are nonspecific. Patient in whom scan suggests "intermediate probability" may require pulmonary angiography to rule in/out pulmonary embolism. Pulmonary angiography is the best diagnostic test and, ideally, should be performed within 24-48 hours.

- Normal results on perfusion scan exclude pulmonary embolism in >95% of cases.
- Intermediate probability scan may necessitate pulmonary angiography.
- Patients in whom pulmonary embolism is strongly suspected should be administered heparin before other diagnostic tests are performed.

Treatment

In acute deep vein thrombosis and/or pulmonary embolism, heparin and warfarin therapy both can be initiated simultaneously unless there is contraindication to the use of warfarin. In uncomplicated and nonrecurrent deep vein thrombosis and/or pulmonary embolism, anticoagulation therapy with warfarin for 6 months should suffice. Recurrent and complicated cases (coagulopathies, etc.) may require life-long anticoagulation therapy. Bleeding complications from heparin are 3%-8% and from warfarin, 4%. Drugs that prolong the effect of warfarin include salicylates, heparin, estrogen, antibiotics, clofibrate, quinidine, cimetidine, etc. Drugs that decrease its effect include glutethimide, rifampin, barbiturates, and ethchlorvynol. Inferior vena cava plication or umbrella insertion is indicated for recurrent deep vein thrombosis if a patient recently had a massive pulmonary embolism, or if there is a bleeding disorder or contraindication to

anticoagulation therapy or failure of anticoagulation therapy. Thrombolytic agents are used in massive pulmonary embolus. They should be given within 24 hours of the pulmonary embolus. Contraindications to thrombolytic agents include recent (within 10 days) surgical procedure, intra-arterial procedures, renal or liver biopsy within 14 days, ulcer disease, recent stroke, hemorrhagic diathesis, and pregnancy. Prophylaxis includes early ambulation postoperatively or after immobilization, intermittent pneumatic compression of the lower extremities, active and passive leg exercises, and low doses (10,000-15,000 units/day) of heparin given subcutaneously.

- In acute deep vein thrombosis and/or pulmonary embolism, heparin and warfarin therapy can be initiated simultaneously.
- Bleeding complications from heparin are 3%-8% and from warfarin, 4%.
- Inferior vena cava plication does not replace anticoagulation therapy; many patients require both.
- Monitor thrombolytic therapy with thrombin time.

Pulmonary Hypertension

Pulmonary hypertension exists when pulmonary artery pressure at rest is >30/10, with a mean of ≥20 mm Hg. It can be classified broadly into primary and secondary forms.

Primary Pulmonary Hypertension

Primary pulmonary hypertension is a rare disease of unknown cause. It is manifested by various degrees of precapillary pulmonary hypertension. By definition, identifiable causes of pulmonary hypertension have to be ruled out before primary pulmonary hypertension can be diagnosed. Normally, it is a disease of young females (female-to-male ratio is from 10:1 to 2:1); nearly 10% of patients with primary pulmonary hypertension are >60 years old. Familial association is fairly common. Dyspnea, fatigue, and frequent syncope are common symptoms. Angina-like pain may be present and Raynaud's phenomenon is occasionally seen. Exercise-induced hypoxemia and decreased diffusing capacity are important findings. Chest radiography shows prominent central pulmonary arteries. Pulmonary artery pressure measurement is most helpful in making the diagnosis. Most patients die within 5-6 years after diagnosis; the mortality rate during pregnancy may be as high as 50%. Right ventricular failure is the primary determinant of prognosis. Vasodilators (calcium channel blockers) and long-term anticoagulation prolong life. Oxygen therapy is necessary to relieve hypoxemia. Lung transplantation is a therapeutic option.

- Primary pulmonary hypertension: young women with normal findings on pulmonary function testing and low diffusing capacity.
- Exertional dyspnea, fatigue, and syncopal episodes.
- Nearly 10% of patients are >60 years old.

Recurrent Pulmonary Embolism

Recurrent pulmonary embolism is a relatively common cause of secondary pulmonary hypertension. Mechanical obstruction of 1/2-2/3 of the pulmonary vascular bed by emboli is necessary for pulmonary hypertension to develop. It is often difficult to distinguish pulmonary hypertension caused by recurrent pulmonary embolus from primary pulmonary hypertension. A significant number (10%) of patients have underlying coagulopathies (deficiencies of antithrombin III, protein S and C, and presence of lupus anticoagulant). The gradual onset of dyspnea and signs of pulmonary hypertension and right ventricular strain are the presenting symptoms.

- Difficult to distinguish pulmonary hypertension caused by pulmonary embolus from primary pulmonary hypertension.
- High incidence (10%) of underlying coagulopathies.
- Surgical thromboendarterectomy is indicated in selected cases.
- Life-long anticoagulation after inferior vena cava interruption is required for many patients.

Pulmonary Veno-Occlusive Disease

Pulmonary veno-occlusive disease is a disease of young men. It is uncommon and has no known cause, although mycoplasma infection, chemotherapy, and toxins may be responsible. Common findings are the gradual onset of exertional dyspnea associated with diffuse mottling and Kerley's B lines on chest radiographs, hypoxemia, and low diffusing capacity. Without lung biopsy, the diagnosis cannot be firmly established. This is a rapidly fatal condition, with death within 2 years after diagnosis. Treatment is symptomatic.

- Pulmonary veno-occlusive disease: young males with rapidly progressive pulmonary hypertension.
- Kerley's B lines and diffuse mottling on chest radiographs.

Other Causes of Pulmonary Hypertension

Mitral stenosis, left atrial myxoma, obstruction to left ventricular outflow, pulmonary arterial tumor emboli, schistosomiasis, severe chronic hypoxemia (COPD, sleep apnea, etc.), mixed connective tissue disease, scleroderma, systemic lupus erythematosus, eosinophilia-myalgia syndrome, chronic liver disease, sickle cell disease, and Raynaud's phenomenon are associated with pulmonary hypertension. Diagnosis of these entities is based on clinical suspicion, and treatment is aimed at the underlying causes.

Pulmonary Vasculitides

The vasculitides are a heterogeneous group of disorders of unknown cause characterized by varying degrees of inflammation and necrosis of the arteries and sometimes veins. Immunologic factors, absence or deficiency of certain chemical mediators in the body, and infectious processes caused by mycoses, particularly *Aspergillus* and *Mucor*, are associated with vasculitis. The common vasculitides and their incidence in North America is as follows: giant cell (temporal) arteritis, 26.5%; polyarteritis nodosa, 14.6%; Wegener's granulomatosis, 10.5%; Henoch-Schönlein purpura, 10.5%; Takayasu's arteritis, 7.8%; and Churg-Strauss syndrome, 2.5%. The rest of the vasculitides are due to collagen diseases and nonspecific causes.

Giant Cell (Temporal) Arteritis

Giant cell arteritis is a vasculitis of unknown cause, but it has been described in association with polymyalgia rheumatica. It usually affects persons of middle age and older. The clinical illness appears gradually, with nonspecific constitutional symptoms (low-grade fever, malaise, and weight loss) followed by specific symptoms such as claudication of the jaw and sudden loss of vision. Headache is the commonest symptom. Pulmonary involvement in giant cell arteritis may present with cough, sore throat, and hoarseness. Nearly 10% of patients with giant cell arteritis have prominent respiratory symptoms, and the respiratory symptoms are the initial manifestation in 4%. Giant cell arteritis should be considered in older patients with a new cough or throat pain without obvious cause. Pulmonary nodules, interstitial infiltrations, pulmonary artery occlusion, and aneurysms have been described.

- Giant cell arteritis: elderly persons with cough, low-grade fever, malaise, weight loss, headache, and polymyalgia.

- Nearly 10% of patients have prominent respiratory symptoms.
- Cough, sore throat, and hoarseness may be the presenting features of giant cell arteritis.

Wegener's Granulomatosis

Wegener's granulomatosis is a distinct type of systemic vasculitis characterized by necrotizing granulomatous vasculitis of the upper and lower respiratory tract, glomerulonephritis, and variable degrees of small vessel vasculitis. The term "limited Wegener's granulomatosis" is used to describe the disease involving the lungs only, but patients with this "limited" form show kidney involvement if renal biopsy specimens are obtained. Histologic features include discrete or confluent granulomatosis, necrotizing granuloma in combination with vasculitis, fibrinoid necrosis, microabscesses, focal vasculitis, thrombosis, and fibrous obliteration of the vascular lumen. Eosinophilic infiltrates are seen in tissue samples, but peripheral blood eosinophilia is not a feature of Wegener's granulomatosis.

- Wegener's granulomatosis is a systemic disease with major respiratory manifestations.
- Renal involvement with focal segmental glomerulonephritis is characteristic.

The mean age at onset of symptoms is 45.2 yr (the male-to-female ratio is 2:1); 91% of the patients are Caucasians. Initial symptoms are nonspecific: fever, malaise, weight loss, arthralgias, and myalgias. The organs affected are the skin (40%-50% of patients), eyes (43%), and central nervous system (25%). Arthralgias occur in 58% of patients and frank arthritis in 28%. ENT symptoms are the initial complaints in 90% of patients (rhinorrhea, purulent or bloody nasal discharge, sinus pain, nasal mucosal drying and crust formation, epistaxis, and otitis media).

- Major organs affected: "ELKS," i.e., **E**NT, **L**ungs, **K**idney, and **S**kin.
- ENT symptoms are the initial complaints in 90% of patients.
- Nasal septal perforation and ulceration of the vomer bone are two important signs.
- Differential diagnosis of "saddle-nose" deformity: Wegener's granulomatosis, relapsing polychondritis, and leprosy.

Ulcerated lesions of the larynx and trachea occur in 30% of untreated patients and subglottic stenosis in 8%-18% of treated patients. The pulmonary parenchyma is affected in more than 60% of patients. Symptoms include cough, hemoptysis, and dyspnea. The clinical manifestations can range from subacute to rapidly progressive respiratory failure. Most patients with pulmonary symptoms have associated nodular infiltrates on chest radiography. Hemoptysis is seen in 98% of patients and radiographic abnormalities in 65%, including unilateral (55% of patients), bilateral (45%), infiltrates (63%), nodules (31%), infiltrates with cavitation (8%), and nodules with cavitation (10%). Chest radiography shows rounded opacities (from a few millimeters to several centimeters large). The nodules are usually bilateral and one-third cavitate. Solitary nodules occur in 30%-40% of patients. Pneumonic infiltrates, lobar consolidation, and pleural effusions are also seen. Typical interstitial infiltrates are uncommon. Massive pulmonary alveolar hemorrhage is occasionally a life-threatening emergency. Benign stenoses of the tracheobronchial tree are more likely in chronic cases and in patients whose disease is stable.

- Hemoptysis in almost all patients.
- Radiographic features: multiple nodules or masses with cavitation in 35% of patients.
- Diffuse alveolar infiltrates indicate alveolar hemorrhage; diffuse alveolar hemorrhage in 5%-45% of biopsy/autopsy-documented cases.
- Tracheobronchial stenosis occurs in 15%.

Laboratory Findings

Laboratory findings in Wegener's granulomatosis include an increased erythrocyte sedimentation rate, normochromic normocytic anemia, thrombocytosis, positive rheumatoid factor, and increase in immunoglobulin and circulating immune complexes. The identification of antineutrophil cytoplasmic antibodies in most of the patients with Wegener's granulomatosis has helped to establish the diagnosis in atypical or unusual cases of systemic vasculitis. Two main patterns of cytoplasmic fluorescence are recognized: granular with central accentuation (cANCA) and perinuclear (pANCA). The granular pattern is reported to be specific for Wegener's granulomatosis. When a restrictive definition of Wegener's granulomatosis is used (i.e., one that requires documented granulomatous inflammation of the lungs), the granular pattern is present in >90% of patients with untreated active diseases. False-positive rates for the granular pattern range from 8% to 12%.

- Wegener's granulomatosis: routine laboratory findings are nonspecific.
- The granular pattern of cytoplasmic fluorescence is reported to be specific for Wegener's granulomatosis; titers of antineutrophil cytoplasmic antibodies correlate with activity of the disease.
- p-ANCA has been noted in other vasculitides and collagen diseases.

Corticosteroids with cyclophosphamide therapy are effective. A complete response is seen in >90% of patients. In milder cases, corticosteroid therapy alone may suffice. Many patients require prolonged treatment with smaller doses of corticosteroid and/or cyclophosphamide. Some physicians have observed resolution of Wegener's granulomatosis after treatment with an antimicrobial agent, trimethoprim-sulfamethoxazole. Subglottic stenosis may require surgical therapy.

- Cyclophosphamide and corticosteroids are effective.

Churg-Strauss Syndrome

Churg-Strauss syndrome, also known as "allergic granulomatosis and angiitis," is separate from hypersensitivity vasculitis and polyarteritis nodosa. It has been portrayed as an overlap syndrome to include hypereosinophilic disease (Löffler's syndrome), systemic vasculitides (hypersensitivity vasculitis and polyarteritis nodosa), and Wegener's granulomatosis. Churg-Strauss syndrome is uncommon and is characterized by pulmonary and systemic vasculitis, extravascular granulomas, and eosinophilia, which occur exclusively in patients with asthma or a history of allergy. Allergic rhinitis, nasal polyps, nasal mucosal crusting, and septal perforation occur in >70% of the patients. Nasal polyposis is a major clinical finding. The chief pulmonary manifestation is asthma, which is noted in almost all patients. Radiographic abnormalities are noted in >60% of patients: patchy and occasionally diffuse alveolar-interstitial infiltrates in the perihilar area, with a predilection for the upper two-thirds of the lung fields. Dramatic response can be expected with high doses of systemic corticosteroids.

- Churg-Strauss syndrome: an uncommon cause of vasculitis.
- Refractory asthma and progressive respiratory distress should suggest Churg-Strauss syndrome.
- Allergic rhinitis, nasal polyps, nasal mucosal crusting,

and septal perforation occur in >70% of patients.
- Tissue and blood hypereosinophilia and elevation of IgE are common.

Behçet's Disease

Behçet's disease is a chronic relapsing multisystemic inflammatory disorder characterized by aphthous stomatitis along with two or more of the following: aphthous genital ulcerations, uveitis, cutaneous nodules or pustules, synovitis, and meningoencephalitis. Occlusion of major vessels and aneurysms have been observed in 10%-37% of the patients. Superficial and deep vein thromboses of the upper and lower extremities and thrombosis of the inferior and superior venae cavae occur in 7%-37% of patients. Pulmonary vascular involvement produces major hemoptysis. Serious hemoptysis, initially responsive to therapy with corticosteroids, tends to recur; death is due to hemoptysis in 39% of patients. Radiography may show lung infiltrates, pleural effusions, prominent pulmonary arteries, and pulmonary artery aneurysms.

- Behçet's disease: major hemoptysis is the cause of death in 39%.
- Fistula between the airway and vascular structures is common.
- High incidence of deep vein thrombosis and pulmonary thromboembolism.

Takayasu's Arteritis

Takayasu's arteritis, or "pulseless disease," is a chronic inflammatory disease of unknown cause that primarily affects the aorta and its major branches, including the proximal coronary arteries and renal arteries and the elastic pulmonary arteries. Pulmonary artery involvement is seen in 50% of cases, with lesions in the medium- and large-sized arteries. Early abnormalities occur in the upper lobes, whereas the middle and lower lobes are involved in later stages of the disease. Perfusion lung scans have shown abnormalities in >75% of patients.

- Takayasu's arteritis: pulmonary artery involvement in >50% of patients.

Urticarial Vasculitis

Urticarial vasculitis is manifested by urticarial lesions, pruritus, and arthralgias in 60% of the patients, arthritis in 28%, abdominal pain in 25%, and glomerulonephritis in

15%. Many of the pulmonary complications described have been in patients with the hypocomplementemic variety of the disease. Pulmonary vasculitis has not been demonstrated in patients with urticarial vasculitis. However, many of these patients have COPD, and up to 62% of patients with hypocomplementemic urticarial vasculitis acquire COPD. Many of these patients have been smokers.

- Higher incidence of COPD in patients with hyper-complementemic urticarial vasculitis.

Eosinophilia Myalgia Syndrome

Dietary ingestion of L-tryptophan tablets was linked to an epidemic of eosinophilia myalgia syndrome in 1989. By April 1990, more than 1,400 cases were reported to the Centers for Disease Control. Eosinophilia myalgia syndrome is a toxic reaction to contaminant(s) in over-the-counter preparations of L-tryptophan that are used for various health reasons. Clinical manifestations of this syndrome include myalgias, fatigue, muscle weakness, arthralgias, edema of the extremities, skin rash, oral and vaginal ulcers, scleroderma-like changes, ascending neuropathy, and peripheral blood eosinophilia. Approximately 60% of the patients have pulmonary complaints. Pulmonary complications consist of pulmonary infiltrates associated with severe pulmonary distress and progressive hypoxemia, pleural effusion, diffuse bilateral reticulonodular infiltrates, and pulmonary hypertension. Lung biopsy reveals changes characteristic of hypersensitivity pneumonitis.

- Eosinophilia myalgia syndrome is caused by contaminant in L-tryptophan preparations.
- Features: pulmonary hypertension, interstitial granulomas, respiratory distress.
- Eosinophilia myalgia syndrome and Spanish toxic oil syndrome have identical causative mechanisms.

Essential Mixed Cryoglobulinemia

Essential mixed cryoglobulinemia is characterized by recurrent episodes of purpura, arthralgias, weakness, and multiorgan involvement. Histologic features are comparable to those of leukocytoclastic vasculitis. Increases in rheumatoid factor and cryoglobulin are frequent findings. Pulmonary insufficiency, Sjögren's syndrome-like illness with lung involvement, fibrosing alveolitis, and bronchiectasis have been described in isolated cases.

Polyarteritis Nodosa

Polyarteritis nodosa is characterized by a necrotizing arteritis of small- and medium-sized muscular arteries that involves multiple organ systems. It is important to recognize that this disease almost never affects the lungs. Although the earlier literature described vasculitis in the bronchial and pulmonary vasculature, many of the patients had granulomatous lesions with eosinophilic infiltrates. In retrospect, it appears that the majority of the patients diagnosed to have pulmonary polyarteritis nodosa indeed had Churg-Strauss syndrome.

Secondary Vasculitis

Many of the rheumatologic diseases (systemic lupus erythematosus, rheumatoid arthritis, scleroderma, etc.) demonstrate secondary vasculitic processes in the tissues involved. Certain infectious processes, particularly mycoses, may cause secondary vasculitis. When confronted with vasculitic lesions, the well-known etiologic agents, such as drugs and chemicals, should be considered.

Alveolar Hemorrhage Syndrome

Diffuse hemorrhage into the alveolar spaces is called "alveolar hemorrhage syndrome." Disruption of the pulmonary capillary lining may result from damage caused by different immunologic mechanisms (Goodpasture's syndrome, renal-pulmonary syndromes, glomerulonephritis, systemic lupus erythematosus, etc.), direct chemical/toxic injury (toxic or chemical inhalation, trimellitic anhydride), physical trauma (pulmonary contusion), and increased vascular pressure within the capillaries (mitral stenosis, severe left ventricular failure). The severity of hemoptysis, anemia, and respiratory distress depends on the extent and rapidity with which bleeding occurs in the alveoli.

- Alveolar hemorrhage syndrome is caused by different mechanisms.
- Hemoptysis is not always present in alveolar hemorrhage syndrome.
- Chest radiography may show a diffuse alveolar process, but this is not always typical.
- Serial measurement of diffusing capacity is not a reliable test for continued intra-alveolar bleeding.
- Detection of hemosiderin-laden macrophages in bronchoalveolar lavage or sputum is not a dependable test for diagnosing alveolar hemorrhage syndrome.

Goodpasture's Syndrome

Goodpasture's syndrome is a classic example of cytotoxic (type II) disease. The Goodpasture antigen (located in the type IV collagen) is the primary target for the autoantibodies of patients with Goodpasture's syndrome or anti-glomerular basement membrane disease. The highest concentration of Goodpasture antigen is in the glomerular basement membrane. The alveolar basement membrane is affected by cross-reactivity to the glomerular basement membrane. Lung biopsy reveals diffuse alveolar hemorrhage and intra-alveolar hemosiderin-laden macrophages. Immunofluorescent microscopy shows linear deposition of IgG and complement (in contrast to the "lumpy-bumpy" deposition seen in systemic lupus erythematosus) along basement membranes. Anti-glomerular basement membrane antibody is positive in >90% of patients with Goodpasture's syndrome. The male-to-female ratio is 7:1, with an average age of 27 years. Recurrent hemoptysis from intra-alveolar hemorrhage, pulmonary insufficiency, renal involvement, and anemia are the main features. Radiography typically shows a diffuse alveolar filling process. Treatment consists of high doses of corticosteroids and plasmapheresis.

- Goodpasture's syndrome: example of a type II (cytotoxic) immune reaction.
- Anti-glomerular basement membrane antibody is present in >90% of patients with Goodpasture's syndrome.
- Anti-glomerular basement membrane antibody is also present in persons exposed to influenza virus, hydrocarbons, and penicillamine and in some patients with systemic lupus erythematosus, polyarteritis nodosa, and Henoch-Schönlein purpura.
- Smoking increases the risk of bleeding.

Glomerulonephritis

Nearly 50% of the patients with alveolar hemorrhage syndromes caused by a renal mechanism do not have anti-glomerular basement membrane antibody. The mechanism of alveolar hemorrhage in these patients is mediated by immune-complex disease. Several vasculitic syndromes belong to this group. The alveolar hemorrhage syndrome in systemic lupus erythematosus and other vasculitides is discussed elsewhere.

Vasculitides

Diffuse alveolar hemorrhage is sometimes seen in patients with vasculitides. Alveolar hemorrhage is rare as an initial symptom of Wegener's granulomatosis and is more common in Churg-Strauss syndrome and Henoch-Schönlein purpura than in Wegener's granulomatosis. Alveolar hemorrhage is much more common in Behçet's disease than in other vasculitides.

Mitral Valve Disease

Diffuse alveolar hemorrhage is a well-known feature of mitral stenosis, even though the possibility is rarely considered in clinical practice. Severe mitral insufficiency can also produce alveolar hemorrhage. In surgically untreated patients, recurrent episodes of alveolar hemorrhage may lead to chronic hemosiderosis of the lungs, fibrosis, and punctate calcification/ossification of the lung parenchyma.

- Mitral stenosis is an important cause of alveolar hemorrhage syndrome.

Idiopathic Pulmonary Hemosiderosis

Idiopathic pulmonary hemosiderosis is a rare disorder of unknown cause. It is manifested as recurrent intra-alveolar hemorrhage, hemoptysis, and secondary iron deficiency anemia. Most cases begin in childhood. Although this disease is often fatal, a prolonged course is common. In childhood, the male-to-female ratio is 1:1; in adults, it is 3:1. Pathologic features include hemosiderin-laden macrophages. No autoimmune phenomena are noted. Some patients have cold agglutinins. The iron content in the lung depends on the duration of the disease. Clinical features are chronic cough with intermittent hemoptysis, iron deficiency anemia, fever, and weight loss. Chest radiography shows transient, blotchy, perihilar alveolar infiltrates in the mid and lower lung fields. Small nodules, fibrosis, and cor pulmonale may also be found. Treatment is repeated blood transfusions, iron therapy, steroids, and possibly cytotoxic agents. A 30% mortality within 5 years after onset has been reported. Idiopathic pulmonary hemosiderosis is a diagnosis of exclusion.

- Idiopathic pulmonary hemosiderosis: chronic cough with intermittent hemoptysis and iron deficiency anemia.
- Generalized lymphadenopathy in 25% of patients, hepatosplenomegaly in 20%, and clubbing in 15%.
- Kidneys are not involved.
- Eosinophilia in 10% of patients.

Toxic Alveolar Hemorrhage

Fumes or dust of trimellitic anhydride (a component of certain plastics, paints, and epoxy resins) act as a hapten to cause acute rhinitis and asthmatic symptoms if exposure is minor. With greater exposure, alveolar hemorrhage probably occurs by a different immunologic mechanism. The trimellitic anhydride-hemoptysis anemia syndrome occurs after "high-dose exposure" to fumes. Antibodies to trimellitic anhydride-human proteins and erythrocytes have been found in these patients. Other toxins known to cause alveolar hemorrhage syndromes are penicillamine and mitomycin C.

LUNGS IN NONPULMONARY DISEASES

Rheumatoid Arthritis

"Rheumatoid lung" indicates diffuse interstitial pneumonitis and fibrosis associated with rheumatoid arthritis. It is the most serious pleuropulmonary complication of rheumatoid arthritis. Chest radiography shows this process in 1.6%-4.5% of patients, whereas the results of pulmonary function tests suggest restrictive lung process in more than 30%. Clinical, physiologic, and histologic features mimic those of idiopathic pulmonary fibrosis. Chest radiography reveals a bibasilar interstitial process, micronodules, or honeycombing (the latter in late stages of the disease).

Rheumatoid (necrobiotic) nodules occur in the lung parenchyma. These are more common in men and in those with seropositive rheumatoid arthritis. They may precede the arthritic symptoms. The rheumatoid nodules produce minimal symptoms. They measure from a few millimeters to several centimeters, are usually bilateral, and occur near pleuropulmonary surfaces. Two-thirds of them cavitate. Rheumatoid pneumoconiosis (Caplan's syndrome) is pneumoconiosis associated with rheumatoid nodules. It is found in persons with silicosis, asbestosis, aluminosis, etc. This syndrome is characterized by pulmonary nodules (1-5 cm in diameter), which evolve rapidly and may undergo cavitation.

Rheumatoid pleurisy is the commonest thoracic manifestation of rheumatoid arthritis. In clinical practice, its incidence is 8% in males and 1.6% in females with rheumatoid arthritis. One-third of the patients with rheumatoid pleurisy remain asymptomatic. Pleural effusion may precede the onset of arthritic symptoms by months. Pleural fluid analysis shows that the effusion is typically an exudate, usually yellow and rarely bloody.

Chronic effusions appear opalescent green due to high cholesterol content ("pseudochylothorax"). The glucose is very low (<30 mg/dL) in >80% of patients.

Obstructive airway disease is seen in one-third of patients with rheumatoid arthritis. Histologic findings include follicular bronchiolitis and bronchitis. The combination of rheumatoid arthritis and smoking is associated with a much higher prevalence of obstructive lung disease than is either of these conditions alone. A genetic predisposition to obstructive lung disease may be a contributing factor.

- Pulmonary manifestations are more common in males with rheumatoid arthritis.
- Pleural involvement occurs in up to 10% of patients.
- Cholesterol pleural effusions.
- Rheumatoid lung mimics idiopathic pulmonary fibrosis.
- Obstructive airway disease is seen in 34% of patients with rheumatoid arthritis.

Systemic Lupus Erythematosus

Pleural involvement is the commonest and often the presenting feature of systemic lupus erythematosus in 50%-83% of patients. Painful pleurisy is observed in 50% of patients. Pleural effusions are small to moderate and bilateral in 50% of patients. The fluid is almost always an exudate, and the glucose level is normal or high. Levels of C50 as well as of C3 and C4 are decreased in 80% of patients. Lupus erythematosus cells have been found in none to >85% of effusions. The presence of these cells is specific for lupus pleuritis. Diffuse interstitial pneumonitis is distinctly uncommon in systemic lupus erythematosus. Patchy and irregular areas of interstitial pneumonitis and fibrosis develop in 15% to 45% of patients with systemic lupus erythematosus. Plate-like or discoid atelectasis is more common and occurs in the lower two-thirds of the lung fields. Infectious processes, particularly in patients receiving immunosuppressive therapy for systemic lupus erythematosus, are the commonest cause of pulmonary parenchymal infiltrates. Pulmonary function tests usually reveal a restrictive dysfunction.

Pulmonary hemorrhage is an important complication that is noted in up to 10% of patients. Renal disease from systemic lupus erythematosus enhances the risk of alveolar hemorrhage. Pulmonary hemorrhage may range from subclinical to massive. Significant hemoptysis is observed in 8%-15% of patients. Chest radiography reveals bibasal, patchy, alveolar infiltrates. The mortality from systemic lupus erythematosus-induced alveolar hemorrhage is in excess of 50%, with patients dying within several days of the onset of hemoptysis.

Pulmonary embolism is more common than in other collagenoses in systemic lupus erythematosus because of the lupus anticoagulant syndrome (manifested by a prolonged APTT, normal clotting and platelet counts, presence of anticardiolipin antibody, and false-positive results on the VDRL test). Long-term anticoagulation therapy is required to prevent venous thromboembolic phenomena. Pulmonary hypertension is rare in systemic lupus erythematosus. Lupus pneumonitis, a very rare feature of systemic lupus erythematosus, is characterized by acute dyspnea, high fever, and cough with occasional hemoptysis. Diaphragmatic dysfunction has been described in some patients, but the clinical significance of this finding is unclear, even though it may account for the "unexplained dyspnea." Drug-induced systemic lupus erythematosus is described above.

- Pleural involvement is common in systemic lupus erythematosus; low complement level in pleural fluid.
- Diffuse pulmonary infiltrates and fibrosis are uncommon.
- Alveolar hemorrhage is seen in 10% of patients; significant hemoptysis in 10%.
- Pulmonary embolism is relatively common (due to lupus anticoagulant).
- Lupus pneumonitis is very rare.
- Pleural effusion is more common with procainamide- and hydralazine-induced systemic lupus erythematosus than with other drug-induced forms of the disease.

Scleroderma (Progressive Systemic Sclerosis)

Diffuse pulmonary fibrosis is seen in up to 80% of patients at post mortem, even though many patients are minimally symptomatic during life. Chronic progressive pulmonary fibrosis is seen in two-thirds of patients and is the commonest respiratory complication. The pathologic features are identical to those of idiopathic pulmonary fibrosis. One-third of patients have abnormal radiographic findings, but >50% complain of exertional dyspnea and exhibit low diffusing capacity. Pulmonary involvement is more severe in the CREST (**C**alcinosis, **R**aynaud's phenomenon, **E**sophageal involvement, **S**clerodactyly, and **T**elangiectasia) variant of scleroderma. The commonest abnormality on pulmonary function testing is the slow but progressive restrictive dysfunction with low diffusing capacity. The earliest abnormality is the decreased

diffusing capacity; this test is an important predictor of mortality. Aspiration pneumonia results from the esophageal dysfunction and reflux that are extremely common in scleroderma. Pulmonary hypertension is common in scleroderma and is a major cause of mortality and morbidity. The pathogenic mechanisms include chronic hypoxemia secondary to pulmonary fibrosis and/or medial hypertrophy of the pulmonary arteries. The latter mechanism, which is independent of the arterial changes caused by hypoxia, is responsible for pulmonary hypertension in 35%-60% of patients. The incidence of pulmonary hypertension is higher in patients with the CREST variant of scleroderma.

- Diffuse lung fibrosis (similar to that of idiopathic pulmonary fibrosis) is seen in most patients.
- Aspiration pneumonia from esophageal dysfunction and reflux.
- Pulmonary hypertension: major cause of morbidity and mortality.
- All pulmonary complications are more severe in CREST syndrome.
- Pleural disease, pleural effusion, obstructive disease, and hemoptysis are uncommon in scleroderma.

Polymyositis-Dermatomyositis

Interstitial pneumonitis and fibrosis, occurring in the basal areas of the lungs, are the most common pulmonary abnormalities and are seen in 5%-10% of patients. Pulmonary disease caused by polymyositis may present as acute pneumonitis with alveolar or mixed alveolar-interstitial infiltrates. There is a lack of relationship between the severity and progression of the myositis and the severity of respiratory disease. Not all patients demonstrate the anti-Jo1 antibody in their serum. However, >50% with this antibody exhibit interstitial pulmonary disease. In 35% of patients, pulmonary disease precedes the skin and/or myopathic features by 1-24 months. Pulmonary disease presents as dyspnea, cough, and hypoxemia; symptoms related to gastroesophageal reflux may be the initial manifestation in some patients. A restrictive type of lung dysfunction is present in nearly 50% of patients. Aspiration pneumonitis is a common feature because of esophageal involvement. Poor cough strength due to weakness of respiratory muscles augments the progression of aspiration pneumonia, which is the cause of death in 10% of patients. Hypoventilation results from proximal myopathy. Progressive hypoventilation and respiratory failure manifested by increasing hypercarbia are poor prognostic signs.

- Polymyositis-dermatomyositis: interstitial pneumonitis and fibrosis in up to 10% of patients.
- Over 50% with anti-Jo1 antibody in their serum have interstitial pulmonary disease.
- Aspiration pneumonia from esophageal dysfunction causes death in 10% of patients.
- Hypoventilation due to proximal myopathy is the leading cause of death.
- Weakness of proximal muscles and a characteristic skin rash (heliotrope hue).
- Paraneoplastic variant of polymyositis-dermatomyositis (see under Lung Cancer) should be differentiated from the idiopathic or autoimmune types of the disease discussed here.
- When elderly patients present with polymyositis-dermatomyositis, an underlying malignancy must be excluded before considering the diagnosis of autoimmune polymyositis-dermatomyositis.

Mixed Connective Tissue Disease

Patients with mixed connective tissue disease have the clinical features of systemic lupus erythematosus, scleroderma, and polymyositis-dermatomyositis and high titers of a specific circulating antibody to an extractable nuclear ribonucleoprotein antigen. Most of the patients are women, and the average age at time of diagnosis is 37 years. Renal disease occurs in 10%-20% of patients, and pulmonary involvement is observed in 20%-80%. Many of the clinical and pathophysiologic pleuropulmonary manifestations are similar to those observed in systemic lupus erythematosus, scleroderma, and polymyositis-dermatomyositis. Abnormal findings on pulmonary function tests and chest radiography have been observed in 69% of asymptomatic patients, impaired diffusing capacity in 67%, and restrictive lung volumes in 50%. Pleurisy is one of the common manifestations of the disease, with an incidence of 6%-40%. Pleural fluid shows the same characteristics as that in systemic lupus erythematosus. The effusions are usually small and resolve spontaneously. Pulmonary hypertension is the most serious complication of mixed connective tissue disease and is noted in up to 67% of patients.

- Mixed connective tissue disease: clinical features of systemic lupus erythematosus, scleroderma, and polymyositis-dermatomyositis.
- Features: pulmonary fibrosis, pleural effusion, aspiration pneumonia, and pulmonary hypertension.

Ankylosing Spondylitis

Ankylosing spondylitis is a chronic disorder of unknown cause characterized by progressive inflammatory disease involving the axial spine and adjacent soft tissues. The sacroiliac, hip, and shoulder joints are commonly affected. It is distinctly a disease of males. Pulmonary involvement is reported in 2%-70% of the patients. Pulmonary problems include chest wall restriction due to ankylosis of costovertebral joints, fibrosis of the lung apices, and, rarely, apical cavitations. The commonest abnormality is the fibrobullous apical lesion, which is noted in 14%-30% of cases. Bullous changes, mycetomas, parenchymal fibrosis, and bronchiectasis are other complications. The cavitated lesions may occasionally become infected by *Aspergillus*, *M. avium* complex, or *M. kansasii*. Pleural effusion is rare. Fixation of the cricoarytenoid with respiratory distress, calcification and ossification of cartilaginous structures in the upper airways, ankylosing hyperostosis of cervical spines, and bilateral vocal cord paralysis with airway obstruction have been described. Costovertebral ankylosis seldom produces pulmonary symptoms even though pulmonary function testing shows diminished total lung capacity, vital capacity, and diffusing capacity. Increased residual volume and functional reserve capacity are common findings.

- In clinical practice, <5% of patients with ankylosing spondylitis have pulmonary problems.
- Fibrobullous lesions are in lung apices; may become secondarily infected.
- Diaphragmatic calcification develops in a small number of patients.

Sjögren's Syndrome

Pulmonary complications are seen in both the primary and secondary forms of Sjögren's syndrome and occur in 1.5%-75% of patients. These complications include desiccation of the upper respiratory tract (xerotrachea), obstructive process involving both large and small airways, localized infiltrates, bronchiectasis, pleurisy, and pleural effusion. The diffuse interstitial process in Sjögren's syndrome (seen in 1% of cases) usually represents lymphocytic interstitial pneumonitis. Both primary and secondary forms of Sjögren's syndrome are associated with lymphoproliferative diseases in the respiratory system. Pulmonary involvement by lymphoma is associated with the syndrome in 15%-20% of patients. Hilar lymphadenopathy or masses should also suggest the likelihood of lymphoma. Most of these lymphomas are of B-cell origin and respond favorably to therapy.

- Sjögren's syndrome: diffuse lung infiltrate usually represents lymphocytic interstitial pneumonitis.
- The most serious complication is lymphoma.
- Cough is common; due to xerotrachea.

Lymphomatoid Granulomatosis

Lymphomatoid granulomatosis is a lymphoproliferative disease and not a vasculitis, even though it is characterized by prominent vascular infiltrates and necrosis along with granulomatosis. The histologic features form a spectrum from benign-appearing lymphocytic interstitial pneumonitis to frank lymphoma in the same patient. Lymphoma develops in more than 50% of patients. Multisystem involvement is common. Radiographic findings are similar to those in Wegener's granulomatosis, with patchy ill-defined infiltrates to multiple nodules. Nearly one-third of the nodules cavitate. Presence of hilar lymphadenopathy suggests lymphomatous changes. Mean age at diagnosis for males is 48 years; the male-to-female ratio is 1.7:1. Cough, dyspnea, hemoptysis, fever, weight loss, malaise, central nervous system symptoms, and peripheral neuropathy are common. Dermal lesions occur in 30% of patients. Prognosis is poor.

- Lymphomatoid granulomatosis: a lymphoproliferative disease and not a vasculitis.
- Clinically resembles Wegener's granulomatosis.

Relapsing Polychondritis

Relapsing polychondritis, a rare disease of unknown cause, affects cartilage throughout the body. It is an autoimmune disease and has been described in association with Wegener's granulomatosis, systemic lupus erythematosus, cryptogenic cirrhosis, and hydralazine therapy. Even though the involvement of the tracheobronchial cartilage is a late phenomenon, >50% of deaths are due to respiratory involvement. Diagnosis is made by noting inflammation of two or more cartilaginous sites. Other manifestations are iritis, episcleritis, hearing deficit, cataracts, aortic valvular insufficiency, anemia, increased erythrocyte sedimentation rate, and liver dysfunction. Treatment with high doses of corticosteroids is reported to be beneficial.

- Relapsing polychondritis: expiratory collapse of the major airways.
- Features: recurrent lung infections and respiratory distress.

Leukemia

The lungs are commonly involved in late leukemia. Infection is the commonest cause of death. Mediastinal and hilar adenopathy are seen in 25% of patients (especially in chronic lymphocytic leukemia), parenchymal involvement in 25% (especially in acute monomyelocytic leukemia, chronic lymphocytic leukemia), pleural effusion in 20%, and pulmonary hemorrhage in 6%.

- Leukemic lung infiltrates are uncommon.
- Commonest cause of infiltrates is infection.
- Leukemia patient receiving chemotherapy and with prolonged (>3 weeks) granulocytopenia is most likely to have disseminated aspergillosis.

Plasma Cell Dyscrasia

Amyloidosis involving the lungs is common in the primary form of amyloidosis. The diffuse type has a poor prognosis. Tracheobronchial amyloidosis produces diffuse submucosal infiltration and hemoptysis. Solitary amyloidoma presents as a lung mass. Myeloma is seen as a direct extension of a rib lesion, plasmacytoma, parenchymal infiltrates (rare), or as a pleural effusion (rare). Waldenström's macroglobulinemia produces effusion in 50% of patients and may also produce parenchymal infiltrates.

- Amyloidosis is also associated with sleep apnea (macroglossia).
- Secondary amyloidosis associated with chronic bronchiectasis and other chronic lung diseases is a pathologic finding with minimal clinical problems.

Transfusion Reactions

Transfusion-related acute lung injury is a form of noncardiogenic pulmonary edema. It is caused by the passive transfer of granulocyte or lymphocyte antibodies in the donor serum. HLA-specific antibodies are identified in the donor sera of 65% of patients who have this reaction. Acute respiratory distress within 4 hours (after 2 hours in most) after transfusion is typical. Clinical manifestations include chills, fever, tachycardia, dry cough, and blood eosinophilia. Chest radiography shows perihilar patchy opacities. Recovery is rapid and complete in almost all patients.

- Consider transfusion-related reaction if radiographic findings suggest pulmonary edema.

Hemoglobinopathies

Sickle cell anemia is the most important entity. Pulmonary infections are seen in >50% of patients; *S. pneumoniae* is frequently implicated. Pulmonary infarctions are common in adults. Lung functions in chronic cases show a restrictive pattern. Recurrent pulmonary embolism and infarction may produce pulmonary hypertension. Pneumovax is indicated in all patients with sickle cell disease.

- Recurrent lung infections (*S. pneumoniae*).
- Pneumovax is important (asplenia or hyposplenia).
- Recurrent pulmonary embolism and secondary pulmonary hypertension.

Methemoglobinemia

Methemoglobinemia occurs when >1% of blood hemoglobin is oxidized to the ferric form. Physicians should check for asymptomatic cyanosis, normal PaO_2, low SaO_2, and a history of drug ingestion.

- Methemoglobinemia: normal PaO_2, low SaO_2.

Renal Diseases

Many pulmonary complications are seen in renal diseases. "Uremic lung" is a form of noncardiogenic pulmonary edema that occurs in acute and chronic renal failure. "Butterfly" shadows (alveolar infiltrates limited to the inner two-thirds of both lungs, with sparing of peripheral areas) seen on chest radiographs should suggest this diagnosis. The radiographic changes are proportional to the degree of azotemia and acidosis in acute renal failure. Pleural effusion is common in acute and chronic renal failure, uremia, and nephrotic syndrome and in patients receiving peritoneal and hemodialysis. In most cases, the fluid is a transudate. Pulmonary calcification occurs in chronic renal failure, especially in patients receiving chronic maintenance hemodialysis, and in secondary hyperparathyroidism. It is due to "metastatic calcification" of the lungs. Chest radiography shows soft infiltrates that resemble pulmonary edema. The diagnosis is made by demonstrating pulmonary uptake of [99]technetium diphosphonate in radionuclide scans. Hypoxemia during dialysis is the result of hypoventilation to compensate for loss of CO_2 through the dialysis membrane. Pulmonary-renal syndromes, sometimes called "lung purpura" consist of those entities in which the lungs and kidneys are affected by the same pathologic process. Examples include Goodpasture's syndrome, Wegener's granulomatosis, polyarteritis nodosa, Henoch-Schönlein purpura, Churg-Strauss syndrome, systemic lupus erythematosus, scleroderma, and drug-induced vasculitis.

- Uremic lung (pulmonary edema) is proportional to degree of azotemia; produces "butterfly" alveolar pattern on chest radiographs.
- Subdiaphragmatic pleural effusions (small transudates) are common in renal diseases.
- Pulmonary calcification occurs with chronic hemodialysis.
- Hypoventilation (thus, low PaO_2) during hemodialysis is due to loss of CO_2 through dialysis membrane.

Gastrointestinal Diseases

It is important to look for hiatal hernia and air-fluid level behind the heart on chest radiography. Check for a history of aspiration. Aspiration pneumonia should be considered in any patient with esophageal problems or symptoms. Peptic ulcer disease and COPD exist together frequently, perhaps because gastric hypersecretion is stimulated by increased arterial PCO_2 and decreased PO_2. Gastrectomy patients have an increased incidence of pulmonary tuberculosis. Celiac sprue is reported in association with pulmonary hemosiderosis and fibrosis. Chronic ulcerative colitis and Crohn's ileitis are associated with increased incidence of asthma, obstructive airway disease, bronchiectasis, and upper airway involvement. Whipple's disease is associated with cough (50% of patients), hilar adenopathy, and pleuropericardial effusions.

- Hiatal hernia and other esophageal problems should be considered in determining the cause of aspiration pneumonia and other lung problems.
- Tuberculosis occurs in postgastrectomy patients.

Hepatic Diseases

Pleural effusion is found in 6% of patients with hepatic cirrhosis; it is usually right-sided and almost always associated with ascites. The fluid is identical in character to ascitic fluid. Uninfected fluid is usually a transudate. A large amount of peritoneal fluid may push both hemidiaphragms superiorly, causing respiratory distress. Unless ascites is adequately treated, pleural fluid continues to accumulate despite repeated thoracentesis. Arterial hypoxemia is common in hepatic cirrhosis and is the result of venoarterial shunting in the basal regions of the lungs. Orthodeoxia (desaturation in upright posture) and platypnea (dyspnea in upright posture) are due to increased right-to-left shunting from gravitational forces. α_1-Antitrypsin deficiency may be associated with cirrhosis of the liver, especially in children.

- Ascites: right-sided pleural effusion; usually transudate.
- Pleural fluid persists unless ascites is adequately treated.
- Dyspnea (platypnea) and hypoxemia (orthodeoxia) are made worse by standing.
- α_1-Antitrypsin deficiency associated with cirrhosis.

Pancreatic Diseases

Acute pancreatitis can produce adult respiratory distress syndrome, pulmonary edema, left-sided pleural effusion, elevation of hemidiaphragm, basal atelectasis, etc. The incidence of pleural effusion is 3%-15%; effusion is left-sided in 95% of patients. The pleural fluid exhibits increased amylase and exudative levels of proteins. Pulmonary edema (adult respiratory distress syndrome) is seen in 20%-50% of patients with acute pancreatitis. It is related to the diminished production of lecithin, the main constituent of the surfactant dipalmitoyl lecithin. Massive effusions and pleurocutaneous fistulae are seen in chronic pancreatitis.

- Adult respiratory distress syndrome is the most serious pulmonary complication of pancreatitis.
- Pleural effusion (exudate) is left-sided in 95% of patients; bloody in 30%.

Endocrine Diseases

Acromegaly is associated with sleep apnea. Thyroid goiter causes tracheal deviation and cough. Stridor and superior vena cava syndrome are rare. Of intrathoracic goiters, 85% are anterior to the trachea and present as anterior mediastinal masses. The other 15% arise from the posterior aspect. Thyrotoxicosis is seen in some patients, but malignant changes are rare. Calcification within the mass is common. Thyrotoxicosis commonly produces exertional dyspnea; this is related to myopathy, increased work of breathing, and increased oxygen uptake. Asthma is difficult to manage in thyrotoxicosis because of more sensitive bronchomotor tone and rapid metabolism of bronchodilators. Myxedema may be associated with pleural effusions that are small and transudates. Both central and obstructive sleep apnea occur in myxedema, and both resolve with treatment of myxedema. Diabetes mellitus is associated with an increased incidence of bron-

chitis, tuberculosis, and mucormycosis. Cushing's syndrome and excessive steroid therapy may produce mediastinal lipomatosis and widening (chest CT is diagnostic). Electrolyte imbalances can affect respiratory function. Severe hypophosphatemia can cause respiratory muscle weakness and respiratory failure. Hypokalemia and hypomagnesemia can also cause respiratory weakness.

- No increased risk of malignant transformation in intrathoracic goiters.
- Thyrotoxic dyspnea is common; related to myopathy and increased work of breathing.
- Obstructive and central sleep apnea are seen in myxedema; both resolve with treatment of myxedema.
- Increased incidence of tuberculosis and mucormycosis in diabetes mellitus.
- Severe hypophosphatemia can cause respiratory failure.
- Severe metabolic alkalosis can present as hypercarbic respiratory acidosis (due to compensatory hypoventilation).

Pregnancy

Dyspnea occurs during the second (in 50% of pregnant women) and third (in 75%) trimesters. Increased resting ventilation is common. Hiatal hernia (moderately symptomatic) occurs in 60% of pregnant women. Pulmonary edema occurs in eclampsia, toxemia, and amniotic fluid embolism and with the use of tocolytics (β_2-agonists). Amniotic fluid embolism accounts for 8% of maternal deaths. Varicella pneumonia and coccidioidomycosis carry higher morbidity and mortality in pregnant women. Sarcoidosis resolves during pregnancy (perhaps because of estrogens) but recurs post partum. Molar pregnancy is associated with trophoblastic embolization into lungs in 10% of women undergoing evacuation of hydatidiform mole. Choriocarcinoma metastasizes to the lung in 65% of cases.

Gynecology

Catamenial (associated with menses) pneumothorax is responsible for 5% of the cases of spontaneous pneumothorax in women ≤50 years. The cause is unclear, although diaphragmatic defects and endometriosis have been proposed. Almost all cases of pneumothorax are right-sided. Thoracic endometriosis may cause hemoptysis, atelectasis, and catamenial pneumothorax. In Meig-Salmon syndrome, ascites and pleural effusion occur in association with ovarian fibroma and other benign tumors. The effusions are frequently right-sided transudates. The effusion resolves with resection of the ovarian tumor.

Neurologic Diseases

Central (neurogenic) hypoventilation is usually from acquired causes such as narcotic overdosage, cerebral edema, central nervous system infections, myxedema, syringomyelia, and, in some cases, Parkinson's disease. Central hyperventilation is a regular, rapid breathing that keeps the rate of respiration in the range of 3-6 times normal for hours or days. Although the arterial oxygen level of these patients is normal, they are reported to have a high mortality rate. Neurogenic pulmonary edema is a complication of catastrophic cerebrovascular accidents, trauma to the head, epileptic seizures, and acute trauma to the spinal cord. This form of noncardiogenic pulmonary edema is thought to occur when increased intracranial pressure stimulates hypothalamic centers that release an excessive α-adrenergic discharge. This reaction produces increased systemic and pulmonary vascular resistance, severe hemodynamic alternations, and pulmonary edema. Chest radiography shows asymmetrical, hazy, diffuse changes that persist even after pulmonary hemodynamics return to normal. Coma and loss of consciousness result in loss of airway protection, which in turn may lead to aspiration and pneumonia. In chronic cases, recurrent pulmonary infections and pulmonary thromboembolism are serious threats to life.

Spinal cord disorders cause several lung problems. In patients with quadriplegia, lung volumes (total lung capacity and vital capacity) may be diminished by 33%-55% of predicted normal values. Most deaths associated with quadriplegia are due to pulmonary complications, such as hypoventilation, aspiration, ineffective cough, recurrent infections, and pulmonary emboli. Neuromyopathies that affect the respiratory system include myasthenia gravis, myasthenic syndrome, amyotrophic lateral sclerosis, polymyositis, periodic paralysis, acid maltase deficiency, hypokalemia, and hypophosphatemia. In myasthenia gravis, the risk of respiratory failure is increased by surgical procedures, infections, corticosteroid therapy, and the use of aminoglycosides. In addition to decreased static lung volumes, patients with neuromyopathies may have decreased inspiratory and expiratory forces. Testing of maximal inspiratory and expiratory pressures is a sensitive way to assess respiratory muscle weakness. Anterior horn cell disorders such as acute febrile polyneuritis (Guillain-Barré syndrome) and acute poliomyelitis produce hypoventilatory respiratory failure. Patients with myotonic dystrophy or progressive muscular dystrophy may have insidious chronic respiratory failure. Autonomic nervous system disorders such as familial dysautonomia can diminish the response to hypoxia and hypercapnia. Autonomic dysfunction due to diabetes mellitus, amyloidosis, and syringomyelia may progress to respiratory failure. Obstructive sleep apnea and central sleep apnea have been reported in autonomic disturbances.

- Neurogenic pulmonary edema is a form of noncardiogenic pulmonary edema caused by increased intracranial pressure.
- Aspiration and pneumonia, recurrent pulmonary infections, and pulmonary thromboembolism occur in comatose and unconscious patients.
- In myasthenia gravis, the risk of respiratory failure is increased by surgical procedures, infections, corticosteroid therapy, and the use of aminoglycosides.
- Measurement of maximal inspiratory and expiratory pressures is a sensitive way to assess respiratory muscle weakness.
- Obstructive sleep apnea and central sleep apnea occur in diseases of the autonomic nervous system.
- In middle-aged or elderly persons with progressive respiratory deterioration, hypercapnia, and aspiration (with or without fasciculations), consider amyotrophic lateral sclerosis.

Diaphragmatic Paralysis

Unilateral diaphragmatic paralysis decreases total lung capacity by 35% and vital capacity and maximal voluntary ventilation by 20%. Bilateral diaphragmatic paralysis diminishes vital capacity by 50% in the upright position and perhaps by 60%-75% in the supine position. In patients with bilateral diaphragmatic paralysis, orthopnea is a major problem. Ipsilateral diaphragmatic dysfunction is frequently associated with hemiplegia. A sniff test (to demonstrate paradoxical motion) or diaphragmatic electromyography may be necessary to document diaphragmatic paralysis.

- Inability to assume supine posture should suggest the possibility of bilateral diaphragmatic paralysis.
- Diaphragmatic fluoroscopy (sniff test) is useful, but 6% of normal subjects have positive findings on this test.

- Chronic diaphragmatic paralysis (>6 months) usually has an idiopathic cause.
- Acute unilateral diaphragmatic paralysis should be evaluated; hilar mass should be excluded.

Skeletal Diseases

Kyphoscoliosis is the commonest spinal deformity associated with pulmonary complications. The causes of scoliosis include congenital, neuropathic (poliomyelitis, cerebral palsy, syringomyelia), myopathic (muscular dystrophy, amyotonia, and Friedreich's ataxia), and traumatic causes. It also occurs in mesenchymal disorders and in association with neurofibromatosis. In practice, idiopathic scoliosis is the commonest variety seen. A familial type is also reported. The curvature or angulation of a scoliotic spine is best measured by Cobb's scoliotic angle. Pulmonary symptoms are noted when the angle is >70 degrees. Angulation increases during younger life, and pulmonary symptoms appear during the fourth and fifth decades. The commonest pulmonary abnormality is a decrease in static lung volumes: total lung capacity and vital capacity. There is an inverse correlation between the angle and vital capacity, total lung capacity, functional reserve capacity, residual volume, and compliance. Although arterial hypoxemia is often present in symptomatic patients, $PaCO_2$ is normal in most cases. Hypoventilation and $\dot{V}/Q$ mismatch are mainly responsible for hypoxia. Pulmonary hypertension and cor pulmonale are serious complications. Pectus excavatum ("funnel chest") is caving in of the sternum and the anterior ends of the cartilages and ribs. It is associated with pulmonary sequestration, Marfan syndrome, and *M. avium* complex infection. Pectus carinatum ("pigeon breast") is the bulging or protruding of the sternum and anterior cartilages and ribs. It is associated with congenital heart disease.

- Pulmonary symptoms begin when scoliotic angle is >70 degrees.
- Respiratory symptoms appear during fourth and fifth decades.
- Although arterial hypoxemia is often present in symptomatic patients, $PaCO_2$ is normal in most cases.
- Static lung volumes are diminished; inverse relationship between scoliotic angle and lung volumes.
- Pectus deformities may be associated with congenital cardiac disorders.

PULMONARY INFECTIONS

Viral Infections

One-third of the upper respiratory tract infections are caused by the rhinovirus group. The common cold is caused by rhinovirus, parainfluenza virus, adenovirus, respiratory syncytial virus, and coxsackievirus A21. Coxsackieviruses are a more frequent cause of viral respiratory tract infections in summer and autumn. The virus cannot be isolated in 40% of respiratory tract infections presumed to be caused by a virus. Ciliary abnormalities with microtubular alterations (dysmorphic cilia) is a common acquired (transient) problem during acute viral illness. Therefore, temporary interference with mucociliary clearance may increase the risk of other infections. Viral respiratory tract infections constitute 83% of all acute infectious problems, and these infections are highly contagious. They have seasonal variation: 50% of people have a viral respiratory tract infection during December-February, and only 20% in June-August.

- Coxsackieviral infections are more frequent in the summer and autumn.
- Ciliary abnormalities are common (acquired and transient) during acute viral illness.

Viral Pneumonia

Viral pneumonia is caused by respiratory syncytial virus; parainfluenza virus types 1, 2, 3; adenovirus types 1, 2, 3, 5, 7; and influenza virus A and B. In adults, it is caused by influenza virus and adenovirus. Respiratory syncytial virus is the common cause of respiratory problems in children, and parainfluenza virus types 1 and 3 cause bronchiolitis. In adults, varicella pneumonia is a severe illness. Resolution of the disease may be followed by nodular pulmonary calcification. Herpesvirus may cause pneumonia in immunocompromised host or patients with extensive burns. Cytomegalovirus, a member of the herpesvirus group, is found in almost all body secretions of infected patients. This virus is seen more commonly in immunocompromised and transplant patients and in cases of lymphoreticular malignancy, cardiopulmonary bypass, and multiple blood transfusions, and in association with *Pneumocystis carinii* infection (AIDS). Cytomegalovirus is the second most common infection in patients with AIDS. Diffuse, small nodular or hazy infiltrates are seen on chest radiography in 15% of cases of pneumonia caused by cytomegalovirus, but interstitial pneumonia due to cytomegalovirus is seen in 50% of bone marrow graft recipients. Findings of inclusion bodies and high titers of cytomegalovirus may help in making the diagnosis.

- Viral pneumonia in nonimmunocompromised adults is caused by influenza virus and adenovirus.
- Varicella (chicken pox) pneumonia is more common in adults than in children; results in diffuse pulmonary calcification.
- Cytomegalovirus infection is more common in immunocompromised patients and in patients with AIDS.
- Isolation of cytomegalovirus from respiratory tract secretions does not always establish infection.

Influenza

Nearly all patients with influenza pneumonia have underlying heart disease, usually rheumatic valvular disease. Clinical features are high fever, dyspnea, cyanosis, fluffy or nodular infiltrates in the mid lung fields, and respiratory failure. Annual (in the autumn) influenza vaccination is recommended for high-risk individuals (COPD, heart disease, diabetes, kidney disease, debilitated condition, >60 years old, and compromised patients, etc.). Overall protection rates are 70%.

- Patients at risk of influenza infection: heart disease, COPD, kidney disease, diabetes, chronic anemia, and immunosuppressed.
- Secondary bacterial pneumonia is common.
- Coxsackievirus B causes pleurodynia (Bornholm disease or "devil's grip"): fever, headache, malaise, and severe pleuritic pain lasting from several days to weeks.

Hantavirus Pulmonary Syndrome

Hantavirus pulmonary syndrome, first recognized in the southwestern U.S. in May 1993, is caused by a hantavirus. The rodent reservoir for this virus is the deer mouse. Through October 1993, 42 cases of this syndrome had been reported to the Centers for Disease Control from 12 states, all west of the Mississippi River. The overall mortality was 62%. Clinical features: median age of patients, 32 years (range, 12-69 years), males (52%), and Native Americans (55%). The illness is characterized by a prodrome of fever, myalgia, headache, abdominal pain, nausea or vomiting (or both), and cough, followed by the abrupt onset of respiratory distress. Bilateral pulmonary infiltrates that occur within 48 hours have been reported

in all patients. Hemoconcentration in 71% and thrombocytopenia in 71%. Fever, hypoxia, and hypotension occur after hospitalization. Poor prognosis in those with shock and lactic acidosis. No sequelae in survivors. Autopsy has routinely revealed serous pleural effusions and heavy edematous lungs with interstitial mononuclear cells in alveolar septa, alveolar edema, focal hyaline membranes, and occasional alveolar hemorrhage. Hantavirus antigens are detected with immunohistochemistry. Serologic (hantavirus-specific immunoglobulin M or increasing titers of IgG), polymerase chain reaction, and other studies are available through the Centers for Disease Control. Ribavirin trials are being conducted.

- Reservoir for hantavirus is the deer mouse.
- More common in southwestern U.S.
- Febrile illness, unexplained respiratory distress, bilateral pulmonary infiltrates, and pleural effusion.
- Hemoconcentration, thrombocytopenia, shock, and hypoxemia.

Mycoplasma

Because humans are the only reservoir for *Mycoplasma*, spread is from person to person. Thus, infections occur in epidemic and endemic form and outbreaks occur in closed populations (military camps, colleges, etc.). Epidemics are more common in the summer and autumn. Illness is more common in school-aged children and young adults. The incubation period is 2-3 weeks. The predilection is for the respiratory tract. Clinical features include fever (85% of patients), coryza, pharyngitis (50%), bullous myringitis (20%), tracheobronchitis, cough (>95%), pleural effusion, hemolytic anemia, erythema multiforme, hepatitis, thrombocytopenia, and Guillain-Barré syndrome. Pneumonia occurs in only 3%-10% of infected persons and is more likely in younger adults (military recruits or summer camps); it causes interstitial pneumonia and acute bronchiolitis. Chest radiography shows unilateral bronchopneumonia, lower lobes (65% of cases), and pleural effusion (5%). Cold agglutinins (>1:64 in 50% of patients) appear during the 2nd or 3rd week after the onset of symptoms and the titer decreases to insignificant levels by 4-6 weeks. Complement fixation serology--fourfold increase in titer noted in 50%-80%. The organism can be cultured from respiratory tract secretions, the middle ear, and the cerebrospinal fluid.

- Epidemic and endemic forms in closed populations.

- Bullous myringitis, hemolytic anemia, erythema multiforme, and Guillain-Barré syndrome.
- Causes interstitial pneumonia and acute bronchiolitis.
- Cold agglutinins (>1:64 in 50% of patients) appear during 2nd or 3rd week.

Bacterial Infections

Sinusitis

Most bacterial infections of sinuses occur after a viral infection of the nasal mucosa. Bacteria in acute (A) and chronic (C) sinusitis are: pneumococci (A, 20%-35% of patients; C, 5%-15%), *H. influenzae* (A, 15%-30%; C, 3%-10%), *Streptococcus* anaerobes and aerobes (A, 5%-35%; C, 10%-25%), *S. aureus* (A, 3%-6%; C, 5%-15%), and no growth (A, 2%-25%; C, 25%-60%). Nearly 10% of the cases of maxillary sinusitis are related to odontogenic infections.

- Sinus involvement is also seen in asthma, chronic bronchitis, bronchiectasis, cystic fibrosis, Kartagener's syndrome, and Wegener's granulomatosis.

Otitis Media

The relationship between otitis media and common viral infections is strong, especially in children. Nearly 10% of children with measles have otitis media. Bacteria are isolated in 70%-80% of patients with otitis media and include pneumococci (25%-75% of patients), *H. influenzae* (15%-30%), anaerobes (peptococci and propionibacteria) (20%-30%), group A streptococci (2%-10%), and *S. aureus* (1%-5%). Ampicillin-resistant *H. influenzae* is found in 15%-40% of the patients.

- Otitis media occurs in severe diabetes and cystic fibrosis.

Pharyngitis

Pharyngitis is caused by group A *S. pyogenes* (>30% of patients), *N. gonorrhoeae*, *C. diphtheriae*, and *M. pneumoniae* (5%). Sore throat is also caused by adenovirus, Epstein-Barr virus, and others.

Pneumonia

Streptococcal Pneumonia

Streptococcus pneumoniae is responsible for 90% of the cases of pneumonia in adults. The incidence peaks in the winter and spring, when carrier rates in the general population may be as high as 70%. People at high risk include those with cardiopulmonary disease (especially pulmonary edema), viral respiratory infections, hemoglobinopathy, and hyposplenism and immune-suppressed patients. Many patients are elderly, alcoholic, or immunocompromised. Bacteremic pneumonia in the elderly is not associated with fever in 30% but is associated with minimal respiratory symptoms in 50%, altered mental state in 50%, and volume depletion in 50%. The incidence of bacteremic pneumonia in hospitalized patients is 25% and carries a mortality rate of 20%. Leukocytosis of 10,000-30,000/mm^3 is common. Sputum may be blood streaked or rusty. Early in the disease, radiographic findings may be normal, but later, they may show classic lobar pneumonia. Pleurisy/effusion is common and cavitation is rare.

- Mortality of about 28% in bacteremic patients >50 years old.
- Pneumovax decreases the incidence of pneumonia by 79%-92%.
- Pneumovax is indicated for patients with COPD, kidney disease, and metabolic disease and for patients in chronic care facilities, convalescing from severe disease, older than 50 years, and postsplenectomy; it is not recommended during pregnancy.
- Those who received pneumovax before 1983 should receive the newer 23-valent vaccine; repeat immunization every 10 years may be indicated.

Staphylococcus Pneumonia

S. aureus occurs in the nasal passages of 20%-40% of normal adults, but pneumonia is uncommon. *S. aureus* pneumonia is more likely to occur in patients with severe diabetes, immunocompromised status, dialysis, drug abusers, and those with influenza or measles. In drug addicts, it may begin as septic emboli with right-sided endocarditis. It is one of the nosocomial types of pneumonia. Consolidation, bronchopneumonia, abscess with air-fluid level, pneumatocele, empyema, and a high mortality characterize staphylococcal pneumonia.

- Present in nasal passages of normal subjects.
- Immunocompromised, diabetics, and drug abusers.
- Lung abscess and pneumatoceles more common.

Pseudomonas aeruginosa

P. aeruginosa is a ubiquitous organism commonly isolated from patients with cystic fibrosis and bronchiectasis. Pneumonia may occur in patients with COPD, congestive heart failure, diabetes, kidney disease, alcoholism, tracheostomy, prolonged ventilation, postoperative status, and compromised hosts. *Pseudomonas* pneumonia results in microabscess, alveolar hemorrhage, and necrotic areas. Chest radiography may show bilateral, patchy infiltrates.

- *P. aeruginosa*: difficult to distinguish colonization from true infection.
- Important organism in cystic fibrosis, bronchiectasis, malignant otitis media, and ventilator patients.

Klebsiella pneumoniae

Pneumonia due to *K. pneumoniae* is more likely in alcoholics, diabetics, and hospitalized patients. Also, it is more common in males. Dependent lobes are affected more frequently. It is a lobar pneumonia with bulging fissure. Complications include abscess and empyema.

- *K. pneumoniae*: more likely to cause pneumonia in alcoholics, diabetics, and hospitalized patients.
- Bulging fissure sign.

Haemophilus influenzae

Unencapsulated strains of *H. influenzae* are present in the sputum of 30%-60% of normal adults and in 58%-80% of patients with COPD. In contrast, bacteremia is almost always associated with encapsulated strains. Both strains cause pulmonary infections and otitis, sinusitis, epiglottitis, and pneumonia. Most patients with pneumonia have underlying COPD or alcoholism, even though *H. influenzae* pneumonia develops in healthy military recruits. The amount of sputum production is significant. Pneumonia is seen in lower lobes more often than in the upper lobes. Chest radiographic findings are typical for bronchopneumonia or lobar pneumonia. Pleural effusions occur in 30% of patients, and cavitation is rare.

- *H. influenzae*: both unencapsulated and encapsulated strains cause lung infections.
- Pleural effusion in 30% of patients with pneumonia; cavitation is rare.
- More common in those with COPD and alcoholism and in military recruits.

Moraxella catarrhalis

M. catarrhalis is a gram-negative diplococcus that is part of the normal flora. It causes sinusitis, otitis, and pneumonia. The latter is more likely in patients with COPD, alcoholism, and immunocompromised status. Infection produces segmental patchy bronchopneumonia in the lower lobes. Cavitation and pleural effusion are rare. These bacteria produce β-lactamase and most are resistant to penicillin and ampicillin.

- *M. catarrhalis*: formerly known as *Branhamella*.
- COPD, immunocompromised status, and alcoholics.
- Most strains produce β-lactamase.

Legionella pneumophila

More than 20 species of *Legionella*, a gram-negative bacillus, have been identified. Water is its natural habitat. Disease results from inhalation of aerosolized organisms. Epidemics have occurred because of contaminated air conditioning cooling towers, construction or excavation in contaminated soil, and contaminated hospital showers. Risk factors include COPD, smoking, cancer, diabetes mellitus, immunosuppression, chronic heart and kidney diseases. Almost all cases of pneumonia are caused by *L. pneumophila* (85% of cases) and *L. micdadei* (10%). Bacteria can be demonstrated in tissue by Dieterle's stain and with fluorescent antibody staining. Most cases occur in summer and early autumn. Men older than 50 years are more likely to be infected than younger people. The incubation period is 2-10 days. Symptoms, in decreasing order of frequency, are: abrupt onset of cough (hemoptysis in 30% of patients), chills, dyspnea, headache, myalgia, arthralgia, and diarrhea. Common signs include fever, relative bradycardia, and change in mental status. The diagnosis is established by fluorescent antibody stain (FA stain), which is positive in the sputum in 20% of serologically positive cases. Bacteria can be cultured from tissue or other samples. Serology takes from 1-3 weeks before a titer of 1:64 is seen; peak titer is reached in 5-6 weeks. A titer of 1:128 is suspicious and a 4x increase in titer is diagnostic.

- COPD, smoking, cancer, diabetes mellitus, immunosuppression, chronic heart and kidney diseases.
- Hyponatremia and hypophosphatemia in 50% of patients, lobar consolidations in 50%, leukocytosis (>10,000) in 60%, proteinuria in 20%, and increased SGOT in 60%.
- False-positive titer can be seen in plague, tularemia, leptospirosis, and adenovirus infections.
- *Legionella* serology titer of 1:128 is suspicious and a 4x increase in titer is diagnostic.

Anaerobic Bacteria

Bacteroides melaninogenicus, Fusobacterium nucleatum, anaerobic cocci, and anaerobic streptococci are responsible for most cases of anaerobic pneumonia. *Bacteroides fragilis* is recovered from 15%-20% of patients with anaerobic pneumonia. Most of these anaerobes reside in the oropharynx as saprophytes. Common factors responsible for aspiration of anaerobes include altered consciousness, tooth extraction, poor dental hygiene, oropharyngeal infections, and drug overdose. Anaerobic bacterial infections may complicate underlying pulmonary problems (cancer, bronchiectasis, foreign body, etc.). Foul-smelling sputum is found in >50% of patients. Patchy pneumonitis in dependent segments may progress to lung abscess and empyema.

- Aspiration of anaerobes associated with: altered consciousness, tooth extraction, poor dental hygiene, oropharyngeal infections, and drug overdose.
- Cavitated lung abscess in dependent lobes and empyema.

Community-Acquired "Atypical" Pneumonia

Organisms causing "atypical" community-acquired pneumonia include *Mycoplasma pneumoniae, Chlamydia psittaci, Chlamydia pneumoniae, Coxiella burnetii,* tularemia, and *Legionella* species. Mycoplasma pneumonia and legionellosis are discussed above.

- Community-acquired "atypical" pneumonia caused by *M. pneumoniae, C. psittaci, C. pneumoniae, C. burnetii,* and *Legionella* species.

Chlamydia pneumoniae (TWAR strain)

Chlamydia pneumoniae is confined to the human respiratory tract; no reservoirs are known. Person-to-person spread occurs among schoolchildren, family members, and military recruits. The incubation period is 10-65 days (mean, 31 days). Reinfection may be common, with cycles of disease every few years. Patients (90%) are asymptomatic or have pharyngitis (1%), sinusitis (5%), bronchitis (5%), or pneumonia (10%). Pharyngeal erythema and wheezing are common. Among older adults, 40% of community-acquired cases of pneumonia are due to *C. psittaci.* Chest radiography shows unilateral segmental patchy opacity. Complement fixation test is not sensitive and nonspecific.

- *C. pneumoniae*: person-to-person spread among schoolchildren, family members, and military recruits.

- Causes pneumonia in 10% of patients, bronchitis in 5%, and pharyngitis in 1%.
- Pneumonia caused by *C. pneumoniae* is separate from psittacosis (see below).

Chlamydia psittaci

C. psittaci causes psittacosis in humans. The organism is found in psittacine birds (parrots, lories), turkeys, pigeons, and other birds. Infected birds develop anorexia, weight loss, diarrhea, ruffled feathers, inability to fly, conjunctivitis, and rhinitis. In humans, the incubation period is 1-6 weeks. Clinical features: myalgias, fever, headache, lethargy, confusion, delirium, and splenomegaly (1%-10%). Pulmonary symptoms are late and mild. Chest radiography shows patchy unilateral or bilateral lower lobe pneumonia and an occasional small pleural effusion. Normal leukocyte count, increased CPK level, 4x increase in complement fixation test over >2 weeks.

- Psittacosis: caused by exposure to sick birds that harbor *C. psittaci.*
- Clinical features: myalgias, fever, headache, lethargy, confusion, delirium, and splenomegaly (1%-10%).
- Pulmonary symptoms are late and mild; radiographically, patchy unilateral or bilateral lower lobe pneumonia and an occasional small pleural effusion.
- Note the differences: chlamydia pneumonia (human-to-human transmission of virus), psittacosis (birds-to-human transmission of virus), and pigeon breeder's or bird fancier's lung (hypersensitivity pneumonitis caused by immune reaction to avian proteins).

Coxiella burnetii

C. burnetii is a rickettsia shed in urine, feces, milk, and birth products of sheep, cattle, goats, and cats. It causes Q fever. Humans are infected by inhalation of dried aerosolized material. The incubation period is 10-30 days. Clinical features: fever, myalgias, chills, nausea, vomiting, chest pain, and cough (late). Radiographic findings may be normal or show unilateral bronchopneumonia and small pleural effusions. Hepatitis and endocarditis can occur. The leukocyte count is normal, but liver enzyme levels may increase; complement fixation serology is positive.

- *C. burnetii*: rickettsial illness (Q fever).
- Inhalation of dried inoculum from urine, feces, milk, and birth products of sheep, cattle, goats, and cats.
- Bronchopneumonia and pleural effusion.

Francisella tularensis

F. tularensis is a gram-negative bacillus transmitted to man from wild rabbits, squirrels, and other wild animals and by bites of ticks or deer flies. The incubation period is 2-5 days. Cutaneous ulcer and lymphadenopathy are common features. Cough, fever, and chest pain are frequent, but many patients are asymptomatic. Chest radiography shows unilateral lower lobe patchy infiltrates (bilateral in 30% of patients), and pleural effusion in 30%. The leukocyte count is normal; the organism is not seen in Gram staining of the sputum. Serology (agglutinins): 4x change; titer <1:160.

- *F. tularensis*: a gram-negative bacteria; causes tularemia.
- Transmitted from wild rabbits, squirrels, and other wild animals.
- Bronchopneumonia and pleural effusion.

Yersinia pestis

Y. pestis is a gram-negative bacillus that causes plague. It is more prevalent in New Mexico, Arizona, Colorado, and California than in other states. It is spread from wild rodents (occasionally, cats), either directly or by fleas, usually in May-September. The incubation period is 2-7 days. Clinical features are fever, headache, bubo (groin or axilla), cough, and tachypnea. Pneumonia occurs in 10%-20% of the patients. Bilateral lower lobe alveolar infiltrates are found on radiographic study. Pleural effusion is common and nodules and cavities can occur. Leukocyte count is 15,000-20,000; the organism is seen with Giemsa staining and in cultures or direct fluorescent antibody from blood, lymph node, sputum. Serology is positive.

- *Y. pestis*: more prevalent in southwestern U.S. (as is coccidioidomycosis).
- It is spread from wild rodents (occasionally, cats) either directly or by fleas.
- Pneumonia in 10%-20% of patients; pleural effusions are common.

Hospital-Acquired (Nosocomial) Pneumonia

Almost 60% of the cases are caused by gram-negative bacilli, 10% by *S. aureus*, 10% by *S. pneumoniae*, and the rest by anaerobes, *Legionella* species, etc. Risk factors include coma, hypotension, shock, acidosis, azotemia, prolonged treatment with antibiotics, major surgical operations, lengthy procedures, mechanical ventilation, and immunosuppressive therapy.

- Hospital-acquired pneumonia: nearly 60% of cases caused by gram-negative bacilli, 10% by *S. aureus*, 10% by *S. pneumoniae*.
- In hospital outbreaks involving a single type of organism, consider contaminated respiratory equipment.

Aspiration Pneumonitis

The two separate types of aspiration pneumonitis are acute and chronic. The acute type usually results from aspiration of a volume >50 mL with a pH <2.4. It produces classic aspiration pneumonia. Predisposing factors include nasogastric tube, anesthesia, coma, seizures, central nervous system problems, diaphragmatic hernia with reflux, tracheoesophageal fistula, etc. Hospitalized patients who develop aspiration pneumonia are infected by *E. coli*, *S. aureus*, *K. pneumoniae*, and *P. aeruginosa*. Community-acquired cases of aspiration pneumonia are caused by infections due to anaerobes (*B. melaninogenicus*, *F. nucleatum*, and gram-positive cocci). Multiple antibiotics may be needed. Use of steroids is a matter of controversy. Preventive measures are important. Chronic aspiration pneumonia results from recurrent aspiration of small volumes. Examples of this type include patients with diaphragmatic hernia and reflux and mineral oil granuloma. Unexplained chronic cough, patchy lung infiltrates, and nocturnal wheeze and cough are the symptoms.

- Acute aspiration pneumonia usually results from aspiration of a volume >50 mL with a pH of <2.4; may cause adult respiratory distress syndrome.
- Chronic aspiration pneumonia results from aspiration of small volumes on a chronic recurrent basis, as in diaphragmatic hernia with reflux and mineral oil granuloma.

Lung Abscess

A parenchymal suppurative process is usually caused by bacteria. Radiographs show a cavitary lesion, often with an air-fluid level. Three clinical groups of lung abscesses are primary, opportunistic, and hematogenous. Primary lung abscesses are associated with oral sepsis; aspiration accounts for up to 90% of all abscesses. Common causes include alcohol, drugs, anesthesia, seizures, stroke, coma, esophageal disorders, endobronchial obstruction (cancer, foreign body), and postpneumonic necrosis. Lung abscesses caused by opportunistic infections are seen in newborn infants with prematurity or congenital cardiopulmonary disorders and in elderly patients with blood dyscrasia and in cancer of the lung or oropharynx. The infections may be nosocomial and occur with steroid therapy and postoperatively. Hematogenous lung abscesses occur with septicemia, septic embolism, and sterile infarcts (3%). History of any of these conditions in association with fever, cough with purulent or blood sputum, weight loss, and leukocytosis suggests the diagnosis. Chest radiography is helpful in making the diagnosis. The abscess may rupture into the pleural space and cause empyema or flood other areas of the lung, causing adult respiratory distress syndrome. Bronchoscopy should be performed in selected patients to obtain cultures, drain abscess, and exclude obstructing lesions. Treatment includes drainage (physiotherapy, postural, and bronchoscopic), antibiotics for 4-6 weeks, and surgical treatment if medical therapy fails.

- Primary lung abscess: associated with oral sepsis; aspiration accounts for up to 90% of all abscesses.
- Opportunistic lung abscesses are more common in elderly patients with blood dyscrasia, cancer of lung or oropharynx, steroid therapy, postoperative status, and nosocomial pneumonia.
- Hematogenous lung abscess is seen in septicemia, septic embolism, and sterile infarcts (3%).
- Bacteria responsible include anaerobic cocci (30%-40%), anaerobic bacilli (30%-50%), aerobic gram-positive cocci (25%), and aerobic gram-negative bacilli (5%-12%).

Mycobacterium tuberculosis

M. tuberculosis causes the commonest type of human-to-human chronic infection by mycobacteria worldwide. Transmission of infection is by inhalation of droplet nuclei from expectorated respiratory secretions. Diagnosis of active infection is by demonstrating the organism in respiratory secretions or other body fluids or tissues. The diagnostic yield from sputum is 25%-30%; induced sputum, 28%-55%; laryngeal swab, 25%; and gastric washings, 10%-34%. Bronchoscopically obtained specimens have 30% more yield compared with induced sputum and gastric washings. Culture of pleural fluid alone has a low yield (<20%), but culture of pleural biopsy specimens has a >70% diagnostic yield.

- Positive tuberculin skin test, using purified protein derivative (PPD), indicates exposure to mycobacteria

and not active infection.
- Diagnosis of active infection is by demonstration of organism in respiratory secretions or other body fluids or tissues.
- Bronchoscopically obtained specimens have 30% more yield compared with induced sputum and gastric washings.

The tuberculin skin test (PPD) is an example of delayed (T-cell-mediated) hypersensitivity reaction. The sensitization process that follows infection with mycobacteria occurs primarily in the regional lymph nodes, derived from the pool of T lymphocytes. After 6-8 weeks, these lymphocytes enter the bloodstream and circulate for long periods of time (months to years). When this pool of cells is depleted by the aging process or loss of immunity, PPD can become negative (false-negative result). A false-negative PPD is seen in infections with viruses, bacteria (typhoid, brucella, leprosy), live virus vaccinations, chronic renal failure, nutritional deficiency, diseases of lymphoid organs (Hodgkin's disease, sarcoid, chronic lymphocytic leukemia), drugs (steroids and immunosuppressive agents), extremes of age (newborn or old), recent or overwhelming infection with mycobacteria, and acute stress. Other factors include tuberculin type, dilutions, improper storage of tuberculin, contamination, technique, etc. The method of administration and the recording of results are also responsible for some false-negative and false-positive results. PPD skin testing should use a 5-TU (intermediate strength) preparation; the widest induration is read at 48 and 72 hours. Bigger reactions usually mean higher chance of active disease.

- PPD reaction represents delayed type of hypersensitivity reaction.
- PPD becomes positive within 4 weeks after exposure to tubercle bacilli.
- False-negative PPD: immunocompromised patients, lymphomas, high dose of corticosteroid therapy, and disseminated tuberculosis.
- 5-TU PPD is recommended; read reaction after 48 and 72 hours.

A reaction of ≥5 mm should be considered positive for persons who have had recent contact with an index case or whose chest radiographic findings suggest tuberculosis and for HIV-infected persons. Indications for PPD include persons with signs and symptoms suggestive of current tuberculous infection, recent contacts with known or suspected cases of tuberculosis, abnormal radiographic findings compatible with past tuberculosis, patients with diseases that increase the risk of tuberculosis (silicosis, gastrectomy, diabetes, immune suppression, HIV infection), and groups at high risk of recent infection with *M. tuberculosis* (immigrants, long-time residents and workers in hospitals, nursing homes, prisons, and inner city or skid-row populations).

- A reaction of ≥5 mm should be considered positive for persons who have had recent contact with an index case, whose radiographic findings suggest tuberculosis, and HIV-infected persons.
- Nearly 25% of patients with active disease show negative PPD reaction.

Prophylactic therapy (standard prophylaxis consists of isoniazid, 300 mg orally once a day for 12 months) is indicated in household and close contacts, positive PPD with abnormal radiographic finding, recent PPD converters, and in those with positive PPD and immune suppression, hematologic malignancies, diabetes, silicosis and postgastrectomy, renal insufficiency, heroin addicts, HIV-positive persons, and patients receiving corticosteroid therapy (>15 mg/day). Contacts to source cases who are receiving 9 months or less of therapy for their disease may be treated with 9 months of preventive therapy with isoniazid, provided they have normal radiographic findings. More vulnerable contacts who presumably have been infected by source case shedding isoniazid-resistant organisms should receive preventive therapy with rifampin for 12 months; for less vulnerable contacts, such treatment is an acceptable option. Twice weekly high-dose (900 mg) preventive therapy with isoniazid should be considered for high-risk subjects who are deemed noncompliant.

Definitive therapy is indicated for all patients with culture-proved tuberculosis. Usually, treatment should include multiple drug (>2 drugs) therapy in all patients with active tuberculosis (see Tables 26-11 and 26-12 for recommendations by the Centers for Disease Control).

- Treatment usually should include multiple drug (>2 drugs) therapy in all patients with active tuberculosis.
- A 9-month regimen of isoniazid and rifampin (may be supplemented during the initial 2 months with ethambutol, streptomycin, or pyrazinamide) is the standard therapy for tuberculosis.

Drug Toxicity

With isoniazid, the incidence of hepatitis is age-dependent: rare in patients <20 years old, 0.3% between 20-34 years, 1.2% between 35-49 years, and 2.3% for those older than 50. Overall incidence is <1%. Hepatic dysfunction develops in 46% of patients within the first 2 months, in 36% during the 2nd month, and in 54% after the 3rd month. Middle-aged and black females are at higher risk. Hepatitis is more likely in rapid acetylators, and neuritis is more likely in slow acetylators. The rate of acetylation is genetically determined. Phenytoin toxicity is higher in slow acetylators. Isoniazid also causes skin rash, purpura, drug-induced systemic lupus erythematosus, and arthritis. Pyridoxine, 6 mg/day, is recommended for patients taking isoniazid. Patients older than 35 years who are receiving preventive therapy with isoniazid should have their liver function monitored, with levels of transaminase being measured at 1, 3, 6, and 9 months; however, tests of liver function should not replace careful clinical assessment. Rifampin has an overall incidence of serious side effects of 1%. Transient increase in SGOT is common. Hepatitis is worse with isoniazid therapy. Rifampin increases metabolism of contraceptive pills, corticosteroids, warfarin, oral hypoglycemic agents, methadone, and digitalis derivatives; therefore, dosages of these drugs may have to be increased. Intermittent rifampin therapy is associated with thrombocytopenia, flu-like syndrome, and hemolytic anemia. Rifampin causes a harmless orange discoloration of body secretions. Ethambutol, in doses >25 mg/kg, causes retrobulbar neuritis in <1% of patients; symptoms are observed usually 2 months after therapy is begun. Because ophthalmoscopic findings are normal in these patients, symptoms are important. Streptomycin causes vestibular toxicity, especially in the elderly. Isoniazid, rifampin, pyrazinamide, streptomycin, and ethionamide are mycobactericidal, whereas ethambutol, aminosalicylate sodium (para-aminosalicylic acid), cycloserine, and capreomycin are bacteriostatic.

- The overall incidence of serious side effects from isoniazid, rifampin, and ethambutol is 1%.
- Liver damage is the most serious complication from isoniazid, rifampin, and pyrazinamide.
- Retrobulbar neuritis results from ethambutol therapy.
- Vestibular toxicity results from streptomycin.

Mycobacterium avium Complex

M. avium complex, a noncontagious mycobacterium,

Table 26-11.--Regimen Options for Initial Treatment of Tuberculosis Among Children and Adults

| TB without HIV infection | | | TB with HIV infection |
Option 1	Option 2	Option 3	
Administer daily INH, RIF, and PZA for 8 weeks followed by 16 weeks of INH and RIF daily or 2-3 times/week* in areas where the INH resistance rate is not documented to be <4%. EMB or SM should be added to the initial regimen until susceptibility to INH and RIF is demonstrated. Continue treatment for at least 6 months and 3 months beyond culture conversion. Consult a TB medical expert if the patient is symptomatic or smear or culture positive after 3 months.	Administer daily INH, RIF, PZA, and SM or EMB for 2 weeks followed by 2 times/week* administration of the same drugs for 6 weeks (by DOT), and subsequently, with 2 times/week administration of INH and RIF for 16 weeks (by DOT). Consult a TB medical expert if the patient is symptomatic or smear or culture positive after 3 months.	Treat by DOT, 3 times/week* with INH, RIF, PZA, and EMB or SM for 6 months.[†] Consult a TB medical expert if the patient is symptomatic or smear or culture positive after 3 months.	Option 1, 2, or 3 can be used, but treatment regimens should continue for a total of 9 months and at least 6 months beyond culture conversion.

DOT, directly observed therapy; EMB, ethambutol; INH, isoniazid; PZA, pyrazinamide; RIF, rifampin; SM, streptomycin; TB, tuberculosis.
*All regimens administered 2 times/week or 3 times/week should be monitored by DOT for the duration of therapy.

[†]The strongest evidence from clinical trials is the effectiveness of all four drugs administered for the full 6 months. There is weaker evidence that SM can be discontinued after 4 months if the isolate is susceptible to all drugs. The evidence for stopping PZA before the end of 6 months is equivocal for the 3 times/week regimen, and there is no evidence of the effectiveness of this regimen with EMB for less than the full 6 months.
From Centers for Disease Control and Prevention: Initial therapy for tuberculosis in the era of multidrug resistance. Recommendations of the Advisory Council for the Elimination of Tuberculosis. MMWR 42(No. RR-7):1-8, 1993.

Table 26-12.--Dosage Recommendation for Initial Treatment of Tuberculosis Among Children* and Adults

| | Dosage | | | | | |
| | Daily | | 2 times/week | | 3 times/week | |
Drugs	Children	Adults	Children	Adults	Children	Adults
Isoniazid	10-20 mg/kg	5 mg/kg	20-40 mg/kg	15 mg/kg	20-40 mg/kg	15 mg/kg
	Max., 300 mg	Max., 300 mg	Max., 900 mg	Max., 900 mg	Max., 900 mg	Max., 900 mg
Rifampin	10-20 mg/kg	10 mg/kg	10-20 mg/kg	10 mg/kg	10-20 mg/kg	10 mg/kg
	Max., 600 mg	Max., 600 mg	Max., 600 mg	Max., 600 mg	Max., 600 mg	Max., 600 mg
Pyrazinamide	15-30 mg/kg	15-30 mg/kg	50-70 mg/kg	50-70 mg/kg	50-70 mg/kg	50-70 mg/kg
	Max., 2 g	Max., 2 g	Max., 4 g	Max., 4 g	Max., 3 g	Max., 3 g
Ethambutol[†]	15-25 mg/kg	5-25 mg/kg	50 mg/kg	50 mg/kg	25-30 mg/kg	25-30 mg/kg
	Max., 2.5 g	Max., 2.5 g	Max., 2.5 g	Max., 2.5 g	Max., 2.5 g	Max., 2.5 g
Streptomycin	20-30 mg/kg	15 mg/kg	25-30 mg/kg	25-30 mg/kg	25-30 mg/kg	25-30 mg/kg
	Max., 1 g	Max., 1 g	Max., 1.5 g	Max., 1.5 g	Max., 1 g	Max., 1 g

*Children ≤12 years old.
[†]Ethambutol is generally not recommended for children whose visual acuity cannot be monitored (<6 years of age). However, ethambutol should be considered for all children with organisms resistant to other drugs, when susceptibility to ethambutol has been demonstrated, or susceptibility is likely.
From Centers for Disease Control and Prevention: Initial therapy for tuberculosis in the era of multidrug resistance. Recommendations of the Advisory Council for the Elimination of Tuberculosis. MMWR 42(No. RR-7):1-8, 1993.

is widely distributed in the environment. The organisms are isolated from older Caucasians, persons living in rural areas, and from patients with underlying COPD, bronchiectasis, prior tuberculosis, reflux esophagitis, or silicosis. *M. avium* complex usually exists as a saprophyte in patients with these conditions, but it may assume a pathogenic role in patients with AIDS and hairy-cell leukemia and in other patients with immunocompromised status. *M. avium* complex is a relatively common cause of noncontagious tuberculosis involving lymph nodes and bone. The organism is isolated from 21% of all mycobacterial pathogens (*M. tuberculosis* is isolated from 65%) and from 61% of all pathogenic nontuberculous mycobacteria. The highest rates of isolation are in Hawaii (10.8%), Connecticut (8.9%), Florida (8.4%), and Kansas (6.8%). In Wisconsin, Minnesota, Nebraska, Montana, and Hawaii, the number of isolates of *M. avium* complex exceeds that of *M. tuberculosis*. Nearly 30% of patients with isolates of *M. avium* complex have active disease. A clinically significant infection from atypical mycobacteria is diagnosed if the same organism is isolated repeatedly from the same source, if clinical features suggest active infection, and if tissue samples show active granuloma formation and organisms. In patients with AIDS, *M. avium* complex has been isolated from bone marrow, sputum/pulmonary tissue, blood, lymph node, gastrointestinal tract, and liver. A marked granulomatous response is not usually seen because of a severe decrease in the number of T lymphocytes. Patients with AIDS suspected to have *M. avium* complex infection should have their blood, bone marrow, lymph nodes, stool, small bowel biopsy, and bronchoscopic specimen tested for these organisms. Lung infection caused by *M. avium* complex may produce patchy nodules or infiltrates; the latter more closely resembles *M. tuberculosis* on chest radiography. Repeated sputum cultures and tissue sampling may be necessary to make the diagnosis of active infection.

- *M. avium* complex can become a pathogen in patients with AIDS, hairy-cell leukemia, silicosis, immunosuppression, and prosthetic devices and in the post-transplant state.
- The organisms exist as saprophytes in older Caucasians and in persons living in rural areas or who have underlying COPD, bronchiectasis, prior tuberculosis, reflux esophagitis, or silicosis.
- Higher incidence of disseminated *M. avium* complex in homosexual Caucasian males with AIDS; *M. tuberculosis* is more common in heroin addicts and Haitians

with AIDS.
- *M. avium* complex: a major cause of mortality and morbidity in patients with AIDS.

M. avium complex infection is highly resistant to medical treatment. For the usual "moderately severe" case of pulmonary disease, initial therapy should consist of isoniazid, rifampin, and ethambutol for 18-24 months, with streptomycin during the initial 2-3 months. For patients (immunologically intact) with a solitary pulmonary nodule, chemotherapy need not be given after resection. For patients with rapidly progressive (particularly AIDS) and highly symptomatic pulmonary disease, a more aggressive initial therapy is indicated-- one using regimens of 5-6 drugs, including ethionamide, cycloserine, and kanamycin as well as the agents listed in Table 26-12 and below. Initial chemotherapy with 5-6 drugs is also indicated for patients with life-threatening disseminated disease. For patients with localized pulmonary disease and adequate cardiorespiratory reserve, resection in combination with chemotherapy may offer a better outcome than chemotherapy alone.

- *M. avium* complex is usually resistant to antituberculous therapy.
- For the usual case, initial therapy should consist of isoniazid, rifampin, and ethambutol for 18-24 months, with streptomycin during the initial 2-3 months.
- For more serious infections, 5-6 drugs for a prolonged time (>18 months) may be required.

Patients with HIV infection and <100 CD4+ T lymphocytes/μL should be administered prophylaxis (rifabutin, 300 mg/day orally) against *M. avium* complex. Prophylaxis should be continued for the patient's lifetime. Disseminated *M. avium* complex infection should be treated with at least two agents, and every regimen should contain either azithromycin or clarithromycin. Therapy should be continued for patient's lifetime.

Other Mycobacteria

M. kansasii is also likely to infect previously damaged lungs. Clinically, it can resemble *M. tuberculosis* infection. The response to 3-drug therapy is good, with cure rates >85%. *M. kansasii* (as well as *M. avium* complex and *M. scrofulaceum*) are most commonly involved in cervical lymphadenopathy. Excision of the nodes is sufficient therapy in most cases.

Mycobacteria that are easy to treat include *M. haemophilum, M. kansasii, M. marianum, M. szulgai, M. ulcerans,* and *M. xenopi.*

Mycobacteria that are difficult to treat: *M. avium* complex, *M. chelonei, M. fortuitum, M. scrofulaceum,* and *M. simiae.*

Rarely pathogenic mycobacteria: *M. asiaticum* and *M. malmoense.*

Nonpathogenic species: *M. flavescens, M. gordonae, M. nonchromogenicum, M. parafortuitum, M. phlei, M. smegmatis, M. terrae* complex, *M. triviale,* and *M. vaccae.*

Pulmonary Mycoses

Serious fungal infections are found at autopsy in 2% of patients overall, in 5%-10% of patients with solid tumors, and in 20%-40% of patients dying of leukemia. Renal transplantation patients (15%) have a fungal infection at some time in their post-transplant course. Almost all mycoses produce granulomas. The saprophytic state of fungi is a common problem, particularly with aspergillus species.

Histoplasma capsulatum causes histoplasmosis. This infection is more common in the Mississippi, Ohio, and St. Lawrence River valleys. Infection is by inhalation of fungal spores. A large number of infectious spores are present in chicken coops, dusty areas, starling roosts, bat-infected caves, and decayed wood. Clinical forms include asymptomatic infection, symptomatic infection (similar to viral upper respiratory tract infection), disseminated (compromised host), chronic cavitary (structural defects), mediastinal granuloma, mediastinal fibrosis, pulmonary nodules, and calcified lesions on chest radiography. Hilar adenopathy may be seen. Skin testing is not useful in clinical practice. More than 80% of the population in endemic areas have positive findings on skin test. Skin test may produce positive serology. Complement fixation titer of >1:32 is not diagnostic but strongly supportive of active disease and may help as a prognostic indicator. Immunodiffusion shows that the H-band is the last to come and the first to go and the M-band is the first to come and the last to go. Recovery of the organism from body fluids, bone marrow, or tissue is diagnostic. The serum level of ACE may be increased in histoplasmosis. There is no need to treat acute disease (self-limiting). Progressive or disseminated disease requires therapy with antifungal agents.

Histoplasmosis: exposure to chicken coops, dusty

areas, starling roosts, bat-infected caves, and decayed wood.

Histoplasmin skin test should not be used to diagnose infection.

Chronic cavitary form clinically mimics chronic tuberculosis.

Mediastinal fibrosis, pulmonary calcification, broncholithiasis, and superior vena cava syndrome.

Commonest cause of mediastinal granuloma.

Coccidioides immitis causes coccidioidomycosis. The endemic zone extends from northern California to Argentina. Infections are more common when dry windy conditions exist, with epidemics occurring in the dry hot months after the rainy season, often after the soil is disturbed. Clinical forms include mildly symptomatic pulmonary infection (flu-like illness in 40% of patients), asymptomatic nodules or thin-walled cavities, coccidioidal pneumonia, chronic cavitary form, disseminated, and "valley fever" (erythema nodosum, erythema multiforme, arthralgia, arthritis, and eosinophilia). Chest radiography may show lobar infiltrates (70% of patients), scattered patchy areas, atelectasis, hilar adenopathy (25%), pleural effusion (3%), cavities (8%), nodules (5%), and normal findings (3%). Filipinos, African-Americans, and Mexicans are at greater risk of dissemination and death. Infection acquired late during pregnancy is associated with higher maternal and fetal mortality. Coccidioidin (mycelial phase) skin test (used previously) does not affect coccidioidomycosis serology but may produce positive serology for histoplasmosis. Thirty percent more cases are diagnosed with spherulin (parasitic phase) skin test (currently used) than with coccidioidin. The incidence of positive skin reaction in disseminated cases is higher (>60%). A violent reaction occurs if given to patients with erythema nodosum. Latex particle agglutination (IgM) serology is positive in 71% of patients within 2 weeks and in 90% within 4 weeks. The false-positive rate is 6%-10%; it has no value in detecting antibody in cerebrospinal fluid. Titer is not helpful in follow-up evaluation. Complement fixation (IgG) serology becomes positive later than the latex test; <10% are positive within first 10 days, 80% become positive in 4-6 weeks. Titer is very helpful in diagnosis and prognosis: a rapidly increasing titer is associated with a poor prognosis; a titer >1:16 is significant, and a titer <1:8 may persist for years. Positive cerebrospinal fluid titer confirms infection in the central nervous system.

- Coccidioidomycosis: southwestern U.S.; epidemics occur in the dry hot months after the rainy season.
- Clinical forms: asymptomatic nodules, thin-walled cavities, coccidioidal pneumonia, chronic cavitary form, and disseminated.
- Spherulin (parasitic phase) skin test (currently used) diagnoses 30% more cases than coccidiodin.
- Complement fixation serology is very helpful in diagnosis and prognosis.

Blastomyces dermatitidis causes blastomycosis. Mini-epidemics have occurred in North Carolina, Minnesota, and Illinois. One mini-epidemic involved campers in Wisconsin, "Namekagon fever." Most cases occur in the southern, south-central, and Great Lakes states. Persons in contact with soil are more likely to be infected. The male-to-female ratio is 10:1. Pulmonary forms are acute pneumonic form (resolution or progressive pulmonary involvement), asymptomatic, and insidious pulmonary or extrapulmonary dissemination. The most characteristic radiographic finding is a perihilar mass that mimics carcinoma. Pleural effusion is seen in <3% of patients with the pneumonic form. The skeletal system (vertebral bodies, ribs, skull, and long bones) is the second common site of dissemination, and the male genitourinary tract (excluding the kidneys) is the third most frequent site. The mucosa, central nervous system, adrenals, and other organs are not commonly involved. No good skin test or serology is available. In self-limiting or asymptomatic blastomycosis, amphotericin B therapy may not be needed. No skin test is available.

- Blastomycosis: contact with soil, manual laborers, and Great Lakes states.
- Most characteristic radiographic finding: a perihilar mass mimicking carcinoma.
- Extrapulmonary dissemination is seen in 65% of cases. Skin is the most frequent site of dissemination.
- Serologic test is available but unreliable.

Cryptococcus neoformans, the only fungus that is not dimorphic (no mycelia), causes cryptococcosis. The organism is widely distributed in the soil, foods, and excreta of pigeons and other animals. In humans, it may exist as a saprophyte in preexisting lung disease, but one-third to one-half of patients with cryptococcosis are immunosuppressed. The lung is the portal of entry, but the commonest clinical presentation is subacute or chronic meningitis (common cause of death). The diseases with which it is commonly associated are Hodgkin's and non-Hodgkin's disease, leukemia, sarcoidosis, and diabetes. The onset of central nervous system symptoms, fever, nausea, and anorexia is insidious. Pulmonary features include cough with scant sputum (15% of patients), chest pain (45%), dyspnea (25%), hemoptysis (7%), and night sweats (25%). Nodular infiltrates with cavitation, especially in the lower lobes, occasional hilar adenopathy, and solitary mass may be found. Diagnosis can be established by positive sputum cultures (35%), bronchoscopic specimens (35%), and open lung biopsy (100%). India ink preparation of the cerebrospinal fluid is positive in 30%-60% of patients. Serology (detects polysaccharide antigen) of the cerebrospinal fluid is positive in 90% of central nervous system infections and in 30% of non-central nervous system infections. Serology should be performed on blood, cerebrospinal fluid, and urine.

- *C. neoformans*: saprophytic or pathogenic state.
- Infection is more common in immunocompromised patients.
- Nodular, cavitary, and patchy infiltrates.
- The cerebrospinal fluid should be examined in almost all patients with organisms in respiratory secretions.

Aspergillus fumigatus, A. flavus, and *A. niger* are responsible for several pulmonary manifestations. The clinical forms include 1) allergic bronchopulmonary aspergillosis (discussed above), 2) hypersensitivity pneumonitis in red cedar wood workers, 3) mycetoma or fungus ball in preexisting lung disease, 4) locally invasive (chronic necrotizing) aspergillosis, 5) disseminated, 6) bronchocentric granulomatosis, and 7) saprophytic. The organism is ubiquitous and frequently colonizes the respiratory tract in patients with lung disease. Invasive aspergillosis in immunosuppressed hosts is the most serious form of infection and occurs mainly in granulocytopenic patients with hematologic malignancies. *Aspergillus* is isolated at autopsy in 10% of patients with acute leukemia. Of all patients with invasive aspergillosis (diagnosed pre or post mortem), 40% have acute lymphocytic leukemia, 20% have acute myelomonocytic leukemia, 10% have chronic myelogenous leukemia, 5% have Hodgkin's disease, and 10% have other hematologic malignancies. The presence of the organism in respiratory secretions is not diagnostic; tissue invasion should be documented. Aspergilloma is a mass of fungal hyphae in preexisting lung cavities. The major symptoms include hemoptysis, cough, low-grade fever, and weight loss.

Fungus ball can be caused by *Candida, Coccidioides, Nocardia,* and *Sporotrichum.* Chest radiographs and tomograms show a meniscus of air around the fungus ball (Monod's sign), almost always in the upper lobes. Skin testing gives positive results in 20% of patients, and serology is positive in >90%. Allergic bronchopulmonary aspergillosis shows positive skin test findings in 100% of patients and positive serology in >75%.

- Granulocytopenia and lung infiltrates in hematologic malignancies almost always mean disseminated aspergillosis.
- Aspergillosis is frequently accompanied by *Pseudomonas* or *Candida.*
- Aspergilloma (fungus ball) occurs in previously damaged lung; hemoptysis is a serious complication.

Zygomycetes includes the order Mucorales (phycomycetes) and causes zygomycosis. The organisms have a worldwide distribution. Serious infections of the lungs, central nervous system, and skin are seen in patients with diabetes, hematologic malignancies, skin or mucosal injuries, and those receiving cytotoxic drugs. The organism invades blood vessels (as does *Aspergillus*) and may cause significant hemoptysis. Chest radiography may show patchy infiltrates, consolidation, cavitation, and effusions. Bronchial stenosis is a peculiar complication of zygomycosis. The diagnosis must be established by biopsy, although sputum culture may suggest it. No serology is available. Zygomycosis is the only nonseptate fungus.

- Immunocompromised and diabetic patients.
- Propensity to invade blood vessels; hemoptysis is common.
- In a poorly controlled diabetic patient with swelling of eyelids and black discharge from the nose, consider zygomycosis.

Candida albicans causes candidiasis and is responsible for about 75% of serious infections. This is a ubiquitous organism that is present in the oropharynx of 30% of normal persons, in the gastrointestinal tract in 65% of normal persons, and in the vagina of 30%-70% of women. Systemic candidiasis is found at autopsy in as many as 25% of patients with leukemia. Other risk factors are diabetes, cancer, cirrhosis, renal failure, blood dyscrasia, cytotoxic therapy, intravenous or urinary catheters, antibiotics given intravenously, prostheses, cachexia, and burns.

Lung involvement is relatively rare, and chest radiography shows patchy or diffuse infiltrates. *Candida* bronchitis, an occupational disease of tea tasters, is manifested by low-grade fever, cough, and patchy infiltrates.

- Candidiasis: more common in patients with hematologic malignancies.
- Prolonged granulocytopenia predisposes to disseminated infection.
- Lung involvement is uncommon; patchy or diffuse lung infiltrates.

Sporothrix schenckii causes sporotrichosis. The organism is a dimorphous fungus that exists as a saprophyte in the soil, plants, wood, straw, sphagnum moss, decaying vegetation, cats, dogs, and rodents. Sporotrichosis is an occupational hazard for farmers, florists, gardeners, horticulturists, and forestry workers. Infection is by cutaneous inoculation. Cutaneous nodules along lymphatics may appear in 75% of patients. Hematogenous dissemination to the lungs is rare, but inhalation-induced pulmonary disease mimics cavitary tuberculosis. The diagnosis is made by tissue examination. Latex agglutination with an increasing titer and a titer of >1:80 suggest active disease. Skin infection may be associated with negative serology.

- Sporotrichosis: florists, horticulturists, and gardeners.
- Lymphangitis of the skin and subcutaneous nodules.
- Pulmonary infection mimics chronic tuberculosis.

Nocardia asteroides (also *N. brasiliensis* and *N. caviae*) causes nocardiosis. *N. asteroides* is a weakly acid-fast organism that is a saprophyte in the soil, dust, plants, and water. The lungs and central nervous system are the two commonly involved organs. Infection is more common in immunosuppressed patients and in patients with pulmonary alveolar proteinosis. Primary infection leads to necrotizing pneumonia with abscess formation. No inflammatory response or granuloma formation occurs. Infection may produce pleural effusion. Lymphohematogenous spread is seen in 20% of patients; nearly all these have brain abscesses. The diagnosis is made at autopsy in 40% of cases. Isolation of the organism from respiratory secretions is not diagnostic of infection, because the saprophytic state is well recognized. No serologic test is available.

- Nocardiosis: immunocompromised patients and those

with pulmonary alveolar proteinosis.
- Necrotizing pneumonia and lung abscess.
- Saprophytic state should be differentiated from pathogenic state.
- Central nervous system involvement common in those with disseminated infection.

Actinomyces israelii or *A. bovis* cause actinomycosis. The organism is a fungus-like bacterium. *Actinomyces* is not found in the soil or vegetation but is easily isolated from scrapings around the teeth, gums, and tonsils. It is an opportunistic infection and becomes invasive with severe caries, tissue necrosis, and aspiration. In tissue, the organism grows into a "sulfur granule" caused by mycelial clumps in a matrix of $CaPO_4$. The disease is more common in rural areas, with a male-to-female ratio of 2:1. Infection is always mixed with anaerobes. Skin abscesses, ulcers, sinus tracts, and cervicofacial node involvement are found in 30%-40% of cases. Pulmonary involvement is seen in 20%, with cough, fever, pulmonary consolidation, pleurisy with effusion, and, eventually, draining sinuses. Serology (agar double-dilution test) is positive in 90% of cases of disseminated disease, and negative in localized infection.

- Actinomycosis: associated with severe dental caries, tissue necrosis, and aspiration; opportunistic infection.
- Sulfur granules from abscesses, fistulas, or wounds.
- Cough, fever, pulmonary lesions, pleural effusion, and fistula and sinus tracts.

Protozoal Infections

Included in protozoal infections are *Pneumocystis carinii*, toxoplasmosis, and amebiasis. *Pneumocystis carinii* is either a protozoan or a fungus with trophozoite and cyst stages. The cyst stains best with methenamine silver nitrate. This organism is seen mainly in immunosuppressed patients and accounts for 40% of the cases of interstitial pneumonia in these patients. The frequency of infection increases in proportion to the intensity of immunosuppressive treatment. *P. carinii* infection is seen in 5% of patients receiving treatment with a single drug, 28% of those receiving four drugs, and 43% of those receiving polychemotherapy and irradiation. Patients with AIDS are in the high-risk group for *P. carinii* infection. Infection causes alveolar and interstitial inflammation and edema, with plasma cell infiltrates. Organisms are found in alveolar macrophages. Clinical features include abrupt onset of fever, tachypnea, hypoxia,

cyanosis, respiratory distress, relatively normal findings on lung examination, and a patchy or diffuse interstitial/alveolar process. Routine laboratory data are unhelpful. The diagnosis can be made with induced sputum, bronchoalveolar lavage, or lung biopsy findings.

- *P. carinii* infection: respiratory symptoms and signs are more serious in non-AIDS patients.
- Induced sputum and bronchoalveolar lavage are excellent methods for diagnosis.
- The number of organisms in tissue preparations from non-AIDS patients is smaller.
- Upper lobe process seen on chest radiography in patients receiving pentamidine aerosol therapy.

Noninfectious Pulmonary Complications in AIDS

Infectious pulmonary complications are discussed in Chapter 20. Noninfectious complications include diffuse interstitial lung disease, lymphocytic interstitial pneumonitis, cystic lung disease, pneumothorax, pulmonary hypertension, Kaposi's sarcoma, and non-Hodgkin's lymphoma.

Nonspecific interstitial pneumonitis is a common occurrence in patients with chronic AIDS and represents 30%-40% of all episodes of lung infiltrates in these patients. More than 25% of patients with this problem have either concurrent Kaposi's sarcoma, previous experimental therapies, or a history of *P. carinii* pneumonia or drug abuse. The clinical features are similar to those of patients with *P. carinii* pneumonia. Histopathologic features of the lung in interstitial pneumonitis associated with AIDS may include varying degrees of edema, fibrin deposition, and interstitial inflammation with lymphocytes and plasma cells. There is no known therapy.

- More than 25% of patients with interstitial pneumonitis have either concurrent Kaposi's sarcoma, previous experimental therapies, or a history of *P. carinii* pneumonia or drug abuse.

Lymphocytic interstitial pneumonitis is caused by pulmonary infiltration with mature polyclonal B lymphocytes and plasma cells. It occurs in children of mothers in groups at high risk for AIDS, Haitians, and patients with AIDS. Systemic corticosteroid therapy may produce significant improvement. Lymphocytic interstitial pneumonitis is a nonspecific entity in adults with AIDS.

- Lymphocytic interstitial pneumonitis is diagnostic of AIDS when it occurs in a child younger than 13 years old with positive HIV serology.
- Pulmonary lymphoid hyperplasia has been reported in 40% of children with AIDS.

Cystic lung disease is more common in patients with *P. carinii* infections and in those receiving aerosolized pentamidine therapy. Cystic lesions are more common in the upper and mid lung zones. Chest CT identifies these small- to medium-sized cystic lesions. Pneumothorax occurs with increasing frequency in patients with *P. carinii* pneumonia and in those receiving pentamidine aerosol therapy. Cystic lesions and pneumothorax may be interrelated.

- Cystic lung disease and pneumothorax are more common in those with *P. carinii* pneumonia and in those receiving aerosolized pentamidine therapy.

Pulmonary hypertension has been found in patients with AIDS. The mechanism is not clear, but HIV is thought to affect directly the endothelium and cause vascular changes. The clinical, physiologic, and pathologic features are identical to those in primary pulmonary hypertension.

- Pulmonary hypertension in AIDS is clinically identical to that in idiopathic pulmonary hypertension.

Kaposi's sarcoma occurs with a greater frequency in homosexuals with AIDS. The incidence of this sarcoma has gradually decreased. Previous or concurrent pulmonary opportunistic infections have been noted in >70% of patients. Pulmonary involvement from Kaposi's sarcoma occurs in 18%-35% of patients with this sarcoma. In most patients, pulmonary Kaposi's sarcoma is established only at autopsy. The diagnostic yield from bronchoscopy is 24% and from lung biopsy is 56%. Hemoptysis is an uncommon complication in Kaposi's sarcoma, although nearly 30% of patients develop endobronchial metastasis. Chest radiography may show the typical nodular infiltrates in a small number (<10%) of patients. The more nodular (as opposed to interstitial) pattern and the rather slow evolution of lung infiltrates from Kaposi's sarcoma are different from the relatively rapidly evolving *P. carinii* pneumonia.

- Pulmonary Kaposi's sarcoma is frequently preceded by cutaneous lesions.
- Pulmonary involvement from Kaposi's sarcoma occurs in 18%-35% of patients with this sarcoma.
- At autopsy, lung involvement is found in nearly 50% of patients with Kaposi's sarcoma.
- Clinically, pulmonary Kaposi's sarcoma is indistinguishable from *P. carinii* pneumonia or opportunistic pneumonia.
- Multiple, discrete, raised, violaceous, or bright red tracheobronchial lesions can be seen with bronchoscopy.
- Endobronchial lesions are also caused by *M. avium* complex.

Non-Hodgkin's lymphoma involving the lungs is seen in a small number (<10%) of patients with AIDS. The lymphoma in these patients is usually extranodal non-Hodgkin's B-cell lymphoma.

Multiple Choice

1. Severe deficiency of α_1-antitrypsin typically produces which of the following pulmonary diseases?
   a. Panlobular emphysema
   b. Chronic bronchitis
   c. Diffuse bronchiectasis
   d. Cystic fibrosis
   e. Centrilobular emphysema

2. Patients with severe anatomical emphysema demonstrate the following:
   a. Decreased residual volume
   b. Decreased total lung capacity
   c. Increased vital capacity
   d. Diminished diffusing capacity for carbon monoxide
   e. Increased arterial carbon dioxide

3. Cystic fibrosis is transmitted by which of the following genetic mechanisms?
   a. Autosomal dominant
   b. Autosomal recessive
   c. Autosomal codominant
   d. X-linked dominant
   e. Unknown mode of inheritance

4. A 26-year-old man presents with a 7-year history of persistent cough with varying amounts of mucus production, occasional wheezing, and mild exertional dyspnea. In addition to clinical examination and chest radiography, initial evaluations of this patient's respiratory illness should include all the following tests except:
   a. Spirometry with bronchodilator
   b. Estimation of α_1-antitrypsin level
   c. Quantitative pilocarpine iontophoresis
   d. Tests to exclude infertility
   e. Quantitation of immunoglobulin levels

5. Which of the following entities is not associated with smoking and/or aggravated by smoking?
   a. Pulmonary alveolar proteinosis
   b. Pulmonary eosinophilic granuloma
   c. Small cell carcinoma
   d. Calcification of asbestos-induced pleural plaques
   e. Pulmonary alveolar microlithiasis

6. Which of the following statements is incorrect about hypersensitivity pneumonitis?
   a. Majority of cases are due to fungal precipitins
   b. Silo-filler's lung disease is a typical example of hypersensitivity pneumonitis
   c. In the acute form, symptoms usually appear 4-6 hours after exposure to antigen(s)
   d. Positive serology is not diagnostic of hypersensitivity pneumonitis
   e. Chronic disease may remain undetected for years and may resemble idiopathic pulmonary fibrosis

7. A 30-year-old woman with no history of smoking or asthma presents with exertional dyspnea and cough. Chest radiography reveals a diffuse bilateral interstitial/nodular process. Pulmonary function tests show moderately severe obstructive dysfunction. These findings are not compatible with which of the following?
   a. Diffuse bronchiectasis
   b. Sjögren's syndrome
   c. Idiopathic pulmonary fibrosis
   d. Pulmonary lymphangioleiomyomatosis
   e. Pulmonary eosinophilic granuloma

8. A 24-year-old white man who is a smoker presents with pain in his left humerus as a result of a solitary cystic lesion in the bone. Evaluations include chest radiography, which shows a bilateral reticulonodular process, most pronounced in the upper two-thirds of both lungs, and an osteolytic lesion of a rib. The most likely diagnosis is:
   a. Sarcoidosis with bone involvement
   b. Hodgkin's lymphoma with pulmonary and skeletal involvement
   c. Acute histoplasmosis with systemic dissemination
   d. Pulmonary eosinophilic granuloma with bone involvement
   e. Scleroderma with lung disease

9. Systemic corticosteroid therapy is not indicated in:
   a. Asymptomatic stage I (type I) sarcoidosis
   b. Berylliosis
   c. Sarcoidosis with persistent hypercalcemia
   d. Acute rheumatoid lung disease
   e. Chronic eosinophilic pneumonia

10. Cytotoxic reaction (autoantibody or type II immune

reaction) is exemplified by which of the following diseases?

a. Goodpasture's syndrome
b. Rheumatoid lung disease
c. Allergic bronchopulmonary aspergillosis
d. Penicillin anaphylaxis
e. Hereditary angioneurotic edema

11. Which of the following statements about uremic pulmonary edema is incorrect?

a. It is seen in acute and chronic renal failure
b. It is commonly due to intra-alveolar bleeding
c. It is caused by pulmonary arterial damage from a uremic process
d. It is usually noncardiogenic in origin
e. Intra-alveolar fluid is usually an exudate

12. Which of the following is the least common manifestation of systemic lupus erythematosus?

a. Diffuse interstitial process
b. Plate-like (discoid) atelectasis
c. Pleural effusion
d. Pulmonary hemorrhage
e. Diaphragmatic dysfunction

13. Diffuse pulmonary disease is more likely to be seen in which of the following?

a. Rheumatoid arthritis
b. Systemic lupus erythematosus
c. Scleroderma
d. Sjögren's syndrome
e. Ankylosing spondylitis

14. A 53-year-old woman presents with chronic progressive dyspnea. Other symptoms and signs include dizziness, thickened skin over fingers, Raynaud's phenomenon, dysphagia, reflux, and telangiectases over the face. Which of the following is least likely to occur in this patient?

a. Pleural effusion
b. Pulmonary hypertension
c. Diffuse interstitial pulmonary process
d. Aspiration pneumonia
e. Cor pulmonale

15. Rheumatoid arthritis may be associated with all the following pulmonary complications except:

a. Obstructive airway disease

b. Aspiration pneumonia from esophageal dysmotility
c. Exudative pleural effusion
d. Bronchiolitis obliterans
e. Multiple pulmonary nodules

16. A 35-year-old man presents with a 2-year history of gradually progressive dyspnea and cough. He has been employed in a pet store where he handles birds. Chest radiography reveals diffuse interstitial process, and pulmonary function tests show restrictive dysfunction with diminished diffusing capacity for carbon monoxide. Which of the following diagnoses is most likely?

a. Pneumonia secondary to *Chlamydia pneumoniae* (TWAR agent)
b. Psittacosis secondary to *Chlamydia psittaci*
c. Cryptococcosis
d. Hypersensitivity pneumonitis
e. Histoplasmosis

17. A 19-year-old woman presents with a 10-day history of fever, sore throat, and cough. She just returned from college. Examination reveals a bullous lesion over the left tympanic membrane and diminished lung sounds over right lower lobe. Chest radiography shows a tiny right pleural effusion. The treatment of choice is:

a. Erythromycin
b. Trimethoprim-sulfamethoxazole
c. Penicillin
d. Amoxicillin
e. Ciprofloxacin

18. A 62-year-old man, a heavy smoker, is hospitalized because of alcohol-induced stupor. After initial treatment, chest radiography shows a large cavity with an air-fluid level in the superior segment of the right lower lobe. Which of the following initial measures is not appropriate?

a. Penicillin by intravenous route
b. Gram's staining and culture of sputum
c. Bronchoscopy to obtain culture material
d. Thoracoscopic drainage of the lung abscess under topical anesthesia
e. Sputum cytology

19. A patient dies of complications from AIDS. Autopsy shows disseminated infection caused by

Mycobacterium avium complex. The 28-year-old woman resident physician who treated the patient develops cough; her chest radiograph shows nodular infiltrate in the left upper lobe, and the tuberculin test elicits a 12-mm induration. The most appropriate next step is to:

a. Immediately begin antituberculous therapy with at least four drugs because *Mycobacterium avium-intracellulare* is resistant to two-drug therapy
b. Obtain sputum and gastric washings for acid-fast bacilli
c. Start prophylactic isoniazid 300 mg/day for 12 months
d. Begin isoniazid and rifampin with plan to treat for 18 months
e. Order HIV serology

20. A 34-year-old man with acute myelocytic leukemia develops progressive respiratory distress, and chest radiography shows diffuse alveolar infiltrates. The patient had completed intensive chemotherapy 6 weeks earlier. The total leukocyte count has remained <900/mm^3 for over 3 weeks. He is currently receiving cephalosporin (3rd generation) intravenously. Which of the following is the most appropriate treatment?

a. Blood transfusion to increase the number of leukocytes in the circulation
b. Antibiotics to cover gram-negative bacteria
c. Amphotericin B given intravenously
d. Antituberculous therapy using at least three drugs
e. Trimethoprim-sulfamethoxazole given intravenously

True/False
21. Diffusing capacity for carbon monoxide is diminished in:
a. Anatomical emphysema
b. During early phase of an asthmatic attack
c. Right-to-left shunt
d. Polycythemia
e. Supine posture
f. Intra-alveolar hemorrhage

22. The following manifestations are relatively common in adult patients with cystic fibrosis:
a. Hemoptysis
b. Pneumothorax
c. Sinusitis and nasal polyposis
d. Pancreatic insufficiency

e. Intussusception and fecal impaction
f. Retrolental fibroplasia

23. Noncaseous granuloma can be seen in the following disease entities:
a. Sarcoidosis
b. Mycobacterial infections
c. Hypersensitivity pneumonitis
d. Berylliosis
e. Tobacco bronchitis
f. Silicosis

24. Bronchoalveolar lavage is helpful in the diagnosis of diffuse pulmonary disease caused by the following diseases:
a. Lymphangitic carcinomatosis
b. Diffuse alveolar sarcoidosis
c. Pulmonary eosinophilic granuloma (histiocytosis X)
d. Hypersensitivity pneumonitis
e. Pneumonia caused by *Pneumocystis carinii*
f. Silicosis

25. A 28-year-old woman complains of progressive dyspnea and abdominal swelling and discomfort. Recently, she had mild hemoptysis and has had two episodes of pneumothorax on the right. Her abdomen is doughy to palpate and ascites is noted. Chest radiography shows diffuse nodular changes and left pleural effusion. Thoracentesis shows chylous fluid. The following is/are likely in this patient:
a. Diabetes insipidus
b. Smooth muscle hyperplasia in lung parenchyma
c. Obstructive pulmonary dysfunction
d. Chylous ascites
e. Potential for therapy with progesterone/oophorectomy
f. Restrictive type of lung dysfunction

26. A 50-year-old woman has gradual onset of dyspnea, difficulty in swallowing, recurrent bouts of aspiration, and difficulty in getting up from a sitting position. The erythrocyte sedimentation rate is 85 mm/hour, and the creatine phosphokinase level is increased to 5x normal level. Which of the following features is/are likely to occur in this patient?
a. Basal interstitial infiltrates
b. Progressive increase in PaCO$_2$

c. Aspiration pneumonia
d. Cor pulmonale
e. Progressive obstructive lung disease
f. Large bilateral pleural effusions

27. The following infections tend to occur in outbreaks among closed populations:
    a. *Mycoplasma* pneumonia
    b. *Haemophilus influenzae* pneumonia
    c. *Moraxella catarrhalis* pneumonia
    d. *Chlamydia pneumoniae* pneumonia
    e. Tularemia
    f. Tuberculosis

28. A 23-year-old pigeon breeder/laborer and nonsmoker has gradual onset of cough and mild exertional dyspnea over a 3-year period. Chest radiography shows mediastinal widening, subcarinal lymphadenopathy with large intranodal calcification, and extrinsic compression of the left main stem bronchus. This patient is at risk for developing:
    a. Bronchogenic carcinoma
    b. Superior vena caval obstruction
    c. Dysphagia
    d. Hemoptysis
    e. Broncholithiasis
    f. Nephrolithiasis

NOTES

CHAPTER 27

RHEUMATOLOGY I

William W. Ginsburg, M.D.

CRYSTALLINE ARTHROPATHIES

Gout and Hyperuricemia

Hyperuricemia has been described in 2%-18% of normal populations, but the prevalence of clinical gouty arthritis ranges from 0.1%-0.4%. There is a family history of gout in 6%-18% of patients. Genetic studies suggest a multifactorial inheritance pattern. Of patients with hyperuricemia whose uric acid level is >9 mg/dL, gout will develop in 5 years in approximately 20%.

- Hyperuricemia occurs in 2%-18% of normal populations.
- Prevalence of gouty arthritis is 0.1%-0.4%.
- 6%-18% of patients have family history of gout.
- In patients with uric acid level >9 mg/dL, gout develops in 20% in 5 years.

Hyperuricemia may result from uric acid overproduction or underexcretion, or both. Overproduction is the cause in ≤10% of patients with primary gout. Of these 10%, about 15% have one of the two X-linked inborn errors of purine metabolism: 1) hypoxanthine-guanine phosphoribosyltransferase (HGPRTase) deficiency (Lesch-Nyhan syndrome) and 2) 5-phosphoribosyl-1-pyrophosphate (PRPP) synthetase overactivity. Of the remaining 90% of patients who have overproduction, most are obese, but the cause of overproduction and the relationship between obesity and overproduction of uric acid remain unknown.

- ≤10% of patients with primary gout have overproduction of uric acid.

Underexcretion of uric acid occurs in approximately 90% of patients with gout. They have reduced filtration of uric acid, enhanced tubular reabsorption, or decreased tubular secretion.

Events leading to initial crystallization of monosodium urate in the joint after approximately 30 years of asymptomatic hyperuricemia are unknown. Trauma with disruption of microtophi in cartilage leads to release of urate crystals into synovial fluid. The urate crystals become coated with immunoglobulin and then complement. They are then phagocytosed by leukocytes with subsequent release of chemotactic protein, activation of the kallikrein system, and disruption of the leukocytes, which release lysosomal enzymes into synovial fluid.

- Events leading to initial crystallization of monosodium urate in joint after years of asymptomatic hyperuricemia are unknown.

Important Enzyme Abnormalities in Uric Acid Pathway

Lesch-Nyhan syndrome is a complete deficiency of hypoxanthine-guanine phosphoribosyltransferase. It is characterized by X-linked disorder in young boys, hyperuricemia, self-mutilation, choreoathetosis, spasticity, growth retardation, and severe gouty arthritis (Fig. 27-1).

- Lesch-Nyhan syndrome characterized by X-linked disorder in young boys, self-mutilation, spasticity, severe gouty arthritis.

5-Phosphoribosyl-1-pyrophosphate (PRPP) synthetase

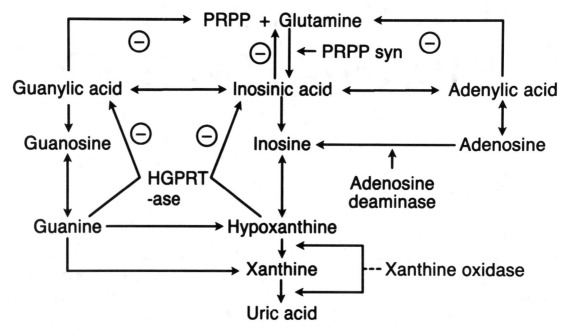

Fig. 27-1. Purine metabolism. HGPRT-ase, hypoxanthine-guanine phosphoribosyltransferase; PRPP, phosphoribosylpyrophosphate; PRPP syn, phosphoribosylpyrophosphate synthetase; ⊖, feedback inhibition.

overactivity is associated with hyperuricemia, X-linked disorder, and gouty arthritis.

Adenosine deaminase deficiency is autosomal recessive. There is a buildup of deoxyadenosine triphosphate in lymphocytes, which is toxic to immature lymphocytes. It is a combined immunodeficiency state with severe T-cell and mild B-cell dysfunction. Features of the disorder are hypouricemia, recurrent infection, chondro-osseous dysplasia, and elevated deoxyadenosine in plasma and urine. Treatment for the disorder is with irradiated frozen red blood cells or marrow transplantation.

- Adenosine deaminase deficiency is combined immunodeficiency state with severe T-cell and mild B-cell dysfunction.
- It is autosomal recessive.
- Features are hypouricemia and recurrent infection.

Xanthine oxidase deficiency is autosomal recessive. It is characterized by hypouricemia, xanthinuria with xanthine stones, and myopathy associated with deposits of xanthine and hypoxanthine.

- Xanthine oxidase deficiency is characterized by hypouricemia.
- It is autosomal recessive.

Causes of Secondary Hyperuricemia

Secondary hyperuricemia can be attributed to increased catabolism (turnover) of purine and decreased renal clearance of uric acid (Table 27-1).

Causes of Hypouricemia

Increased urinary excretion of uric acid contributes to hypouricemia. It can develop in healthy persons with an isolated defect in tubular reabsorption of uric acid. It is also related to diminished reabsorption of urate, such as in Fanconi syndrome, Fanconi syndrome associated with Wilson's disease, carcinoma of the lung, acute myelogenous leukemia, light-chain disease, and use of outdated tetracycline. Malignant neoplasms, such as carcinoma, Hodgkin's disease, and sarcoma, are also associated with increased uric acid excretion. Hypervolemia caused by inappropriate secretion of antidiuretic hormone can also be a factor. Drugs involved in increased uric acid excretion are high-dose aspirin, probenecid and other uricosuric agents, and glyceryl guaiacolate. Radiographic contrast agents that can cause hypouricemia are iopanoic acid (Telopaque), iodipamide meglumine (Cholografin), and diatrizoate sodium (Hypaque). It can also occur in severe liver disease.

- Causes of increased urinary excretion of uric acid are isolated defect in tubular reabsorption of uric acid, Fanconi syndrome, carcinoma of lung, acute myelogenous leukemia, drugs (high-dose aspirin, probenecid), radiographic contrast agents, and severe liver disease.

Table 27-1.--Causes of Secondary Hyperuricemia

Increased catabolism (turnover) of purine
  Myeloproliferative disorders
    Polycythemia, primary or secondary
    Myeloid metaplasia
    Chronic myelocytic leukemia
  Lymphoproliferative disorders
    Chronic lymphatic leukemia
    Multiple myeloma
  Disseminated carcinoma and sarcoma
  Sickle cell anemia and other forms of chronic hemolytic
    anemia
  Psoriasis (uncommon)
  Cytotoxic drugs
Decreased renal clearance of uric acid
  Intrinsic disease of the kidney
    Chronic renal insufficiency of diverse cause
    Saturnine gout (lead nephropathy)
    Sickle cell anemia
  Functional impairment in tubular transport of uric acid--
    mostly a decrease in secretion
    Drug-induced: thiazide diuretics, furosemide,
      ethacrynic acid, ethambutol, pyrazinamide, low doses
      of aspirin, cyclosporine
    Hyperlactic acidemia: lactic acidosis, ethanolism,
      preeclampsia, glycogen storage disease type I, chronic
      beryllium disease
    Hyperketoacidemia (acetoacetic and β-hydroxybutyric
      acids): diabetic ketoacidosis, starvation, glycogen
      storage disease type I
    Congenital vasopressin-resistant diabetes insipidus
    Bartter's syndrome (hyperaldosteronism and
      hypokalemic alkalosis)
    Down's syndrome

Decreased synthesis of uric acid can also cause hypouricemia. The drug allopurinol inhibits the enzyme xanthine oxidase, causing hypouricemia. The decrease can also be caused by congenital deficiencies in enzymes involved in purine biosynthesis: 5-phosphoribosyl-1-pyrophosphate synthetase deficiency, adenosine deaminase deficiency, purine nucleoside phosphorylase deficiency, and xanthine oxidase deficiency (xanthinuria). Acquired deficiency in xanthine oxidase activity (metastatic adenocarcinoma of lung) can also cause decreased synthesis of uric acid, as can acute intermittent porphyria.

- Decreased synthesis of uric acid caused by congenital deficiency in enzymes involved in purine biosynthesis.

Predisposing Factors to Gout and Pseudogout

The following can predispose to an attack of gout or pseudogout: trauma, operation (3 days after), major medical illness (myocardial infarction, cerebrovascular accident, pulmonary embolus), fasting, alcohol use, and infection.

- Factors that precipitate gout and pseudogout: trauma, operation, alcohol.

Treatment of Acute Gouty Arthritis

Do not administer allopurinol or probenecid until the acute attack completely subsides. Because of severe gastrointestinal side effects, oral colchicine is rarely used any more for acute attack. Intravenously administered colchicine (1-2 mg) has no gastrointestinal side effects. It causes increased toxicity in patients with elevated creatinine values. In patients with a history of heart failure or gastric or duodenal ulcers, this is drug of choice. It can cause severe extravasation if it infiltrates into subcutaneous tissues.

- Colchicine: severe gastrointestinal side effects with oral form, no gastrointestinal side effects with intravenous administration.

Indomethacin (or other nonsteroidal anti-inflammatory drugs) is one of the drugs of choice when used for 7- to 10-day course and when there is no contraindication to its use. Do not use it in patients with congestive heart failure or gastric ulcer. It can have marked sodium retention properties. It should not be used in patients with nasal polyps and aspirin sensitivity because indomethacin may cause bronchospasm. Frontal headache is an uncommon side effect.

- Avoid indomethacin in patients with congestive heart failure or peptic ulcer.
- Avoid indomethacin in patients with nasal polyps and aspirin allergy.

Intra-articular or oral corticosteroids are other treatments.

Treatment of Intercritical Period

Probenecid is a uricosuric. It inhibits tubular reabsorption of filtered and secreted urate, thereby increasing urinary excretion of uric acid. Colchicine, 0.6 mg twice a day, is given prophylactically for 6-12 months to prevent exacerbation of acute gout. It should not be used if the patient has a history of kidney stones or if 24-hour urine uric acid value is >1,000 mg (normal, <600 mg/day). Probenecid delays renal excretion of indomethacin and thereby increases its blood level. Probenecid delays the renal excretion of acetylsalicylic acid (ASA), and ASA completely blocks the uricosuric effect of probenecid. ASA also blocks tubular secretion of urates. Do not use probenecid with methotrexate because probenecid increases methotrexate blood levels, which increase toxicity from methotrexate.

- Probenecid inhibits tubular reabsorption of filtered and secreted urate.
- Not used if patient has a history of kidney stones or if 24-hour uric acid value is >1,000 mg/day.
- Delays renal excretion of indomethacin.
- Delays renal excretion of ASA.
- Do not use with methotrexate.

Allopurinol is a xanthine oxidase inhibitor. It can precipitate acute gout, so colchicine, 0.6 mg twice a day, is given for 6-12 months. It is the drug of choice if the patient has a history of renal stones or renal insufficiency. If allopurinol is used, the dose of 6-mercaptopurine or azathioprine needs to be reduced by 25%. Allopurinol and probenecid are usually not used simultaneously unless the patient has extensive tophaceous gout with good renal function. Allopurinol can cause rash and a severe toxicity syndrome consisting of eosinophilia, fever, hepatitis, decreased renal function, and an erythematous desquamative rash. This usually occurs in patients with decreased renal function. Allopurinol should be given in the lowest dose possible to keep the uric acid value <6 mg/dL.

- Allopurinol is xanthine oxidase inhibitor.
- It can precipitate gout.
- It is drug of choice if patient has history of renal stones or renal insufficiency.
- Can cause severe toxicity syndrome: eosinophilia, fever, hepatitis, decreased renal function, erythematous desquamative rash.

The indications for allopurinol rather than probenecid for lowering the uric acid level are tophaceous gout, gout complicated by renal insufficiency, uric acid excretion >1,000 mg/day, history of uric acid calculi, use of cytotoxic drugs, allergy to uricosuric agents, and secondary hyperuricemia with overproduction of uric acid. Allo-

purinol should be used before treatment of rapidly proliferating tumors. The nucleic acid liberated with cytolysis is converted to uric acid and can cause renal failure secondary to precipitation of uric acid in collecting ducts and ureters (acute tumor lysis syndrome). Patients should also have adequate hydration and alkalinization of the urine before chemotherapy.

- Indications for allopurinol: tophaceous gout, gout complicated by renal insufficiency, history of uric acid calculi, use of cytotoxic drugs.

Renal Disease and Uric Acid

Renal function is not necessarily adversely affected by an elevated serum urate concentration. The incidence of interstitial renal disease and renal insufficiency is no greater than that in patients of comparable age with similar degrees of hypertension, arteriosclerotic heart disease, diabetes, and primary renal disease. Correction of hyperuricemia (to ≤10 mg /dL) has no apparent effect on renal function. Most rheumatologists do not treat asymptomatic hyperuricemia if the uric acid level is <10.0 mg/dL (normal, to 8.0). When hyperuricemia is associated with a urinary uric acid >1,100 mg/24 hours, which increases the risk of uric acid stones, renal function should be observed closely. Excessive exposure to lead may contribute to the renal disease found in some patients with gout.

- Renal function not adversely affected by elevated serum urate concentration.
- Correction of hyperuricemia (to ≤10 mg/dL) has no apparent effect on renal function.

Miscellaneous Points of Importance

- Positive diagnosis of a crystalline arthritis requires identification of crystal by polarization microscopy.
- Uric acid crystals are strongly negatively birefringent (needle-shaped).
- 30% of patients with chronic tophaceous gout will be positive for rheumatoid factor (usually weakly positive).
- 10% of patients with acute gout will be positive for rheumatoid factor (usually weakly positive).
- 5%-10% of patients will have simultaneous gout and pseudogout attack.
- 50% of synovial fluids aspirated from first metatarsophalangeal joints of asymptomatic patients with gout have crystals of monosodium urate.

- Gout in premenopausal female is very unusual.
- There have been many recent reports of superimposed gout occurring in Heberden's and Bouchard's nodes in older women taking diuretics.
- A septic joint can trigger a gout or pseudogout attack in a predisposed person. Always obtain synovial fluid analysis for crystals, Gram stain, and culture. The frequency of gout in patients who have had cardiac transplantation is high (25%). Both cyclosporine and diuretics cause hyperuricemia.

Calcium Pyrophosphate Deposition Disease

Etiologic Classification

Calcium pyrophosphate deposition disease (CPPD) is classified as idiopathic, hereditary, or associated with metabolic disease. The associated diseases include hyperparathyroidism, hemochromatosis-hemosiderosis, hypothyroidism, gout (5% of patients have gout and pseudogout simultaneously), hypomagnesemia, hypophosphatasia, Wilson's disease, and ochronosis.

Pseudogout

When CPPD causes an acute inflammatory arthritis, the term "pseudogout" is applied. CPPD crystals are weakly positively birefringent and are rhomboid-shaped. Pseudogout rarely involves the first metatarsophalangeal joint. It most commonly affects knees, but wrists, elbows, ankles, and intervertebral disks may be involved. It usually occurs in older individuals. Most patients with pseudogout have chondrocalcinosis on radiography. The presence of chondrocalcinosis does not necessarily mean that a patient will have pseudogout or even CPPD. Dicalcium phosphate dihydrate apatite (calcium hydroxyapatite) also can cause chondrocalcinosis to be seen on radiography, although less frequently. Persons on dialysis in whom acute arthritis or periarthritis develops frequently have calcium hydroxyapatite-induced disease. Gout, pseudogout, calcium oxalate, and infection are also possibilities in patients who undergo dialysis.

- Pseudogout is acute inflammatory arthritis caused by CPPD.
- CPPD crystals are weakly positively birefringent.
- Most commonly affects knees; wrist, elbows, ankles, and intervertebral disks can be affected.
- Chondrocalcinosis is found on radiographs in most patients with pseudogout.
- Chondrocalcinosis does not mean that patient will have pseudogout or even CPPD.

Treatment of Pseudogout

For treatment of acute attacks, nonsteroidal anti-inflammatory drugs or injection of a steroid preparation can be used. Intravenously administered colchicine is effective for acute attacks, but oral administration is not consistently effective. Prophylactic oral colchicine (0.6 mg twice to three times daily) can lead to a decrease in frequency and severity of pseudogout attacks. In patients with underlying metabolic disease, the frequency of acute attacks of pseudogout does not decrease with treatment of the underlying disease (e.g., hypothyroidism, hyperparathyroidism).

- Treatment of acute attacks of pseudogout: nonsteroidal anti-inflammatory drugs, injection of steroid preparation, or colchicine given intravenously.
- Prophylactic oral colchicine can lead to decrease in frequency and severity of attacks.

Hydroxyapatite Deposition Disease

Presentation

Clinical presentations include 1) acute inflammation (calcific tendinitis, osteoarthritis with inflammatory episodes, periarthritis/arthritis dialysis syndrome, rupture of calcinotic deposits in scleroderma) and 2) chronic inflammation (osteoarthritis and Milwaukee shoulder--glenohumeral osteoarthritis, rotator cuff tear, noninflammatory joint fluid containing hydroxyapatite).

- Hydroxyapatite deposition disease can present as acute or chronic inflammation.

Diagnosis and Treatment

Individual crystals cannot be seen on routine polarization microscopy (Table 27-2). Small, round (shiny coin) bodies 0.5 to 100 μm are seen. On electron microscopy, these represent lumps of needle-shaped crystals. Positive identification requires transmission electron microscopy or elemental analysis. Alizarin red stain showing calcium staining provides a presumptive diagnosis (if CPPD is excluded). Treatment involves nonsteroidal anti-inflammatory drugs and intra-articular steroids.

- Individual crystals not seen on polarization microscopy.
- Positive identification requires transmission electron microscopy.

Table 27-2.--Differential Diagnosis According to Results of Synovial Fluid Analysis

Diagnosis	Leukocyte count, /mm^3	Differential	Polarization microscopy
Degenerative joint disease	<1,000	Mononuclear cells	Negative
Rheumatoid arthritis	5,000-50,000	PMNs	Negative
Gout	5,000-75,000	PMNs	Monosodium urate
Pseudogout	5,000-75,000	PMNs	CPPD
Hydroxyapatite	5,000-75,000	PMNs	Negative
Septic arthritis	≥100,000	PMNs	Negative

CPPD, calcium pyrophosphate deposition disease; PMN, polymorphonuclear leukocytes.

Calcium Oxalate Arthropathy

This disorder occurs in patients with primary oxalosis and patients on chronic hemodialysis. It can cause acute inflammatory arthritis. Crystals are large, bipyramidal, and birefringent. Calcium oxalate can cause chondrocalcinosis or large soft tissue calcifications.

- Calcium oxalate arthropathy occurs in patients with primary oxalosis and patients on chronic hemodialysis.

SPONDYLOARTHROPATHIES

Conditions that form the spondyloarthropathies include ankylosing spondylitis, Reiter's syndrome, reactive arthritis, enteropathic spondylitis, and psoriatic arthritis.

Spondyloarthropathies are characterized by involvement of sacroiliac joints (uncommon in rheumatoid arthritis), peripheral arthritis (usually asymmetric oligoarticular), absence of rheumatoid factor, and an association with HLA-B27; they are enthesopathic disorders.

The human leukocyte antigen (HLA) region of the 6th chromosome contains genes of the human histocompatibility complex. Every person has two 6th chromosomes, one inherited from each parent. On each of these there is an HLA-A and HLA-B allele. Therefore, everyone has two HLA-A types and two HLA-B types. With regard to inheritance, an offspring has a 50% chance of acquiring a specific HLA-A or HLA-B antigen from a parent (Fig. 27-2). Siblings have a 25% chance of being identical for all four HLA-A and HLA-B alleles.

Frequency of HLA-B27 in control populations is as follows: whites (United States), 8%; African blacks, 0%; Orientals, 1%; Haida (North American Indian), 50%.

The rheumatic diseases associated with HLA-B27 are ankylosing spondylitis (HLA-B27 in >90%), Reiter's syndrome or reactive arthritis (>80%), enteropathic spondylitis (approximately 75%), and psoriatic spondylitis (approximately 50%).

- Ankylosing spondylitis associated with HLA-B27 in >90% of cases.

Many theories have been proposed to explain the association between HLA-B27 and the spondyloarthropathies: B27 may act as a receptor site for an infective agent; B27 is a marker for an immune response gene that determines susceptibility to an environmental trigger; and B27 may

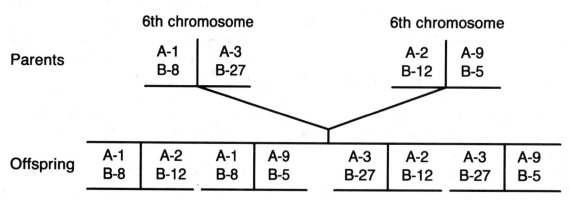

Fig. 27-2. Inheritance of HLA antigens.

induce tolerance to foreign antigens with which it cross-reacts.

An offspring of a person with HLA-B27 has a 50% chance of carrying the antigen. In randomly selected persons with HLA-B27, the chance of developing disease is 2%-10%. In B27-positive relatives of B27-positive patients with ankylosing spondylitis, the risk of developing disease is 25%-50%.

Ankylosing Spondylitis

New York Criteria of 1966

Clinical criteria include 1) limitation of motion of the lumbar spine in all three planes (anterior flexion, lateral flexion, extension), 2) history of or the presence of pain at the dorsolumbar junction or in the lumbar spine, and 3) limitation of chest expansion to 1 inch (2.5 cm) or less measured at the level of the fourth intercostal space.

Grading

Ankylosing spondylitis is graded as follows: definite ankylosing spondylitis is 1) grade 3-4, bilateral sacroiliitis with at least one clinical criterion; 2) grade 3-4 unilateral or grade 1 bilateral sacroiliitis with clinical criterion 1 (limitation of back movement in all three planes) or with both clinical criteria 2 and 3 (back pain and limitation of chest expansion). Probable ankylosing spondylitis is grade 3-4 bilateral sacroiliitis with no clinical criteria.

Features

Characteristic features of low back pain in ankylosing spondylitis are age at onset usually between 15-40 years, insidious onset, duration >3 months, morning stiffness, improvement with exercise, family history, involvement of other systems, and diffuse radiation of back pain.

- Features of low back pain in ankylosing spondylitis: age at onset between 15-40 years, insidious onset, improvement with exercise.

Findings of ankylosing spondylitis on physical examination are listed in Table 27-3.

Table 27-3.--Findings in Ankylosing Spondylitis

Characteristic	
Scoliosis	Absent
Decrease of range of movement	Symmetric
Tenderness	Diffuse
Hip flexion with straight-leg raising	Normal
Pain with sciatic nerve stretch	Absent
Hip involvement	Frequently present
Neurodeficit	Absent

Other physical findings in ankylosing spondylitis are listed in Table 27-4.

The radiographic findings in ankylosing spondylitis are 1) sacroiliac involvement (erosions, "pseudowidening" of joint space, sclerosis [both sides of sacroiliac joint; this finding is needed for diagnosis], fusion); and 2) spine involvement (squaring of superior and inferior margins of vertebral body, syndesmophytes, bamboo spine).

- Radiographic findings in ankylosing spondylitis: erosions, syndesmophytes, bamboo spine.

Table 27-4.--Results of Testing in Ankylosing Spondylitis

Test	Method	Results
Schober	Make a mark on the spine at level of L-5 and one at 10 cm directly above with the patient standing erect. Patient then bends forward maximally and the distance between the two marks is measured	An increase of <5 cm indicates early lumbar involvement
Chest expansion	Measure maximal chest expansion at nipple line	Chest expansion of <5 cm is clue to early costovertebral involvement
Sacroiliac compression	Exert direct compression over sacroiliac joints	Tenderness or pain suggests sacroiliac involvement

Laboratory Findings

The erythrocyte sedimentation rate may be elevated, there may be an anemia of chronic disease, rheumatoid factor is absent, and 95% of white patients are positive for HLA-B27.

Extraspinal Involvement

Enthesopathic involvement distinguishes spondyloarthropathies from rheumatoid arthritis and consists of plantar fasciitis, Achilles' tendinitis, and costochondritis. Hip and shoulder involvement are common (up to 50%), but peripheral joints can be affected, usually asymmetric involvement of the lower extremities. Some patients diagnosed with juvenile rheumatoid arthritis, especially male adolescents, really have juvenile ankylosing spondylitis in which peripheral arthritis preceded the low back pain.

- Enthesopathic involvement in ankylosing spondylitis: plantar fasciitis, Achilles' tendinitis, costochondritis.
- Hip and shoulder involvement common (up to 50%).
- Some patients diagnosed with juvenile rheumatoid arthritis, especially male adolescents, have juvenile ankylosing spondylitis.

Extraskeletal Involvement

Other findings in active disease include 1) fatigue, 2) weight loss, 3) low-grade fever, and 4) iritis (25% of patients). Iritis is an important clinical clue in the diagnosis of spondyloarthropathies. It is not found in adults with rheumatoid arthritis.

- Iritis is important clue to diagnosis of spondyloarthropathies; not found in adults with rheumatoid arthritis.

Late complications can include 1) cord compression due to traumatic spinal fracture, 2) cauda equina syndrome (symptoms include neurogenic bladder, fecal incontinence, leg pain), 3) fibrotic changes in upper lung fields (cavities can develop and aspergillomas have been reported), 4) aortic insufficiency, 5) complete heart block, and 6) amyloidosis.

- Late complications of ankylosing spondylitis: cord compression due to traumatic spinal fractures, cauda equina syndrome, fibrotic changes in upper lung fields, aortic insufficiency.

Ankylosing Spondylitis in Men and Women

Ankylosing spondylitis has been thought to be a disease primarily of men, but it is now recognized that the incidence in women is similar, although they have less tendency for spinal ankylosis. Women more frequently have osteitis pubis and peripheral joint involvement.

Differential Diagnosis

The differential diagnosis includes diffuse hypertrophic skeletal hyperostosis (DISH), osteitis condensans ilii, fusion of sacroiliac joint in paraplegia, osteitis pubis, and degenerative joint disease. The clinical symptoms of DISH are "stiffness" of spine and relatively good preservation of spine motion. Patients with DISH can have dysphagia related to cervical osteophytes. It generally affects middle-aged and elderly men. Criteria for DISH are "flowing" ossification along the anterolateral aspect of at least four contiguous vertebral bodies, preservation of disk height, absence of apophyseal joint involvement, absence of sacroiliac joint involvement, and extraspinal ossifications, including ligamentous calcifications.

Osteitis condensans ilii usually affects young to middle-aged females with normal sacroiliac joints. Radiography shows sclerosis on iliac side of sacroiliac joint only. The sacroiliac joint can also be involved with 1) tuberculosis, 2) metastatic disease, 3) gout, 4) Paget's disease, or 5) infection (*Brucellosis, Serratia, Staphylococcus*).

- Osteitis condensans ilii usually affects young to middle-aged females; radiography shows sclerosis on iliac side of sacroiliac joint only.
- Sacroiliac joint can be involved with metastatic disease, gout, Paget's disease, infection (*Brucella, Serratia, Staphylococcus*).

Treatment

Treatment involves physical therapy (posture very important), exercise (swimming), cessation of smoking, genetic counseling, and drug therapy with nonsteroidal anti-inflammatory drugs such as indomethacin; aspirin is not effective.

Reiter's Syndrome

This is a seronegative asymmetric arthropathy (predominantly affects lower extremities). One or more of the following conditions also occurs: 1) urethritis, 2) dysentery, 3) inflammatory eye disease (conjunctivitis), and 4) mucocutaneous disease (balanitis, oral ulcerations, or keratoderma). In addition, approximately 80% of patients are HLA-B27 positive. Another finding is keratoderma blennorrhagicum (characteristic skin and mucous membrane findings (skin lesions are painless). It is *indistinguishable* clinically and histologically from psoriasis. Joint predilection is for the toes and asymmetric large joints in the lower extremities. It can cause "sausage"-toe-like psoriasis. The distal interphalangeal joints in the hands can be affected also. Cardiac conduction disturbances and aortitis can develop. Because most patients are HLA-B27 positive, sacroiliitis (sometimes unilateral) and iritis can occur. Antibiotics for nonspecific urethritis do not alter the course of the disease. Long-term studies indicate that the disease remains episodically active in 75% of patients and that disability is a frequent outcome.

- Reiter's syndrome: seronegative asymmetric arthropathy with urethritis, dysentery, inflammatory eye disease, mucocutaneous disease.
- 80% of patients are HLA-B27 positive.
- Cardiac conduction disturbances and aortitis can develop.
- Antibiotics for nonspecific urethritis do not alter course.

Treatment is with nonsteroidal anti-inflammatory drugs (indomethacin), gold, and methotrexate.

Reactive Arthritis

This is an aseptic arthritis induced by a host response to an infectious agent rather than direct infection. HLA-B27 is associated in 80% of cases. The condition develops after infections with *Salmonella* organisms, *Shigella flexneri*, *Yersinia enterocolitica*, and *Campylobacter jejuni*, which cause diarrhea, and *Chlamydia* and *Ureaplasma urealyticum*, which cause nonspecific urethritis. In addition to polyarthritis, clinical features of Reiter's syndrome, including sacroiliitis, may develop. Patients usually have self-limited disease. Joint destruction is *not* common. The condition is usually managed with nonsteroidal anti-inflammatory drugs.

- Reactive arthritis: aseptic arthritis induced by host response to infectious agent rather than direct infection.
- HLA-B27 associated in 80% of cases.
- Develops after infections with *Salmonella*, *Shigella flexneri*, *Yersinia enterocolitica*, *Campylobacter jejuni*, *Chlamydia*, *Ureaplasma urealyticum*.

- Clinical features of Reiter's syndrome may develop.

Arthritis Associated With Inflammatory Bowel Disease

Two distinct types of arthritis are associated with chronic inflammatory bowel disease: 1) a nondestructive oligoarthritis of peripheral joints tending to come and go in time with the activity of the bowel disease and 2) ankylosing spondylitis (enteropathic spondylitis). The spondylitis is not a complication of the bowel disease. It is often diagnosed many years before the onset of bowel symptoms, and its subsequent progress bears little relationship to the bowel disease. Approximately 75% of patients with ankylosing spondylitis and inflammatory bowel disease are HLA-B27 positive. Patients with inflammatory bowel disease alone do not have an increased frequency of HLA-B27 and are not at increased risk for development of spondylitis.

- Patients with inflammatory bowel disease alone do not have increased frequency of HLA-B27.

Psoriatic Arthritis

Psoriatic arthritis develops in 7% of patients with psoriasis. Pitting of nails is strongly associated with joint disease. Patients with more severe skin disease are at higher risk for development of arthritis. Hyperuricemia is present in 15% of all patients with psoriasis whether or not they have arthritis. A "sausage" finger or toe is characteristic of psoriatic arthritis and is very uncommon in rheumatoid arthritis. Radiographic evidence of involvement of the distal interphalangeal joint with erosions is common in psoriasis and uncommon in rheumatoid arthritis. Psoriatic arthritis also can cause a characteristic "pencil-in-cup" deformity of the distal interphalangeal and proximal interphalangeal joints on radiography.

- Psoriatic arthritis develops in 7% of patients with psoriasis.
- Pitting of nails strongly associated with joint disease.
- Hyperuricemia present in 15% of all patients with psoriasis.
- "Sausage" finger or toe is characteristic.
- "Pencil-in-cup" deformity of distal and proximal interphalangeal joints is radiographic finding.

There are five clinical groups of psoriatic arthritis: 1) predominant distal interphalangeal joint involvement, 2) arthritis mutilans, 3) symmetrical polyarthritis-like rheumatoid arthritis but negative for rheumatoid factor, 4) asymmetrical oligoarthritis, and 5) psoriatic spondylitis (HLA-B27 positive in 50%-75% of cases). Treatment is with nonsteroidal anti-inflammatory drugs, gold, hydroxychloroquine, methotrexate, and azathioprine.

LYME DISEASE

Lyme disease is a tick-borne spirochetal illness with acute and chronic manifestations affecting the skin, heart, joints, and nervous system primarily. Diagnosis is important because treatment with appropriate antibiotics at an early stage of disease can prevent chronic sequelae. Even some chronic symptoms are treatable. Endemic areas in the United States include Connecticut, Delaware, Maryland, Massachusetts, New Jersey, New York, Pennsylvania, Rhode Island, Minnesota, Wisconsin, California, Nevada, Oregon, and Utah.

- Lyme disease is tick-borne spirochetal illness.
- Acute and chronic manifestations affect skin, heart, joints, nervous system.

The Tick

Ticks that transmit Lyme disease include *Ixodes dammini* in the northeastern and midwestern United States and *Ixodes pacificus* in the western United States. *Amblyomma americanum* ("Lone Star" tick) is a possible vector in the eastern, southern, and western United States. *Ixodes scapularis* is the common deer tick. It has a wide distribution. Humans are accidental hosts.

The Spirochete

Borrelia burgdorferi was an unknown organism until isolated initially from ticks by Burgdorfer in 1983. It is similar to an organism causing relapsing fever. It apparently exists only in the digestive tract of tick vectors.

Clinical Stages of Lyme Disease

Signs and symptoms occur in stages that may overlap. Later stages may occur *without* evidence of previous disease.

Stage I

About 50% of patients experience erythema chronicum migrans. Flu-like symptoms, including fever, headache, malaise, and adenopathy, can occur. They usually occur several days to a month after the tick bite.

- In stage I, 50% of patients experience erythema chronicum migrans.

Stage II

Symptoms begin weeks to months after the initial symptoms in stage I. Disseminated infection develops and can include symptoms of the skin, musculoskeletal system, heart, and nervous system. In approximately 15% of patients, neurologic symptoms develop, including Bell's palsy, meningoencephalitis, and sensory and motor radiculoneuritis. Approximately 5% of patients have cardiac abnormalities, including heart block. About 30%-50% of patients have arthritis. This usually affects large joints, primarily the knee, and joint fluid analysis shows a leukocytosis similar to that in rheumatoid arthritis. Baker's cysts may form early and are prone to rupture in patients who have arthritis of the knees.

- In stage II, symptoms begin weeks to months after initial symptoms of stage I.
- Disseminated infection develops.
- 15% of patients have neurologic symptoms.
- 5% of patients have cardiac abnormalities.
- 30%-50% of patients have arthritis.

Stage III

This usually occurs several years after the initial onset of illness. Episodes of arthritis can develop and become chronic. Histologically, the synovium resembles that in rheumatoid arthritis, although a unique feature of Lyme arthritis is the finding of an obliterative endarteritis. Spirochetes are occasionally seen in and around the blood vessels. Patients in whom chronic joint disease develops have increased frequency of HLA-DR4, often in combination with HLA-DR2. Patients with chronic arthritis have a poor response to antibiotics.

- Stage III occurs several years after initial onset of illness.
- Episodes of arthritis can be chronic.
- Synovium resembles that in rheumatoid arthritis.
- Unique feature of Lyme arthritis is obliterative endarteritis in the synovium.
- Patients with chronic joint disease have increased frequency of HLA-DR4, often in combination with HLA-DR2.

Diagnosis

Culturing the organism is difficult and of low yield.

Antibody to spirochete can be measured by several techniques. The enzyme-linked immunosorbent (ELISA) assay is most commonly performed, but this is not standardized and there is significant frequency of false-positive and false-negative results. Patients with other autoimmune diseases can have false-positive results. Also, such results may occur in syphilis, relapsing fever, and Rocky Mountain spotted fever. Although patients with syphilis have false-positive Lyme serologic results by ELISA, patients with Lyme disease have negative results of VDRL test. Up to 25% of patients with lupus and rheumatoid arthritis have false-positive results of Lyme test by ELISA. It is important to remember that test results remain negative for up to 4 to 6 weeks after infection. Also, if patients are treated early with tetracycline or another antibiotic, the results might never be positive, although symptoms of chronic Lyme disease can result. The Western blot assay for Lyme disease is now being used as a confirmatory test if the ELISA test result is positive.

- In Lyme disease, culturing organism is difficult and of low yield.
- ELISA assay is commonly performed but is not standardized.
- Significant frequency of false-positive results with ELISA.
- False-positive results may occur in syphilis, relapsing fever, Rocky Mountain spotted fever.
- Up to 25% of patients with lupus and rheumatoid arthritis have false-positive results of Lyme test by ELISA.
- Patients treated early with tetracycline or other antibiotic may never have positive results.

Treatment

For early treatment of Lyme disease, either oral tetracycline or doxycycline, or amoxicillin in children, can prevent later complications. The optimal treatment for patients with chronic symptoms is unclear but can include the use of penicillin G, 20 million units intravenously daily for 14 days, or ceftriaxone, 2 g intravenously daily for 14 days. Patients with Lyme disease can experience worsening of symptoms analogous to the Jarisch-Herxheimer reaction and can be treated with acetaminophen.

- Early treatment of Lyme disease is either oral tetracycline or doxycycline (amoxicillin in children).

HYPERTROPHIC PULMONARY OSTEOARTHROPATHY

This syndrome is characterized by an oligoarthritis or polyarthritis that can have a presentation similar to that of rheumatoid arthritis. Patients have associated clubbing, and periosteal new bone formation at the end of long bones is noted on radiography. This finding is very unusual in rheumatoid arthritis. This syndrome is usually associated with carcinoma of the lung, but it can occur with other types of cancer. It also occurs in severe cystic fibrosis and in congenital heart disease when hypoxia is present.

- Hypertrophic pulmonary osteoarthropathy has associated clubbing.
- Radiography shows periosteal new bone formation at end of long bones.
- Syndrome is usually associated with carcinoma of lung.

OSTEOID OSTEOMA

Osteoid osteoma is a benign bone tumor. It usually occurs between the ages of 5 and 30 years in males and females with equal frequency. The classic symptom is bone pain at night, which is relieved completely with aspirin or another nonsteroidal anti-inflammatory agent. Diagnosis is made by routine radiography, but often this is negative and a bone scan is needed to locate the tumor, and tomography or computed tomography can then be done for better visualization. Radiography shows a small nidus, usually less than 1 cm, varying from radiolucent to radiopaque, depending on the age of the lesion. There is usually a lucent ring around the nidus and adjacent bone sclerosis. Treatment includes excision, which is curative.

- Osteoid osteoma is benign bone tumor.
- Bone pain at night relieved by aspirin or other nonsteroidal anti-inflammatory agent.
- Diagnosed with routine radiography.
- Treatment includes excision, which is curative.

NEUROPATHIC ARTHRITIS

This occurs because of loss of proprioception of affected joints. The most common cause of a neuropathic (Charcot) joint is diabetes, which characteristically affects the ankle, tarsal bones, and metatarsophalangeal joints. Tabes dorsalis affects the spine and knees, and syringomyelia characteristically affects the shoulders and elbows. Most patients experience some pain, but not as much as would be expected in a patient with degenerative arthritis without superimposed neuropathy. Radiographic changes usually show marked destruction of affected joints.

- Neuropathic arthritis occurs because of loss of proprioception of affected joints.
- Most common cause of neuropathic (Charcot) joint is diabetes.
- Diabetes characteristically affects the ankle, tarsal bones, metatarsophalangeal joints.
- Tabes dorsalis affects spine and knees.
- Syringomyelia affects shoulder and elbows.

BYPASS ARTHRITIS

This occurs in patients who have undergone intestinal bypass operations, including jejunocolic or jejunoileal. The arthritis may be acute or subacute, is usually intermittent, and can last occasionally for short periods only to recur. The most commonly affected joints include the metacarpophalangeal, proximal interphalangeal, wrists, knees, and ankles. It is commonly associated with a dermatitis, which can be pustular in nature. Circulating immune complexes composed of bacterial antigens have been found in both the circulation and the synovial fluid and are thought to be the cause of this disorder. Treatment entails nonsteroidal anti-inflammatory agents and antibiotics such as tetracycline, but many times reanastomosis may be necessary for resolution of symptoms.

- Bypass arthritis occurs in patients who have had intestinal bypass operations.
- Most commonly affected joints: metacarpophalangeal, proximal interphalangeal, wrists, knees, ankles.
- Commonly associated with a dermatitis.

AVASCULAR NECROSIS OF BONE

Many conditions are associated with spontaneous avascular necrosis. Common associated conditions include alcoholism, steroid use, connective tissue diseases (especially lupus), and hemoglobinopathies. Other conditions include diabetes, fat embolism, gout, hyperlipidemia, immunosuppressive therapy, radiation therapy, pancreatitis, thermal injuries including burns, electrical injuries and frostbite, compression syndrome (caisson's disease),

and hematopoietic disorders including hemophilia, histiocytosis, polycythemia, and Gaucher's disease. The most commonly affected joints include the hips, shoulders, and knees.

- Conditions associated with avascular necrosis of bone: alcoholism, steroid use, connective tissue diseases (especially lupus), hemoglobinopathies.
- Most commonly affected joints: hips, shoulders, knees.

Increased interosseous pressure has been noted. Because of this, core decompression of the hip reportedly prevents further progression, but proof of this outcome has not been established. Many times, patients with avascular necrosis have bilateral disease, although they have symptoms on only one side. Early in the disease radiographs may be normal. A radiolucent crescent line can occasionally be seen; this represents a plane of cleavage or fracture. Magnetic resonance imaging is the most sensitive test to demonstrate avascular necrosis, but bone scanning can also be used. Standard treatment includes non-weight-bearing of the affected joint.

- Magnetic resonance imaging is most sensitive test for demonstrating avascular necrosis; bone scanning can also be used.

SYSTEMIC LUPUS ERYTHEMATOSUS

Systemic lupus erythematosus (SLE) is a chronic inflammatory disease of unknown cause with a wide spectrum of clinical manifestations and variable course. Antibodies that react with nuclear and cytoplasmic antigens commonly are found in patients with the disease. Genetic, hormonal, and environmental factors seem to be important in the cause. Multiple organs may be affected, and the disease course is variable and characterized by exacerbations and remissions.

- Genetic, hormonal, and environmental factors seem important in cause of SLE.
- SLE characterized by exacerbations and remissions.

Diagnosis

Four of the following findings are needed for diagnosis of SLE: malar rash; discoid lupus; photosensitivity; oral ulcers; arthritis; proteinuria (protein, >0.5 g/day) or cellular casts; seizures or psychosis; pleuritis or pericarditis; hemolytic anemia, leukopenia, lymphopenia, or thrombocytopenia; antibody to nDNA, antibody to Sm (Smith) or LE cells, or false-positive results of VDRL test; and positive results of fluorescent antinuclear antibody test.

Epidemiology

The female:male ratio is 9:1, particularly during the reproductive years. The first symptoms usually occur between the second and fourth decades of life. The disease seems to be less severe in the elderly. The frequency of SLE is increased in American blacks, Native Americans, and Orientals.

- Female:male ratio in SLE is 9:1.
- Increased frequency of SLE in American blacks, Native Americans, Orientals.

Etiology

Type C oncornavirus is present in NZB/W mice, and both viral protein and antibody to protein are found in mouse glomeruli. Direct causal relationship has *not* been established. In human disease, viral-like particles in glomeruli of patients with SLE are also seen in other kinds of kidney damage. Attempts to isolate viruses have been unsuccessful. Patients with SLE have elevated antibody titers to a wide range of antigens without much sign of specificity for a particular viral agent.

- In SLE, elevated antibody titers to a wide range of antigens without much sign of specificity for a particular viral agent.

Genetics

Among relatives of patients with SLE, 20% have an immunologic disease. Another 25% have antinuclear antibodies, circulating immune complexes, antilymphocyte antibodies, or a false-positive result on VDRL test without clinical disease. Concordance among monozygotic twins is much greater than among dizygotic twins. Genetic and environmental factors are both important in development of SLE. Immune complex levels are much higher in persons with close contact to patient than in unexposed consanguineous relatives. The frequency of HLA-DR2 and HLA-DR3 is increased.

- 20% of relatives of patients with SLE have "immunologic" disease.
- In SLE, frequency of HLA-DR2 and HLA-DR3 is increased.

Immune System

There is a decrease in the cellular immune system with an absolute decrease in T-suppressor cells. There is an increase in the humoral immune system with a relative increase in helper T cells.

- In SLE, absolute decrease in T-suppressor cells, relative increase in helper T cells.

Pathogenesis

Circulating immune complexes (anti-nDNA) are responsible for glomerulonephritis and probably skin disease. Immune complexes bind complement, which initiates inflammatory process. Organ-specific autoantibodies are 1) antierythrocyte, 2) antiplatelet, 3) antileukocyte, and 4) antithyroid.

- Circulating immune complexes (anti-nDNA) are responsible for glomerulonephritis.

Late complications of SLE are related to vascular damage in relative absence of active immunologic disease. Damage to intima during active disease probably results in premature deterioration of vasculature and various thrombotic, ischemic, and hypertensive manifestations.

Clinical Manifestations

Arthritis is characteristically nondeforming and nonerosive. Avascular necrosis of bone occurs, and not only in patients taking steroids. Navicular, femoral head, and tibial plateau are most commonly affected.

Fever in SLE is usually caused by the disease, but infection *must* be ruled out. Shaking chills and leukocytosis strongly suggest infection. Subacute cutaneous LE is a subset of SLE that primarily has skin involvement with psoriasiform or annular erythematous lesions. Patients may be negative for antinuclear antibodies but frequently are positive for antibodies to the extractable nuclear antigen SS-A (Ro).

- Fever in SLE usually caused by disease, but infection must be ruled out.

Central nervous system lupus is a most variable and unpredictable phenomenon. Manifestations such as impaired organic psychiatric function, seizures, long tract signs, cranial neuropathies, and migraine-like attacks occur with little apparent relationship to each other or to other systemic manifestations. Immune complexes in the choroid plexus are *not* specific for central nervous system disease. They also occur in patients without central nervous system disease. There is no specific laboratory abnormality. Patients may have increased cerebrospinal fluid protein (IgG) and pleocytosis. C4 levels in cerebrospinal fluid are not helpful.

- Central nervous system lupus is a most variable and unpredictable phenomenon.
- Immune complexes in choroid plexus are *not* specific for central nervous system disease.

Electroencephalography can be abnormal. Brain scanning is of no help. Magnetic resonance imaging usually shows areas of increased signal in the periventricular white matter, similar to that found in multiple sclerosis. Magnetic resonance imaging findings are nonspecific and can be seen in patients who have SLE without central nervous system manifestations. Pathologic examinations of autopsy specimens usually reveal microinfarcts, nerve cell loss, vasculitis, or no detectable abnormalities. Psychosis caused by steroid therapy is probably rarer than previously thought. When in doubt about the cause of the psychosis, the steroid dose can be increased and the patient observed. Patients can have isolated central nervous system involvement and normal results of cerebrospinal fluid examination and no other organ involvement.

- Electroencephalography can be abnormal in SLE.
- Brain scanning is not helpful.
- Magnetic resonance imaging findings are nonspecific.
- Psychosis caused by steroid therapy probably rarer than thought.

Women with SLE who become pregnant have a high prevalence of spontaneous abortion. Because abortion itself may lead to a flare of disease, therapeutic abortion ordinarily is not recommended after first trimester. Flares of disease should be treated with steroids, particularly during the postpartum period.

- High prevalence of spontaneous abortion in SLE.
- Therapeutic abortion not recommended after first trimester.

Infants of mothers with SLE can develop thrombocytopenia and leukopenia from passive transfer of anti-bodies. They also can develop transient cutaneous lesions and transient complete heart block. Mothers usually have anti-SS-A (Ro), which crosses the placenta and is transiently present in the infant. Mothers usually are HLA-B8/DR3, but there is no HLA association in the child. In some affected infants, no clinical disease is present in the mother although antibodies are present.

Renal Involvement

Types of renal disease in SLE are 1) mesangial, 2) focal glomerulonephritis, 3) membranous glomerulonephritis, 4) diffuse proliferative glomerulonephritis, 5) interstitial nephritis with defects in renal tubular handling of K^+, and 6) renal vein thrombosis with nephrotic syndrome.

Treatment of renal disease depends in part on the results of renal biopsy. Patients with mesangial changes alone do not require aggressive therapy. Patients with active diffuse proliferative glomerulonephritis are treated with high-dose steroids with or without immunosuppressive agents. Immunosuppressive agents are steroid-sparing and lower the incidence of renal failure in patients with diffuse proliferative glomerulonephritis but do not improve overall survival. Appropriate treatment for focal proliferative glomerulonephritis and membranous glomerulonephritis is controversial because the prognosis is favorable. Renal biopsies can be helpful in directing therapy. Patients with high activity indices such as active inflammation, proliferation, necrosis, and crescent formation are considered for aggressive therapy. Patients with high chronicity indices such as tubular atrophy, scarring, and glomerulosclerosis are less likely to respond to aggressive therapy.

- Patients with mesangial changes alone do not require aggressive therapy.
- Active diffuse proliferative glomerulonephritis is treated with high-dose steroids with or without immunosuppressive agents.
- Renal biopsies helpful for directing therapy.

Laboratory Findings

Anemia of chronic disease and hemolytic anemia (Coombs' positive) can occur. Leukopenia usually does not predispose to infection. Antilymphocyte antibodies cause lymphopenia in SLE. In Felty's syndrome, infection is common as a result of granulocytopenia. Idiopathic thrombocytopenic purpura with presence of platelet antibodies can be the initial manifestation of SLE. Polyclonal gammopathy secondary to hyperactivity of humoral immune system is common. The erythrocyte sedimentation rate usually correlates with disease activity.

- Hemolytic anemia (Coombs' positive) can occur in SLE.
- Idiopathic thrombocytopenic purpura can be the initial manifestation of SLE.

A low total hemolytic complement value usually correlates with active disease. A low value on CH_{50} assay with increased anti-nDNA antibodies usually implies renal disease (or skin disease). A total complement value too low to measure but normal C3 and C4 values suggest a hereditary complement deficiency. Familial C2 deficiency is the most common complement deficiency in SLE, but C1r, C1s, C5, C6, C7, and C8 deficiencies also have been reported.

- Low total hemolytic complement value usually correlates with active disease.
- Low value on CH_{50} assay with increased anti-nDNA antibodies usually implies renal disease (or skin disease).

Patients with SLE may have false-positive results of VDRL test as a result of antibody to phospholipid, which cross-reacts with VDRL. Among patients with false-positive results on VDRL test, 80% have circulating anticoagulant. Patients with SLE also can have false-positive results of fluorescent treponemal antibody test, but this is usually of the "beaded pattern" of fluorescence. LE cells are present in approximately 70% of patients

with SLE. They are caused by antibody to deoxyribonucleoprotein (DNP). Testing for this is not performed in many centers. Anti-DNP is also detected by the fluorescent antinuclear antibody test in a homogeneous pattern.

- 80% of patients with false-positive results on VDRL test have a circulating anticoagulant.
- LE cells present in about 70% of patients with SLE.

Anti-nDNA levels fluctuate with disease activity, whereas levels of other autoantibodies (i.e., ribonucleoprotein, Sm, antinuclear antibody) show no consistent relationship to levels of anti-nDNA or disease activity. Methods used to measure anti-nDNA are 1) an immunofluorescent method using *Crithidia luciliae*, an organism with a kinetoplast that contains helical native DNA free of other nuclear antigens--therefore, there is no single-stranded DNA contamination; and 2) radioimmunoassay and other techniques, which suffer from the difficulty of maintaining DNA in its native double-stranded state and so are contaminated with single-stranded DNA. All patients with lupus should have positive results of antinuclear antibody test. A positive result is by no means specific for lupus. Antinuclear antibody patterns are outlined in Table 27-5. Other autoantibodies and disease associations are outlined in Table 27-6.

- Anti-nDNA levels fluctuate with disease activity.
- Positive result of antinuclear antibody test is by no means specific for lupus.

Table 27-5.--Antinuclear Antibody Patterns

Fluorescent pattern	Antigen	Disease association
Rim, peripheral, shaggy	nDNA	SLE
Homogeneous	DNP	SLE, others
Speckled	ENA	MCTD, SLE, others
Nucleolar	RNA	Scleroderma

DNP, deoxyribonucleoprotein; ENA, extractable nuclear antigens; MCTD, mixed connective tissue disease; RNA, ribonucleic acid.

Treatment

Treatment should match the activity of SLE in the individual patient. Serial monitoring of organ function and appropriate immunologic evaluation (anti-nDNA, C3, erythrocyte sedimentation rate) allow rapid recognition and treatment of flares and appropriate tapering of steroid

dose during periods of disease quiescence. Table 27-7 provides guidelines for treatment, and Table 27-8 outlines the complications of treatment.

Outcome

The 10-year survival rate is 75%. Prognosis is worse

Table 27-6.--Autoantibodies in Rheumatic Diseases

Antibody	Disease association
Anti-ssDNA	SLE, 100%
	High frequency in other CTD; also chronic infection, CAH, interstitial lung disease
Anti-nDNA	SLE, 50%-60%
Anti-Sm (Smith)	SLE, 30%
Anti-RNP (ribonuclear protein)	MCTD, 100% high titer
	SLE, 30% titer
	Scleroderma, low frequency, low titer
Anti-SS-A	Sjögren's, 70%
	SLE, 35%
	Scleroderma + MCTD, low frequency, low titer
Anti-SS-B	Sjögren's, 60%
	SLE, 15%
Antihistone	Drug-induced SLE, 95%
	SLE, 70%
	RA, 20%
Anti-Sc1-70	Scleroderma, 25%
Anticentromere	CREST, 70%-90%
	Scleroderma, 10%-15%
Anti-PM1	PM, 50%
Anti-Jo1 (histidyl-tRNA synthetase)	PM, 30%

CAH, chronic active hepatitis; CREST, syndrome of *c*alcinosis cutis, *R*aynaud's phenomenon, *e*sophageal dysmotility, *s*clerodactyly, *t*elangiectasia; CTD, connective tissue disease; MCTD, mixed connective tissue disease; PM, polymyositis; RA, rheumatoid arthritis.

in blacks and Hispanics than in whites. Prognosis is worse in patients with creatinine values >3.0 mg/dL. The major causes of death are 1) renal disease, 2) infection, and 3) vascular disease (e.g., myocardial infarction).

- The 10-year survival rate in SLE is 75%.
- Prognosis worse in blacks and Hispanics.

DRUG-INDUCED LUPUS

Many drugs have been implicated in drug-induced lupus. The most common drugs are listed in Table 27-9. One must differentiate between the clinical syndrome of drug-induced lupus and only a positive antinuclear antibody result without clinical symptoms. Many drugs can cause a positive antinuclear antibody result without ever causing the clinical syndrome of drug-induced lupus. Only hydralazine and procainamide have been strongly

Table 27-7.--Treatment of Manifestations of Systemic Lupus Erythematosus

Manifestation	Treatment
Arthritis, fever, mild systemic symptoms	ASA, NSAID
Photosensitivity, rash	Avoidance of sun, use of sunscreens
Rash, arthritis	Hydroxychloroquine (Plaquenil)
Significant thrombocytopenia, hemolytic anemia	Steroids
Renal disease, CNS disease, pericarditis, other significant organ involvement	Steroids
Rapidly deteriorating renal function	? Pulse therapy
CNS, renal disease	? Cytotoxic agents
Renal disease	? Plasmapheresis

ASA, acetylsalicylic acid; CNS, central nervous system; NSAID, nonsteroidal anti-inflammatory drug.

Table 27-8.--Complications of Treatment for Systemic Lupus Erythematosus

Treatment	Complication
Ibuprofen	Aseptic meningitis (headache, fever, stiff neck, CSF pleocytosis)
NSAID	Decreased renal blood flow
ASA	Salicylate hepatitis (common), benign
Cyclophosphamide	Hemorrhagic cystitis, alopecia, opportunistic lymphomas, infection, increased incidence of lymphomas (CNS)
Hydroxychloroquine (Plaquenil)	Retinal toxicity

ASA, acetylsalicylic acid; CNS, central nervous system; CSF, cerebrospinal fluid; NSAID, nonsteroidal anti-inflammatory drug.

implicated in drug-induced lupus. Approximately 5% of persons taking hydralazine will develop a drug-induced lupus syndrome, and approximately 15%-25% of those who take procainamide for more than a year will develop drug-induced lupus. Virtually all patients taking procainamide for 1 year will have a positive result of antinuclear antibody test.

- Only hydralazine and procainamide are strongly implicated in drug-induced lupus.

- Virtually all patients taking procainamide for 1 year have positive antinuclear antibody test.

Table 27-9.--Implicated Agents in Drug-Induced Lupus

Definite	Probable
Common	Phenytoin
Procainamide	Carbamazepine
Hydralazine	Ethosuximide
Uncommon	Propylthiouracil
Isoniazid	Penicillamine
Methyldopa	Sulfasalazine
Chlorpromazine	Lithium carbonate
Quinidine	Acebutolol

Clinical Features

The clinical manifestations of drug-induced lupus are arthralgias and polyarthritis, which occur in approximately 80% of cases. Malaise is common, and fever has been reported in up to 40% of cases. Cardiopulmonary involvement is common, and approximately 30% of patients have pleural-pulmonary manifestations as their presenting symptoms. Pericarditis has been reported in approximately 20% of cases. Diffuse interstitial pneumonitis has been noted. Asymptomatic pleural effusions may be found on routine chest radiography. A few cases of pericardial tamponade have been reported. In contrast to SLE, the incidence of renal and central nervous system involvement is low in drug-induced lupus. Therefore, it is regarded as more benign than SLE. Clinical differences include a lower incidence of skin manifestations, lymphadenopathy, and myalgias in drug-induced disease.

- In drug-induced lupus, arthralgias and polyarthritis occur in about 80% of cases.
- Malaise is common; fever occurs in up to 40% of cases.
- About 30% of patients have pleural-pulmonary manifestations.
- Pericarditis reported in about 20% of cases.
- Incidence of renal and central nervous system involvement is low.

Other differences between drug-induced lupus and SLE include age and sex distribution. SLE is predominantly a disease of premenopausal females, whereas drug-induced disease has an almost equal sex distribution and

occurs in an older population. This disparity in age reflects the use of hydralazine and procainamide in primarily an older population.

Laboratory Abnormalities

Virtually all patients with SLE and drug-induced lupus have antinuclear antibodies. Although patients with SLE and drug-induced lupus are serologically similar in many respects, there are notable differences. Antibodies to native DNA are found in only a small percentage of cases of drug-induced lupus but in approximately 60% of cases of SLE. Serum total hemolytic complement is usually normal in drug-induced disease, in contrast to SLE. However, antibodies such as anti-Sm, SS-B, and ribonucleoprotein are also unusual in drug-induced lupus. The frequency of antihistone antibodies in drug-induced lupus is high (>95% of cases), but these also occur in approximately 60% of cases of SLE. Other laboratory abnormalities in drug-induced lupus can include a positive LE prep, positive Coombs' test, positive rheumatoid factor, false-positive result of serologic test for syphilis, circulating anticoagulants, and cryoglobulins.

Metabolism

Drugs involved in drug-induced lupus have different chemical structures, but three of them--isoniazid, procainamide, and hydralazine--contain a primary amine or hydralazine that is acetylated by the hepatic N-acetyltransferase system. Persons who are taking one of these drugs and who are slow acetylators have a much higher incidence of serologic abnormalities and clinical disease than rapid acetylators. These manifestations also occur over a shorter period in slow acetylators than in rapid acetylators.

- Slow acetylators have a much higher incidence of serologic abnormalities and clinical disease.

Treatment

When possible, patients with drug-induced lupus should stop using the offending drug. Symptoms will usually subside within several weeks, although the duration for complete resolution varies depending on the drug. Serologic abnormalities can remain for years after resolution of clinical symptoms. Patients taking procainamide are most likely to have a rapid remission once use of the drug is stopped, but patients taking hydralazine might have prolonged clinical manifestations. Treatment depends on the clinical manifestations and could include aspirin or other nonsteroidal anti-inflammatory agents or possibly prednisone if needed.

ANTIPHOSPHOLIPID SYNDROME

Systemic lupus erythematosus is an autoimmune disease that is characterized by the formation of many autoantibodies. Recently, much attention has been focused on antiphospholipid antibodies, including the lupus circulating anticoagulant and various anticardiolipin antibodies that have been associated with recurrent arterial and venous thrombosis. Several studies have shown that the lupus anticoagulant is an antiphospholipid antibody of either the IgG or the IgM immunoglobulin class. The hallmark of the lupus anticoagulant is prolongation of all phospholipid-dependent coagulation tests. The anticoagulant acts at the level of the prothrombin activator complex of the clotting cascade. The complex that consists of factor V, factor Xa, calcium, and phospholipids is necessary for the conversion of prothrombin to thrombin. The lupus anticoagulant antibody is thought to interact with the phospholipid portion of the complex, interfering with the calcium-ion-dependent binding of prothrombin factor Xa to the phospholipid. The failure of normal plasma to correct the prolonged clotting time distinguishes the lupus anticoagulant from antibodies directed against specific clotting factors and from clotting factor deficiencies. In the usual coagulation screening tests, the lupus anticoagulant results in prolongation of the activated partial thromboplastin time with or without slight prolongation of the prothrombin time (Table 27-10).

- Lupus anticoagulant is antiphospholipid antibody of either IgG or IgM immunoglobulin class.
- Prolongation of all phospholipid-dependent coagulation tests is hallmark of lupus anticoagulant.
- Anticoagulant acts at level of prothrombin activator complex of clotting cascade.
- Activated partial thromboplastin time is prolonged.

Table 27-10.--Coagulation Tests Characterizing the Lupus Anticoagulant

Screening tests
  Prothrombin time (PT) normal or prolonged
  Partial thromboplastin time (PTT) prolonged
  Plasma clot time prolonged
Tests identifying the lupus anticoagulant
  Prolonged PTT not corrected by adding normal plasma

Various other tests are reported to be sensitive for detection of lupus anticoagulants, including the plasma clot time, kaolin clotting time, a platelet neutralization procedure, and modified Russell's viper venom time.

Given 1) the long-recognized association of the lupus anticoagulant with a chronic biologic false-positive serologic test for syphilis (reagin), 2) the identification of cardiolipin (a phospolipid) as the principal antigen in the test for reagin, and 3) the demonstration of cross-reactivity of lupus anticoagulant antibodies with phospholipids, sensitive solid-phase radioimmunoassays and enzyme-linked immunosorbent assays have been developed for the detection of anticardiolipin antibodies. Anticardiolipin antibodies can be of either the IgG or the IgM immunoglobulin class. Many, but not all, patients with the lupus anticoagulant have elevated IgG or IgM anticardiolipin antibody levels. Like the lupus anticoagulant, anticardiolipin antibodies cross-react with several negatively charged phospholipids.

- Anticardiolipin antibodies can be of either the IgG or the IgM immunoglobulin class.
- Many, but not all, patients with lupus anticoagulant have elevated IgG or IgM anticardiolipin antibody levels.

The lupus anticoagulant and anticardiolipin antibodies are most commonly associated with systemic lupus erythematosus, but they have also been reported in various other autoimmune, malignant, infectious, and drug-induced diseases. Other diseases include Sjögren's syndrome, rheumatoid arthritis, idiopathic thrombocytopenic purpura, Behçet's syndrome, myasthenia gravis, and mixed connective tissue disease. The antibodies can also be found in persons who have no apparent disease but who develop recurrent thrombosis.

- Lupus anticoagulant and anticardiolipin antibodies have also been reported in various other autoimmune, malignant, infectious, and drug-induced diseases.

In contrast to the earliest reports of patients with lupus anticoagulants in which an association with hemorrhagic disorders has been noted, subsequent studies have shown that the risk of bleeding is rare and when bleeding is present it is usually due to associated thrombocytopenia or prothrombin deficiency. There is a paradoxical association between the presence of the lupus anticoagulant and anticardiolipin antibodies and recurrent venous or arterial thrombosis. Thrombotic events described have included stroke, transient ischemic attacks, myocardial infarctions, brachial artery thrombosis, deep venous thrombophlebitis, retinal vein thrombosis, hepatic vein thrombosis resulting in Budd-Chiari syndrome, and pulmonary hypertension. Other manifestations include recurrent fetal loss, thrombocytopenia, positive results of Coombs' test, migraines, chorea, epilepsy, chronic leg ulcers, livedo reticularis, and progressive dementia resulting from cerebrovascular accidents. Recently, acquired valvular heart disease, especially aortic insufficiency, has been described. The mechanism or mechanisms by which antiphospholipid antibodies are associated with thromboembolic manifestations remain unclear. Blocking of the production of prostacyclin from vascular endothelial cells, inhibition of prekallikrein activity and fibrinolysis, and decreased plasminogen activator release have all been described.

- Risk of bleeding is rare; when present, it is usually due to associated thrombocytopenia or prothrombin deficiency.
- Paradoxical association between the presence of the lupus anticoagulant and anticardiolipin antibodies and recurrent venous or arterial thrombosis.
- Other manifestations: recurrent fetal loss, thrombocytopenia, positive Coombs' test, migraines, chorea, epilepsy, chronic leg ulcers, livedo reticularis, progressive dementia from cerebrovascular accidents.
- Acquired valvular heart disease, especially aortic insufficiency, has been described.

Although many patients with lupus and other diseases can have a lupus anticoagulant or anticardiolipin antibodies, of either the IgG or the IgM class, they will not necessarily develop thrombosis. In general, patients with the highest levels of anticardiolipin antibodies are more prone to thrombosis than those with lower levels. Also, the IgG anticardiolipin antibody is much more strongly associated with recurrent thrombosis than is the IgM anticardiolipin antibody. If there is no history of thrombosis, most physicians are reluctant to treat the patient for a lupus anticoagulant or elevated anticardiolipin antibodies alone without clinical manifestations.

- Patients with highest levels of anticardiolipin antibodies are more prone to thrombosis.
- IgG anticardiolipin antibody is more strongly associated with recurrent thrombosis than is IgM anticardiolipin antibody.

Treatment

Treatment of patients with the lupus anticoagulant and anticardiolipin antibodies is unclear. For most patients who have recurrent thrombosis, warfarin (Coumadin) is prescribed and will need to be taken for life. Treatment with steroids decreases the lupus anticoagulant activity, but no studies suggest that they prevent recurrent thrombosis; this possibility is still undetermined.

RAYNAUD'S PHENOMENON

This is biphasic or triphasic color changes (pallor, cyanosis, erythema) accompanied by pain and numbness in hands or feet. Cold is a common precipitating agent. Associated factors are listed in Table 27-11.

- Cold is common precipitating agent for Raynaud's phenomenon.

Table 27-11.--Causes of Secondary Raynaud's Phenomenon

Chemotherapeutic agents
Bleomycin
Vinblastine
Toxins
Vinyl chloride
Vibration-induced injuries
Jackhammer use
Vascular occlusive disorders
Thoracic outlet obstruction
Atherosclerosis
Vasculitis
Connective tissue diseases
Scleroderma, 90%-100%
Mixed connective tissue disease, 90%-100%
Systemic lupus erythematosus, 15%
Rheumatoid arthritis, <10%
Polymyositis
Miscellaneous
Cryoglobulinemia
Cold agglutinins
Increased blood viscosity

Raynaud's phenomenon is a possible abnormality of microvasculature with intimal fibrosis. Male patients with Raynaud's phenomenon, a rare occurrence, often develop a connective tissue disease. Although Raynaud's phenomenon is common in females, it usually is not associated with a connective tissue disease unless the patient has positive results for antinuclear antibody, which suggest that a connective tissue disease is likely to develop in the future.

Skin capillary microscopy reveals tortuous, dilated capillary loops in systemic sclerosis, mixed connective tissue disease, and polymyositis. They also may be present in patients with Raynaud's phenomenon who will go on to develop systemic sclerosis, polymyositis, or mixed connective tissue disease.

Treatment involves smoking cessation, wearing gloves, biofeedback, 2% nitrol paste, and antihypertensives (methyldopa, prazosin, dibenzyline, nifedipine). Stellate ganglion block is used if ischemia is severe. β-Adrenergic blockers increase spasm and so are not used.

To differentiate primary Raynaud's phenomenon from the secondary form (resulting from a connective tissue disease) clinical features are considered. In primary Raynaud's disease, females are usually affected, the onset is at menarche, usually all digits are involved, and attacks are very frequent. The severity of symptoms is mild to moderate, and they can be precipitated by emotional stress. Digital ulceration and finger edema are rare, as is periungual erythema. Livedo reticularis is frequent. In persons with Raynaud's phenomenon secondary to a connective tissue disease, both males and females are affected. The onset of Raynaud's phenomenon is in the mid-20s or later. If often begins in a single digit, and attacks are usually infrequent (zero to five a day). The severity is moderate to severe, and it is not precipitated by emotional stress. Digital ulceration occurs in 30%-50% of cases, and finger edema and periungual erythema are frequent. Livedo reticularis is uncommon.

SYSTEMIC SCLEROSIS

For diagnosis of systemic sclerosis, one major criterion or two or more minor criteria need to be present. The major criterion is symmetric induration of skin of fingers and skin proximal to metacarpophalangeal or metatarsophalangeal joints. The minor criteria are sclerodactyly, digital pitting scars or loss of substance from the finger pad, and bibasilar pulmonary fibrosis.

- Systemic sclerosis characterized by symmetric induration of skin of fingers and skin proximal to metacarpophalangeal or metatarsophalangeal joints and by bibasilar pulmonary fibrosis.

Clinical Manifestations

Skin

Patients are at risk for developing rapidly progressive acral and trunk skin thickening and early visceral abnormalities. Skin and visceral changes tend to parallel each other in severity, but not always. Some patients have rapid progression for 2-3 years and then arrestment or some improvement of the disorder.

Raynaud's Phenomenon

Raynaud's phenomenon occurs in almost all patients. It usually occurs more than 2 years before skin changes. The vasospasm in the hands can be associated with reduced perfusion to heart, lungs, kidneys, and gastrointestinal tract. If Raynaud's phenomenon is not present, but skin findings are suggestive of scleroderma, another disease such as eosinophilic fasciitis should be considered.

Articular

Nondeforming symmetrical polyarthritis similar to rheumatoid arthritis may precede cutaneous manifestations by 12 months. Patients can develop both articular erosions and nonarticular bony resorptive changes of ribs, mandible, radius, ulna, and distal phalangeal tufts which are unique to systemic sclerosis. Up to 60% of patients have "leathery" crepitation of tendons of wrist.

Pulmonary

Significant decrease in CO diffusion can be present with normal chest radiograph. Diffuse interstitial fibrosis occurs in approximately 70% of patients and is most common pulmonary abnormality. Pleuritis (with effusion) is very rare. Pulmonary hypertension is more common in patients with CREST variant (see page 795).

- Significant decrease in CO diffusion can be present with normal chest radiograph.
- Diffuse interstitial fibrosis occurs in about 70% of patients.
- Pleuritis very rare.

Cardiac Manifestations

Cardiac abnormalities occur in up to 70% of patients. Conduction defects and supraventricular arrhythmias are most common. Pulmonary hypertension with cor pulmonale is most serious problem.

- Cardiac abnormalities in up to 70% of patients.
- Pulmonary hypertension with cor pulmonale is most serious problem.

Gastrointestinal

Esophageal dysfunction is the most frequent gastrointestinal abnormality. It occurs in 90% of patients and often is asymptomatic. Lower esophageal sphincter incompetence with acid reflux may produce esophageal strictures or ulcers. Antacids or cimetidine may help. Reduced esophageal motility may respond to therapy with metoclopramide, nifedipine, and methacholine alone or in combination. Small bowel hypomotility may be associated with bacterial overgrowth and malabsorption. Treatment with tetracycline may be helpful.

- Esophageal dysfunction is most frequent gastrointestinal abnormality.
- Lower esophageal sphincter incompetence with acid reflux may produce esophageal strictures or ulcers.
- Small bowel hypomotility may be associated with bacterial overgrowth.

Renal

Renal involvement frequently results in fulminant hypertension, renal failure, and death if not treated aggressively. Proteinuria, newly diagnosed *mild* hypertension, microangiopathic hemolytic anemia, vascular changes on renal biopsy, and rapid progression of skin thickening may precede overt clinical findings of renal crisis. Association of renal involvement with hyperreninemia prompted use of suppressors of renin synthesis and release (propranolol) and of angiotensin converting enzyme inhibitors. Aggressive early antihypertensive therapy can extend life expectancy.

Laboratory Findings

Antiscleroderma antibody (anti-Scl70) is found in approximately 25% of patients, and anticentromere antibody occurs in 10%-20%.

Treatment

No remissive or curative therapy is available. Retrospective studies suggest that D-penicillamine (750 mg daily) may decrease skin thickness, prevent or delay internal organ involvement, and prolong life expectancy.

- No remissive or curative therapy available.

CREST SYNDROME

This is characterized by *c*alcinosis cutis, *R*aynaud's phenomenon, *e*sophageal dysmotility, *s*clerodactyly, and *t*elangiectasias. Skin involvement progresses slowly and is limited to extremities. Development of internal organ involvement is delayed. Lung involvement occurs in 70% of patients. Diffusing capacity is low, and pulmonary hypertension can develop. The latter is more common in CREST than in diffuse scleroderma. Onset of Raynaud's phenomenon occurs before skin changes (less than 2 years before skin changes). Anticentromere antibody is found in 70%-90% of patients and antiscleroderma-70 antibody in 10%. The incidence of primary biliary cirrhosis is increased.

- In CREST syndrome, 70% of patients have lung involvement.
- Diffusing capacity low, and pulmonary hypertension can develop.
- Anticentromere antibody in 70%-90% of patients.
- Increased incidence of primary biliary cirrhosis.

SCLERODERMA-LIKE SYNDROMES

Disorders Associated With Occupation or Environment

This group includes polyvinyl chloride disease, jackhammer disease, silicosis, silicone implants (still a questionable association), and toxic oil syndrome.

Eosinophilic Fasciitis

Clinical features of this disorder are 1) tight bound-down skin of extremities characteristically sparing the hands and feet. Peau d'orange skin changes can develop. Onset after vigorous exercise is common. Raynaud's phenomenon does not occur, and there is no visceral involvement. Flexion contractures and carpal tunnel syndrome can develop.

- Eosinophilic fasciitis characterized by tight bound-down skin of extremities, usually sparing hands and feet.
- No visceral involvement.

Laboratory findings are peripheral eosinophilia, increased sedimentation rate, and hypergammaglobulinemia. The diagnosis is based on the findings of inflammation and thickening of fascia on deep fascial biopsy.

Treatment is with prednisone (40 mg daily). The response is usually good. Associated conditions are aplastic anemia and thrombocytopenia (both antibody-mediated) and leukemias and myeloproliferative diseases.

- Lab findings include peripheral eosinophilia.
- Treatment with prednisone provides good response.

Disorders With Metabolic Causes

This group includes porphyria, amyloidosis, carcinoid, and diabetes mellitus (flexion contractures of tendons in hands can develop).

Others

As a manifestation of *graft-versus-host disease*, skin induration develops in up to 30% of patients who receive bone marrow transplant. *Drug-induced disorders* are caused by carbidopa and bleomycin. *Eosinophilic myalgia syndrome* is associated with ingestion of L-tryptophan. Patients develop eosinophilia, myositis, skin induration, fasciitis, and peripheral neuropathy. Skin changes are similar to those of eosinophilic fasciitis. A contaminant rather than L-tryptophan itself is thought to be the cause. There is a poor response to steroids. *Scleredema* frequently occurs after streptococcal upper respiratory tract infection in children. It is usually self-limiting. Swelling of the head and neck is common. In adults, diabetes mellitus is often associated. *Scleromyxedema* is associated with IgG monoclonal protein.

INFLAMMATORY MYOPATHIES

Inflammatory myopathies can be classified into several categories, including polymyositis, dermatomyositis, myositis associated with malignancy, childhood-type, and overlap connective tissue disease. Polymyositis is an inflammatory myopathy characterized by proximal muscle weakness. Patients with dermatomyositis can have an associated rash that includes a heliotrope hue of the eyelids, a rash on the metacarpophalangeal and proximal interphalangeal joints (Gottron papules), and photosensitivity dermatitis of the face. Most patients have an elevated creatine kinase level, a characteristic electromyogram, and a characteristic muscle biopsy.

- Polymyositis is inflammatory myopathy characterized by proximal muscle weakness.
- Feature of dermatomyositis is rash that includes heliotrope hue of eyelids.

The electromyogram is characteristic but not diagnostic of inflammatory myopathies. It shows decreased amplitude and increased spike frequency, it is polyphasic, and conduction speed is normal. Fibrillation is not specific for inflammatory myopathies, but when present it indicates active disease. Loss of fibrillation usually means the inflammatory myopathy is under control, but if the electromyogram is still myopathic, it suggests an associated steroid myopathy caused by treatment. The muscle biopsy, which is mandatory in all patients with inflammatory myopathy, shows degeneration, necrosis, and regeneration of myofibrils and lymphocytic plus monocytic infiltrate in a perivascular or interstitial distribution.

- Electromyogram is characteristic but not diagnostic of polymyositis.

The association of polymyositis and dermatomyositis with malignancy is controversial. In patients older than 40 years, perhaps 10% of those with polymyositis and 30% with dermatomyositis have an associated malignancy. The antibody anti-Jo1 is associated with polymyositis and dermatomyositis in approximately 25% of cases. This antibody is associated with inflammatory arthritis, interstitial lung disease, and increased mortality primarily due to respiratory failure.

- Perhaps 10% of patients >40 years with polymyositis and 30% with dermatomyositis have associated malignancy.
- Anti-Jo1 associated with polymyositis and dermatomyositis in about 25% of cases.

Treatment of polymyositis includes prednisone (60 mg daily), usually for 1 to 2 months, until the muscle enzyme values normalize. The dosage is slowly reduced thereafter, and the clinical course and creatine kinase values are monitored. In steroid-resistant cases, either azathioprine (1-2 mg/kg per day) or methotrexate can be used.

Aspiration pneumonia can occur as a result of pharyngeal weakness. If so, a liquid diet, feeding tube, or feeding gastrostomy is needed until there is clinical improvement.

With regard to the differential diagnosis, inclusion body myositis needs to be considered. This usually occurs in the older age group. The onset of weakness is more insidious, occurring over many years. The creatine kinase value often is only minimally to several times elevated, and distal weakness and proximal weakness occur. The electromyogram, besides showing a myopathic picture, can also have an associated neuropathic picture. Diagnosis of inclusion body myositis is made from biopsy. Histopathology is indistinguishable from that of polymyositis except for the presence of eosinophilic inclusions and rimmed vacuoles with basophilic enhancement. Inclusion body myositis responds poorly to prednisone

and immunosuppressive therapy, and the course is one of slow progressive weakness.

- Inclusion body myositis usually occurs in older age group.
- Diagnosis is made from biopsy.
- It responds poorly to prednisone.

QUESTIONS
(See "Answers" section)

Multiple Choice

1. A 45-year-old woman presents with a 1-month history of a facial rash, arthritis, and pleurisy. Urinalysis reveals 40-50 erythrocytes per high-power field with erythrocyte casts and +2 protein. Testing for which of the following best corresponds to the renal involvement?
   a. Anti-SS-A
   b. Antihistone
   c. Anti-ssDNA
   d. Anti-nDNA
   e. Anticardiolipin antibodies

2. A 47-year-old white man develops proximal muscle weakness and dysphagia. The creatine kinase value is 10,000 U/L (normal, 50-250). Which of the following would be the most likely cause of death during the first 3 months of illness?
   a. Pericardial tamponade
   b. Renal disease
   c. Aspiration pneumonia
   d. Pulmonary fibrosis
   e. Myoglobinuria

3. In a patient with Raynaud's phenomenon, which one of the following findings would be most helpful in making a diagnosis?
   a. Positive antinuclear antibody test
   b. History of L-tryptophan use
   c. Elevated eosinophil count
   d. Sclerodactyly
   e. Abnormal esophageal motility

4. An 85-year-old man has been taking procainamide for >1 year for a cardiac arrhythmia. He is feeling well. Antinuclear antibody testing is positive at 1:640. Which of the following is an appropriate course of action?
   a. Stop use of procainamide
   b. Obtain other serologic evidence for systemic lupus erythematosus, including anti-nDNA and complement determinations
   c. Prescribe steroids, 10 mg daily
   d. Prescribe prednisone, 60 mg daily, and stop use of procainamide
   e. Continue use of current medication and observe

5. A 53-year-old white woman has a 15-year history of systemic lupus erythematosus. Multiple flares of her disease during the past several years have necessitated high-dose prednisone. She now presents with a 3-week history of pain in the left groin with ambulation. She denies fever, chills, or other symptoms that she has equated with a flare in the past. Routine radiography of her pelvis, including hips, is normal. Which one of the following would be most helpful in determining the cause of her symptoms?
   a. Electromyography
   b. Sedimentation rate and anti-nDNA determinations
   c. Magnetic resonance imaging of the hips
   d. Empiric trial of a corticosteroid injection into the hip under fluoroscopy
   e. Bone scanning

6. A 63-year-old white man has had recurrent episodes of gout. The uric acid value is 8.2 mg/dL (normal, <8.0). Radiographs of his feet reveal erosive changes of the first metatarsophalangeal joints, and tophi are apparent

on physical examination. He is asymptomatic at examination. A 24-hour urinary uric acid value is 300 mg (normal, <1,000). Which of the following would be most appropriate in the treatment of this patient?

a. Continued observation and treatment of the acute attacks when they occur
b. Indomethacin, 50 mg four times a day with food
c. Begin use of allopurinol
d. Begin use of probenecid
e. Begin use of allopurinol in conjunction with colchicine

7. A 48-year-old man presents for a general medical examination. He is not taking any medications and considers himself in good health. There is no history of kidney stones or gout. On routine laboratory evaluation, his serum uric acid value is 10 mg/dL (normal, <8.0). A 24-hour urine uric acid value is 300 mg (normal, <1,000). Renal function is normal. Which of the following is the most appropriate treatment?

a. Begin use of allopurinol
b. Begin use of probenecid
c. Begin use of allopurinol in conjunction with colchicine
d. Observe
e. Begin use of colchicine

8. A 42-year-old hunter from Connecticut presents with a 1-week history of an erythematous skin lesion and associated "flu-like" symptoms. He does not recall a tick bite. He considers himself otherwise healthy. Laboratory studies reveal negative results of Lyme serology, both by enzyme-linked immunosorbent assay and Western blot. Which of the following is the most appropriate course of action?

a. Tests for antinuclear antibody and rheumatoid factor
b. Skin biopsy of the lesion for immunofluorescence
c. Empiric trial of tetracycline
d. Observe
e. Repeat the Lyme serology study in 4-6 weeks

9. A 21-year-old white man has recurrent episodes of iritis and a 12-month history of low back pain with morning stiffness. The most useful testing for establishing a diagnosis would be which of the following?

a. Rheumatoid factor
b. Antinuclear antibody
c. HLA-B27

d. Antineutrophilic cytoplasmic antibodies
e. Radiograph of pelvis

10. A 37-year-old white man presents with an acutely swollen right ankle. He had severe, self-limiting diarrhea on a recent foreign trip. The most likely diagnosis is:

a. Reactive arthritis
b. Gout
c. Ankylosing spondylitis
d. Arthritis of inflammatory bowel disease
e. Rheumatoid arthritis

True/False

11. Drug-induced lupus is characterized by:

a. Renal disease
b. High-titer anti-nDNA
c. Pleuropericardial disease
d. Arthritis
e. Antihistone antibodies
f. Seizures

12. The following laboratory findings or history could be suggestive of the antiphospholipid antibody syndrome:

a. False-positive VDRL result
b. History of recurrent spontaneous miscarriage
c. Thrombocytopenia
d. Leukopenia
e. Budd-Chiari syndrome
f. Prolonged activated partial thromboplastin time not corrected with normal plasma

13. The following conditions can be a manifestation of ankylosing spondylitis:

a. Iritis
b. Scleromalacia perforans
c. Complete heart block
d. Secondary amyloidosis
e. Neurogenic bladder
f. Osteitis pubis

14. Gout can be precipitated by the following:

a. Fasting
b. Initiation of allopurinol therapy
c. Surgery
d. Hypothyroidism
e. Joint infection
f. Treatment with diuretics

CHAPTER 28
RHEUMATOLOGY II

Robert M. Valente, M.D.

RHEUMATOID ARTHRITIS

Rheumatoid arthritis is a chronic systemic inflammatory disease characterized by joint destruction. It affects 0.03%-1.5% of the population worldwide. Its incidence peaks between the ages of 35 and 45; however, the age-related prevalence continues to increase even past age 65.

Pathophysiology

The presentation of an unknown antigen to immunologically susceptible persons is believed to trigger rheumatoid arthritis. Several viruses have been implicated in chronic arthritis, including Epstein-Barr virus, HTLV-1 virus, rubella virus, cytomegalovirus, herpes simplex virus, parvovirus, and arbovirus. Mycobacterium, heat-shock proteins, and autoimmunity to such endogenous components as immunoglobulin, proteoglycans, and collagen are also implicated.

There is an immunogenetic predisposition to developing rheumatoid arthritis. Class II major histocompatibility complex (MHC) molecules on the surface of antigen-presenting cells are responsible for initiating cellular immune responses and for stimulating the differentiation of B lymphocytes into plasma cells that produce antibody. Most patients with rheumatoid arthritis have class II MHC type HLA-DR4 or HLA-DR1 or both. HLA-DR4 can be divided into five subtypes, two of which independently promote susceptibility to rheumatoid arthritis. Compared with controls, patients with HLA-DR2 are less likely to have rheumatoid arthritis. Rheumatoid arthritis patients with HLA-DR3 may have low-titer rheumatoid factor and increased toxicity to gold and D-penicillamine.

- Most patients with rheumatoid arthritis have class II MHC type HLA-DR4 or HLA-DR1 or both.
- 6x increase in concordance of rheumatoid factor-positive rheumatoid arthritis among dizygotic twins.
- 30x increased risk of rheumatoid arthritis in a monozygotic twin when sibling has the disease.
- There is a 3x-5x increased risk of rheumatoid arthritis in white Americans with HLA-DR4.

The earliest pathologic changes in the disease are microvascular injury that leads to increased vascular permeability and the accumulation of inflammatory cells (CD4 lymphocytes, polymorphonuclear leukocytes, and plasma cells) in the perivascular space. Cytokines, lymphokines, and various anaphylatoxins and chemoattractants are released. Angiogenesis occurs in the synovial membrane. Patients have swelling, pain, and joint stiffness with the onset of angiogenesis and vascular injury. The warmth, swelling, pain, and limitation of motion worsen as the synovial membrane proliferates and the inflammatory reaction builds. Mediators of inflammation promote synovial cell proliferation, the accumulation of neutrophils in synovial fluid, and the maturation of B cells into plasma cells. The local immune response becomes self-perpetuating.

- Rheumatoid factor is an immunoglobulin (usually IgM) that binds other immunoglobulins (usually IgG) at their Fc components, forming immune complexes.
- Plasma cells in the joint locally synthesize IgM and IgG rheumatoid factor.

The immune complexes activate the complement system, releasing chemotactic factors and promoting vascular permeability and opsonization. Increased phagocytosis leads to increased lysosomal enzyme release and the digestion of collagen, cartilage matrix, and elastic tissues. The release of oxygen free radicals injures cells. Damaged cell membranes release phospholipids that fuel the arachidonic acid cascade and promote the local inflammatory response. Proliferating synovium polarizes into a centripetally invasive pannus, destroying the weakened cartilage and subchondral bone. Chondrocytes, stimulated in the inflammatory milieu, release their own proteases and collagenases.

Clinical Features

The joints most commonly involved (>85% of patients) in rheumatoid arthritis are the metacarpophalangeal and proximal interphalangeal joints and the wrists. The distribution of involvement is symmetrical; predominantly small joints are involved. Ultimately, the knees (80% of patients), ankles (80%), shoulders (60%), elbows (50%), hips (50%), acromioclavicular joints (50%), cervical spine (40%), and temporomandibular joints (30%) can be involved. The sternoclavicular joints, cricoarytenoid joints, and the ear ossicles are infrequently affected.

- The joints most commonly involved are the metacarpophalangeal and proximal interphalangeal joints and the wrists (>85% of patients).

Musculoskeletal Complications of Rheumatoid Arthritis

Characteristic deformities include:

- Boutonnière deformity of the finger, with hyperextension of the distal interphalangeal joint and flexion of the proximal interphalangeal joint.
- Swan-neck deformity of the finger, with hyperextension at the proximal interphalangeal joint and flexion of the distal interphalangeal joint .
- Ulnar deviation of the metacarpophalangeal joints; it can progress to complete volar subluxation of the proximal phalanx from the metacarpophalangeal head.
- Compression of the carpal bones and radial deviation at the carpus.
- Subluxation at the wrist.
- Valgus of the ankle and hindfoot.
- Pes planus.
- Forefoot varus and hallux valgus.

- Cock-up toes from subluxation at the metatarsophalangeal joints.

Cervical Spine

One-half of all seropositive rheumatoid arthritis patients have involvement of the cervical spine. It is diagnosed with cervical flexion and extension radiographs that demonstrate subluxation. One-half of these patients have subluxation at the atlantoaxial level, and the rest have subaxial subluxations, typically at two or more levels. The cervical instability is usually asymptomatic; however, patients may have pain and stiffness in the neck, occiput, shoulder, or interscapular areas. Patients may present with syncope, light-headedness, paresthesias of the face or limbs, or nystagmus. Occasionally the first sign of cervical instability may be sudden ataxia, weakness of the limbs, or frank tetraplegia. Interference with blood flow in the vertebral arteries (vertebrobasilar insufficiency) explains some of the cranial nerve symptoms and the blackouts. New neurologic symptoms mandate urgent neurologic evaluation and consideration of surgical intervention. However, cervical subluxation does not usually progress to neurologic or vascular compromise. Indications for surgery include neurologic or vascular compromise and intractable local symptoms. In active patients, prophylactic cervical spine stabilization is recommended when there is evidence of extreme (>8 mm) subluxation of C-1 over C-2. The probability of cervical involvement is predicted by the severity of peripheral arthritis.

- One-half of all seropositive rheumatoid arthritis patients have involvement of the cervical spine.
- Patients may present with syncope, light-headedness, paresthesias of face and limbs, or nystagmus.
- New neurologic symptoms mandate urgent neurologic evaluation and consideration of surgical intervention.

Popliteal Cyst

Flexion of the knee markedly increases the interarticular pressure of a swollen joint. This pressure produces an out-pouching of the posterior components of the joint space that is termed a "popliteal" or a "baker's" cyst. The cyst can rupture down into the calf or, rarely, superiorly into the posterior thigh. Rupture of the popliteal cyst with dissection into the calf may resemble acute thrombophlebitis and is called "pseudophlebitis." Fever and leukocytosis can occur with the rupture. Ultrasonographic examination of the popliteal space can be diagnostic. Popliteal cysts should be distinguished from a popliteal artery aneurysm, lymphadenopathy, and (more rarely) benign or malignant tumors. Treatment of an acute rupture includes bed rest, elevation of the leg, ice massage, and an intra-articular injection of corticosteroid.

- Popliteal cyst is a "baker's" cyst.
- Rupture of popliteal cyst: may resemble acute thrombophlebitis, is called "pseudophlebitis."
- Ultrasonographic exam can be diagnostic.
- Distinguish them from popliteal artery aneurysm, lymphadenopathy, tumors.

Tenosynovitis

Tenosynovitis of the finger flexor tendon sheaths is common. It presents with diffuse swelling between the joints or a palpable grating within the flexor tendon sheaths in the palm with passive movement of the digit. Other tenosynovial syndromes in rheumatoid arthritis include de Quervain's and wrist tenosynovitis. Persistent inflammation can produce stenosing tenosynovitis, loss of function, and, ultimately, rupture of hand extensor tendons. Treatment of acute tenosynovitis includes immobilization, warm soaks, nonsteroidal anti-inflammatory drugs, and local injections of corticosteroid.

- Tenosynovitis of the finger is common.
- Other syndromes: de Quervain's and wrist tenosynovitis.
- Treatment: immobilization, warm soaks, nonsteroidal anti-inflammatory drugs, local injections of corticosteroids.

Carpal Tunnel Syndrome

Rheumatoid arthritis is the second most common cause of carpal tunnel syndrome (pregnancy is the number one cause). This syndrome causes paresthesias of the hand in a typical median nerve distribution. Discomfort may radiate up the forearm or into the upper arm. The symptoms worsen with prolonged flexion of the wrist and at night. Late complications include thenar muscle weakness and atrophy and permanent sensory loss. Other nerve entrapment syndromes, including tarsal tunnel syndrome, affect patients with rheumatoid arthritis. Treatment includes resting splints, control of inflammation, and local injection of corticosteroid. Surgical release is recommended for persistent symptoms.

- Rheumatoid arthritis: second most common cause of carpal tunnel syndrome.
- Tarsal tunnel syndrome affects patients with rheumatoid arthritis.

Constitutional Features

Fatigue initially affects up to 40% of patients, and weight loss, muscle pain, excessive sweating, or low-grade fever occurs in 20% of patients presenting with rheumatoid arthritis. Most patients with active arthritis have more than 1 hour of morning stiffness.

- Most patients have more than 1 hour of morning stiffness.

Extra-Articular Complications of Rheumatoid Arthritis

Extra-articular complications typically are seen in patients who have high titers of rheumatoid factor. In general, the number and severity of the extra-articular features vary with the duration and severity of disease.

- Extra-articular complications: typically in patients with high titers of rheumatoid factor.

Rheumatoid Nodules

From 20% to 35% of patients have rheumatoid nodules, which occur over extensor surfaces and at pressure points. They also occur in the lungs, heart, kidney, and dura mater. Rheumatoid nodules have a characteristic histopathology. A central area of necrosis encircled by palisading fibroblasts is surrounded by a collagenous capsule and a perivascular collection of chronic inflammatory cells. Breakdown of the skin over nodules, with ulcers and infection, can be a major source of morbidity. The infection can spread to local bursae, infect bone, or spread hematogenously to joints. Endarteropathy (a form of vasculitis) is responsible for nodule formation.

- 20%-35% of patients have rheumatoid nodules.
- They occur over extensor surfaces and at pressure points.
- They have a characteristic histopathology.
- Endarteropathy (a form of vasculitis) is responsible for nodule formation.

Rheumatoid Vasculitis

Rheumatoid vasculitis usually occurs in patients who have severe deforming arthritis and a high titer of rheumatoid factor. Vasculitis is mediated by the deposition of circulating immune complexes on the vessel wall, with activation of complement. At its most benign, it can occur with rheumatoid arthritis nodulosis and include infarcts on the nodules and at the cuticles. Proliferation of the vascular intima and media causes this obliterative endarteropathy, which has little association with inflammation. It is best managed by controlling the underlying arthritis. Leukocytoclastic or small vessel vasculitis produces palpable purpura or cutaneous ulceration, particularly over the malleoli of the lower extremities. This can cause pyoderma gangrenosum or peripheral sensory neuropathy. Secondary polyarteritis, which is clinically and histopathologically identical to polyarteritis nodosa, can result in mononeuritis multiplex. Occasionally, the vasculitis appears after the joint disease appears "burned out." Corticosteroids do not promote vasculitis in cases of rheumatoid arthritis.

- Vasculitis is mediated by deposition of circulating immune complexes on vessel wall.
- Rheumatoid vasculitis: an obliterative endarteropathy.
- Leukocytoclastic or small vessel vasculitis.

Neurologic Manifestations

Neurologic manifestations include mild peripheral sensory neuropathy. Sensory-motor neuropathy suggests vasculitis or nerve entrapment (e.g., carpal tunnel syndrome). Cervical vertebral subluxation can cause myelopathy. Erosive changes may promote basilar invagination of the odontoid process of C-2 into the underside of the brain, causing cord compression and death.

Lung Disease

The commonest form of lung disease in patients with rheumatoid arthritis is mild obstructive change on pulmonary function testing. The prevalence of obstructive change increases with duration of disease. It is associated with keratoconjunctivitis sicca. Pleural disease has been noted in 40% of autopsies of cases of rheumatoid arthritis. Clinically significant pleural disease is less frequent. Characteristically, rheumatoid pleural effusions are asymptomatic until they become large enough to interfere mechanically with respiration. The pleural fluid is an exudate. Pleural fluid glucose is low (10-50 mg/dL) because of impaired transport of glucose into the pleural space. The pleural effusion in rheumatoid arthritis has a mononuclear cell predominance and usually less than

5,000 cells/μL. Pulmonary nodules appear singly or in clusters in the lung. Single nodules have the appearance of a coin lesion. Nodules typically are pleural-based and may cavitate and create a bronchopleural fistula. Pneumoconiosis in rheumatoid arthritis, "Caplan's syndrome," is synergistic, producing a violent fibroblastic reaction and large nodules. Acute interstitial pneumonitis is a rare complication that progresses to alveolitis, respiratory insufficiency, and death. Interstitial fibrosis has physical findings of diffuse dry crackles on lung auscultation. A reticular or reticular nodular radiographic pattern affects both lung fields, initially in the lung bases. A decrease in the diffusing capacity of the lung for carbon dioxide and a restrictive pattern on pulmonary function testing complicate symptomatic interstitial fibrosis. Interstitial changes are highly associated with smoking. Interstitial lung disease may be a complication of treatment with penicillamine or gold. Bronchiolitis obliterans with or without organizing pneumonia may occur with rheumatoid arthritis or its treatment.

- Pleural disease noted in 40%.
- Caplan's syndrome.
- Acute interstitial pneumonitis is rare.
- Bronchiolitis obliterans.

Cardiac Complications

Pericarditis has been noted in 50% of autopsies of cases of rheumatoid arthritis. Rheumatoid nodules can occur in the pericardium. However, patients rarely present with pericardial symptoms. Effusive pericarditis uncommonly produces cardiac tamponade. Recurrent effusive pericarditis without symptoms occasionally evolves to chronic constrictive pericarditis. Untreated, constrictive pericarditis has a 70% 1-year mortality. Rheumatoid arthritis carditis includes conduction abnormalities in the myocardium. Valve dysfunction and coronary vasculitis have also been described. Granulomatous inflammation can spread to involve the base of the aorta.

- Patients rarely present with pericardial symptoms.
- Untreated, constrictive pericarditis has a 70% 1-year mortality.

Liver Abnormalities

Patients with rheumatoid arthritis can have increased levels of liver enzymes, particularly alkaline phosphatase. Increased levels of aspartate aminotransferase, gamma glutamyl transferase, and acute-phase proteins and decreased levels of albumin and prealbumin also occur in active rheumatoid arthritis. Liver biopsy shows nonspecific changes of inflammation or nodular regenerative hyperplasia, which may cause portal hypertension and hypersplenism. Many medications used to treat rheumatoid arthritis increase liver enzyme levels.

- Liver biopsy shows nonspecific changes.
- Many medications used to treat rheumatoid arthritis increase liver enzyme levels.

Ophthalmic Abnormalities

Keratoconjunctivitis sicca, or secondary Sjögren's syndrome, is the commonest ophthalmic complication. Episcleritis and scleritis also occur independent of the joint inflammation and are usually treated topically. Severe scleritis progressing to scleromalacia perforans causes blindness. Infrequent ocular complications of rheumatoid arthritis include episcleral nodules, palsy of the superior oblique muscle caused by tenosynovitis of its tendon sheath (Brown's syndrome), and uveitis. Retinopathy is infrequently a complication of the use of antimalarial medication.

- Keratoconjunctivitis sicca, or secondary Sjögren's syndrome, is the commonest ophthalmic complication.
- Episcleritis and scleritis are usually treated topically.

Laboratory Findings

Nonspecific alterations in many laboratory values are common. Normocytic anemia (hemoglobin in the 10-g/dL range), leukocytosis, thrombocytosis, hypoalbuminemia, and hypergammaglobulinemia are common. Rheumatoid factor (IgM) occurs in 90% of patients, but its presence may not be detected for months to years after the initial joint symptoms are noted. Rheumatoid factor is a marker of immune stimulation and occurs in various connective tissue diseases and infections, including subacute bacterial endocarditis and lymphoproliferative disorders. Five percent of the normal population have a low titer of rheumatoid factor.

- Normocytic anemia and leukocytosis are common.
- Rheumatoid factor is neither specific nor sensitive for the diagnosis of rheumatoid arthritis.
- Five percent of the normal population have a low titer of rheumatoid factor.

Cryoglobulins and antinuclear antibodies are common.

Eosinophilia occurs in up to 30% of patients with rheumatoid arthritis and may complicate treatment with intramuscular injections of gold. It may be a marker for future gold toxicity, and it may accompany rheumatoid vasculitis.

- Cryoglobulins and antinuclear antibodies are common.
- Eosinophilia occurs in up to 30% of patients.

C-reactive protein correlates with disease activity, but it is not more helpful than the erythrocyte sedimentation rate. Rheumatoid arthritis patients with active disease have low iron-binding capacity, low plasma levels of iron, and low erythropoietin levels unless they are iron deficient.

- C-reactive protein correlates with disease activity, but it is not more helpful than the erythrocyte sedimentation rate.

Synovial fluid is cloudy and light yellow, with poor viscosity, and typically contains 10,000-75,000 leukocytes/μL (60%-75% polymorphonuclear neutrophils). Synovial fluid levels of glucose are low, and microscopic crystals are absent. Ragocytes, phagocytic cells with intercellular immunoglobulin and cholesterol crystals, may be found.

- Synovial fluid levels of glucose are low, and microscopic crystals are absent.

Diseases in bold type in Table 28-1 are most likely to have high titers of rheumatoid factor.

The radiographic findings in early rheumatoid arthritis are normal or show soft tissue swelling. Later, the characteristic changes of periarticular osteoporosis, symmetrical narrowing of the joint space, and marginal bony erosions become obvious. Radiographic changes at end-stage rheumatoid arthritis include subluxation and other deformities, joint destruction, fibrous ankylosis, and, rarely, bony ankylosis.

- Later, the characteristic changes of periarticular osteoporosis, symmetrical narrowing of the joint space, and marginal bony erosions become obvious.

Diagnosis

To make the diagnosis of rheumatoid arthritis, symptoms must be present for ≥6 weeks in persons ≥16 years old. Four of the seven criteria of the American Rheumatism Association listed in Table 28-2 must be satisfied for the diagnosis to be made.

Table 28-1.--Diseases That May Have Positive Rheumatoid Factor

Rheumatoid arthritis
Sjögren's syndrome
Systemic lupus erythematosus
Scleroderma
Sarcoidosis
Idiopathic pulmonary fibrosis
Mixed cryoglobulinemia
Hypergammaglobulinemic purpura
Asbestosis
Malignancies
Infectious mononucleosis
Influenza
Chronic active hepatitis
Vaccinations
Tuberculosis
Syphilis
Subacute bacterial endocarditis
Brucellosis
Leprosy
Salmonellosis
Malaria
Kala-azar
Schistosomiasis
Filariasis
Trypanosomiasis

Table 28-2.--American Rheumatism Association Criteria for Making the Diagnosis of Rheumatoid Arthritis[*]

One or more hours of morning stiffness in and around the
  joints
Arthritis of three or more joint areas involved simultaneously
Arthritis of at least one area in the wrist,
  metacarpophalangeal, or proximal interphalangeal joints
Symmetrical arthritis involving the same joint areas on both
  sides of the body
Rheumatoid nodules
Serum rheumatoid factor
Radiographic changes typical of rheumatoid arthritis,
  including periarticular osteoporosis, joint-space narrowing,
  and marginal erosions.

[*]1987 revision

Natural History

More than one-half of patients with rheumatoid arthritis have insidious onset of the joint disease occurring over weeks to months. In one-third of the patients, the onset is rapid, occurring in days or weeks. Early in the course of the disease, most patients have oligoarthritis. Their disease becomes polyarticular with time. From 10% to 20% of patients have progressive arthritis. The course may be slow, fluctuating, or rapid, but the endpoint is the same--disabling, destructive arthritis. The group that does not respond to therapy is small (<5% of all patients with seropositive rheumatoid arthritis). Patients with polycyclic disease have flares interrupted by partial or complete remissions. They account for 70% of all rheumatoid arthritis patients. Spontaneous remissions in the polycyclic or progressive group almost never occur after 2 years of disease.

- The majority of disability is determined within the first several years of disease.
- The relationship between disease duration and inability to work is nearly linear.
- After 15 years of rheumatoid arthritis, 15% of patients are completely disabled.
- Mortality is predicted by age, disease severity, comorbid cardiovascular disease, and functional status.
- The life span of men with rheumatoid arthritis is reduced by 7.5 years and 3.5 years for women, in comparison with their normal counterparts.
- Mortality is also influenced by educational level and socioeconomic factors.

Patients who meet the 1987 American Rheumatism Association modified criteria for rheumatoid arthritis, including wrist and metacarpophalangeal involvement, are at high risk for progressive rheumatoid arthritis. Choosing predictive features for progressive rheumatoid arthritis has obvious implications for the amount and timing of medical therapy for the disease.

Seronegative Rheumatoid Arthritis

Rheumatoid factor-negative (seronegative) rheumatoid arthritis in patients younger than 60 usually is not associated with extra-articular manifestations of the disease. However, the arthritis can still be destructive and deforming.

Seronegative Rheumatoid Arthritis of the Elderly

A subgroup of patients older than 60 with seronegative rheumatoid arthritis may have milder arthritis. This subgroup suddenly develops polyarticular inflammation that is best controlled with low doses of prednisone. Minimal destructive changes and deformity occur. An additional group of elderly seronegative arthritis patients (men in their 70s) present with acute polyarthritis and pitting edema of the hands and feet. They have a prompt and gratifying response to low doses of prednisone.

- Patients >60 suddenly develop polyarticular inflammation best controlled with low doses of prednisone.

Adult-Onset Still's Disease

Systemic-onset juvenile rheumatoid arthritis is known as "Still's disease." It has quotidian or double quotidian high spiking fevers, arthralgia, arthritis, seronegativity (negative rheumatoid factor and antinuclear antibody), leukocytosis, macular evanescent rash, serositis, lymphadenopathy, splenomegaly, and hepatomegaly. Fever, rash, and arthritis are the classic triad of Still's disease.

Adult-onset Still's disease has a slight female predominance. Its onset commonly occurs between the ages of 16 and 35. Fever greater than 39°C in a quotidian or double quotidian pattern occurs in 96% of the patients. The rash has a typical appearance--a macular salmon-colored eruption on the trunk and extremities. The transient rash is usually noticed at the time of increased temperature. Arthritis occurs in 95% of these patients, and in about one-third of the patients, the joint disease is progressive and destructive. Adult-onset Still's disease has a predilection for the wrist, shoulders, hips, and knees. Weight loss and abdominal pain are not uncommon, and 60% of patients complain of sore throat, which can confuse the diagnosis with rheumatic fever. Lymphadenopathy occurs in two-thirds of the patients and hepatosplenomegaly in approximately one-half. Pleurisy and pneumonitis occur in less than one-third of the patients.

- Its onset commonly occurs between ages 16 and 35.
- Fever > 39°C occurs in 96% of the patients.
- The rash has a typical appearance--a macular salmon-colored eruption on the trunk and extremities.
- Arthritis occurs in 95% of these patients.
- Adult-onset Still's disease has a predilection for the wrist, shoulders, hips, and knees.
- Lymphadenopathy occurs in two-thirds of the patients.

Treatment of adult-onset Still's disease includes high doses of aspirin or indomethacin. Corticosteroids may be needed to control the systemic symptoms. Half of the patients require gold salts, immunosuppressive agents, or D-penicillamine to control the systemic and articular features.

- Treatment of adult-onset Still's disease includes high doses of aspirin or indomethacin.
- Half of the patients require gold salts, immunosuppressive agents, or D-penicillamine.

Felty's Syndrome

Felty's syndrome has the classic triad of rheumatoid arthritis, leukopenia, and splenomegaly. (Classic Felty's syndrome usually occurs after 12 years or more of rheumatoid arthritis.) It occurs in less than 1% of patients with rheumatoid arthritis. Splenomegaly either may not be clinically apparent or may be manifested only after the arthritis and leukopenia have been present for some time. Other features of Felty's syndrome are listed in Table 28-3. Patients with this syndrome frequently have bacterial infections, particularly of the skin and lungs. Infection related to the cytopenia is the major cause of mortality. High titers of rheumatoid factor are the rule, and a positive antinuclear antibody occurs in two-thirds of the patients. Hypocomplementemia often occurs with active vasculitis. Rarely, the hematologic abnormalities in Felty's syndrome spontaneously remit. Shortened erythrocyte survival related to the splenomegaly aggravates inflammatory-block anemia. In 40% of patients, thrombocytopenia is caused by splenic sequestration. The leukocyte count typically is less than 3,500/µL. An absolute neutropenia occurs with granulocyte counts between 500 and 1,000/µL. Bone marrow studies usually document myeloid hyperplasia, with an excess of immature granulocyte precursors suggesting maturation arrest. The marrow is rarely hypocellular. Patients often die of sepsis despite vigorous antibacterial treatment.

- Felty's syndrome has the classic triad of rheumatoid arthritis, leukopenia, and splenomegaly.
- Splenomegaly may not be apparent.
- High titers of rheumatoid factor are the rule.
- Antinuclear antibody occurs in two-thirds of the patients.
- In 40% of patients, thrombocytopenia is caused by splenic sequestration.

Table 28-3.--Features of Felty's Syndrome

Classic triad
Nodular, erosive polyarthritis
Leukopenia
Splenomegaly
Other features
Recurrent fevers with and without infection
Weight loss
Lymphadenopathy
Skin hyperpigmentation
Lower extremity ulcers
Vasculitis
Neuropathy
Keratoconjunctivitis sicca
Xerostomia
Other cytopenias

Treatment includes use of corticosteroids, gold, methotrexate, lithium, and splenectomy. There is considerable variability in the response to therapy. Recurrent infection, life-threatening infection, or life-threatening hemolytic anemia are indications for splenectomy. Felty's syndrome must be distinguished from a neoplastic disorder, large granular lymphocytosis, and nodular regenerative hyperplasia of the liver with hypersplenism and portal hypertension.

● Recurrent infection, life-threatening infection, or life-threatening hemolytic anemia are indications for splenectomy.

Treatment of Rheumatoid Arthritis
The management of patients with rheumatoid arthritis requires making the correct diagnosis, determining the functional status of the patient, and selecting goals of management with the patient.

Goals of management include relieving inflammation and pain and maintaining function. The principles emphasized by physical medicine include bed rest or rest periods, improving nonrestorative sleep, and joint protection (including modification of activities of daily life, range of motion exercises, orthotics, and splints, if they help the pain).

● Goals of management include relieving inflammation and pain and maintaining function.

Exercise should begin with range of motion and stretch-ing to overcome contracture. Strengthening and conditioning exercises should be carefully prescribed, depending on the activity of the patient's disease.

● Strengthening and conditioning exercises should be carefully prescribed.

Classically, initial treatment is with a nonsteroidal anti-inflammatory drug given at anti-inflammatory doses. If the response is inadequate at 3-4 weeks, a trial of a second nonchemically related nonsteroidal anti-inflammatory drug is used.

Disease-modifying agents of rheumatic disease are also known as second-line agents, slow-acting antirheumatic drugs, or remittive agents. Short-term studies with disease-modifying agents of rheumatic disease confirm improved quality of life. They are used sequentially. The classic indications for adding a disease-modifying or second-line agent include the correct diagnosis, failure to respond to a nonsteroidal anti-inflammatory agent, and sufficient disease to justify the therapeutic risk. Six months of uninterrupted treatment with one of these agents is usually required to assess its efficacy. They augment the response to concomitantly used nonsteroidal anti-inflammatory agents or corticosteroids given in low doses. Disease-modifying agents of rheumatic disease include:

● Methotrexate.
● Antimalarial drugs.
● Intramuscular injections of gold.
● Cyclophosphamide.
● Azathioprine.
● Sulfasalazine.

Patients receiving one of these disease-modifying agents will take it, on average, for 3-5 years before the lack of efficacy or toxicity forces discontinuation of its use. A second disease-modifying agent is substituted for the first one when a therapeutic or toxic roadblock is reached. Failure to respond to one of these agents does not predict a negative response or intolerance to the other ones. Clinical trials of combinations of disease-modifying agents do not have a favorable benefit-to-toxicity ratio.

● A second disease-modifying agent is substituted for the first one when a therapeutic or toxic roadblock is reached.

To anticipate or to attempt to achieve complete symptomatic relief in every patient is an unrealistic and impossible goal.

Sjögren's syndrome

Sjögren's syndrome has a triad of clinical features: keratoconjunctivitis sicca (with or without lacrimal gland enlargement), xerostomia (with or without salivary gland enlargement), and connective tissue disease (usually rheumatoid arthritis).

- Sjögren's syndrome triad of clinical features: keratoconjunctivitis sicca (with or without lacrimal gland enlargement), xerostomia (with or without salivary gland enlargement), and connective tissue disease (usually rheumatoid arthritis).

Idiopathic Sjögren's syndrome is diagnosed predominantly in middle-aged women. Histologically, it is characterized by CD4 lymphocytic infiltration and destruction of lacrimal salivary glands. Clinically, it is manifested by dry eyes, dry mouth, and a waxing and waning polyarthritis. Most patients with Sjögren's syndrome have a polyclonal hypergammaglobulinemia. Autoantibodies typically are present, including rheumatoid factor, antinuclear antibodies, and antibodies to extractable nuclear antigens (SSA and SSB).

Less commonly, systemic lupus erythematosus, scleroderma, polyarteritis nodosa, or polymyositis accompanies Sjögren's syndrome. Patients can present with primary Sjögren's syndrome without any additional connective tissue disease. The primary syndrome typically has an episodic and nondeforming arthritis. There is no perfect definition for Sjögren's syndrome, and no test is completely diagnostic. Simple dry eyes of the aged must be distinguished from Sjögren's syndrome. Features of primary Sjögren's syndrome are listed in Table 28-4.

- There is no perfect definition for Sjögren's syndrome.

When focal central nervous system abnormalities occur in Sjögren's syndrome, vasculitis or demyelinating processes similar to that of multiple sclerosis are suspected.

Patients with Sjögren's syndrome have an increased risk of developing non-Hodgkin's lymphoma. Transient episodes of lymphocytic pneumonitis, lymphocytic pulmonary infiltrates, and episodes of pleuritic pain may be prominent features in a subset of patients. Some patients

Table 28-4.--Features of Sjögren's Syndrome

Malaise
Fatigue
Arthralgias
Myalgias
Low-grade episodic polyarthritis
Raynaud's phenomenon
Renal tubular acidosis
Cutaneous vasculitis
Central nervous system abnormalities
Peripheral neuropathy
Sensory
Autonomic

have diffuse interstitial pulmonary fibrosis.

Treatment of primary Sjögren's syndrome is mainly symptomatic. In addition to hydration, systemic therapy is indicated if there is evidence of systemic inflammation. A Sjögren-like syndrome has been described in patients with HIV infection.

- Treatment is mainly symptomatic.
- A Sjögren-like syndrome has been described in patients with HIV infection.

Osteoarthritis

Osteoarthritis is the failure of articular cartilage associated with degenerative changes in subchondral bone, bony joint margins, synovium, and para-articular fibrous and muscular structures. Osteoarthritis is the commonest rheumatic disease; 80% of the patients have some limitation of their activities, and 25% are unable to perform major activities of daily living. More than 10% of the population older than 60 have osteoarthritis. Half a million new patients annually develop symptomatic hip or knee osteoarthritis.

- Osteoarthritis is the commonest rheumatic disease.
- 25% are unable to perform major activities of daily living.
- More than 10% of the population older than 60 have osteoarthritis.

The radiographic features of osteoarthritis do not always predict the amount of symptoms. Common radiographic features include: osteophyte formation, asymmetrical joint-space narrowing, subchondral bony sclerosis, subchondral cysts, and buttressing of angle joints. Later bony changes include malalignment and deformity. In the spine, the radiographic findings called "spondylosis" include anterolateral spinous osteophytes, degenerative disk disease with disk-space narrowing, and facet sclerosis. A defect in the bony structure of the posterior neural arch produces spondylolysis. With bilateral spondylolysis, subluxation of one vertebra on another may occur, "spondylolisthesis." The causes of spondylolisthesis include trauma, osteoarthritis, and congenital etiologies.

Pathogenesis of Osteoarthritis

Two principal changes associated with osteoarthritis are the progressive focal disintegration of articular cartilage and the formation of new bone in the floor of the cartilage lesion at the joint margins (osteophytes). Not all the mechanisms causing osteoarthritis have been identified. Current theories include: 1) changes in proteoglycan synthesis by chondrocytes, 2) enzymatic degradation of cartilage, 3) changes in the collagen framework of cartilage, 4) change in subchondral bone resilience, 5) crystal deposition in cartilage, and 6) abnormality of the bone and cartilage interface.

Primary Osteoarthritis

Primary osteoarthritis is cartilage failure without a known cause that would predispose to osteoarthritis. It is divided into several clinical patterns (1-6 below).

- Primary osteoarthritis almost never affects the shoulders, metacarpophalangeal joints, or ulnar side of the wrist.

1. Generalized osteoarthritis involves the distal interphalangeal joints, proximal interphalangeal joints, first carpometacarpal joints, hips, knees, and spine. It occurs more frequently in middle-aged postmenopausal women. Many of the patients have joint hypermobility.

- In women, incidence and severity of generalized osteoarthritis involving knees is related to obesity.

2. Isolated nodal osteoarthritis is primary osteoarthritis affecting only the distal interphalangeal joints. It occurs predominantly in women and has a familial predisposition.

- Isolated nodal osteoarthritis is primary osteoarthritis affecting only the distal interphalangeal joints.

3. Isolated hip osteoarthritis is more common in men.

It has no clear association with obesity or activity.

- Isolated hip osteoarthritis is more common in men.

4. Mucous cysts are gelatinous cysts that form on the dorsolateral or dorsomedial aspect of the distal interphalangeal joints in osteoarthritis. Fluid aspirated from these cysts contains hyaluronic acid. The cyst communicates with the distal interphalangeal joint space and can regress spontaneously or rupture. Joint sepsis can occur after cyst rupture. Surgical removal usually requires removal of the associated osteophyte; otherwise, the mucous cyst will return.

- Fluid aspirated from mucous cysts contains hyaluronic acid.
- Cysts can regress spontaneously or rupture.

5. Erosive osteoarthritis affects only the distal and proximal interphalangeal joints. Patients with erosive osteoarthritis have episodes of local inflammation. Mucous cyst formation is common. Painful flare-up of the disease recurs for years. Symptoms usually begin about the time of menopause. Bony erosions and collapse of the subchondral plate--features not usually seen in primary osteoarthritis--are markers for this erosive osteoarthritis. Joint deformity can be severe. In many cases, bony ankylosis develops. Ankylosis is usually associated with relief of pain. The synovium is intensely infiltrated with mononuclear cells. This condition may be confused with rheumatoid arthritis. Up to 15% of the patients may later develop more classic features of rheumatoid arthritis.

- Erosive osteoarthritis affects only the distal and proximal interphalangeal joints.
- Mucous cyst formation is common.
- Joint deformity can be severe.
- Ankylosis is usually associated with pain relief.

6. Diffuse idiopathic skeletal hyperostosis is a variant of primary osteoarthritis. It occurs chiefly in men older than 50 years. It is also known as "Forestier disease," "ankylosing hyperostosis of the spine," "spondylitis ossificans ligamentosa," and "spondylosis hyperostotica." The diagnosis requires finding characteristic, exuberant, flowing osteophytosis that connects four or more vertebrae, with preservation of the disk space. Diffuse idiopathic skeletal hyperostosis must be distinguished from

typical osteoarthritis of the spine with degenerative disk disease and from ankylosing spondylitis. Extraspinal sites of disease involvement include calcification of the pelvic ligaments, exuberant osteophytosis at the site of peripheral osteoarthritis, well-calcified bony spurs at the calcaneus, and heterotopic bone formation after total joint arthroplasty. Patients with diffuse idiopathic skeletal hyperostosis are often obese, and 60% have diabetes or glucose intolerance. Symptoms include mild back stiffness and occasionally back pain. Pathologically and radiologically, diffuse idiopathic skeletal hyperostosis is distinct from other forms of primary osteoarthritis.

- Patients with diffuse idiopathic skeletal hyperostosis are often obese.

Secondary Osteoarthritis

Secondary osteoarthritis is cartilage failure caused by some known disorder, trauma, or abnormality. Congenital hip dysplasia, slipped capital epiphysis, multiple epiphyseal dysplasia, and other congenital bony abnormalities lead to premature secondary osteoarthritis. Metabolic abnormalities, including ochronosis, hemochromatosis, Wilson's disease, and acromegaly, are complicated by secondary osteoarthritis. Any patient with an unusual distribution of osteoarthritis or widespread chondrocalcinosis should be considered to have secondary osteoarthritis.

- Osteoarthritis involving the shoulder or metacarpophalangeal joints should prompt physicians to look for secondary causes of osteoarthritis.

1. Alkaptonuria/ochronosis is a rare disorder of tyrosine metabolism. Deficiency of the enzyme homogentisic acid oxidase leads to excretion of large amounts of homogentisic acid in the urine. Oxidized, polymerized homogentisic acid pigment collects in connective tissues ("ochronosis"). The diagnosis may go unrecognized until middle life. The first manifestation can be secondary osteoarthritis. The patient's urine darkens when allowed to stand or with addition of NaOH. Ochronotic arthritis affects the large joints, e.g., the hips, knees, and shoulders. The radiographic finding of calcified intervertebral disks at multiple levels is characteristic of ochronosis. Other manifestations include grayish brown scleral pigment and generalized darkening of the ear pinnae.

- Alkaptonuria/ochronosis is a rare disorder of tyrosine metabolism.

- First manifestation can be secondary osteoarthritis.
- Ochronotic arthritis affects large joints (hips, knees).
- Calcified intervertebral disks at multiple levels are characteristic of ochronosis.

2. Hemochromatosis--Arthropathy affects up to 50% of patients with hemochromatosis and generally resembles osteoarthritis; however, it involves joints not typically affected by generalized primary osteoarthritis. Hemochromatosis arthropathy involves the metacarpophalangeal joints and shoulders. Attacks of acute pseudogout arthritis may occur in relation to deposition of calcium pyrophosphate dihydrate crystals. Chondrocalcinosis is commonly superimposed on chronic osteoarthritic change in hemochromatosis. The pathogenesis of joint degeneration in hemochromatosis is not clear. Iron is present in very low quantities in the affected cartilage. Treatment is symptomatic; the underlying iron accumulation is also treated.

- Arthropathy affects up to 50% of patients with hemochromatosis and generally resembles osteoarthritis.
- Attacks of acute pseudogout arthritis may occur.

3. Wilson's disease--Arthropathy occurs in 50% of adults with Wilson's disease. Arthropathy is unusual in children. The radiologic appearance varies somewhat from that of primary osteoarthritis. There are more subchondral cysts, sclerosis, cortical irregularities, and radiodense lesions, which occur centrally and at the joint margins. Focal areas of bone fragmentation occur, but they are not related to neuropathy. Although chondrocalcinosis occurs, calcium pyrophosphate dihydrate crystals have not been observed in the synovial fluid.

- Arthropathy occurs in 50% of adults with Wilson's disease.

4. Apatite microcrystals are associated with degenerative arthritis and are found in patients with hypothyroidism, hyperparathyroidism, and acromegaly. They occur without an associated endocrinopathy. The role of microcrystalline disease and the progression of osteoarthritis are not clear, especially in the absence of acute recurrent flares of pseudogout.

- Apatite microcrystals are found in patients with hypothyroidism, hyperparathyroidism, and acromegaly.

5. Neuroarthropathy or Charcot's joints commonly affect patients with diabetes. Men and women are equally affected. Patients with diabetic neuroarthropathy have had their diabetes an average of 16 years. Frequently, the diabetes is poorly controlled. Neuroarthropathy is a consequence of the peripheral neuropathy responsible for blunted pain perception and poor proprioception. Repeated microtrauma, overt trauma, and, occasionally, small vessel occlusive disease (diabetes) contribute to the cause. The foot is most commonly involved in diabetics. Involvement of the knee, lumbar spine, and upper extremity is uncommon. Classically, hip and spinal neuroarthropathy is caused by tertiary syphilis, and shoulder neuroarthropathy is associated with syringomyelia. Patients can present with an acute arthritic condition that includes swelling, erythema, and warmth. Callus formation occurs at the site of bony damage, and the callus subsequently blisters and ulcerates. Patients usually describe some pain and walk with an antalgic limp. Osteomyelitis frequently complicates diabetic neuroarthropathy. Infection can spread from skin ulcers to the bone.

- Neuroarthropathy or Charcot's joints commonly affect patients with diabetes.
- The foot is most commonly involved in diabetics.
- Classically, hip and spinal neuroarthropathy is caused by tertiary syphilis.
- Shoulder neuroarthropathy is associated with syringomyelia.

6. Diabetic neuroarthropathy--The classic form begins with trauma-induced fragmentation of bone and cartilage. The tarsometatarsal joint is most often affected. There is disorganization of the normal joint architecture. Bone and cartilage fragments later coalesce to form characteristic sclerotic loose bodies. With joint destruction and disorganization, there is attempt at reconstruction with new bone formation. This periosteal new bone is inhibited by small vessel ischemic change in some diabetics. Diabetic osteopathy is a second form of neuroarthropathy. Osteopenia of para-articular areas, particularly the distal metacarpals and proximal phalanges, results in rapidly progressive osteolysis and juxta-articular cortical defects. As in classic neuroarthropathy, this can be associated with osteomyelitis.

7. Post-traumatic osteoarthritis--Stress from repeated impact loading can weaken subchondral bone. Isolated large joint involvement is a clue to post-traumatic osteoarthritis. Internal joint derangement with ligamentous laxity or meniscal damage alters the normal mechanical alignment of the joint.

8. Avascular or aseptic necrosis of the bone may lead to collapse of the articular surface and subsequent osteoarthritis. It usually is seen in the hip after femoral neck fracture. Aseptic necrosis of the bone has various causes, including alcoholism, sickle cell disease, systemic lupus erythematosus, trauma, and caisson disease. Systemic corticosteroid therapy increases the risk of aseptic necrosis. Rare causes of osteonecrosis include Gaucher's syndrome, atherosclerotic vascular disease, and fat emboli. No underlying cause can be identified in 10%-25% of cases.

- Avascular or aseptic necrosis usually is seen in the hip after femoral neck fracture.
- Aseptic necrosis of the bone has various causes, including alcoholism, sickle cell disease, systemic lupus erythematosus.

9. Hemophilic arthropathy--Patients with hemophilia and recurrent hemarthroses are at risk for hemophilic arthropathy, a type of progressive degenerative arthropathy that is more destructive than primary osteoarthritis. Widening of the intercondylar notch of the knees is an early radiographic feature suggesting the diagnosis of this condition.

- Hemophilic arthropathy is more destructive than primary osteoarthritis.

Therapy

Therapeutic goals include relieving pain, preserving joint motion and function, and preventing further cartilage injury and wear. Weight loss (important in knee osteoarthritis), use of canes or crutches, correction of postural abnormalities, and proper shoe support are helpful measures. Isometric or isotonic range of motion exercises and muscle strengthening provide para-articular structures with extra support and help reduce symptoms. Relief of muscle spasm with local application of heat or cold to reduce pain can help.

Initial drug therapy should be analgesics, such as acetaminophen (1 g 4 times daily as needed). Nonsteroidal anti-inflammatory drugs are beneficial for inflammatory flares of osteoarthritis and usually do not need to be taken every day. Rarely, depot corticosteroids offer some temporary relief. Joint arthroplasty may relieve pain, stabilize joints, and improve function. Osteotomy redistributes joint forces. Arthroscopy removes loose bodies and trims torn menisci to correct joint lockup or give way. Herniated disks or spinal stenosis may require decompression.

- Nonsteroidal anti-inflammatory drugs usually do not need to be taken every day.

Total joint arthroplasty is very successful at the knee or hip. Table 28-5 describes the indications for total joint arthroplasty in a patient with radiographically advanced osteoarthritis. Surgical treatment for osteoarthritis of the shoulder is usually reserved for patients with intractable pain. The functional outcome in total shoulder arthroplasty is less predictable.

Table 28-5.--Indications for Total Joint
Arthroplasty

Radiographically advanced osteoarthritis
Night pain that cannot be modified by changing position
Lockup or give way of the weight-bearing joint associated with falls or near falls
Joint symptoms compromise activites of daily living

Arthritis in Chronic Renal Failure

Up to 75% of patients undergoing chronic renal dialysis have musculoskeletal complaints after 4 years of dialysis.

- Up to 75% of patients undergoing chronic renal dialysis have musculoskeletal complaints.

Erosive symmetrical polyarthritis occurs in patients who have received maintenance dialysis for more than 10 years. It can affect the interphalangeal joints, metacarpophalangeal joints, wrists, shoulders, and knees. Symmetrical joint-space narrowing and para-articular osteoporosis are prominent. There is no osteophytosis to confuse this condition with osteoarthritis. The synovial fluid is noninflammatory, and the synovitis on biopsy is nonspecific.

Destructive arthropathy of large joints frequently affects the hip, knee, shoulder, and wrist. Rapid progression to complete joint-space loss occurs over a 3- to 12-month period. Subchondral cysts and erosions usually precede the narrowing of the joint space by 2-4 years. Beta$_2$-microglobulin amyloid is frequently found in the synovium and in the cysts. Ischemic necrosis occasionally causes problems with large joints.

Amyloid Caused by Renal Failure

After 10 years of hemodialysis, 65% of patients have pathologic or radiologic evidence of amyloid deposition. The amyloid is composed of beta$_2$-microglobulin, which has a high affinity for Congo red and is permanganate sensitive. It is arthrotropic. Serum concentrations of beta$_2$-microglobulin are 60 times higher in long-term hemodialysis patients than in normal persons. Patients receiving peritoneal dialysis have similar elevations in beta$_2$-microglobulin. Shoulder pain and stiffness syndrome and carpal tunnel syndrome are strongly related to amyloid deposition. Currently, treatment is aimed at relieving the symptoms.

- 65% of patients have pathologic or radiologic evidence of amyloid deposition.
- Shoulder pain, stiffness syndrome, and carpal tunnel syndrome are strongly related to amyloid deposition.

Septic Arthritis

Gonococcal Arthritis

Any new acute inflammatory arthritis should be considered septic or related to microcrystalline inflammation until proved otherwise.

Approximately 0.2% of all patients with gonorrhea develop disseminated gonococcal infection (male-to-female ratio of 3:1). Females present with acute gonococcal arthritis during pregnancy or within 1 week after onset of menses (related to the pH of the vaginal secretions). Typically, the patient is between 15 and 30 years old. The two distinct forms of gonococcal arthritis are the first, or bacteremic, form (also called the "dermatitis tenosynovitis" form) and the second, or nonbacteremic, form. Patients with the first form have inflammatory tenosynovitis, dermatitis, and fever. About one-half of them present with a migratory inflammatory arthritis/arthralgia of the knee, wrist, or ankle. Synovial fluid effusions are uncommon. In the second form, constitutional features, rash/pustules, or tendonitis are not noted. Blood cultures are typically negative. This form begins as a migratory polyarthralgia that subsequently localizes in one or more joints.

- Any new acute inflammatory monarthritis in a sexually

active person should be considered related to gono-coccal infection until proved otherwise.

- When gonococcal infection is suspected, it is essential that specimens from the throat, joint, anorectum, blood, and genitourinary tract be cultured.

Among patients with known disseminated gonococcal infections, synovial cultures are positive in 30% of them. Culture of a skin papule/pustule is positive for gonococcus in 40%-60% of cases. The leukocyte count in joint fluid is often 5,000-10,000/μL, which is lower than in other septic arthropathies. The articular manifestations of disseminated gonococcal infections more often are related to a reactive or postinfectious arthritis than to a classic septic arthritis. This hypersensitivity reaction in the joint may explain why cultures are frequently negative and synovial fluid leukocyte counts can be quite low.

- The leukocyte count in joint fluid is often 5,000-10,000/μL.
- The articular manifestations are related more often to a reactive arthritis than to a classic septic arthritis.

Therapy--Patients with a purulent arthropathy or who are noncompliant should be hospitalized for intravenous administration of antibiotics for 24-48 hours, after which they may receive therapy as outpatients. Daily aspiration of the joint or joints may be required until clinical recovery is documented. A decreasing leukocyte count in the synovial fluid and decreasing joint effusion are markers for good clinical recovery. Patients who have recurrent disseminated gonococcal infection may have an associated terminal complement component deficiency. Occasionally, antibiotic prophylaxis is required. Gonococcal arthritis due to penicillin-resistant organisms has been described.

- The association of migratory oligoarticular arthritis and tenosynovitis suggests disseminated gonococcal infection rather than meningococcal disease.
- A decreasing leukocyte count in the synovial fluid and decreasing joint effusion are markers for good clinical recovery.

Nongonococcal Bacterial Arthritis

Nongonococcal bacterial arthritis is caused by hematogenous spread of bacteria, direct inoculation, or extension of soft tissue infection or osteomyelitis into the joint space. The joints most commonly affected are the knees, hips, shoulders, ankles, wrists, elbows, fingers, and toes. Patients with cancer, diabetes, chronic renal failure, liver disease, or sickle cell anemia are predisposed to septic arthropathy. Patients with chronic inflammatory and degenerative arthritis also are at increased risk for septic arthritis. The possibility of septic arthritis should always be considered in a patient with polyarthritis who has a single joint flare that is out of proportion to the rest of the joint symptoms. Patients who are taking immunosuppressive agents and intravenous drug abusers are also at increased risk for septic arthritis. In any patient with a septic joint, the possibility of infectious endocarditis, other septic joints, or disk-space infection should be considered.

- The joints most commonly affected are the knees, hips, shoulders, ankles, wrists, elbows, fingers, and toes.
- A single joint flare that is out of proportion to the rest of the joint symptoms.
- Patients who are taking immunosuppressive agents are also at increased risk for septic arthritis.

Bony destruction is not seen for 10 days to 3 weeks after the disease starts; therefore, radiographic findings may lag considerably behind clinical symptoms. Early features include osteoporosis, marginal erosions, and secondary osteomyelitis with periostitis. Nongonococcal septic arthritis is a rheumatologic medical emergency. Delay in either the diagnosis or the treatment of infection increases the risk of permanent disability and joint destruction. Cultures of the blood and other areas should be performed as clinically indicated. Synovial fluid should be harvested immediately. Gram staining of centrifuged synovial fluid should also be performed. Typically, patients with nongonococcal septic arthritis have more than 50,000/μL leukocytes in the synovial fluid. Synovial fluid levels of glucose and lactic acid are not helpful in making the diagnosis of infectious arthritis. Organisms involved in nongonococcal bacterial arthritis include *Staphylococcus aureus*, *Streptococcus* species, gram-negative bacilli, *Staphylococcus epidermidis*, *Diplococcus pneumoniae*, and *Haemophilus influenzae*. In sickle cell anemia, *Salmonella* is the organism usually causing septic arthritis. The portal of entry can predict the organism. Rheumatoid nodule breakdown and ulcer formation predispose the patient with rheumatoid arthritis to staphylococcal septic arthritis.

- Organisms involved in nongonococcal bacterial arthritis include *Staphylococcus aureus*, *Streptococcus* species, gram-negative bacilli, *Staphylococcus epidermidis*, *Diplococcus pneumoniae*, and *Haemophilus influenzae*.

- In sickle cell anemia, *Salmonella* is the organism usually causing septic arthritis.

Broad-spectrum antibiotics should be used until culture results are available. The infected joint must be drained as completely as possible. Repeated aspirations may be necessary. Progress can be monitored with serial studies of the synovial fluid. The number of leukocytes in the synovial fluid should progressively decrease over a 5-7-day period, along with a decrease in the amount of synovial fluid formed. If this pattern is not observed at 5-7 days, orthopedic open drainage must be considered. Orthopedic drainage is usually indicated in joints such as the hip that are not readily accessible with closed needle drainage. Duration of treatment depends on the virulence of the organism. Antibiotics should be given intravenously for at least 2 weeks and until clinical recovery (synovial fluid does not reaccumulate) is obvious.

- The infected joint must be drained as completely as possible.

Mycobacterial Joint Infections

Mycobacteria and fungi are responsible for chronic bone and joint infections. Many months pass before focal areas of osteopenia or articular erosions develop. In weight-bearing joints, the joint space is preserved for some time after erosive changes occur. A negative PPD rules out *Mycobacterium tuberculosis* monarticular arthropathy in well-fed, nonsuppressed patients. A synovial biopsy from a mycobacterial joint infection documents granulomas, with or without caseation. The absence of granulomas does not rule out fungal or mycobacterial infection.

- Mycobacteria and fungi are responsible for chronic bone and joint infections.
- A negative PPD rules out *Mycobacterium tuberculosis* monarticular arthropathy.
- The absence of granulomas does not rule out fungal or mycobacteria infection.

Rheumatic Fever and Poststreptococcal Reactive Arthritis

The incidence of acute rheumatic fever in the U.S. has

been declining steadily, although scattered outbreaks have occurred among U.S. school children and armed forces personnel. It is important to consider rheumatic fever with any new polyarthritis. One-third of patients with acute rheumatic fever deny any antecedent sore throat.

- Consider rheumatic fever with any new polyarthritis.

Arthritis affects two-thirds of all patients with rheumatic fever. In adults, arthritis occurs more frequently and may be the only feature of acute rheumatic fever. Although any joint may be affected, the arthritis usually involves the large joints, particularly the knees, ankles, elbows, and wrists. It is accompanied by the signs and symptoms of an acute febrile illness. Each joint remains inflamed for no more than 1 week, and the entire course of polyarthritis is usually severe for about 1 week. By the end of 4 weeks, it usually subsides. Flare-ups may occur in a small percentage of patients when treatment with salicylates or corticosteroids is withdrawn. Rheumatic fever never causes permanent joint damage. However, repeated attacks of rheumatic fever may result in a particular type of deformity called "Jaccoud's deformity," in which the metacarpophalangeal joints are no longer aligned correctly but are in ulnar deviation.

- Arthritis affects two-thirds of all patients with rheumatic fever.
- The arthritis usually involves the large joints, particularly the knees, ankles, elbows, and wrists.
- It is accompanied by the signs and symptoms of an acute febrile illness.
- Rheumatic fever never causes permanent joint damage.

Therapy--Patients with mild arthralgias and no carditis can be treated with analgesics. Corticosteroids are more potent than salicylates in suppressing acute inflammation and may be required for patients who do not respond to salicylates. Rebounds of rheumatic activity may appear when anti-inflammatory therapy is discontinued. Rebounds do not occur more than 6 weeks after stopping anti-inflammatory therapy. Doses of salicylates are typically 6-9 g/day in patients weighing ≥70 kg.

Viral Arthritis

Arthritis accompanies several common viral diseases in humans. Viruses commonly associated with arthralgia or arthritis include HIV, hepatitis B, rubella, and parvovirus and, less commonly, mumps virus, adenovirus, herpesvirus, and enterovirus. Most viral-related arthritides have joint symptoms that occur quite suddenly, are of brief duration, and do not recur. In most cases, the arthritis is nondestructive and does not lead to any currently recognized form of chronic joint disease.

- Viruses commonly associated with arthralgia or arthritis include HIV, hepatitis B, rubella, parvovirus, and, less commonly, mumps virus, adenovirus, herpesvirus, and enterovirus.
- Joint symptoms that occur quite suddenly, are of brief duration, and do not recur.

Patients with arthritic symptoms related to hepatitis B infection develop an earlier than usual antibody response. Similar musculoskeletal involvement has not been demonstrated in patients with type A or type C hepatitis. Up to 25% of those with hepatitis B infection have a prodromal polyarthralgia/arthritis. Joint symptoms persist from several days to weeks before resolving with the onset of jaundice.

- Similar musculoskeletal involvement has not been demonstrated in patients with type A or type C hepatitis.
- 25% of those with hepatitis B infection have a prodromal polyarthralgia/arthritis.

Rubella-associated arthritis usually occurs in women 20-40 years old. Joint symptoms may occur as early as 6 days before or as long as 6 days after the appearance of the characteristic macular, papular rash of rubella. Symptoms usually evolve over a 2-week period. Arthralgias have been reported to be present for more than 1 year. A live virus vaccine for rubella has also been associated with transient arthralgia and arthritis.

NONARTICULAR RHEUMATISM

Fibromyalgia

Fibromyalgia is a uniform syndrome characterized by chronic diffuse musculoskeletal pain. Other names for this condition are fibrositis, tension myalgias, generalized nonarticular rheumatism, psychogenic rheumatism, and benign myalgic encephalomyelitis. For the diagnosis, the pain should be present for at least 3 months and should involve areas on both sides of the body above and below the waist and some part of the axial skeleton. A high tender point count is an additional obligatory criterion for classification of fibromyalgia. Fibromyalgia affects up to 5% of all Americans and 15% of all general medical patients seen by internists; 75%-95% of all the patients are women. It is unusual for the diagnosis to be made in a person younger than 12 or for a first episode to occur after age 60. Of the patients (or their parents), 60% recall childhood growing pains or leg pains. Fibromyalgia is the second commonest reason (after the common cold) for lost work days. In the U.S., the diagnosis of fibromyalgia is not sufficient for disability pension.

- The pain should be present for at least 3 months.
- A high tender point count is an additional obligatory criterion.
- 75%-95% of all the patients are women.
- Fibromyalgia is the second commonest reason for lost work days.

Symptoms

The patients typically describe pain all over the body and use qualitatively different descriptions of the pain and discomfort than used by patients with rheumatoid arthritis. Patients localize the pain poorly, referring it to muscle attachment sites or muscles. The discomfort is worse in the morning and can be associated with stiffness. Physical activity or changes in the weather typically aggravate the symptoms. Most patients describe nonrestorative, nonrestful sleep. Anxiety is common. Active depression is not seen more commonly in these patients than in the general population. Articular symptoms can be prominent. Patient complaints include subjective joint swelling, hand and joint pain, prolonged morning stiffness, Raynaud-like vasospasm, and dry eyes. Headaches, paresthesias, numbness, and pseudosciatica-like pains are also common. Approximately one-third of the patients have visceral symptoms, including urinary urgency, severe pelvic pain unexplainable as dysmenorrhea or endometriosis, and irritable bowel syndrome. The onset of fibromyalgia occurs in more than half of the patients after an acute illness, typically a viral syndrome. In some patients, symptoms develop after trauma, such as injury on the job or motor vehicle accidents. Conditions associated with the onset of fibromyalgia are listed in Table 28-6.

- Patients localize the pain poorly.
- The discomfort is worse in the morning.

- Most patients describe nonrestorative, nonrestful sleep.
- Anxiety is common.

Table 28-6.--Conditions Associated With the Onset of Fibromyalgia

Viral syndrome
Trauma
Exposure to noxious substances
New systemic rheumatic disease
Hypothyroidism
Hyperthyroidism
Corticosteroid withdrawal
Family disharmony
Substance abuse/withdrawal
Emotional stress

Diagnosis

Fibromyalgia is a diagnosis of exclusion. Detailed physical examination will exclude most inflammatory and neurologic diseases. The finding of painful, tender points at muscle attachment sites supports the diagnosis of fibromyalgia. Laboratory evaluation includes performing a complete blood cell count, erythrocyte sedimentation rate, and thyroid function studies and determining levels of electrolytes, creatinine, calcium, and phosphorus. In selected cases, creatine kinase values and pelvic and spine radiographic findings are helpful in excluding other diseases. No diagnostic test confirms the diagnosis of fibromyalgia. Muscle biopsies, electromyographic and sleep studies, and magnetic resonance imaging (MRI) are not necessary for the diagnosis.

- The finding of painful, tender points at muscle attachment sites supports the diagnosis of fibromyalgia.

Natural History

Fibromyalgia is a chronic waxing and waning prob-lem. Patients have periods of pain and dysfunction alternating with variable periods of feeling reasonably well. Over a period of years, patients' symptoms and concerns can shift considerably from musculoskeletal concerns to fatigue to headaches or to irritable bowel. There is no progressive disability in patients who have had fibromyalgia for longer periods of time in comparison with patients in whom the diagnosis is recent. The factors that may affect the presentation and perpetuation of fibromyalgia are listed in Table 28-7.

- Fibromyalgia is a chronic waxing and waning problem.
- There is no progressive disability.

Treatment

Treatment includes reassurance and education, ensuring an adequate night's sleep, establishing a cardiovascular fitness program, and better flexibility and posture. Nonsteroidal anti-inflammatory drugs have a slight synergistic effect with sedating medications.

Low Back Pain

One-third of all people over age 50 have acute low back pain. Chronic low back pain is the number-one compensable work-related injury. The many causes of low back pain include mechanical, neurologic, inflammatory, infectious, neoplastic, and metabolic causes and referred pain from the viscera. Only 3% of patients presenting with acute low back pain have an organic cause not apparent after initial interview and physical examination. More than 80% find relief on their own or with the help of their physician or chiropractor within the first 2 weeks of symptoms.

- Low back pain: only 3% have an organic cause.

Diagnosis

The possibility of severe spinal cord or cauda equina

Table 28-7.--Factors That May Influence the Presentation and Perpetuation of Fibromyalgia Syndrome

Neurophysiology	Personal traits	External factors
Poor spinal postures	Personality type	Lack of physical fitness
Sleep disorder	Self-esteem	Job satisfaction
Activated deep pain system	Cultural beliefs	Family dysfunction
	Coping skills	Substance abuse
	Pain language	Loss of control over life options

compromise should be considered on the initial evaluation of acute low back pain. Objective weakness or numbness in the legs or bladder and bowel dysfunction are indications for more extensive physical examination, consideration of urgent lumbar myelography, and possible surgical decompression. Historical features may help sort out the causes of the backache. An insidious onset with prominent morning stiffness suggests an inflammatory axial arthropathy. Pain that worsens with coughing, straining, or sneezing suggests irritation of the dura mater. Radiating pain, weakness, or numbness in an extremity implicates spinal root irritation. Significant weight loss or pain that interferes with sleep suggests a neoplastic or infectious process. Referred pain from an abdominal, pelvic, or hip area suggests an extra-axial cause. Exertional calf or thigh cramping but normal peripheral pulses suggests pseudoclaudication or symptomatic lumbar stenosis. Pseudoclaudicant symptoms improve with leaning over a cart or with sitting (not standing still).

- An insidious onset with prominent morning stiffness suggests an inflammatory axial arthropathy.
- Pain that worsens with coughing, straining, or sneezing suggests irritation.

The radiographic findings of spondylosis, single disk degeneration, facet osteoarthritis, transitional lumbosacral segments, Schmorl's nodes, spina bifida occulta, mild scoliosis, and increased lumbosacral angle are not relevant to a patient's complaints of acute back pain. In the absence of specific historical or physical examination findings, laboratory or plain radiograph findings would not suggest malignancy, infection, systemic illness, or neurologic compromise. The use of bone scans, electromyography, computed tomography (CT), or MRI is not necessary to evaluate acute low back pain. The indications for spinal radiography in patients with acute low back pain are listed in Table 28-8.

- Clinical suspicion of lumbar stenosis and pseudoclaudication requires performing either MRI or CT with myelography.

Treatment

The treatment of acute nonspecific low back pain begins with reassuring the patient, because 80% of all patients with acute low back pain have significant improvement in 2 weeks. Of the 20% that continue to have significant symptoms, 80% will have improvement in another 2

Table 28-8.--Indications for Spinal Radiography in Patients With Acute Low Back Pain

First episode of acute back pain is after age 50
History of back disease
History of back surgery
History of neoplasm
Acute history of direct trauma to the back
Fever
Weight loss
Severe pain unrelieved in any position
Neurologic symptoms or signs

weeks. Bed rest should be prescribed for all cases of acute nonspecific low back pain. Short-term use of narcotic analgesics can supplement the use of acetaminophen, nonsteroidal anti-inflammatory drugs, and muscle relaxants such as cyclobenzaprine. Physical therapy measures include local heat and ice massage. Pelvic traction and TENS add little to the management of acute nonspecific low back pain. Corticosteroids injected epidurally are best suited to acute disk herniation, although their role is controversial. Injections into the facets are helpful occasionally, particularly if patients describe a locking or catching as part of their pain syndrome.

Bursitis

A bursa is a closed sac containing a small amount of synovial fluid and lined with a membrane similar to that surrounding a diarthrodial joint. Bursae are present in the areas where tendons and muscles move over bony prominences. Additional bursae form in response to irritative stimuli. Trauma to a bursal area may lead to an inflammatory response. Chronic overuse or irritation can aggravate bursal inflammation. Greater trochanteric bursitis is aggrevated by tight ileotibial bands, hard mattresses, and a waddling gait. Systemic disorders such as rheumatoid arthritis or gout cause bursitis.

Septic bursitis may occur secondary to puncture wounds or cellulitis or after a local injection. At least half of the time there is no portal of entry for infection in septic superficial bursitis (olecranon and prepatellar bursae). The organisms frequently responsible for infection are staphylococci (*aureus* and *epidermidis*) and streptococci. Patients with septic superficial bursitis present with localized pain and swelling. Erythema may be present, but it does not necessarily suggest infection. Warmth about the area of the superficial bursa should raise the possibility of a septic bursa. When in doubt, the bursa should be aspirated with strict aseptic technique. The needle should be passed through uninvolved skin.

- Septic bursitis may occur secondary to puncture wounds.
- Organisms frequently responsible for infection are staphylococci (*aureus* and *epidermidis*) and streptococci.

When infection is suspected, patients should be treated empirically with antistaphylococcal and antistreptococcal oral antibiotics, pending the microbiologic results. Gram stains are positive in only 40%-60% of cases. The number of leukocytes in infected bursal fluid can be quite low compared with that in infected joint fluid. This may be due to the modest blood supply of the bursae compared with that of joints. Patients with more severe infections or with associated cellulitis frequently do not respond to outpatient management. They should be hospitalized and given antibiotics intravenously, and the affected part should be immobilized for 3-4 days. Repeated aspirations may be necessary until the fluid stops accumulating. Occasionally, incision and drainage are required, and in chronic cases refractory to antibiotics, bursectomy is indicated.

- Gram stains are positive in only 40%-60% of cases.
- Number of leukocytes in infected bursal fluid can be quite low.
- Patients with more severe infections should be hospitalized.

Treatment of aseptic bursitis involves strict immobilization, ice compresses, nonsteroidal anti-inflammatory drugs, bursal aspiration, and corticosteroid injections. Corticosteroids should not be given when there is a clinical suggestion of sepsis. All bursal fluid should be cultured and evaluated for crystals. Acute trochanteric bursitis responds to reduced activity (especially walking), the use of a walking stick in the opposite hand, a foam mattress pad, and local modalities described above.

- Treatment of aseptic bursitis involves strict immobilization.
- All bursal fluid should be cultured and evaluated for crystals.

Polymyalgia Rheumatica

Polymyalgia rheumatica is a clinical syndrome usually characterized by the sudden onset of aching and morning stiffness in the proximal musculature. The definition includes an elevated erythrocyte sedimentation rate. Results of rheumatologic studies, including rheumatoid factor, antinuclear antibody, and complement levels, are negative or normal. In 1%-3% of cases, patients can present with a normal erythrocyte sedimentation rate. The presence of other specific diseases such as rheumatoid arthritis, chronic infection, inflammatory myositis, or malignancy excludes the diagnosis of polymyalgia rheumatica. Some definitions of polymyalgia rheumatica require a rapid response to small doses of prednisone (10-15 mg daily). This condition is more common in whites and has a moderate female predominance. It almost never occurs in persons younger than 50. It is endemic in the population of people over age 50, with as many as 50 new cases each year per 100,000 population.

- Elevated erythrocyte sedimentation rate.
- Results of rheumatologic studies are negative or normal.
- Presence of other specific diseases such as rheumatoid arthritis, chronic infection, inflammatory myositis, or malignancy excludes the diagnosis of polymyalgia rheumatica.
- This condition is more common in whites.
- It almost never occurs in persons younger than 50.

Features and Differential Diagnosis

Patients with polymyalgia rheumatica complain of stiffness more than pain. This stiffness is most prominent in the mornings and after prolonged sitting. Because the patients have difficulty raising their arms over their heads when they awaken, they characteristically roll to the edge of the bed and allow their feet to drop when getting out of bed. They occasionally have mild constitutional symptoms, including sweats, fevers, anorexia, and weight loss. Prominent constitutional features should suggest associated giant cell arteritis. Oligoarticular synovitis can occur, particularly at the knees, wrists, and shoulders. Polyarticular small joint arthritis is not a feature. Table 28-9 summarizes the rheumatic syndromes and other diseases that occasionally present with a polymyalgia rheumatica-like syndrome. Depression must be considered in patients with atypical features. Clinical evaluation and screening laboratory tests usually distinguish polymyalgia rheumatica from these other conditions.

- Stiffness is most prominent in the mornings.

- Prominent constitutional features should suggest associated giant cell arteritis.
- Oligoarticular synovitis can occur.
- Depression must be considered in patients with atypical features.

Table 28-9.--Systemic Illnesses Presenting With a Polymyalgia-Like Syndrome

Rheumatic syndromes	Other systemic illnesses
Systemic vasculitis	Paraneoplastic syndromes
Myositis	Systemic amyloidosis
Systemic lupus erythematosus	Infectious endocarditis
Seronegative rheumatoid arthritis	Hyperthyroidism
	Hypothyroidism
Polyarticular osteoarthritis	Hyperparathyroidism
Fibromyalgia	Osteomalacia
Remitting seronegative, symmetric synovitis and peripheral edema	Depression

Pathogenesis and Relationship to Giant Cell Arteritis

The pathogenesis of polymyalgia rheumatica is unknown. Clinicians appreciate the close relationship between giant cell arteritis and polymyalgia rheumatica. Familial aggregation and increased incidence in patients of northern European background suggest a genetic predisposition. HLA-DR4 is associated with these conditions more commonly than would be expected by chance. Polymyalgia rheumatica patients without vasculitis may have granulomatous myocarditis and hepatitis. Radionuclide joint scans in patients with active polymyalgia rheumatica confirm hip and shoulder synovitis. Muscles from these patients show normal tissue or mild type II muscle fiber atrophy.

- Up to 15% of patients with polymyalgia rheumatica also have giant cell arteritis.
- 40%-50% of patients with active giant cell arteritis have symptoms of polymyalgia rheumatica.
- Polymyalgia rheumatica can begin before, appear simultaneously with, or develop after the symptoms of giant cell arteritis.

Treatment

All patients with polymyalgia rheumatica should respond completely after 3-5 days of treatment with pred-

nisone, 20 mg/day. After giant cell arteritis has been excluded, most patients can be managed initially with prednisone doses of 15 mg/day or less. Follow the patients clinically, and when necessary, determine the erythrocyte sedimentation rate to confirm the clinical suspicion of a disease flare. Other acute-phase reactants are not superior to the erythrocyte sedimentation rate. Polymyalgia rheumatica is thought to be a self-limited disease. Prednisone treatment is discontinued in more than half the patients within 2 years.

- All patients respond completely after 3-5 days of treatment with prednisone.
- Determine the erythrocyte sedimentation rate to confirm the clinical suspicion of a disease flare.

ANTIRHEUMATIC DRUG THERAPIES

Nonsteroidal Anti-Inflammatory Drugs

Nonsteroidal anti-inflammatory drugs are among the most commonly prescribed medications in the world. There are no clear guidelines for selecting a particular nonsteroidal anti-inflammatory drug on the basis of toxicity or efficacy. Patients vary in their responsiveness to different drugs. The variety of these drugs available permits individualization of therapy. All of them are equivalent to acetylated salicylates with regard to efficacy. They are all potent cyclooxygenase inhibitors or pro-drugs of cyclooxygenase inhibitors. No clinical study has consistently found greater efficacy or tolerance for any one of these medications. Nonsteroidal anti-inflammatory drugs are used to treat all types of arthritis and many types of soft tissue rheumatism.

- There are no clear guidelines for selecting a particular nonsteroidal anti-inflammatory drug on the basis of toxicity or efficacy.
- They are all potent cyclooxygenase inhibitors or pro-drugs of cyclooxygenase inhibitors.

Mechanism of Action

The mechanism of the action of nonsteroidal anti-inflammatory drugs is poorly understood. They reduce prostaglandin synthesis by inhibiting cyclooxygenase conversion of arachidonic acid to prostaglandin precursors. Prostaglandins cause vasodilatation, mediate pain, and potentiate the inflammatory effects of histamines and kinase. Furthermore, prostaglandins act as immunomodulators, influencing cellular and humoral immune responses.

- They reduce prostaglandin synthesis by inhibiting cyclooxygenase conversion of arachidonic acid to prostaglandin precursors.
- Prostaglandins cause vasodilatation, mediate pain, and potentiate the inflammatory effects of histamines and kinase.

Nonsteroidal anti-inflammatory drugs have potent analgesic effects that are related to their suppression of prostaglandin synthesis. Decreased levels of prostaglandin decrease the sensitivity of peripheral nerve receptors and may affect pain transmission. Acetaminophen is not a potent prostaglandin inhibitor in peripheral tissue. However, it does affect prostaglandin concentrations in neural tissue. This may explain the analgesic effect of acetaminophen. Acetaminophen, salicylates, and other nonsteroidal anti-inflammatory drugs are potent antipyretic medications.

- Nonsteroidal anti-inflammatory drugs have potent analgesic effects that are related to their suppression of prostaglandin synthesis.
- Acetaminophen is not a potent prostaglandin inhibitor in peripheral tissue.

Mechanism of Toxicity of Nonsteroidal Anti-Inflammatory Drugs

Toxic reactions are primarily due to inhibition of prostaglandin production. Prostaglandins protect the gastric mucosal barrier from autodigestion. Patients with renal insufficiency or liver or cardiac disease may have prostaglandin-dependent renal blood flow. They have further decrease of renal function when nonsteroidal anti-inflammatory drugs inhibit prostaglandins. Also, nonsteroidal anti-inflammatory drugs interfere with the synthesis of thromboxane, which influences platelet aggregation and hemostasis. Blocking cyclooxygenase with nonsteroidal anti-inflammatory drugs augments conversion of arachidonic acid to leukotrienes. Leukotrienes (previously known as "slow-reacting substance of anaphylaxis") aggravate asthma, rhinitis, hives, and nasal polyps.

- Toxic reactions are primarily due to inhibition of prostaglandin production.
- Prostaglandins protect the gastric mucosal barrier from autodigestion.
- Nonsteroidal anti-inflammatory drugs interfere with the synthesis of thromboxane.

Nonsteroidal anti-inflammatory drugs are extensively bound to plasma proteins. Protein binding has obvious implications for other medications that are also protein bound. Phenylbutazone and aspirin inhibit the metabolism of oral hypoglycemic agents and increase the risk of hypoglycemia. Indomethacin, diclofenac, and piroxicam decrease lithium excretion. Nonsteroidal anti-inflammatory drugs can also influence methotrexate toxicity at high doses (>50 mg/week) by interfering with the renal clearance of methotrexate.

- Nonsteroidal anti-inflammatory drugs are extensively bound to plasma proteins.
- Phenylbutazone and aspirin inhibit the metabolism of oral hypoglycemic agents.
- Indomethacin, diclofenac, and piroxicam decrease lithium excretion.
- Nonsteroidal anti-inflammatory drugs at high doses interfere with the renal clearance of methotrexate.

Most nonsteroidal anti-inflammatory drugs *attenuate the effects of antihypertensive medications*. Diuretics, β-blockers, and angiotensin-converting enzyme inhibitors are the drugs affected most by the influence of nonsteroidal anti-inflammatory drugs on renal prostaglandins. Aspirin irreversibly inhibits cyclooxygenase. The effect of all the other nonsteroidal anti-inflammatory drugs on cyclooxygenase is reversible. All these drugs prolong the bleeding time. The use of aspirin needs to be discontinued for up to 10 days before the bleeding time returns to normal. Nonsteroidal anti-inflammatory drugs should be discontinued at least 4-drug half-lives before an invasive procedure. Nonsteroidal anti-inflammatory drugs with a short half-life are best when an acute effect (e.g., treatment of acute gout) is required. The half-life is proportional to the onset of maximal clinical benefit.

- Most nonsteroidal anti-inflammatory drugs *attenuate the effects of antihypertensive medications*.
- Aspirin irreversibly inhibits cyclooxygenase.

The common effects of nonsteroidal anti-inflammatory drugs are listed in Table 28-10.

Table 28-10.--Common Side Effects of Nonsteroidal Anti-Inflammatory Drugs

Gastrointestinal
  Nausea
  Abdominal pain
  Constipation or diarrhea
  Occult blood loss and iron deficiency anemia
  Peptic ulcer disease
  Colitis and colonic hemorrhage
Renal
  Reduced renal blood flow
  Reduced glomerular filtration rate
  Increased creatinine clearance
  Pyuria
  Interstitial nephritis
  Papillary necrosis
  Nephrotic syndrome
  Hyperkalemia and type IV renal tubular acidosis
  Fluid retention
Hematologic
  Bone marrow suppression
    Agranulocytosis
    Aplastic anemia
  Iron deficiency anemia
  Platelet aggregating defect
Neurologic
  Delirium/confusion
  Headache
  Dizziness
  Blurred vision
  Mood swings
  Aseptic meningitis
Dermatologic
  Urticaria
  Erythema multiforme
  Exfoliative syndromes (toxic epidermal necrolysis)
  Oral ulcers
  Dermatitis
Pulmonary
  Pulmonary infiltrates
  Noncardiac pulmonary edema (aspirin toxicity)
  Anaphylaxis and bronchospasm
  Nasal polyps
Drug interactions
  Augment hemostatic defect of warfarin
  Attenuate antihypertensive effect of diuretics, β-blockers, angiotensin-converting enzyme inhibitors
  Influence drug metabolism
    Methotrexate (high doses only)
    Lithium
    Oral hypoglycemic agents

Gastrointestinal Side Effects

Twenty percent of chronic users of nonsteroidal anti-inflammatory drugs have gastric ulcer noted on endoscopy, and 15%-35% report dyspepsia, but this complaint does not appear to be related to abnormal findings on endoscopy. Nausea and abdominal pain are described in up to 40% of users of nonsteroidal anti-inflammatory drugs. Stomach upset/pain forces discontinuation of these drugs in more than 10% of patients. Gastrointestinal blood loss related to these drugs is most often occult and can result in iron deficiency anemia. The true incidence of significant gastrointestinal bleeding requiring hospitalization or operation or resulting in death is unknown. However, the elderly are at greatest risk for significant gastrointestinal toxicity related to nonsteroidal anti-inflammatory drugs. Patients with significant comorbid factors--such as cardiovascular disease, previous stomach ulcer, and diabetes--and those taking corticosteroids are at higher risk. Alcohol and tobacco use also predisposes to the development of gastrointestinal toxicity.

- Twenty percent of chronic users of nonsteroidal anti-inflammatory drugs have gastric ulcer noted on endoscopy.
- Nausea and abdominal pain are described in up to 40% of users.
- Gastrointestinal blood loss related to these drugs is most often occult.
- The elderly are at risk for significant gastrointestinal toxicity related to nonsteroidal anti-inflammatory drugs.

Other Toxic Effects of Nonsteroidal Anti-Inflammatory Drugs

Bone marrow toxicity, including agranulocytosis and aplastic anemia, can occur with all nonsteroidal anti-inflammatory drugs, most frequently with phenylbutazone. This drug should be used only by physicians comfortable with monitoring for its toxicity. Central nervous system symptoms such as headaches, dizziness, mood alterations, blurred vision, and confusion are reported most frequently with the use of indomethacin. Ibuprofen, tolmetin, and sulindac have been associated with aseptic meningitis in patients with systemic lupus erythematosus. All the central nervous system effects resolve when the use of nonsteroidal anti-inflammatory drugs is discontinued. Rashes, urticaria, exfoliative dermatitis, erythema multiforme, and scalded skin syndrome or toxic epidermal necrolysis all occur with the use of different nonsteroidal anti-inflammatory drugs. Easy bruisability is a common complaint of chronic users of these drugs. Patients may develop dependent petechiae if their platelet function is already compromised. Pulmonary infiltrates, bronchospasm, and anaphylaxis may occur with all nonsteroidal anti-inflammatory drugs, including aspirin. Although it is not IgE-mediated, it is seen most commonly in patients who have the classic triad of asthma, nasal polyps, and aspirin sensitivity.

- Bone marrow toxicity can occur most frequently with phenylbutazone.
- Central nervous system symptoms are reported most frequently with the use of indomethacin.
- Easy bruisability is a common complaint.
- Pulmonary infiltrates, bronchospasm, and anaphylaxis may occur with all nonsteroidal anti-inflammatory drugs, including aspirin.

Combination therapy with nonsteroidal anti-inflammatory drugs should be avoided. Whereas toxicity is additive, there is no evidence that the therapeutic effect is additive.

- Combination therapy with nonsteroidal anti-inflammatory drugs should be avoided.

Nonacetylated Salicylates

Careful studies have not identified significant differences in efficacy of nonacetylated salicylates compared with nonsteroidal anti-inflammatory drugs. Nonacetylated salicylates minimally inhibit prostaglandin production. Although their use reduces the incidence of gastrointestinal bleeding, they do not prevent many of the gastrointestinal symptoms that influence patient compliance. Tinnitus remains a potential problem. Nonacetylated salicylates do not interfere with renal blood flow, and they do not inhibit platelet function. Also, they can usually be prescribed for patients with aspirin allergy. Because nonacetylated salicylates also are tightly protein bound, they can influence the metabolism of other medications.

- Nonacetylated salicylates minimally inhibit prostaglandin production.
- Nonacetylated salicylates also are tightly protein bound.

Disease-Modifying Antirheumatic Drugs

Antimalarial Compounds (Hydroxychloroquine)

Open and randomized placebo-controlled studies have confirmed the benefit of hydroxychloroquine in the management of rheumatoid arthritis and systemic lupus erythematosus. The drug collects in pigmented tissues, including the pigment layer of the retina and skin. The dose typically does not exceed 4.5 mg/kg daily.

Retinopathy is the major toxic effect associated with the use of hydroxychloroquine. The risk of irreversible retinopathy is quite small (<3%) in patients taking ≤4.5 mg/kg daily. The elderly may be at somewhat increased risk. Regular eye examinations can identify the premaculopathy stage of the toxic reaction, which is reversible. Permanent symptomatic retinopathy is preventable when patients have eye examinations every 6 months.

- Retinopathy is the major toxic effect associated with the use of hydroxychloroquine.

In rheumatoid arthritis, the clinical response to hydroxychloroquine does not appear before 8 weeks. Improvement may not occur until after 6 months of continuous therapy. Approximately 40%-60% of patients with rheumatoid arthritis may respond (based on established criteria for response). It is most commonly used in combination with nonsteroidal anti-inflammatory drugs or low doses of corticosteroids in patients with early or mild polyarthritis. The use of hydroxychloroquine in combination with other disease-modifying antirheumatic drugs has not been completely studied.

- In rheumatoid arthritis, the clinical response to hydroxychloroquine does not appear before 8 weeks.
- Improvement may not occur until after 6 months of continuous therapy.

Gold Salts

There are three preparations of gold salts: gold sodium thiomalate I.M. (Myochrysine, given intramuscularly), aurothioglucose (Solganal, given intramuscularly), and auranofin (Ridaura, given orally). Intramuscular injections of gold salts, started in the first few years of disease, can reduce the number of tender and swollen joints and improve grip strength. Gold treatment decreases the erythrocyte sedimentation rate and typically reduces the rheumatoid factor titer. Gold may work partly by influencing macrophage function. Adding intramuscular injections of gold to the treatment within the first 2 years of rheumatoid arthritis increases the potential for complete remission by approximately one-third over patients not treated with a disease-modifying antirheumatic drug. Gold given intramuscularly is also prescribed to patients with HLA-B27-associated peripheral arthritis. It has no effect on axial inflammatory arthritis. Intramuscular injections of gold may cause disease flares in systemic lupus erythematosus.

- Intramuscular injections of gold salts can reduce the number of tender and swollen joints.
- Gold treatment decreases the erythrocyte sedimentation rate and typically reduces the rheumatoid factor titer.
- It has no effect on axial inflammatory arthritis.

Gold therapy may be initiated if there is no history of previous gold toxicity, and the results of complete blood cell count and urinalysis are normal or stable. Gold therapy should be continued until at least 1,000 mg have been administered before a lack of response prompts discontinuation. It is important to check for any potential toxic reaction with each intramuscular injection. A complete blood cell count and urinalysis are usually performed before each injection. Patients should be questioned regarding any new symptoms. Adverse experiences in patients treated with injections of gold are responsible for 1-year toxicity dropout rates approaching 35%. Vasomotor responses (nitritoid reaction) occur more commonly with gold sodium thiomalate than with aurothioglucose. The nitritoid reaction occurs shortly after injection and is characterized by weakness, dizziness, nausea, vomiting, sweating, and facial flushing. Aurothioglucose does not cause these symptoms as often as the other gold salts.

- It is important to check for any potential toxic reaction with each intramuscular injection.
- The nitritoid reaction occurs and is characterized by weakness, dizziness, nausea, vomiting, sweating, and facial flushing.

Common reactions to intramuscular injections of gold include stomatitis and rashes. More than 50 types of rashes occur with gold injections. Often, the mucocutaneous reaction can be managed by changing the gold preparation or holding and later rechallenging with a lower dose. Gold therapy causes membranous glomerulonephropathy with proteinuria and nephrotic syndrome. Of the patients receiving intramuscular injections of gold, 40% have to discontinue use of the medication because of nephropathy. Hematologic disturbances occur in <2% of all patients receiving gold injec-

tions. Immunothrombocytopenia, agranulocytosis, and aplastic anemia can be life-threatening conditions.

- Common reactions to intramuscular injections of gold include stomatitis and rashes.
- The mucocutaneous reaction can be managed by changing the gold preparation.
- Hematologic disturbances occur in <2% of all patients.

Auranofin is an orally administered gold compound. About 25% of the dose is rapidly absorbed; the majority of the medication is eliminated in the feces. The medication should be continued for at least 4-6 months to assess its therapeutic potential. Meta-analysis suggests auranofin is less effective than other disease-modifying antirheumatic drugs, including gold (intramuscularly) or methotrexate. The most frequent toxic effect is diarrhea.

- Auranofin is an orally administered gold compound.
- The majority of the medication is eliminated in the feces.
- Auranofin is less effective than other disease-modifying antirheumatic drugs.
- The most frequent toxic effect is diarrhea.

D-Penicillamine

The mechanism of action of D-penicillamine is not completely understood. It does reduce immune complex formation. Penicillamine is a treatment for systemic sclerosis or scleroderma. Penicillin allergy is not a contraindication to the use of penicillamine. The adage "go low, go slow" emphasizes dosing increments that reduce the toxic effects associated with penicillamine, which is the only rheumatologic medication that needs to be taken on an empty stomach, 1 hour before or 2 hours after meals. The medication should be tried for at least 6 months if tolerated to assess its potential for therapeutic benefit. Its toxicity profile is similar to that of intramuscular injections of gold, including the mucocutaneous reactions, nephropathy, and hematologic abnormalities. Several autoimmune phenomena have been described, including myasthenia gravis, polymyositis, systemic lupus erythematosus-like syndrome, and a Goodpasture-like syndrome. Penicillamine causes skin fragility and poor wound healing by inhibiting collagen synthesis.

- The mechanism of action of D-penicillamine is not completely understood.

- Penicillin allergy is not a contraindication to the use of penicillamine.
- Penicillamine needs to be taken on an empty stomach.
- Several autoimmune phenomena.

Sulfasalazine

Enteric-coated tablets of sulfasalazine (Azulfidine) have reduced some of the immediate gastrointestinal upset associated with this drug. The metabolites of sulfasalazine include 5-aminosalicylic acid and sulfapyridine. The mechanism of its action is unknown. Short-term randomized trials report significant efficacy in mild-to-moderate rheumatoid arthritis. Rheumatologists also recommend treatment with sulfasalazine for seronegative spondyloarthropathies and psoriatic arthritis. The benefit of this drug in rheumatoid arthritis is equal to that of intramuscular injections of gold but with fewer toxic effects. Sulfasalazine treatment is usually reserved for milder cases of inflammatory polyarthritis. Although the onset of efficacy occurs as early as 8 weeks, the effect may not be documented for as many as 6 months. The toxic effects include nausea, vomiting, gastric ulcers, and, more rarely, hepatitis or cholestasis. Ten percent of patients complain of headache or sense of fatigue. Currently, this drug does not have FDA approval for management of rheumatoid arthritis.

- The mechanism of its action is unknown.
- The benefit of this drug in rheumatoid arthritis is equal to that of intramuscular injections of gold.

Methotrexate

Methotrexate is a structural analogue of folic acid and is considered an antimetabolite rather than a cytotoxic agent. It is used extensively in rheumatoid arthritis and also has a place in the treatment of psoriatic arthritis and peripheral arthritis of seronegative spondyloarthropathies. Methotrexate may have a role in the treatment of some aspects of systemic lupus erythematosus and scleroderma. Its mechanism of action in rheumatoid arthritis and other systemic inflammatory conditions is not completely known. It has both immunomodulator and anti-inflammatory effects. Its strongest effect is on rapidly dividing cells, particularly those in the S phase of the cell cycle. Methotrexate is unique among disease-modifying antirheumatic drugs because its antirheumatic effect occurs within 4-6 weeks. Oral, subcutaneous, and intramuscular and/or intravenous routes are equally effective for low dosages.

- Methotrexate is a structural analogue of folic acid.
- Its mechanism of action is not completely known.

In the management of rheumatoid arthritis and with appropriate dose titration, 80% of patients have a significant improvement in their condition within the first year of therapy. At 5 years, it is estimated that at least 35% of patients treated with methotrexate still take it. No other disease-modifying antirheumatic drug has this combination of efficacy and tolerability. Most patients with rheumatoid arthritis have a severe flare of their disease within 3 weeks after discontinuation of methotrexate therapy. This drug should not be used in patients with significant renal dysfunction (creatinine >2.0 mg/dL). Coadministration of trimethoprim sulfa antibiotics and methotrexate increases hematologic toxicity.

- 80% of patients have a significant improvement in their condition within the first year of therapy.
- No other disease-modifying antirheumatic drug has this combination of efficacy and tolerability.
- Most patients with rheumatoid arthritis have a severe flare of their disease within 3 weeks.
- Should not be used in patients with significant renal dysfunction.

Gastrointestinal toxic reactions are the common side effects of methotrexate. Nausea and vomiting may persist for 24-48 hours after ingestion. Stomatitis and diarrhea prove to be insurmountable problems for some patients. Methotrexate treatment should be withheld from patients with significant gastric ulceration until their ulcers have healed. Increased liver enzyme levels suggest subclinical hepatic toxic effect due to methotrexate. Persistent increase in aspartate aminotransferase levels or decreasing albumin levels are markers for developing hepatic fibrosis and, potentially, cirrhosis. Cryptic cirrhosis may develop without liver enzyme abnormalities being detected. Stomatitis and the less common hematologic abnormalities such as leukopenia, thrombocytopenia, and pancytopenia may respond to folic acid supplementation. Pulmonary abnormalities, including chemical pneumonitis and insidious pulmonary fibrosis, may occur with methotrexate treatment. In 50% of cases, acute pneumonitis due to methotrexate is associated with eosinophilia. Neurologic features such as headache and seizure are uncommon. Methotrexate is teratogenic and should be withheld for 3 months before the patient attempts to conceive.

- Gastrointestinal toxic reactions are the common side effects of methotrexate.
- Cryptic cirrhosis may develop without liver enzyme abnormalities being detected.
- Pulmonary abnormalities, including chemical pneumonitis and insidious pulmonary fibrosis, may occur with methotrexate treatment.

Azathioprine

Azathioprine and its metabolites are purine analogues. It is considered a cytotoxic agent. Azathioprine is metabolized by xanthine oxidase and thiopurine methyltransferase (TMPT). Allopurinol, an inhibitor of xanthine oxidase, delays the metabolism of azathioprine and can lead to toxic reactions if the dose of azathioprine is not reduced by 50%-66%. Thiopurine methyltransferase can be assayed; low levels of this enzyme predict the 1 in 300 patients who will develop a severe hematologic reaction to azathioprine. Controlled studies document the efficacy of azathioprine in the treatment of rheumatoid arthritis and, to a lesser extent, systemic lupus erythematosus.

- Azathioprine is considered a cytotoxic agent.
- Allopurinol can lead to toxic reactions if the dose of azathioprine is not reduced by 50%-66%.

The most common problem with azathioprine is gastrointestinal toxic effects. An idiosyncratic, acute pancreatitis-like attack is an absolute contraindication to further treatment with this drug. Cholestatic hepatitis is rare, but if it occurs, it generally does so within the first several weeks of drug administration. If tolerated initially, hematologic toxic effects become the most significant concern. In patients who have undergone organ transplant, azathioprine treatment increases the risk of neoplasia, particularly lymphomas, leukemias, and skin and cervical malignancies. Azathioprine does not alter fertility, but it may have some teratogenic potential. For pregnant women, azathioprine should be reserved for those with severe or life-threatening rheumatic diseases.

- The most common problem with azathioprine is gastrointestinal toxic effects.
- An idiosyncratic, acute pancreatitis-like attack is an absolute contraindication to further treatment with this drug.

Cyclophosphamide

Cyclophosphamide is a potent alkylating agent. It acts on dividing and nondividing cells, interfering with cellular DNA function. It depletes T cells and B cells, causing considerable immunosuppression. Oral cyclophosphamide is well absorbed and completely metabolized within 24 hours, and most of its metabolites are excreted in the urine. Allopurinol increases the risk of leukopenia in patients receiving cyclophosphamide. Short-term studies document significant efficacy of this drug in the treatment of rheumatoid arthritis at doses of 1-2 mg/kg per day. Unequivocal healing and arresting of erosive change occur. The considerable toxicity associated with chronic administration of cyclophosphamide has raised questions about whether it should be used in rheumatoid arthritis. It is the treatment used for many patients with Wegener's granulomatosis. Intravenous administration of cyclophosphamide is efficacious in managing severe systemic lupus erythematosus and diffuse proliferative nephritis. Short-term advantages of intravenous pulse of cyclophosphamide in lupus nephritis patients may include fewer bladder toxic effects and perhaps a lower risk of infection.

- Cyclophosphamide is a potent alkylating agent interfering with cellular DNA function.
- It depletes T cells and B cells.
- It is the treatment used for Wegener's granulomatosis.

Dose-related bone marrow suppression is common in patients receiving cyclophosphamide and requires close laboratory monitoring. Immune suppression from treatment with cyclophosphamide increases the risk of infection. Herpes zoster infection occurs in most patients receiving the drug orally. Cyclophosphamide directly affects ovarian and testicular function. Premature ovarian failure frequently occurs in premenopausal lupus patients taking the drug. Spermatogenesis can also be affected by this drug, which causes seminiferous tubule atrophy. Cyclophosphamide has teratogenic potential. Alopecia, stomatitis, cardiomyopathy (with drug doses used to treat cancer), and pulmonary fibrosis may complicate cyclophosphamide therapy. The metabolites of this drug, including acrolein, accumulate in the bladder. Acrolein has direct mucosal toxic effects and causes hemorrhagic cystitis. This complication is potentially life-threatening. The chronic use of cyclophosphamide taken orally is associated with increased risk of neoplasia, including hematologic and bladder malignancies. The risk of malignancy with intravenous pulse therapy has not been established.

- Dose-related bone marrow suppression is common.
- Immune suppression increases the risk of infection.
- Cyclophosphamide directly affects ovarian and testicular function.
- Cyclophosphamide has teratogenic potential.
- Acrolein has direct mucosal toxic effects and causes hemorrhagic cystitis.
- This complication is potentially life-threatening.
- The chronic use of cyclophosphamide taken orally is associated with increased risk of neoplasia.

Glucocorticosteroids

The role of corticosteroids in the treatment of rheumatoid arthritis is a controversial matter. Pulse or bolus therapy cannot be recommended for the routine management of flairs of rheumatoid arthritis. High doses of corticosteroids (1-2 mg of prednisone per kilogram of patient body weight) may be required for life-threatening or serious complications of inflammation. Low doses of corticosteroids (<10 mg of prednisone/day) are frequently used in the day-to-day management of the articular manifestations of rheumatoid arthritis. At least one-third of all patients with rheumatoid arthritis take corticosteroids chronically. These drugs have many side effects, which are not idiosyncratic but actually unwanted effects of the medication. The longer patients receive corticosteroids and the higher the dose that is used determine how fast an unwanted effect appears. Many patients with rheumatoid arthritis tolerate prednisone doses in the 1-5 mg/day range for years without having serious side effects. Patient concerns about corticosteroids include weight gain from increased appetite, water retention, and hirsutism. Longer term concerns include thinning of the skin, bruising easily, progressive osteoporosis (unclear if this happens with physiologic doses of prednisone) and compression fractures, high blood pressure, glucose intolerance, cataract formation, and aggravation of glaucoma. The psychoactive potential of high doses of corticosteroids is an additional factor in treating older patients. Corticosteroid psychosis can complicate the diagnosis of neuropsychiatric lupus.

SURGERY IN THE TREATMENT OF RHEUMATOID ARTHRITIS

Synovectomy of the wrist and nearby tendon sheaths is beneficial when medication alone fails to control the synovitis. The operation preserves joint function and prevents the lysis of extensor tendons that can result in a loss of function. Synovectomy of the knee, either open or through an arthroscope, can delay the progression of rheumatoid arthritis from 6 months to 3 years. Removal of nodules and treatment for local nerve entrapment syndromes are also important surgical treatments for rheumatoid arthritis. Arthroplasty is reserved for patients in whom medical management has failed and in whom intractable pain or compromise in function developed because of a destroyed joint. Arthroplasty, arthrodesis (wrist), and synovectomy are important components of well-balanced rheumatology treatment programs. Joint replacement surgery has had a major impact on patient disability.

- Synovectomy preserves joint function.
- Synovectomy of the knee can delay the progression of rheumatoid arthritis.
- Arthroplasty is reserved for patients in whom medical management has failed.

VASCULITIC SYNDROMES

Introduction

Vasculitis or angiitis is an inflammatory disease of blood vessels. It often causes damage to the vessel wall and stenosis or occlusion of the vessel lumen by thrombosis and progressive intimal proliferation of the vessel. The pathologic consequences of vasculitis are directly related to the ischemic consequences of vascular occlusion. The distribution of the vascular lesions and the size of the blood vessels involved vary considerably in different vasculitic syndromes and in different patients with the same syndrome. Vasculitis can be transient, chronic, self-limited, or progressive. It can be the primary abnormality or secondary to another systemic process. Histopathologic classification does not distinguish local from systemic illness or secondary from primary insult. The key clinical features suggestive of vasculitis are listed in Table 28-11. Vasculitis "look-alikes" or simulators are listed in Table 28-12. These diseases and conditions should be considered whenever the patient's condition suggests vasculitis. A scheme for diagnosing vasculitis is outlined in Table 28-13. The ability to recognize characteristic clinical patterns of involvement is very helpful to the diagnosis of vasculitis.

Table 28-11.--Clinical Features That Suggest Vasculitis

Constitutional features
  Fatigue, fever, weight loss, and anorexia
Skin lesions
  Palpable purpura, necrotic ulcers, livedo reticularis, urticaria, nodules, and digital infarcts
Arthralgia or arthritis
Myalgia or prominent fibrositis
  Polymyalgia rheumatica symptoms
Claudication or phlebitis
Headache
Cerebrovascular accident
Neuropathy
  Mononeuritis multiplex
Hypertension
Abnormal renal sediment
Pulmonary abnormalities
  Pulmonary hemorrhage, pulmonary nodules with cavities
Abdominal pain or intestinal hemorrhage
Nonspecific indicators of inflammation
  Anemia, thrombocytosis, low levels of albumin, elevated erythrocyte sedimentation rate, increased levels of liver enzymes, or eosinophilia

Table 28-12.--Syndromes That Mimic Vasculitis

Cardiac myxoma with embolization
Infective endocarditis
Thrombotic thrombocytopenic purpura
Atheroembolism: cholesterol or calcium emboli
Ergotism
Pseudoxanthoma elasticum
Ehlers-Danlos type 4
Neurovasculopathy secondary to antiphospholipid syndrome
Arterial coarctation or dysplasia
Infectious angiitis
  Lyme disease
  Rickettsial infection
  HIV infection

Specific Vasculitic Syndromes

Giant Cell Arteritis

Giant cell arteritis, also known as "temporal arteritis," predominantly affects persons over age 50. The prevalence exceeds 223 cases per 100,000 persons over age 50. It is most common in people of northern European ancestry. Females outnumber males by a ratio of 3:1.

Table 28-13.--The Diagnostic Approach to Vasculitis

Proper clinical suspicion for vasculitis[*]
Consider conditions that mimic vasculitis
Recognize clinical pattern of involvement
Define the extent and severity of disease
Narrow the diagnostic possibilities with laboratory tests
Select the confirmatory study
  Efficient (highest yield study)
  Safe as possible
Weigh urgency of diagnosis with risk of
  Diagnostics
  Therapeutics

[*]Table 28-11.

There is considerable morbidity with this disease; however, the rate of blindness is declining. The mortality rate for patients with giant cell arteritis is similar to that for the general population.

- Giant cell arteritis predominantly affects persons older than 50.

Pathology--Giant cell arteritis involves the blood vessels originating from the arch of the aorta. However, any artery, and occasionally veins, can be affected, but it is unusual for the intracranial arteries to be involved. Giant cell arteritis affects arteries in a segmental or patchy fashion. Histopathologically, extensive disruption of all layers of the vessel wall occurs, with intimal thickening and a prominent mononuclear and histiocytic infiltrate. Multinucleated giant cells infiltrate the vessel wall in 50% of cases. The other characteristic feature--fragmentation and disintegration of the internal elastic membrane--is closely associated with the accumulation of giant cells.

- Giant cell arteritis involves the blood vessels originating from the arch of the aorta, but it is unusual for the intracranial arteries to be involved.
- Giant cell arteritis affects arteries in a segmental or patchy fashion.

Clinical features--Early clinical features of giant cell arteritis include temporal headache, polymyalgia rheumatica symptoms, fatigue, and fever. The classic features of this disease are included in Table 28-14. Polymyalgia rheumatica symptoms may develop in 40%-50% of all patients with giant cell arteritis. Up to 15% of patients with polymyalgia rheumatica have temporal artery biopsies positive for giant cell arteritis.

- Clinical features of giant cell arteritis include temporal headache, polymyalgia rheumatica symptoms, fatigue, and fever.
- Up to 15% of patients with polymyalgia rheumatica have temporal artery biopsies positive for giant cell arteritis.

Table 28-14.--Classic Clinical Features of Giant Cell Arteritis

---

Fever, weight loss, fatigue
Polymyalgia rheumatica symptoms
Temporal headache
Jaw or tongue claudication
Ocular symptoms
   Blindness
   Diplopia
   Ptosis
Scalp tenderness
Dry cough
Peripheral large vessel vasculitis (10%)

Arteritis of the branches of the ophthalmic or posterior ciliary arteries causes blindness because of ischemia of the optic nerve (ischemic optic neuritis). Less often, retinal arterioles are occluded. After the visual deficit is established, it is usually permanent. When blindness occurs in an untreated person, it often occurs bilaterally within 1-2 weeks. Blindness occurs in less than 15% of patients. Large peripheral artery involvement in giant cell arteritis occurs in about 10% of patients. Extremity claudication, Raynaud's phenomenon, aortic dissection, decreased pulses, and vascular bruits suggest large peripheral vessel involvement. Patients with this involvement do not differ from those with more classic giant cell arteritis, either histologically or with regard to laboratory findings.

- Arteritis of the branches of the ophthalmic or posterior ciliary arteries causes blindness.
- The visual deficit is usually permanent.
- Blindness occurs in less than 15% of patients.

Diagnosis--The diagnosis of giant cell arteritis is made on the basis of:

- Characteristic clinical presentation.
- Markedly elevated erythrocyte sedimentation rate.
- Temporal artery biopsy documenting the typical histopathologic picture.

The diagnostic criteria for giant cell arteritis are given in Table 28-15.

Table 28-15.--Diagnostic Criteria for Giant Cell Arteritis

Temporal artery biopsy findings positive for classic giant cell arteritis

or

Four of the five following criteria:
   Tender, swollen temporal artery
   Jaw claudication
   Blindness
   Polymyalgia rheumatica symptoms
   Rapid response to corticosteroids

Positive temporal artery biopsy findings make a search for occult malignancy unnecessary and document the long-term need for corticosteroid therapy. This is important when corticosteroid therapy toxicity becomes an issue, particularly in elderly patients. The temporal artery biopsy should be 3-5 cm in length to compensate for patchy involvement. Multiple histologic sections should be taken of the pathologic specimen. In 15% of cases, the biopsy is positive on the other side if that on the initial side is negative. Typical laboratory abnormalities in acute active giant cell arteritis include a markedly elevated erythrocyte sedimentation rate, moderate normochromic anemia, and thrombocytosis. Mild increase in liver enzymes, most typically alkaline phosphatase, occurs in one-third of the patients. Liver biopsies performed in selected cases have documented granulomatous hepatitis. The erythrocyte sedimentation rate can be normal in patients with active giant cell arteritis. This occurs in <2% of all cases.

- The temporal artery biopsy should be 3-5 cm in length.
- In 15% of cases, the biopsy is positive on the other side if that on the initial side is negative.
- Liver biopsies performed in selected cases have documented granulomatous hepatitis.

Treatment--Treatment is initiated with corticosteroids when the diagnosis is entertained and the biopsy requested. A temporal artery biopsy specimen remains positive for disease even after 3-4 days of corticosteroid treatment. Treatment includes prednisone, typically 40-60 mg per day in a divided dose. Corticosteroids can be given parenterally in case of visual or life-threatening symptoms. Most symptoms of giant cell arteritis begin to respond within 24 hours after initiating corticosteroid therapy. Visual changes that are present for more than a few hours are invariably irreversible. Alternate-day administration of corticosteroids does not control symptoms in at least half of the patients.

- Treatment is initiated with corticosteroids when the diagnosis is entertained.
- Corticosteroids can be given parenterally in case of visual or life-threatening symptoms.
- Most symptoms of giant cell arteritis begin to respond within 24 hours.

Outcome--Giant cell arteritis typically has a self-limited course over a period of 1-2 years. In 24 months, half the patients are able to discontinue their treatment with corticosteroids. Except for penicillamine and azathioprine, the use of steroid-sparing agents has not been systematically studied. Methotrexate and cyclophosphamide may be considered in patients not responding to or intolerant of corticosteroids.

- Giant cell arteritis typically has a self-limited course over a period of 1-2 years.

Takayasu's Arteritis

Takayasu's arteritis is also known as "aortic arch syndrome" or "pulseless disease." Each year, approximately 2.6 new cases per 1,000,000 population occur. By definition, all patients are between the ages of 15 and 40. At least 80% of them are female. This disease is more common in the Orient, Latin America, and Eastern Europe. Microscopically, its pathologic features cannot be distinguished from those of giant cell arteritis. Takayasu's arteritis affects the aorta and its primary branches. The arterial wall is irregularly thickened, with luminal narrowing, dilatations, aneurysms, and distortions. The aortic valve and coronary ostia can be involved.

- All patients are between the ages of 15 and 40.
- 80% of them are female.
- Is more common in the Orient, Latin America, and Eastern Europe.

- Takayasu's arteritis affects the aorta and its primary branches.

Clinical and laboratory features--The constitutional features of fever, weight loss, fatigue, and arthralgia can precede symptoms of ischemia to the brain or claudication of the extremities. Renovascular hypertension, pulmonary hypertension, and coronary artery insufficiency can complicate Takayasu's arteritis. Cutaneous vasculitis, erythema nodosum, and synovitis occasionally occur in cases of active Takayasu's arteritis. Compromise of the cerebral vasculature can lead to dizziness, blurry or fading vision, syncope, and, occasionally, stroke. Physical examination findings confirm vascular bruits, absence of peripheral pulses, and, occasionally, fever. When the disease is active, abnormal values of laboratory studies reveal increased erythrocyte sedimentation rate, normochromic anemia, and thrombocytosis.

- Constitutional features of fever, weight loss, fatigue, and arthralgia can precede symptoms of ischemia to the brain.
- Renovascular hypertension, pulmonary hypertension, and coronary artery insufficiency can complicate Takayasu's arteritis.
- Physical examination findings confirm vascular bruits, absence of peripheral pulses, and, occasionally, fever.

Treatment and outcome--Corticosteroid therapy alone is usually adequate for controlling the inflammation. On average, patients receive corticosteroids for about 2 years. In about half of the cases, the pulse returns. Late stenotic complications are amenable to vascular surgery and bypass grafting. Survival is excellent, >90% at 10 years. Congestive heart failure from previous coronary artery involvement and cerebral vascular accidents are major causes of mortality.

- Corticosteroid therapy alone is usually adequate.
- In about half of the cases, the pulse returns.
- Survival is excellent, >90% at 10 years.

Polyarteritis

Polyarteritis is a systemic necrotizing vasculitis of medium and small muscular arteries. It occurs either by itself or in association with several diseases (secondary). When it occurs as a primary vasculitis, it is called "polyarteritis nodosa." A necrotizing vasculitis that is indistinguishable from polyarteritis nodosa occurs in association with rheumatoid arthritis, systemic lupus erythematosus, other connective tissue diseases, cryoglobulinemia, hepatitis-B infection, hairy-cell leukemia, and other malignant conditions. Histopathologically, polyarteritis is a focal transmural inflammation of small muscular arteries marked by fibrinoid necrosis and a pleomorphic, neutrophil-predominant infiltration. Elastic laminae are disrupted, producing a characteristic "blow out" of the vessel wall and microaneurysms. The coexistence of normal, active, and healed areas in the same vessel is unique to polyarteritis. Polyarteritis nodosa occurs in one patient per year per 100,000 population. Males outnumber females 2:1. The peak incidence occurs in ages 40 to 60, although all age groups are affected. If untreated, the systemic form of polyarteritis has <15% survival at 5 years.

- It occurs either by itself or in association with several diseases.
- Males outnumber females 2:1.
- Peak incidence occurs in ages 40 to 60.
- Untreated, the systemic form of polyarteritis has <15%

survival at 5 years.

Clinical features--Polyarteritis is usually a systemic illness associated with prominent constitutional features, including fever, fatigue, weight loss, and, occasionally, myalgia or arthralgia. Other common features are listed in Table 28-16.

Patients can have temporal artery involvement with jaw claudication. Occasionally, polyarteritis is limited to a single organ or found incidentally associated with cancer at the time of surgery. In such cases, patients may have a prognosis different from that of those with multi-system disease. Polyarteritis limited to the kidney parenchyma is called "microscopic polyarteritis nodosa" and is one cause of acute renal failure. Occasionally, patients with microscopic polyarteritis nodosa have positive antineutrophil cytoplasmic antibody (ANCA), usually with a perinuclear staining pattern (p-ANCA) or myeloperoxidase-antineutrophil cytoplasmic antibody.

- Patients can have temporal artery involvement with jaw claudication.

Table 28-16.--Clinical Features of Polyarteritis

Common features	Uncommon features
Fever, fatigue, weight loss	Coronary arteritis
Arthralgia, arthritis	Myocardial infarction
Myalgia	Congestive heart failure
Mononeuritis multiplex	Central nervous system abnormalities
Focal necrotizing glomerular nephritis	Seizures
Abnormal renal sediment	Cerebrovascular accident
Hypertension	Lung (interstitial pneumonitis)
Skin abnormalities	Eye (retinal hemorrhage)
Palpable purpura	Testicular pain
Livedo reticularis	
Cutaneous infarctions	
Abdominal pain/ischemic bowel	
Liver enzyme abnormalities	

Diagnosis--Abnormal laboratory findings include normocytic anemia, increased erythrocyte sedimentation rate, and thrombocytosis. Evaluation should document the extent and severity of the condition. The confirmatory test typically is angiography or biopsy of involved tissue showing vasculitis. The biopsy should be of accessible symptomatic tissue. The sensitivity of confirmatory tests in symptomatic and asymptomatic sites is listed in Table 28-17.

Visceral angiography, including views of the renal and mesenteric arteries, shows saccular or fusiform aneurysm formation coupled with smooth, tapered stenosis alternating with normal or dilated blood vessel. Angiography distinguishes polyarteritis from atherosclerosis.

Treatment--The cornerstone of treatment is early diagnosis and corticosteroid therapy. Cytotoxic and antimetabolite drugs such as cyclophosphamide, chlorambucil, methotrexate, and azathioprine are often used in

Table 28-17.--Sensitivity of Confirmatory Tests for Polyarteritis Nodosa

Test	Symptomatic, % positive	Asymptomatic, % positive
Nerve biopsy		20
(+/- neuropathy)	70	
Testicular biopsy		20
(+/- testicular pain)	70	
Muscle biopsy		29
(+/- myalgia and positive EMG findings)	66	
Liver biopsy		-
(abnormal findings on liver enzyme tests)	20	
Kidney biopsy		-
(+ active sediment)	20	
Visceral angiography		-
(+ abdominal pain/infarction)	60	

combination with corticosteroids. The role of these agents in the management of polyarteritis includes control of the cellular immune response and inhibition of the proliferative response to inflammatory changes in the blood vessel. They act as steroid-sparing agents. When confronted with possible progression of disease, consider superimposed infection and noninflammatory proliferative vasculopathy. The role of antivasospastic medication and antiplatelet agents has not been well established, but they may be helpful in the vasculopathic or healing phase of polyarteritis.

Outcome--In the first year after diagnosis of polyarteritis, deaths are related to the extent of disease activity, particularly gastrointestinal ischemia and renal insufficiency. After 1 year, complications of treatment, including infections in the immune-compromised patient, contribute most to mortality rates. Polyarteritis survival at 5 years with active treatment is between 55%-60%. This does not seem to be influenced by the addition of cytotoxic agents to corticosteroid treatment.

- In the first year after diagnosis of polyarteritis, deaths are related to the extent of disease activity.
- After 1 year, complications of treatment contribute most to mortality rates.
- Survival at 5 years with active treatment is between 55%-60%.

Churg-Strauss Vasculitis

Churg-Strauss vasculitis, or Churg-Strauss syndrome, is similar to polyarteritis and usually accounts for 6%-30% of series that combine polyarteritis and Churg-Strauss syndrome. The median age at onset is about 38 years (range, 15 to 69 years). Churg-Strauss vasculitis is defined by 1) a history of or current symptoms of asthma, 2) peripheral eosinophilia ($>1.5 \times 10^9$ eosinophils/L), and 3) systemic vasculitis of at least two extrapulmonary organs. There is a slight male predominance. The histopathology of the disease includes eosinophilic extravascular granulomas and granulomatous or nongranulomatous small vessel necrotizing vasculitis. It typically involves the small arteries, veins, arterioles, and venules.

- The median age at onset is about 38 years.
- Churg-Strauss vasculitis is defined by a history of or current symptoms of asthma, peripheral eosinophilia.

There are three clinical stages of Churg-Strauss syndrome. Patients need not progress in an orderly manner from one stage to another. Usually there is a prodrome of allergic rhinitis, nasal polyposis, or asthma. Later, peripheral blood and tissue eosinophilia suggest Löffler's syndrome. Chronic eosinophilic pneumonia and gastroenteritis may remit or recur over years. The final stage is life-threatening vasculitis. Transient, patchy, pulmonary infiltrates or nodules, pleural effusions, pulmonary angiitis and cardiomegaly, eosinophilic gastroenteritis, extravascular necrotizing granulomata of the skin, mononeuritis multiplex, and polyarthritis can complicate Churg-Strauss syndrome.

Treatment and outcome--One-year survival with Churg-Strauss syndrome is somewhat better than for polyarteritis and is >90%. There is more cardiac involvement but fewer renal deaths than in polyarteritis. Treatment relies on corticosteroids with or without the addition of cytotoxic agents. The eosinophilia resolves with treatment. Typically, cytotoxic agents are reserved for patients with disease not controlled by corticosteroids or for those requiring a steroid-sparing agent.

Buerger's Disease

Buerger's disease, or thromboangiitis obliterans, occurs almost exclusively in young adult smokers, who typically present with claudication of the instep and loss of digits from ischemic injury. They occasionally require amputation of an affected limb. Buerger's disease affects the small- and medium-sized arteries and veins of the extremities. Acute vasculitis in Buerger's disease is accompanied by characteristic intraluminal thrombus-containing microabscesses. Usually, the disease is arrested when smoking is stopped.

- Buerger's disease occurs almost exclusively in young adult smokers.
- Claudication of the instep and loss of digits from ischemic injury.
- Buerger's disease affects the small- and medium-sized arteries and veins of the extremities.
- The disease is arrested when smoking is stopped.

Primary Angiitis of the Central Nervous System

Primary angiitis of the central nervous system, once thought to be rare, has a chronic fluctuating and progressive course. The average age of patients presenting with this disease is 45 years. It has a slight male predominance. Forty percent of the patients present with <4 weeks of symptoms; another 40% present with symptoms that have been noted for >3 months. The commonest symptom is headache (mild or severe) associated with nausea or vomiting. Nonfocal neurologic abnormalities (including confusion, dementia, drowsiness, or coma) may interrupt prolonged periods of apparent remission. Acute stroke-like focal neurologic presentations are increasingly described, particularly in young, previously healthy women. Cerebral hemorrhage occurs in <4% of cases. Focal and nonfocal neurologic abnormalities coexist in half of the patients. Systemic features--fever, weight loss, arthralgia, and myalgia--are uncommon and occur in <20% of the patients; seizures occur in about 25%.

- The average age of patients presenting with this disease is 45 years.
- The commonest symptom is headache.

- Nonfocal neurologic abnormalities may interrupt prolonged periods of apparent remission.
- Cerebral hemorrhage occurs in <4%.
- Seizures occur in about 25%.

Diagnosis--There are no reliable noninvasive tests for making the diagnosis. The mainstays of diagnosis are cerebral angiography and biopsy of central nervous system tissues, including the leptomeninges. Nearly 40% of all cases with positive biopsy findings (pathologically documented) have normal arteriographic results. At least one in four patients with angiographically documented vasculitis have false-negative biopsy findings. The typical pathologic feature of primary angiitis of the central nervous system is a granulomatous inflammatory process centered around small veins and arterioles that is more prominent in the leptomeninges than in the underlying cortex. In 15% of cases, there is no granulomatous change. Inflammation is patchy, which may explain the biopsy sampling error. Cerebrospinal fluid examination is highly sensitive for the disease. The cerebrospinal fluid is abnormal in >90% of those patients with pathologically documented primary angiitis of the central nervous system. CT examinations of the head are not specific or sensitive for the condition. MRI examinations may be sensitive but do not distinguish this primary angiitis from other vasculopathic or demyelinating lesions of the brain. MRI is not useful in following the condition. Patients with a chronic progressive course are more likely to have the diagnosis made pathologically and have abnormal results on examination of the cerebrospinal fluid.

- No reliable noninvasive tests for making the diagnosis.
- Nearly 40% of all cases with positive biopsy findings have normal arteriographic results.
- A granulomatous inflammatory process centered around small veins and arterioles.
- Cerebrospinal fluid examination is highly sensitive for the disease.
- Cerebrospinal fluid is abnormal in >90%.
- CT examinations of the head are not specific or sensitive.

Treatment--The treatment for primary angiitis of the central nervous system may be influenced by the clinical subset. Younger patients with acute disease in whom the diagnosis was made with angiography have a benign course and typically respond well to a short course of corticosteroid treatment and calcium channel blockers to prevent vasospasm. Patients with a protracted course and diagnosis made with biopsy are best treated with combination therapy, including corticosteroids and cytotoxic agents. If untreated, this clinical subset has high mortality. The angiitis of the central nervous system associated with HIV infection is discussed below.

Rheumatologic syndromes that may produce a clinical picture similar to that of primary angiitis of the central nervous system include Cogan's syndrome (nonsyphilitic keratitis and vestibular dysfunction), Behçet's syndrome (uveitis, oral and genital ulcers, meningitis, and vasculitis), systemic lupus erythematosus, and polyarteritis. Drug-induced, particularly cocaine, vasculopathy, demyelinating disease, HIV infection, Lyme disease, syphilis, carcinomatous meningitis, angiocentric immunoproliferative lesions, and antiphospholipid antibody syndrome are also part of the differential diagnosis of patients presenting with a syndrome suggesting primary angiitis of the central nervous system.

Wegener's Granulomatosis

Wegener's granulomatosis is a well-recognized pathologic triad of upper and lower respiratory tract necrotizing granulomatous inflammation and focal segmental necrotizing glomerulonephritis. Wegener's granulomatosis occurs in <1 person annually per 100,000 population. Peak incidence of the disease occurs in the fourth and fifth decades of life. There is a slight male predominance. Eighty-five percent of the patients have generalized disease, including glomerulonephritis; 15% can present with local inflammation involving only the upper respiratory tract or the kidneys. The clinical features of this disease are summarized by the mnemonic ELKS: involvement of Ear/nose/throat, Lung, Kidney, and Skin. Lung involvement most commonly includes thick-walled, centrally cavitating pulmonary nodules. Alveolitis and pulmonary hemorrhage occur in up to 20% of patients. Biopsy in the patients with renal involvement shows focal segmental necrotizing glomerulonephritis and, occasionally, granulomatous vasculitis. Skin involvement may include urticaria, petechiae, papules, vesicles, ulcers, pyoderma, and livedo reticularis. Inflammatory arthritis is uncommon. Wegener's granulomatosis arthritis can appear like rheumatoid arthritis. However, the arthritis is usually oligoarticular and transient, occurring early in the clinical presentation. Nervous system involvement includes distal sensory neuropathy, mononeuritis multiplex, and cranial nerve palsies. Conjunctivitis, uveitis, and proptosis

are not unusual. Neurosensory hearing loss has been described together with serous otitis and inner ear vasculitis. Wegener's granulomatosis-associated subglottic tracheal stenosis secondary to chondritis should be distinguished from primary polychondritis.

- Peak incidence of the disease occurs in the fourth and fifth decades of life.
- ELKS: involvement of Ear/nose/throat, Lung, Kidney, and Skin.
- Most commonly includes thick-walled, centrally cavitating pulmonary nodules.
- Pulmonary hemorrhage occurs in up 20% of patients.
- Focal segmental necrotizing glomerulonephritis.

Diagnosis--Relevant laboratory findings in active Wegener's granulomatosis include nonspecific increase in the erythrocyte sedimentation rate and platelet count, normocytic anemia, and low levels of albumin. The recent recognition of the antineutrophil cytoplasmic antibody has helped with making the diagnosis. Antineutrophil cytoplasmic antibody with cytoplasmic staining (c-ANCA) is directed against proteinase 3, a serine protease from azurophilic granules. c-ANCA occurs in >90% of active cases of generalized Wegener's granulomatosis, in 75% of the cases of disease without renal involvement, and in 10%-50% of syndromes similar to Wegener's granulomatosis. These syndromes include idiopathic crescentic glomerulonephritis (30% of cases), microscopic polyarteritis nodosa (50%), and Churg-Strauss syndrome (10%). The antibody titer correlates loosely with disease activity, although the titers can remain elevated despite clinical improvement. p-ANCA is directed against myeloperoxidase and other neutrophil cytoplasmic constituents. p-ANCA (myeloperoxidase) is found in idiopathic crescentic glomerulonephritis (70% of cases), microscopic polyarteritis nodosa (50%), Churg-Strauss syndrome (70%), Wegener's granulomatosis (20%), and systemic lupus erythematosus. p-ANCA directed against leukocyte elastase, lactoferrin, and other antigens can occur in patients with various vasculitic syndromes, primary sclerosing cholangitis, ulcerative colitis, primary biliary cirrhosis, rheumatoid arthritis, and in 5% of normal subjects.

- c-ANCA occurs in >90% of active cases of generalized Wegener's granulomatosis, in 75% of the cases of disease without renal involvement.
- p-ANCA is found in idiopathic crescentic glomeru-

lonephritis, microscopic polyarteritis nodosa, Churg-Strauss syndrome, Wegener's granulomatosis, and systemic lupus erythematosus.

Histopathology and biopsy diagnosis of Wegener's granulomatosis--The diagnosis of Wegener's granulomatosis requires finding characteristic pathologic features in biopsy specimens. Biopsy of the upper respiratory tract suggests the diagnosis in 55% of cases, but only 20% show granulomata and/or vasculitis associated with necrosis. The finding of acute and chronic inflammation and necrosis without granulomata may be adequate to make the diagnosis if the rest of the clinical picture is classic. An open lung biopsy has a higher diagnostic yield than transbronchial biopsy. Renal biopsies usually document only a focal segmental necrotizing glomerulonephritis. Infrequently, a renal biopsy shows vasculitis. Further refinement in the c-ANCA test may simplify diagnosis. Currently, the c-ANCA test alone is not adequate to make the diagnosis of Wegener's granulomatosis.

Treatment and outcome--If untreated, generalized Wegener's granulomatosis has a mean survival of 5 months and 95% mortality in 1 year. More than 95% of patients eventually have a clinical remission with oral cyclophosphamide treatment. Intravenously given cyclophosphamide does not maintain remission as well as the drug given orally. Corticosteroids are useful initially but can be tapered quickly after the disease is controlled. The median time to achieve remission after initiating therapy is 12 months, but 50% of the patients achieving remission have a relapse. Mortality in the first year of disease is related primarily to the inflammatory process, with pulmonary hemorrhage or renal failure. In subsequent years, drug toxicity may dominate, with opportunistic infection and increasing risk of neoplasm and hemorrhagic cystitis related to the use of cyclophosphamide.

- If untreated, generalized Wegener's granulomatosis has a mean survival of 5 months.
- Corticosteroids are useful initially but can be tapered quickly after the disease is controlled.
- Median time to achieve remission is 12 months.
- 50% of the patients achieving remission have relapse.

Nonsystemic Small Vessel Vasculitis

Small vessel vasculitis complicates many primary and connective tissue disease-related systemic vasculitides. Uncommonly, small vessel vasculitis involves internal organs and nerves. Mononeuritis multiplex, diffuse pul-

monary hemorrhage, and renal vasculitis are complications of systemic small vessel vasculitis. More commonly, however, the disease is a nonsystemic process. It occurs in the skin and may be manifested by urticaria, palpable purpura, livedo reticularis, or skin ulceration. It can be associated with peripheral neuropathy, arthralgia, or synovitis.

- It occurs in the skin and may be manifested by urticaria, palpable purpura, livedo reticularis, or skin ulceration.
- It can be associated with peripheral neuropathy, arthralgia, or synovitis.

Histopathologically, a neutrophilic- or (uncommonly) lymphocytic-predominant infiltrate surrounds small arteries, veins, arterioles, or venules. Immune complexes deposit in vessel walls, along with fibrin deposition, endothelial cell swelling and necrosis, and a polymorphonuclear leukocytoclasis with scattering of nuclear fragment or nuclear dust. This histopathologic picture is called "leukocytoclastic vasculitis." It is a pathologic diagnosis and does not predict the clinical condition. Palpable purpura is the classic clinical correlate of leukocytoclastic vasculitis. However, many other cutaneous presentations of leukocytoclastic vasculitis occur. Small vessel vasculitis occurs with many illnesses; a partial listing is given in Table 28-18. These various conditions are distinguished clinically and pathologically. For instance, Schönlein-Henoch vasculitis has IgA deposition in vessel walls and normal complement levels. Mixed cryoglobulinemia has circulating cryoglobulins and low complement levels. Hypersensitivity vasculitis is almost always a nonsystemic small vessel vasculitis temporally related to infection, ingestion of drugs, or, less commonly, malignancy.

- This histopathologic picture is called "leukocytoclastic vasculitis." It is a pathologic diagnosis.

Diagnosis--The results of laboratory studies are nonspecific. The leukocyte count and platelet count may be increased. Complement levels, especially C4, may be low transiently in hypersensitivity vasculitis. Eosinophilia may be present. The erythrocyte sedimentation rate is usually increased. The diagnosis is made on the basis of the presence of vasculitis on skin biopsy and identification of a potential inciting agent or associated condition.

- Results of laboratory studies are nonspecific.

- Complement levels may be low transiently in hypersensitivity vasculitis.
- Eosinophilia may be present.

Table 28-18.--Conditions With Small Vessel
Vasculitis

Systemic small vessel vasculitis
    Systemic vasculitis
        Wegener's granulomatosis
        Polyarteritis (primary and secondary)
        Churg-Strauss vasculitis
        Takayasu's arteritis
        Schönlein-Henoch purpura/vasculitis
    Serum sickness
    Goodpasture's syndrome
Nonsystemic small vessel vasculitis
    Hypocomplementemic vasculitis
    Leukocytoclastic vasculitis related to:
        Rheumatoid arthritis
        Sjögren's syndrome
        Systemic lupus erythematosus
        Other connective tissue diseases
    Drug-induced and postinfectious angiitis
    Mixed cryoglobulinemia
    Malignancy-associated vasculitis
    Inflammatory bowel disease
    Organ transplant-associated vasculitis

Treatment and outcome--Typically, the outcome of nonsystemic small vessel vasculitis is good. Control of the infection or discontinuation of the offending drug may be all that is required. In other cases, corticosteroids or nonsteroidal anti-inflammatory agents are beneficial. Hypersensitivity vasculitis is usually self-limited, but it may recur with repeated exposure to the antigen or drug. Control of the concomitant systemic inflammation is important. Better control of rheumatoid arthritis, lupus, or other connective tissue diseases may be required.

- The outcome of nonsystemic small vessel vasculitis is good.
- Corticosteroids or nonsteroidal anti-inflammatory agents are beneficial.
- Hypersensitivity vasculitis is usually self-limited.

Cryoglobulinemia
Cryoglobulins are immunoglobulins that reversibly precipitate at reduced temperatures. They are grouped into two major categories. Type I cryoglobulins are aggregates of a single monoclonal immunoglobulin and are generally associated with multiple myeloma, Waldenström's macroglobulinemia, and lymphomas. They are usually found in high concentration (1- 5 g/dL). Type I cryoglobulins are often asymptomatic. Symptoms related to type I cryoglobulins are usually related to increased viscosity and include headaches, visual disturbances, nosebleeds, Raynaud's phenomenon, and ischemic ulceration from occlusion of arterioles and venules by precipitated immune complex. Vasculitis is rare.

- Type I cryoglobulins are aggregates of a single monoclonal immunoglobulin.
- Type I cryoglobulins are often asymptomatic.
- Symptoms related to type I cryoglobulins are usually related to increased viscosity.
- Vasculitis is rare.

Type II cryoglobulins consist of more than one class of immunoglobulin. Type II cryoglobulinemia (or mixed cryoglobulinemia) can occur alone (primary) or secondary to another disease. Commonly, type II cryoglobulinemia involves an IgM molecule with anti-immunoglobulin specificity (rheumatoid factor). However, not all rheumatoid factors are cryoglobulins. Other components of the immune complexes formed include hepatitis B antigen, other infectious agents, cellular/nuclear antigens, and complement. These immune complexes precipitate slowly and are present in smaller quantities (50-500 mg/dL) than type I cryoglobulins. This is the reason that cooled specimens must be kept for up to 3 days to identify type II cryoglobulins. Type II cryoglobulins have been further divided into those complexes in which one immunoglobulin is a monoclonal protein (monoclonal-mixed cryoglobulinemia). This distinction appears to have little clinical or prognostic usefulness.

- Type II cryoglobulinemia can occur alone or secondary to another disease.

Type II cryoglobulins are frequently associated with chronic infections and autoimmune disorders. The infecting agent or autoimmune antigen complexed with IgG antibody probably presents an antigenic aggregate and stimulates IgM production. When these infections resolve, the cryoglobulins disappear. The immune complexes that form precipitate on endothelial cells in peripheral blood vessels and fix complement, promoting vasculitic inflammation. The size of immune complexes, ability to fix complement, persistent IgM production, and many other factors may influence the clinical presentation of mixed cryoglobulinemia. The typical presentation is that of nonsystemic small vessel vasculitis with palpable purpura, urticaria, and cutaneous ulceration. Peripheral neuropathy, arthralgia, and arthritis are common. Less commonly, systemic small vessel vasculitis occurs with hepatosplenomegaly, pneumonitis or pulmonary hemorrhage, focal segmental necrotizing glomerulonephritis, serositis (pleurisy, pericarditis), and thyroiditis.

- Type II cryoglobulins are frequently associated with chronic infections and autoimmune disorders.
- The typical presentation is that of nonsystemic small vessel vasculitis with palpable purpura, urticaria, and cutaneous ulceration.
- Peripheral neuropathy, arthralgia, and arthritis are common.

Laboratory studies--Nonspecific indicators of inflammation are usually found in laboratory studies, including an increased erythrocyte sedimentation rate. Immunoglobulin levels are elevated, rheumatoid factor is positive (usually in high titers), and complement levels are low. Evidence of previous hepatitis infection (particularly hepatitis C) is frequently identified. For cryoglobulin testing, it is important to draw blood into a warmed syringe and to keep it warm until transferred to a cryocrit tube. Serum protein electrophoresis, immunoelectrophoresis, and quantitative immunoglobulin determinations can be helpful in some cases. Hepatitis C and other viral serologies may elucidate the nature of the disease and help in decisions about therapy (therapy is discussed above in the section on small vessel vasculitis).

- Immunoglobulin levels are elevated, rheumatoid factor is positive, and complement levels are low.
- Previous hepatitis infection is frequently identified.

Outcome--The clinical course of nonsystemic vasculitis is mild and prolonged. In systemic small vessel vasculitis caused by mixed cryoglobulinemia, the course and prognosis depend on the organs involved. Progressive renal disease is most common. Pulmonary hemorrhage is life-threatening. Some patients with mixed cryoglobulinemia eventually develop cirrhosis or a lymphoproliferative disorder.

- The clinical course is mild and prolonged.
- Progressive renal disease is most common.
- Pulmonary hemorrhage is life-threatening.

Vasculitis Associated With Connective Tissue Disease

Vascular involvement in rheumatoid arthritis can have various presentations. A positive rheumatoid factor is invariably present in patients with vasculitis related to rheumatoid arthritis. Digital nail fold and nodule infarcts occur in some patients with active rheumatoid arthritis. Histopathologically, this is a bland, obliterative endarteropathy with intimal proliferation. Managing the rheumatoid arthritis itself is all that is needed, because these vasculopathic changes require no other therapy. Small vessel vasculitis or leukocytoclastic vasculitis with palpable purpura and systemic vasculitis (polyarteritis) can occur with severe seropositive nodular rheumatoid arthritis.

- Digital nail fold and nodule infarcts occur in some patients with active rheumatoid arthritis.
- Small vessel vasculitis or leukocytoclastic vasculitis can occur with severe seropositive nodular rheumatoid arthritis.

A process similar to that of obliterative endarteropathy occurs in scleroderma. Systemic lupus erythematosus can present with obliterative endarteropathy, leukocytoclastic vasculitis, or a polyarteritis-like picture. Sjögren's syndrome uncommonly includes small vessel vasculitis, with either a polymorphonuclear leukocyte or lymphocyte predominance. This vasculitis may cause peripheral neuropathy and some of the central nervous system features of Sjögren's syndrome.

- Obliterative endarteropathy occurs in scleroderma.
- Sjögren's syndrome uncommonly includes small vessel vasculitis.

Aortitis, an inflammation of the aortic root with dilatation and aortic insufficiency, occurs in a minority of patients with HLA-B27-associated spondyloarthropathies. Type II cryoglobulins and vasculitis may complicate many different connective tissue diseases. Cryoglobulins should be assayed in any patient with a formal autoimmune disease who develops vasculitis.

- Aortitis occurs in a minority of patients with HLA-B27-associated spondyloarthropathies.

Atypical Vasculitic Syndromes: Differential Diagnosis

Patients may present with the classic features of one of the vasculitic syndromes described above. When they do not, a diagnostic approach to what type of vasculitis is present may prove more difficult. Other patterns of disease and their differential diagnoses are listed in Tables 28-19 and 28-20.

Table 28-19.--Acute Pulmonary-Renal Syndrome: Differential Diagnosis

Common	Uncommon
Wegener's granulomatosis	Schönlein-Henoch vasculitis
Churg-Strauss syndrome	Connective tissue diseases with associated vasculitis
Systemic lupus erythematosus	Rheumatoid arthritis
Cryoglobulinemic vasculitis	Mixed connective tissue disease
Goodpasture's syndrome	Polychondritis
Systemic small vessel vasculitis	Behçet's syndrome
	Thrombotic thrombocytopenic purpura
	Thromboembolic disease
	Infectious pneumonia
	Streptococcus
	Mycoplasma
	Legionella

Table 28-20.--Palpable Purpura: Differential Diagnosis

Polyarteritis
Churg-Strauss vasculitis
Wegener's granulomatosis
Leukocytoclastic vasculitis (classic)
Schönlein-Henoch vasculitis
Connective tissue disease-associated vasculitis
Cryoglobulinemia
Hypersensitivity to drugs, infection, and malignancy

Palpable Purpura

Palpable purpura almost always suggests leukocytoclastic vasculitis, but this pathologic diagnosis does not define the clinical syndrome. Table 28-20 outlines the differential diagnosis of palpable purpura. Nodules or papules diagnosed as necrotizing granuloma on biopsy occur in Churg-Strauss syndrome, Wegener's granulomatosis, rheumatoid arthritis, and, occasionally, systemic lupus erythematosus. Other nodules or papules without necrotizing granulomata can be the sign of angiocentric lymphoproliferative disorders or sarcoid or they may be related to inflammatory bowel disease. Urticarial or pustular lesions complicate hypocomplementemic vasculitis, inflammatory bowel arthritis syndrome, and Behçet's syndrome. Livedo reticularis, which is associated with proliferative endarteropathy, occurs in connective tissue diseases and antiphospholipid antibody syndrome and in association with cholesterol emboli and many systemic necrotizing vasculitides.

- Palpable purpura almost always suggests leukocytoclastic vasculitis.

Included in the differential diagnosis of sinusitis and presumed vasculitis are Wegener's granulomatosis, Churg-Strauss syndrome, relapsing polychondritis, angiocentric lymphoproliferative disorders, sarcoid, nasopharyngeal carcinoma, and, occasionally, systemic bacterial or fungal infection.

Figure 28-1 is an algorithm for diagnosing the condition associated with focal segmental glomerulonephritis. Vasculitis presenting with only overt renal disease is sufficiently common that this scheme is very useful.

ACQUIRED IMMUNODEFICIENCY SYNDROME AND RHEUMATIC DISEASE

Many musculoskeletal conditions are associated with HIV infection, and several of them may be the first manifestations of this infection. HIV infection may be confused with diseases such as systemic lupus erythematosus and Sjögren's syndrome. The implications for the correct diagnosis are obvious. Rheumatic syndromes in

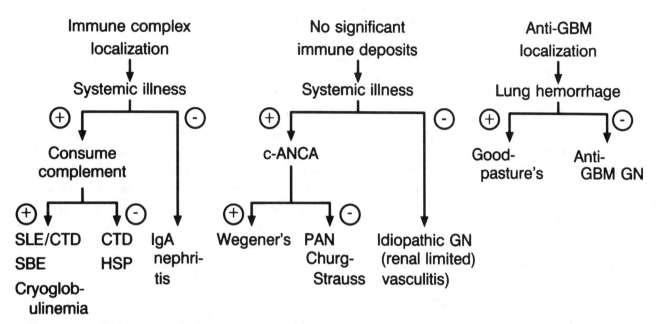

Fig. 28-1. Diagnostic approach to vasculitis. Disease pattern recognition. Focal segmental necrotizing glomerulonephritis (kidney biopsy). GBM, glomerular basement membrane; GN, glomerulonephritis; HSP, Henoch-Schönlein purpura; PAN, polyarteritis nodosa; SLE, systemic lupus erythematosus; CTD, connective tissue diseases; SBE, subacute bacterial endocarditis. Modified from Rosen S, Falk RJ, Jennette JC: Polyarteritis nodosa, including microscopic form and renal vasculitis. *In* Systemic Vasculitides. Edited by A Churg, J Churg. New York, IGAKU-SHOIN Medical Publishers, 1991, pp 57-77. By permission of publisher.

patients with HIV infection have significant prognostic implications. The morbidity associated with these syndromes is considerable and often requires treatments and monitoring not typically required by their non-HIV infected counterparts. Epidemiologic studies have not concluded whether HIV infection predisposes to arthritis or whether viral or immune mechanisms associated with HIV infection have a role in the pathogenesis of arthritis.

Specific Rheumatologic Manifestations of HIV Infection

Reiter's Syndrome and Undifferentiated Spondyloarthropathy

A spectrum from classic psoriatic or Reiter's syndrome to more nonspecific spondyloarthropathies with no cutaneous or mucous membrane involvement occurs in the HIV-infected population. The prevalence of these conditions in HIV-infected patients varies from 0.5% to 10% of reported populations. Except for several cases of very mild sacroiliitis, axial involvement does not occur in HIV-associated arthritides. These HIV-associated spondyloarthropathies have a predisposition for HLA-B27 and frequently have severe enthesopathy and dactylitis. The foot and ankle are the common sites of inflammation/enthesopathy in Reiter's syndrome. Sometimes the "AIDS

foot" features are so severe as to be almost diagnostic. The arthritis of Reiter's syndrome in HIV infection can be additive and ultimately destructive and disabling; however, it more commonly is episodic and associated with remissions. Conjunctivitis in this population is unusual. Most HIV-positive patients with Reiter's syndrome have clinical features such as urethritis, keratoderma blennorrhagicum, circinate balanitis, or painless oral ulcers, thus fulfilling the diagnostic criteria for Reiter's syndrome. Genitourinary tract infection with *Ureaplasma* or *Chlamydia* is uncommon. However, in one-third of the cases, the onset of HIV-associated Reiter's syndrome was linked to a documented infection with enteric organisms known to precipitate reactive arthritis.

- These HIV-associated spondyloarthropathies have a predisposition for HLA-B27.
- Foot and ankle are the common sites of inflammation/enthesopathy in Reiter's syndrome.
- Most HIV-positive patients with Reiter's syndrome have clinical features fulfilling the diagnostic criteria for Reiter's syndrome.
- The signs and symptoms of Reiter's syndrome occur before or simultaneously with the onset of "full blown" AIDS in approximately two-thirds of reported cases.
- The inflammation of Reiter's syndrome may activate latent HIV infection.

Systemic Lupus Erythematosus-Like Illness in HIV Infection

Many of the features of systemic lupus erythematosus are similar to those found in HIV infections. These similarities can lead to diagnostic difficulties. HIV infection should be considered when the diagnosis of systemic lupus erythematosus is considered in men or in patients who practice high-risk behaviors for HIV. Antinuclear antibodies in titers >1:80 have not been observed in HIV infection, and antibodies to anti-double-strand DNA are absent in HIV infection.

- Many of the features of systemic lupus erythematosus are similar to those found in HIV infections.
- HIV infection should be considered when the diagnosis of systemic lupus erythematosus is considered in men or in patients who practice high-risk behaviors for HIV.

- Patients with systemic lupus erythematosus and rheumatoid arthritis have had resolution of their inflammatory symptoms after HIV infection.

HIV-Associated Vasculitis

Many vasculitic syndromes have been described in association with HIV infection. The common ones are primary angiitis of the central nervous system and angiocentric lymphoproliferative lesions related to lymphomatoid granulomatosis. It has to be proved whether the association of vasculitis and HIV infection is coincidental, related to comorbid factors (drugs or other infections), or represents a direct pathogenic role for HIV. Patients with primary angiitis of the central nervous system and lymphoproliferative angiocentric vasculopathies should be tested for HIV. Furthermore, any person with known HIV infection who presents with new mononeuritis should be evaluated for vasculitis.

QUESTIONS
(See "Answers" section)

Multiple Choice

1. Erosive osteoarthritis presents:
   a. In large weight-bearing joints
   b. In the spines of elderly type-II diabetic men
   c. In the distal and proximal interphalangeal joints of perimenopausal women
   d. As a complication of tophaceous gout
   e. Is never associated with joint inflammation or swelling

2. The arthropathy of hemochromatosis is:
   a. Indistinguishable from that of primary osteoarthritis
   b. Commonly affects the metacarpophalangeal joints
   c. Is always associated with calcium pyrophosphate dihydrate crystals
   d. Affects the same joints as erosive osteoarthritis
   e. Never affects the shoulders

3. Classic manifestations of Felty's syndrome include:
   a. Dry eyes, dry mouth, and arthritis
   b. Neutropenia, splenomegaly, and rheumatoid arthritis
   c. Fever, arthritis, and rash
   d. Large granular lymphocyte proliferation
   e. Edema, symmetrical polyarthritis, and steroid responsiveness

4. Which potential toxic effect of nonsteroidal anti-inflammatory agents is shared by nonacetylated salicylates?
   a. Aggravation of hypertension
   b. Gastrointestinal tract upset
   c. Increased risk of peptic ulcer
   d. Bleeding time prolongation
   e. Dependent edema

5. Which of the following slow-acting antirheumatic agents requires no routine monitoring of hemoglobin concentration, white blood cell count, and platelet count?
   a. Methotrexate
   b. Sulfasalazine
   c. Penicillamine

d. Hydroxychloroquine

e. Azathioprine

6. Which of the following facts and features about septic superficial bursitis is true?

a. A portal of entry is almost always found if the bursa is infected

b. Gram staining of the infected bursal fluid is almost always positive

c. The leukocyte count from the synovial fluid of the superficial septic bursa helps predict an infection

d. Septic prepatellar bursitis should always be treated with antibiotics

e. The warmth of an inflamed superficial bursa suggests the presence of infection

7. Which treatment is not effective in the management of fibromyalgia?

a. Reassurance and education

b. Prednisone

c. Flexibility exercises

d. Ensuring an adequate night's sleep

e. Cardiovascular fitness program

f. Tricyclic antidepressants

8. Which of the following statements about polymyalgia rheumatica is correct?

a. Polymyalgia rheumatica frequently presents with a normal erythrocyte sedimentation rate

b. Peripheral joint synovitis rules out the possibility of polymyalgia rheumatica

c. Polymyalgia rheumatica is almost always associated with giant cell arteritis

d. Initial doses of prednisone required to treat polymyalgia rheumatica are between 40 and 60 mg per day

e. Fifty percent of polymyalgia rheumatica patients have remission within the first 2 years of their disease

9. Sudden wrist drop and hand numbness in a patient with seropositive rheumatoid arthritis is most likely due to:

a. Cervical subluxation and myelopathy

b. Wrist extensor tendon rupture due to proliferative tenosynovitis

c. A flare of rheumatoid arthritis with carpal tunnel syndrome

d. Vasculitis

e. Gold toxicity

10. Which of the following vasculitic syndromes is commonly associated with complement consumption and low complement levels?

a. Giant cell arteritis

b. Schönlein-Henoch purpura

c. Wegener's granulomatosis

d. Cryoglobulinemia with hepatitis C

e. Buerger's disease

True/False

11. Which of the following are associated with rheumatoid factor-positive rheumatoid arthritis?

a. Cervical radiculopathy

b. Constrictive pericarditis

c. Nodular regenerative hyperplasia of the liver

d. Episcleritis

e. Pulmonary interstitial fibrosis

f. Felty's syndrome

12. Appropriate actions when suspecting acute septic arthritis after aspirating a joint include:

a. Initiating treatment with antibiotics after a microorganism has been identified

b. Consider other foci of infection, including disk space, heart valves, and other joints

c. Stop antibiotic therapy if plain radiographs of the affected joints show no infection

d. Aspirating the affected joint as long as fluid reaccumulates

e. Treat all patients with a minimum of 4 weeks of antibiotics given intravenously

13. Which of the following diseases can be associated with a positive rheumatoid factor?

a. Subacute bacterial endocarditis

b. Sjögren's syndrome

c. Mixed cryoglobulinemia

d. Adult-onset Still's syndrome

e. Wegener's granulomatosis

f. Polymyalgia rheumatica

14. Common causes of acute pulmonary and renal failure syndrome include:

a. Wegener's granulomatosis

b. Goodpasture's syndrome

c. Systemic lupus erythematosus

d. Polyarteritis nodosa

e. Systemic small vessel vasculitis

f. Takayasu's arteritis

NOTES

CHAPTER 29
VASCULAR DISEASES

Thom Rooke, M.D.

ANEURYSMS

Abdominal Aortic Aneurysms

Although congenital or acquired aneurysms can affect any blood vessel in the body, abdominal aortic aneurysms are the ones most commonly encountered by the general medical practitioner. In autopsy series or studies in which unselected adult patients are screened with ultrasonography, the frequency of abdominal aortic aneurysms (usually defined as a vessel diameter ≥3 cm) ranges from 1.5%-3.2%. In high-risk patients, such as those with coronary or peripheral vascular disease, the rate may be as high as 5%-10%. The growth rate of these aneurysms is typically 0.3-0.5 cm per year, and 95% are located below the origin of the renal arteries. Five percent of all aneurysms are the so-called inflammatory type. For a patient with an abdominal aortic aneurysm, the chance that a first-degree relative also has one is approximately 20%.

- Abdominal aortic aneurysms are the most common aneurysm encountered by general practitioner.
- Frequency (vessel diameter ≥3 cm) is 1.5%-3.2%.
- In high-risk patients, frequency is as high as 5%-10%.
- Growth rate is 0.3-0.5 cm per year.
- 95% are below origin of renal arteries.
- Chance that first-degree relative has aneurysm is about 20%.

Cause

Most aneurysms are associated with atherosclerosis and hypertension, but predisposing factors such as connective tissue disease (Marfan syndrome, Ehlers-Danlos syndrome, pseudoxanthoma elasticum), infection, trauma, vasculitis, and others may also be involved.

- Most abdominal aortic aneurysms are associated with atherosclerosis and hypertension.
- Other predisposing factors: connective tissue disease (Marfan syndrome, Ehlers-Danlos syndrome), infection.

Rupture

The overall mortality rate with ruptured abdominal aortic aneurysm is 80%, and 50% of patients die before they reach the hospital. Of those who survive to reach the hospital, 25% die before operation can be performed, and 40% die during or after operation. The risk of rupture is directly related to aneurysm size. For aneurysms of 5.0, 6.0, or 7.0 cm in diameter, the yearly rate of rupture is <5%, 5%-10%, and 20%, respectively.

- Overall mortality rate with ruptured abdominal aortic aneurysm is 80%.
- 50% of patients die before they reach hospital.
- Of survivors to hospital, 25% die before operation.
- 40% of patients die during or after operation.
- Risk of rupture is related to aneurysm size.

Treatment

In the series with the best results, surgical mortality rate for elective aneurysm resection is 3%-5%. If the operation is performed on high-risk patients, on elderly patients (>80 years), or in hospitals not specializing in vascular surgery, the mortality rate doubles to 7%-10%. A reasonable approach to management is based on the size of the aneurysm: <4.5 cm in diameter, observe; 4.5-6.0 cm, operate electively if the patient is a good surgical risk; and >6.0 cm, consider operation even if the patient is a poor surgical risk.

- Surgical mortality rate for elective resection of abdominal aortic aneurysm: 3%-5%.
- Rate in high-risk patients is 7%-10%.
- Management based on aneurysm size: <4.5 cm, observe; 4.5-6 cm, operate electively; >6.0 cm, consider operation even if poor risk.

Other Aneurysms

Other aneurysms that are occasionally encountered by the internist include popliteal aneurysms (these typically thrombose rather than rupture, and when they do so they may cause limb-threatening embolizations or acute ischemia); splenic aneurysms (these often appear in the left upper quadrant as calcified masses on radiographs of chest or abdomen); iliac aneurysms (almost always seen in conjunction with abdominal aortic aneurysm); and thoracic aortic aneurysms (ascending or descending). Whenever an aneurysm is detected, it is essential that the clinician screen for the presence of occult aneurysms.

- Popliteal aneurysms typically thrombose rather than rupture.
- May cause limb-threatening embolization.
- When aneurysm is detected, clinician must screen for occult aneurysms.

ACUTE ARTERIAL OCCLUSION

Cause

Most cases of acute arterial occlusion can be attributed to one of three causes: thrombosis, emboli, and dissection.

Thrombosis

Thrombosis in situ usually occurs at the site of an underlying vascular abnormality such as an atherosclerotic lesion (plaque rupture) or within an aneurysm. Clotting disorders are only rarely the cause of spontaneous arterial thrombosis. Both antiplatelet and anticoagulant agents may be useful in preventing arterial thrombosis.

- Thrombosis in situ that causes acute arterial occlusion occurs at site of atherosclerotic lesion or within aneurysm.
- Antiplatelet and anticoagulant agents may prevent arterial thrombosis.

Emboli

Emboli large enough to occlude relatively large arteries usually (in >95% of cases) have a cardiac source. The most common abnormalities producing cardiac-derived emboli include ventricular mural thrombus (typically caused by an infarct or cardiomyopathy), valvular disease (native or prosthetic), and atrial disorders such as chronic or paroxysmal atrial fibrillation. Mural tumors such as atrial myxoma rarely embolize. Other unusual causes of large arterial emboli include paradoxic emboli, in which a thrombus originating in the deep venous system passes through an atrial septal defect or patent foramen ovale and enters the arterial system.

- Emboli large enough to occlude large arteries usually have cardiac source.
- Cardiac-derived emboli result from ventricular mural thrombus, valvular disease, paroxysmal atrial fibrillation.
- Unusual cause of emboli is paradoxic emboli: thrombus passes through atrial septal defect or patent foramen ovale and enters arterial system.

Dissection

Dissections are usually associated with hypertension, atherosclerosis, aneurysms, or certain degenerative or connective tissue disorders. As invasive diagnostic and therapeutic cardiovascular interventions have become more popular, iatrogenic dissection has markedly increased in frequency. Trauma (blunt or penetrating) also accounts for a significant number of dissections.

- Dissections usually associated with hypertension, atherosclerosis, aneurysms, certain degenerative or connective tissue disorders.
- Iatrogenic dissection has increased in frequency.

Clinical Manifestations

Remember the six P's: 1) pulseless, 2) polar (cool), 3) pallor, 4) pain, 5) paresthesias, and 6) paralysis. It is essential to remember that when acute arterial occlusion occurs, the first abnormalities noted include pulselessness, limb coolness, and limb pallor; although these are important findings, they do not necessarily imply serious ischemia, and the limb can generally be watched as long as necessary. When pain and paresthesia occur, revascularization is necessary and should be performed at the earliest convenient opportunity. However, when motor weakness or paralysis begins to develop in a patient with acute arterial occlusion, the potential for limb loss is high, and revascularization should be performed immediately (within 2 or 3 hours if possible).

- Six P's of acute arterial occlusion: 1) pulselessness, 2) polar (cool), 3) pallor, 4) pain, 5) paresthesias, and 6) paralysis.
- When motor weakness or paralysis begins to develop, potential for limb loss is high; immediate revascularization needed.

Treatment

Specific forms of treatment depend on the cause of the occlusion and are largely beyond the scope of this chapter. Thrombosis may be treated surgically or with lytic agents. Emboli may be treated surgically, including percutaneous removal with a Fogarty balloon catheter. Dissection typically requires operation, although in some situations a dissection may heal with conservative therapy. In most cases, anticoagulation, control of hypertension, and limb protection are indicated.

VASCULITIS (SMALL AND MEDIUM-SIZED VESSELS)

Cause

Several processes may produce vasculitis of small and medium-sized vessels; although none of these are individually common, as a group they are encountered by the internist on a regular basis. In general, immunologic or autoimmune phenomena are thought to be involved in the production of most vasculitides, although the exact mechanism(s) by which this occurs is poorly understood.

Specific Vasculitides

The most commonly encountered types of vasculitis are described.

Polyarteritis Nodosa

This is an acute, necrotizing vasculitis (Fig. 29-1) that affects primarily medium-sized and small arteries. It is a systemic disorder that may involve the kidneys, joints, skin, nerves, and various other tissues. The diagnosis is usually made with biopsy (the affected tissues generally show necrotizing changes and disruption within blood

vessels) or angiography (focal stenoses and microaneurysms are typical). Corticosteroids and cytotoxic agents (such as cyclophosphamide and azathioprine) are frequently effective for treatment.

- Polyarteritis nodosa: acute, necrotizing vasculitis that affects medium-sized and small arteries.
- It is a systemic disorder.
- Diagnosis is made with biopsy and angiography.
- Corticosteroids and cytotoxic agents are effective therapy.

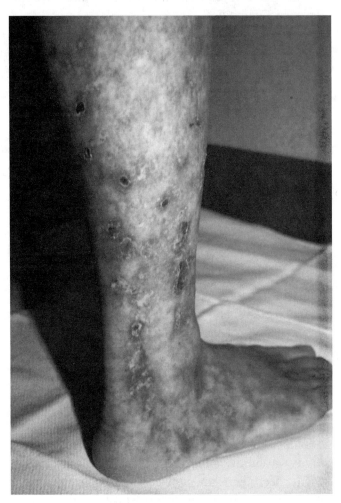

Fig. 29-1. Necrotizing vasculitis. The constellation of findings shown here (ulcerations, livedo, petechial skin lesions) are typical of many vasculitic processes that affect small or medium-sized vessels.

Wegener's Granulomatosis

This granulomatous, necrotizing process can affect blood vessels in the respiratory tract and kidneys. In severe cases, surrounding structures, including the skin, may be involved. The syndrome is typically fatal without treatment. The diagnosis has been aided in recent years by the ability to test for antineutrophil cytoplasmic antibodies; although they are present in many vasculitides, a typical granular pattern is seen in Wegener's granulomatosis. Treatment consists of prednisone, cyclophosphamide, and, in some cases, trimethoprim-sulfamethoxazole.

- Wegener's granulomatosis can affect blood vessels in respiratory tract and kidneys.
- Syndrome is typically fatal without treatment.
- Diagnosis is aided by testing for antineutrophil cytoplasmic antibodies.
- Treatment consists of prednisone and cyclophosphamide.

Rheumatoid Vasculitis

Blood vessels are frequently involved in rheumatoid and other collagen vascular diseases. The findings frequently resemble those of polyarteritis nodosa, although the skin is affected more often. In the United States, rheumatoid vasculitis is the third most common cause of chronic leg ulcers, after atherosclerosis and venous disorders. Prednisone is usually effective, with or without other immunosuppressive agents.

- Rheumatoid vasculitis is similar to polyarteritis nodosa, except skin is affected more often.
- It is third most common cause of chronic leg ulcers in United States.
- Prednisone is usually effective treatment.

Other Vasculitides

A wide variety of other vasculitides may affect small and medium-sized vessels. These include allergic angiitis (Churg-Strauss syndrome), cryoglobulinemia, Schönlein-Henoch purpura, various forms of hypersensitivity vasculitis, serum sickness, and numerous nonspecific necrotizing and nonnecrotizing vasculitides. In general, most of these can be treated with corticosteroids or a steroid-sparing immunosuppressant.

BUERGER'S DISEASE

Cause

The cause of Buerger's disease (thromboangiitis obliterans) remains unknown, but its association with smoking is powerful and well known. Few, if any, cases occur in the absence of tobacco use. Pathologically, the disease resembles a vasculitis; the vessel is typically throm-

bosed and infiltrated with inflammatory cells. Granuloma formation and microabscesses are common.

- Cause of Buerger's disease unknown.
- Association with smoking is powerful and well known.
- Granuloma and microabscesses are common.

Clinical Manifestations

The disease usually affects the small distal arteries first and progresses proximally if smoking is continued. Veins are also often involved; the first manifestation of Buerger's disease may be superficial phlebitis. If smoking is discontinued, the process is frequently arrested; if smoking continues, the disease almost always progresses. Interestingly, whereas other vasculitides typically demonstrate an elevated erythrocyte sedimentation rate, in Buerger's disease it is often minimally elevated or normal.

- Buerger's disease affects small distal arteries first.
- Veins are also involved.
- First manifestation may be superficial phlebitis.
- Erythrocyte sedimentation rate is minimally elevated or normal.

Diagnosis

The diagnosis is usually made on the basis of the history. The patient is typically <40 years old, has distal disease (Fig. 29-2), and has a history of cigarette use. Men were once thought to be primarily affected, but in recent years the number of women with this diagnosis has increased. Angiography shows typical findings that can aid in the diagnosis, and definitive pathologic findings can often be obtained on appropriate biopsy.

- Typical patient with Buerger's disease: <40 years, has distal disease, has history of cigarette use.

Treatment

Cessation of smoking is an absolute necessity. Other treatments (such as pentoxifylline and sympathectomy) are of unknown benefit.

- Cessation of smoking is a necessity in Buerger's disease.

ERGOTISM

Mechanism of Action

Ergotamine and ergot derivatives are potent arterial vasoconstrictors. They are thought to produce vasocon-

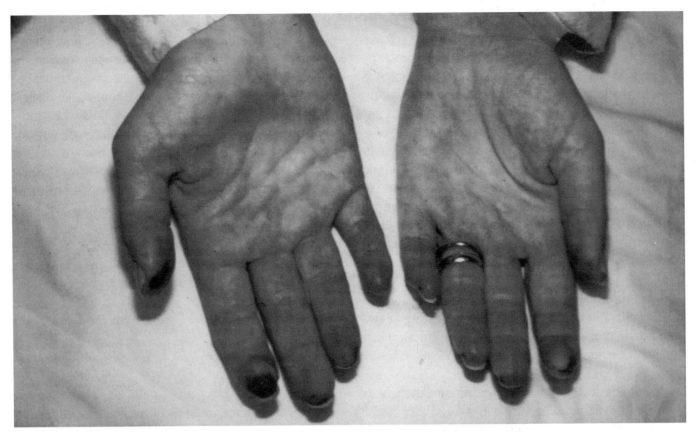

Fig. 29-2. Buerger's disease. Distal portions of digits are severely ischemic. Bilateral ischemia affecting multiple digits is suggestive of either Buerger's disease or embolic disease.

striction by cross-reacting with α-adrenergic (and to a lesser extent, serotonergic) receptors in the blood vessel wall. These compounds are typically given either orally or by suppository. Their major indication is for the treatment of vasomotor (migraine) headache.

- Ergotamine and ergot derivatives are potent arterial vasoconstrictors.
- They cross-react with α-adrenergic receptors in blood vessel wall.

Clinical Manifestations

The typical patient with ergotism is a young female with a history of headaches. The patient may complain of vasospastic phenomena such as Raynaud's disease or Prinzmetal's angina. However, the vasospasm may be so persistent and severe that it mimics or leads to arterial occlusion. Myocardial infarction, mesenteric insufficiency or infarction, limb ischemia, neurologic findings, cutaneous infarctions, and other ischemic syndromes may result from its use.

- Typical patient with ergotism: young female with his-

tory of headaches.
- Vasospastic phenomena may be present, such as Raynaud's disease or Prinzmetal's angina.

Diagnosis

The diagnosis of ergot toxicity is almost always made from the history and by exclusion. It is often difficult to elicit a history of ergot use from patients, many of whom use the compound unknowingly, fail to recognize the significance of its use, or use it in an intentionally abusive way.

- Diagnosis of ergot toxicity is almost always made from history and by exclusion.

Treatment

Discontinuing the use of ergot usually leads to relief of symptoms. Occasionally, vasodilator therapy is indicated. Sodium nitroprusside is generally effective in this regard, although calcium or α-adrenergic blockers may also be useful.

- Discontinuing use of ergot leads to relief of symptoms.
- Sodium nitroprusside is generally effective.

THORACIC OUTLET SYNDROME

Cause

Thoracic outlet syndrome occurs when the brachial plexus, subclavian artery, or subclavian vein becomes compressed in the region of the thoracic outlet. Symptoms are thought to result from nerve compression in 90%-95% of cases; only a small number are clearly due to venous or arterial compression. Thoracic outlet syndrome is the most common cause of acute arterial occlusion in the upper extremity of adults <40 years. Repetitive trauma to the artery can lead to intimal damage, embolization, aneurysm formation, or acute thrombosis. Thoracic outlet syndrome is also the most common cause of upper extremity acute venous occlusion in the young adult. "Stress" thrombosis, which occurs during periods of intense upper extremity activity such as lifting heavy weights, is typically the consequence of intermittent venous occlusion.

- Symptoms of thoracic outlet syndrome are thought to result from nerve compression in 90%-95% of cases.
- Thoracic outlet syndrome is most common cause of acute arterial occlusion in upper extremity of adults <40 years.
- Thoracic outlet syndrome is most common cause of upper extremity acute venous occlusion in young adults.

Diagnosis

When arterial compression is present, obliteration of the radial pulse is a strong indication of thoracic outlet syndrome. Nerve involvement is much more difficult to determine; electromyography and nerve conduction studies have not proved consistently useful for diagnosis. Intermittent venous compression is also difficult to document, and when it is found (on ultrasound duplex scan or magnetic resonance imaging) its significance is uncertain. One of the most useful clinical tests is the elevated arm stress test (EAST), in which the patient raises his or her hands above the head and clenches and unclenches the fist for 1 or 2 minutes. The appearance of typical symptoms, with or without signs of vascular involvement such as delayed capillary refilling, is suggestive of the syndrome.

- Indication of thoracic outlet syndrome: obliteration of radial pulse.
- Nerve involvement difficult to determine.
- Useful test is elevated arm stress test.

Treatment

Conservative measures should be tried first. These include exercise, stretching activities, and avoidance of aggravating factors. When conservative measures fail and symptoms warrant, surgical resection of the first rib is curative in 80%-85% of patients. In those with significant arterial involvement (such as intimal damage or aneurysm formation), the involved section of arteries should be replaced with a graft. Patients with recent venous thrombosis can have the clot cleared preoperatively with thrombolytic therapy.

- For thoracic outlet syndrome, conservative measures should be tried first.
- Surgical resection of first rib is curative in 80%-85% of cases.

MICROEMBOLI

Cause (Fig. 29-3)

Whereas macroemboli most frequently originate in the heart, microemboli more commonly originate from the peripheral vessels, although cardiac sources can occur. The most common variety are atheroemboli, which are small thrombi or cholesterol particles given off by fragmenting atherosclerotic plaques. Malfunctioning cardiac valves (native or prosthetic), dissection flaps, intracardiac tumors, and a host of other lesions can also spawn microemboli. Plaque rupture may occur spontaneously, but it is increasingly found as a complication of invasive (catheter) procedures.

- Microemboli commonly originate from peripheral vessels.
- Most common variety are atheroemboli.
- Plaque rupture may occur spontaneously or as complication of invasive procedure.

Clinical Manifestations

Microemboli may produce livedo, rubor, petechia, focal cutaneous necrosis, or organ ischemia or infarction. These findings depend on the distribution and extent of embolization. Diffuse microembolization from a source proximal to the renal or mesenteric vessels is a catastrophic occurrence that can lead to visceral and renal infarction and severe peripheral ischemia.

- Microemboli may produce livedo, rubor, petechia,

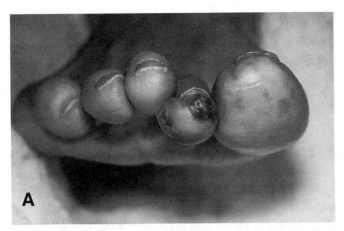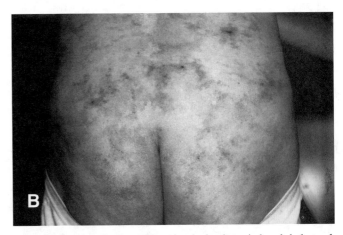

Fig. 29-3. Embolic disease. *A*, Distal infarcts and petechia. *B*, Emboli to buttocks after aortic catheterization. This patient had catheter-induced cholesterol microemboli that caused small infarctions and petechiae over back and buttocks.

focal cutaneous necrosis, or organ ischemia or infarction.

Treatment

The only reliable treatment for persistent microemboli is identification and removal of the embolic source. Because atherosclerosis is a diffuse process, the search for an embolic source often demonstrates widespread disease for which no simple surgical repair is readily apparent. Medical therapy, such as aspirin or anticoagulation, may help but often does not. Indeed, there is a well-recognized syndrome in which warfarin triggers or exacerbates atheroemboli. The exact mechanism of this phenomenon remains uncertain. Dipyridamole has been advocated by some, but it remains of unproven value.

- Only reliable treatment for microemboli is identification and removal of embolic source.
- There is a syndrome in which warfarin triggers or exacerbates atheroemboli.

DISSECTION

Cause

Dissection, like aneurysm formation, is a degenerative condition that can affect most large or medium-sized arteries. Dissection occurs when the intima or media separates from the remainder of the artery creating a "flap" that can obstruct the lumen of the vessel. Aneurysm formation or rupture of the weakened wall may occur. Marfan syndrome, Ehlers-Danlos syndrome, "cystic medial necrosis," and a host of other conditions can predispose to dissection. Hypertension is frequently present.

The aorta is the artery most frequently affected by dissection. Iatrogenic dissection may occur because of, for example, invasive diagnostic or therapeutic intravascular procedures, blunt trauma, or deceleration injuries.

- Dissection is degenerative condition affecting most large or medium-sized arteries.
- Marfan syndrome, Ehlers-Danlos syndrome, and "cystic medial necrosis" predispose to dissection.
- Hypertension is frequently present.
- Aorta is most frequently affected by dissection.

Classification

The two most common systems for classifying aortic dissection are the Stanford and the DeBakey systems, defined as follows:

Stanford A: any dissection involving the ascending aorta regardless of the site of primary intimal tear or distal extent of propagation

Stanford B: any dissection confined entirely to the distal aorta (i.e., distal to the aortic arch)

DeBakey type 1: equivalent to Stanford A

DeBakey type 2: a dissection limited to the ascending portion of the aorta

DeBakey type 3: equivalent to Stanford B.

Diagnosis

The sudden onset of "tearing" chest, scapular, or abdominal pain should alert the clinician to the possibility of aortic dissection. The pain commonly migrates as the dissection extends. Evidence of arterial occlusion to the limbs may be present if the dissection flap causes vascular obstruction. Care must be taken to avoid misdiagnosing dissection as myocardial infarction because the administration of thrombolytics in this setting is potentially lethal. Several tests may be used to screen for or confirm the diagnosis of dissection. Aortography is the historical standard, although computed tomography (conventional and ultrafast) and transesophageal echocardiography are rapidly emerging as equivalent or possibly superior technologies. Magnetic resonance imaging, digital subtraction angiography, transthoracic or abdominal duplex ultrasonography, and other similar tests are less desirable because of their limited ability to visualize the flap and their increased expense.

- Symptoms of aortic dissection: "tearing" chest, scapular, or abdominal pain.
- Pain commonly migrates as dissection extends.
- Misdiagnosis as myocardial infarction needs to be avoided.
- Aortography is standard test.

Treatment

Dissections involving the ascending aorta (Stanford A, DeBakey type 1 or 2) should be treated with emergency operation. The mortality rate for patients in this group who are treated medically is >90%. Operation can usually be performed with a perioperative mortality rate ≤20%. When the dissection involves the aortic valve, replacement or repair of the valve is necessary. Dissections involving the descending aorta (Stanford B or DeBakey type 3) may be treated either medically or surgically. Generally, medical therapy can be attempted first (β-adrenergic blockade, reduction of blood pressure as much as tolerated), and if the pain resolves promptly the patient can be followed. Operation should be performed if pain persists or recurs, aneurysms develop or enlarge, or limb or abdominal ischemia occurs. Regardless of the treatment used, serial follow-up with computed tomography should be performed to look for enlargement or resolution of the dissection and integrity of the graft anastomosis.

- Dissections of ascending aorta should be treated with emergency operation.
- Mortality rate with medical treatment of dissection of ascending aorta is >90%.
- Dissection of descending aorta may be treated medically or surgically.
- Operation for dissection of descending aorta is needed if pain persists or recurs, aneurysms develop, or limb or abdominal ischemia occurs.

Other Dissections

Dissections of the coronary artery can result from diagnostic catheterization or interventional therapeutic procedures such as percutaneous transluminal coronary angioplasty. Spontaneous carotid dissection can occur and is manifested by a constellation of symptoms that include unilateral headache, focal cerebral ischemic symptoms, and pulsatile tinnitus. Although there is no surgical option for this condition, spontaneous resolution is the rule. In contrast, spontaneous renal dissection is usually treated surgically. Iliofemoral dissections are usually the result of diagnostic or therapeutic catheter procedures performed through groin puncture sites.

- Carotid dissection resolves spontaneously.
- Renal dissection is usually treated surgically.

FIBROMUSCULAR DYSPLASIA

Background

Fibromuscular dysplasia (FMD) is a dysplastic disease affecting medium-sized and small arteries. Women are affected much more frequently than men. Most patients with FMD have renovascular involvement (60%-70%), and about 30% have cerebrovascular involvement. FMD can affect any layer of the arterial wall (intima, media, adventitia); the pathologic classification of this disease is usually based on the site of involvement. The most common form of FMD is medial (medial fibroplasia), which represents 70%-95% of all forms of FMD.

- FMD is dysplastic disease of medium-sized and small arteries.
- Renovascular involvement occurs in 60%-70% of cases.
- Cerebrovascular involvement occurs in about 30% of cases.

Diagnosis

In patients with renovascular hypertension or arterial occlusive disease, an FMD-related cause can be determined by angiography. In the most common forms of dysplasia the artery has a "string-of-beads" appearance (Fig. 29-4). These beads typically represent alternating stenotic and aneurysmal regions of blood vessels. Examination of biopsy specimens, when available, can aid in the diagnosis of FMD. Pathogenetically, FMD can produce stenotic lesions that may limit or occlude blood flow. It can also predispose to aneurysm formation or dissection.

- FMD diagnosed with angiography.
- Artery has "string-of-beads" appearance.
- FMD can produce stenotic lesions or predispose to aneurysm formation or dissection.

Treatment

FMD is best treated, when possible, by percutaneous transluminal angioplasty (PTA). Nearly two-thirds of patients with renovascular FMD will be "cured" by PTA alone. Operation should be reserved for patients in whom PTA fails, or in whom aneurysm or dissection is present. In certain patients, particularly those in whom PTA has failed and who are poor surgical risks, drug therapy alone may be adequate.

- FMD is best treated by percutaneous transluminal angioplasty.
- Almost two-thirds of patients are "cured" by angioplasty alone.
- Operation is used when angioplasty fails or when aneurysm or dissection is present.

GIANT CELL ARTERITIS

Background

Giant cell arteritis is a granulomatous vasculitic process of unknown cause. The large arteries are primarily affected. The two major syndromes of giant cell arteritis are Takayasu's arteritis and temporal arteritis.

- Giant cell arteritis is a granulomatous vasculitic process.
- Two major syndromes: Takayasu's arteritis and temporal arteritis.

Takayasu's Arteritis

Takayasu's arteritis affects primarily the aorta and its major branches, particularly those of the aortic arch. It is more common in females than in males. Also known as "pulseless disease," it frequently leads to complete occlusion of the brachiocephalic vessels. Patients are almost always <50 years old. Affected arteries may occasionally form aneurysms. The diagnosis is usually made from the history, examination, and arteriography. Angiographic findings include tapered narrowings (such as the "string" sign) of the brachiocephalic vessels; these occasionally go on to produce occlusion. When necessary,

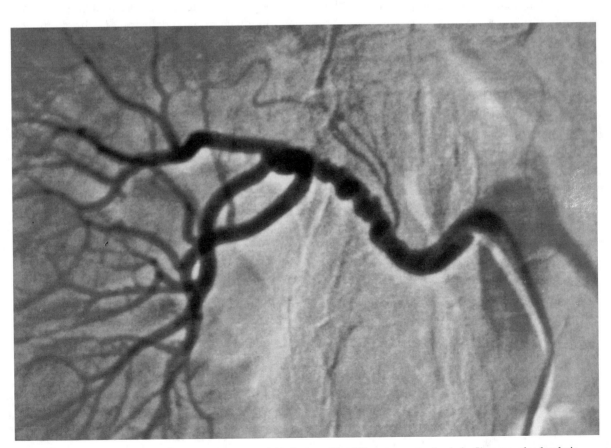

Fig. 29-4. Fibromuscular dysplasia. This typical angiographic "string-of-beads" appearance is classic for fibromuscular dysplasia.

or when tissue is available, the diagnosis can be made from biopsy. The erythrocyte sedimentation rate is almost always elevated in patients with active Takayasu's arteritis, and it can serve as an index of disease activity. Other acute-phase reactants, such as C-reactive protein, are occasionally useful.

- Takayasu's arteritis is more common in females.
- Patients are almost always <50 years old.
- Diagnosis made from history, examination, arteriography.

Therapy primarily involves the use of prednisone. High-dose prednisone (50-100 mg daily in single dose or divided doses) is usually instituted for 3-6 weeks, or until the sedimentation rate has stabilized in the normal range. Slow taper (2.5-5.0 mg every 2-4 weeks) is the rule, with the taper slowing to as little as 1 mg per month once the daily dose reaches 10 mg. The rate of taper should be modified according to the sedimentation rate and the clinical picture. In some cases, low-dose prednisone may be needed for prolonged periods or even indefinitely. Occasionally, vessels that were stenotic during the active phase of the disease will "reopen" during treatment. When surgical correction is necessary, effort should be made to hold off until the disease has been adequately treated, or preferably until it is "burned out."

- Treatment of Takayasu's arteritis is with high-dose prednisone that is slowly tapered.

Temporal Arteritis

Temporal arteritis primarily affects people >50 years old. It predominantly affects secondary or tertiary branches from the aorta. Like Takayasu's arteritis, its systemic manifestations may include fatigue, malaise, fever, and myalgias. It is pathologically indistinguishable from Takayasu's arteritis. Temporal arteritis should be suspected in any patient with systemic symptoms and pain or tenderness localized to the temporal arteries. As with Takayasu's arteritis the erythrocyte sedimentation rate is typically elevated, and the degree of elevation can be used to monitor the activity of the disease. Although angiography can be used to make the diagnosis, biopsy is much more commonly used because of the accessibility of the temporal artery. Biopsy should utilize as long a piece of the temporal artery as possible, and it may need to be performed bilaterally before the disease can be excluded.

- Temporal arteritis primarily affects people >50 years old.

- Systemic manifestations: fatigue, malaise, fever, myalgias.
- Temporal arteritis is pathologically indistinguishable from Takayasu's arteritis.
- Diagnosis should be suspected in any patient with pain or tenderness localized to temporal arteries.

Like Takayasu's arteritis, the treatment of temporal arteritis involves the use of corticosteroids. A typical program is 50-100 mg of prednisone per day, and treatment is usually maintained for 3-6 weeks or until the erythrocyte sedimentation rate has stabilized in the normal range. The relapse rate during taper is higher than that for Takayasu's arteritis, and in some series it approaches 50%. Longer-term, higher-dose corticosteroid programs may be necessary.

If the diagnosis of temporal arteritis is being seriously considered, treatment with prednisone should begin immediately. This approach prevents the sudden, unexpected complication of blindness due to occlusion of the central retinal artery. Biopsy results remain accurate if biopsy is performed within several days after starting treatment with corticosteroids.

- For temporal arteritis, treatment with prednisone should begin immediately to prevent sudden, unexpected blindness due to occlusion of central retinal artery.

RAYNAUD'S PHENOMENON

Background

Raynaud's phenomenon refers to any inappropriate or excessively intense episode of cutaneous, digital, or limb vasoconstriction. It most commonly affects the upper limb. Females are affected far more commonly than males. Attacks are usually triggered by exposure to the cold or by emotional stress. The disease can be divided into two categories, primary and secondary, depending on cause.

- Raynaud's phenomenon is inappropriate or excessively intense episode of cutaneous, digital, or limb vasoconstriction.

Primary Raynaud's Phenomenon

The cause of primary Raynaud's phenomenon is unknown. Episodes are usually bilateral. Digital ulcerations are rare but may occur occasionally. The symptoms are usually stable and may be related to abnormalities in adrenergic function, blood viscosity, or endothelial disorders.

- Episodes of primary Raynaud's phenomenon are usually bilateral.
- Digital ulcerations are rare.

Secondary Raynaud's Phenomenon

This refers to Raynaud's phenomenon occurring as the result of some other underlying abnormality. Predisposing factors include atherosclerosis, arteritis, cancer, collagen vascular disease, thoracic outlet syndrome, embolic occlusions, occupational disease, certain drugs (β-adrenergic blocker, nicotine, ergotamine), and various other conditions. Secondary Raynaud's phenomenon is occasionally unilateral (perhaps affecting a single digit) and may produce skin breakdown.

- Secondary Raynaud's phenomenon is result of some other underlying abnormality.

Diagnosis

The diagnosis of Raynaud's phenomenon is made primarily on clinical grounds. Provocative testing to document and assess normal vasoconstriction is often of limited value because of the difficulty in reliably reproducing symptoms in the laboratory setting.

- Diagnosis of Raynaud's phenomenon is made on clinical grounds.

Treatment

The treatment of Raynaud's phenomenon is often difficult. In cases of secondary Raynaud's phenomenon, treatment of the underlying condition should be attempted whenever possible. Simple conservative measures such as dressing warmly, avoiding unnecessary exposure to the cold, and intermittent hand warming may improve the condition substantially. Biofeedback is effective in certain cases. Drugs with a potential for causing vasoconstriction should be avoided. Occasionally it is necessary to move to a warmer climate to achieve complete relief. Certain vasodilators, especially nifedipine, prazosin, and other calcium or α-adrenergic blockers, may help in selected cases. Interruption of the sympathetic nerves, either through ganglionic injection or surgical sympathectomy, is often useful in patients with severe symptoms.

- Simple treatment for Raynaud's phenomenon: dressing warmly, avoiding exposure to cold, intermittent hand warming.
- Certain vasodilators may help in selected cases.

ACUTE DEEP VENOUS THROMBOSIS

Cause

The factors predisposing to deep venous thrombosis (DVT) include those of Virchow's triad: stasis, trauma, and hypercoagulability. Underlying conditions that can predispose to DVT include cancer, inflammatory bowel disease, pregnancy or estrogen use, obesity, age, surgery or trauma, congestive heart failure, previous DVT, and a host of others.

- Factors in DVT include Virchow's triad: stasis, trauma, hypercoagulability.

Clinical Manifestations

Acute DVT is notoriously difficult to diagnose on clinical grounds only. Swelling, pain, discoloration, positive Homans' sign, cord palpation, and other typical features can suggest the diagnosis but are frequently misleading. In many cases extensive DVT may be minimally symptomatic or even nonsymptomatic, whereas in others the proximal DVT is so massive that the leg becomes mottled, cyanotic, markedly tender, and ischemic; this condition is referred to as phlegmasia cerulea dolens.

- DVT is notoriously difficult to diagnose on clinical grounds only.

Diagnosis

Venography has long been the standard method for definitively diagnosing DVT, but duplex scanning (with or without color flow) is rapidly emerging as an equivalent method for the diagnosis of proximal DVT. Nonimaging (functional) methods such as impedance plethysmography and continuous-wave Doppler remain reliable, cost-efficient methods for detecting proximal DVT. They are unreliable for excluding below-knee thrombus. Fortunately, the embolic potential of below-knee thrombus is extremely low, and in many clinical situations it is safe to follow patients who have negative results of functional studies such as impedance plethysmography.

- Venography is standard method to diagnose DVT.
- Duplex scanning is equivalent method for diagnosis of proximal DVT.

Treatment

Patients with acute, proximal DVT should be hospitalized and treated with intravenously administered heparin for 5-7 days. The activated partial thromboplastin should be kept at 2.0-2.5 times the control value throughout heparinization. In the past, warfarin was not given until 5-7 days into treatment; newer programs are now administering warfarin at the time of admission and discontinuing the use of heparin when the prothrombin time is therapeutic and stable. In any case, the patient should remain hospitalized until the prothrombin time is therapeutic (1.5-2.0 times control value) and the patient is able to ambulate without pain. Use of warfarin should be maintained for at least 3 months. In most cases of DVT, an elastic compression stocking should be prescribed and worn during treatment with warfarin.

- Treatment for DVT: hospitalization, intravenously administered heparin for 5-7 days.
- Patient is hospitalized until prothrombin time is therapeutic.
- Warfarin is used for at least 3 months.

Unprecipitated DVT

In patients with unprecipitated DVT, be sure to search for an underlying, occult disorder that may be predisposing the patient to clot formation.

- For unprecipitated DVT, search for underlying disorder.

PULMONARY EMBOLISM

Background

Pulmonary embolism is a major cause of death in the United States and may cause as many as 250,000 fatalities per year. It is estimated that up to 80% of significant pulmonary emboli escape detection and that 50% of patients suspected of having pulmonary emboli on clinical grounds actually do not. The mortality rate is between 20% and 35% for untreated pulmonary emboli, and it is 8% when the condition is properly diagnosed and treated.

- Mortality rate with untreated pulmonary emboli: 20%-35%.

Pathophysiology

The risk factors for pulmonary emboli are the same as those for deep venous thrombosis (see page 851). Emboli are most likely to originate in the large, deep veins of the lower extremity (iliofemoral system), although 10% of pulmonary emboli seem to come from the upper extremity. Thrombi in the superficial veins or deep venous system distal to the knee do not commonly embolize.

- Emboli most likely to originate in large, deep veins of lower extremity.
- 10% of emboli come from upper extremity.

Signs and Symptoms

There is generally poor correlation among symptoms, clinical findings, and the presence or absence of pulmonary emboli. Most pulmonary emboli occur silently. When signs and symptoms occur, they are highly variable. In the Urokinase Pulmonary Embolism Trial, the most common signs and symptoms included tachypnea (respiration rate >16 per minute), 92%; dyspnea, 85%; pleuritic chest pain, 74%; apprehension, 59%; rales, 58%; and cough, 53%. Phlebitis was clinically apparent in only 32%. Other common findings included an accentuated second heart sound, tachycardia, fever, hemoptysis, diaphoresis, and syncope. Massive pulmonary embolism may cause syncope, cor pulmonale, cardiogenic shock, and cardiac arrest with electromechanical dissociation. Chronic pulmonary emboli may lead to pulmonary hypertension and the development of cor pulmonale.

- Correlation is poor among symptoms, clinical findings, and presence or absence of pulmonary emboli.
- Most pulmonary emboli occur silently.
- Chronic pulmonary emboli may lead to pulmonary hypertension.

Screening Tests

The most common electrocardiographic abnormality noted in pulmonary embolism is sinus tachycardia. "Classic" electrocardiographic findings such as an S_1, Q_3, T_3 pattern, right bundle-branch block, right-axis deviation, and increased P wave are present in only one-fourth of patients. Chest radiography is likewise nonspecific; findings include pleural effusion in 50%, right-sided cardiomegaly, pulmonary infarction, elevation of the hemidiaphragm, and atelectasis. The arterial blood gas may show decreased P_{O_2} and P_{CO_2}.

Specific Tests

Ventilation-perfusion scanning is one of the most widely used tests to screen for pulmonary embolism. It should be viewed as a useful test when the findings suggest either a high probability or normal results. Intermediate- or low-probability results should be viewed as nondiagnostic. Pulmonary angiography remains the standard diagnostic method. Computed tomography, especially ultrafast, is also a useful diagnostic tool.

- Ventilation-perfusion scanning is widely used to screen for pulmonary embolism.
- Pulmonary angiography is standard diagnostic method.

Treatment

Anticoagulation is the mainstay of treatment for acute pulmonary embolism. It should be started immediately with heparin, which is given for 5-10 days. The regimen is then switched to warfarin, which should be maintained for 3-6 months. In cases of massive pulmonary embolism, thrombolytic therapy should be considered. Streptokinase, urokinase, and tissue-plasminogen activator are all potentially useful agents. In patients with massive, life-threatening pulmonary embolism who have contraindications to thrombolytic therapy or who have not responded to an attempt at lysis, or in whom severe, chronic pulmonary embolism is present, surgical embolectomy can be considered. Patients who cannot tolerate anticoagulation should be considered for a caval filter to prevent recurrent, possibly lethal, pulmonary embolism.

CHRONIC DEEP VENOUS INSUFFICIENCY (POSTPHLEBITIC SYNDROME)

Background

Chronic deep venous insufficiency (DVI) is the second most common cause of leg ulcer in the United States. The condition develops when veins become chronically obstructed, or when venous valvular incompetence develops. These recurrences are usually caused by deep venous thrombosis. Although the exact mechanism by which venous insufficiency produces chronic changes is unknown, it appears that chronically elevated venous pressure is the culprit.

- DVI is second most common cause of leg ulcer in United States.

- Recurrences are usually caused by deep venous thrombosis.

Clinical Manifestations

DVI may lead to limb swelling, pigmentation (from hemosiderin deposition in the perivascular tissues), induration and cellulitis, dermatitis, and ulceration. The most commonly affected area of the leg is the medial malleolus, although any portion of the lower part of the leg may be involved.

- DVI most often affects medial malleolus.

Diagnosis

The diagnosis is made from the clinical history, physical findings, and objective testing. Specific tests for DVI include continuous-wave Doppler (with or without duplex imaging), various types of plethysmographic studies, and descending venography.

Treatment

DVI is treated primarily with measures to control swelling. The leg should be elevated whenever possible, and long periods of standing or sitting should be avoided. Elastic compression, either in the form of stockings or wrap, is essential. The compression must be graduated and of sufficient magnitude to prevent swelling. If stockings are to be used, the swelling should be maximally reduced before fitting. Additional compression can be supplied by the use of elastic pads. Dermatitis and other forms of inflammation are often improved by the use of corticosteroid cream. Antibiotics should be reserved for situations in which infection is apparent. Anticoagulation is not necessary unless recurrent clotting has developed or is likely. Venous stripping or perforator ligation may be useful in a limited number of cases with refractory ulcers. The stripping of superficial veins should be avoided if deep venous obstruction is present, because the superficial veins may be acting as collaterals. Occasionally a chronic arteriovenous fistula may mimic DVI. This possibility should be considered when penetrating trauma, surgical procedures, or other causes of fistula are present.

- Elastic compression is essential for DVI.
- Venous stripping or perforator ligation is useful in limited number of cases.
- Chronic arteriovenous fistula may mimic DVI.

LYMPHEDEMA

Background

Lymphedema is the result of hypoplasia, dysfunction, or obstruction of the lymphatic vessels. As a result, lymphatic fluid accumulates in the interstitial space and the extremity becomes swollen. Pitting edema is present early in the disease, but in chronic cases the subcutaneous tissues become fibrotic and hyperplastic, producing woody "nonpitting" edema.

- Lymphedema results from hypoplasia, dysfunction, or obstruction of lymphatic vessels.
- Pitting edema occurs early in disease.

Cause

Lymphedema may be primary (due to a congenital abnormality or predisposition) or secondary (due to trauma, infection, cancer, and other disorders). Primary lymphedema most commonly becomes manifest at puberty (lymphedema praecox) and may be familial in about 15% of cases. Secondary lymphedema is a worldwide problem of major proportion. In tropical countries, the most common causes of lymphedema are filarial disorders, and the lymphedema produced can be severe (elephantiasis). In Western or industrialized countries, tumor (such as breast, prostate, gynecologic) and recurrent infections are the most common cause. The treatment of breast cancer commonly produces edema of the upper extremity. The likelihood and severity of lymphedema depend on the type and extent of operation and the use of adjuvant therapy such as radiation or chemotherapy.

- Primary lymphedema manifests at puberty (lymphedema praecox) and may be familial.
- In tropical countries, common causes of lymphedema are filarial disorders.
- In Western countries, tumor and recurrent infections are most common cause of lymphedema.

Diagnosis

The diagnosis of lymphedema can usually be made from the history and physical examination. When a confirmatory study is necessary, the best technique is lymphoscintigraphy. In this test, a small amount of radiolabeled colloid is injected in the web space between the digits, where its progress through the lymphatics is followed with nuclear scanning. The patency of lymphatics can thus be determined. Lymphangiography has been considered the standard, but it should be avoided whenever possible because of its invasive nature and tendency to cause lymphangitis, which may worsen lymphedema.

- Lymphoscintigraphy is best diagnostic technique for lymphedema.
- Lymphangiography should be avoided because of its invasive nature.

Treatment

In most cases, lymphedema is incurable but treatable. Good hygiene and protection from trauma are among the most important elements of care. The limb should be elevated as often as possible to drain the tissue and keep swelling to a minimum. Elastic compression stockings (often with pressures as high as 50 or 60 mm Hg) are the mainstay of treatment. Sequential compression pumps capable of generating pressures of 80-100 mm Hg can be used to "milk" lymphatic fluid out of the legs. Antibiotics should be used liberally to treat or provide prophylaxis against bacterial infection. In some cases, surgical techniques to reduce the size of the limb or bypass blocked lymphatics are possible.

- Elastic compression stockings are mainstay of treatment for lymphedema.

ARTERIOVENOUS MALFORMATION OR FISTULA

Background

Arteriovenous malformation or fistula (Fig. 29-5) may be acquired or congenital. Acquired ones are generally due to penetrating trauma, iatrogenic processes such as surgery or catheterization, or spontaneous degeneration of blood vessels. Congenital malformation or fistula may involve primarily arterial, venous, capillary, or lymphatic tissues; at times the lesions are mixed and involve elements of all four.

- Arteriovenous malformations may be acquired or congenital.

Consequences

Arteriovenous malformations may be of cosmetic significance only, or they can produce pain, tissue destruction, or limb hypertrophy, especially when the flow is high. In some patients, congestive heart failure has occurred as a result of the high demand for blood flow associated with these lesions.

Treatment

The treatment of many arteriovenous malformations is difficult because the malformation may involve deep or vital structures and make resection impossible; vessels feeding or draining the lesion may be difficult to identify, reach, and ligate; the lesion has a propensity to redevelop after resection; and successful treatment may produce ischemia in regions distal to the malformation. Thus, conservative measures are frequently used. When pain, swelling, congestive heart failure, the possibility of malignancy, or other problems force a consideration of interventional therapy, surgery or embolization is usually attempted. Catheter-directed embolization is showing increasing utility in this regard.

- Treatment of arteriovenous malformation is difficult.

ULCERS

Types

Vascular ulcers can be divided into four categories: ischemic, venous, arteriolar, and neurotrophic.

Ischemic

Ischemic ulcers (Fig. 29-6) result from arterial occlusive disease (large or small vessels) that reduces blood flow below the level necessary for maintaining skin viability. The ulcers tend to be distal (digits or foot) and may be triggered by trauma, including mild abrasion from shoes. They often become infected. Ischemic ulcers are usually painful unless associated neuropathy is present.

- Ischemic ulcers result from arterial occlusive disease.
- Ischemic ulcers tend to be distal (digits or foot).
- Ulcers are usually painful.

Venous

Venous ulcers (Fig. 29-7) were discussed on page 853. They result from skin breakdown associated with chronic venous insufficiency. Other signs or symptoms of venous stasis are usually present around the ulcer, including swelling, pigmentation, and indurated cellulitis. Trauma is often a precipitating factor. The ulcers are usually located over the medial malleolus, but they may occur

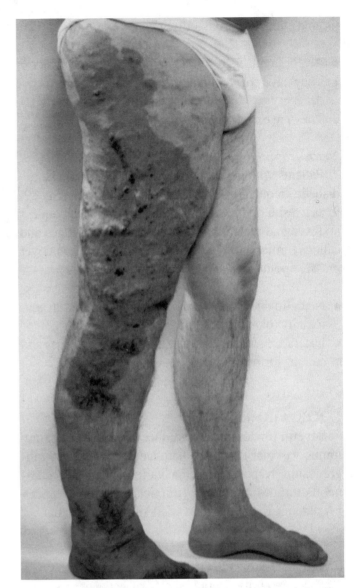

Fig. 29-5. Arteriovenous malformation. This extensive congenital malformation has led to venous volume and pressure overload. As a result, many of the clinical findings are similar to those of chronic venous insufficiency. If blood flow is high enough, heart failure may develop.

on any part of the leg. They are typically painful, but not as painful as ulcers caused by ischemia.

- Venous ulcers are associated with chronic venous insufficiency.
- Venous ulcers are not as painful as ischemic ulcers.

Arteriolar

Also known as "hypertensive" ulcers, arteriolar ulcers (Fig. 29-8) result from small-vessel occlusion. They tend to have punched-out or irregular (serpiginous) borders and are usually extremely painful. A wide variety of processes can lead to the small-vessel occlusion producing arteriolar ulcers; these include hypertension, vasculitis, and collagen vascular diseases.

- Arteriolar ulcers result from small-vessel occlusion.
- They have punched-out or irregular (serpiginous) borders.
- They are extremely painful.

Neurotrophic

Patients with neuropathy, particularly those who are diabetic, frequently develop neurotrophic ulcers (Fig. 29-9) as a result of chronic trauma. The ulcers are painless and pale and typically have associated thick edges and callous formation. They are almost always present over pressure points or sites of repetitive trauma.

- Neurotrophic ulcers often develop in patients with neuropathy (diabetes).
- Ulcers are painless and pale and have thick edges and callous formation.

LOOK-ALIKES

Several processes can produce leg ulcers that may mimic vascular lesions. These include pyoderma gangrenosum, Kaposi's sarcoma, various infections, cutaneous tumors, lipedema (mimicking lymphedema), myxedema, trauma, and a variety of other problems.

WARFARIN NECROSIS

This rare entity occurs in <1% of patients receiving the medication. It usually develops 3-6 days after initiation of therapy (more often in women) and is characterized by the sudden development of erythematous or hemorrhagic skin lesions. These eventually become gangrenous, and the overlying skin sloughs. Areas of skin with underlying fatty deposits (e.g., breasts, buttocks) are most commonly affected. The exact cause of this reaction is unknown, but a decreased level of protein C may be involved. When it occurs, the use of warfarin should be discontinued immediately.

- Warfarin necrosis occurs in <1% of patients receiving the medication.
- It develops 3-6 days after therapy.
- It is characterized by erythematous or hemorrhagic skin lesions that become gangrenous.
- Use of warfarin should be discontinued immediately.

HEPARIN-INDUCED THROMBOCYTOPENIA

The frequency of heparin-induced thrombocytopenia is probably 1% or 2%, but estimates as high as 30% have been reported. It typically begins 5-10 days after the initiation of heparin therapy. Patients with this condition are frequently asymptomatic but may develop hemorrhagic or thrombotic complications. The cause probably involves an antigen/antibody interaction, but the exact mechanism is poorly understood. Treatment consists of discontinuing use of heparin when the problem is identified.

- Heparin-induced thrombocytopenia occurs in 1% or 2% of patients receiving the medication.
- It begins 5-10 days after initiation of therapy.
- Cause involves antigen/antibody interaction.

IATROGENIC VASCULAR DISEASE AND TRAUMA

Vascular trauma is an increasingly common occurrence. Interventional procedures such as catheterization can produce occlusion, dissection, or bleeding. Other common sources of trauma include penetrating injuries, acceleration injuries, and blunt trauma.

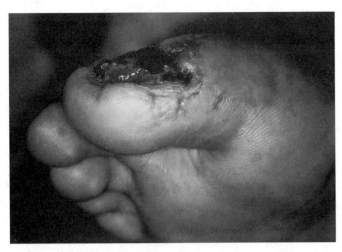

Fig. 29-6. Ischemic ulcer located distally on foot. There was poor wound granulation, and the ulcer was very painful.

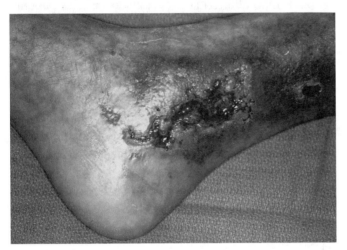

Fig. 29-7. Venous ulcer. Note location over medial malleolus and surrounding hyperpigmentation and cellulitis.

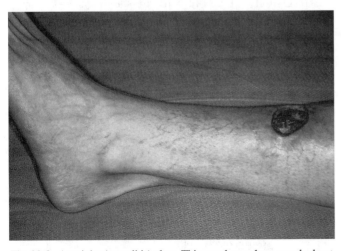

Fig. 29-8. Arteriolar (vasculitis) ulcer. This case has a clean, punched-out appearance.

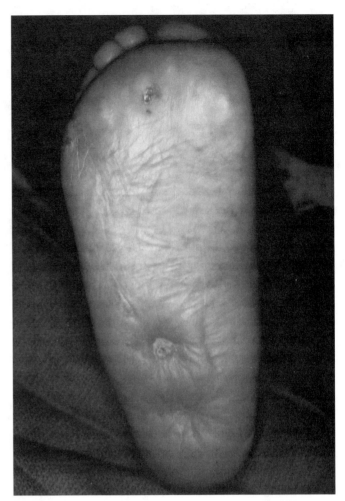

Fig. 29-9. Neurotrophic ulcers over pressure points on insensitive foot.

QUESTIONS
(See "Answers" section)

Multiple Choice

1. Which of the following statements about aneurysms is false?
   a. Popliteal aneurysms are more likely to thrombose and occlude than they are to rupture
   b. Abdominal aortic aneurysms should be operated on before they reach 4.5 cm in maximal diameter because the risk of rupture increases sharply at that point
   c. Patients with popliteal aneurysms have a relatively high incidence of associated abdominal aortic aneurysms
   d. Aortic aneurysms are usually associated with atherosclerosis
   e. Fibromuscular dysplasia may predispose to aneurysm formation

2. Which of the following statements about lymphedema is false?
   a. The most common secondary cause of lymphedema worldwide is filarial disease
   b. Penicillin is usually adequate to treat or prevent cellulitis associated with lymphedema
   c. Elastic compression usually helps to control the swelling of lymphedema
   d. Cancer is the most common secondary cause of lymphedema in the United States
   e. The swelling of lymphedema is usually painful

3. Which of the following statements about thoracic outlet syndrome (TOS) is false?
   a. TOS may cause subclavian vein thrombosis
   b. TOS may cause arterial damage and aneurysm formation
   c. TOS can cause arterial embolization
   d. Nerve compression is relatively rare in TOS
   e. Surgery is unnecessary in most cases of symptomatic TOS

4. Which of the following statements about thromboembolic disease is true?
   a. Duplex scanning is as accurate as venography for the diagnosis of femoropopliteal deep venous thrombosis
   b. Fatal pulmonary emboli usually come from the deep calf veins
   c. Deep venous thrombosis and pulmonary embolism can be reliably diagnosed on clinical grounds
   d. Ventilation-perfusion scanning is as accurate as pulmonary angiography for the diagnosis of pulmonary embolism
   e. Warfarin therapy should be routinely maintained for a full year after most deep venous thromboses or pulmonary emboli

5. Which of the following statements about giant cell arteritis is false?
   a. Temporal arteritis almost always affects patients >50 years old
   b. Takayasu's arteritis almost always affects patients <50 years old
   c. Patients with suspected symptomatic temporal arteritis should be given corticosteroids immediately to prevent sudden blindness
   d. The erythrocyte sedimentation rate is typically increased in temporal arteritis but is usually normal in Takayasu's arteritis
   e. The diagnosis of temporal arteritis or Takayasu's arteritis can usually be made by biopsy or angiography

True/False

6. Patients with Raynaud's phenomenon:
   a. Almost always require vasodilation therapy
   b. Usually have connective tissue disease
   c. Usually progress to develop digital ulcerations
   d. May worsen if given β-adrenergic blockers
   e. Should stop smoking
   f. May be helped by sympathetic nerve block

7. Factors that predispose to deep venous thrombosis include:
   a. Obesity
   b. Hip fracture
   c. Ergotamine
   d. Estrogen
   e. Pregnancy
   f. β-Adrenergic blockers

ANSWERS

Chapter 2   ALLERGY
(Questions--pages 25-26)

1. Answer a.

The histopathology of airways in patients with severe asthma includes mucosal infiltration with eosinophils, mucosal edema, damage to airway epithelium, hypertrophy of airway smooth muscle, and hyperplasia of mucous glands. IgE immune complex deposition, deposition of mast cell histamine, and pollen in the airway lumen are not found in fatal asthma.

2. Answer d.

Important adverse effects of aerosol corticosteroids include dysphonia and oral candidiasis. Systemic corticosteroids can cause aseptic necrosis of the hip; theophylline can cause seizures; inhaled or oral β-agonists can cause tremor.

3. Answer e.

Immunotherapy is effective in selected asthma patients who are sensitive to grass pollen, ragweed pollen, dust mites, mold, and animal dander. Immunotherapy for *Candida*, smoke, bacteria, and *Trichophyton* has never been shown to be effective.

4. Answer d.

Environmental precautions for dust mite allergy should include encasing pillows and mattresses in dust-proof casings, removing carpeting, using an efficient air filter on high-volume ventilation systems, and killing dust mites with high temperatures. Humidification actually increases dust mite proliferation.

5. Answer b.

Fatal asthma is associated with overuse of β-agonist inhalers as well as frequent hospitalizations for asthma, recent intubation for severe asthma, tapering schedule of systemic glucocorticoids, and psychiatric disease. Tapering inhaled glucocorticoids, allergy to animal dander, recent allergy skin tests, and the use of anticholinergic agents are not associated with asthma fatality.

6. Answer a.

Patients with anaphylactic hypersensitivity to honeybee stings should learn to use self-administered epinephrine and may benefit from honeybee venom immunotherapy. Allergen immunotherapy is allergen-specific, so that yellow jacket venom treatment would not benefit a patient sensitive to honeybees. Also, whole body extracts are not effective immunotherapy reagents for anaphylaxis; honeybee venom immunotherapy is the treatment of choice for honeybee sensitivity.

7. Answer c.

Medical conditions that can cause year-round rhinitis include dust mite allergy, rhinitis medicamentosa, and structural problems such as nasal polyposis and nasal septal deviation. Ragweed pollen allergy causes a seasonal rhinitis.

8. Answer d.

Erythema multiforme, exfoliative dermatitis, and the Stevens-Johnson syndrome are potentially life-threatening drug reactions. Patients who develop such drug reactions should not be rechallenged with the offending drug or related agents. β-Lactam antibiotics have no structural similarity with sulfamethoxazole. There are no accurate allergy skin tests for sulfa drugs.

9. Answer c.

Asthma, helminth infections, allergic bronchopulmonary aspergillosis, and Churg-Strauss vasculitis are closely associated with peripheral blood eosinophilia. Patients with sensitivity to radiocontrast media do not show eosinophilia.

10. Answer b.

Terminal component complement deficiencies (C5, C6, C7, C8) are associated with increased susceptibility to infection with *Neisseria*. This increased susceptibility to infection is not seen in the hypereosinophilia syndrome, allergic bronchopulmonary aspergillosis, C1 esterase inhibitor deficiency, or systemic mastocytosis.

11. a, false; b, false; c, true; d, true; e, false; f, true.

β-Adrenergic agonists such as albuterol, terbutaline, and pirbuterol inhibit the early phase bronchial response to aerosolized antigen in sensitive patients. Inhaled glucocorticoids such as beclomethasone and triamcinolone inhibit the late phase bronchial response. Aerosol cromolyn sodium inhibits both the early and late phase responses.

12. a, true; b, true; c, true; d, false; e, true; f, false.

Patients with aspirin idiosyncrasy often show cross-sensitivity to other nonsteroidal anti-inflammatory agents that inhibit the cyclooxygenase enzyme. Aspirin idiosyncrasy, asthma, and nasal polyposis are closely associated. Oral desensitization to aspirin can be accomplished in aspirin-sensitive patients who must take aspirin for other medical indications, but the desensitization procedure is hazardous and should be conducted only by specialists. There are no accurate skin tests for aspirin sensitivity.

13. a, true; b, true; c, true; d, false; e, true; f, false.

Cystic fibrosis and asthma and aspirin sensitivity are associated with nasal polyposis. Symptoms of nasal polyps include chronic and nasal congestion and recurrent sinusitis.

14. a, false; b, true; c, false; d, true; e, true; f, false.

Many patients with selective IgA deficiency are asymptomatic. Some patients with selective IgA deficiency may also have IgG subclass deficiency, and these patients may demonstrate increased susceptibility to infection. Selective IgA deficiency is the commonest immunoglobulin deficiency state. Patients with selective IgA deficiency are at risk for transfusion reactions caused by anti-IgA antibodies. Intravenous gamma globulin contains only trace amounts of IgA. Although gamma globulin is relatively contraindicated in selective IgA deficiency because of the risk of transfusion reactions, patients with selective IgA deficiency and IgG subclass deficiency may benefit from intravenously administered gamma globulin under special circumstances.

Chapter 3   BLOOD GASES
(Questions--pages 37-38)

1. Answer e.

This patient's arterial hypoxemia has been corrected by oxygen therapy, suggesting that the cause is ventilation-perfusion mismatch or ventilation-diffusion mismatch rather than right-to-left shunt.

2. Answer b.

By definition, the patient does not have hypoventilation because her $PaCO_2$ is normal. She has a right-to-left shunt, probably intrapulmonary, which should be caused by perfusion of unventilated lung, which in turn is usually caused by obstruction of a bronchus (as might occur with an endotracheal tube, mucous plug, or foreign body) or by the filling of alveoli with liquid (as occurs with adult respiratory distress syndrome, left-sided heart failure, pneumonia, or near drowning as with aspiration of gastric contents).

3. Answer d.

The $PaCO_2$ is 60 mm Hg, which is the same as the last two digits of the pH. This is the upper limit of compensation for simple primary metabolic alkalosis. When patients breathe air, if the $PaCO_2$ increases much higher, the PaO_2 declines to a level that will stimulate respiration by causing a hypoxic drive, thus limiting the compensation. Compensation thus tends to be less pronounced in patients with lung diseases who have an increase in alveolar to arterial oxygen tension difference or in patients who are studied at higher altitudes. This constraint to compensation is removed when oxygen supplementation is given.

4. Answer b.

The most common cause for combined primary respiratory alkalosis and primary metabolic acidosis with an increased anion gap resulting in a normal pH in a child is salicylate poisoning.

5. a, true.

Lactic acidosis is the most common cause of a rapid-onset, high anion gap metabolic acidosis.

b, true.

Carboxyhemoglobinemia is more common than cyanide poisoning as a cause for lactic acidosis in fires. Cyanide poisoning is not uncommon when isocyanate materials are burned and is a common problem in patients trapped in burning aircraft, but in these patients carbon monoxide poisoning is usually present also.

c, true.

The oxygen therapy is indicated to speed the reversal of carboxyhemoglobinemia.

6. False.

This is a commonly asked board question. Although the Pa_{O_2} is in the normal range, for a normal Pa_{CO_2}, the Pa_{O_2} in this patient is distinctly low for this Pa_{CO_2}. Remember that when the Pa_{CO_2} is abnormal you should calculate an alveolar to arterial oxygen tension difference (in this example, if the patient were at sea level, breathing an inspired P_{O_2} of 150, the alveolar P_{O_2} would be 124, and the alveolar to arterial oxygen tension difference would be 42 mm Hg).

7. a, false.

The alveolar P_{O_2} is 54 mm Hg, the arterial is 50; therefore, the alveolar to arterial oxygen tension difference is normal.

b, false.

When the pH decreases from 7.0 to 7.15, one would expect the serum potassium value to increase by about 1.2 mEq/L. In this patient, if the pH were corrected to 7.40, one would expect the serum potassium value to be 4.5 mEq/L.

c, false.

When the Pa_{CO_2} increases from 40 to 80 with acute respiratory acidosis, the bicarbonate value should increase by 4 mEq/L simply by hydration and dissociation of the increased Pa_{CO_2} and subsequent buffering of the hydrogen ion alone.

Chapter 4   CARDIOLOGY I
(Questions--pages 66-68)

Part I

1. Answer b.

Randomized trials have shown that β-blockers, thrombolytic therapy, and aspirin are all useful in decreasing mortality and preserving left ventricular function in patients with large anterior myocardial infarction. Also, in those with anterior myocardial infarction and cardiogenic shock, emergency percutaneous transluminal coronary angioplasty decreases mortality. Calcium channel blockers are not known to be effective in this situation.

2. Answer c.

Streptokinase, tissue-plasminogen activator, and urokinase are all thrombolytic agents that are useful in myocardial infarction but must be given as prolonged infusions. However, anisoylated plasminogen streptokinase activator complex can be given as an isolated intravenous bolus.

Intravenous nitroglycerin is very short acting and must be given as a continuous infusion.

3. Answer c.

Heart rate, contractility, afterload, and wall tension are all components of myocardial oxygen demand. Coronary perfusion pressure is a component of myocardial oxygen supply.

4. Answer d.

The optimal therapy for this patient consists of an appropriate dosage of thrombolytic therapy (1.5×10^6 U of streptokinase). Aspirin and β-blockers should be used concomitantly to improve mortality. Angiotensin-converting enzyme inhibitors given acutely or calcium channel blockers given acutely are contraindicated in this situation.

5. Answer c.

By Bayes' theorem, this patient, on the basis of his medical history, has known coronary artery disease. The treadmill exertion test should not be used for diagnosis of coronary artery disease. However, the excellent work load portends a good prognosis.

6. a, false; b, false; c, true; d, false; e, false.

Catheter-based interventions are effective in decreasing the severity of a stenosis in coronary artery lesions. With current technology, the immediate success rate approaches 90%. However, percutaneous transluminal coronary angioplasty has a high restenosis rate and, thus, does not decrease the incidence of myocardial infarction or reduce mortality. It should not necessarily be performed on all high-grade lesions after thrombolytic therapy for myocardial infarction. Other technologies, such as laser angioplasty and atherectomy, do not produce a lower restenosis rate.

7. a, true; b, false; c, true; d, false; e, false.

Several large randomized trials have shown that coronary artery bypass grafting prolongs survival in patients with left main coronary artery disease and in those patients with three-vessel disease and depressed left ventricular function. It is more effective than percutaneous transluminal coronary angioplasty in relieving symptoms of angina. However it will not prevent myocardial infarction, improved left ventricular function, or effectively treat sustained ventricular tachycardia.

Part II

8. Answer d.

Dilated cardiomyopathy has abnormalities of systolic and diastolic function. Mitral regurgitation is frequently present because of a dilated annulus. An apical thrombus is frequently present. Dynamic left ventricular outflow tract obstruction is seen in patients with hypertrophic cardiomyopathy.

9. Answer d.

In multiple trials, only the angiotensin-converting enzyme inhibitors have decreased mortality in severely symptomatic patients with dilated cardiomyopathy. In one trial, the combination of nitrates and hydralazine was shown to decrease mortality, but the intolerance to these medications was high. No study has shown that prazosin or a 48-hour infusion of dobutamine improves mortality. Currently, a large randomized trial is being conducted to determine whether digoxin decreases mortality in these patients.

10. Answer c.

Digoxin, angiotensin-converting enzyme inhibitors, nitrates, and hydralazine are all useful in symptomatic patients with dilated cardiomyopathy. Warfarin should be given if there is no contraindication to prevent future embolic events. Milrinone, a phosphodiesterase inhibitor, actually increases mortality in these patients.

11. Answer c.

A selective α_1-blocker and an angiotensin-converting enzyme inhibitor reduce afterload and, thus, increase stroke volume. A β_1-agonist and digoxin directly increase contractility of the left ventricle. A long-acting nitrate actually reduces preload and can decrease stroke volume.

12. Answer e.

Diastolic dysfunction is a primary pathophysiologic mechanism in patients with restrictive cardiomyopathy. Systolic function may be normal in these patients.

13. a, true; b, true; c, true; d, false; e, true; f, false.

In multiple trials, angiotensin-converting enzyme inhibitors have been shown to prolong life in severely symptomatic patients with dilated cardiomyopathy. Recent studies have shown that they also prevent ventricular dilatation after anterior myocardial infarction and decrease future hospitalization in the asymptomatic patients with dilated cardiomyopathy. They are not more effective than nitrates and hydralazine in decreasing symptoms but are better tolerated. They do not prevent sudden death in these patients.

14. a, true; b, true; c, true; d, true; e, false; f, true.

All these cardiac diseases have a hereditary component except mitral stenosis, which is an acquired defect due to rheumatic fever.

Chapter 5 CARDIOLOGY II
(Questions--pages 91-95)

1. Answer e.

Coronary angiography is not the most important test at this time because the patient had excellent exercise performance on a thallium test with no evidence of ischemia. Echocardiography can give information concerning ventricular function but is not the most critical test at this time in the patient's evaluation because he has no symptoms to suggest congestive heart failure. A 24-hour ambulatory electrocardiographic monitoring is not the best choice. The patient has already had cardiac arrest in the absence of acute myocardial infarction. He requires further evaluation whether or not there was complex ventricular ectopy on the Holter monitor. The patient has already had ventricular fibrillation and therefore does not need signal-averaged electrocardiography to predict whether he is at risk for ventricular fibrillation. In addition, this test cannot be interpreted accurately in the presence of left bundle-branch block. Electrophysiology study would be the appropriate test because the patient has a significant risk for recurrent ventricular fibrillation and cardiac arrest. This risk can be markedly reduced by a systematic approach to managing his ventricular arrhythmias, and electrophysiologic testing is the initial test to help direct the clinician to appropriate rhythm management.

2. Answer b.

Sinoatrial exit block is incorrect. For sinoatrial exit block to be present, the P-P interval encompassing the pause needs to be exactly 2 times the basic P-P interval, indicating the P wave fails to be generated because of exit block from the sinus node but the sinus node itself is firing on time. Nonconducted atrial premature complex is the correct answer. The P wave can be seen to fuse with the preceding T wave, resulting in a peaked T wave representing the nonconducted atrial premature complex. In regard to atrioventricular nodal Wenckebach and Mobitz II block at the level of atrioventricular node, there is no evidence of a P wave occurring on time that fails to conduct the ventricle. Carotid sinus hypersensitivity would not cause the deformity of the T wave, which is a hallmark of a nonconducted atrial premature complex.

3. Answer c.

Signal-averaged electrocardiography is not necessary in this patient because he has already demonstrated a life-threatening ventricular arrhythmia. Signal-averaged electrocardiography is used to predict future risk of arrhythmia but is not necessary in a patient already demonstrating arrhythmia. The patient has ischemia with angina provoked by standard treadmill testing; thallium testing is not necessary in this case to establish the diagnosis of myocardial ischemia. Coronary angiography is the appropriate test because the patient had a positive treadmill test with life-threatening polymorphic ventricular tachycardia, and the presence of a high-grade coronary artery lesion needs to be assessed. Initiation of β-adrenergic blocker therapy and dismissal from hospital would not be appropriate therapy without at least repeating the exercise test to make certain the therapy prevented ischemia and the polymorphic ventricular tachycardia. Because there is day-to-day variability between exercise tests in patients with exercise-induced ventricular tachycardia, it would be best to proceed with coronary angiography. In regard to amiodarone, see comments for β-adrenergic blocker therapy above.

4. Answer b.

The blood pressure does not help decide whether a tachycardia is supraventricular or ventricular in origin because there is great overlap with well-tolerated ventricular tachycardia, having minimal effect on blood pressure and poorly tolerated supraventricular tachycardia associated with hypotension. QRS morphology similar to sinus rhythm supports the presence of supraventricular tachycardia. Patients with preexisting bundle-branch block who have the same conduction pattern during a wide complex tachycardia almost always have supraventricular tachycardia as the mechanism. The presence of atrioventricular dissociation suggests ventricular tachycardia. The prior history of myocardial infarction suggests a wide complex tachycardia is ventricular in origin, not supraventricular. In regard to a QRS width of 0.18 second, a wide complex tachycardia >0.14 second with a right bundle morphology, or >0.16 second with a left-bundle morphology, is almost always ventricular in origin.

5. Answer c.

Adequate control of hypertension has not been demonstrated to prevent episodes of atrial fibrillation, although it is a known risk factor for atrial fibrillation. The patient is at risk for thromboembolism and therefore requires antithrombotic therapy and not merely observation. Warfarin would be the appropriate choice of therapy because the patient has a history of hypertension and therefore increased risk for thromboembolism, which is helped by treatment with warfarin. Although aspirin, 81 mg daily, is an effective antithrombotic therapy, it is not as useful as warfarin in a patient with a history of hypertension. The same is true for aspirin, 5 g daily.

6. Answer d.

Adenosine is not appropriate because it will only slow the ventricular rate for 10 seconds before the drug was cleared. Verapamil is not appropriate because the drug causes peripheral vasodilatation, reflex increase in catecholamines, and acceleration of the rate of conduction over the accessory pathway. Lidocaine does not help terminate atrial fibrillation or slow conduction over the accessory pathway. Procainamide has the benefit of converting atrial fibrillation and slowing conduction over the accessory pathway if atrial fibrillation persists. Digoxin shortens refractoriness of the accessory pathways and will accelerate conduction over the accessory pathway during atrial fibrillation, creating risk of rapid ventricular response.

7. Answer a.

Empirical use of quinidine has not been demonstrated to prevent recurrence of sudden cardiac death. Coronary angiography could be considered to assess for life-threatening coronary disease as the cause of the patient's cardiac death. Electrocardiography and cardiac enzyme tests would be appropriate to determine whether the patient had an acute myocardial infarction as the cause of the sudden cardiac death. Patients with sudden cardiac death related to an acute myocardial infarction have low risk for recurrent sudden cardiac death, assuming their coronary artery disease is treated appropriately. Electrophysiologic testing to guide management should be considered in any patient surviving sudden cardiac death in the absence of myocardial infarction or reversible cause such as abnormal electrolytes or proarrhythmic effect of a drug. Use of the implantable defibrillator in patients with no inducible arrhythmia at electrophysiologic testing is an appropriate approach to treatment because such patients continue to have a high risk for sudden cardiac death despite the negative results of electrophysiologic study.

8. Answer a.

The ECG demonstrates an acute inferior myocardial infarction with Mobitz I (Wenckebach) atrioventricular block. Observation is the correct answer because the arrhythmia usually does not progress to a further degree of block and does not require treatment when the patient is asymptomatic. Adenosine will aggravate the block by worsening conduction through the atrioventricular node. Atropine will improve the conduction but will also increase sinus rate and therefore oxygen demand, which is an appropriate step in the management of a patient with an acute myocardial infarction who is asymptomatic from arrhythmia. Temporary pacing is not used because the patient is asymptomatic. This would be the appropriate therapy if the patient was symptomatic as a result of bradycardia. β-Adrenergic blocker therapy will aggravate conduction through the atrioventricular node and worsen the degree of block. This therapy should be initiated once the atrioventricular conduction block has resolved.

9. Answer b.

The arrhythmia demonstrated is an accelerated idioventricular arrhythmia that is seen in patients with acute myocardial infarction. The arrhythmia is usually asymptomatic and resolves spontaneously. The current arrhythmia is asymptomatic and does not degenerate to ventricular tachycardia and therefore does not require atropine treatment. Observation is the approach used because the arrhythmia is asymptomatic and does not degenerate to ventricular tachycardia and therefore does not require specific therapy. Lidocaine will suppress this arrhythmia but has the risk of toxicity and therefore should not be used because the patient is not asymptomatic and this is not a serious arrhythmia. Magnesium is not the best approach for treatment of this arrhythmia. Magnesium is a medication being used for myocardial infarction but has not been shown to specifically control episodes of idioventricular rhythm. Overdrive pacing is not correct because it is unnecessary to expose the patient to the risk of temporary pacing because she is asymptomatic and this is not a serious arrhythmia.

10. a, false; b, false; c, true; d, true; e, false; f, true.

Mobitz II is not the mechanism because there clearly is prolongation of the P-R interval before the nonconducted P wave. For Mobitz II to be present, the P-R interval before and after the nonconducted P wave should be equal. The arrhythmia is not the most likely cause of the patient's syncope. Mobitz I rarely causes symptoms, and a pause of this duration should not cause symptoms other than a sensation of a skipped beat. Mobitz I is not a serious rhythm problem and in itself does not require evaluation or treatment. The P-R interval before the nonconducted P wave is significantly longer than the P-R interval after the nonconducted P wave, consistent with Mobitz I Wenckebach block. The tracing shows progressive P-R prolongation before the P wave that fails to conduct. Mobitz I is most often due to delay in conduction in the atrioventricular node, especially in the presence of a narrow QRS complex, and only rarely leads to complete heart block or need for permanent pacing. The arrhythmia can be due to an inferior myocardial infarction. With an inferior infarction, there may be ischemia of the septum, which will result in delayed conduction through the atrioventricular node and Mobitz I block.

11. a, true; b, false; c, true; d, false; e, true; f, true.

Quinidine is useful for preventing atrial fibrillation in approximately 50% of patients at 1 year. Mexiletine has no beneficial effect on preventing atrial fibrillation. Propafenone prevents paroxysmal atrial fibrillation in approximately 50% of patients followed for 1 year. Digoxin does not help to prevent episodes of atrial fibrillation but only to slow the ventricular rate. Sotalol helps to prevent atrial fibrillation in 50%-60% of patients at 1 year. Amiodarone helps to prevent atrial fibrillation in approximately 60% of patients at 1 year.

12. a, true; b, true; c, true; d, true; e, true; f, true.

Amiodarone alters iodine uptake and conversion of thyroxine to triiodothyronine and therefore can cause either hyperthyroidism or hypothyroidism. Skin photosensitivity occurs in approximately 15% of patients. It manifests as easy sun burning, and approximately 1%-2% of patients develop a bluish discoloration of their skin. Hepatitis is a known complication of amiodarone therapy, occurring in 1%-2% of patients. Amiodarone will cause pulmonary fibrosis, clinically apparent on chest radiography in 5%-10% of patients and associated with a nonproductive cough in approximately 10% of patients. A small percentage of patients will develop neurologic problems manifested as ataxia as a result of amiodarone therapy. Hypothyroidism also occurs (see above).

13. a, true; b, true; c, true; d, false; e, false; f, false.

A wide QRS complex supports the finding of ventricular tachycardia. Atrioventricular dissociation is present on the electrocardiogram where P waves are seen to march through the wide QRS complexes. This is diagnostic of ventricular tachycardia and is seen in approximately 25% of patients with a wide QRS tachycardia. The fifth beat from the beginning and the fourth beat from the end are narrow beats that are fusion beats comprised of conduction from the atrium and ventricle. Retrograde conduction cannot be observed and is not diagnostic of either supraventricular or ventricular tachycardia. Northwest axis implies a marked left-axis deviation and therefore should be negative in lead II. Concordance indicates the QRS complexes are pointing the same direction in the chest leads and cannot be diagnosed with only a single lead, as presented in this case.

14. a, false; b, true; c, true; d, false; e, false; f, true.

The mechanism is not atrial fibrillation because the arrhythmia is a ventricular arrhythmia termed torsades de pointes. The mechanism is torsades de pointes because the rhythm shows the typical twisting point morphology of torsades de pointes with associated Q-T interval prolongation. This is a known complication of quinidine. This arrhythmia can occur after the first dose of quinidine and can occur early into quinidine therapy in patients who are sensitive to the medication. Procainamide would not be useful to prevent occurrence because it is a IA antiarrhythmic agent such as quinidine and has the associated risk of torsades de pointes. The arrhythmia is related to quinidine. Quinidine has a 1%-2% chance of causing torsades de pointes associated with Q-T prolongation. Isoproterenol would be useful to prevent recurrence because it helps to shorten the Q-T interval. This medication can be given intravenously to allow time for the offending medication to be metabolized or the electrolyte disturbance to be corrected. An alternative therapy would be pacing or magnesium.

Chapter 6   CARDIOLOGY III
(Questions--pages 120-122)

1. Answer d.

This is a classic radiograph of mitral stenosis with a big left atrium, prominent pulmonary artery, and straight left heart border. A systolic ejection murmur should not be heard with mitral stenosis. A diastolic decrescendo murmur would be heard with aortic or pulmonary regurgitation. The first heart sound is loud in mitral stenosis because the high left atrial-left ventricular pressure gradient forces the valve leaflets together abruptly, producing a loud first sound. A diastolic rumble is heard with mitral stenosis, and the longer the rumble the more severe the stenosis. A holosystolic murmur is not associated with mitral stenosis.

2. Answer e.

With handgrip, an outflow murmur decreases because there is an increase in peripheral resistance. On standing, the murmur increases because there is a decrease in venous return and a smaller left ventricular cavity size. Amyl nitrite, which causes vasodilatation, increases the murmur, and Valsalva increases the intrathoracic pressure and decreases the ventricular filling and, therefore, increases the murmur associated with hypertrophic cardiomyopathy. After a premature ventricular complex, there is a prolonged compensatory pause and a longer time for diastolic filling, and so the heart is "moved up" on the Starling curve, producing increased force of contraction and increasing the murmur.

3. Answer c.

The valve is still often pliable when a patient reaches 30 years of age. The shorter the interval from second heart sound to opening snap, the more severe the stenosis because the high left atrial-left ventricular pressure gradient forces the valve open earlier. Percutaneous valvotomy provides good palliation in properly selected patients when the valve and subvalve apparatus are pliable and noncalcified. Mitral stenosis is more common in females. The first heart sound is loud.

4. Answer d.

The new American Heart Association guidelines suggest that no antibiotic prophylaxis is necessary for an uncomplicated vaginal delivery. A patient with an isolated secundum atrial septal defect does not require antibiotic prophylaxis. A patent ductus arteriosus, once ligated, implies cure and patients do not need endocarditis prophylaxis. Irrespective of whether the valve is stenotic or regurgitant, patients with bicuspid aortic valves all require antibiotic prophylaxis. Cardiac catheterization should be a sterile procedure and, therefore, endocarditis prophylaxis is not needed.

5. Answer c.

Electrical alternans relates to altering position of the heart in a pericardial fluid space and is commonly present in patients with tamponade. Kussmaul's sign (increased venous pressure with inspiration) may occur with tamponade and also with pericardial constriction. Pulsus alternans, when the systolic pressure alternates more than 20 mm Hg, is caused by severe impairment of left ventricular function. Pulsus paradoxus and narrow pulse pressure are both very common with tamponade.

6. Answer b.

Because of increased cardiac output during pregnancy and a decrease in peripheral resistance, bounding pulses and a systolic ejection murmur are very common. The murmur is never louder than grade 3/6. A physiologic third heart sound is also common, and 80% of pregnant women have peripheral edema because of increased venous pressure in the lower extremities.

7. Answer a.

The radiograph shows classic appearances of a secundum atrial septal defect with cardiomegaly, prominent pulmonary artery, and pulmonary plethora. The ejection systolic murmur arises from the pulmonary outflow due to increased flow. The right ventricular lift occurs because of right ventricular volume overload. A fixed split second sound is a classic feature of atrial septal defect, and a tricuspid diastolic rumble occurs when the shunt is large and is due to increased flow across the tricuspid valve.

8. Answer b.

There is no association of coarctation with mitral valve prolapse. Most coarctations are detected in childhood. It usually occurs distal to the subclavian artery. Despite good surgical repair, premature death is common because of problems with an associated bicuspid aortic valve, rupture or dissection of the aorta, stroke, systemic hypertension, and aneurysms in the circle of Willis.

9. Answer b.

All other carcinomas frequently metastasize to the heart.

10. Answer d.

This patient is in a precarious situation, but with an infarcted bowel needs urgent surgery, and there is not time to perform any other investigation. Hemodynamic monitoring will facilitate optimal fluid control and medical management of her congestive heart failure.

11. a, true; b, false; c, false; d, false; e, false; f, false.

With standing, there is a decrease in venous return and a decrease in stroke volume; thus, with diminished ventricular filling, the click and murmur of mitral valve prolapse occur earlier after first heart sound. For the same reason, the murmur of hypertrophic obstructive cardiomyopathy gets louder. Because venous return and ventricular filling are decreased, the jugular venous pressure does not increase on standing. Postural maneuvers do not permit distinction between diastolic sounds. Because venous return is decreased, pulmonary flow murmurs get softer. Because venous return is diminished, and stroke volume is decreased, the murmur of mitral regurgitation does not get louder.

12. a, true; b, false; c, true; d, true; e, true; f, true.

In the presence of impaired right ventricular function, the jugular venous pressure will be elevated. Septic shock associated with hypotension does not produce elevated jugular venous pressure. Constrictive pericarditis and pericardial tamponade by impairing venous return elevate the jugular venous pressure, as does any obstruction of the superior vena cava. Severe tricuspid regurgitation produces a cv wave in the jugular venous pulse.

13. a, false; b, false; c, false; d, true; e, true; f, false.

Verapamil can be used safely during pregnancy. Propranolol in large doses can be associated with intrauterine growth retardation, but in general can be used safely. Digoxin causes no problem during pregnancy. Captopril and all angiotensin converting enzyme inhibitors should be avoided because they cause renal dysgenesis. Warfarin has profound teratogenic effects and is associated with, for example, optic atrophy, nasal hypoplasia, and bony stippling. Quinidine can be used safely if necessary.

14. a, false; b, true; c, false; d, true; e, true; f, true.

A loud systolic murmur is not heard with Eisenmenger ventricular septal defect because the pressure in both ventricles is the same and there is very little flow between the two chambers. An ejection click is common from the dilated pulmonary artery. A thrill is never heard because there are no high flows in any chamber. A right ventricular lift is common, owing to the elevated right-sided pressures. A decrescendo diastolic murmur is often heard due to pulmonary regurgitation, and a loud P2 is a sign of pulmonary hypertension.

Chapter 7 CHEST X-RAY
(Questions--page 140-143)

1. Answer c.
Metastatic breast cancer to right paratracheal node. The two least expensive steps you can take are to get old chest x-rays and ask to review an abnormality you have noted on a chest x-ray with a radiologist. There is right paratracheal adenopathy that subsequently proved to be metastatic breast cancer. A chest CT would certainly see this but would not be diagnostic. Bronchoscopy with paratracheal needle aspiration for cytology would give a positive result in about 80% of patients, and, if that were negative, mediastinoscopy would be positive in 100% of patients.

2. Answer e.
Coarctation with tortuous aorta and rib notching. In addition to a poststenotic aortic aneurysm, note the inferior rib notching consistent with a diagnosis of coarctation of the aorta. A thorough physical examination would note diminished-to-absent pulses in the lower extremities.

3. Answer b.
Infrapulmonic left pleural effusion. Note the distance between the gastric bubble and the supposed top of the left hemidiaphragm, which is actually infrapulmonic effusion. Why in some persons a meniscus does not form when pleural effusion is present is unknown.

4. Answer a.
Scar carcinoma. The calcified nidus is eccentric and, thus, not one of the characteristic calcifications of benign lesions, namely bull's eye, laminated, or popcorn calcification. The air bronchograms within the lesion are quite characteristic for bronchoalveolar cell carcinoma, with this being a scar carcinoma.

5. Answer e.
Histiocytosis X with right pneumothorax. Spontaneous pneumothoraces occur in up to 25% of patients with histiocytosis X. Note the honeycombing evident in the interstitial pattern. More than 85% of adult patients with histiocytosis X have been or are smokers. In spite of extensive parenchymal changes, histiocytosis X is one of those interstitial lung conditions in which the chest x-ray frequently looks worse than the patient's complaints. Obstructive features in this patient could be from smoking or from histiocytosis X involving the airways.

6. Answer a.
Silicosis. This chest x-ray shows pulmonary silicosis with typical nodular distribution greater in the upper two-thirds of the lung fields; it is fairly typical for the patient to be relatively asymptomatic in spite of changes of this extent. No drug or familial disease will produce this picture. Miliary tuberculosis would show nodular infiltrates greater in the lower lung fields and would not be asymptomatic. Also, the nodules usually are not this big.

7. Answer e.
Any smoker or recent smoker within the last 10 years should have any suspicious lesion considered a possible primary lung cancer until proved otherwise. Waiting 1 year is too long for lung cancer even though it has only been growing slowly over 2 years' time, because it may already have metastasized in the absence of symptoms.

8. False.
Wegener's cavitary lesions. There are many possible causes of cavitary lesions in the lung and, when multiple like this, Wegener's granulomatosis should be suspected. Other possibilities include paragonimiasis, hydatid lung disease, and septic emboli with cavitation in some. Pulmonary infarction rarely cavitates, and when it does, it is usually a solitary process, although there may be other abnormalities noted in the lung fields. Some fungi will cavitate, but rarely are they multiple nodules like this.

9. True.
Kartagener's syndrome of dextrocardia with bronchiectasis. Note that the "left marker" (*arrow*) is at the upper left portion of the screen, meaning the chest x-ray was viewed improperly and should be flipped so that dextrocardia is evident. In about 20% of patients with dextrocardia (isolated as well as totalis), it is associated with dysmotile cilia syndrome and, in turn, bronchiectasis and sinusitis. This patient has left middle lobe bronchiectasis, which is best defined by high-resolution CT rather than bronchography which is almost never done anymore. Note azygous lobe left apex.

10. False.

Arteriovenous malformation of hereditary hemorrhagic telangiectasia (Rendu-Osler-Weber syndrome). The pulmonary artery and vein can be seen coming and going from this right lower lobe lesion. There were also smaller lesions present in other parts of the lung, especially in the left lower lobe. Currently, the preferred treatment is insertion of coils into the pulmonary artery to block the flow to these malformations, rather than a surgical procedure, because in this patient the lesions are multiple and would require bilateral thoracotomies. It is also likely that more lesions will develop in this patient in the future. Again these will best be treated with the radiologist inserting coils.

Chapter 8 CLINICAL PHARMACOLOGY AND TOXICOLOGY
(Questions--page 159)

1. Answer c.

The anticholinergic syndrome can occur in overdoses of atropine, antihistamines, antiparkinsonian medications, tricyclic antidepressants, and phenothiazines. The pupils are dilated; therefore, miosis does not occur.

2. Answer a.

Both ethylene glycol ingestion and methanol ingestion produce profound anion gap metabolic acidosis. Only ethylene glycol, however, produces calcium oxalate crystalluria.

3. Answer e.

Although an elevated anion gap metabolic acidosis is commonly associated with aspirin overdose, the *first* metabolic abnormality to occur is respiratory alkalosis. A metabolic alkalosis does not occur.

4. Answer b.

Any patient who has a serious aspirin overdose and deteriorates after appropriate therapy should be considered a candidate for hemodialysis. In addition, patients who have pulmonary edema or renal failure are also appropriate for hemodialysis.

5. Answer a.

Tricyclic antidepressant overdose remains one of the most deadly overdoses. Stomach evacuation by gastric lavage is indicated if patient arrives in the emergency department within 1-2 hours. Gastric lavage should be performed after endotracheal intubation if patient has had a seizure, is unconscious, or has a poor gag reflex. Ipecac is not indicated in tricyclic overdose because patients can deteriorate rapidly

6. a, false; b, true; c, true; d, false; e, false; f, true.

Hemodialysis is effective for substances that are of low molecular weight, have limited protein and lipid binding, and are water soluble. Digoxin and tricyclic antidepressants have large V_d and are highly protein-bound and are thus poor candidates for hemodialysis. Hemodialysis is not indicated in the vast majority of ethanol intoxications.

7. a, true; b, true; c, true; d, false; e, false; f, false.

Activated charcoal does not bind alcohols, small ionic compounds, or metals well. It is also not indicated in caustic injections.

Chapter 9 CRITICAL CARE
(Questions--page 175)

1. Answer c.

Of the choices listed, a maximal expiratory pressure of -15 cm H_2O is the most severe abnormality. The normal inspiratory pressure should be greater than -150 cm H_2O. The shunt fraction of 0.08 is slightly elevated. The other choices are close to normal values.

2. Answer d.

The question describes an attempt to ventilate a patient with severe airway obstruction at 20 L/min. This would be expected to cause dynamic hyperinflation or breath stacking, with increased intrathoracic pressure and decreased cardiac output. Treatment should be directed at the underlying airway obstruction and at decreasing the degree of air trapping. Of the options listed, dopamine is the least appropriate in a patient with normal or hyperdynamic cardiovascular function. Although treatment with steroids would take several hours to become effective, early treatment is appropriate. Saline given intravenously may be useful to increase preload.

3. Answer b.

After recovery from adult respiratory distress syndrome, mild impairment of gas exchange can usually be shown. Severe restrictive or obstructive disease typically is not found.

4. Answer d.

The hemodynamic values describe low-normal filling pressures with increased cardiac output and relatively high-mixed venous oxygen saturation for a hypotensive patient. These findings are typical for early sepsis.

5. Answer e.

Each of the options listed may be associated with multiorgan failure, but this severe complication is associated most often with sepsis.

6. a, false; b, true; c, true; d, true; e, false; f, true.

The arterial blood gases show a pattern of hypoxemia due to hypoventilation with a normal alveolar-arterial gradient. The hypoventilation also explains the pure respiratory acidosis. Given the normal alveolar-arterial gradient, there is no evidence for another cause of ventilation-perfusion mismatch such as aspiration pneumonia. The treatment should include supplemental oxygen and assisted ventilation. Correcting the respiratory disorder will correct the pH, and bicarbonate would be inappropriate.

7. a, true; b, false; c, true; d, false; e, true; f, false.

Adult respiratory distress syndrome is characterized by diffuse pulmonary infiltrates with decreased lung compliance and hypoxemia due to intrapulmonary shunting. Increased numbers of neutrophils have been found in lavage fluid. Loss of type II pneumocytes contributes to surfactant deficiency and alveolar collapse. Overall survival is approximately 50%. Steroids have not been shown to be beneficial.

Chapter 10   DERMATOLOGY
(Questions--pages 201-202)

1. Answer a.

Acrodermatitis enteropathica is either an acquired disorder in chronic diarrheal states or an autosomal recessive disorder. The clinical features are diarrhea, diffuse alopecia, and periorificial and acral eruptions.

2. Answer c.

All of the porphyrias may present with cutaneous abnormalities with the exception of acute intermittent porphyria.

3. Answer d.

Pseudoporphyria may occur in patients on hemodialysis or may be induced by nonsteroidal anti-inflammatory drugs.

4. Answer a.

The clinical associations are between pemphigus erythematosus and thymoma, ichthyosis and lymphoma, acute febrile neutrophilic dermatosis and acute myeloid leukemia, erythema gyratum repens and carcinoma of the breast, and dermatitis herpetiformis and, rarely, intestinal lymphoma.

5. Answer e.

Subacute cutaneous lupus erythematosus is characterized by photosensitivity with the development of annular scaly lesions, circulating anti-Ro antibodies, a negative antinuclear antibody, and negative lupus band test.

6. Answer c.

Sézary syndrome is characterized by a proliferation of T cells, and the histology of the skin is similar to that of mycosis fungoides.

7. Answer d.

In pemphigus foliaceus, the antibody is directed against a proponent of the intracellular substance, and the split is in the intraepidermal region.

8. Answer b.

Dermatitis herpetiformis is an intensely pruritic eruption characterized by the deposition of IgA in the dermal papillae on direct immunofluorescence studies. Many patients have an associated gluten-sensitive enteropathy. Therapy is with dapsone with or without a gluten-free diet.

9. Answer b.

Erythema nodosum may occur with all of the entities listed, but streptococcal pharyngitis is the most common association.

10. Answer a.

Allergic contact dermatitis is mediated by Langerhans cells, which are involved in antigen presentation. Paraphenylenediamine is present in solutions used for hair permanents, thiuram is present in rubber and may be a component of shoes, and chromate is present in cement.

11. a, true; b, false; c, false; d, true; e, true; f, false.

The following associations are recognized: angiokeratomas with renal insufficiency (Fabry's disease), acanthosis nigricans with carcinoma of the stomach, Paget's disease with intraductal breast carcinoma, pyoderma gangrenosum with leukemia, and sebaceous adenomas with colonic carcinoma (Muir-Torre syndrome). Bullous pemphigoid has not been associated with an increased incidence of underlying malignancy.

12. a, true; b, true; c, true; d, false; e, true; f, true.

The following are specific syndromes: osteomas and adenocarcinoma of the colon (Gardner's syndrome), macular pigmentation of the lips and intestinal polyposis (Peutz-Jeghers syndrome), trichilemmomas and breast carcinoma (Cowden's syndrome), palmoplantar keratoderma and carcinoma of the esophagus (Howel-Evans' syndrome), café-au-lait spots and acoustic neuromas (neurofibromatosis), and zinc deficiency and perineal dermatitis (acrodermatitis enteropathica).

13. a, true; b, true; c, false; d, false; e, true; f, true.

In addition to hypertriglyceridemia, sticky skin, teratogenicity, and conjunctivitis, leukopenia may occur in patients receiving 13-cis-retinoic acid therapy. Hyperostosis may also occur in long-term systemic retinoid therapy.

14. a, false; b, true; c, true; d, true; e, false; f, true.

Kaposi's sarcoma occurs typically on the trunk and head and neck in patients with HIV. Unfortunately, syphilis in HIV-infected patients is resistant to conventional first-line therapy.

Chapter 11 ENDOCRINOLOGY
(Questions--pages 298-300)

1. Answer b.

Dopamine is a known stimulant of GH secretion, and L-dopa stimulation test is a very effective provocative test for assessing GH reserve. Oral glucose somatostatin and dexamethasone suppress GH secretion. Metyrapone has no effect on GH secretion.

2. Answer a.

Bitemporal hemianopsia is the commonest effect of compression of the optic chiasm. Compression of the pituitary stalk may result in the so-called stalk-effect

hyperprolactinemia because of interference with the access of dopamine, the prolactin-inhibitory hormone, to the pituitary lactotrophes.

3. Answer c.

The characteristic triad in MEN I are tumors of the pituitary, parathyroids, and endocrine pancreas. Pheochromocytoma and medullary carcinoma of the thyroid may be an integral part of the syndrome in MEN IIA and MEN IIB. The other options do not occur in MEN.

4. Answer a.

The sine qua non for the diagnosis of active acromegaly is the absence of normal growth hormone suppressibility to <2 ng/mL during a glucose tolerance test. An increased somatomedin C (IGF I) is universally present in active acromegaly and is a useful confirmatory test.

5. Answer c.

The thyroid gland in a patient with TSH hypersecretion is diffusely hyperplastic and enlarged, and ^{131}I uptake is increased. Endocrine ophthalmopathy and high levels of thyroid-stimulating immunoglobulins are characteristic of Graves' disease.

6. Answer d.

Subacute thyroiditis is characterized by a painful tender goiter, high erythrocyte sedimentation rate, and a suppressed ^{131}I uptake. Hyperthyroidism may occur in about 50% of patients in the acute phase and is self-limiting. It is followed by transient hypothyroidism in a significant number of patients. Permanent hypothyroidism occurs in <5% of patients; recovery of euthyroidism is the rule.

7. Answer a.

Magnesium deficiency is a common cause of functional hypoparathyroidism. Magnesium depletion interferes with parathyroid hormone secretion and biologic effect. Magnesium repletion corrects the functional hypoparathyroid state. All the other listed options are true of hypoparathyroidism.

8. Answer c.

Medullary carcinoma of the thyroid may be sporadic or familial. The familial form may be isolated or a part of MEN IIA or MEN IIB. Serum calcitonin level is characteristically high and shows an abnormal response to pentagastrin. Hypercalcitonemia is usually silent; hypocalcemia is exceedingly rare. Ectopic humoral syndromes may be seen with medullary carcinoma of the thyroid; Cushing's syndrome, if present, is due to ectopic ACTH--not cortisol--overproduction. Serum thyroglobulin level is a marker of functioning thyroid-follicle cancers (papillary and follicular cancers) and not of medullary carcinoma of the thyroid.

9. Answer c.

In silent thyroiditis, ^{131}I uptake is suppressed, antimicrosomal antibody titers are usually normal, and the hypothyroidism seen as a late phase in the illness is usually transient and reversible. High levels of thyroid-stimulating immunoglobulins are characteristic of Graves' disease.

10. Answer d.

Decreased serum level of T_3 is characteristic of the euthyroid sick syndrome and is due to decreased T_4 to T_3 conversion by the peripheral tissues. All other options are correct.

11. Answer b.

Gestational diabetes is the detection of diabetes mellitus during pregnancy in a woman without a history of diabetes in the nonpregnant state (this same patient may have had gestational diabetes in a previous pregnancy). The risk of development of non-insulin-dependent diabetes mellitus in these patients approaches 60% in 15 years. If diagnosed, it should be treated with diet and insulin.

12. Answer c.

Fasting hyperglycemia in such a patient may be caused by either insufficient insulin and the dawn's phenomenon (due to increase in the anti-insulin growth hormone) or to Somogyi's phenomenon with rebound from early a.m. hypoglycemia. Measurement of blood glucose at 3:00 a.m. is critical in making the distinction; in this patient a value of 120 mg/dL indicated insufficient insulin effect and dictates an increase in the infusion rate.

13. Answer c.

The presence of hyperinsulinemia and increased C peptide in a hypoglycemic patient indicates endogenous hyperinsulinemia. The most important differential diagnosis is between insulinoma and the use of sulfonylureas, often surreptitiously in those with access to the medication (e.g., pharmacists). Determining the plasma level of sulfonylurea is essential in the differential diagnosis.

14. Answer c.

The usual therapeutic step-up in such a patient would be diet, diet plus sulfonylurea, and, finally, diet plus insulin.

15. Answer a.

Aldosterone secretion is stimulated by decreased blood volume and serves as a homeostatic response to this challenge. Hypokalemia and angiotensin-converting enzyme inhibitors suppress aldosterone secretion. Metyrapone and dexamethasone have no significant effects on aldosterone production.

16. Answer c.

Classic Klinefelter's syndrome is characterized by a 47,XXY karyotype, hyalinization of the seminiferous tubules, small firm testes, hypergonadotropism, and irreversible infertility.

17. Answer d.

Anosmia and hypogonadotropic hypogonadism are characteristic of Kallmann's syndrome. A short vagina and absence of female internal genitalia are seen in complete testicular feminization. Precocious isosexual puberty and shortness of stature which responds to therapy with estrogen are not true of 45/XO syndrome.

18. Answer b.

In Addison's disease, the adrenal cortex is unresponsive to any secretory stimulus. The secretory defect usually involves all the hormones of the adrenal cortex, including cortisol, aldosterone, and the adrenal androgens. The commonest cause in the U.S. is an autoimmune disorder that may also affect other endocrine glands.

19. Answer a.

Kallmann's syndrome is characterized by hypogonadotropism due to absence of GnRH-producing cells and anosmia due to absence of the olfactory bulbs. The karyotype is normal for the patient phenotype. Other pituitary functions are normal; the testes are normal prepubertal testes. MR images of the hypothalamus are normal.

20. a, true; b, true; c, false; d, false; e, true.

Insulin-dependent diabetes mellitus accounts only for about 10% of all the diabetic population. Familial incidence is definitely and significantly increased in non-insulin-dependent diabetes mellitus. The concordance rate in an identical twin of a patient with insulin-dependent diabetes mellitus is about 40%-50%.

21. False.

Cortisol is necessary for the ability to excrete a water load. The development of hypocortisolinism in a patient with central diabetes insipidus leads to amelioration of the symptoms because of impairment of renal excretion of water.

22. False.

Primary hypothyroidism may lead to hyperprolactinemia and a sellar mass consisting of hyperplastic thyrotroph cells. Such hyperprolactinemia and sellar mass regress after the institution of thyroid hormone replacement therapy. Determining the serum level of TSH is a necessary diagnostic step in the evaluation of hyperprolactinemia to rule out primary hypothyroidism as the cause.

23. True.

Chronic ingestion of supraphysiologic doses of T_3 suppresses TSH secretion: the gland atrophies, the uptake of ^{131}I is reduced, and the production of T_4 and T_3 is inhibited.

24. False.

Familial hypocalciuric hypercalcemia is parathyroid-dependent and characterized by absence of chronic complications of hypercalcemia.

25. a, true; b, false; c, true; d, false; e, true; f, true.

Sulfonylureas are contraindicated in pregnancy and are of no use in the management of patients with insulin-dependent diabetes mellitus because of absence of insulin secretory reserve in these patients. The risk of hypoglycemia with sulfonylureas is significant, particularly in elderly patients with reduced food intake.

26. a, true; b, true; c, true; d, true; e, false; f, false.

Symptoms of hypoglycemia alone are not sufficient to make the diagnosis; for the diagnosis, all features of Whipple's triad have to be fulfilled. The symptoms of hypoglycemia are the same whether or not the hypoglycemia is insulin-mediated.

27. True.

In hypogonadotropism, the testes are basically normal but unstimulated. Providing the gonadotropin stimulus leads to a normal testicular response.

28. False.

In Cushing's syndrome due to an adrenal adenoma, pituitary ACTH secretion is suppressed; thus, the hyper-cortisol state is not high-dose dexamethasone suppressible.

Chapter 12   ETHICS IN MEDICINE
(Questions--pages 307-308)

1. Answer b.

Immediate cardiopulmonary resuscitation should be undertaken in the absence of other information regarding this patient.

2. Answer a.

The primary physician is responsible for providing the correct answer to the patient who poses a specific question. The responsibility cannot be shifted to others.

3. Answer d.

In the case of a minor, the courts have ruled that parents or religious beliefs cannot interfere with appropriate therapy in life-threatening situations. Please check your local and state laws regarding the definition of a "mature minor."

4. Answer b.

Irrespective of the patient's other medical and psychiatric problems, the primary physician should provide information when the patient asks for it. If the primary physician is not familiar with the procedure, then the physician who recommended the procedure should provide the information.

5. Answer a.

Most patients do not strictly adhere to all medical recommendations. The primary physician should reevaluate her or his own method of treating this patient before terminating the relationship. Some medical associations and societies have recommendations regarding the handling of noncompliant patients.

6. a, true; b, false; c, false; d, true; e, false; f, false.

The true answers apply to medical practice in Minnesota, particularly in regard to answer "d." Please check your own state health guidelines regarding this situation.

7. a, false; b, true; c, false; d, false; e, true; f, false.

Please check the text for details on moral surrogates, informed consent, living will, and definition of maleficence.

Chapter 13 GASTROENTEROLOGY I
(Questions--pages 353-355)

1. Answer d.

The conditions that predispose to esophageal (squamous) cancer include achalasia, lye stricture, Plummer-Vinson syndrome, tylosis, smoking, and alcohol. Diffuse esophageal spasm is not a premalignant syndrome.

2. Answer c.

Oropharyngeal dysphagia is the result of faulty transfer of the food bolus from the oropharynx to the esophagus. It can be caused by structural causes or by neurologic or muscular disorders. This symptom complex presents as high esophageal dysphagia associated with coughing, choking (aspiration), or nasal regurgitation. It is not associated with epigastric pain.

3. Answer e.

Many dietary substances, including fat, chocolate, caffeine (coffee), theophylline (tea), and carminatives (spearmint, peppermint), decrease lower esophageal sphincter pressure. A protein meal increases lower esophageal sphincter pressure. Of the many drugs that decrease lower esophageal sphincter pressure, anticholinergic agents, calcium channel blockers, and nitrates are the most important.

4. Answer d.

Medications commonly associated with medication-induced esophagitis include tetracycline, doxycycline, quinidine, potassium, ferrous sulfate, and ascorbic acid. Anticholinergic agents have not been implicated in medication-induced esophagitis, but they commonly aggravate gastroesophageal reflux disease.

5. Answer c.

Aspirin and nonsteroidal anti-inflammatory drugs are associated with an increased frequency of peptic ulcer disease. The effect of corticosteroids is controversial, and no clear-cut increased risk has been demonstrated. The incidence of peptic ulcers is higher if there is associated chronic lung disease, cirrhosis, or chronic renal failure.

6. Answer a.

Clinical entities that have an osmotic mechanism for diarrhea include lactase deficiency, food containing sorbitol, saline cathartics, and antacids. Surreptitious laxative ingestion is the commonest cause of unexplained, chronic watery diarrhea of a secretory mechanism.

7. Answer c.

In malabsorption syndrome, edema and muscle wasting are caused by decreased protein absorption. Bone pain is caused by decreased calcium absorption. Easy bruisability and petechiae result from vitamin K malabsorption, and night blindness and hyperkeratosis, from decreased vitamin A absorption. Alopecia is not commonly seen in malabsorption.

8. Answer a.

Extraintestinal manifestations of inflammatory bowel disease include arthritis, skin lesions (erythema nodosum, pyoderma gangrenosum, aphthous ulcer), eye lesions (episcleritis, uveitis), primary sclerosing cholangitis, and renal stones. Celiac sprue is not associated with inflammatory bowel disease.

9. Answer c.

The indications for colonoscopy in inflammatory bowel disease include evaluation of the extent of disease, to evaluate a stricture, to evaluate a filling defect, to differentiate Crohn's disease from ulcerative colitis, and to obtain biopsy specimens to evaluate for dysplasia or precancerous changes. Iron deficiency anemia is not an indication for colonoscopy in active inflammatory bowel disease.

10. Answer e.

Conditions associated with the development of pseudomembranous colitis include intestinal obstruction, uremia, ischemia, intestinal surgery, and all antibiotics except vancomycin. Foreign travel is associated with a number of intestinal infections but not with the overgrowth of *Clostridium difficile*, which produces pseudomembranous colitis.

11. Answer e.

Adenomatous polyps are premalignant polyps, and the risk of cancer increases with increasing size (>1 cm) and increasing villous architecture. Gardner's syndrome and familial polyposis are associated with adenomatous polyps. Juvenile polyposis is associated with hamartomatous polyps, which are not premalignant.

12. Answer a.

Causes of toxic megacolon include aerophagia, opiates, anticholinergic agents, hypokalemia, and barium enema. Proctoscopic examination can be performed safely in a patient with suspected acute colitis to confirm the diagnosis.

13. Answer b.

The diagnosis of chronic pancreatitis is documented by structural abnormalities (pancreatic calcifications, ductal abnormalities by endoscopic retrograde cholangiopancreatography, or scarring on biopsy), endocrine insufficiency (diabetes), or exocrine insufficiency (malabsorption). Abdominal pain is commonly present with chronic pancreatitis, but it does not confirm the diagnosis.

14. Answer a.

Drugs that have been firmly associated with acute pancreatitis include azathioprine, 6-mercaptopurine, L-asparaginase, hydrochlorothiazide diuretics, sulfonamide, sulfasalazine, tetracycline, furosemide, estrogens, valproic acid, pentamidine, and the antiretroviral drug dideoxyinosine (ddI). The evidence that corticosteroids, nonsteroidal anti-inflammatory drugs, methyldopa, procainamide, chlorthalidone, ethacrynic acid, phenformin, nitrofurantoin, enalapril, erythromycin, metronidazole, and aminosalicylates cause pancreatitis is less convincing.

15. Answer d.

Nonpulmonary features of cystic fibrosis include exocrine pancreatic insufficiency (malabsorption), endocrine pancreatic insufficiency (diabetes), rectal prolapse, a distal small-bowel obstruction from thick secretions (meconium ileus equivalent), and focal biliary cirrhosis. Celiac sprue is not associated with cystic fibrosis.

16. a, false; b, true; c, true; d, true; e, false; f, true.

Helicobacter pylori occurs in 10% of the general population younger than age 30 and in 60% of the population older than age 60. Many of these people are asymptomatic without peptic ulcer disease. *H. pylori* is the commonest cause of histologic gastritis and is an important factor in the development of type B antral gastritis, duodenal ulcers, gastric ulcers, and gastric adenocarcinoma. If *H. pylori* is eradicated, the healing of active duodenal ulcers is accelerated and the rate of recurrence of both duodenal ulcers and gastric ulcers decreases.

17. a, true; b, true; c, true; d, false; e, true; f, false.

The organisms that cause infectious diarrhea have been associated with certain foods. *Bacillus cereus* is associated with fried rice from oriental restaurants; *Salmonella*, with poultry; and *Vibrio parahaemolyticus*, with shellfish ingestion. The only infectious diarrhea for which antibiotics shorten the duration of illness is *Vibrio cholerae*. In *Salmonella* infection, antibiotics may prolong the carrier state and do not affect the course of disease. Antibiotics are indicated in *Salmonella* infection only if the blood cultures are positive. In traveler's diarrhea, treatment is supportive unless there is high fever and toxicity, bloody stools, or positive blood cultures.

18. a, true; b, false; c, true; d, false; e, true; f, true.

Risk factors for colorectal cancer include an age older than 40 years, a medical history of colon adenomatous polyps, a family history of colon cancer, inflammatory bowel disease, and a history of female genital or breast cancer. Hyperplastic polyps are not premalignant and diverticulosis is not associated with colon cancer.

19. a, false; b, true; c, true; d, true; e, false; f, false.

Corticosteroids are useful for suppressing active inflammation, but because of cumulative toxicity, they have little role in maintenance therapy for inflammatory bowel disease. Left-sided ulcerative colitis may be treated with steroid or aminosalicylate enemas. Severe attacks of acute ulcerative colitis usually require high doses of corticosteroids. To minimize the steroid side effects, immunosuppressive agents may be effective for chronically active steroid-dependent patients. Bowel rest has not been shown to be more effective than elemental diet, and antibiotics are more effective in Crohn's disease with perineal involvement than in ulcerative colitis.

20. a, true; b, false; c, true; d, false; e, false; f, true.

The presence of oil droplets and undigested meat fibers in the stool suggests pancreatic insufficiency but not intestinal disease as a cause for malabsorption. Vitamin B_{12} is bound to R protein. In pancreatic disease, this bond may not be cleaved. Thus, vitamin B_{12} cannot bind to intrinsic factor. Therefore, vitamin B_{12} deficiency may be seen in pancreatic insufficiency. Iron is absorbed in the proximal small bowel and is abnormal in small bowel disease but not in pancreatic insufficiency. Blunted small bowel villi are compatible for celiac sprue but may occur in many other conditions and are not diagnostic of celiac sprue. Response to a gluten-free diet is diagnostic of celiac sprue. In Whipple's disease, the characteristic findings on small bowel biopsy are PAS-positive organisms in macrophages.

Chapter 14   GASTROENTEROLOGY II
(Questions--pages 372-373)

1. Answer d.
This patient has ascending cholangitis. Ultrasonographic findings are often normal in patients with an acute obstruction.

2. Answer a.
Patients with long-standing chronic hepatitis B are at risk for the development of hepatocellular carcinoma. An elevated alpha-fetoprotein value should prompt imaging of the liver.

3. Answer c.
Thirty to fifty percent of patients with chronic hepatitis C infection have no identifiable risk factors.

4. Answer d.
Cardiomyopathy is not a complication of cholestatic liver disease but can be seen in genetic hemochromatosis

5. Answer a.
This patient has acute hepatitis, likely superimposed on chronic liver disease. A search for a cause as well as treatment for encephalopathy is appropriate.

6. a, false; b, true; c, false; d, false; e, true; f, false.
Seventy to eighty percent of patients with primary sclerosing cholangitis have inflammatory bowel disease, usually ulcerative colitis. Only 4%-5% of patients with inflammatory bowel disease have primary sclerosing cholangitis. Patients with primary sclerosing cholangitis may develop steatorrhea and are at increased risk for the development of bile duct cancer.

7. a, true; b, false; c, true; d, false; e, false; f, false.
A serum-ascites albumin gradient >1.1 is characteristic of the ascites due to portal hypertension. Those patients with ascitic protein levels <1.1 g/dL are at higher risk for the development of spontaneous bacterial peritonitis.

Ascites due to congestive heart failure and malignancy usually has protein concentrations >2.5 g/dL. One episode of spontaneous bacterial peritonitis in a cirrhotic patient does not mandate a search for a gastrointestinal source of the infection. Patients with hepatocellular carcinoma can have ascites as part of their underlying liver disease or because of venous outflow obstruction; cytologic results are usually negative.

Chapter 15   GENERAL INTERNAL MEDICINE
(Questions--page 389)

1. Answer b.

		Disease present	Disease absent	
Diagnostic test result	Positive	75 a	180 b	255 a+b
	Negative	c 25	d 720	c+d 745
		a+c	b+d	a+b+c+d
	Total	100	900	1,000

2. Answer e.
The above diagram correctly fills in the numbers for questions 1 and 2. Question 1 asks you to determine the positive predictive value of the test, or a/(a+b), i.e., 75/255 = 29%. Question 2 asks you to determine the negative predictive value of the test, or d/(c+d), i.e., 720/745 = 97%.

3. Answer a.
Generally, the use of preoperative medications such as atenolol should be continued in the perioperative period. Aspirin irreversibly affects platelets and, thus, its use needs to be discontinued 5-7 days preoperatively to be sure of decreasing the bleeding risk. The use of insulin should be continued at one-half the preoperative dose (fasting state). Finally, the physician should not recommend a particular type of anesthesia to an anesthesiologist; furthermore, spinal anesthesia is not associated with decreased surgical risk.

4. Answer e.
LDL cholesterol = (total cholesterol - HDL cholesterol - triglycerides/5), or 180 mg/dL. Answers b, c, and d are obviously true. Finally, a bile acid sequestrant is not the

best first-line treatment for a patient with increased cholesterol and triglycerides, because it may increase the triglyceride level. A medication such as nicotinic acid or gemfibrozil would be more appropriate.

5. Answer b.

Of the answers listed, only acetaminophen is not associated with increased risk of bleeding.

6. a, true; b, true; c, false; d, false; e, false; f, false.

Upper abdominal surgery increases risk for pulmonary complication (decreases breathing and cough). No test should be routinely performed in all patients receiving general anesthesia. Chest radiography should be performed only if indicated. Diastolic blood pressure >110 mm Hg is associated with increased surgical risk, but mild hypothyroidism is not.

7. a, true; b, true; c, true; d, false; e, false; f, true.

Answers a, b, and c accurately state the advantages for using the International Normalized Ratio (INR). The INR only applies to warfarin anticoagulation. Heparin anticoagulation still relies on an activated partial thromboplastin time value compared with control value. Mechanical heart valve patients should have an INR of at least 2.5-3.5.

Chapter 16 GENETICS
(Questions--pages 417-418)

1. Answer b.

The risk after having one affected child is low, but increased over the general population risk of 1 in 800.

2. Answer c.

Venous thrombosis is characteristic of patients with homocystinuria, who have a body habitus similar to that of persons with Marfan syndrome.

3. Answer d.

The inheritance is autosomal dominant.

4. Answer c.

On average, 50% of daughters will be carriers but most will be clinically healthy.

5. Answer a.

Without a detectable mutation in another family member it would be impossible to exclude a mutation in fetal DNA.

6. a, false; b, true; c, false; d, false; e, false.

There are no mitochondria in the portion of the sperm that enters the egg. The egg contains many mitochondria. Heteroplasmy (a mix of mitochondria with different DNA patterns) is common. Mutations can be inherited, and they can be clinically silent.

7. a, true; b, true; c, true; d, false; e, true.

Renal cancers are characteristics of von Hippel-Lindau disease, not neurofibromatosis.

Chapter 17 GERIATRICS
(Questions--pages 430-431)

1. Answer a.

This is an easy, inexpensive, minimally invasive test that can be performed to help rule out overflow incontinence. Little useful medical history is available from this patient. Because the prostate is enlarged on physical examination, overflow incontinence is a possibility.

Cystometry, fluoroscopy, and electromyography are tests that may help in evaluating incontinence, but they are expensive, invasive, and not the first tests to consider for patients with incontinence. A trial of oxybutynin may improve detrusor overactivity, but it could worsen overflow incontinence. Because a diagnosis has not been established, oxybutynin should not be used.

2. Answer c.

Medicare covers very little of the nursing home expenses--less than 5%. One must meet strict criteria to qualify, including the requirement for needing skilled services and not custodial care.

Life span has not increased significantly in the last 50 years; more people are living to the end of the life span (about 100-110 years), resulting in increased life expectancy. Only about 5% of the population lives in a nursing home, a much smaller number than most people realize. The majority live independently. Those over the age of 85 represent the fastest growing segment of the population. Their care costs more than that of any other segment of the population.

3. Answer e.

Pilocarpine is an effective treatment for glaucoma;

however, it causes pupilloconstriction rather than pupillodilatation. With pupilloconstriction, the trabecular meshwork pores open. This increases the drainage of aqueous humor.

Symptoms of chronic open-angle glaucoma develop insidiously. Patients usually present with a reduction in the peripheral vision of which they may be unaware. Patients whose chronic open-angle glaucoma is well-controlled with medication can often be given medications with anticholinergic effects. Anticholinergics do have the potential to precipitate an attack of angle-closure glaucoma in those with narrow angles. Acute angle-closure glaucoma is associated with symptoms such as eye pain and blurred vision.

4. Answer a.

Most patients with temporal arteritis have an increased erythrocyte sedimentation rate. An occasional patient, especially one who is quite elderly, may not have an elevated rate.

The pathologic changes of temporal arteritis are spotty. Therefore, a large piece of temporal artery should be obtained to make the pathologic diagnosis. At least 4-5 cm should be taken, first from the symptomatic side and, if negative, from the contralateral side. Treatment with high doses of steroids (40-60 mg/day) should be initiated as soon as the disease is suspected. The initiation of treatment will not affect the pathologic changes if the biopsy is performed in the next 1-2 days. Temporal arteritis may coexist with polymyalgia rheumatica; however, a biopsy should be performed only in those with symptoms of temporal arteritis. Patients with polymyalgia rheumatica should be watched closely because temporal arteritis may eventually develop. The treatment for polymyalgia rheumatica is not adequate for temporal arteritis. Temporal arteritis is more common in women than in men.

5. Answer d.

There is no highly effective treatment for Alzheimer's disease. Some patients may improve with antidepressants, which probably reflects the coexistence of depression in this population. Depression may cause many of the same symptoms as dementia, and one must be careful not to overlook it as a cause of cognitive impairment.

Patients with Alzheimer's disease have large amounts of neurofibrillary tangles and senile plaques; however, these are not specific to Alzheimer's disease and occur in other types of dementias as well as in normal aged persons (but in smaller numbers). CT of the head should be part of the evaluation of demented persons, not to look for cerebral atrophy but rather to rule out structural lesions such as tumor, hematoma, or normal-pressure hydrocephalus. Various neurotransmitters are lost in Alzheimer's disease but not specifically dopamine. (Specific loss of dopamine is associated with Parkinson's disease.) There is evidence for genetic transmission of Alzheimer's disease. It is most significant in families with multiple members affected at an early age.

6. True.

All three of these substances decrease sleep latency and reduce the time it takes a person to fall asleep. However, none of these substances are useful when used nightly for treatment of chronic insomnia. Benzodiazepines may produce impaired cognition and can contribute to falls; some persons develop tolerance to the sedating effects. Antihistamines have anticholinergic effects and may cause disturbing adverse effects of dry mouth, constipation, or urinary retention. Alcohol acts as a diuretic and may also suppress the deep stages of sleep, causing frequent nighttime awakenings.

7. False.

Cystometry is most useful in helping to establish a diagnosis in patients with detrusor overactivity. It can detect early detrusor contractions characteristic of the syndrome. In urinary stress incontinence, the diagnosis can usually be established with a thorough medical history. Cystometry would not be of much help. If a urodynamic test were necessary for stress incontinence, it would need to assess internal sphincter resistance.

Chapter 18 HEMATOLOGY
(Questions--pages 475-477)

1. Answer d.

High erythropoietin levels are present in marrow hypoproliferative states (such as pure red blood cell aplasia), deficiency states (such as iron deficiency), autonomous production (such as hepatocellular carcinoma), and high altitude.

2. Answer b.

Each cell and its volume and hemoglobin are measured variables on the complete blood cell count. The other variables of the complete blood count are calculated, including hematocrit, mean corpuscular volume, mean corpuscular hemoglobin, mean corpuscular hemoglobin concentration, and red cell distribution width.

3. Answer b.

In an acute hemolytic state, the glucose-6-phosphate dehydrogenase level may be normal. Normally, the half-life of glucose-6-phosphate dehydrogenase is 62 days, but it is 124 days in reticulocytes and 31 days in aged cells.

4. Answer c.

Hereditary spherocytosis is a Coombs' negative hemolytic anemia with positive findings on osmotic fragility test. The inheritance pattern is autosomal dominant, and it is essential to study family members.

5. Answer b.

Disseminated intravascular coagulopathy and not thrombotic thrombocytopenic purpura is characterized by a prolonged prothrombin time, positive fibrin D-dimer, and an elevated partial thromboplastin time. An increased creatinine level occurs in <20% of patients with thrombotic thrombocytopenic purpura.

6. Answer b.

This patient has pathologic stage IA Hodgkin's disease. The treatment of choice is radiation therapy in the mantle and para-aortic fields.

7. Answer e.

A low leukocyte alkaline phosphatase score may be present in chronic myelogenous leukemia, aplastic anemia, paroxysmal nocturnal hemoglobinuria, and infectious mononucleosis.

8. Answer a.

This patient has a monoclonal protein of undetermined significance, not multiple myeloma. This disorder should be observed and not treated.

9. Answer c.

Patients with chronic lymphocytic leukemia and a gamma spike of <0.3 g/dL are at increased risk of infection. Prophylactic gamma globulin is the treatment of choice.

10. Answer c.

The strategies for the management of chronic lymphocytic leukemia are distinguished by staging systems.

Patients with a hemoglobin <11 g/dL and a platelet count <100,000 have Rai stage IV disease or International Workshop Classification stage C disease and should receive treatment.

11. Answer e.

Drugs that antagonize warfarin include cholestyramine, which reduces the absorption of warfarin. The drugs that increase the clearance of warfarin include barbiturates, carbamazepine, and rifampin. Phenylbutazone, metronidazole, sulfapyrazone, trimethoprim/sulfamethoxazole, and disulfiram all potentiate warfarin.

12. Answer b.

Hemophilia A is characterized by an abnormal factor VIIIC and normal bleeding time, factor VIII ristocetin, factor IX, and fibrinogen levels.

13. Answer d.

Patients with mild von Willebrand's disease may have significant bleeding at the time of a surgical procedure.

14. Answer e.

Fresh frozen plasma contains all coagulation factors. More specific treatment is indicated in von Willebrand's disease.

15. Answer d.

Prothrombin time is normal in von Willebrand's disease.

16. Answer a.

Hepatitis non-A, non-B, non-C, and hepatitis A are the most common forms of hepatitis associated with aplastic anemia.

17. Answer c.

The transferrin saturation is >62% early in life in hemochromatosis. 2-4/1,000 are affected in the general population, and this entity is inherited as an autosomal recessive trait; 50% of patients are diabetic at presentation. Features not altered by chelation include arthropathy, hypogonadism, development of hepatocellular carcinoma, and hepatic cirrhosis.

18. Answer d.

The platelet count in hemophilia A without HIV infection is normal.

19. Answer c.

This patient presents with superior vena cava syndrome. It is essential to establish a diagnosis before initiating treatment. Mediastinoscopy offers the safest approach to obtaining a histologic diagnosis.

20. Answer d.

Drugs that may precipitate an attack of acute intermittent porphyria include sulfa, griseofulvin, phenytoin, progesterone, estrogen, barbiturates, and ergot preparations.

21. a, false; b, false; c, false; d, false; e, false; f, false.

Iron deficiency anemia typically has a microcytic anemia, decreased ferritin, red blood cell count $<5.10^{12}/L$, and red cell distribution width >16, and transferrin saturation $<9\%$. Hemoglobin A_2 is $>4\%$ in β-thalassemia trait.

22. a, true; b, false; c, true; d, true; e, true; f, true.

Aplastic anemia occurs as a complication in 5%-10% of patients with paroxysmal nocturnal hemoglobinuria.

23. a, false; b, true; c, false; d, true; e, true; f, false.

The major criteria in the diagnosis of polycythemia rubra vera are splenomegaly, normal oxygen saturation, and increased red blood cell mass. The minor criteria are platelet count $>400,000$, white blood cell count $>12,000$, leukocyte alkaline phosphatase score >100, and vitamin $B_{12} >900$.

24. a, true; b, false; c, true; d, true; e, true; f, true.

The International Non-Hodgkin's Lymphoma Prognostic Factor Project identified the following as poor risk factors: age older than 60; serum LDH ≥ 1x normal; performance status of 2, 3, or 4; stage III and IV; or >1 extranodal site of disease.

25. a, true; b, true; c, true; d, true; e, false; f, false.

Heparin forms a complex with antithrombin III. Warfarin is contraindicated in the management of deep venous thrombosis in pregnancy.

26. a, true; b, true; c, true; d, true; e, false; f, true.

Bleeding time is normal in hemophilia A and abnormal in von Willebrand's disease.

27. a, false; b, false; c, false; d, true; e, true; f, false.

Related donors should not be used in aplastic anemia because they may expose the patient to minor histocompatibility antigens. The survival rates for patients not receiving transfusion who undergo an allogeneic bone marrow transplantation are significantly better than for those who had transfusion. The treatment of choice in HLA-matched patients with aplastic anemia younger than 40 is allogeneic bone marrow transplantation. Spontaneous remissions are not common.

28. a, true; b, true; c, true; d, true; e, true; f, true.

Females are at higher risk for acute hemolytic transfusion reactions, transfusion-associated adult respiratory distress syndrome, delayed hemolytic transfusion reactions, and febrile transfusion reactions because of previous pregnancies and transfusions.

Chapter 19 HYPERTENSION
(Questions--pages 498-499)

1. Answer b.

Primary aldosteronism is usually associated with mild hypernatremia and hypokalemia. Thus, answers a and e are incorrect. Although answers c and d demonstrate mild hypernatremia and hypokalemia, urinary potassium excretion is reduced; so there is no evidence for inappropriate kaluresis, which is also a characteristic of primary aldosteronism.

2. Answer c.

Methyldopa is the drug usually used initially in the treatment of hypertension during pregnancy. Although there are some theoretical concerns with the use of labetalol, hydralazine, and hydrochlorothiazide, none of these drugs are absolutely contraindicated. Angiotensin-converting enzyme inhibitors such as lisinopril can induce serious fetal abnormalities and are the only class of drugs absolutely contraindicated for the treatment of hypertension during pregnancy.

3. Answer c.

Thiazide diuretics decrease urinary calcium excretion. This is the rationale for their use in the treatment of idiopathic calcium nephrolithiasis. They often cause mild hypercalcemia.

4. Answer b.

Unlike methyldopa, guanabenz is not known to cause hemolytic anemia.

5. Answer d.

True hypertensive crisis is a medical emergency and requires hospitalization, usually in an intensive care unit.

6. a, false; b, false; c, true; d, true; e, false; f, false.

Norepinephrine is further metabolized to epinephrine only in the adrenal gland. Thus, increase of both plasma and urinary norepinephrine and epinephrine levels would be more suggestive of a tumor located in the adrenal glands. The medical treatment for pheochromocytoma is alpha-blockade. β-Blockers are only used for suppression of tachycardia, which occasionally occurs after alpha-blockade. Pheochromocytoma can be associated with von Hippel-Lindau disease, neurofibromatosis, and multiple endocrine neoplasia syndrome type II. Although labetalol is a combination of an α-blocker and β-blocker, its β-blocking effect may be dominant and, thus, it should not be used as initial therapy for pheochromocytoma. Untreated patients with pheochromocytoma are often characterized by extracellular volume contraction.

7. a, true; b, false; c, false; d, true; e, false; f, true.

Fibromuscular dysplasia should always be considered in a young female with new onset hypertension, especially if a bruit is noted on abdominal examination. Renovascular hypertension is often associated with secondary aldosteronism and associated hypokalemia. A characteristic bruit is noted on abdominal examination in only 50% of patients with renovascular hypertension. Because angiotensin II is often required for the maintenance of glomerular filtration rate in kidneys with high-grade renal artery stenoses, the use of an angiotensin-converting enzyme inhibitor can result in sudden reductions in renal function. The longer the duration of hypertension before diagnosis of renovascular disease, the greater the likelihood of nephrosclerosis and vascular changes that will result in persistence of hypertension even after correction of renal artery stenosis. Although there are many screening tests to detect the presence of renovascular disease, the captopril radionuclide renal scan is thought to be the most sensitive and specific by many.

Chapter 20   INFECTIOUS DISEASES
(Questions--pages 579-583)

1. Answer d.

Bacterial pneumonia occurring after influenza virus infection is usually due to *Streptococcus pneumoniae* or *Staphylococcus aureus*. The chest radiographic finding of pneumatoceles strongly suggests *Staphylococcus aureus* pneumonia.

2. Answer b.

None of the cephalosporins are active against *Enterococcus*.

3. Answer d.

Spontaneous bacteremias due to *Pseudomonas* often develop in patients with profound leukopenia. The skin finding described suggests ecthyma gangrenosum, which can be caused by the *Pseudomonas* infection.

4. Answer d.

Pasteurella multocida is part of the normal feline flora. It causes a rapidly progressing cellulitis.

5. Answer e.

No specific toxins or virulence factors have been identified for the organism *Streptococcus mitis*. Of the other organisms listed, both *Staphylococcus* and *Streptococcus* produce exotoxins that facilitate their tissue invasion. Many of the disease manifestations caused by *Clostridium tetani* and *Corynebacterium diphtheriae* are related to their toxin production.

6. Answer d.

There is no known viral or other infectious cause of chronic fatigue syndrome.

7. Answer a.

JC virus, a polyoma virus, causes progressive multifocal leukoencephalopathy in immunocompromised hosts. This should not be confused with the Creutzfeld-Jakob agent, which causes a spongiform encephalopathy.

8. Answer c.

Tularemia can be transmitted by insect bite (ticks or deer flies) and by exposure to infected animals such as rabbits. The patient described has ulceroglandular fever.

9. Answer c.

Ascariasis is the only parasite listed which causes intraluminal intestinal infection.

10. Answer a.

Toxoplasma gondii, a protozoan parasite, can be transmitted by eating raw or undercooked meat and is also shed in the intestinal tracts of young cats. Transmission by heart transplantation and disease in patients with AIDS are well described. Fish do not harbor this organism.

11. Answer c.

Streptococcus pneumoniae is far and away the most common cause of acute bacterial meningitis in a previously healthy adult.

12. Answer d.

Endocarditis caused by *Streptococcus mutans* (a type of viridans streptococcus) can be reliably cured by a 2-week course of penicillin plus gentamicin or by 4 weeks of penicillin alone. The addition of gentamicin for a full 4 weeks may result in unnecessary toxicity.

13. Answer d.

Gonococcal septic arthritis continues to be a not uncommon problem, especially in the young, sexually active population.

14. Answer b.

The penicillins are the preferred drugs for treating syphilis. Primary syphilis can be adequately treated with a single dose of a long-acting penicillin.

15. Answer d.

Bacteroides fragilis can be associated with chronic sinusitis, but the other organisms listed are far more common as causes of acute sinusitis.

16. Answer c.

Nafcillin is metabolized by the liver primarily.

17. Answer d.

Empiric therapy for fever in a neutropenic patient requires antimicrobials directed against aerobic gram-negative rods, including *Pseudomonas aeruginosa*. All of the regimens listed are active against *Pseudomonas* except the combination of cefoxitin and vancomycin.

18. Answer c.

Acyclovir can cause nephrotoxicity by precipitating in the renal tubules. This effect can be avoided by ensuring that the patient is well hydrated and that the acyclovir is infused slowly.

19. Answer a.

None of the available quinolones is reliably active against *Streptococcus pneumoniae*. For this reason, most experts do not recommend using quinolones such as ciprofloxacin for treating community-acquired respiratory infections.

20. Answer d.

Many drugs can interfere with theophylline metabolism. Of the listed drugs, only erythromycin has significant effects. Additional antimicrobial agents that affect theophylline levels include ciprofloxacin, norfloxacin, and rifampin.

21. Answer c.

Although inhaled pentamidine decreases the risk of developing *Pneumocystis carinii* pneumonia (PCP), it is not nearly as effective as prophylaxis with trimethoprim-sulfamethoxazole. For cases in which PCP develops while patient is taking pentamidine, the involved areas are usually the upper lobes, and the diagnosis may be difficult because of small numbers of cysts present in the lung.

22. Answer c.

Tuberculosis is one of the few infections in patients with AIDS which can be cured with appropriate antimicrobial agents.

23. Answer d.

Toxoplasma seronegativity and prophylaxis with trimethoprim-sulfamethoxazole make cerebral toxoplasmosis an unlikely diagnosis. The situation described could be due to any number of causes, including lymphoma, bacterial, fungal, and mycobacterial infections.

24. Answer a.

This is a case of *Listeria* meningitis. None of the cephalosporins are active against this organism. Penicillins, with or without an aminoglycoside, are the drugs of choice.

25. Answer b.

Because of the increasing incidence of resistance in tuberculosis, a four-drug regimen is often recommended as initial therapy until susceptibilities are known.

26. a, true; b, false; c, true; d, true; e, true; f, true.

Neutropenic patients are susceptible to bacteremia with *Pseudomonas* without an identifiable source. This can result in ecthyma gangrenosum, which is a necrotic skin lesion. Hot tubs that are inadequately chlorinated provide ideal culture media for growing *Pseudomonas*. Hospitalized patients are susceptible to infection with resistant gram-negative organisms such as *Pseudomonas*, especially when they are receiving broad-spectrum antibiotics or are intubated for prolonged periods. Patients with cystic fibrosis often have respiratory tracts that are colonized with *Pseudomonas aeruginosa*. *Pseudomonas* is not known to cause an enteric infection.

27. a, true; b, true; c, false; d, true; e, true; f, true.

Health care workers are at increased risk for tuberculosis because of increased exposure. HIV infection, silicosis, and diabetes all increase the risk of tuberculosis because of impaired host immunity. Previous gastrectomy is a risk factor in areas of the world where bovine tuberculosis still exists. There is no increased risk of tuberculosis from slaughtering animals.

28. a, false; b, true; c, true; d, false; e, true; f, true.

Actinomyces, an anaerobic organism, is part of normal flora in the mouth and tonsils of humans. It causes an indolent infection when aspirated into the lungs or introduced into the bloodstream. It often causes a draining lesion as extension from the primary source of infection.

29. a, false; b, false; c, true; d, false; e, false; f, true.

Coccidioidomycosis occurs in the desert southwest around Arizona, southern California, and northern Mexico. Primary infection usually manifests as an acute, flu-like respiratory infection and resolves spontaneously. It can be associated with erythema nodosum, but when this occurs it is almost always a limited disease. If coccidioidomycosis meningitis develops, it is virtually impossible to cure and requires maintenance therapy with amphotericin B or fluconazole. Ketoconazole is effective, but because it does not achieve adequate levels in the spinal fluid it cannot be used to treat central nervous system disease. Tissue biopsy of infected material reveals a spherule, usually with endospores rather than invasive hyphae.

30. a, false; b, true; c, false; d, false; e, true; f, false.

Toxic shock syndrome can occur with virtually any *Staphylococcus aureus* infection in which the organism grows in a localized area. It is almost never associated with bacteremia. It is a clinical diagnosis that can be assisted by isolation of the organisms.

31. a, false; b, false; c, true; d, true; e, false; f, false.

The most common cause of early prosthetic valve endocarditis is coagulase-negative staphylococci. The most important indication for surgical intervention is acute heart failure resulting from valvular dysfunction. Recent use of antimicrobials can obscure the detection of the bacteremia associated with endocarditis. *Streptococcus bovis* endocarditis has been associated with up to 50% rate of colonic lesions. Although several regimens have been described for empiric treatment of culture-negative endocarditis, imipenem is not listed in any of them. Although injection drug users are at risk for endocarditis due to *Candida* and gram-negative bacilli, *Staphylococcus aureus* is the most common organism to cause this condition.

32. a, true; b, false; c, false; d, true; e, true; f, true.

Amphotericin B is associated with several toxic and metabolic abnormalities. However, hypocalcemia and pancreatitis are not among these.

33. a, false; b, true; c, false; d, true; e, false; f, true.

The β-lactamase inhibitors generally expand the spectrum of the penicillins to include anaerobic organisms such as *Bacteroides* and penicillinase-producing *Staphylococcus aureus*. The β-lactamase produced by *Pseudomonas aeruginosa* is generally not inhibited by these agents. Organisms that acquire their resistance by altered penicillin-binding proteins such as methicillin-resistant *Staphylococcus aureus* and penicillin-resistant *Streptococcus pneumoniae* are also not affected by these β-lactamase inhibitors. *Legionella pneumophila* is not susceptible to any β-lactam agents.

34. a, false; b, true; c, false; d, true; e, true; f, true.

Mycobacterium avium complex is usually a late manifestation of very advanced AIDS. It can cause widespread infection and be detected in tissue, blood, sputum, and stool. Symptoms often manifest as fever, weight loss, and sweats. The organisms tend to be resistant to standard antimycobacterial agents.

35. a, false; b, true; c, false; d, true; e, false; f, false.

Time of seroconversion after primary infection with HIV varies but can range from 2 weeks to 6 months. Although most patients are symptomatic with their primary acquisition of HIV, there is often a mononucleosis-like syndrome associated. Aseptic meningitis can occur but is not the most common presentation. Even a very sensitive and specific test like the HIV ELISA will have a low positive predictive value when used to screen populations with a low prevalence of HIV infection. The mean time to development of AIDS is up to 10 years.

Chapter 21 NEPHROLOGY
(Questions--pages 610-612)

1. Answer c.

Rhabdomyolysis may be due to carbon monoxide poisoning. Acute hypocalcemia is a common accompaniment of acute renal failure due to rhabdomyolysis. Because there is no hemolysis, the haptoglobin is normal, as is the appearance of the serum. The findings on urine benzidine dipstick test are positive due to myoglobulinuria.

2. Answer c.

Acetoacetate can increase the serum creatinine levels independently of decreases in the glomerular filtration rate. This is often seen in diabetic ketoacidosis. The other agents have no effect on serum creatinine independently of decreases in GFR.

3. Answer d.

Patients with syndrome of inappropriate antidiuretic hormone have plasma hypotonicity despite urine that is not maximally dilute. Water restriction corrects the hyponatremia, and there must be an absence of hypocortisolism and hypothyroidism. Urinary sodium excretion is equal to dietary intake.

4. Answer c.

Of the agents listed, aspirin is the only one that does not increase the osmolar gap. The osmolar gap (measured plasma osmolality minus the calculated plasma osmolality) is >10 in these ingestions except for aspirin.

5. Answer a.

In vomiting, the urine chloride is a common accompaniment of hypokalemia. The urine chloride is a useful clinical measure to determine which forms of metabolic alkalosis may be saline-responsive (low urine chloride) versus saline-unresponsive (high urine chloride).

6. Answer a.

All the listed ingestions are associated with a high anion gap metabolic acidosis except for isopropyl alcohol, which is metabolized to acetone.

7. Answer c.

The American Diabetes Association recommends all diabetics be screened on an annual basis for microalbuminuria, which is the number one predictor of eventual diabetic nephropathy.

8. Answer e.

Focal glomerulosclerosis has been definitely associated with HIV infection, reflux nephropathy, heroin use, and massive obesity. Hodgkin's disease is associated with minimal change disease and may represent a T-cell lymphokine disorder.

9. Answer a.

Streptococcal glomerulonephritis, IgA nephropathy, polyarteritis nodosa, and Goodpasture's syndrome all represent glomerular injury that may result in red blood cell cast formation. Amyloidosis is generally associated with proteinuria alone, and red blood cell casts are not seen.

10. Answer d.

Of the renal diseases listed, the hemolytic uremic syndrome is the least likely to respond to corticosteroid therapy. There is good evidence that all the other glomerular lesions may respond to this therapy.

11. Answer d.

Lithium may induce a nephrogenic diabetes insipidus. Ethylene glycol and its metabolite oxalate cause acute renal failure. Lead ingestion can produce nephropathy and gout (saturine gout). Hypercalcemia interferes with urinary concentration and results in nephrogenic diabetes insipidus. Patients with tumor lysis syndrome have a urine uric acid-to-urine creatinine ratio >1.

12. Answer d.

Adult polycystic kidney disease is an autosomal dominantly inherited disorder that does not necessarily result in end-stage renal disease. There is no association of deafness with adult polycystic kidney disease, and it has been associated with up to 10% of all end-stage renal disease patients in the U.S. Patients with polycystic kidney disease often have a relative excess of erythropoietin production and, thus, do not develop as severe anemia as other, comparable patients with chronic renal failure due to other causes.

13. Answer e.

An acid urine is necessary to form renal stones composed of uric acid. Alkalinization of the urine makes it possible to dissolve these stones.

14. Answer d.

Most patients with struvite stones have underlying stone-forming tendency, and after surgical removal of the stone material, long-term antibiotic suppressive therapy is necessary to clear the infection of the urease-producing bacteria.

15. Answer a.

Stone formers with idiopathic hypercalciuria who do not respond to fluid intake alone are best treated with thiazide diuretics to decrease the urine level of calcium. This will be effective only if the patients also limit their sodium intake.

16. Answer e.

Renal osteodystrophy is commonly associated with hyperphosphatemia. Osteitis fibrosa cystica (hyperparathyroidism), osteomalacia (vitamin D deficiency), osteoporosis, and growth retardation are all components of renal osteodystrophy.

17. Answer e.

Hemodialysis patients often have a low total thyroxine with normal thyroid function. Growth hormone levels are increased. Hypergastrinemia and impaired fertility are also common accompaniments. Patients receiving hemodialysis often have high prolactin levels that are not clinically significant.

18. Answer e.

Dietary phosphorus restriction is the principal, initial treatment for renal osteodystrophy. Later in the course of chronic renal failure, phosphate binders such as calcium carbonate and acetate are useful, and 1,25 vitamin D may be necessary in advanced renal osteodystrophy.

19. Answer b.

The metabolic acidosis due to early chronic renal failure is secondary to decreased ammonia production by the renal tubule. The metabolic acidosis of early chronic renal failure is not associated with a high anion gap.

20. Answer c.

Patients with chronic hypertension, analgesic abuse, and chronic renal parenchymal disease often have small kidneys at the time they advance toward chronic renal failure. Polycystic kidney disease patients have enlarged kidneys, and only diabetics have relatively preserved renal size as they develop chronic renal failure.

21. a, false; b, true; c, false; d, true; e, true.

Oliguria due to acute tubular necrosis commonly lasts <8 weeks. During treatment, maintaining the BUN <100 improves patient outcome. Although hypocalcemia can accompany acute renal failure, it rarely requires treatment. Ethylene glycol poisoning and its metabolite, oxalate, may cause acute intrarenal obstruction in renal failure. A clue to atheroembolic-induced renal failure is eosinophilia.

22. a, false; b, true; c, true; d, false; e, true.

Of the diuretics listed, acetazolamide's effects are principally in the proximal tubule, where carbonic anhydrase is in its highest concentration. Ethacrynic acid is a loop diuretic, as is furosemide. Thiazide diuretics act in the distal tubule and spironolactone in the collecting duct.

23. a, true; b, true; c, true; d, true; e, true.

Multiple myeloma is associated with pseudohyponatremia if the M-protein concentrations are high. This also is a cause of low anion gap. Hypercalcemia is a common accompaniment of multiple myeloma. Type II or proximal renal tubular acidosis is one component of Fanconi's syndrome, which can be associated with multiple myeloma. Patients are often heavily proteinuric and develop nephrotic syndrome.

24. a, true; b, true; c, true; d, false; e, false.

Polyarteritis nodosa and Wegener's granulomatosis are not associated with hypocomplementemia, but the other listed glomerular diseases are. Poststreptococcal glomerulonephritis generally is associated with hypocomplementemia for a limited period of time (6-8 weeks).

25. a, false; b, true; c, true; d, true; e, false.

Aspirin alone and acetaminophen alone have not been associated with analgesic nephropathy. Anemia, hypertension, and rarely multicentric transitional cell carcinomas occur with analgesic nephropathy.

26. a, true; b, false; c, false; d, false; e, false.

Of the listed cystic renal diseases, only medullary cystic disease is inherited. The other cysts are all acquired and have no known genetic inheritance.

27. a, true; b, true; c, true; d, true; e, true.

All the agents listed require a decrease in dose in chronic renal failure. Angiotensin-converting enzyme inhibitors have the added disadvantage of causing hyperkalemia. Magnesium and digoxin toxicities may be serious if the doses of medications are not adjusted. Acyclovir can precipitate in the renal tubule and cause acute renal failure. Long-acting calcium channel blockers can cause complete heart block if the doses are not decreased in chronic renal failure.

28. a, false; b, true; c, true; d, false; e, true.

Recombinant human erythropoietin therapy has not been associated with allergic reactions or decreased hemodialysis efficiency. Hypertension, improved appetite, and reticulocytosis are associated with the initiation of therapy.

Chapter 22   NEUROLOGY
(Questions--pages 640-641)

1. Answer d.

In the elderly, many signs seen in the neurologic examination are not considered pathologic. These include small pupils, impairment of upward gaze, difficulty with tandem gait and balancing on one leg, difficulty with rapid alternating movements, decrease in muscle bulk, decreased ankle reflexes, decreased vibratory sensation in the legs, increase in motor tone, and even the presence of unusual reflexes such as snouting, palmomental, rooting, and sucking. There is decrease in the special sensations of vision, hearing, smell, and taste. However, paratonia and grasping reflexes in the hands and feet in an awake elderly person are abnormal.

2. Answer e.

Dementia leads to cognitive impairments but does not cause impairment in the level of awareness. In other words, a demented patient has lost his/her cognitive functions but is awake and alert.

3. Answer a.

Lumbar puncture is contraindicated whenever there is a mass lesion, regardless of the nature of the mass. The only time it is safe to perform a lumbar puncture with increased intracranial pressure is in the syndrome of idiopathic intracranial hypertension or pseudotumor cerebri. A cerebral abscess can be diagnosed on the basis of the medical history and with MRI or CT of the head.

4. Answer a.

Although cluster headache is classified as a vascular headache, it does not cause pulsatile headache. It does cause a unilateral headache, but the pain is of a boring, steady, deep aching nature, usually centered around the eye and the frontal temporal areas.

5. Answer c.

This type of "dizziness" is common among the elderly and is actually a problem with standing and walking. The patient feels secure if he or she can have the support of another person, a wall or furniture, or a cane. This syndrome is referred to as the "multisensory deficit" syndrome, because the patient usually has a combination of mild impairment in many modalities such as vision, hearing, proprioception, and tactile sensation and perhaps even mild vestibular and mild baroreceptor dysfunction. Extensive studies and drugs are not needed.

6. a, true; b, true; c, true; d, false; e, false; f, true.

Acute confusional states are a group of disorders that can be caused by systemic problems, neurologic problems, and even psychophysiologic problems. Elderly patients are especially prone to acute confusional states. Acute confusional states cause impairment of cognitive function and impairment of the state of awareness as well as fluctuations in these functions. Paratonic rigidity is common in elderly confused patients and has no localizing value; however, unusual movements such as blepharospasm and hemifacial spasm are not part of the acute confusional state.

7. a, false; b, false; c, true; d, false; e, false; f, true.

A partial simple or a partial complex seizure denotes a focal structural problem in the brain, but because metabolic encephalopathy causes diffuse problems, one would expect that any seizure that occurs would be of a generalized tonic-clonic type. Most seizures can be treated effectively with monotherapy rather than polypharmacy, which usually leads to more serious side effects. Blood levels of anticonvulsants should only be used as guidelines and never as the basis for changing the dose of the anticonvulsant. The decision to change the dose or to change to another anticonvulsant is based on the clinical situation. Toxicity is a clinical phenomenon and not a laboratory phenomenon, and patients can do well with levels above and below the therapeutic range. If the patient has good seizure control and is not clinically toxic, it does not matter what the blood level of the anticonvulsant is, and, therefore, one need not determine the level. Status epilepticus can be treated with a benzodiazepine, but a long-acting anticonvulsant has to be added because the benzodiazepines work only for a short time. Pseudoseizures are very difficult to diagnose and can occur in both epileptic and nonepileptic patients. Several of these types of spells can mislead the treating physician to think that the patient is "intractable." These spells are best diagnosed at special centers with EEG telemetry and video/monitoring. Although intractable epilepsy may be helped by various surgical procedures performed at specialty centers, surgical treatment is under-used.

Chapter 23   ONCOLOGY
(Questions--pages 662-664)

1. Answer d.

With mammography, the false-negative rate is 8%-10%. Thus, a suspicious palpable nodule should be excised despite a negative mammogram. A wire localization biopsy is used for mammographically determined, nonpalpable lesions.

2. Answer b.

Adjuvant tamoxifen has been shown to reduce recurrences of breast cancer in both node-positive and node-negative disease. Tamoxifen acts as an agonist on bone and endometrium. Consequently, there is endometrial hyperplasia but no loss of bone density. The rate of thromboembolic events with tamoxifen is approximately 1%, and hot flashes are common.

3. Answer c.

The patient is premenopausal and has node-positive disease. Standard adjuvant therapy for this patient remains six cycles of adjuvant chemotherapy.

4. Answer b.

Major risk factors for breast cancer (relative risk >4.0) include family history of premenopausal breast cancer, atypia, and older age. Late menopause and nulliparity are also risk factors for this disease. Numerous studies have explored the relationship between use of oral contraceptives and breast cancer, and there is no clear consensus on their relationship.

5. Answer d.

Optimal surgical debulking, by a gynecologic oncologist, is critical to outcome in ovarian cancer.

6. Answer c.

Numerous studies have confirmed that the depth of invasion of the primary lesion is the best predictor of outcome in melanoma.

7. Answer d.

Right-sided heart failure with tricuspid regurgitation describes carcinoid heart disease, a complication of the carcinoid syndrome. This does not occur with small cell carcinoma of the lung. Small cell carcinoma of the lung is known to elaborate antidiuretic hormone and adrenocorticotropic hormone and to generate cross-reacting antibodies that have serious neurologic sequelae.

8. Answer b.

Squamous cell carcinoma of the lung is most commonly associated with hypercalcemia, secondary to the parathyroid hormone-related peptide. Adrenal carcinomas may elaborate cortisol but not adrenocorticotropic hormone. They may also elaborate aldosterone or androgens. There is no "pituitoma," and prostate cancer has only rarely been associated with ectopic adrenocorticotropic hormone production.

9. Answer e.

Although smoking has clearly been shown to be of etiologic importance in several cancers, this does not appear to be the case with breast cancer.

10. Answer d.

Patients with severe hypercalcemia are dehydrated. Rehydration, before the institution of a diuretic, is the first step in their management.

11. a, true; b, false; c, false; d, true.

α-Fetoprotein is never expressed in seminomas. β-Human chorionic gonadotropin level is elevated in approximately 10% of patients with seminoma. Increased levels of markers in testicular cancer are taken as evidence of disease progression, even in the absence of physical or radiographic abnormalities. Approximately 85% of nonseminomas elaborate one of the tumor markers.

12. a, false; b, false; c, false; d, true.

In a young man with a midline mass, a germ cell tumor must be considered. α-Fetoprotein and β-human chorionic gonadotropin should be determined in this setting. Carcinoembryonic antigen value is very nonspecific and would not be helpful in evaluation. Determination of CA-125 is used primarily in ovarian cancer. This presentation would be most unusual for prostate cancer, and hence the prostate-specific antigen value would not be of value.

13. a, false; b, false; c, false; d, true; e, false; f, false.

Axillary node dissection is necessary for all patients with invasive breast cancer because it provides important prognostic information. Lumpectomy followed by close observation is associated with an unacceptably high, approximately 40%, recurrence rate in the breast. Breast conservation therapy, namely, lumpectomy, breast irradiation, and axillary dissection, has been shown in numerous clinical trials to be the therapeutic equivalent of mastectomy. Studies of lumpectomy in women with tumors of 4- to 5-cm in size have reported successful results. Generally, chemotherapy follows the local treatment for breast cancer ("neoadjuvant" is a term used to describe preoperative chemotherapy).

14. a, true; b, true; c, true; d, false; e, true; f, true.

Chemotherapy's "selectivity" is largely based on the presence of dividing cells. Therefore, nondividing cells are relatively resistant to therapy. Any mechanism that decreases drug concentration within the tumor cells, such as decreased uptake or increased efflux, can mediate resistance. Certain drugs are administered in "prodrug" forms and require activation by tumor cell enzymes. Increased drug activation would not be a form of resistance to therapy. Enhanced DNA repair processes have been described in cancers and obviously counteract the desired effect of DNA-damaging chemotherapeutics.

Chapter 24 PREVENTIVE MEDICINE
(Questions--pages 677-678)

1. Answer d.

Primary prevention is done *before* the existence of disease; secondary prevention is done *after* disease occurs but before it is symptomatic; and tertiary prevention is done after the diagnosis and treatment of initial clinical disease. Thus, answer a, a risk factor, is primary prevention; answer b, tamoxifen treatment, is tertiary prevention; answer c, refers to primary prevention; and answer e, immunizations, is primary prevention.

2. Answer a.

As a rate, incidence requires a number of events over a length of time, typically, new diagnoses per year. Answer b has no time element; answer c does not have a length of time and is an example of "prevalence"; answer d lacks a time element; and answer e refers to the measure "potential years of life lost."

3. Answer d.

Ideally, a screenable disease has a long period during which it is detectable but remains confined or of low virulence--the "window of opportunity" for screening. Additionally the disease should be relatively common and serious, thus posing a "burden" on the population being screened. Screening should "salvage" sufficient years of life to justify the cost. Knowledge of the natural history of the disease is important to avoid "length bias"--detection, by screening, of only the slow growing relatively benign forms of the disease.

4. Answer d.

Lung cancer, the leading cause of cancer death for men and women, has not proved to be a good screening disease. Even with aggressive screening measures, early detection does not improve survival. With current technology, lung cancer screening is not recommended.

5. Answer b.

Many aspects of breast cancer screening remain controversial, such as mammographic screening in 40- to 49-year-old women. However, based on demonstrated effectiveness in multiple randomized controlled trials, there is agreement that annual mammography should be performed in women between the ages of 50 and 65. The additional benefit of clinical breast examination is less clearly demonstrated, but it appears to detect additional disease and is recommended.

6. a, true; b, false; c, false; d, true; e, true; f, false.

a) The tetanus vaccine should be updated every 10 years; b) by virtue of her age, she is considered to be immune on the basis of likely childhood exposure (certain high-risk persons such as health care workers might benefit from revaccination); c) lung cancer screening is not effective; d) because she is older than 50, she should receive mammography yearly; e) fecal occult blood test effectively reduces mortality from colorectal cancer in those older than 50; f) ovarian cancer screening would be very expensive and has not yet been tested for effectiveness.

7. a, true; b, true; c, false; d, false; e, true; f, false.

The commonly administered live virus vaccines include measles, mumps, rubella, and oral polio virus OPV (though inactivated forms can be given). Smallpox vaccine is a live vaccinia virus but is no longer used (smallpox is believed to have been eradicated). Yellow fever vaccine is a live attenuated viral vaccine for use in travelers to endemic areas, such as equatorial Africa, Panama, and South America. A live attenuated varicella zoster vaccine for use in chicken pox prevention in children may soon be available.

8. a, false; b, true; c, true; d, true; e, false; f, false.

a) Colon cancer screening should begin at age 50. The only screening method currently demonstrated to reduce mortality is occult blood screening. b) His wound is a high-risk wound, and he has not had the primary series of tetanus vaccination. Passive (and immediate) immunity is achieved by injecting 250 units of tetanus immune globulin (TIG) intramuscularly. d) He has never had a primary series of tetanus vaccine (or diantheria vaccine). The first dose of this series should be given in the emergency room, with a different syringe and at a different intramuscular site than used for the TIG. The primary series is completed by giving a second dose 4 weeks or more later and a third dose 6-12 months later. The combined tetanus and diptheria toxoid should be used to protect against both diseases. d) Smoking is the single biggest threat to health in the U.S. Smoking cessation counseling is probably the most cost-effective treatment a health care provider can give. Every reasonable opportunity should be taken to counsel patients. e) Polio vaccination is not recommended to adults unless they are traveling to high-risk areas of the world or are health care workers. f) Emergency health care should, in general, be provided without reference to compensation. In this case, safety counseling may prevent a future need for an emergency room visit.

Chapter 25 PSYCHIATRY
(Questions--pages 695-696)

1. Answer d.

Confabulation refers to filling gaps in memory with detailed accounts of factitious events that the person believes to be true. This most often occurs in the organic mental disorder, Korsakoff's syndrome.

2. Answer d.

Anorexia nervosa occurs more commonly in persons younger than age 40 and would not be a primary source of decreased appetite in the age group of this patient.

3. Answer b.

Patients with schizophrenia or other psychotic disorders are not more prone to developing delirium. The other choices do represent high-risk groups for developing delirium.

4. Answer e.

Drug-induced psychosis is the common form of psychosis diagnosed in hospitalized medical/surgical patients.

5. Answer d.

Electroconvulsive therapy is most effective for the treatment of depression.

6. a, true; b, true; c, true; d, false; e, true; f, true.

The specific quantities of alcohol used and frequency of use per week are much less important in diagnosing alcoholism than the other features listed in the question.

7. a, false; b, true; c, true; d, true; e, false; f, true.

See Table 25-5. Renal excretion of lithium is influenced by changes in sodium balance and glomerular filtration rate. Lithium is reabsorbed in the proximal tubule to the same degree that sodium and water are. A low sodium diet can lead to a negative sodium balance and, therefore, increase lithium reabsorption and potentially increased plasma lithium levels. Caffeine and theophylline both potentially decrease lithium levels because of increased lithium excretion. Thiazide diuretics, angiotensin-converting enzyme inhibitor antihypertensives, and nonsteroidal anti-inflammatory drugs decrease renal lithium clearance, thereby leading to increased plasma levels of lithium. The use of these drugs or low sodium diet with lithium is not absolutely contraindicated, but when used with lithium, the plasma lithium levels need to be closely monitored.

Chapter 26   PULMONARY DISEASES
(Questions--pages 770-773)

1. Answer a.

Basal panlobular emphysema is typical in patients with α_1-antitrypsin deficiency. Centrilobular emphysema is more common in chronic smokers and is seen mostly in upper lung zones.

2. Answer d.

Loss of alveolocapillary interphase from emphysematous destruction of lung parenchyma diminishes capillary volume which is an important factor in estimating the diffusing capacity for carbon monoxide. Patients with anatomical emphysema demonstrate diminished total lung capacity and vital capacity and increased residual volume. An increase in arterial carbon dioxide is not seen until late in disease.

3. Answer b.

Cystic fibrosis is the commonest autosomal recessive disease among Caucasians in the 2nd and 3rd decades of life.

4. Answer d.

See text for differential diagnoses of chronic lung disease in young subjects. In this patient, infertility is not a complaint and does not require testing in the initial evaluation. Excluding infertility does not rule in or rule out a specific disease.

5. Answer e.

The cause of alveolar microlithiasis is unknown, although familial cases have been described. Smoking is strongly associated with pulmonary alveolar proteinosis, pulmonary eosinophilic granuloma, and calcification of asbestos-induced pleural plaques.

6. Answer b.

Silo-filler's lung is caused by inhalation of nitrogen dioxide; the lesion is secondary to gaseous injury. Farmer's lung disease represents hypersensitivity pneumonitis.

7. Answer c.

Obstructive pulmonary function can be seen in all the listed conditions except for idiopathic pulmonary fibrosis. The latter typically produces restrictive dysfunction in a nonsmoker.

8. Answer d.

Histiocytosis X (eosinophilic granuloma) causes solitary cystic lesions in long bones. Pulmonary involvement is more common in upper lung zones. Sarcoid bone disease involves distal phalanges and not long bones. Hodgkin's lymphoma, acute histoplasmosis with systemic dissemination, and scleroderma with lung disease seldom affect bones.

9. Answer a.

Progressive stage II or III sarcoidosis and/or involvement of the eyes, myocardium, central nervous system, and hypercalcemia are indications for corticosteroid therapy in sarcoidosis. Berylliosis, acute rheumatoid lung disease, and chronic eosinophilic pneumonia should be treated with high doses of corticosteroids.

10. Answer a.

Goodpasture's syndrome is a typical example of cytotoxic (autoantibody or type II) immune reaction. Rheumatoid lung disease is thought to represent type III (antigen-antibody) reaction. Allergic bronchopulmonary aspergillosis may result from both type I and type III reactions. Penicillin anaphylaxis is caused by type I allergic reaction. Hereditary angioneurotic edema is caused by hereditary deficiency or absence of C1-esterase inhibitor.

11. Answer b.

Uremic pulmonary edema is noncardiogenic in origin and may be seen in both acute and chronic renal failure. Intra-alveolar fluid is always an exudate.

12. Answer a.

Diffuse interstitial process, as in scleroderma or rheumatoid lung disease, is extremely uncommon in systemic lupus erythematosus. Multiple areas of plate-like atelectasis, pleural effusion, pulmonary hemorrhage, and diaphragmatic dysfunction are more common.

13. Answer c.

Of the choices listed, scleroderma is most likely to cause diffuse pulmonary disease. Clinical, radiographic, and pulmonary function abnormalities are similar to those in idiopathic pulmonary fibrosis.

14. Answer a.

This patient has typical CREST variant of scleroderma. Pleural involvement is uncommon in scleroderma; one publication reported an incidence of <5%.

15. Answer b.

Esophageal involvement is not a feature of rheumatoid arthritis. Bronchiolitis and resultant obstructive airways disease are well-known complications, as are pleural effusion and rheumatoid lung nodules.

16. Answer d.

Gradually progressive dyspnea over a 2-year period, chest radiographic, and pulmonary function abnormalities are typical of hypersensitivity lung disease (bird-breeder's lung). Pneumonia secondary to *C. pneumoniae* and psittacosis secondary to *C. psittaci* produce acute illness. Clinical data provided are not compatible with cryptococcosis and histoplasmosis.

17. Answer a.

The clinical features are typical of mycoplasma infection (i.e., college student, bullous myringitis, small pleural effusion).

18. Answer d.

Initial measures include all except thoracoscopic drainage of the lung abscess under topical anesthesia. Initial treatment of lung abscess is conservative. Bronchoscopy helps obtain cultures, assist in drainage, and, more importantly, excludes postobstructive abscess from a tumor in this heavy smoker.

19. Answer b.

The patient had a noncontagious type of tuberculosis. Therefore, immediate antituberculous therapy is improper. The physician may have converted her PPD from exposure to another patient with *M. tuberculosis*. Prophylactic isoniazid therapy in the presence of positive PPD and abnormal chest radiographic findings is improper.

20. Answer c.

Prolonged granulocytopenia in a patient with hematologic malignancy treated with chemotherapy predisposes to disseminated aspergillosis. Infection caused by *P. carinii* is uncommon in this patient population.

21. a, true; b, false; c, true; d, false; e, false; f, false.

See answer to question 2. Early phase of an asthmatic attack, polycythemia, supine posture, and intra-

alveolar hemorrhage tend to either maintain normal diffusing capacity for carbon monoxide or to increase it slightly.

22. a, true; b, true; c, true; d, true; e, true; f, false.

Even though pancreatic insufficiency is common in adults with cystic fibrosis, most of them are relatively asymptomatic.

23. a, true; b, true; c, true; d, true; e, false; f, true.

Noncaseous granuloma can be seen in the early phase of tubercle formation in tuberculosis.

24. a, true; b, false; c, true; d, false; e, true; f, false.

Bronchoalveolar lavage is diagnostic in >60% of patients with lymphangitic pulmonary malignancy. Special staining for OKT6 helps in the diagnosis of pulmonary eosinophilic granuloma. The clinical role of bronchoalveolar lavage in establishing the diagnosis of sarcoidosis, hypersensitivity pneumonitis, silicosis, and asbestosis remains unproved.

25. a, false; b, true; c, true; d, true; e, true; f, false.

Lymphangioleiomyomatosis produces all the features described in the question. Chylous effusion and chylous ascites are not seen in histiocytosis X. Diabetes insipidus is seen in histiocytosis X.

26. a, true; b, true; c, true; d, true; e, false; f, false.

This patient has dermatopolymyositis. Obstructive lung disease and pleural effusions are not seen in this disease. Hypercarbia is secondary to weakness of respiratory muscles and signifies poor prognosis.

27. a, true; b, false; c, false; d, true; e, false; f, true.

See text for details about infections in closed populations (schools and colleges, nursing homes, military camps, etc.).

28. a, false; b, true; c, true; d, true; e, true; f, false.

The duration of symptoms in this young non-smoker is too long for primary bronchogenic carcinoma. Calcification of lymph nodes suggests a chronic process. This patient has histoplasmosis-induced complications (mediastinal fibrosis, intranodal calcification, possible broncholithiasis, and esophageal obstruction caused by mediastinal fibrosis). Nephrolithiasis is not a complication of histoplasmosis.

Chapter 27   RHEUMATOLOGY I
(Questions--pages 797-798)

1. Answer d.

Anti-nDNA titers correlate with renal involvement in systemic lupus erythematosus, especially diffuse proliferative glomerulonephritis. A high anti-nDNA titer associated with a low complement value is the hallmark of renal involvement. Anti-nDNA levels and complement values fluctuate with disease activity.

2. Answer c.

The most likely cause of death is aspiration pneumonia. The upper third of the esophagus is skeletal muscle, and this can become weak in polymyositis; the weakness leads to aspiration pneumonia. Patients with polymyositis do not commonly develop renal disease or pericardial tamponade.

3. Answer d.

The finding of sclerodactyly would help establish a diagnosis. The patient could have either CREST syndrome or systemic sclerosis, depending on the rest of the physical findings. These diseases can have an associated positive antinuclear antibody test, but this does not establish a diagnosis. Sclerodactyly is a criterion for both CREST syndrome and scleroderma. The esophageal motility test can also be abnormal in patients with Raynaud's phenomenon, but it does not establish a precise diagnosis. Patients who have used L-tryptophan develop an eosinophilic myalgia syndrome but not Raynaud's phenomenon.

4. Answer e.

Virtually 100% of patients taking procainamide for >1 year will have positive results of antinuclear antibody testing. This finding does not mean that they will develop drug-induced lupus. Approximately 20% of patients taking procainamide will develop drug-induced lupus, but this cannot be prognosticated on the basis of a positive antinuclear antibody test alone. Therefore, if procainamide is clinically indicated, its use should be continued unless a patient develops symptoms of drug-induced lupus such as fever, arthritis, pleurisy.

5. Answer c.

The most helpful test would be magnetic resonance imaging of the hips. This patient has two risk factors for avascular necrosis of the hip: 1) systemic lupus erythematosus and 2) prednisone use. Although bone scanning would be positive, this does not provide a precise diagnosis, whereas magnetic resonance imaging does.

6. Answer e.

Although the patient is asymptomatic at the time of examination, radiographs of his feet do reveal erosive changes, and tophi are present on physical examination. Either one of these findings would be sufficient to begin therapy to lower his uric acid with either allopurinol or probenecid. When use of these drugs is initiated they can precipitate gout, and thus they are used in conjunction with colchicine (0.6 mg twice a day) until the tophi have completely resolved. The colchicine does provide some protection in preventing an acute attack of gout.

7. Answer d.

There is no history of kidney stones or gout. The urinary uric acid value is normal, as is renal function. Although he does have an elevated serum uric acid value, this does not predict whether he will ever have an attack of gouty arthritis. Also, an elevated serum uric acid value alone will not have a deleterious effect on the kidneys.

8. Answer c.

The patient is presumed to have Lyme disease. Although he has a negative Lyme serology result, testing was performed shortly after the onset of the skin lesion and flu-like symptoms. It can take up to 4-6 weeks for the results to be positive. The erythematous skin lesion and flu-like symptoms suggest active disease, and treatment with tetracycline should be initiated.

9. Answer e.

The history of low back pain, morning stiffness, and iritis suggests an underlying spondyloarthropathy such as ankylosing spondylitis. One of the criteria for ankylosing spondylitis is sacroiliitis, which can be seen on radiography. An HLA-B27 is associated with ankylosing spondylitis, but this is not one of the criteria for diagnosing ankylosing spondylitis or another spondyloarthropathy.

10. Answer a.

Reactive arthritis usually occurs in patients who are HLA-B27 positive. The self-limiting diarrhea suggests that the patient did not have the arthritis of inflammatory bowel disease.

11. a, false; b, false; c, true; d, true; e, true; f, false.

Drug-induced lupus is usually characterized by pleuropericardial disease and arthritis and is associated with antihistone antibodies. Patients usually do not develop high-titer anti-nDNA titers and, therefore, usually do not develop renal disease. Central nervous system disease is rare.

12. a, true; b, true; c, true; d, false; e, true; f, true.

A false-positive VDRL result can occur in the antiphospholipid antibody syndrome because the antigen in the test is a phospholipid. Patients with the antiphospholipid antibody syndrome can have a history of recurrent spontaneous miscarriages, possibly due to placental infarction. Also, they can have thrombosis of the hepatic vein leading to a Budd-Chiari syndrome. An occasional patient with this syndrome can develop thrombocytopenia because of antibodies to the platelet cell wall, which contains a phospholipid. Leukopenia is not associated with this syndrome. A prolonged activated partial thromboplastin time not corrected with normal plasma is the characteristic finding with a coagulation survey. The patient's serum will neutralize the normal plasma because of antibodies to phospholipid, which is the cause of the prolonged activated partial thromboplastin time. In a patient with a clotting deficiency, normal plasma should correct a prolonged time.

13. a, true; b, false; c, true; d, true; e, true; f, true.

Approximately 25% of patients with ankylosing spondylitis will develop iritis. Complete heart block is a late manifestation of the disease, as is secondary amyloidosis, which can cause a nephrotic syndrome. Cauda equina syndrome can also occur in ankylosing spondylitis as a late complication, and this can lead to a neurogenic bladder. Patients with ankylosing spondylitis can also have osteitis pubis documented by radiography. Scleromalacia perforans does not occur with the spondyloarthropathies but more commonly with rheumatoid arthritis and Wegener's granulomatosis.

14. a, true; b, true; c, true; d, false; e, true; f, true.

Gout is not precipitated by hypothyroidism. There is an association between hypothyroidism and pseudogout. Gout is commonly precipitated by surgery, usually occurring approximately 3 days after the surgical procedure. Diuretics and fasting can increase uric acid and precipitate gout. Also, joint infections and the initiation of allopurinol therapy can precipitate gout in patients who have had previous gouty arthritis.

Chapter 28   RHEUMATOLOGY II
(Questions--pages 838-839)

1. Answer c.

Erosive osteoarthritis is a unique proliferative degenerative arthritis associated with erosions beginning in the central portion of the distal and proximal interphalangeal joints. It is seen predominantly in perimenopausal women. Erosive osteoarthritis is commonly, though transiently, associated with joint inflammation and swelling, which is another distinguishing feature from primary osteoarthritis.

2. Answer b.

The arthropathy of hemochromatosis is a secondary osteoarthritis and is distinguishable from primary osteoarthritis by the distribution of joint involvement. In particular, primary osteoarthritis almost never affects the metacarpophalangeal joints or shoulders. Anytime osteoarthritis occurs in these joints without a history of trauma, one should think of secondary osteoarthritis.

3. Answer b.

Felty's syndrome occurs in 1% of all seropositive rheumatoid arthritis patients. The classic triad of neutropenia, splenomegaly, and rheumatoid arthritis defines the syndrome. It is also associated with cutaneous vasculitis, hyperpigmentation, and usually chronic, severe, and, sometimes, burned-out rheumatoid arthritis. Many patients with Felty's syndrome die of the complications of neutropenia and infection. Dry eyes, dry mouth, and arthritis make up the triad of Sjögren's syndrome. Fever, arthritis, and rash are the triad described in Still's disease. Elderly patients with seronegative rheumatoid arthritis may have a variant that includes peripheral edema, symmetrical small joint polyarthritis, and steroid responsiveness.

4. Answer b.

Nonacetylated salicylates do not inhibit prostaglandins to any meaningful degree. They do not cause prostaglandin inhibition in the kidney or at the gastric mucosal border. Patients with nonacetylated salicylates would not have worsening of blood pressure, increased risk of peptic ulcer, bleeding time abnormalities, or water retention. However, up to one-third of patients taking nonacetylated salicylates have dyspepsia unrelated to gastric ulcer. It should be noted that dyspepsia has no predictive value for the presence of significant gastric ulcer related to nonsteroidal anti-inflammatory drug therapy.

5. Answer d.

Toxicity monitoring for hydroxychloroquine includes eye examinations for retinopathy, usually twice a year. All the other mentioned medications have the potential to affect hematopoiesis.

6. Answer e.

Superficial bursae have a poor blood supply. Warmth in a superficial bursa is enough of a clinical clue to begin treatment for presumed septic superficial bursitis. In 40%-50% of cases, Gram staining of the bursal fluid gives negative results and leukocyte counts are typically quite low for an infectious process. Prepatellar septic bursitis is difficult to treat with oral antibiotics, and it is almost always a good idea to give antibiotics intravenously for 24-48 hours.

7. Answer b.

Anti-inflammatory agents generally do not have much effect for the pain of fibromyalgia. The pain is not caused by inflammation. Prednisone is absolutely contraindicated. In double blinded control studies, nonsteroidal anti-inflammatory drugs have not been beneficial. However, in combination with tricyclic antidepressants, they may offer additional pain control.

8. Answer e.

Between 1% and 3% of all patients with polymyalgia rheumatica present with a normal erythrocyte sedimentation rate. It is not uncommon to have an oligoarticular inflammatory arthritis as part of polymyalgia rheumatica. Polymyalgia rheumatica is associated with giant cell arteritis in only 15% of cases. The initial dose of prednisone to treat polymyalgia rheumatica is never more than 20 mg/day. Unlike many other rheumatic diseases, polymyalgia rheumatica remits in the majority of cases within the first 2 years of disease and requires no further therapy.

9. Answer d.

A combination of a loss of motor function and sensory abnormalities in the same nerve distribution can only be a mononeuritis. This is a peripheral nerve lesion and would not be caused by cervical subluxation. A wrist extensor tendon rupture would not be associated with numbness. Carpal tunnel syndrome affects only the muscles in the thenar prominence of the hand, and gold toxicity is a very unusual cause of mononeuritis.

10. Answer d.

This is an immune complex-associated vasculitis. The immune complex is deposited on the vessel wall, can fix complement, and will cause vessel damage. The other vasculitides mentioned are distinguished by their lack of complement consumption.

11. a, false; b, true; c, true; d, true; e, true; f, true.

Cervical myelopathy is the consequence of severe rheumatoid arthritis affecting the cervical spine. The resulting instability can cause a cervical myelopathy. Instability occurs most commonly at C-1/C-2 without associated radiculopathy. The other conditions are all complications of seropositive rheumatoid arthritis. Nodular regenerative hyperplasia of the liver is an uncommon cause of cryptic portal hypertension and hypersplenism. It would need to be distinguished from classic Felty's syndrome.

12. a, false; b, true; c, false; d, true; e, false.

If a joint is thought to be septic, treatment with antibiotics should be started immediately. Considerable loss of joint function may occur if therapy is delayed even 12 hours. It is important to consider other foci of infection whenever there is a septic joint. Findings on plain radiographs lag 8-10 days behind the initiation of the infectious process. Therefore, normal plain radiographs are not adequate to rule out an infection if the symptoms are less than 2 weeks in duration. Because this is a closed space infection, it is important to drain the fluid, just as in draining an abscess until the fluid no longer accumulates. Another indicator of therapeutic adequacy is a serial drop in the white cell count in the synovial fluid with each subsequent joint aspiration. The duration of antibiotic therapy depends on the virulence of the organism and the joint involved. Joints infected with organisms that have low virulence and have oral antibiotic sensitivity can be treated with 2 weeks of intravenous antibiotic therapy.

13. a, true; b, true; c, true; d, false; e, true; f, false.

Any disease that causes circulating immune complexes, particularly chronic infectious diseases, is associated with positive rheumatoid factors. Subacute bacterial endocarditis is a classic example. It is not unusual to find complement consumption in this situation. Sjögren's syndrome can have the highest titers of rheumatoid factor found in any connective tissue disease. By definition, adult-onset Still's disease is rheumatoid factor and antinuclear antibody negative. Wegener's granulomatosis can have a positive rheumatoid factor in up to one-third of all cases. By definition, polymyalgia rheumatica is rheumatoid factor negative. Genetic studies suggest that patients who have rheumatoid arthritis are protected from getting polymyalgia rheumatica and vice versa.

14. a, true; b, true; c, false; d, true; e, false; f, false.

Polyarteritis nodosa almost never affects the lungs. Whereas Takayasu's arteritis can affect pulmonary arteries and cause pulmonary hypertension, pulmonary failure and hemorrhage are not part of that syndrome.

Chapter 29   VASCULAR DISEASES
(Questions--page 858)

1. Answer b.

The risk of rupture for abdominal aortic aneurysms is minimal when they are <4.5 cm in maximal diameter and is probably less than the risk of surgery. For this reason, they are usually observed when small.

2. Answer e.

Although the swelling of lymphedema may cause disfigurement and even immobility, it is rarely painful.

3. Answer d.

Nerve compression is the most common cause of symptoms in thoracic outlet syndrome.

4. Answer a.

For proximal deep venous thrombosis, duplex scanning is now considered as accurate as venography.

5. Answer d.

The erythrocyte sedimentation rate is usually increased in both temporal arteritis and Takayasu's arteritis.

6. a, false; b, false; c, false; d, true; e, true; f, true.

Patients with Raynaud's phenomenon may worsen in response to β-adrenergic blockers, smoking, and an assortment of other pharmacologic or physiologic stimuli. A sympathetic nerve block (or sympathetic-blocking drugs) may help these symptoms.

7. a, true; b, true; c, false; d, true; e, true; f, false.

Obesity, hip fracture, estrogen, pregnancy, and a host of other conditions may predispose to deep venous thrombosis. In contrast, ergotamine is often used as a prophylactic agent. β-Adrenergic blockers have no known predisposing effect.

NOTES

NOTES

NOTES

NOTES